Tintinalli's
Emergency Medicine Manual

Notice

Tintinalli's Emergency Medicine Manual 8th Edition

Rita K. Cydulka, MD, MS
Professor, Department of Emergency Medicine
Associate Professor, Department of Biostatistics and Epidemiology
Case Western Reserve University
MetroHealth Medical Center
Cleveland, Ohio

Michael T. Fitch, MD, PhD
Professor and Vice Chair for Academic Affairs
Department of Emergency Medicine
Wake Forest School of Medicine
Winston-Salem, North Carolina

Scott A. Joing, MD
Associate Professor
Department of Emergency Medicine
University of Minnesota Medical School
Faculty Physician
Hennepin County Medical Center
Minneapolis, Minnesota

Vincent J. Wang, MD, MHA
Professor of Clinical Pediatrics
Keck School of Medicine of the University of Southern California
Associate Division Head
Division of Emergency Medicine
Children's Hospital Los Angeles
Los Angeles, California

David M. Cline, MD
Professor and Director of Departmental Research
Department of Emergency Medicine
Wake Forest School of Medicine
Winston-Salem, North Carolina

O. John Ma, MD
Professor and Chair
Department of Emergency Medicine
Oregon Health & Science University
Portland, Oregon

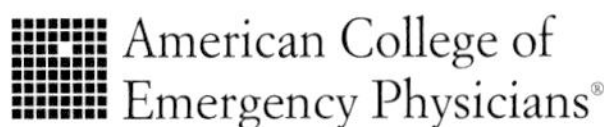

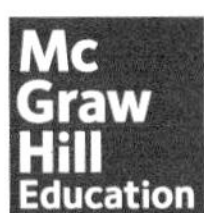

New York Chicago San Francisco Athens London Madrid Mexico City
Milan New Delhi Singapore Sydney Toronto

Tintinalli's Emergency Medicine Manual, 8th Edition

8 9 DSS 24

ISBN 978-0-07-183702-6
MHID 0-07-183702-7

This book was set in Times by MPS Limited.
The editors were Brian Belval and Christie Naglieri.
The production supervisor was Catherine H. Saggese.
Project management was provided by Poonam Bisht, MPS Limited.

Library of Congress Cataloging-In-Publication Data

Names: Cydulka, Rita K., editor.
Title: Tintinalli's emergency medicine manual / [edited by] Rita K. Cydulka, David M. Cline, O. John Ma, Michael T. Fitch, Scott Joing, Vincent J. Wang.
Other titles: Emergency medicine manual
Description: 8th edition. | New York : McGraw-Hill Education, 2017. | Includes bibliographical references and index.
Identifiers: LCCN 2017009768 | ISBN 9780071837026 (pbk.) | ISBN 0071837027 (pbk.)
Subjects: | MESH: Emergency Medicine—methods | Emergencies | Emergency Treatment
Classification: LCC RC86.7 | NLM WB 105 | DDC 616.02/5—dc23 LC record available at https://lccn.loc.gov/2017009768

Contents

Contributors xi
Preface xix

Section 1 Resuscitation Techniques 1
1 Advanced Airway Support *Darren Braude* 1
2 Management of Cardiac Rhythm Disturbances *James K. Takayesu* 10
3 Resuscitation of Children and Neonates *Marc F. Collin* 29
4 Fluids, Electrolytes, and Acid-Base Disorders *Benjamin W. Wachira* 37
5 Therapeutic Approach to The Hypotensive Patient *Saurin P. Bhatt* 60
6 Anaphylaxis, Acute Allergic Reactions, and Angioedema *Alix L. Mitchell* 64

Section 2 Analgesia, Anesthesia, and Sedation 67
7 Acute Pain Management and Procedural Sedation *Michael S. Mitchell* 67
8 Chronic Pain *David M. Cline* 77

Section 3 Emergency Wound Management 81
9 Evaluating and Preparing Wounds *Timothy J. Reeder* 81
10 Methods for Wound Closure *Corey R. Heitz* 85
11 Lacerations to The Face and Scalp *J. Hayes Calvert* 96
12 Injuries to the Arm, Hand, Fingertip, and Nail *John Pettey Sandifer* 101
13 Lacerations to the Leg and Foot *Moira Davenport* 108
14 Soft Tissue Foreign Bodies *Michael T. Fitch* 112
15 Puncture Wounds and Bites *Michael T. Fitch* 115
16 Postrepair Wound Care *Eugenia B. Quackenbush* 121

Section 4 Cardiovascular Diseases 125
17 Chest Pain: Cardiac or Not *Andrew Nyce* 125
18 Acute Coronary Syndromes: Myocardial Infarction and Unstable Angina *Maame Yaa A. B. Yiadom* 131
19 Cardiogenic Shock *Brian Hiestand* 138
20 Low-Probability Acute Coronary Syndrome *David A. Wald* 141
21 Syncope *Jo Anna Leuck* 146
22 Acute Heart Failure *Lori J. Whelan* 149
23 Valvular Emergencies *Boyd Burns* 152
24 The Cardiomyopathies, Myocarditis, and Pericardial Disease *Lorraine Thibodeau* 160
25 Venous Thromboembolism *Christopher Kabrhel* 167
26 Systemic and Pulmonary Hypertension *Michael Cassara* 175
27 Aortic Aneurysms and Aortic Dissection *David E. Manthey* 181
28 Arterial Occlusion *Carolyn K. Synovitz* 187

Section 5 Pulmonary Emergencies 191
29 Respiratory Distress *Baruch S. Fertel* 191
30 Bronchitis, Pneumonia, and Novel Respiratory Infections *Jeffrey M. Goodloe* 199
31 Tuberculosis *Amy J. Behrman* 204
32 Spontaneous and Iatrogenic Pneumothorax *Mike Cadogan* 208
33 Hemoptysis *Nilesh Patel* 211
34 Asthma and Chronic Obstructive Pulmonary Disease *Stacey L. Poznanski* 213

Section 6 Gastrointestinal Emergencies 217

35 Acute Abdominal Pain *Bryan E. Baskin* 217
36 Nausea and Vomiting *Jonathan A. Maisel* 222
37 Disorders Presenting Primarily with Diarrhea *Jonathan A. Maisel* 225
38 Acute and Chronic Constipation *Thomas E. Carter* 233
39 Gastrointestinal Bleeding *Mitchell C. Sokolosky* 237
40 Esophageal Emergencies *Mitchell C. Sokolosky* 239
41 Peptic Ulcer Disease and Gastritis *Teresa Bowen-Spinelli* 244
42 Pancreatitis and Cholecystitis *Rita K. Cydulka* 247
43 Acute Appendicitis *Charles E. Stewart* 252
44 Diverticulitis *James O'Neill* 256
45 Intestinal Obstruction and Volvulus *Olumayowa U. Kolade* 259
46 Hernia in Adults and Children *Louise Finnel* 262
47 Anorectal Disorders *Chad E. Branecki* 265
48 Jaundice, Hepatic Disorders, and Hepatic Failure *Cem Oktay* 273
49 Complications of General Surgical Procedures *Daniel J. Egan* 282

Section 7 Renal and Genitourinary Disorders 287

50 Acute Kidney Injury *Sum Ambur* 287
51 Rhabdomyolysis *Annet Alenyo Ngabirano* 292
52 Emergencies in Renal Failure and Dialysis Patients *Jonathan A. Maisel* 296
53 Urinary Tract Infections and Hematuria *David R. Lane* 299
54 Acute Urinary Retention *Casey Glass* 303
55 Male Genital Problems *Gavin R. Budhram* 306
56 Urologic Stone Disease *Geetika Gupta* 312
57 Complications of Urologic Procedures and Devices *Steven Go* 316

Section 8 Gynecology and Obstetrics 319

58 Vaginal Bleeding and Pelvic Pain in the Nonpregnant Patient *Joelle Borhart* 319
59 Ectopic Pregnancy and Emergencies in The First 20 Weeks of Pregnancy *Robert Jones* 323
60 Comorbid Diseases in Pregnancy *Abigail D. Hankin* 328
61 Emergencies After 20 Weeks of Pregnancy and The Postpartum Period *Kathleen Kerrigan* 335
62 Emergency Delivery *Stacie Zelman* 340
63 Vulvovaginitis *Robert R. Cooney* 344
64 Pelvic Inflammatory Disease *Abigail D. Hankin* 347
65 Complications of Gynecologic Procedures *Robert R. Cooney* 350

Section 9 Pediatrics 353

66 Fever and Serious Bacterial Illness in Children *Todd P. Chang* 353
67 Common Neonatal Problems *Lance Brown* 361
68 Common Infections of the Ears, Nose, Neck, and Throat *Yu-Tsun Cheng* 366
69 Upper Respiratory Emergencies—Stridor and Drooling *Christopher S. Cavagnaro* 372
70 Wheezing in Infants and Children *Richard J. Scarfone* 379
71 Pneumonia in Infants and Children *Ameer P. Mody* 385
72 Pediatric Heart Disease *Garth D. Meckler* 388
73 Vomiting and Diarrhea in Infants and Children *Stephen B. Freedman* 395
74 Pediatric Abdominal Emergencies *Janet Semple-Hess* 400
75 Pediatric Urinary Tract Infections *Marie Waterhouse* 407
76 Seizures and Status Epilepticus in Children *Ara Festekjian* 409
77 Altered Mental Status and Headache in Children *Carlo Reyes* 412
78 Syncope and Sudden Death in Children and Adolescents *Derya Caglar* 417

79 Hypoglycemia and Metabolic Emergencies in Infants and Children *Teresa J. Riech* 420
80 Diabetes in Children *Adam Vella* 425
81 Fluid and Electrolyte Therapy in Infants and Children *Ron L. Kaplan* 428
82 Musculoskeletal Disorders in Children *Mark X. Cicero* 432
83 Rashes in Children *Lance Brown* 443
84 Sickle Cell Anemia in Children *Ilene Claudius* 455
85 Hematologic-Oncologic Emergencies in Children *Ilene Claudius* 461
86 Renal Emergencies in Infants and Children *Saranya Srinivasan* 468

Section 10 Infectious and Immunologic Diseases 473
87 Sexually Transmitted Infections *Jennifer L. Hannum* 473
88 Toxic Shock Syndromes *Sorabh Khandelwal* 480
89 Sepsis *John E. Gough* 484
90 Soft Tissue Infections *Jon Femling* 491
91 Serious Viral Infections *Matthew J. Scholer* 497
92 HIV Infection and AIDS *Sarah Battistich* 505
93 Infective Endocarditis *Kristin M. Berona* 513
94 Tetanus and Rabies *Michael T. Fitch* 517
95 Malaria *Jennifer L. Hannum* 523
96 Foodborne and Waterborne Diseases *Benjamin Weston* 527
97 Zoonotic Infections *David Gordon* 531
98 World Travelers *Bret A. Nicks* 540
99 The Transplant Patient *Sarah E. Unterman* 546

Section 11 Toxicology and Pharmacology 555
100 General Management of the Poisoned Patient *L. Keith French* 555
101 Anticholinergic Toxicity *O. John Ma* 564
102 Psychopharmacologic Agents *Shan Yin* 566
103 Sedatives and Hypnotics *Shan Yin* 574
104 Alcohols *Michael Levine* 580
105 Drugs of Abuse *D. Adam Algren* 584
106 Analgesics *Joshua N. Nogar* 591
107 Xanthines and Nicotine *Robert J. Hoffman* 598
108 Cardiac Medications *Michael Levine* 602
109 Anticonvulsants *Robert J. Hoffman* 613
110 Iron *O. John Ma* 617
111 Hydrocarbons and Volatile Substances *Allyson A. Kreshak* 621
112 Caustics *Jennifer Cullen* 624
113 Pesticides *Charles W. O'Connell* 626
114 Metals and Metalloids *D. Adam Algren* 631
115 Industrial Toxins *Landen Rentmeester* 637
116 Vitamins and Herbals *Janna H. Villano* 643
117 Dyshemoglobinemias *Chulathida Chomchai* 646

Section 12 Environmental Injuries 649
118 Cold Injuries *Gerald (Wook) Beltran* 649
119 Heat Emergencies *Eric Kraska* 655
120 Bites and Stings *Michael Levine* 658
121 Trauma and Envenomation from Marine Fauna *Christian A. Tomaszewski* 666
122 High-Altitude Disorders *Shaun D. Carstairs* 670
123 Dysbarism and Complications of Diving *Christian A. Tomaszewski* 673
124 Near Drowning *Richard A. Walker* 675
125 Thermal and Chemical Burns *Sandra L. Werner* 678
126 Electrical and Lightning Injuries *Norberto Navarrete* 686

127 Carbon Monoxide *Jon B. Cole* 692
128 Mushroom and Plant Poisoning *Chulathida Chomchai* 695

Section 13 Endocrine Emergencies 701
129 Diabetic Emergencies *Michael P. Kefer* 701
130 Alcoholic Ketoacidosis *Michael P. Kefer* 709
131 Thyroid Disease Emergencies *Aziz Darawsha* 711
132 Adrenal Insufficiency *Michael P. Kefer* 715

Section 14 Hematologic and Oncologic Emergencies 719
133 Evaluation of Anemia and the Bleeding Patient *Rita K. Cydulka* 719
134 Acquired Bleeding Disorders *Alisheba Hurwitz* 726
135 Hemophilias and von Willebrand Disease *Colin G. Kaide* 729
136 Sickle Cell Disease and Other Hereditary Hemolytic Anemias *Colleen Fant* 734
137 Transfusion Therapy *Özlem Köksal* 739
138 Anticoagulants, Antiplatelet Agents, and Fibrinolytics *Jessica L. Smith* 745
139 Emergency Complications of Malignancy *Ross J. Fleischman* 751

Section 15 Neurology 759
140 Headache *Steven Go* 759
141 Stroke Syndromes and Spontaneous Subarachnoid Hemorrhage *Steven Go* 765
142 Altered Mental Status and Coma *C. Crawford Mechem* 775
143 Ataxia and Gait Disturbances *Ross J. Fleischman* 781
144 Acute Vertigo *Steven Go* 784
145 Seizures and Status Epilepticus in Adults *C. Crawford Mechem* 792
146 Acute Peripheral Neurologic Lesions *Nicholas E. Kman* 796
147 Chronic Neurologic Disorders *Michael T. Fitch* 800
148 Central Nervous System and Spinal Infections *Michael T. Fitch* 806

Section 16 Eye, Ear, Nose, Throat, and Oral Emergencies 813
149 Eye Emergencies *Steven Go* 813
150 Face and Jaw Emergencies *Jeffrey G. Norvell* 826
151 Ear, Nose, and Sinus Emergencies *Michael E. Vrablik* 831
152 Oral and Dental Emergencies *Steven Go* 838
153 Neck and Upper Airway Disorders *Rebecca Kornas* 845

Section 17 Disorders of the Skin 851
154 Dermatologic Emergencies *Jason P. Stopyra* 851
155 Other Dermatologic Disorders *Jason P. Stopyra* 856

Section 18 Trauma 865
156 Trauma in Adults *Rita K. Cydulka* 865
157 Trauma in Children *Matthew Hansen* 869
158 Trauma in the Elderly *O. John Ma* 873
159 Trauma in Pregnancy *John Ashurst* 877
160 Head Trauma *O. John Ma* 880
161 Spine Trauma *Jeffrey Dan* 886
162 Facial Injuries *Gerald (Wook) Beltran* 892
163 Neck Injuries *Steven Go* 897
164 Cardiothoracic Injuries *Paul Nystrom* 903
165 Abdominal Injuries *O. John Ma* 909
166 Penetrating Trauma to The Flank and Buttocks *Sum Ambur* 914
167 Genitourinary Injuries *Thomas Dalton* 916

168 Trauma to The Extremities *Amy M. Stubbs* 920

Section 19 Injuries to the Bones, Joints, and Soft Tissue 923
169 Initial Evaluation and Management of Orthopedic Injuries *Gregory M. Johnston* 923
170 Hand and Wrist Injuries *Robert R. Cooney* 929
171 Forearm and Elbow Injuries *Sandra L. Najarian* 934
172 Shoulder and Humerus Injuries *Sandra L. Najarian* 942
173 Pelvis, Hip, and Femur Injuries *Jeffrey G. Norvell* 949
174 Knee and Leg Injuries *Sandra L. Najarian* 956
175 Ankle and Foot Injuries *Sarah Elisabeth Frasure* 961
176 Compartment Syndrome *Sandra L. Najarian* 966

Section 20 Nontraumatic Musculoskeletal Disorders 969
177 Neck and Back Pain *Amy M. Stubbs* 969
178 Shoulder Pain *Andrew D. Perron* 975
179 Hip and Knee Pain *Augusta Czysz* 979
180 Acute Disorders of The Joints and Bursae *Andrew D. Perron* 983
181 Emergencies in Systemic Rheumatic Diseases *Nicholas Genes* 988
182 Nontraumatic Disorders of The Hand *Michael P. Kefer* 995
183 Soft Tissue Problems of The Foot *Gavin R. Budhram* 998

Section 21 Psychosocial Disorders 1003
184 Clinical Features of Behavioral Disorders *Leslie S. Zun* 1003
185 Emergency Assessment and Stabilization of Behavioral Disorders *Leslie S. Zun* 1007
186 Panic and Conversion Disorders *Kimberly Nordstrom* 1010

Section 22 Abuse and Assault 1013
187 Child and Elderly Abuse *Jonathan Glauser* 1013
188 Sexual Assault and Intimate Partner Violence and Abuse *Mary Hancock* 1016

Section 23 Special Situations 1021
189 Palliative Care *Kate Aberger* 1021

Index *1025*

Contributors

Kate Aberger, MD FACEP, Medical Director, Palliative Care Division, St. Joseph's Regional Medical Center, Paterson, New Jersey; Associate Professor of Emergency Medicine, New York Medical College

D. Adam Algren, MD, Associate Professor of Emergency Medicine and Pediatrics, Truman Medical Center/Children's Mercy Kansas City, University of Missouri; Kansas City School of Medicine, University of Kansas Hospital Poison Control Center, Kansas City, Kansas

Sum Ambur, MD, FACEP, FAAEM, Emergency Medicine Faculty, Hennepin County Medical Center, Abbott Northwestern Hospital Intensivist, Minneapolis, Minnesota

John Ashurst, DO, MSc, Kingman Regional Medical Center, Kingman, Arizona

Bryan E. Baskin, DO, FAAEM, Assistant Professor, Department of Emergency Medicine, Case Western Reserve University School of Medicine; Associate Clinical Operations Director, Department of Emergency Medicine, MetroHealth Medical System, Cleveland, Ohio; Attending Physician, Department of Emergency Medicine, MetroHealth Medical Center, Cleveland, Ohio

Sarah Battistich, MD, MSc, DTM&H, Assistant Professor, Liaison, Program for the Survivors of Torture, Bellevue Hospital, University Department of Emergency Medicine, New York

Amy J. Behrman, MD, FACOEM, FACP, Associate Professor, Department of Emergency Medicine, Perelman University of Pennsylvania School of Medicine, Philadelphia, Pennsylvania

Gerald (Wook) Beltran, DO, MPH, FACEP, FAEMS, Chief, Department of Emergency Medicine, Division of Prehospital and Disaster Medicine, Baystate Health Systems, Springfield, Massachusetts

Kristin M. Berona, MD, Department of Emergency Medicine, Keck School of Medicine of USC, LAC + USC Medical Center, Los Angeles, California

Saurin P. Bhatt, MD, Center for Emergency Medicine, Cleveland Clinic, Cleveland, Ohio

Joelle Borhart, MD, FACEP, FAAEM, Assistant Program Director, Assistant Professor of Emergency Medicine, Department of Emergency Medicine, Georgetown University Hospital & Washington Hospital Center, Washington, DC

Chad E. Branecki, MD, FACEP, University of Nebraska Medical Center, Omaha, Nebraska

Darren Braude, MD, MPH, FACEP, FAEMS, Chief, Division of Prehospital, Austere and Disaster Medicine, Professor of Emergency Medicine, EMS and Anesthesiology, University of New Mexico Health Sciences Center, Albuquerque, New Mexico

Lance Brown, MD, MPH, Professor of Emergency Medicine and Pediatrics, Loma Linda University School of Medicine, Chief, Division of Pediatric Emergency Medicine, Loma Linda University Medical Center, Loma Linda University Children's Hospital, Loma Linda, California

Gavin R. Budhram, MD, Director, Emergency Ultrasound Fellowship, Associate Professor of Emergency Medicine, Department of Emergency Medicine, Baystate Medical Center, University of Massachusetts Medical School

Boyd Burns, DO, FACEP, FAAEM, George Kaiser Family Foundation, Chair in Emergency Medicine, Associate Professor & Program Director, Department of Emergency Medicine, University of Oklahoma School of Community Medicine, Tulsa, Oklahoma

Mike Cadogan, FACEM, FFSEM, Emergency Physician, Sir Charles Gairdner Hospital, Perth, Australia

Derya Caglar, MD, Associate Professor, Department of Pediatrics, University of Washington School of Medicine; Attending Physician, Seattle Children's Hospital, Seattle, Washington

J. Hayes Calvert, DO, Department of Emergency Medicine, Wake Forest School of Medicine, Winston-Salem, North Carolina

Shaun D. Carstairs, MD, FACEP, FACMT, Division of Medical Toxicology, Department of Emergency Medicine, University of California, San Diego, California

Thomas E. Carter, MD, FACEP, Emergency Consultant, Palmerston North Hospital, Palmerston North, New Zealand; Clinical Associate Professor, Ohio University Heritage College of Osteopathic Medicine

Michael Cassara, DO, MSEd, FACEP, CHSE, Associate Professor of Emergency Medicine, Hofstra Northwell Health School of Medicine; Director of Simulation/Core Faculty, Department of Emergency Medicine, North Shore University Hospital; Associate Professor of Nursing, Hofstra Northwell School of Graduate Nursing and Physician Assistant Studies; Adjunct Associate Professor, Department of Specialized Programs in Education, Hofstra University School of Education; Medical Director, Northwell Health Patient Safety Institute/Emergency Medical Institute, Marcus Avenue Suite, Lake Success, New York

Christopher S. Cavagnaro, MD, Attending Physician, Division of Pediatric Emergency Medicine, Children's Hospital at Montefiore; Assistant Professor, Albert Einstein College of Medicine, Bronx, New York

Todd P. Chang, MD, MAcM, Director of Research & Scholarship, Pediatric Emergency Medicine; Associate Fellowship Director, Children's Hospital Los Angeles; Associate Professor of Clinical Pediatrics (Educational Scholar), University of Southern California, Los Angeles, California

Yu-Tsun Cheng, MD, Rady Children's Hospital San Diego, University of California, San Diego, California

Chulathida Chomchai, MD, Associate Professor of Pediatrics, Mahidol University International College, Bangkok, Thailand

Mark X. Cicero, MD, Departments of Pediatrics and Emergency Medicine, Yale University School of Medicine

Ilene Claudius, MD, Associate Professor, Department of Emergency Medicine, LAC+USC, Los Angeles, California

David M. Cline, MD, Professor of Emergency Medicine, Wake Forest School of Medicine, Winston-Salem, North Carolina

Jon B. Cole, MD, FACEP, FACMT, Department of Emergency Medicine, Hennepin County Medical Center; Medical Director, Minnesota Poison Control System; Associate Professor of Emergency Medicine, University of Minnesota Medical School

Marc F. Collin, MD, Associate Professor of Pediatrics, Department of Pediatrics, Case Western Reserve University School of Medicine; NICU Medical Director, MetroHealth Medical Center, Cleveland, Ohio

Robert R. Cooney, MD, MSMedEd, RDMS, FAAEM, FACEP, Associate Program Director, Emergency Medicine Residency Program, Geisinger Medical Center, Danville, Pennsylvania

Jennifer Cullen, MD, Emergency Medicine Physician, Tri-City Medical Center, San Diego, California

Rita K. Cydulka, MD, MS, Professor, Department of Emergency Medicine, Case Western Reserve University, Cleveland, Ohio

Augusta Czysz, MD, Conemaugh Memorial Medical Center, Franklin St, Johnstown, Pennsylvania

Thomas Dalton, MD, Clinical Assistant Professor, Department of Emergency Medicine, Stanford Medical Center, Standford, California

Jeffrey Dan, MD, Adjunct Professor, Baystate Medical Center, Tufts University School of Medicine, Baystate Medical Center, Springfield, Massachusetts

Aziz Darawsha, MD, Head of Emergency Medicine Department Hadassah University Hospital, Ein Kerem Jerusalem, Israel

Moira Davenport, MD, Departments of Emergency Medicine and Orthopaedic Surgery, Allegheny General Hospital, Pittsburgh, Pennsylvania; Associate Professor, Temple University School of Medicine

Daniel J. Egan, MD, Associate Professor of Emergency Medicine, Icahn School of Medicine at Mount Sinai; Residency Program Director, Mount Sinai St. Lukes and Roosevelt, New York

Colleen Fant, MD, MPH, Emergency Medicine Fellow, Ann and Robert H. Lurie Children's Hospital of Chicago, Chicago, Illinois

Jon Femling, MD, PhD, Department of Emergency Medicine, University of New Mexico, Albuquerque, New Mexico

Baruch S. Fertel, MD, MPA, FACEP, Assistant Professor of Medicine, Center for Emergency Medicine; Medical Director Clinical Systems Office, Cleveland Clinic, Cleveland, Ohio

Ara Festekjian, MD, MS, Assistant Professor of Clinical Pediatrics, Keck School of Medicine, University of Southern California, Division of Emergency & Transport Medicine, Children's Hospital Los Angeles, Los Angeles, California

Louise Finnel, MD, Fellow of the Australasian College for Emergency Medicine (FACEM), West Melbourne, Victoria, Australia

Michael T. Fitch, MD, PhD, Professor and Vice Chair for Academic Affairs Department of Emergency Medicine, Wake Forest School of Medicine, Winston-Salem, North Carolina

Ross J. Fleischman, MD, MCR, Department of Emergency Medicine, Harbor-UCLA Medical Center, Torrance, California

Sarah Elisabeth Frasure, MD, Clinical Instructor, Department of Emergency Medicine, Harvard Medical School, Brigham and Women's Hospital, Boston, Massachusetts

Stephen B. Freedman, MDCM, MSc, Associate Professor of Pediatrics, Alberta Children's Hospital, Foundation Professor in Child Health and Wellness, Alberta Children's Hospital, Theme Lead, Alberta Children's Hospital Research Institute, Cumming School of Medicine, University of Calgary, Calgary, Albarta, Canada

L. Keith French, MD, Adjunct Professor, Oregon Health & Science University, Oregon Poison Center, Portland, Oregon

Nicholas Genes, MD, PhD, FACEP, Associate Professor, Department of Emergency Medicine, Icahn School of Medicine at Mount Sinai, New York, New York

Casey Glass, MD, Assistant Professor, Department of Emergency Medicine, Wake Forest School of Medicine, Winston-Salem, North California

Jonathan Glauser, MD, FACEP, MBA, Professor, Emergency Medicine, Case Western Reserve University, Faculty Residency Program in Emergency Medicine, MetroHealth Medical Center, Cleveland, Ohio

Steven Go, MD, Associate Professor of Emergency Medicine, Department of Emergency Medicine, University of Missouri, Kansas City School of Medicine, Kansas City, Missouri

Jeffrey M. Goodloe, MD, NRP, FACEP, FAEMS, Professor & EMS Section Chief Director, Department of Emergency Medicine, Oklahoma Center for Prehospital & Disaster Medicine, The University of Oklahoma, Norman, Oklahoma

David Gordon, MD, Associate Professor, Division of Emergency Medicine, Department of Surgery, Duke University, Durham, North Carolina

John E. Gough, MD, Professor, Department of Emergency Medicine, East Carolina University, Greenville, North Carolina

Geetika Gupta, MD, Core Clinical Faculty, St Joseph Mercy Health System, Emergency Medicine Department, University of Michigan Emergency Medicine Residency, Ann Arbor, Michigan

Mary Hancock, MD, Attending Physician, Emergency Services Institute, Cleveland Clinic, Euclid Ave, Cleveland, Ohio

Abigail D. Hankin, MD, MPH, Assistant Professor, Emergency Medicine, Emory University, Atlanta, Georgia

Jennifer L. Hannum, MD, FACEP, Assistant Professor, Department of Emergency Medicine, Wake Forest School of Medicine, Winston-Salem, North Carolina

Matthew Hansen, MD, MCR, Assistant Professor of Emergency Medicine and Pediatrics, Oregon Health & Science University, Portland, Oregon

Corey R. Heitz, MD, Associate Professor of Emergency Medicine, Carilion Clinic, Virginia Tech Carilion School of Medicine, Roanoke, Virginia

Janet Semple-Hess, MD, Clinical Assistant Professor of Pediatrics, Keck School of Medicine, University of Southern California, Division of Emergency Medicine, Children's Hospital Los Angeles, Los Angeles, California

Brian Hiestand, MD, MPH, FACEP, Professor and Vice Chair of Clinical Operations, Department of Emergency Medicine, Wake Forest School of Medicine, Winston-Salem, North Carolina

Robert J. Hoffman, MD, MS, Attending Physician, Division of Emergency Medicine Sidra Medical and Research Center, Doha, Qatar

Alisheba Hurwitz, MD, Clinical Assistant Professor of Emergency Medicine, Thomas Jefferson University, Philadelphia, Pennsylvania

Gregory M. Johnston, MD, MS, FACEP, FAAEM, Staff Physician, Department of Emergency Medicine, Hunter Holmes McGuire VA Medical Center, Richmond, Virginia

Robert Jones, DO, FACEP, Director, Emergency Ultrasound, Director, Emergency Ultrasound Fellowship, MetroHealth Medical Center, Cleveland, Ohio; Associate Professor, Case Western Reserve University, Cleveland, Ohio

Christopher Kabrhel, MD, MPH, Director, Department of Emergency Medicine, Center for Vascular Emergencies, Massachusetts General Hospital; Associate Professor of Emergency Medicine, Harvard Medical School, Boston, Massachusetts

Colin G. Kaide, MD, FACEP, FAAEM, UHM, Associate Professor of Emergency Medicine, Department of Emergency Medicine, Board-Certified Specialist in Hyperbaric Medicine, Wexner Medical Center, The Ohio State University, Columbus, Ohio

Ron L. Kaplan, MD, Associate Professor, Department of Pediatrics, University of Washington School of Medicine; Attending Physician, Emergency Department, Seattle Children's Hospital, Seattle, Washington

Michael P. Kefer, MD, Attending Physician, Summit Medical Center, Oconomowoc, Wisconsin

Kathleen Kerrigan, MD, FACEP, FACOG, Assistant Professor, Department of Emergency Medicine, Baystate Medical Center, Tufts University School of Medicine, Springfield, Massachusetts

Sorabh Khandelwal, MD, Samuel J Kiehl Professor in Emergency Medicine, Residency Program Director, Department of Emergency Medicine, Director of the Patient Care Competency, College of Medicine, The Ohio State University, Columbus, Ohio

Nicholas E. Kman, MD, FACEP, Director, Part 3, Med 4 Academic Program, Clinical-Associate Professor of Emergency Medicine, Department of Emergency Medicine, Wexner Medical Center, The Ohio State University, Columbus, Ohio

Olumayowa U. Kolade, MBBS, FISQua, Fellow, International Society for Quality in Healthcare (ISQua), Dublin, Ireland; Liaison to Nigeria, American College of Emergency Physician (ACEP); Medical Officer, University College Hospital, Ibadan, Oyo State, Nigeria

Rebecca Kornas, MD, Emergency Medicine Specialist, S.C. Milwaukee, Wisconsin; Division of Medical Toxicology, Department of Emergency Medicine, San Diego School of Medicine, University of California, La Jolla, California

Eric Kraska, MD, CEP America, St Alphonsus Regional Medical Center, Boise, Idaho

Allyson A. Kreshak, MD, FACEP, FACMT, Assistant Clinical Professor, Emergency Medicine, University of California, San Diego, California

David R. Lane, MD, FACEP, Associate Professor of Emergency Medicine, Georgetown University School of Medicine; Vice Chairman, Department of Emergency Medicine, MedStar Southern Maryland Hospital Center, Clinton, Maryland

Jo Anna Leuck, MD, FACEP, Vice Chair of Academics and the Program Director for the Department of Emergency Medicine, John Peter Smith Health System in Fort Worth, Texas

Michael Levine, MD, Division of Medical Toxicology, Department of Emergency Medicine, University of Southern California, Los Angeles, California

O. John Ma, MD, Professor and Chair, Department of Emergency Medicine, Oregon Health & Science University, Portland, Oregon

Jonathan A. Maisel, Associate Residency Director, Department of Emergency Medicine, Yale EM Residency, Yale University, New Haven, Connecticut

David E. Manthey, MD, FACEP, FAAEM, Professor of Emergency Medicine, Wake Forest School of Medicine, Winston-Salem, North Carolina

C. Crawford Mechem, MD, Professor, Department of Emergency Medicine, Perelman School of Medicine at the University of Pennsylvania Hospital, University of Pennsylvania, Philadelphia, Pennsylvania

Garth D. Meckler, MD, MSHS, Associate Professor and Division Head, Pediatric Emergency Medicine, University of British Columbia/BC Children's Hospital, Vancouver, British Columbia

Alix L. Mitchell, MD, Attending Physician, MetroHealth Medical Center, Cleveland, Ohio; Assistant Professor, Case Western Reserve University, Cleveland, Ohio

Michael S. Mitchell, MD, Assistant Professor of Emergency Medicine, Section of Pediatric Emergency Medicine, Wake Forest University School of Medicine, Winston-Salem, North Carolina

Ameer P. Mody, MD, MPH, FAAP, Clinical Assistant Professor of Pediatrics, Keck School of Medicine, University of Southern California, Division of Emergency Medicine, Children's Hospital Los Angeles, Los Angeles, California

Sandra L. Najarian, MD, Assistant Professor, Department of Emergency Medicine, MetroHealth Medical Center, Cleveland, Ohio

Norberto Navarrete, MD, MSc, Emergency Physician, Clinical Epidemiology, Burn Intensive Care Unit, Hospital Simón Bolívar, Bogotá, Colombia

Annet Alenyo Ngabirano, MD, Emergency Medicine Registrar, Stellenbosch University, Cape Town, South Africa

Bret A. Nicks, MD, MHA, Professor, Department of Emergency Medicine, Wake Forest School of Medicine, Winston-Salem, North Carolina

Joshua N. Nogar, MD, Assistant Professor, Emergency Medicine, Assistant Fellowship Director, Medical Toxicology, Northwell Health, NSUH/LIJ, Hofstra NSUH/LIJ School of Medicine, Hempstead, New York

Kimberly Nordstrom, MD, JD, Medical Director, Office of Behavioral Health, School of Medicine, University of Colorado Denver, Denver, Colorado; Immediate Past-President, American Association for Emergency Psychiatry, Parker, Colorado

Jeffrey G. Norvell, MD, Assistant Professor, Division of Emergency Medicine, University of Kansas School of Medicine, Kansas City, Kansas

Andrew Nyce, MD, Associate Professor of Emergency Medicine, Cooper Medical School of Rowan University, Camden, New Jersey

Paul Nystrom, MD, Assistant Professor of Emergency Medicine, University of Minnesota Medical School, Department of Emergency Medicine, Hennepin County Medical Center, Minneapolis, Minnesota

Charles W. O'Connell, MD, Clinical Professor, Division of Medical Toxicology, Department of Emergency Medicine, University of California, San Diego, Scripps Clinical Medical Group, San Diego, California

Cem Oktay, MD, Akdeniz University School of Medicine, Antalya, Turkey

James O'Neill, MD, Associate Professor, Department of Emergency Medicine, Wake Forest School of Medicine, Winston-Salem, North Carolina

Özlem Köksal, MD, PhD, Associate Professor, Department of Emergency Medicine, School of Medicine, Uludag University, Bursa, Turkey

Nilesh Patel, DO, FAAEM, FACOEP, Assistant Professor, Clinical Emergency Medicine, New York Medical College; Program Director, Emergency Medicine, St. Joseph's Regional Medical Center, Paterson, New Jersey

Andrew D. Perron, MD, FACEP, Professor and Residency Program Director, Department of Emergency Medicine, Maine Medical Center, Portland, Maine

Stacey L. Poznanski, DO, Med, Associate Professor, Boonshoft School of Medicine, Wright State University, Dayton, Ohio

Eugenia B. Quackenbush, MD, FACEP, Assistant Professor, Department of Emergency Medicine, UNC-Chapel Hill School of Medicine, Chapel Hill, North Carolina

Timothy J. Reeder, MD, MPH, Vice Chair for Clinical Operations, Department of Emergency Medicine, Brody School of Medicine East Carolina University; Clinical Director, Emergency Department, Vidant Medical Center, Greenville, North Carolina

Landen Rentmeester, MD, Emergency Medicine Specialist, S.C. Milwaukee, Wisconsin; Division of Medical Toxicology, Department of Emergency Medicine, San Diego School of Medicine, University of California, La Jolla, California

Carlo Reyes, MD, Esq, FACEP, FAAP, Vice Chief of Staff, Assistant Medical Director, Department of Emergency Medicine, Los Robles Hospital and Medical Center, Thousand Oaks, California

Teresa J. Riech, MD, MPH, Emergency Medicine/Pediatrics, Medical Director, Pediatric Emergency Department, OSF St. Francis Medical Center, Peoria, Illinois

John Pettey Sandifer, MD, Associate Professor, Associate Program Director, Department of Emergency Medicine, University of Mississippi Medical Center, Jackson, Mississippi

Richard J. Scarfone, MD, Associate Professor of Pediatrics, Perelman School of Medicine, University of Pennsylvania; Medical Director, Disaster Preparedness, The Children's Hospital of Philadelphia, Philadelphia, Pennsylvania

Matthew J. Scholer, MD, PhD, FACEP, Assistant Professor, Department of Emergency Medicine, University of North Carolina, Chapel Hill, North Carolina

Jessica L. Smith, MD, FACEP, Residency Program Director, Department of Emergency Medicine, Alpert Medical School of Brown University, Rhode Island Hospital/The Miriam Hospital, Providence, Rhode Island

Mitchell C. Sokolosky, MD, FACEP, Associate Dean, Graduate Medical Education, ACGME Designated Institutional Official, Associate Chief Medical Officer, Associate Professor of Emergency Medicine, Wake Forest Baptist Medical Center, Winston-Salem, North Carolina

Teresa Bowen-Spinelli, MD, Clinical Assistant Professor, Department of Emergency Medicine, NYU Lutheran Medical Center, Brooklyn, New York

Saranya Srinivasan, MD, Assistant Professor of Pediatrics, Baylor College of Medicine, Pediatric Emergency Medicine Attending, Texas Children's Hospital; Pediatric Emergency Medicine Attending, Memorial Hermann Hospital; Assistant Medical Director, Houston Fire Department, Houstan, Texas

Charles E. Stewart, MD, EMDM, MPH, Emergency Physician, Tulsa, Oklahoma

Jason P. Stopyra, MD, FACEP, FAEMS, Assistant Professor of Emergency Medicine, Department of Emergency Medicine, Wake Forest School of Medicine, Winston-Salem, North Carolina

Amy M. Stubbs, MD, Assistant Professor, Residency Program Director, Department of Emergency Medicine, Truman Medical Center - Hospital Hill, University of Missouri-Kansas City School of Medicine, Kansas City, Missouri

Carolyn K. Synovitz, MD, MPH, FACEP, Clinical Associate Professor, Department of Emergency Medicine, University of Oklahoma School of Community Medicine, Tulsa, Oklahoma

James K. Takayesu, MD, MS, Assistant Residency Director, Harvard-Affiliated Emergency Medicine Residency at BWH/MGH; Clerkship Co-Director, MGH, Departmental Simulation Officer; Assistant Professor of Emergency Medicine, Harvard Medical School, Boston, Massachusetts

Lorraine Thibodeau, MD, Director of Undergraduate Medical Education, Department of Emergency Medicine, Albany Medical Center, Albany, New York

Christian A. Tomaszewski, MD, MS, MBA, FACEP, FACMT, FIFEM, Professor of Clinical Emergency Medicine, Chief Medical Officer, El Centro Regional Medical Center; Attending in Emergency Medicine, Medical Toxicology, and Hyperbarics, University of California San Diego Health Department of Emergency Medicine, San Diego, California

Sarah E. Unterman, MD, Chief of Emergency Medicine, Jesse Brown VA Medical Center, Chicago, Illinois; Clinical Assistant Professor, University of Illinois Hospital and Health Sciences System, University of Illinois at Chicago, Chicago, Illinois

Adam Vella, MD, Associate Professor, Department of Emergency Medicine, Mount Sinai Medical Center, New York, New York

Janna H. Villano, MD, Department of Emergency Medicine, Sharp Chula Vista Medical Center, University of California, San Diego, California

Michael E. Vrablik, DO, Division of Emergency Medicine, University of Washington School of Medicine, Seattle, Washington

Benjamin W. Wachira, MD Dip PEC(SA), FCEM(SA), Assistant Professor, The Aga Khan University, Nairobi; Director, Emergency Medicine Kenya Foundation, Executive Committee Member, African Federation for Emergency Medicine, Nairobi, Kenya, Africa

David A. Wald, DO, Professor of Emergency Medicine, Lewis Katz School of Medicine, Philadelphia, Pennsylvania

Richard A. Walker , MD, FACEP, FAAEM, Associate Professor of Emergency Medicine University of Nebraska Medical Center Omaha, Nebraska

Marie Waterhouse, MD, Clinical Assistant Professor of Pediatrics, Keck School of Medicine, University of Southern California, Division of Emergency Medicine, Children's Hospital Los Angeles, Los Angeles, California

Sandra L. Werner, MD, FACEP, Clinical Operations Director, Associate Director, Emergency Medicine Residency Program, Associate Professor, Case Western Reserve School of Medicine, MetroHealth Medical Center, Cleveland, Ohio

Benjamin Weston, MD, MPH, Assistant Professor, Section of EMS and Disaster Medicine, Department of Emergency Medicine, Medical College of Wisconsin, Milwaukee, Wisconsin

Lori J. Whelan, MD, Vice Chair, OU Department of Emergency Medicine, Associate Professor & Director of Ultrasound, Associate Program Director, University of Oklahoma School of Community Medicine, Tulsa, Oklahoma

Maame Yaa A. B. Yiadom, MD, MPH, VEMRT-NHLBI K12 Emergency Care Scholar, Director, The ED Operations Study Group, Assistant Professor, Emergency Medicine, Vanderbilt University, Nashville, Tennessee

Shan Yin, MD, MPH, Assistant Professor of Pediatrics, Division of Emergency Medicine, Cincinnati Children's Hospital, University of Cincinnati School of Medicine; Medical Director, Drug and Poison Information Center, Cincinnati, Ohio

Stacie Zelman, MD, FACEP, Assistant Professor, Department of Emergency Medicine, Wake Forest Baptist Medical Center, Winston-Salem, North Carolina

Leslie S. Zun, MD, MBA, President, American Association for Emergency Psychiatry; Professor and Chair, Department of Emergency Medicine, Professor, Department of Psychiatry, Chicago Medical School, Rosalind Franklin University of Medicine and Science, North Chicago, Illinois; System Chair, Department of Emergency Medicine, Sinai Health System, Chicago, Illinois

Preface

Prior to the spring of my third year of medical school, I hadn't heard of the specialty emergency medicine. I didn't know where in the medical center our "emergency room" (ER)[1] was and I didn't know that we had a combined emergency medicine (EM)/internal medicine (IM) residency program. Apparently, they didn't promote the program much among the medical students. One day, shortly before I was to begin my final year of medical school, an EM/IM resident enlightened me and convinced me to squeeze an EM elective into my upcoming schedule. Fast forward a few months, I began my EM rotation and was hooked. On September 21,1979, three weeks into my EM elective, emergency medicine (EM) was recognized as the 23rd American specialty. Yes, I'm that old and so is our specialty.

I prepared for my initial EM certification board exams using the first edition of *The Study Guide*. It was well written, easy to read, and much shorter than the current eighth edition of *Tintinalli's Emergency Medicine Manual*, which is derived from the eighth edition of *Tintinalli's Emergency Medicine: A Comprehensive Study Guide*. What a great honor it has been to work with Dr. Tintinalli and to contribute to both her namesake textbook and manual.

While a single editor compiled Tintinalli's first *Study Guide*, the eighth edition of *Tintinalli's Emergency Medicine Manual* includes contributors from across the globe, including several African nations where emergency medicine is an emerging specialty. The eighth edition includes "Palliative Care," which was certainly not on emergency medicine's radar in 1979, but is now recognized as a subspecialty of our discipline. We continue to publish the *Manual* in multiple languages for our readers around the world and hope that the *Manual* and its online version at *accessemergencymedicine.mhmedical.com* continues to serve the daily needs of medical students, residents, advanced practice providers, and practicing emergency physicians.

The co-editors Michael T. Fitch, Scott Joing, Vincent Wang, David M. Cline, O. John Ma, and I would like to thank all the authors for their excellent efforts in writing and updating chapters while also maintaining busy clinical schedules. Thanks, too, to the hardworking crew at McGraw Hill Education for their guidance in taking this project from draft to publication: Brian Belval, Christie Naglieri, Jessica Gonzalez, Juanita Thompson, and Poonam Bisht. Finally, I am grateful to have had such wonderful team of editors with whom to work. They made publishing this handbook a delight. Thanks Michael, Scott, Vincent, David, and John.

RKC dedicates this book to Marc, Matthew, Lissy, and Noah, as well as to emergency care providers around the world; MF dedicates this book to Missy, Mira, and Maya, and in memory of Dr. John Marx; SJ dedicates this book to wonderful Elizabeth, Micah, Owen, Britta, and Emmy along with the outstanding Hennepin County Medical Center EM faculty and residents; VW dedicates this book to Esther, Elijah, and Evaline; DMC dedicates this book to family: home, church, and professional; OJM dedicates this book to everyone dedicated to advancing quality of care and patient safety in emergency medicine.

[1]Prior to becoming known as the Emergency Department (ED), the area was known as the emergency room.

SECTION 1

Resuscitation Techniques

CHAPTER 1 Advanced Airway Support

Darren Braude

Airway assessment and management is one of the most critical interventions that emergency physicians perform. Intubation is not always necessary, however, and rushing into invasive airway management before initial resuscitation can be problematic.

RAPID AIRWAY ASSESSMENT

Perform a rapid clinical airway assessment which includes noting the patient's level of responsiveness, skin color, respiratory rate, and depth of respirations. Obtain oxygen saturation and capnography unless the patient is in impending or actual cardiac arrest. The goal is to determine if the patient is maintaining and protecting their airway and meeting critical oxygenation and ventilation goals. Nothing should be placed in the pharynx to assess gag reflex. Emergent and immediate decisions on airway management may proceed before obtaining blood gases and x-rays.

IMPENDING/ACTUAL CARDIAC ARREST

Open the airway and initiate low-volume ventilation unless following cardiocerebral resuscitation protocols. The primary focus of initial cardiopulmonary resuscitation is on establishing quality chest compressions and evaluating for a shockable rhythm. Once these priorities are addressed, the airway can be further managed with an extraglottic device or endotracheal intubation.

BASIC AIRWAY MANAGEMENT

Position the patient to open the airway, drain secretions and maximize oxygenation and ventilation, while maintaining cervical stabilization precautions if indicated. Place conscious patients in a sitting position, if possible, and unconscious patients on their side unless they require urgent invasive procedures. Patients who are unable to maintain an open airway should have one or two properly sized nasal trumpets placed if they are not anticoagulated or at risk for mid-face fractures; an oral airway may be used instead of, or in addition to, the nasal airways if no gag reflex present. Provide supplemental oxygen if the room air saturation is below 94% with the goal of increasing saturation to above 94%; high flow oxygen should be avoided when possible.

NONINVASIVE POSITIVE PRESSURE VENTILATION

If ventilation is adequate but oxygenation is poor, consider immediate initiation of noninvasive ventilation. Noninvasive positive pressure ventilation (NIPPV) may be used as a temporizing measure while other treatments are initiated (e.g., nitrates in acute cardiogenic pulmonary edema), for preoxygenation prior to intubation in any medical condition, or as an alternative to invasive airway management in some cases, such as in patients with DNR or DNI status. NIPPV for emergency situations is commonly delivered via a full-face mask using either continuous positive airway pressure (CPAP) or bilevel positive airway pressure (BPAP) using a ventilator, stand-alone reusable device, or a disposable device (CPAP only). CPAP provides the same amount of pressure support during inspiration and positive end-expiratory pressure (PEEP) during exhalation—usually 5 to 10 mmHg—while BPAP allows for increasing pressure support up to 15 mm Hg without overwhelming the patient with expiratory resistance, which may remain at 5 to 10 mm Hg. There are no studies showing a significant advantage to one system over another.

MASK VENTILATION

Begin mask ventilation for patients with poor respiratory effort. Patients should be placed in a sniffing or ramped position with airway adjuncts as previously discussed. Apply a properly fitted mask with one provider dedicated to maintaining a tight seal while a second provider or mechanical ventilator provides just enough volume to raise the chest. Two different hand grips are described to achieve a mask seal during two-person mask ventilation with the "T-E" preferred over the "E-C" in most cases (Fig. 1-1). If you are unable to achieve a tight mask seal consider placing an extraglottic device *if there is no gag reflex or other contraindication.* If good chest rise is noted but saturations remain poor despite supplemental oxygen, add PEEP.

EXTRAGLOTTIC DEVICES

Extraglottic devices (EGDs) are placed blindly and fit into the following category: (1) supraglottic devices that include a mask that sits internally over the glottic opening or (2) retroglottic, dual-balloon devices that sit within the proximal esophagus and include distal and proximal balloons to direct the ventilation that occurs through holes between the two balloons into the airway. Supraglottic devices include, but are not limited to, the Ambu Auragain®, LMA Supreme®, LMA Protector®, LMA Fastrach, Intersurgical iGel®, and CookGas AirQ. Retroglottic devices include the Esophageal-Tracheal Combitube, the Rusch EasyTube, and the King Laryngeal Tube®. Many of these devices now include a channel for gastric decompression (theoretically lessens the risk of aspiration) and some facilitate blind or endoscopic intubation.

Extraglottic devices are most commonly used in the ED after a failed airway but may also be used primarily during cardiac arrest, for difficult mask

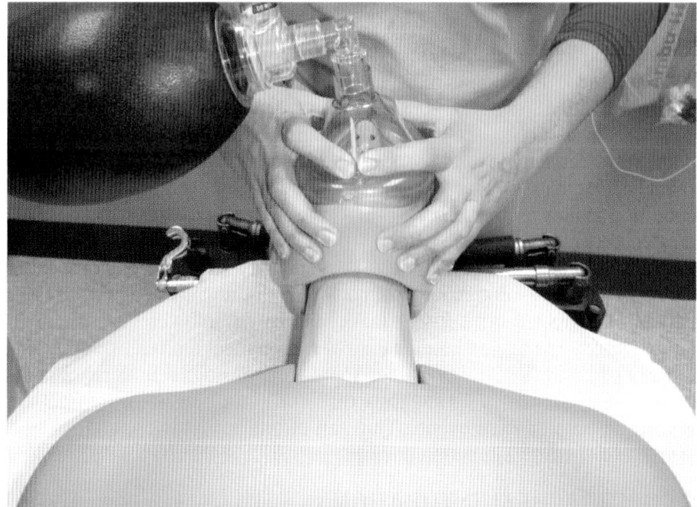

A

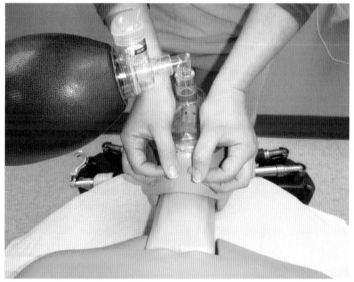

B

FIGURE 1-1. Mask ventilation: traditional "E-C" hand grip (A) and modified "T-E" hand grip (B).

ventilation or as part of rapid sequence airway procedures. It is critical to always have an appropriately sized EGD available during airway management to place the device in case difficulties are encountered but do not rely on an EGD to the exclusion of surgical airway when critical hypoxemia is encountered.

INTUBATION

Intubate patients in cardiac arrest after other critical resuscitation steps have been assured. Intubation is indicated for unconscious, nonarrested patients unless a rapidly correctable situation is suspected, such as an opioid overdose or simple postictal state. Consider intubation for conscious patients with refractory hypoxemia or a deteriorating clinical course. Rapid sequence intubation (RSI) technique should be used unless the patient's condition makes it unnecessary (i.e., cardiac arrest) or when it is contraindicated because of an anticipated difficult airway. RSI includes the simultaneous administration of an induction agent and a neuromuscular blocking agent to facilitate orotracheal intubation in the nonarrested/peri-arrested patient. Anticipated difficulty in mask ventilation, intubation, rescue with an extraglottic device and surgical airway placement are relative contraindications to RSI; awake techniques should be considered in these circumstances. Current evidence suggests that multiple intubation attempts are associated with adverse events. Thus, all efforts should be made to set up success on the first intubation attempt.

OROTRACHEAL INTUBATION

1. Prepare equipment, personnel, and drugs before attempting intubation. Assess airway difficulty and anticipate required airway rescue. Assemble and place suction, bag-valve-mask, and rescue devices within easy reach. Sufficient personnel should be present at the bedside to assist. Assign all the tasks in advance, including medication administration, cervical spine stabilization, external laryngeal manipulation, etc. *Use of a checklist is strongly encouraged.*
2. Ensure adequate ventilation and oxygenation and monitoring while preparing equipment. Preoxygenate with a non-rebreather oxygen mask at maximal oxygen flow rates, NIPPV, or mask ventilation if the patient is not ventilating adequately. Place a nasal cannula with up to 15 L/min of oxygen flow under the mask to provide for apneic oxygenation. *An inability to achieve an oxygen saturation of greater than 93% with these maneuvers places the patient at risk for critical desaturation after apnea is induced*; be prepared to perform controlled positive pressure mask ventilation.
3. Optimize physiology prior to intubation *if at all possible* to lessen the risk of peri-intubation complications. This may include administration of IV fluid boluses, inotropes, and/or vasopressors in addition to oxygenation as above.
4. Select, connect, and test the laryngoscope and blade. Video laryngoscopy (VL) is a good first choice if the operator is familiar with this technique. Direct laryngoscopy (DL) is a reasonable option if the operator has more experience with this technique. Select and test the endotracheal tube, commonly 7.5 mm in women and 8 mm in men. Use a stylet with a "straight-to-cuff" configuration for DL/nonhyperangulated VL blades; hyperangulated VL blades often come with proprietary stylets that include an optimal bend (Fig. 1-2).
5. Position the patient in the sniffing or ramped position to align the external ear canal and sternal notch (Fig. 1-3). If C-spine injury is suspected, maintain the head and neck in a neutral position with an assistant performing inline stabilization and a jaw thrust maneuver.

6. Evidence is mixed on whether pretreatment improves outcomes and is no longer routinely recommended. **Fentanyl,** 3 µg/kg, may be considered in normotensive patients with possible raised intracranial pressure, cardiac ischemia, or aortic dissection.

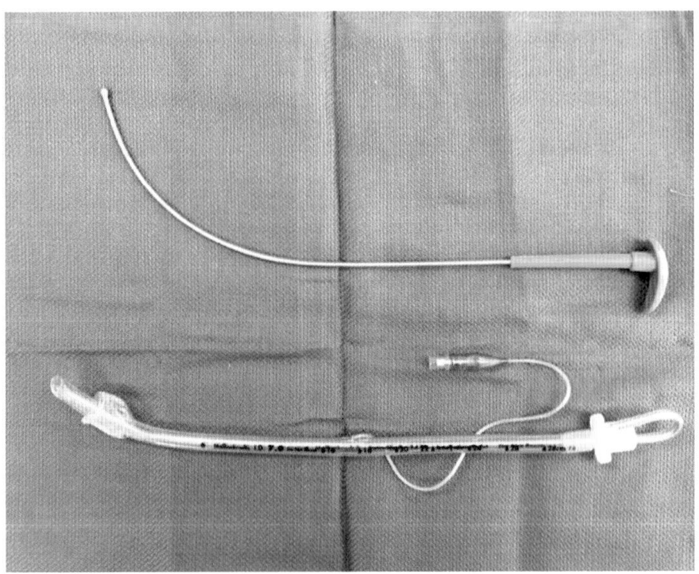

FIGURE 1-2. Top shows a stylet from Intubrite® intended for the hyperangulated video blade. Bottom demonstrates straight-to-cuff stylet shape for direct laryngoscopy.

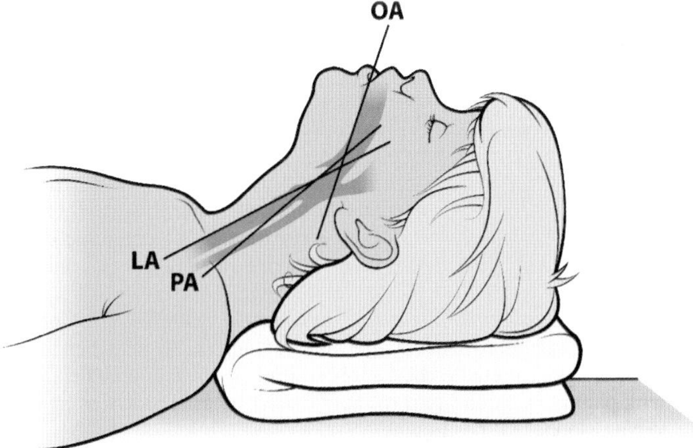

FIGURE 1-3. Sniffing position for optimal mask ventilation and intubation when cervical precautions not indicated. With permission from The Difficult Airway Course™ (www.theairwaysite.com).

7. Administer an intravenous induction agent via rapid push. **Etomidate,** 0.3 mg/kg, is an excellent choice in most circumstances. **Ketamine,** 1 to 2 mg/kg, has become a popular alternative and is generally safe, although cases of hypotension and hypertension have been reported. **Propofol,** 0.5 to 1.5 mg/kg, is another option in patients who are not at risk for hypotension.
8. The induction agent is immediately flushed with a paralytic agent. **Succinylcholine,** 1 to 2 mg/kg of total body weight, is commonly used unless there is risk of serious hyperkalemia (e.g., renal failure, neuromuscular disorders, subacute spinal cord injury, crush injury or burns). **Rocuronium,** 1 to 1.5 mg/kg of ideal body weight, is an increasingly common alternative.
9. Cricoid pressure is no longer recommended due to limited evidence of benefit and clear evidence of worsening laryngoscopic view.
10. Wait for paralysis to occur to diminish the risk of vomiting and aspiration. **Succinylcholine** usually takes effect in 30 to 45 seconds and **rocuruonium** in 60 seconds. Oxygenation should continue via non-rebreather or gentle mask ventilation during this interval.
11. Insert hyperangulated VL blades in the midline. Insert traditional curved blades (whether direct or video) on the right side of the mouth and sweep tongue to the left. Both blades are advanced into the valeculla to trigger to the hyoepiglottic ligament. *Do not over-insert hyperangulated blades*; keep the blade as shallow as possible with the airway visualized in the top half of the screen. Insert straight blades on the right side of the tongue and maintain this "paraglossal" position without sweeping the tongue and gently advance blade as far as it will go. Withdraw the blade slowly until the epiglottis drops into view and then lift it with the tip of the blade. Lift all the blades along the axis of the laryngoscope handle to avoid levering the blade on the teeth and causing dental trauma.
12. If only the epiglottis is visible, use an intubating stylet (aka Bougie) and/or perform external laryngeal manipulation of the thyroid cartilage with the operator's right hand on top of an assistant's hand (Fig. 1-4) to help bring the cords into view.
13. Once the vocal cords or posterior cartilages are visualized, gently pass the tube between the cords (or anterior to the posterior cartilages) until the balloon completely disappears and remove the stylet. When using a hyperangulated blade stylet, it helps to withdraw the stylet 2 to 3 cm once the tip of the tube just enters the airway, before advancing further. Advance tubes in adult females to approximately 21 cm at the corner of the mouth and in adult males to approximately 23 cm and then remove the stylet.
14. Confirm tracheal tube placement immediately with ETCO2. Confirm appropriate depth by listening for bilateral lung sounds and then secure tube. Obtain a portable chest x-ray to further evaluate tube depth and lung pathology. A chest x-ray should never be used to assess tracheal versus esophageal positioning.
15. *Abort the intubation attempt early if oxygen saturation is dropping* and begin immediate mask ventilation. Consider an additional attempt when saturations are maintained in the normal range with appropriate

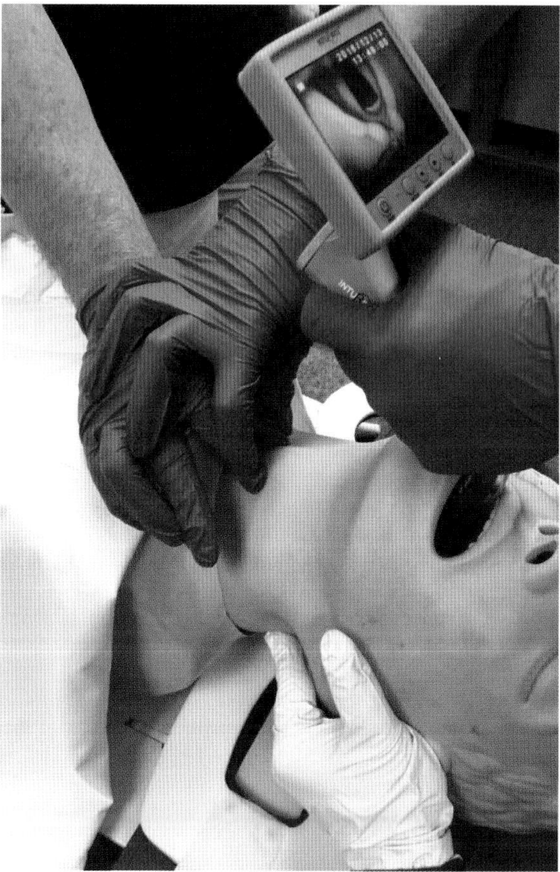

FIGURE 1-4. External laryngeal manipulation with the intubator's right hand placed on top of assistant's hand which is holding the laryngeal cartilage. Another assistant is maintaining in-line cervical stabilization and providing a jaw thrust.

modification to the operator, laryngoscope and blade selection, patient positioning, use of bougie, etc. If unable to maintain saturations with mask ventilation, insert an EGD while preparing for a possible surgical airway. If saturations are maintained but intubation is unsuccessful within three attempts, or deemed unlikely to be successful at any point, place an EGD.

Surgical Airway

A surgical airway is performed either when intubation via the mouth or nose is not considered a reasonable clinical option or when intubation has failed and critical oxygen saturation cannot be maintained via other means.

A surgical airway is contraindicated in children younger than 10 years of age in whom transtracheal jet ventilation is the preferred subglottic technique. Although several surgical techniques have been described, the bougie-aided technique is described here. There are kits available for Seldinger-based and other "less invasive" techniques but these are not reviewed here.

1. Use sterile technique if possible.
2. Palpate the cricothyroid membrane and stabilize the larynx.
3. With a scalpel, make a vertical, 3- to 4-cm incision starting at the superior border of the thyroid cartilage. Incise caudally toward the suprasternal notch (Fig. 1-5).
4. Identify the cricothyroid membrane using blunt dissection if necessary and make a 2-cm horizontal incision. Immediately withdraw and secure the blade while inserting a gloved finger into the incision.
5. Place an adult bougie into the incision with the coude tip directed distally. The bougie should pass easily without resistance until hold-up is appreciated in the smaller airways, generally confirming tracheal placement.
6. Pass a 6.0-cuffed endotracheal tube or #4 cuffed tracheostomy tube over the bougie and into the airway (Fig. 1-6). If using an endotracheal tube stop advancing as soon the cuff is completely within the airway. Inflate cuff.
7. Confirm with capnography and easy chest rise with bilateral breath sounds.
8. Secure the tube.

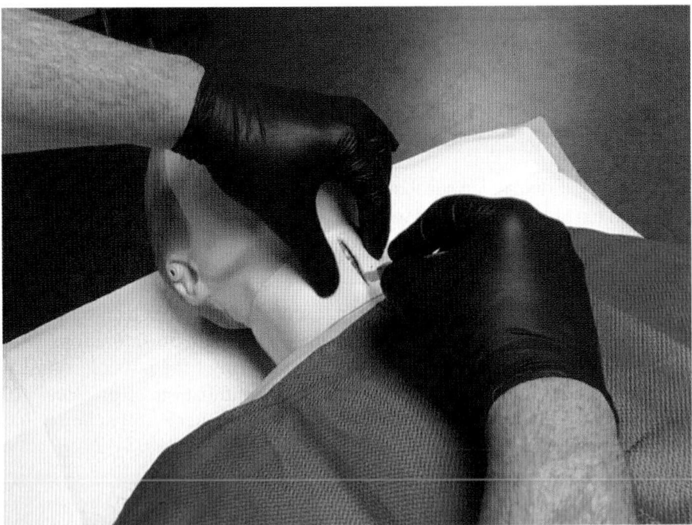

FIGURE 1-5. A 3- to 4-cm vertical midline incision overlying the cricothyroid membrane while the laryngeal cartilage is stabilized.

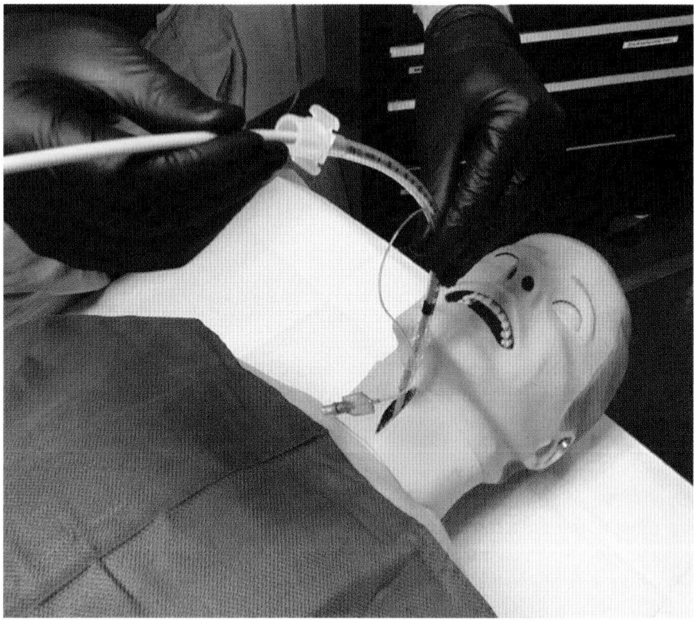

FIGURE 1-6. Passing a 6-0 endotracheal tube over a bougie that has been placed into the trachea through the cricothyroid membrane incision.

FURTHER READING

For further reading in *Tintinalli's Emergency Medicine: A Comprehensive Study Guide*, 8th ed., see Chapter 28, "Noninvasive Airway Management," by Jestin N. Carlson and Henry E. Wang; Chapter 29, "Intubation and Mechanical Ventilation," by Robert J. Vissers and Daniel F. Danzl; and Chapter 30, "Surgical Airways," by Michael D. Smith and Donald M. Yealy.

CHAPTER 2

Management of Cardiac Rhythm Disturbances

James K. Takayesu

NONTACHYCARDIC IRREGULAR DYSRHYTHMIAS

Sinus Arrhythmia

Some variation in the sinoatrial (SA) node discharge rate is common; however, if the variation exceeds 120 milliseconds between the longest and shortest intervals, sinus arrhythmia is present. The electrocardiogram (ECG) characteristics of sinus arrhythmia are (*a*) normal sinus P waves and PR intervals, (*b*) 1:1 atrioventricular (AV) conduction, and (*c*) variation of at least 120 milliseconds between the shortest and longest P–P interval (Fig. 2-1). If two or more different P wave morphologies are present, atrial ectopy, wandering atrial pacemaker, or another competing nonsinus focus may be present. Sinus arrhythmias are affected primarily by respiration and are most commonly found in children and young adults, disappearing with advancing age. Occasional junctional escape beats may be present during very long P–P intervals. No treatment is required.

Premature Atrial Contractions

Premature atrial contractions (PACs) have the following ECG characteristics: (*a*) the ectopic P wave appears sooner (premature) than the next expected sinus beat; (*b*) the ectopic P wave has a different shape and direction; and (*c*) the ectopic P wave may or may not be conducted through the AV node (Fig. 2-2). Most PACs are conducted with typical QRS complexes, but some may be conducted aberrantly through the infranodal system, typically with a right bundle branch block pattern. When the PAC occurs during the absolute refractory period, it is not conducted. Since the sinus node is often depolarized and reset, the interval between normal P waves before and after the PAC will not be twice the existing P to P interval, creating a shorter pause than a fully compensatory pause (unlike that seen after most premature ventricular contractions). PACs are associated with stress, fatigue, alcohol use, tobacco, coffee, chronic obstructive pulmonary disease (COPD), digoxin toxicity, and coronary artery disease, and may occur after adenosine-converted paroxysmal supraventricular tachycardia (PSVT). Patients may complain of palpitations or an intermittent "sinking" or "fluttering" feeling in the chest. PACs are common in all ages, often in the

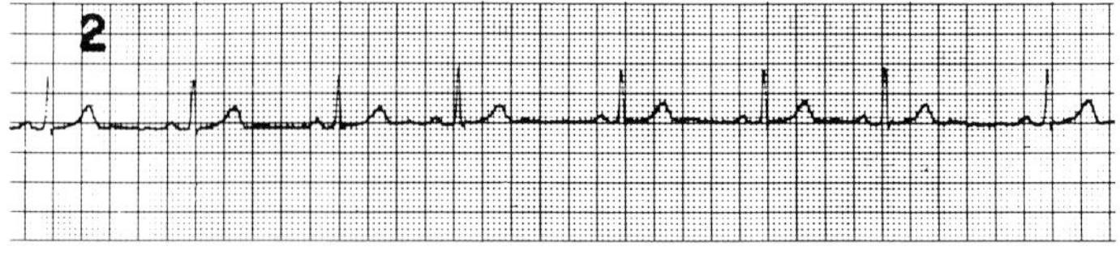

FIGURE 2-1. Sinus arrhythmia.

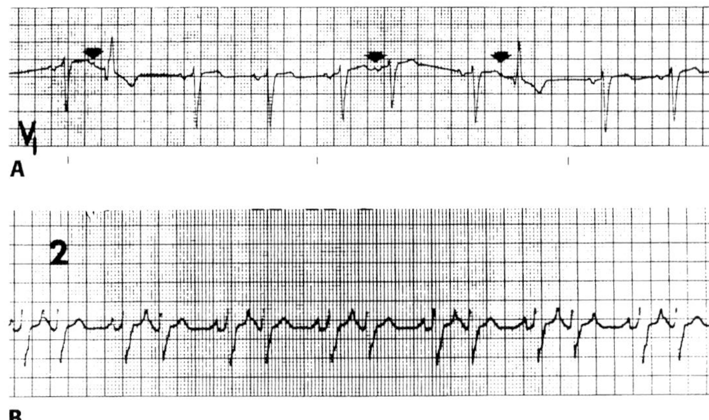

FIGURE 2-2. Premature atrial contractions (PACs). **A.** Ectopic P′ waves (arrows). **B.** Atrial bigeminy.

absence of significant heart disease, but can precipitate sustained atrial tachycardia, flutter, or fibrillation under certain circumstances.

Emergency Department Care and Disposition

1. Discontinue precipitating drugs (alcohol, tobacco, or coffee) or toxins.
2. Treat underlying disorders (stress or fatigue).

Premature Ventricular Contractions

Clinical Features

Premature ventricular contractions (PVCs) are due to impulses originating from single or multiple areas in the ventricles. The ECG characteristics of PVCs are as follows: (*a*) a premature and wide QRS complex; (*b*) no preceding P wave; (*c*) the ST segment and T wave of the PVC are directed opposite the preceding major QRS deflection; (*d*) most PVCs do not affect the sinus node, so there is usually a fully compensatory postectopic pause, or the PVC may be interpolated between two sinus beats; (*e*) many PVCs have a fixed coupling interval (within 40 milliseconds) from the preceding sinus beat; and (*f*) many PVCs are conducted into the atria, thus producing a retrograde P wave (Fig. 2-3). If three or more PVCs occur in a row, patients are considered to have nonsustained ventricular tachycardia.

PVCs are very common, occurring in most patients with ischemic heart disease and acute myocardial infarction (MI). Other common causes of PVCs include digoxin toxicity, congestive heart failure (CHF), hypokalemia, alkalosis, hypoxia, and sympathomimetic drugs. Pooled data and meta-analyses have found no reduction in mortality from suppressive or prophylactic treatment of PVCs. Ventricular parasystole occurs when the ectopic ventricular focus fires frequently enough to compete with the SA node and is associated with cardiac ischemia, electrolyte imbalance, and hypertensive or ischemic heart disease.

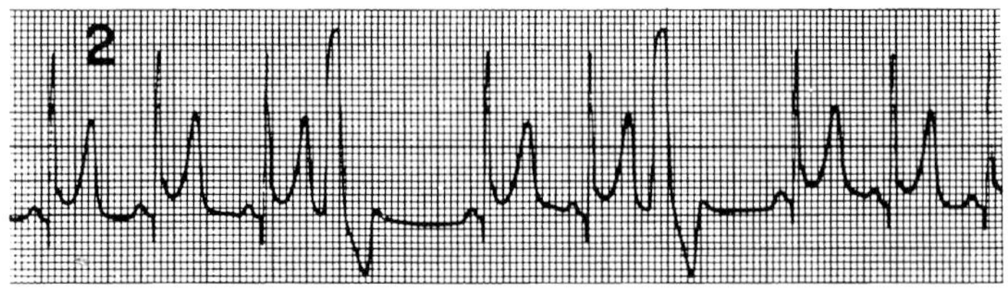

A

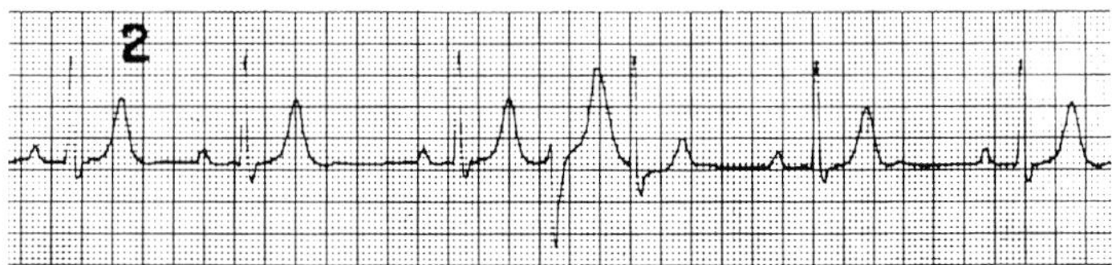

B

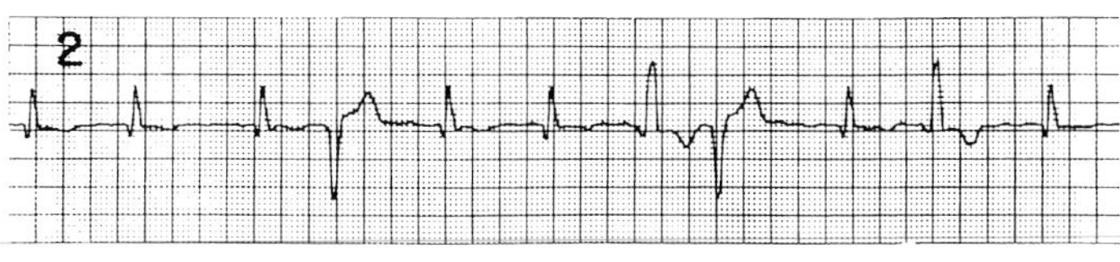

C

FIGURE 2-3. Premature ventricular contractions (PVCs). **A.** Unifocal PVC. **B.** Interpolated PVC. **C.** Multifocal PVCs.

Emergency Department Care and Disposition

1. Stable patients require no treatment.
2. Patients with three or more sequential PVCs should be managed as non-sustained VT.
3. Potential causes such as hypoxia, drug effect, or electrolyte disturbances should be treated.

BRADYDYSRHYTHMIAS

Sinus Bradycardia

Clinical Features

Sinus bradycardia occurs when the SA node rate becomes slower than 60 beats/min. The ECG characteristics of sinus bradycardia are (*a*) normal sinus P waves and PR intervals, (*b*) 1:1 AV conduction, and (*c*) atrial rate slower than 60 beats/min. Sinus bradycardia represents a suppression of the sinus node discharge rate, usually in response to three categories of stimuli: (*a*) physiologic (vagal tone), (*b*) pharmacologic (calcium channel blockers, β-blockers, or digoxin), and (*c*) pathologic (acute inferior myocardial infarction (MI), increased intracranial pressure, carotid sinus hypersensitivity, hypothyroidism, or sick sinus syndrome).

Emergency Department Care and Disposition

Sinus bradycardia usually does not require specific treatment unless the heart rate is slower than 50 beats/min and there is evidence of hypoperfusion.

1. **Transcutaneous cardiac pacing** is the only Class I treatment for unstable patients.
   a. Attach the patient to the monitor leads of the external pacing device.
   b. When placing transcutaneous pacing pads, place the anterior pad over the left lateral precordium and the posterior pad at the level of the heart in the right infrascapular area. Do not use multifunction pacing defibrillation pads unless the patient is unconscious as the pads cause a lot of discomfort.
   c. Slowly increase the pacing output from 0 mA to the lowest point where capture is observed, usually at 50 to 100 mA, but may be up to 200 mA. A widened QRS after each pacing spike denotes electrical capture.
   d. If needed, administer a sedative, such as lorazepam, 1 to 2 mg IV, or an opiate, such as morphine, 2 to 4 mg IV, for pain control.
2. **Atropine** is a Class IIa treatment for symptomatic bradycardia. The dose is 0.5 mg IV push, repeated every 3 to 5 minutes as needed up to a total of 3 mg IV. If given via endotracheal tube, increase the dose by 2 to 2.5 times over the IV dose. Slow administration or lower doses may cause paradoxical bradycardia. Atropine may not be effective in cardiac transplant patients since the heart is denervated and has no vagal stimulation.
3. **Epinephrine**, 2 to 10 μg/min IV, or **dopamine**, 3 to 10 μg/kg/min IV, may be used if external pacing is not available.
4. Permanent pacemaker placement is indicated in the patient with symptomatic recurrent or persistent sinus bradycardia due to sick sinus syndrome.
5. Glucagon 3 to 10 mg IV over 1 to 2 minutes, followed by an infusion of 1 to 5 mg/h may be used in β-blocker or calcium channel blocker toxicity.

Junctional Rhythms

Clinical Features

In patients with sinus bradycardia, SA node exit block, or AV block, junctional escape beats may occur, usually at a rate between 40 and 60 beats/min, depending on the level of the rescue pacemaker within the conduction system. Junctional escape beats may conduct retrogradely into the atria, but the QRS complex usually will mask any retrograde P wave (Fig. 2-4). When alternating rhythmically with the SA node, junctional escape beats

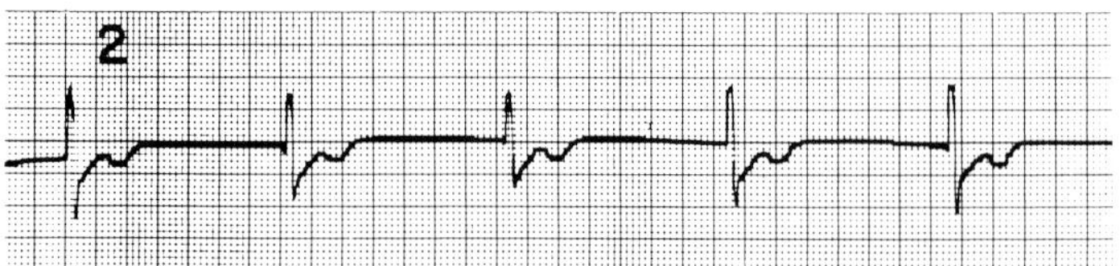

FIGURE 2-4. Junctional escape rhythm, rate 42.

may cause bigeminal or trigeminal rhythms. Sustained junctional escape rhythms may be seen with CHF, myocarditis, acute MI (especially inferior MI), hyperkalemia, or digoxin toxicity ("regularized Afib"). If the ventricular rate is too slow, myocardial or cerebral ischemia may develop. In cases of enhanced junctional automaticity, junctional rhythms may be accelerated (60 to 100 beats/min) or tachycardic (≥100 beats/min), thus overriding the SA node rate.

Emergency Department Care and Disposition

1. Isolated, infrequent junctional escape beats usually do not require specific treatment.
2. If sustained junctional escape rhythms are producing symptoms, treat the underlying cause.
3. In unstable patients, give **atropine** 0.5 mg IV every 5 minutes to a total of 3 mg. This will accelerate the SA node discharge rate and enhance AV nodal conduction.
4. Use transcutaneous or transvenous pacing in unstable patients not responsive to atropine.
5. Manage patients with digoxin toxicity as discussed for SVT.

Idioventricular Rhythm

Clinical Features

The ECG characteristics of idioventricular rhythm (IVR) are (*a*) wide and regular QRS complexes; (*b*) a rate between 40 and 100 beats/min, often close to the preceding sinus rate; (*c*) mostly runs of short duration (3 to 30 beats/min); and (*d*) an AIVR often beginning with a fusion beat (Fig. 2-5). This condition is found most commonly with an acute MI or in the setting of reperfusion after successful thrombolysis.

Emergency Department Care and Disposition

Treatment is not necessary unless the patient is unstable or pulseless. On occasion, especially after reperfusion therapy, the IVR may be the only functioning pacemaker, and suppression with lidocaine can lead to cardiac asystole.

If the patient is hypotensive or in arrest, treatment includes identifying contributing mechanical factors (e.g., aggressive volume resuscitation) and α-adrenergic agents.

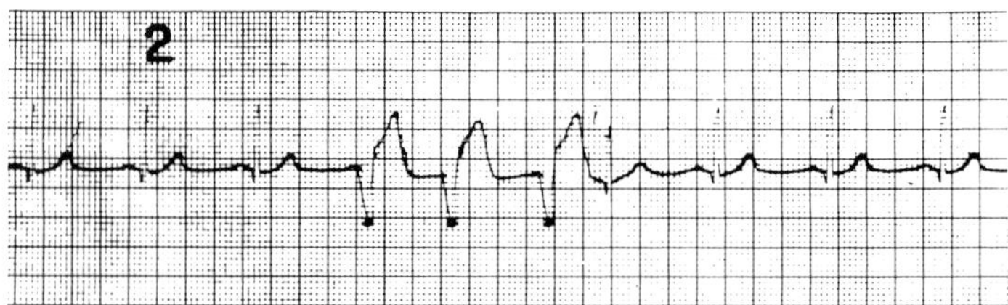

FIGURE 2-5. Accelerated idioventricular rhythms (AIVRs).

Sick Sinus Syndrome

Clinical Features

Otherwise known as tachy-brady syndrome, sick sinus syndrome consists of a variety of abnormalities in impulse generation and conduction, leading to various supraventricular tachycardic rhythms as well as bradycardia due to sinus arrest and SA block. It can be seen in myocardial ischemia, myocarditis, rheumatologic disease, cardiomyopathies, or metastatic disease. Conditions that increase vagal tone such acute abdominal pain, thyrotoxicosis, and hypo- or hyperkalemia exacerbate this condition.

Emergency Department Care and Disposition

Treatment should be based on the presenting rhythm depending on the heart rate and patient instability. Temporary pacing may be needed and admission for permanent pacemaker placement is frequently indicated.

ATRIOVENTRICULAR BLOCKS

First-Degree Atrioventricular (AV) Block

First-degree AV block is characterized by a delay in AV conduction, manifested by a prolonged PR interval (>200 milliseconds). It can be found in normal hearts and in association with increased vagal tone, digoxin toxicity, inferior MI, amyloid, and myocarditis. First-degree AV block needs no treatment. Second-degree AV block is characterized by intermittent AV nodal conduction: some atrial impulses reach the ventricles, whereas others are blocked, thereby causing "grouped beating." These blocks can be subdivided into nodal blocks which are typically reversible and infranodal blocks which are due to irreversible conduction system disease. Third-degree AV block is characterized by complete interruption in AV conduction with resulting AV dissociation.

Second-Degree Mobitz I (Wenckebach) AV Block

Clinical Features

Mobitz I AV block is a nodal block causing a progressive prolongation of conduction through the AV node until the atrial impulse is completely blocked. Usually, only one atrial impulse is blocked at a time. After the dropped beat, the AV conduction returns to normal and the cycle usually repeats itself with the same conduction ratio (fixed ratio) or a different conduction ratio (variable ratio). Although the PR intervals progressively lengthen before the dropped beat, the increments by which they lengthen *decrease* with successive beats causing a progressive *shortening* of each successive R–R interval before the dropped beat (Fig. 2-6). This block is

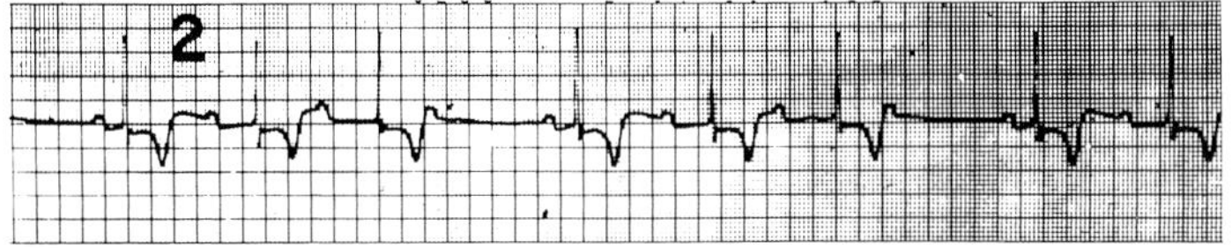

FIGURE 2-6. Second-degree Mobitz I (Wenckebach) AV block 4:3 AV conduction.

often transient and usually associated with an acute inferior MI, digoxin toxicity, or myocarditis or can be seen after cardiac surgery. Because the blockade occurs at the level of the AV node itself rather than at the infranodal conducting system, this is usually a stable rhythm.

Emergency Department Care and Disposition

1. Specific treatment is not necessary unless slow ventricular rates produce signs of hypoperfusion.
2. In cases associated with acute inferior MI, provide adequate volume resuscitation before initiating further interventions.
3. Administer **atropine** 0.5 mg IV repeated every 5 minutes. Titrate to the desired heart rate or until the total dose reaches 3 mg.
4. Although rarely needed, transcutaneous pacing may be used.

Second-Degree Mobitz II AV Block

Clinical Features

Mobitz II AV block is typically due to infranodal disease, causing a constant PR interval with intermittent nonconducted atrial beats (Fig. 2-7). One or more beats may be nonconducted at a single time. This block indicates significant damage or dysfunction of the infranodal conduction system; therefore, the QRS complexes are usually wide coming from the low His–Purkinje bundle or the ventricles. Type II blocks are more dangerous than type I blocks because they are usually permanent and may progress suddenly to complete heart block, especially in the setting of an acute anterior MI, and almost always require permanent cardiac pacemaker placement. When second-degree AV block occurs with a fixed conduction ratio of 2:1, it is not possible to differentiate between a Mobitz type I (Wenckebach) and Mobitz type II block.

Emergency Department Care and Disposition

1. **Atropine** 0.5 to 1 mg IV bolus repeated every 5 minutes as needed up to 3 mg total dose is first-line treatment for symptomatic patients but

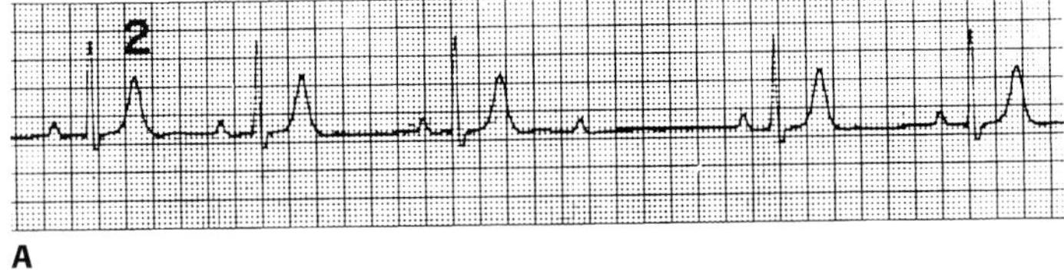

A

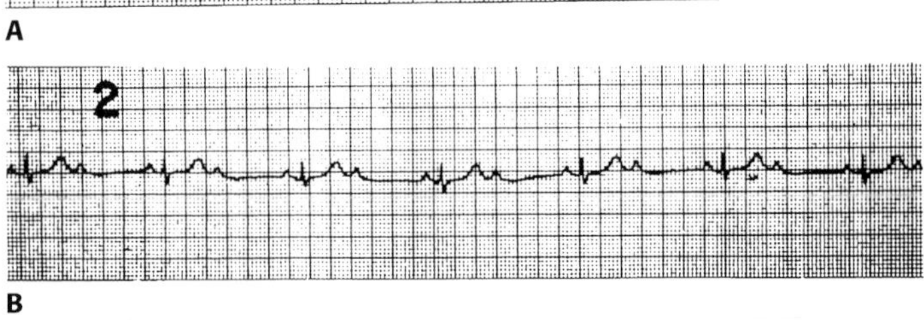

B

FIGURE 2-7. **A.** Second-degree Mobitz II AV block. **B.** Second-degree AV block with 2:1 AV conduction.

may be ineffective. All patients should have transcutaneous pacing pads positioned and ready for use in the case of further deterioration into complete heart block.

2. Initiate transcutaneous cardiac pacing (see section on sinus bradycardia) in patients unresponsive to atropine.
3. If transcutaneous pacing is unsuccessful, initiate transvenous pacing (0.2 to 20 mA at 40 to 140 beats/min via a semi-floating or balloon-tipped pacing catheter).

Third-Degree (Complete) AV Block

Clinical Features

In third-degree AV block, there is no AV conduction. The ventricles are paced by an escape pacemaker from the AV node or the infranodal conduction system at a rate slower than the atrial rate (Fig. 2-8). When third-degree AV block occurs at the AV node, a junctional escape pacemaker takes over with a ventricular rate of 40 to 60 beats/min, and because the rhythm originates from above the bifurcation of the His bundle, the QRS complexes are narrow. Nodal third-degree AV block may develop in up to 8% of acute inferior MIs and it is usually transient, although it may last for several days.

When third-degree AV block occurs at the infranodal level, the ventricles are driven by a ventricular escape rhythm at a rate slower than 40 beats/min. Third-degree AV block located in the bundle branch or the Purkinje system invariably has an escape rhythm with a wide QRS complex. Like Mobitz type II block, this indicates structural damage to the infranodal conduction system and can be seen in acute anterior MIs. The ventricular escape pacemaker is usually inadequate to maintain cardiac output and is unstable with periods of ventricular asystole.

Emergency Department Care and Disposition

1. Perform transcutaneous cardiac pacing in unstable patients until a transvenous pacemaker can be placed.
2. In stable patients, apply transcutaneous pacing pads. Treat the same as second-degree Mobitz II AV block.

FASCICULAR BLOCKS

Conduction blocks may arise in one or more of the three infranodal conduction pathways. Blockage of either of the left fascicles does not prolong the QRS duration, but will change the QRS axis. Left anterior fascicular block (LAFB) causes left axis deviation with qR complex seen in aVR, while the

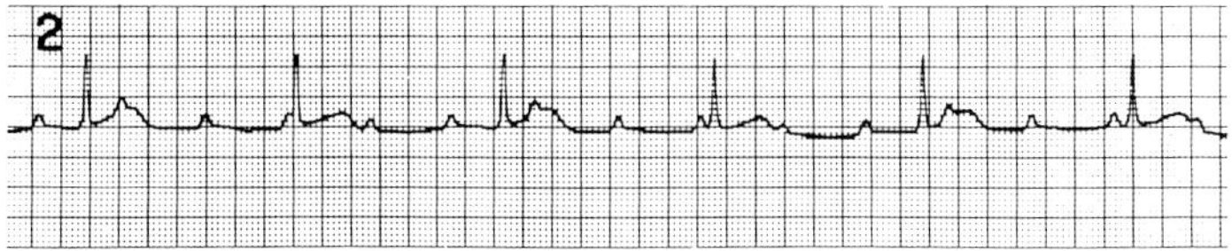

FIGURE 2-8. Third-degree AV block.

much less common left posterior fascicular block (LPFB) causes right axis deviation. Right bundle branch block (RBBB) will prolong the QRS duration (>120 milliseconds) and cause an RSR', or "rabbit ears," in the early precordial leads (V1–2). Bifascicular block denotes a combination of any two of these fascicles, the most notable of which is left bundle branch block (LAFB + LPFB). Trifascicular block denotes the presence of first degree AV block in the presence of a bifascicular block and is indicative of significant conduction system disease that includes the AV node, thus increasing the risk of Mobitz II or third-degree AV block and the potential need for permanent pacemaker placement.

NARROW COMPLEX TACHYCARDIAS

Sinus Tachycardia

Clinical Features

The ECG characteristics of sinus tachycardia are (*a*) normal sinus P waves and PR intervals and (*b*) an atrial rate usually between 100 and 160 beats/min. Sinus tachycardia is in response to one of three categories of stimuli: (*a*) physiologic (pain or exertion), (*b*) pharmacologic (sympathomimetics, caffeine, or bronchodilators), or (*c*) pathologic (fever, hypoxia, anemia, hypovolemia, pulmonary embolism, or hyperthyroidism). In many of these conditions, the increased heart rate is an effort to increase cardiac output to match increased circulatory needs.

Emergency Department Care and Disposition

Since sinus tachycardia is a compensatory rhythm, the focus should be on diagnosing and treating the underlying condition.

Atrial Flutter

Clinical Features

Atrial flutter is a rhythm that originates from a small area within the atria. ECG characteristics of atrial flutter are (*a*) a regular atrial rate between 250 and 350 beats/min; (*b*) "saw tooth" flutter waves directed superiorly and most visible in leads II, III, and aV_F; and (*c*) AV block, usually 2:1, but occasionally greater or irregular (Fig. 2-9). One-to-one conduction may occur if a bypass tract is present. Carotid sinus massage or Valsalva maneuvers are useful techniques to slow the ventricular response by increasing the degree of AV block, which can unmask flutter waves in uncertain cases.

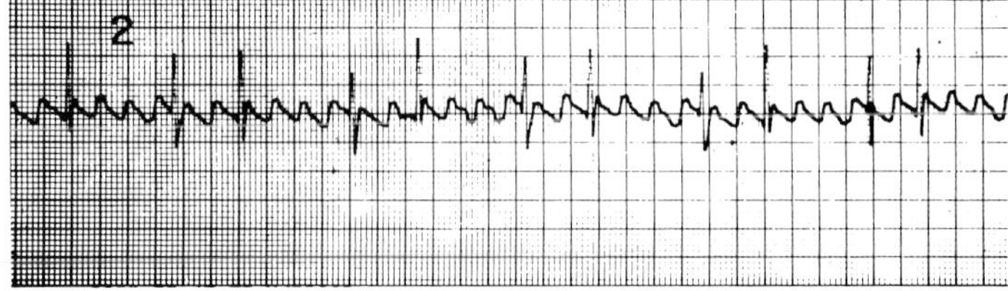

FIGURE 2-9. Atrial flutter.

Atrial flutter is seen most commonly in patients with ischemic heart disease as well as CHF, acute MI, pulmonary embolus, myocarditis, blunt chest trauma, and digoxin toxicity. Atrial flutter may be a transitional arrhythmia between sinus rhythm and atrial fibrillation. Consider anticoagulation in patients with an unclear time of onset or duration longer than 48 hours before conversion to sinus rhythm due to increased risk of atrial thrombus and embolization.

Emergency Department Care

The treatment is the same as atrial fibrillation and is discussed below.

Atrial Fibrillation

Clinical Features

Atrial fibrillation (Afib) occurs when there are multiple, small areas of atrial myocardium continuously discharging in a disorganized fashion. This results in loss of effective atrial contraction and decreases left ventricular end-diastolic volume, which may precipitate CHF in patients with impaired cardiac function. The ECG characteristics of Afib are (*a*) fibrillatory waves of atrial activity, best seen in leads V_1, V_2, V_3, and aV_F; and (*b*) an irregular ventricular response, usually between 170 and 180 beats/min in patients with a healthy AV node (Fig. 2-10).

Afib may be paroxysmal (lasting for less than 7 days), persistent (lasting for more than 7 days), or chronic (continuous). Afib can be idiopathic (lone Afib) or may be found in association with longstanding hypertension, ischemic heart disease, rheumatic heart disease, alcohol use ("holiday heart"), COPD, and thyrotoxicosis. Patients with LV dysfunction who depend on atrial contraction may suffer acute CHF with Afib onset. Rates of greater than 300 beats/min with a wide QRS complex are concerning for a preexcitation syndrome such as Wolff–Parkinson–White (WPW) (Fig. 2-11).

Patients with Afib who are not anticoagulated have a yearly embolic event rate as high as 5% and a lifetime risk greater than 25%. Conversion from atrial fibrillation of 12 hours duration or less to sinus rhythm carries a 0.3% risk of arterial embolism compared to a risk of 1% for durations of 12 to 48 hours. Patients with heart failure and diabetes mellitus are particularly at risk with embolic rates as high as 9.8%. Anticoagulation for 3 weeks is required before cardioversion in patients with atrial fibrillation for longer than 48 hours duration and in those patients with an uncertain time of onset who are not on anticoagulation therapy.

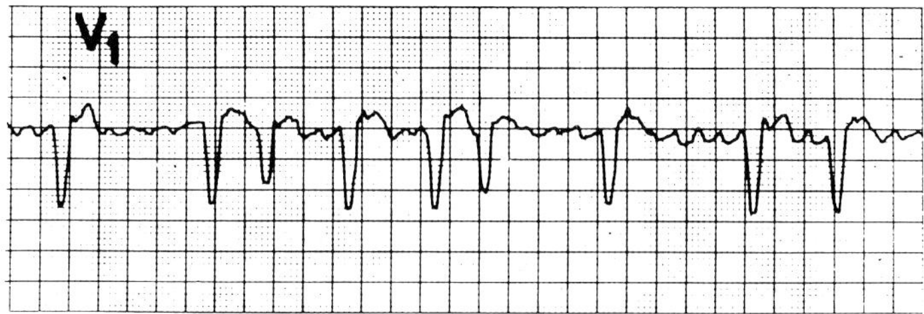

FIGURE 2-10. Atrial fibrillation.

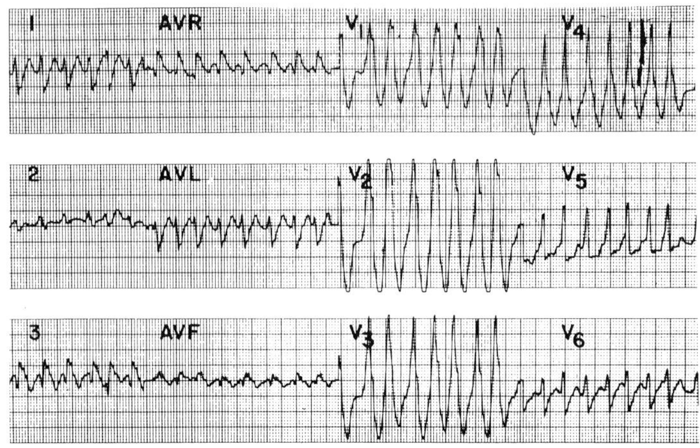

FIGURE 2-11. Atrial fibrillation in Wolff–Parkinson–White syndrome.

Emergency Department Care and Disposition

1. Treat unstable patients with synchronized cardioversion (150 to 200 J).
2. Stable patients with Afib for longer than 48 hours should be anticoagulated before cardioversion. Consider a transesophageal echocardiogram to rule out atrial thrombus before cardioversion.
3. Control rate with diltiazem. Administer 15 to 20 mg (or 0.25 mg/kg) IV over 2 minutes followed by a continuous IV infusion, 5 to 10 mg/h, to maintain rate control. Give a second dose of 25 mg (0.35 mg/kg) in 15 minutes if the first dose fails to control the rate. Alternative rate control agents for patients with normal cardiac function include **verapamil** 2.5 to 5 mg IV or **metoprolol** 5 to 10 mg IV. Treat patients with preexcitation syndromes (e.g., WPW) with **procainamide** 15 to 17 mg/kg IV over 30 minutes followed by an infusion of at 1 to 4 mg/min up to 50 mg/kg or until 50% QRS widening is noted. Avoid β-adrenergic or calcium channel blockers (i.e., verapamil) due to the risk of causing degeneration to VF.
4. In patients with impaired cardiac function (EF <40%), use **amiodarone** 5 mg/kg IV over 30 minutes, followed by 1200 mg over 24 hours (contraindicated in patients with iodine or shellfish allergy; increased risk of rhabdomyolysis if coadministered with simvastatin).
5. Patients with Afib with a clear duration less than 48 hours may be considered for chemical or electrical cardioversion in the emergency department. **Ibutilide** has the highest success rate and is dosed at 0.01 mg/kg IV up to 1 mg, infused over 10 minutes. Median time to conversion is 20 to 30 minutes. Ibutilide should not be administered to patients with known structural heart disease, hypokalemia, prolonged QTc intervals, hypomagnesemia, or CHF because of the possibility of provoking torsades de pointes. Monitor for 4 to 6 hours after giving ibutilide. Patients with impaired cardiac function may be cardioverted with amiodarone or electrically.

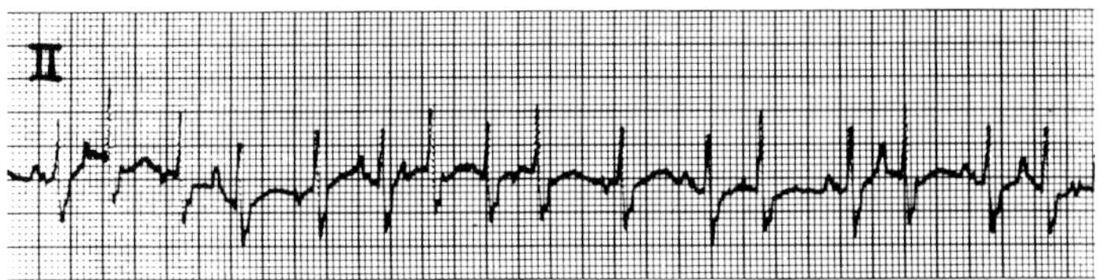

FIGURE 2-12. Multifocal atrial tachycardia (MFAT).

Multifocal Atrial Tachycardia

Clinical Features

Multifocal atrial tachycardia (MAT) is defined as at least three different sites of atrial ectopy. The ECG characteristics of MAT are (*a*) three or more differently shaped P waves; (*b*) changing PP, PR, and RR intervals; and (*c*) atrial rhythm usually between 100 and 180 beats/min (Fig. 2-12). Because the rhythm is irregularly irregular, MAT can be confused with atrial flutter or atrial fibrillation (AFib). MAT is found most often in elderly patients with decompensated COPD, but it also may be found in patients with CHF, sepsis, methylxanthine toxicity, or digoxin toxicity.

Emergency Department Care and Disposition

1. Treat the underlying disorder.
2. Specific antiarrhythmic treatment is not indicated.
3. **Magnesium sulfate** 2 g IV over 60 seconds followed by a constant infusion of 1 to 2 g/h may decrease ectopy and convert MAT to sinus rhythm in some patients.
4. Replete potassium levels to greater than 4 mEq/L to increase myocardial membrane stability.

Paroxysmal Supraventricular Tachycardia

Clinical Features

Supraventricular tachycardia (SVT) is a regular, rapid rhythm that arises from impulse reentry or an ectopic pacemaker above the bifurcation of the His bundle. The reentrant variety is the most common (Fig. 2-13). Patients often present with acute, symptomatic episodes termed paroxysmal supraventricular tachycardia (PSVT). Atrioventricular nodal reentrant tachycardia (AVnRT) can occur in a normal heart or in association with rheumatic heart disease, acute pericarditis, MI, mitral valve prolapse, or preexcitation syndromes. In patients with atrioventricular bypass tracts (AVRT), reentry can occur in either direction, usually (80% to 90% of patients) in a direction that goes down the AV node and up the bypass tract producing a narrow QRS complex (orthodromic conduction). In the remaining 10% to 20% of patients, reentry occurs in the reverse direction (antidromic conduction). Ectopic SVT usually originates in the atria, with an atrial rate of 100 to 250 beats/min and may be seen in patients with acute MI, chronic lung disease, pneumonia, alcohol intoxication, or digoxin toxicity. There is a high incidence of tachyarrhythmias in patients with preexcitation syndromes including PSVT (40% to 80%), atrial fibrillation (10% to 20%), and atrial flutter (about 5%).

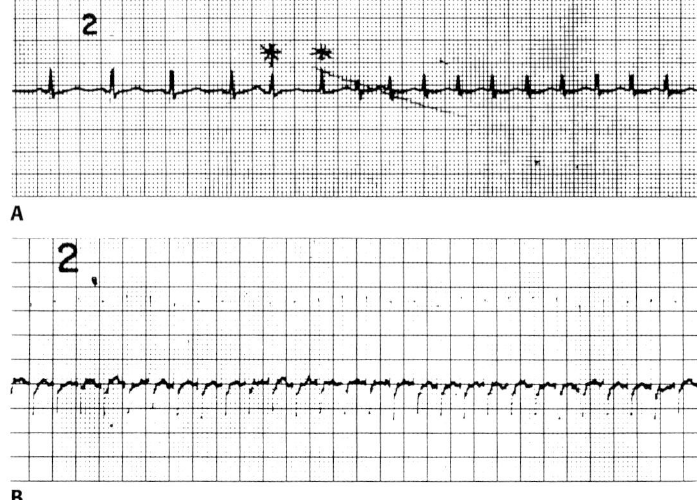

FIGURE 2-13. Reentrant supraventricular tachycardia (SVT). **A.** Second asterisk (*) initiates run of PAT. **B.** SVT, rate 286.

Emergency Department Care and Disposition

1. Perform synchronized cardioversion in any unstable patient (e.g., hypotension, pulmonary edema, or severe chest pain).
2. In stable patients, the first intervention should be vagal maneuvers, including:
   a. Valsalva maneuver: While in the supine position, ask the patient to strain for at least 10 seconds. The legs may be lifted to increase venous return and augment the reflex.
   b. Diving reflex: Have the patient immerse the face in cold water or apply a bag of ice water to the face for 6 to 7 seconds. This maneuver is particularly effective in infants.
   c. Carotid sinus massage: Auscultate to ensure that there is no carotid bruit and massage the carotid sinus against the transverse process of C6 for 10 seconds at a time, first on the side of the nondominant cerebral hemisphere. This should never be done simultaneously on both sides.
3. Administer **adenosine**, 6 mg rapid IV bolus, into a large vein followed by a 20-mL normal saline rapid flush. If there is no effect within 2 minutes, give a second dose of 12 mg IV. Most patients experience distressing chest pain, flushing, or anxiety lasting less than 1 minute. Ten percent of patients may experience transient atrial fibrillation or flutter after conversion. This is first-line treatment for WPW-associated SVT with a narrow QRS complex (orthodromic conduction) but is ineffective in cases of anterograde conduction over an accessory pathway. Adenosine may induce bronchospasm in asthmatics requiring treatment with bronchodilators.
4. Patients with wide complex SVT (antidromic conduction across accessory pathway) should be approached as presumed ventricular tachycardia

(VT; see Ventricular Tachycardia) unless there is a known history of WPW syndrome. Patients with this type of tachycardia are at risk for rapid ventricular rates and degeneration into VF; therefore, agents that preferentially block the AV node such as β-blockers, calcium channel blockers, and digoxin should not be used. Treat stable patients with **procainamide**, 15 to 17 mg/kg IV over 30 minutes up to 50 mg/kg, or until 50% QRS widening is noted (contraindicated in patients with myasthenia gravis since it may increase weakness).

WIDE COMPLEX TACHYCARDIAS

Ventricular Tachycardia

Clinical Features

VT is the occurrence of three or more successive beats from a ventricular ectopic pacemaker at a rate faster than 100 beats/min. The ECG characteristics of VT are (*a*) a wide QRS complex, (*b*) a rate faster than 100 beats/min (most commonly 150 to 200 beats/min), (*c*) a regular rhythm, although there may be some initial beat-to-beat variation, and (*d*) a constant QRS axis (Fig. 2-14). The most common causes of VT are ischemic heart disease and acute MI, accounting for approximately 50% of all cases of symptomatic VT.

Other etiologies include hypertrophic cardiomyopathy, mitral valve prolapse, drug toxicity (digoxin, antiarrhythmics, or sympathomimetics), hypoxia, hypokalemia, and hyperkalemia. In general, all wide complex tachycardia should be treated as VT regardless of clinical symptoms or initial vital signs. Adenosine appears to cause little harm in patients with VT; therefore, stable patients with wide complex tachycardia due to suspected SVT with aberrancy (see previous section) may be treated safely with adenosine when the diagnosis is in doubt. Atypical VT (torsade de pointes, or twisting of the points) occurs when the QRS axis swings from a positive to a negative direction in a single lead at a rate of 200 to 240 beats/min (Fig. 2-15). Drugs that further prolong repolarization—quinidine, disopyramide, procainamide, phenothiazines, and tricyclic antidepressants—exacerbate this arrhythmia.

Emergency Department Care and Disposition

1. Defibrillate pulseless VT with unsynchronized cardioversion starting at 150 to 200 J. Treat unstable patients who are not pulseless with synchronized cardioversion.
2. Treat hemodynamically stable patients with **amiodarone** 150 mg IV over 10 minutes with repeated boluses every 10 minutes up to a total of 2 g. Alternatively, an infusion of 0.5 mg/min over 18 hours may be given

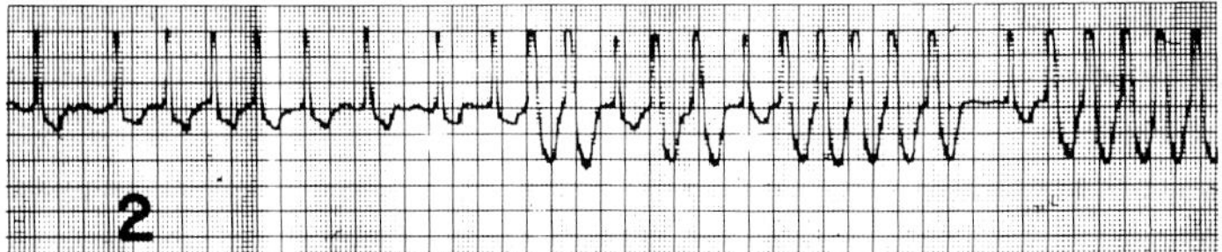

FIGURE 2-14. Ventricular tachycardia.

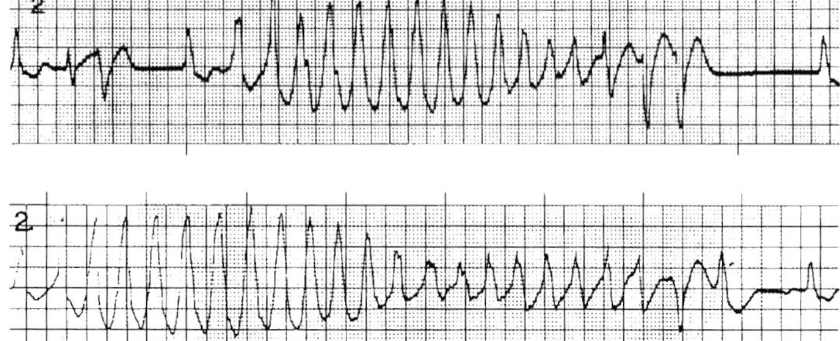

FIGURE 2-15. Two examples of short runs of atypical ventricular tachycardia showing sinusoidal variation in amplitude and direction of the QRS complexes: "Le torsade de pointes" (twisting of the points). Note that the top example is initiated by a late-occurring PVC (lead II).

after the initial bolus. Second-line agents include procainamide (in patients without suspected MI or LV dysfunction) and lidocaine.

3. For patients with torsades de pointes: Try overdrive pacing set at 90 to 120 beats/min to terminate torsades de pointes.
4. **Magnesium sulfate** 1 to 2 g IV over 60 to 90 seconds followed by an infusion of 1 to 2 g/h can be effective.
5. **Isoproterenol**, 2 to 10 μg/min IV infusion, is also used in refractory torsades but carries a risk of increased myocardial oxygen demand.

Undifferentiated Wide Complex Tachycardia

Patients with wide complex tachycardia should be approached as having VT until proven otherwise. Age over 35 years, a history of MI, CHF, or coronary artery bypass grafting strongly favor VT. ECG signs favoring VT include AV dissociation, fusion beats, precordial lead QRS concordance, and a QRS duration longer than 0.14 second. It is a misconception that patients with VT are typically unstable. At the bedside, one should assume any new and symptomatic wide complex tachycardia is ventricular in origin and focus on treating the rhythm as VT, as well as any contributing cause, especially in the unstable patient.

Ventricular Fibrillation

Clinical Features

VF is the totally disorganized depolarization and contraction of small areas of ventricular myocardium during which there is no effective ventricular pumping activity. The ECG shows a fine-to-coarse zigzag pattern without discernible P waves or QRS complexes (Fig. 2-16). VF is seen most commonly in patients with severe ischemic heart disease, with or without an acute MI. It also can be caused by digoxin or quinidine toxicity, hypothermia, chest trauma, hypokalemia, hyperkalemia, or mechanical stimulation (e.g., catheter wire). Primary VF occurs suddenly, without preceding hemodynamic deterioration, and usually is due to acute ischemia or peri-infarct

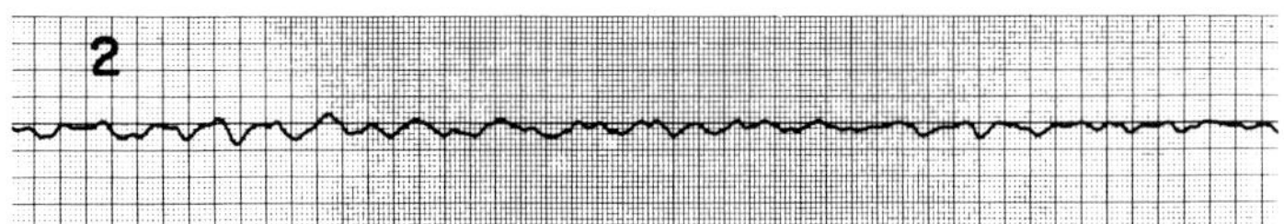

FIGURE 2-16. Ventricular fibrillation.

scar reentry. Secondary VF occurs after a prolonged period of hemodynamic deterioration due to left ventricular failure or circulatory shock.

Emergency Department Care and Disposition

1. Perform immediate electrical defibrillation (unsynchronized) at 200 J (biphasic) and 360 J (monophasic) along with immediate vigorous chest compressions to augment coronary perfusion. Keep defibrillation pads on the patient and in the same location because, with successive countershocks, transthoracic impedance decreases.
2. If the initial two cycles of cardiopulmonary resuscitation (CPR) and defibrillation are unsuccessful, administer antiarrhythmic treatment using **amiodarone** 300 mg IV push. **Lidocaine** is second-line and is dosed at 1.5 mg/kg IV followed by 0.75 mg/kg IV for two more doses. Repeat the CPR-defibrillation cycle.
3. If no pulse is present after the third CPR-defibrillation cycle, give **epinephrine** 1 mg IV push, or **vasopressin** 40 units IV push (one time only), followed by a 20-mL normal saline flush and immediate resumption of the CPR-defibrillation cycle.
4. In refractory VF, administer **magnesium sulfate** 1 to 2 g IV over 60 to 90 seconds followed by an infusion of 1 to 2 g/h.

DYSRHYTHMIA-ASSOCIATED CONDUCTION ABNORMALITIES

Wolff–Parkinson–White (WPW) Syndrome

WPW syndrome is the most common form of ventricular preexcitation involving an accessory conduction pathway that bypasses the AV node (Fig. 2-17). The ventricles are activated by an impulse from the atria sooner than would be expected if the impulse were transmitted down the normal conducting pathway. This premature activation causes initial fusion beat morphology with slurring of initial QRS complex, causing the pathognomonic delta wave. Among patients with WPW–PSVT, 80% to 90% will conduct in the orthodromic direction and the remaining 10% to 20% will conduct in the antidromic direction. ECG findings of atrial fibrillation or flutter with antidromic conduction down the bypass tract show a wide QRS complex that is irregular with a rate faster than 180 to 200 beats/min (see Atrial Fibrillation).

Emergency Department Care and Disposition

1. Treatment of the tachydysrhythmia should be based on the QRS duration and regularity of the rhythm. All unstable patient should be cardioverted (synchronized) at 150 to 200 J.

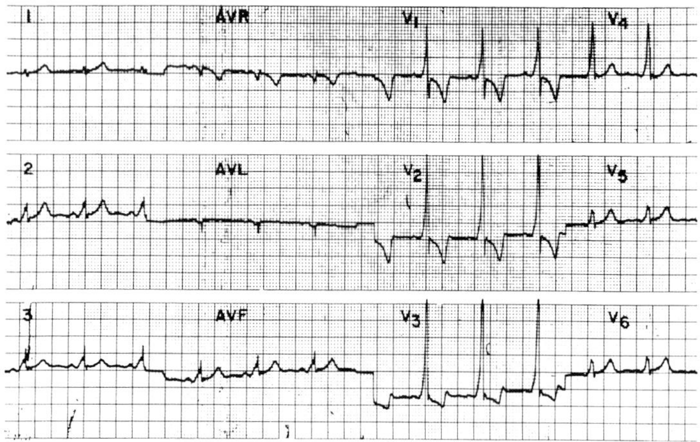

FIGURE 2-17. Type A Wolff–Parkinson–White syndrome.

2. Patients with a narrow regular tachycardia should be treated as SVT (orthodromic conduction) using vagal maneuvers followed by adenosine, if ineffective. Refractory cases may require **procainamide**, 15 to 17 mg/kg IV over 30 minutes up to 50 mg/kg, or until 50% QRS widening is noted.
3. All patients with wide QRS tachycardias, whether regular (SVT with antidromic conduction) or irregular (atrial fibrillation with antidromic conduction), should be treated with procainamide.
4. Nodal blocking agents such as β-blockers and calcium channel blockers should be avoided due to the risk of enhancing conduction across the bypass tract.
5. Patients with stable recurrent episodes may be monitored after cardioversion and discharged to outpatient follow-up. Instability, loss of consciousness, or other concerning features warrant observation on monitoring for recurrence. Asymptomatic patients with WPW, found incidentally, warrant outpatient referral to a cardiologist for further evaluation.

Brugada Syndrome and Long-QT Syndrome

Brugada syndrome and long-QT syndrome increase the risk of spontaneous VT/VF and require evaluation for implantable cardiac defibrillator placement when diagnosed. Brugada syndrome is a genetic disorder of fast sodium channels causing an RBBB pattern in the early precordial leads (V1–2) with a pathognomonic J-point elevation and saddle-shaped or sloped ST segment (Fig. 2-18). Long-QT syndrome is characterized by a QT interval greater than 470 milliseconds in men and greater than 480 milliseconds in women and may be congenital or acquired, leading to an increased risk of torsades de pointes. The risk of arrhythmia increases significantly with QTc durations greater than 500 milliseconds.

Emergency Department Care and Disposition

1. Recognition of the ECG pattern should prompt close outpatient follow-up with a cardiologist, especially in stable symptomatic patients.

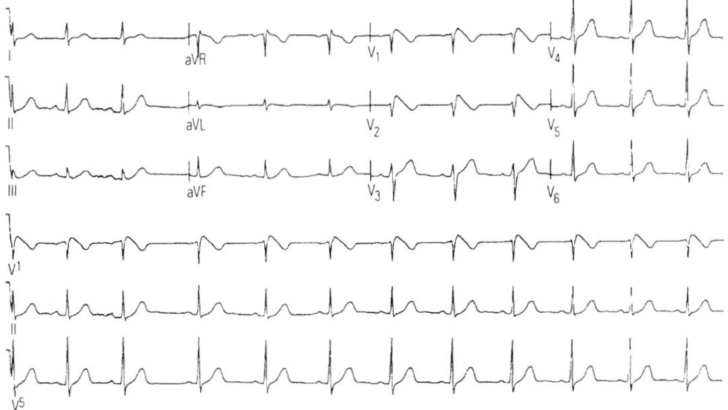

FIGURE 2-18. Brugada syndrome.

2. Patients presently with unstable rhythms or concerning clinical presentations (e.g., drop attacks) should be admitted for monitoring and cardiology consultation.
3. Patients should be advised to avoid any medications that may potentially worsen QT prolongation (http://www.brugadadrugs.org). Patients with long-QT syndrome should be advised to avoid strenuous exercise, particularly swimming, which can increase the chance of sudden death.

PRETERMINAL RHYTHMS

Pulseless Electrical Activity

Pulseless electrical activity is the presence of electrical complexes without accompanying mechanical contraction of the heart. Potential mechanical causes should be diagnosed and treated, including severe hypovolemia, cardiac tamponade, tension pneumothorax, massive pulmonary embolus, MI, and toxic ingestions (e.g., tricyclic antidepressants, calcium channel blockers, β-blockers). In addition, profound metabolic abnormalities such as acidosis, hypoxia, hypokalemia, hyperkalemia, and hypothermia also should be considered and treated.

After intubation and initiating CPR, administer **epinephrine** 1 mg IV/IO (1:10,000 solution) every 3 to 5 minutes. If giving via endotracheal tube, increase the dose 2 to 2.5 times and follow with several rapid ventilations to disperse the drug. Treatment is guided by rapid identification and treatment of the underlying cause. Use agents with α-adrenergic activity, such as norepinephrine and phenylephrine, to improve vascular tone when indicated. Electrical pacing is not effective.

Asystole (Cardiac Standstill)

Asystole is the complete absence of cardiac electrical activity and carries a grim prognosis. Treatment is the same as that for pulseless electrical activity.

CARDIAC PACEMAKERS AND AUTOMATED INTERNAL CARDIAC DEFIBRILLATORS (AICDS)

Pacemakers, AICDs, or combination units may be used in patients with a history of sudden death, heart failure, or cardiomyopathy. Malfunction can occur at any level of the device, including infection or hematoma in the pocket housing the device, lead infection/displacement, failure to pace, failure to sense, overpacing, or inappropriate defibrillation. Most pacemakers will have a magnetic switch which, when triggered by magnet application to the unit, will cause the pacemaker to function in a fixed asynchronous mode.

Emergency Department Care and Disposition

1. Evaluation should include an ECG, electrolytes, and chest x-ray to assess lead position and integrity. Arrangements should be made for electrical interrogation of the unit.
2. Patients with pacing failure may require treatment based on their underlying rhythm and associated symptoms.
3. Patients with overpacing may require magnet application to convert the pacemaker to asynchronous mode pacing at a lower rate.

FURTHER READING

For further reading in *Tintinalli's Emergency Medicine: A Comprehensive Study Guide*, 8th ed., see Chapter 18, "Cardiac Rhythm Disturbances," by William J. Brady, Thomas S. Laughrey, and Chris A. Ghaemmaghami; Chapter 19, "Pharmacology of Antiarrhythmics and Antihypertensives" by Sara Shields, Rachel M. Holland, R. Dustin Pippin, and Benjamin Small; Chapter 20, "Pharmacology of Vasopressors and Inotropes" by Sara Shields and Rachel M. Holland.

Resuscitation of Children and Neonates

Marc F. Collin

Children primarily develop cardiac arrest secondary to hypoxia from respiratory arrest or shock syndromes. Because of age and size differences among children, equipment sizes also differ (Table 3-1).

PEDIATRIC CARDIOPULMONARY RESUSCITATION

Securing the Airway

The airway in infants and children is smaller, variable in size, and higher and more anterior than that in the adult. The prominent occiput and relatively large tongue and epiglottis may lead to obstruction when the child is in the supine position.

Mild extension of the neck in the sniffing position opens the airway. This may be maintained by placing a towel beneath the shoulders. Chin lift or jaw thrust maneuvers may relieve obstruction of the airway related to the tongue. Oral airways are not commonly used in pediatrics but may be useful in the unconscious child who requires continuous jaw thrust or chin lift to maintain airway patency. Oral airways are inserted by direct visualization with a tongue blade.

A bag-valve-mask system is commonly used for ventilation. Minimum volume for ventilation bags for infants and children is 450 mL. The tidal volume necessary to ventilate children is 8 to 10 mL/kg. Observation of chest rise and auscultation of breath sounds will ensure adequate ventilation.

Endotracheal intubation usually is performed with a Miller straight blade with a properly sized tube. Resuscitation measuring tapes have been found to be the most accurate for determining tube size. The formula 16 plus age in years divided by 4 calculates approximate tube size. Uncuffed tubes are commonly used in children up to 8 years, but cuffed tubes can be used in younger children as well.

Respiratory rates should be started at 20 breaths/min for infants beyond the neonatal period, 15 breaths/min for young children, and 10 breaths/min for adolescents unless hyperventilation is required.

Rapid Sequence Intubation

Rapid sequence intubation is the administration of an intravenous (IV) anesthetic with a neuromuscular blocking agent to facilitate endotracheal intubation, and is associated with the highest success and lowest complication rates, compared to other methods. See Table 3-2 for common medications for rapid sequence intubation.

1. All equipment and supplies must be prepared. A well-functioning IV line must be in place. A cardiac monitor and oximetry should be used, and if available, noninvasive capnometry as well. The laryngoscope light source must be checked. Suction equipment should be turned on and immediately available.

TABLE 3-1 Length-Based Equipment Chart (Length = Centimeters*)

Item	54–70	70–85	85–95	95–107	107–124	124–138	138–155
Endotracheal tube size (mm)	3.5	4.0	4.5	5.0	5.5	6.0	6.5
Lip–tip length (mm)	10.5	12.0	13.5	15.0	16.5	18.0	19.5
Laryngoscope	1 straight	1 straight	2 straight	2 straight or curved	2 straight or curved	2–3 straight or curved	3 straight or curved
Suction catheter	8F	8F–10F	10F	10F	10F	10F	12F
Stylet	6F	6F	6F	6F	14F	14F	14F
Oral airway	Infant/small child	Small child	Child	Child	Child/small adult	Child/adult	Medium adult
Bag-valve mask	nfant	Child	Child	Child	Child	Child/adult	Adult
Oxygen mask	Newborn	Pediatric	Pediatric	Pediatric	Pediatric	Adult	Adult
Vascular access (gauge)							
Catheter	22–24	20–22	18–22	18–22	18–20	18–20	16–20
Butterfly	23–25	23–25	21–23	21–23	21–23	21–22	18–21
Nasogastric tube	5F–8F	8F–10F	10F	10F–12F	12F–14F	14F–18F	18F
Urinary catheter	5F–8F	8F–10F	10F	10F–12F	10F–12F	12F	12F
Chest tube	10F–12F	16F–20F	20F–24F	20F–24F	24F–32F	28F–32F	32F–40F
Blood pressure cuff	Newborn/infant	Infant/child	Child	Child	Child	Child/adult	Adult

Directions for use: (1) measure patient length with centimeter tape; (2) using measured length in centimeters, access appropriate equipment column.

TABLE 3-2 Common Rapid-Sequence Intubation Medications in Children*

Medication	Dose†	Comments
Induction agents		
Etomidate	0.3 mg/kg	Preserves hemodynamic stability; may suppress adrenal axis even in a single dose; short acting, requires anxiolysis or analgesia after intubation
Ketamine	1–2 mg/kg	Bronchodilator, preserves respiratory drive, cardiovascular stimulant; drug of choice for intubation for asthma and sepsis
Propofol	1–2 mg/kg	Rapid push, higher dose in infants, may cause hypotension; short acting, requires ongoing anxiolysis or analgesia after intubation
Paralytics		
Rocuronium	1 mg/kg	Nondepolarizing agent; longer duration than succinylcholine
Succinylcholine	<10 kg: 1.5–2.0 mg/kg >10 kg: 1.0–1.5 mg/kg	Shorter duration than rocuronium; better intubating conditions at 60 s; may cause bradycardia in children and hyperkalemic cardiac arrest in children with undiagnosed neuromuscular disease
Sedatives		
Midazolam	0.1 mg/kg	Short-acting sedative
Lorazepam	0.1 mg/kg	Longer-acting sedative
Analgesics		
Fentanyl	1–2 μg/kg	Short-acting analgesic; preserves hemodynamic stability
Morphine	0.1–0.2 mg/kg	Longer-acting analgesic; may cause histamine release

*Premedication is no longer routinely recommended in children due to a lack of supporting evidence.

†Rapid-sequence intubation medications can be given IO when IV access cannot be obtained.

2. Preoxygenate with 100% oxygen.
3. Cricoid pressure may not be needed because it has been associated with difficulty with intubation and bag-mask ventilation, and in children, cricoid pressure can occlude the pliable trachea. If cricoid pressure is applied, release pressure if laryngoscopy and intubation are difficult. Visualization may or may not be enhanced by the Backward-Upward-Rightward-Pressure on the thyroid cartilage (the "BURP" maneuver), moving the cords into better view.
4. **Atropine** 0.02 mg/kg (minimum dose 0.1 mg; maximum dose 1 mg) may be used if symptomatic reflex bradycardia occurs.
5. The trachea should be intubated, proper placement confirmed, and the tube secured.

Vascular Access

Vascular access is obtained in the quickest, least invasive manner possible; peripheral veins (antecubital, hand, foot, or scalp) are tried first. Intraosseous access is also a quick, safe, and reliable route for resuscitation medications, especially in the critically ill infant or child suffering from hypovolemia or shock. Percutaneous access of the femoral vein or saphenous vein cutdown may be attempted, but is more time consuming. Airway management is paramount in pediatric arrest, and should not be delayed while obtaining vascular access.

The technique for insertion of the intraosseous line is as follows: the bone most commonly used is the proximal tibia. The anterior tibial tuberosity is palpated with the index finger. The cannulation site is 1 to 3 cm below this tuberosity and in the middle of the anteromedial surface of the tibia. Manual and powered devices are commonly used. If a bone marrow needle is not available, an 18-G spinal needle can be used but is prone to bending. With sterile technique, the needle is inserted in a slightly caudal direction until the needle punctures the cortex. The stylet is removed, and marrow is aspirated to confirm placement. If no marrow is aspirated but the needle is thought to be in place, flushing the needle may be attempted. Fluids or drugs (including glucose, epinephrine, dopamine, anticonvulsants, and antibiotics) may then be administered as with a standard IV.

Fluids

In hypotension or frank shock, IV isotonic fluid (i.e., normal saline solution) boluses of 20 mL/kg should be given as rapidly as possible and potentially repeated, depending on the clinical response. If hypovolemia has been corrected and shock or hypotension persist, a pressor agent should be considered.

Drugs

The indications for resuscitation drugs are the same for children as for adults; the exception is epinephrine, which is considered first-line therapy in children with bradycardia (Table 3-3).

Proper drug dosages in children require knowledge of the patient's weight. The use of a length-based system for estimating the weight of a child in an emergency situation reduces dosage errors when an exact weight is unavailable and cannot be safely obtained due to the patient's medical condition.

The rule of 6s may be used to quickly calculate continuous drug infusions of drugs such as dopamine and dobutamine. The calculation is 6 mg times weight in kilograms: fill to 100 mL with 5% dextrose in water. The infusion rate in milliliters per hour equals the microgram per kilogram per minute rate (i.e., an infusion running at 1 mL/h = 1 μg/kg/min, or 5 mL/h = 5 μg/kg/min).

Epinephrine is indicated in pulseless arrest and in hypoxia-induced bradycardia unresponsive to oxygenation and ventilation. The initial dose is 0.01 mg/kg (0.1 mL/kg of 1:10,000 solution) IV/IO or 0.1 mg/kg (0.1 mL/kg) of 1:1,000 solution by endotracheal route. Subsequent doses of epinephrine are at the same dose and concentration and may be administered every 3–5 minutes.

TABLE 3-3 Drugs for Pediatric Resuscitation

Drug	Pediatric Dosage	Remarks
Adenosine	IV/IO: 0.1 mg/kg, followed by 2–5 mL NS bolus Double dose and repeat once, if needed	Maximum single dose: 6 mg first dose, 12 mg second dose.
Amiodarone	IV/IO: 5 mg/kg over 20–60 min; then 5–15 μg/kg/min infusion	Maximum bolus repetition to 15 mg/kg/d. Use lowest effective dose. Bolus may be given more rapidly in shock states.
Atropine	IV/IO: 0.02 mg/kg, repeat in 5 min (minimum single dose is 0.1 mg) Endotracheal: 0.04–0.06 mg/kg diluted with NS to 3–5 mL	Maximum single dose: 0.5 mg (child) and 1 mg (adolescent). Maximum cumulative dose: 1 mg (child) and 2 mg (adolescent).
Calcium chloride (10%)	IV/IO: 20 mg/kg (maximum dose 2 g)	*Not routinely recommended.* Use in documented hypocalcemia, calcium channel blocker overdose, hypermagnesemia, or hyperkalemia. Administer slowly.
Epinephrine	Bradycardia: IV/IO: 0.01 mg/kg (0.1 mL/kg of 1:10,000) Endotracheal: 0.1 mg/kg (0.1 mL/kg of 1:1000) Pulseless arrest: IV/IO: 0.01 mg/kg (0.1 mL/kg of 1:10,000) Endotracheal: 0.1 mg/kg (0.1 mL/kg of 1:1000)	Maximum dose: 1 mg IV/IO; 2.5 mg ETT. Unlike other agents, epinephrine per endotracheal tube is 10 × the IV dose. Follow endotracheal dose with several positive pressure ventilations. Maximum dose: 1 mg IV/IO; 2.5 mg ETT. No evidence for high-dose parenteral epinephrine (may worsen outcomes).
Glucose	IV/IO: Newborn: 2 mL/kg $D_{10}W$ Infants and children: 2 mL/kg $D_{25}W$ Adolescents: 1 mL/kg $D_{50}W$	
Lidocaine	IV/IO: 1 mg/kg bolus Endotracheal: double IV dose and dilute with NS to 3–5 mL	
Naloxone	IV/IO: If <5 years or ≤20 kg: 0.1 mg/kg If >5 years and >20 kg: 2.0 mg	Titrate to desired effect.
Sodium bicarbonate	IV/IO: 1 mEq/kg (1 mEq/mL)	*Not routinely recommended.* Infuse slowly and use only if ventilation is adequate for tricyclic antidepressant overdose and hyperkalemia.

Abbreviation: $D_{10}W$, 10% dextrose in water; $D_{25}W$, 25% dextrose in water; $D_{50}W$, 50% dextrose in water; ETT, endotracheal tube; NS, normal saline.

Sodium bicarbonate is no longer recommended as a first-line resuscitation drug. It is recommended only with persistent acidosis after the establishment of effective ventilation, administration of epinephrine, and performance of chest compressions to ensure adequate circulation.

Calcium also is not recommended in routine resuscitation but may be useful in hyperkalemia, hypocalcemia, and calcium-channel blocker overdose. Calcium may be given as calcium chloride, 20 mg/kg (0.2 mL/kg of 10% solution) or calcium gluconate, 60–100 mg/kg (0.6–1 mL/kg of 10% solution) via IV or IO route.

Dysrhythmias

Dysrhythmias in infants and children are most often the result of respiratory insufficiency or hypoxia, not of primary cardiac causes, as in adults. Careful attention to oxygenation and ventilation therefore are cornerstones of dysrhythmia management in children.

The most common rhythm seen in pediatric arrest situations is bradycardia leading to asystole. Oxygenation and ventilation are often sufficient therapy in this situation. Epinephrine may be useful if the child is unresponsive to this respiratory intervention.

The next most common dysrhythmia in children is supraventricular tachycardia (SVT), which presents with a narrow-complex tachycardia with rates between 250 and 350 beats/min. On EKG, p waves are either absent or abnormal. **Adenosine** 0.1 mg/kg given via rapid IV push followed by a normal saline flush through a well-functioning IV line as close to the central circulation as possible is the recommended treatment for stable SVT in children. This dose may be doubled if the first dose is unsuccessful. Treatment of unstable SVT is **synchronized cardioversion** at 0.5–1 J/kg. If not effective, increase to 2 J/kg. Sedation prior to cardioversion is recommended.

It may be difficult to distinguish between a fast sinus tachycardia and SVT. Young infants may have sinus tachycardia with rates as fast as 200–220 beats/min. The presence of normal p waves is strongly suggestive of sinus tachycardia rather than SVT. Patients with sinus tachycardia may have a history of fever, dehydration, or shock, while SVT is usually associated with a vague, nonspecific history.

Defibrillation and Cardioversion

Ventricular fibrillation and ventricular tachycardia are rare in children. When present, immediate **defibrillation** at 2 J/kg is recommended. Immediately after defibrillation, give 2 minutes of high-quality uninterrupted CPR (five cycles of 15:2 compressions and ventilations) to restore coronary perfusion and improve oxygen delivery to the myocardium before additional attempts at defibrillation. If the first defibrillation attempt is unsuccessful, the energy is doubled to 4 J/kg for each subsequent attempt. Epinephrine may also be given and oxygenation and acid–base status should be reassessed. **Synchronized cardioversion** is used to treat unstable tachydysrhythmias at a dose of 0.5 J/kg. Double the energy level to 1 J/kg if the first attempt is unsuccessful.

The largest paddles that still allow contact of the entire paddle with the chest wall are used. Electrode cream or paste is used to prevent burns. One paddle is placed on the right of the sternum at the second intercostal space, and the other is placed at the left midclavicular line at the level of the xiphoid.

NEONATAL RESUSCITATION

Most newborns do not require specific resuscitation after delivery, but about 6% of newborns require some form of life support in the delivery room. Emergency departments, therefore, must be prepared to provide neonatal resuscitation in the event of delivery in the emergency department.

1. The first step in neonatal resuscitation is to maintain body temperature. The infant should be dried and placed on a radiant warmer. Very-low-birth-weight newborns (<1500 g) may also be better maintained in a normothermic state by placement of their torso and limbs in polyethylene bags that have been developed for that purpose. Pulse oximetry or ECG monitoring is now recommended as an adjunct to newborn resuscitation.
2. The airway may be cleared by suctioning the mouth followed by the nose with a bulb syringe or mechanical suction device. It is now recommended that suctioning immediately following birth should be reserved for babies who have obvious obstruction to spontaneous breathing or who require positive-pressure ventilation. Routine deep suctioning is no longer recommended due to the potential for vagally induced bradycardia.
3. While aspiration of meconium-stained amniotic fluid may result in both morbidity and mortality, current evidence indicates that tracheal intubation and suctioning does not help, even in the nonvigorous newborn.
4. The examiner should then assess heart rate, respiratory effort, color, and activity quickly over the next 5–10 seconds. If the infant is apneic or the heart rate is slow (<100 beats/min), positive-pressure ventilation should be administered with bag-mask ventilation. New research suggests that initiating resuscitation with room air may actually result in less morbidity and mortality than 100% oxygen. If the baby is bradycardic (HR <60 beats/minute) after 90 seconds of resuscitation in room air (or with blended oxygen), the oxygen concentration should be increased to 100% until normalization of the heart rate is accomplished. Assisted ventilation rates of 40–60 breaths/min are recommended. Inflation pressure should begin at 20–25 cm H_2O with PEEP of 5 cm H_2O. If chest rise is inadequate and the baby is not responding, pressures as high as 30–40 cm H_2O may be required initially in some term infants. Utilization of high pressures should be undertaken with extreme caution, however, especially in preterm infants due to the possibility of pneumothoraces. In mildly depressed infants, a prompt improvement in heart rate and respiratory effort usually occurs.
5. Resuscitation of newborns less than 35 weeks gestation should be initiated with 21–30% oxygen during positive-pressure ventilation due to concerns for oxygen toxicity. Free-flow oxygen should begin with 30% oxygen. If labored breathing or oxygen desaturations persist even after increasing to 100% oxygen, a trial of CPAP should be instituted.

6. If no heart rate improvement is noted after 15 seconds of bag-mask ventilation, then continue PPV for another 15 seconds. If the heart rate is not improving and/or chest rise is inadequate, initiate corrective actions as follows: Mask adjustment, Reposition head, Suction mouth and nose, Open mouth, increase Pressure, and consider Alternate airway (acronym =MR SOPA). If still no improvement, endotracheal intubation and ventilation should be performed. End tidal CO_2 detectors may aid in determining whether the baby is properly intubated, but it should be noted that CO_2 detector color change indicating intratracheal placement is also dependent on adequate circulation. Proper tube placement can also be determined by noting good chest rise, visualization of vapor steam in the endotracheal tube, and auscultation.
7. If the heart rate is still slower than 60 beats/min after intubation and assisted ventilation for at least 30 seconds, cardiac massage should be started with 90 chest compressions and 30 breaths each minute (3:1 ratio). The "2 thumbs-encircling hands" technique is superior to the "2-finger" technique when performing chest compressions.
8. If there is no improvement in heart rate after these efforts, drug therapy should be initiated. Most neonates respond to appropriate airway management; therefore, drug therapy is rarely needed. Vascular access may be obtained peripherally or via the umbilical vein. The most expedient procedure in the neonate is to place an umbilical catheter in the umbilical vein and advance to 10–12 cm or until free flow of blood is seen in the catheter.
9. **Epinephrine** 0.01–0.03 mg/kg of 1:10,000 solution IV push, which equals 0.1–0.3 mL/kg, may be used if the heart rate is still slower than 60 beats/min despite adequate ventilation and oxygenation for at least 30 seconds and an additional 60 seconds of chest compressions. Repeat every 3–5 minutes if necessary. New data suggests that intratracheal epinephrine is inferior to the IV route.
10. Volume expansion should be considered if hypovolemia is suspected. This may be the result of blood loss and associated with pallor, slow capillary refill time, weak pulses, and inadequate response to the other resuscitative measures. An initial dose of 10–20 mL/kg of normal saline (or Type O/Rh negative blood, if available) is recommended. Lactated Ringer's solution is not recommended.
11. **Sodium bicarbonate** during neonatal resuscitation is now generally contraindicated during initial resuscitation. A dose of 1 mEq/kg of a 4.2% solution (0.5 mEq/mL) IV may be given if there is a significant metabolic acidosis; this therapy should be guided by blood gas values.
12. Naloxone is no longer recommended in the resuscitation for newborns with respiratory depression.

FURTHER READING

For further reading in *Tintinalli's Emergency Medicine: A Comprehensive Study Guide*, 8th Edition, see Chapter 109, "Resuscitation of Children" by William E. Hauda, II; Chapter 108, "Resuscitation of Neonates" by Marc F. Collin; Chapter 111, "Intubation and Ventilation in Infants and Children" by Robert J. Vissers and Nathan W. Mick; and Chapter 112, "Intravenous and Intraosseous Access in Infants and Children" by Matthew Hansen.

Fluids, Electrolytes, and Acid-Base Disorders

Benjamin W. Wachira

Management of fluids, electrolytes, and acid-base disorders in the emergency department (ED) involves immediate correction of life-threatening abnormalities, identification and treatment of the underlying disorder, and eventual restoration of normal tissue homeostasis.

FLUIDS

Crystalloid fluids for human administration have three general components: water, electrolytes, and glucose (Table 4-1).

Because the osmolarity of normal saline (NS) and Lactated Ringer's solution matches that of serum, they are excellent fluids for volume replacement. Dextrose solutions are hypotonic and should never be used to replace volume but may be given as maintenance fluids with or without potassium.

Hypovolemia and Hypervolemia

Hypovolemia or hypervolemia can be determined entirely from the history and physical examination. History of bleeding, vomiting, diarrhea, fever, and/or findings of dry mucous membranes with features of poor perfusion, for example, decreased capillary refill, reduced urine output, and altered

TABLE 4-1 Electrolyte Concentrations of Fluids (mEq/L)

Solution	Plasma	Normal Saline	Lactated Ringer's Solution
Cations			
Sodium	142	154	130
Potassium	4	–	4
Magnesium*	2	–	–
Calcium†	5	–	3
Total cations	153	154	137
Anions			
Chloride	104	154	109
Lactate‡	–	–	28
Phosphates	2	–	–
Sulfates	1	–	–
Bicarbonate	27	–	–
Proteins	13	–	–
Organic adds	6	–	–
Total anions	153	154	137

*Multiply by 0.411 to convert to International System of Units (SI) units in mmol/L.

†Multiply by 0.25 to convert to SI units in mmol/L.

‡Multiply by 0.323 to convert to SI units in mmol/L.

level of consciousness are suggestive of hypovolemia. Lethargy and coma are more ominous signs and may indicate a significant comorbid condition. Risk factors for hypervolemia include renal, cardiovascular, and liver diseases. Edema (central or peripheral), respiratory distress (pulmonary edema), and jugular venous distention (in congestive heart failure) are clinical features of hypervolemia.

Blood pressure and heart rate do not necessarily correlate with volume status alone and laboratory values are not reliable indicators of fluid status. Bedside ultrasound can be used to assess the volume status as an adjunct to, not a replacement for, the physical exam. Measurements of the IVC and following changes in size and respiratory dynamics over time with fluid challenges effectively determine the vascular volume status.

ELECTROLYTE DISORDERS

Management of electrolyte disorders is guided by two variables: severity of symptoms and rate of onset. If the clinical picture and the laboratory data conflict, repeat the lab test prior to initiating therapy. Abnormalities should be corrected at the same rate they develop; however, slower correction is usually safer unless in life-threatening situations which warrant rapid or early intervention.

Hyponatremia ($[Na^+]$ <138 mEq/L)

Hyponatremia is a condition of excess water relative to $[Na^+]$.

Clinical Features

Symptomatic hyponatremia rarely occurs until $[Na^+]$ falls below 135 mEq/L or lower. Symptoms can be divided into moderately severe ($[Na^+]$ <130 mEq/L)—headache, nausea, disorientation, confusion, agitation, ataxia, and areflexia, and severe ($[Na^+]$ <120 mEq/L)—intractable vomiting, seizures, coma, and ultimately respiratory arrest due to brainstem herniation.

Diagnosis and Differential

Evaluate volume status plus measure and calculate plasma osmolality. The formula to calculate effective osmolality is

$$2 \times [\mathrm{Na}^+] + \mathrm{Glucose}/18 \text{ (Normal range, } 275 - 290 \text{ mOsm/L)}$$

If values are in SI units (e.g., mmol/L), do not divide by their molecular weight.

In true hyponatremia, plasma osmolality is reduced; in factitious hyponatremic states, for example, in the presence of hyperproteinemia and hyperlipidemia, it is normal or increased due to the displacement of serum water by elevated concentration of lipids or protein creating laboratory misinterpretation of normal $[Na^+]$.

The diagnosis of hyponatremia and its subtypes is based on the clinical findings of volume status in association with specific laboratory values including serum $[Na^+]$, serum osmolality, volume status, urinary sodium ($U_{Na}{}^+$), and urine osmolality (U_{osm}) (Table 4-2).

TABLE 4-2 Classification, Differential Diagnosis, and Features of Hyponatremia According to Volume Status

	Clinical Conditions	Orthostatic Hypotension	Edema
Hypervolemic hyponatremia	CHF Cirrhosis Nephrotic syndrome Acute and chronic kidney disease	Absent	Yes
Normovolemic hyponatremia	Psychogenic polydipsia Glucocorticoid deficit Hypokalemia Drugs SIADH	Absent	No
Renal hypovolemic hyponatremia	Diuretics Mineralocorticoid deficit Salt-losing nephropathy	Normally present	No
Extrarenal hypovolemic hyponatremia	Vomiting Diarrhea	Normally present	No

Abbreviations: CHF, congestive heart failure; SIADH, syndrome of inappropriate ADH secretion.

Two important hyponatremic disorders are the syndrome of inappropriate ADH secretion (Table 4-3) and the less common cerebral salt-wasting syndrome. Both conditions are diagnoses of exclusion after dismissing other causes of hyponatremia.

Methylenedioxymethamphetamine (MDMA or Ecstasy) induces inappropriate secretion of ADH and causes increased gut water absorption, and intoxication may lead to profound hyponatremia (see also Chapter 105, "Drugs of Abuse").

Emergency Department Care and Disposition

1. Infuse **3% hypertonic saline (Table 4-4)** when $[Na^+]$ is less than 120 mEq/L, the patient presents with severe neurologic symptoms, and hyponatremia is acute.
2. After clinical improvement in severe symptoms, stop the 3% hypertonic saline and either reduce its rate or use a different saline solution, for example, isotonic (0.9%) saline.

TABLE 4-3 Syndrome of Inappropriate Secretion of Antidiuretic Hormone Diagnostic Criteria

Hypotonic hyponatremia with (P_{osm} <275 mOsm/kg H_2O)

Inappropriately elevated urinary osmolality (usually >200 mOsm/kg)

Elevated urinary $[Na^+]$ (typically >20 mEq/L)

Clinical euvolemia

Normal adrenal, renal, cardiac, hepatic, and thyroid functions

TABLE 4-4 Treatment for Hyponatremia Symptomatic with Seizures or Coma

Step 1	Assess for indication for 3% hypertonic saline: severe symptoms of hyponatremia such as seizures or coma with suspected impending brainstem herniation in setting of acute* or chronic† hyponatremia
Step 2	Infuse 100 mL of 3% hypertonic saline IV over 10–15 min‡
Step 3	Measure serum sodium level after each 3% hypertonic saline infusion
Step 4	Stop infusion when symptoms improve, or a target of 5 mEq/L (range 4–6 mEq/L) increase in serum sodium concentration is achieved.
Step 5	May repeat 100 ml of 3% hypertonic saline up to three total doses, or a total of 300 ml IV of 3% hypertonic saline.
Step 6	Keep the IV line open with minimal volume of 0.9% normal saline until cause-specific treatment is started. Limit increase in sodium level to no more than 8 mEq/L during the first 24 hours.

*Both European guidelines and U.S. expert panel recommend 3% hypertonic saline infusion for acute life-threatening hyponatremia, which is most commonly due to self-induced water intoxication during endurance exercise, psychiatric illness, in association with ethylenedioxymethamphetamine intoxication, or intracranial pathology or increased intracranial pressure.

†European guidelines state that regardless of onset of acute or chronic hyponatremia, presence of seizures or coma is an indication for brief infusion of hypertonic saline to improve symptoms.

‡European guidelines recommend a prompt 150-mL 3% hypertonic saline infusion over 20 minutes, then checking the serum sodium concentration after 20 minutes while repeating an infusion of 150 mL 3% hypertonic saline for the next 20 minutes, repeating this sequence up to twice more, and stopping with clinical improvement or when target sodium level is reached.

3. Calculate the volume of a saline solution required to raise the serum sodium to the desired amount using the following formula:

$$\text{Expected change in serum}\,\text{Na}^+(\text{mEq/L}) = \text{Infusate}\,\text{Na}^+(\text{mEq/L}) - \text{Serum}\,\text{Na}^+(\text{mEq/L})/(\text{TBW} + 1)$$

TBW estimates are based on age, sex, and weight of the patient. In children and adult males <65 years old, TBW is 60% of the weight; in adult females <65 years old and elderly males, TBW is 50% of the weight, in elderly females, TBW is 45% of weight. Three percent hypertonic saline contains 513 mEq/L of sodium while isotonic (0.9%) saline contains 154 mEq/L of sodium.

4. For chronic hyponatremia [Na^+], do not exceed 6 mEq/24 h in high-risk patients ([Na^+] <120 mEq/L, chronic heart failure, alcoholism, cirrhosis, hypokalemia, malnutrition, and treatment with vasopressin antagonists, [e.g., tolvaptan]) or 12 mEq/24 h in low-risk patients. Rapid correction of hyponatremia (>12 mEq/L/24 h) may cause a neurologic disorder referred to as osmotic demyelination syndrome.

Hypernatremia ([Na^+] >145 mEq/L)

Hypernatremia is defined as serum or plasma [Na^+] >145 mEq/L and hyperosmolality (serum osmolality >295 mOsm/L).

Clinical Features

History may reveal nausea and vomiting, lethargy, weakness, increased thirst, low water intake, salt intake, and polyuria (>3000 mL of urine per 24 hours). Hypotension, tachycardia, orthostatic blood pressures, sunken eyes, dry mucous membranes (symptoms of hypovolemia), altered mental status, poor skin turgor, or edema in hypervolemic hypernatremia may be present on physical examination. Without intervention, coma, seizures, and shock may occur.

Diagnosis and Differential

Based on volume status, hypernatremia may be classified as hypervolemic hypernatremia (increased total body Na^+ with normal or increased TBW), normovolemic hypernatremia (near normal total body Na^+ and decreased TBW), or hypovolemic hypernatremia (decreased TBW and total body Na^+ with a relatively greater decrease in TBW) (Table 4-5).

Emergency Department Care and Disposition

1. Treat shock, hypoperfusion, or volume deficits with **isotonic (0.9%) saline or Lactated Ringer's solution.**
2. Treat any existing underlying cause, such as diabetes insipidus, vomiting, diarrhea, or fever.
3. Correct the patient's free water deficit (FWD) using the following formula:

$$\text{Free water deficit} = \text{TBW} \times P_{osm} - 285/P_{osm}$$

TABLE 4-5 Hypernatremia Classification and Features According to Volume Status

	Clinical Conditions	Orthostatic Hypotension	Edema
Hypervolemic hypernatremia	Cushing's syndrome Primary hyperaldosteronism Salt water intake Iatrogenic	Absent unless treated with diuretics	Yes
Normovolemic hypernatremia	DI Central DI Partial DI Gestational DI Nephrogenic DI Hypodipsia	Absent	No
Renal hypovolemic hypernatremia	Osmotic diuretics Loop diuretics Postobstructive diuresis	Normally present	No
Extrarenal hypovolemic hypernatremia	Vomiting Diarrhea GI fistulas Sweating Burns	Normally present	No

Abbreviation: DI, diabetes insipidus.

where TBW is calculated based on age and sex (see hyponatremia treatment section for scale), $P_{osm} = 2 \times [Na^+] + \text{glucose}/18$, and 285 is used as normal plasma osmolality. In an alert patient capable of safely drinking water, give two-thirds free water orally and one-third IV in the form of D5W.

In acute hypernatremia (onset over less than 48 hours), correct at a rate of 1 mEq/L/h. In cases of a lethal sodium chloride ingestion/load (0.75 to 3.0 g/kg) <6 hours prior to presentation, FWD may be replaced rapidly with no reported adverse events. In cases of chronic hypernatremia, correct (lower) the sodium level at a rate of **no more than 0.5 mEq/L/h or 10 to 12 mEq/24 h** to avoid the risk of cerebral edema.

4. Hemodialysis may be used as an alternative or as a supplement to D5W to replace FWD in life-threatening acute cases of salt ingestion.

Hypokalemia ($[K^+]$ <3.5 mEq/L)

Clinical Features

Symptoms of hypokalemia (Table 4-6) usually start when serum concentrations reach 2.5 mEq/L, although they may appear sooner with rapid decreases in concentration or appear later (i.e., at even lower [K+]) for chronic depletion.

Diagnosis and Differential

The most frequent causes of hypokalemia are listed in Table 4-7.

Emergency Department Care and Disposition

1. In stable patients with mild hypokalemia (>3.0 mEq/L) who are able to tolerate oral intake, replacement of K^+ should be done orally using

TABLE 4-6 Symptoms and Signs of Hypokalemia

Cardiovascular	Hypertension Orthostatic hypotension Potentiation of digitalis toxicity Dysrhythmias (usually tachyarrhythmias) T-wave flattening, QT prolongation, U waves, ST depression
Neuromuscular	Malaise, weakness, fatigue Hyporeflexia Cramps Paresthesias Paralysis Rhabdomyolysis
GI	Nausea, vomiting Abdominal distension Ileus
Renal	Increased ammonia production Urinary concentrating defects Metabolic alkalemia, paradoxical aciduria Nephrogenic diabetes insipidus
Endocrine	Glucose intolerance

TABLE 4-7 Causes of Hypokalemia

Transcellular shifts	Alkalosis* Increased plasma insulin (treatment of diabetic ketoacidosis) β-Adrenergic agonists
Decreased intake	Fasting Alcoholism (worsened by hypomagnesemia) Eating disorders
GI loss	Vomiting*, nasogastric suction Diarrhea* (including laxative, enema abuse) Malabsorption Enteric fistula
Renal loss	Diuretics (carbonic anhydrase inhibitors, loop diuretics, and thiazide-like diuretics)* Primary hyperaldosteronism Secondary hyperaldosteronism Renal tubular acidosis Osmotic diuresis
Sweat loss	Heavy exercise Heat stroke Fever
Other	Hypomagnesemia Acute leukemia and lymphomas Hypothermia (accidental or induced)

*Frequently encountered etiologies in the ED.

foods rich in K^+ (fruits, dried fruits, vegetables) as well as salt substitutes or K^+ supplements.

2. When giving IV, use **KCl** (maximum recommended [K^+] in 500 mL of a saline solution is 40 mEq, to be infused in 4 to 6 hours) in a peripheral line. If a more aggressive correction is needed, an identical solution can be administered in a second peripheral line. Higher concentrations can be administered through a central line, but infusion rates should never exceed 20 mEq/h).
3. ECG monitoring is recommended.
4. In most cases, hypokalemic patients are also hypomagnesemic. **Mg^{2+}** 20 to 60 mEq/24 h may be added to the infusion both to optimize tubular reuptake of potassium and to contrast proarrhythmic effect of hypokalemia

Hyperkalemia ([K^+] >5.5 mEq/L)

Clinical Features

Cardiac dysrhythmias, such as ventricular fibrillation, sinoatrial and atrioventricular blocks until complete heart block, and asystole, may occur. Death from hyperkalemia is usually the result of diastolic arrest or ventricular fibrillation. Other common symptoms include neuromuscular dysfunctional weakness, paresthesias, areflexia, ascending paralysis, and GI effects (nausea, vomiting, and diarrhea).

TABLE 4-8 Causes of Hyperkalemia

Pseudohyperkalemia	Tourniquet use Hemolysis (in vitro)* Leukocytosis Thrombocytosis
Intra- to extracellular potassium shift	Acidosis* Heavy exercise β-Blockade Insulin deficiency Digitalis intoxication
Potassium load	Transfusion of aged blood Hemolysis (in vivo) GI bleeding Cell destruction after chemotherapy Rhabdomyolysis/crush injury* Extensive tissue necrosis
Decreased potassium excretion	Renal failure* Drugs—potassium-sparing diuretics* Aldosterone deficiency*

*Frequent or important ED diagnostic considerations.

Diagnosis and Differential

Appropriate tests for management include an ECG, electrolytes, and blood gases. The most common cause is factitious hyperkalemia due to release of intracellular potassium caused by hemolysis during phlebotomy. Other causes are listed in Table 4-8.

Emergency Department Care and Disposition

1. A stat ECG and continuous ECG monitoring is essential in all hyperkalemic patients. If ECG changes are present (Table 4-9), with or without electrolyte levels, emergency treatment of hyperkalemia should start immediately.
2. Emergency treatment is divided into three modalities administered sequentially in rapid succession: membrane stabilization (calcium chloride (10%) or gluconate (10%)) (crucial for cardiac tissue, must be done immediately), intracellular shift of K^+ ($NaHCO_3$, albuterol, insulin, and glucose), and removal/excretion of K^+ from the body (furosemide, sodium polystyrene sulfonate, patiromer, hemodialysis) (Table 4-10).
3. If acidotic, correct the underlying cause of the acid-base imbalance.

TABLE 4-9 ECG Changes Associated with Hyperkalemia

$[K^+]$ (mEq/L)	ECG Changes*
6.5–7.5	Prolonged PR interval, tall peaked T waves, short QT interval
7.5–8.0	Flattening of the P wave, QRS widening
10–12	QRS complex degradation into a sinusoidal pattern

*In chronic or slowly developing hyperkalemia, ECG changes may not occur until higher $[K^+]$ levels are reached.

TABLE 4-10 Emergency Therapy of Hyperkalemia

Therapy	Dose and Route	Onset of Action	Duration of Effect
Calcium chloride (10%)*	5–10 mL IV	1–3 min	30–50 min
Calcium gluconate (10%)*	10–20 mL IV	1–3 min	30–50 min
$NaHCO_3$	50–150 mEq IV	5–10 min	1–2 h
Albuterol (nebulized)	10–20 mg in 4 mL of normal saline, nebulized over 10 min	15–30 min	2–4 h
Insulin† and glucose‡	5–10 units regular insulin IV Glucose 25 g (50% solution) IV	30 min	4–6 h
Furosemide	40–80 mg IV	Varies	Varies
Sodium polystyrene sulfonate	25–50 g PO or PR	1–2 h	4–6 h
Patiromer	8.4 g PO	4–7 h	24 h
Hemodialysis	—	Minutes	Varies

*Calcium chloride has three times the elemental calcium when compared to calcium gluconate. 10% calcium chloride = 27.2 mg [Ca]/mL; 10% calcium gluconate = 9 mg [Ca]/mL. Due to its short duration, calcium administration (both chloride and gluconate) can be repeated up to four times per hour.

†Reduce dose of insulin in patients with renal failure.

‡Glucose infusion should be administered after initial bolus to prevent hypoglycemia. Glucose should not be administered in hyperglycemic patients.

4. Consider calcium administration in association with antidigoxin antibodies in severe hyperkalemia secondary to digitalis intoxication with advanced intraventricular conduction impairment (wide, low-voltage QRS complexes).

Hypomagnesemia

Clinical Findings

Hypomagnesemia may present with a wide variety of neuromuscular, GI, and cardiovascular effects (Table 4-11).

Diagnosis and Differential

Table 4-12 lists the different causes of hypomagnesemia.

Hypokalemia, hypocalcemia, and hypophosphatemia are often present with severe hypomagnesemia and must be monitored carefully. Hypocalcemia does not develop until [Mg^{2+}] falls below 1.2 mg/dL.

Emergency Department Care and Disposition

1. Treat or stop the cause of the hypomagnesemia.
2. For asymptomatic patients (including ECG changes), administer magnesium supplements orally.

TABLE 4-11 Symptoms and Signs of Hypomagnesemia

Neuromuscular	Tetany Muscle weakness Chvostek and Trousseau signs Cerebellar (ataxia, nystagmus, vertigo) Confusion, obtundation, coma Seizures Apathy, depression Irritability Paresthesias
GI	Dysphagia Anorexia, nausea
Cardiovascular	Heart failure Dysrhythmias Hypotension
Miscellaneous	Hypokalemia Hypocalcemia Anemia

3. In life-threatening conditions (torsade de pointes, eclampsia), give **magnesium sulfate ($MgSO_4$)** 1 to 4 gm or 8 to 32 mEQ diluted in at least 100 mL of 5% dextrose or normal saline (0.9%) solution in 10 to 60 minutes under continuous monitoring: ECG (risk of hypokinetic arrhythmias),

TABLE 4-12 Causes of Hypomagnesemia

Redistribution	IV glucose Correction of diabetic ketoacidosis Acute pancreatitis
Extrarenal loss	Profuse sweating, burns, sepsis Intestinal or biliary fistula Diarrhea
Decreased intake	Alcoholism (cirrhosis) Malnutrition, poor intake Malabsorption (steatorrhea)
Renal loss	Ketoacidosis Saline or osmotic diuresis Potassium depletion Phosphorus depletion
Drugs	Loop diuretics Aminoglycosides Alcohol Theophylline Proton pump inhibitors
Endocrine disorders	Syndrome of inappropriate antidiuretic hormone secretion Hyperthyroidism Hyperparathyroidism Hypercalcemic states

TABLE 4-13 Symptoms and Signs of Hypermagnesemia

Level (mEq/L)	Clinical Manifestations
2.0–3.0	Nausea
3.0–4.0	Somnolence
4.0–8.0	Loss of deep tendon reflexes
8.0–12.0	Respiratory depression
12.0–15.0	Hypotension, heart block, cardiac arrest

noninvasive blood pressure (risk of hypotension), and ventilatory pattern (risk of respiratory depression, usually preceded by areflexia, that can be monitored as an alarm sign). As a minor side effect, flushing due to vasodilatation is common.

Hypermagnesemia

Clinical Findings

Magnesium decreases the transmission of neuromuscular messages and thus acts as a CNS depressant and decreases neuromuscular activity (Table 4-13).

Diagnosis and Differential

Serum [Mg^{2+}] is usually diagnostic. Consider hypermagnesemia in patients with hyperkalemia or hypercalcemia. Hypermagnesemia also should be suspected in patients with renal failure, particularly in those who are taking magnesium-containing antacids or laxatives (Table 4-14).

Emergency Department Care and Disposition

1. Immediately cease Mg^{2+} administration.
2. If renal failure is not evident, dilution by IV fluids followed by furosemide (40 to 80 mg IV) may be indicated.

TABLE 4-14 Causes of Hypermagnesemia

Renal Failure	Acute or Chronic
Increased magnesium load	Magnesium-containing laxatives, antacids, or enemas* Treatment of pre-eclampsia/eclampsia (mothers and neonates) Diabetic ketoacidosis (untreated)* Tumor lysis Rhabdomyolysis*
Increased renal magnesium absorption	Hyperparathyroidism Familial hypocalduric hypercalcemia Hypothyroidism Mineralocorticoid deficiency, adrenal insufficiency (Addison's disease)

*Most likely presentation relevant to the ED.

3. In severe symptomatic hypermagnesemia, give **10% $CaCl_2$** 10 ML IV over 2 to 3 minutes. Further infusion of 40 to 60 mL during the next 24 hours can be administered.
4. Patients with renal failure may benefit from dialysis.

Hypocalcemia (ionized [Ca^{2+}] level <2.0 mEq/L (<4 mg/dL or <1.1 mmol/L))

Clinical Features

The severity of signs and symptoms depends greatly on the rapidity of the decrease in [Ca^{2+}] (Table 4-15).

Diagnosis and Differential

Table 4-16 lists the most common causes of hypocalcemia and the primary mechanism of each.

Emergency Department Care and Disposition

1. If a patient is asymptomatic or if the hypocalcemia is not severe or prolonged for more than 10 to 14 days, give **oral Ca^{2+}therapy** 500 to 3000 mg of elemental calcium daily, in one dose or up to three divided doses, with or without vitamin D.
2. In severe acute hypocalcemia (ionized [Ca^{2+}] <1.9 mEq/L or <0.95 mmol/L), give **10% $CaCl_2$** 10 ml or 10 to 30 mL of 10% Ca^{2+} gluconate IV over 10 to 20 minutes and repeat every 60 minutes until symptoms resolve or follow with a continuous IV infusion of **10% $CaCl_2$** at 0.02 to 0.08 mL/kg/h (1.4 to 5.6 mL/h in a 70-kg patient).
3. Replace magnesium before, or in conjunction with, Ca^{2+}.

TABLE 4-15 Symptoms and Signs of Hypocalcemia

Muscular	Weakness, fatigue Spasms, cramps
Neurologic	Tetany Chvostek sign, Trousseau sign Circumoral and digital paresthesias Impaired memory, confusion Hallucinations, dementia, seizures Extrapyramidal disorders
Dermatologic	Hyperpigmentation Coarse, brittle hair Dry, scaly skin
Cardiovascular	Heart failure Ventricular arrhythmias, torsade de pointes Vasoconstriction
Skeletal	Osteodystrophy Rickets Osteomalacia
Miscellaneous	Dental hypoplasia Cataracts Decreased insulin secretion

TABLE 4-16 Some Causes of Hypocalcemia

Decreased calcium absorption
Vitamin D deficiency
Malabsorption syndromes
Increased calcium excretion/reduced bone resorption
Alcoholism
Hypoparathyroidism
Pseudohypoparathyroidism
Hypomagnesemia
Drugs, e.g., phenytoin, phenobarbital, loop diuretics, antibiotics, magnesium sulfate, etc.
Sepsis
Acute pancreatitis
Massive transfusions
Rhabdomyolysis

Hypercalcemia (total $[Ca^{2+}]$ >10.5 mg/dL or an ionized $[Ca^{2+}]$ >2.7 mEq/L)

Clinical Features

Hypercalcemic patients with plasma total $[Ca^{2+}] < 12.0$ mg/dL are usually asymptomatic, but higher levels can cause a wide variety of symptoms (Table 4-17).

A mnemonic sometimes used for the signs and symptoms of hypercalcemia is stones (renal calculi), bones (osteolysis), moans (psychiatric disorders), and groans (peptic ulcer disease, pancreatitis, and constipation).

On ECG, hypercalcemia may be associated with depressed ST segments, widened T waves, and shortened ST segments and QT intervals. Bradyarrhythmias may occur, with bundle-branch patterns that may progress to second-degree block or complete heart block. Levels of $[Ca^{2+}]$ above 20 mg/dL may cause cardiac arrest.

Diagnosis and Differential

A corrected calcium level should be calculated if albumin is not in the normal range:

$$\text{Corrected}\,Ca^{2+}(\text{mg/dL}) = \\ \text{Measured total}\,Ca^{2+}(\text{mg/dL}) + 0.8(4.0 - \text{Serum albumin}[\text{g/dL}])$$

where 4.0 represents the average albumin level in g/dL.

If the reference lab reports values in mmol/L, use the following formula:

$$\text{Corrected}\,Ca^{2+}(\text{mmol/L}) = \\ \text{Measured total}\,Ca^{2+}(\text{mmol/L}) + 0.02(40 - \text{Serum albumin}[\text{grams/L}])$$

where 40 represents the average albumin level in g/L.

More than 90% of occurrences are associated with hyperparathyroidism or malignancy, the latter being the most likely presentation in the ED (Table 4-18).

TABLE 4-17 Signs and Symptoms of Hypercalcemia

• *General* Malaise, weakness Polydipsia, dehydration
• *Neurologic* Confusion Apathy, depression, stupor Decreased memory Irritability Hallucinations Headache Ataxia Hyporeflexia, hypotonia Mental retardation (infants)
• *Metastatic calcification* Band keratopathy Conjunctivitis Pruritus
• *Skeletal* Fractures Bone pain Deformities
• *Cardiovascular* Hypertension Dysrhythmias Vascular calcifications ECG abnormalities QT shortening Coving of ST-T wave Widening of T wave Digitalis sensitivity
• *Gastrointestinal* Anorexia, weight loss Nausea, vomiting Constipation Abdominal pain Peptic ulcer disease Pancreatitis
• *Urologic* Polyuria, nocturia Renal insufficiency Nephrolithiasis

Emergency Department Care and Disposition

1. For symptomatic patients or asymptomatic patients with [Ca^{2+}] levels >14 mg/dL, give **0.9% normal saline** at 500 to 1000 mL/h for 2 to 4 hours as tolerated by the patient. In general, 3 to 4 L should be given over the first 24 hours, then 2 to 3 L per 24 hours until a urine output of 2 L/d is achieved.

TABLE 4-18 Causes of Hypercalcemia

Hypercalcemia due to increased bone Ca^{2+} resorption Primary hyperparathyroidism Malignancy Pseudohyperparathyroidism Renal failure Addison's disease Hyperthyroidism Immobilization
Hypercalcemia due to decreased urinary Ca^{2+} excretion Familial hypercalcemic hypocalciuria Thiazides
Hypercalcemia due to increased GI Ca^{2+} absorption Granulomatous diseases (sarcoidosis, tuberculosis, coccidioidomycosis, histoplasmosis) Milk (calcium)-alkali syndrome Vitamin D intoxication

2. **Furosemide** 20 to 40 mg is recommended to promote a diuresis of 150 to 200 mL/h, which increases the calciuric effect.
3. Decreased mobilization of [Ca^{2+}] from bone through reduction of osteoclastic activity can be obtained with corticosteroids, such as **prednisone** 1 to 2 mg/kg PO, or **hydrocortisone,** 200 to 300 mg IV initial dose, in Addison's disease or in steroid-responsive malignancies. For hypercalcemia associated with malignancy, give intravenous bisphosphonates (pamidronate or zoledronate (zoledronic acid)). **Zoledronic acid** 4 mg IV as a single dose over 15 minutes is recommended for a corrected [Ca^{2+}] level of 12 mg/dL or higher. **Calcitonin** 4 U/kg SC or IM works more rapidly than bisphosphonates.
4. In very severe cases, initiate hemodialysis.

Hypophosphatemia ([PO_4^{3-}] <2.5 mg/dL)

Clinical Features

Severe symptoms may not occur until the [PO_4^{3-}] level drops to <1 mg/dL (Table 4-19).

TABLE 4-19 Symptoms and Signs of Hypophosphatemia

- *Hematologic*
  Reduced survival and function of platelets and red and white blood cells
  Impaired macrophage function
- *Neuromuscular*
  Weakness, tremors, circumoral and fingertip paresthesias, decreased deep tendon reflexes, decreased mental status, anorexia
- *Cardiac*
  Impaired myocardial function
- *Metabolic*
  Insulin resistance

TABLE 4-20 Causes of Hypophosphatemia

Shift from ECF to ICF without depletion of [PO_4^{3-}]	Glucose Insulin Catecholamines Respiratory alkalosis
Shift from ECF to ICF with depletion of [PO_4^{3-}]	Hyperalimentation Refeeding syndrome
Decreased intestinal absorption	Low intake Malabsorption Chronic use of calcium acetate or bicarbonate, aluminum hydroxide Vitamin D deficiency
Increased renal loss	Hyperparathyroidism Tubular acidosis Fanconi's syndrome Hypokalemia Hypomagnesemia Polyuria Acidosis
Miscellaneous causes	Alcoholism (poor intake, vitamin D deficiency) Diabetic ketoacidosis (osmotic diuresis) Toxic shock syndrome
Drugs	Osmotic diuretics, loop diuretics, carbonic anhydrase inhibitor, acyclovir, acetaminophen, tyrosine kinase inhibitors, bisphosphonates, aminoglycosides, tetracyclines, valproic acid, cyclophosphamide, cisplatin, and corticosteroids

Abbreviations: ECF, extracellular fluid; ICF, intracellular fluid.

Diagnosis and Differential

Causes of hypophosphatemia are listed in Table 4-20.

Emergency Department Care and Disposition

1. When symptomatic, correct both orally and IV (Table 4-21).
2. In asymptomatic or mildly symptomatic patients, give 50 mmol/d orally for 7 to 10 days
3. In severe hypophosphatemia, higher doses may be necessary.

TABLE 4-21 IV [PO_4^{3-}] Replacement Dose (6 to 72 hours)

Serum [PO_4^{3-}] (mg/dL)	Dose (mmol/kg)	Duration (hours)
<1	0.6	6–72
1–1.7	0.3–0.4	6–72
1.8–2.2	0.15–0.2	6–72

Hyperphosphatemia ([PO_4^{3-}] >4.5 mg/dL)

Clinical Features

The acute symptoms are due to renal failure, hypocalcemia, and hypomagnesemia.

Diagnosis and Differential

The causes of hyperphosphatemia can be divided into three groups according to mechanism (Table 4-22).

Emergency Department Care and Disposition

Phosphate binders such as calcium carbonate or calcium acetate may be used. In very high [PO_4^{3-}] levels, institute hemodialysis.

ACID-BASE DISORDERS

Acid-base disturbances are classified as respiratory or metabolic. Respiratory acid-base disorders are due to primary changes in PCO_2, and metabolic acid-base disorders reflect primary changes in [HCO_3^-].

Clinical Features

History should emphasize events that may result in the gain or loss of acid or base, such as vomiting, diarrhea, medications, or ingestions of toxins, and seek evidence of dysfunction of the organs of acid-base homeostasis—the liver, kidneys, and lungs.

Diagnosis and Differential

Diagnosis and differential must begin with defining the nature of the acid-base disorder and then determining the most likely etiology. Determine blood gases (pH, PCO_2, and [HCO_3^-]) from an arterial puncture, though venous or capillary blood may also be used. Evaluate electrolytes ([Na^+], [K^+], [Cl^-], and [HCO_3^-]), and other factors that affect the patient's acid-base status (albumin, lactic acid, creatinine, BUN, drug levels of suspected

TABLE 4-22 Causes of Hyperphosphatemia

Decrease in renal excretion of [PO_4^{3-}]	Acute and chronic renal failure* Hypoparathyroidism, pseudohypoparathyroidism
Shift of [PO_4^{3-}] from ICF to ECF	Hemolysis* Rhabdomyolysis* Tumor lysis syndrome Respiratory acidosis Diabetic ketoacidosis
Addition of [PO_4^{3-}] exogenous to the ECF	Oral or IV treatment of hypophosphatemia Phosphate-containing laxatives, antacids*
Drugs	Excess of vitamin D Growth hormone Bisphosphonates

*Most likely presentation relevant to the ED.

ingestions, such as salicylate). Based on current history and physical and past medical history, consider the need for calcium, magnesium, phosphate, serum ketones and glucose, serum osmolality, and urine electrolytes, osmolality, and glucose.

Defining the Nature of the Acid-Base Disorder (Figure 4-1)

Use the patient's pre-illness values as a baseline if available; the normal pH range is 7.35 to 7.45 (95% CI), the normal PCO_2 range is 35 to 45 mm Hg (95% CI), and the normal $[HCO_3^-]$ is usually 21 to 28 mEq/L (95% CI). However, a patient's values may all fall within the "normal range" and still have significant acid-base disturbances.

1. Examine the pH for acidosis (pH <7.35) or alkalosis (pH >7.45).
2. Establish the primary mechanism by evaluating the $[HCO_3^-]$ and PCO_2.

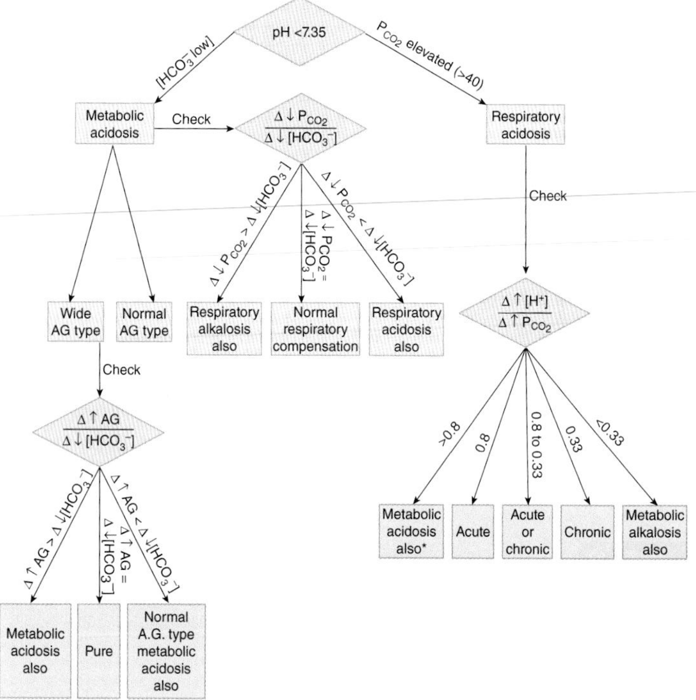

FIGURE 4-1. **A.** Algorithm for determination of type of acidosis. AG, anion gap = $[Na^+] - ([HCO_3^-] + [Cl^-])$ (normal value 12 ± 4 mEq/L). **B.** Algorithm for determination of type of alkalosis. **C.** Algorithm to check for acid-base disturbances when pH is within the "normal" range. ΔAG, delta gap, is a relative change in the AG which may be more important than the actual AG value. Virtually all AG values >15 mEq/L can be considered abnormal, even when there are no previous comparison values available.

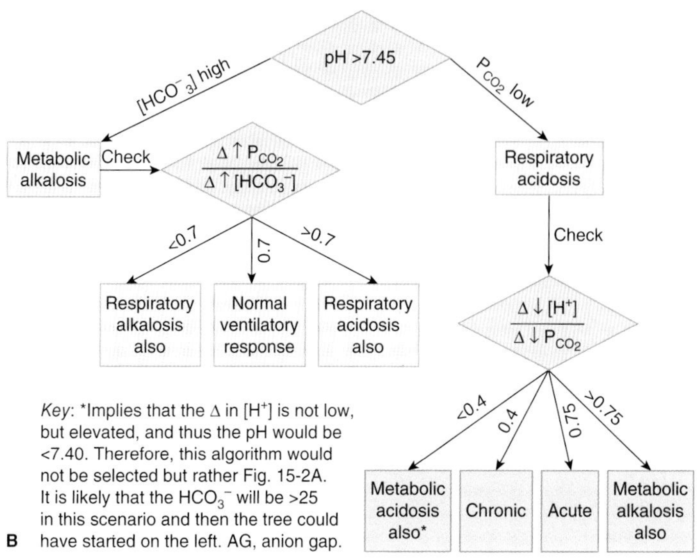

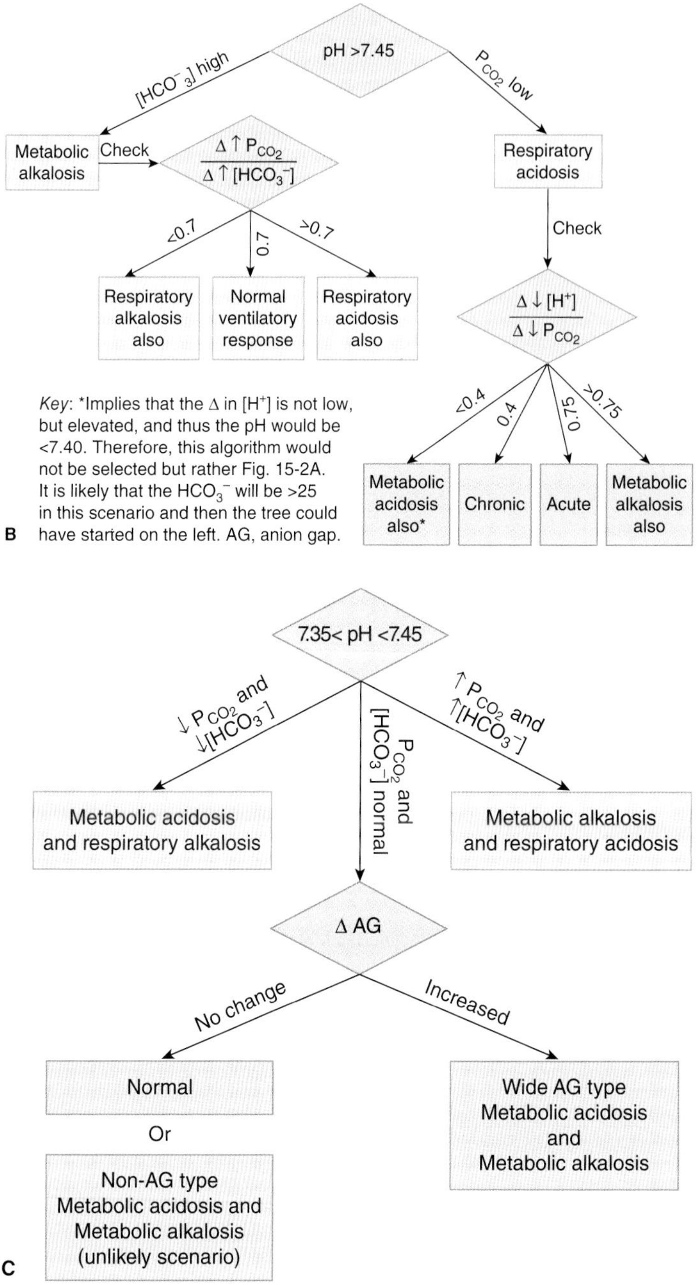

pH >7.45
[HCO$_3^-$] high
P_{CO_2} low
Metabolic alkalosis
Check
$\Delta \uparrow P_{CO_2} / \Delta \uparrow [HCO_3^-]$
<0.7
0.7
>0.7
Respiratory alkalosis also
Normal ventilatory response
Respiratory acidosis also
Respiratory acidosis
Check
$\Delta \downarrow [H^+] / \Delta \downarrow P_{CO_2}$
<0.4
0.4
0.75
>0.75
Metabolic acidosis also*
Chronic
Acute
Metabolic alkalosis also
Key: *Implies that the Δ in [H$^+$] is not low, but elevated, and thus the pH would be <7.40. Therefore, this algorithm would not be selected but rather Fig. 15-2A. It is likely that the HCO$_3^-$ will be >25 in this scenario and then the tree could have started on the left. AG, anion gap.
B
7.35< pH <7.45
$\downarrow P_{CO_2}$ and $\downarrow [HCO_3^-]$
P_{CO_2} and [HCO$_3^-$] normal
$\uparrow P_{CO_2}$ and $\uparrow [HCO_3^-]$
Metabolic acidosis and respiratory alkalosis
Metabolic alkalosis and respiratory acidosis
Δ AG
No change
Increased
Normal
Or
Non-AG type Metabolic acidosis and Metabolic alkalosis (unlikely scenario)
Wide AG type Metabolic acidosis and Metabolic alkalosis
C

FIGURE 4-1. Continued

TABLE 4-23 Causes of Elevated Anion Gap Metabolic Acidosis

Renal failure (uremia)
Ketoacidosis Diabetic Alcoholic Starvation
Lactic acidosis* Sepsis Cardiac arrest Liver failure Iron Metformin Cyanide Carbon monoxide Thiamine deficiency
Exogenous poisoning* Methanol Ethylene glycol (EG) Salicylate Isoniazid

*This is not an exhaustive list; several other causes exist.

Metabolic Acidosis

Metabolic acidosis may be divided into elevated AG acidosis (Table 4-23) and normal AG acidosis (Table 4-24).

Clinical Features

Patients may complain of abdominal pain, headache, nausea with or without vomiting, and generalized weakness, and because acidosis stimulates the respiratory center, the patient may complain of dyspnea.

TABLE 4-24 Causes of Normal Anion Gap Metabolic Acidosis

With a Tendency to Hyperkalemia	With a Tendency to Hypokalemia
Subsiding diabetic ketoacidosis	Renal tubular acidosis, type I (classical distal acidosis)
Early uremic acidosis	Renal tubular acidosis, type II (proximal acidosis)
Early obstructive uropathy	Acetazolamide
Renal tubular acidosis, type IV	Acute diarrhea with losses of HCO_3^- and K^+
Hypoaldosteronism (Addison's disease)	Ureterosigmoidostomy with increased resorption of $[H^+]$ and $[Cl^-]$ and losses of HCO_3^- and K^+
Infusion or ingestion of HCl, NH_4Cl, lysine-HCl, or arginine-HCl	Obstruction of artificial ileal bladder
Potassium-sparing diuretics	Dilution acidosis (may occur with 0.9% NaCl infusion)

Diagnosis and Differential

The differential diagnoses to be considered in emergency practice fall into four broad categories: renal failure (uremia), ketoacidosis (diabetic ketoacidosis, alcoholic ketoacidosis, starvation ketoacidosis), lactic acidosis, and ingestions (methanol, ethylene glycol, salicylates, and many others). Lactic acidosis is not a diagnosis, but a syndrome with its own differential diagnosis (Table 4-23).

Emergency Department Care and Disposition

1. Treat the underlying disorder with particularly emphasis on restoration of normal tissue perfusion and oxygenation.
2. Determine whether there is a respiratory component to the acidosis (i.e., a primary respiratory acidosis). With normal respiratory compensation, PCO_2 decreases by 1 mm Hg for every 1 mEq/L net decrease in $[HCO_3^-]$. If there is inadequate respiratory compensation, correct the respiratory problem.
3. Address electrolyte disturbances.
4. Administer antidotes for toxins as appropriate, and initiate treatment for underlying causes such as sepsis (see Chapter 88, "Toxic Shock") or diabetic ketoacidosis (see Chapter 129, "Diabetic Emergencies").
5. Use of bicarbonate therapy for cardiac arrest, diabetic ketoacidosis, and lactic acidosis, has not shown any benefit. Pediatric patients with diabetic ketoacidosis treated with bicarbonate have an increased rate of development of cerebral edema. The goal of bicarbonate and dialysis therapy in lactic acidosis may be to "bridge" the patient physiologially to definitive treatment of the etiology of the acidosis. Bicarbonate therapy may be appropriate for limited indications (Table 4-25).

TABLE 4-25 Potential Indications for Bicarbonate Therapy in Metabolic Acidosis

Indication	Rationale
Severe hypobicarbonatemia (<4 mEq/L)	Insufficient buffer concentrations may lead to extreme increases in academia with small increases in acidosis.
Severe acidemia (pH <7.00–7.15)* in cases of wide anion gap acidosis, with signs of shock or myocardial irritability that has not responded to supportive measures including adequate ventilation and fluid resuscitation as indicated by the patient's clinical characteristics	Therapy for the underlying cause of acidosis depends on adequate organ perfusion.
Severe hyperchloremic acidemia†	Lost bicarbonate must be regenerated by kidneys and liver, which may require days.

*Presented as a range because recommendations differ among authors; data do not support a specific threshold for treatment.

†No specific threshold indication by pH exists. The presence of serious hemodynamic insufficiency despite supportive care should guide the use of bicarbonate therapy for this indication.

When given, HCO_3^- be dosed 0.5 mEq/kg for each milliequivalent per liter rise [HCO_3^-] desired. The goal is to restore adequate buffer capacity ([HCO_3^-] >8 mEq/L) or to achieve clinical improvement in shock or dysrhythmias. Bicarbonate should be given as slowly as the clinical situation permits. Seventy-five milliliters of 8.4% sodium bicarbonate in 500 mL of dextrose 5% in water produces a nearly isotonic solution for infusion.

Metabolic Alkalosis

Metabolic alkalosis results from gain of bicarbonate or loss of acid. It is typically classified as [Cl^-] sensitive and [Cl^-] insensitive.

Clinical Features

Patients may complain of generalized weakness, dizziness, myalgia, palpitations, nausea with or without vomiting, paresthesia, and possibly muscle spasm or twitching. Neurologic abnormalities, especially tetany, neuromuscular instability, and seizures, are common.

Diagnosis and Differential

Conditions producing "chloride-responsive alkalosis" result in chloride loss, for example, vomiting (which also causes acid loss), diarrhea, diuretic therapy, and chloride-wasting diseases (e.g., cystic fibrosis and chloride-wasting enteropathy), which tend to reduce serum chloride concentration and extracellular volume. Conditions producing "chloride-unresponsive alkalosis" and hypertension include renal artery stenosis, renin-secreting tumors, adrenal hyperplasia, hyperaldosteronism, Cushing's syndrome, Liddle's syndrome, and exogenous mineralocorticoids (e.g., licorice, fludrocortisone). Chloride-unresponsive alkalosis caused by Bartter's and Gitelman's syndromes is usually associated with normotension. Alkalosis results in reductions in ionized calcium, potassium, magnesium, and phosphate levels.

Emergency Department Care and Disposition

1. Treat the underlying cause with careful supportive care.
2. If alkalosis is severe ([HCO_3^-] >45 mmol/L) and associated with serious signs or symptoms not responsive to supportive care, consider IV hydrochloric acid.

Respiratory Acidosis

Respiratory acidosis is defined by alveolar hypoventilation and is diagnosed when the PCO_2 is greater than the expected value.

Clinical Features

The clinical picture usually is dominated by the underlying disorder. Typically, respiratory acidosis depresses the mental function, which may progressively slow the respiratory rate. Patients may be confused, somnolent, and, eventually, unconscious.

Diagnosis and Differential

Inadequate ventilation most frequently results from head trauma, chest trauma, lung disease, or excess sedation. The chronic hypoventilation seen in extremely obese patients is often referred to as the Pickwickian Syndrome. Patients with severe chronic obstructive pulmonary disease have increased dead space and frequently also have decreased minute ventilation. Pulse oximetry may be misleading, making arterial blood gases essential for the diagnosis.

Emergency Department Care and Disposition

1. Improve alveolar ventilation.
2. Ventilatory assistance (intubation or noninvasive ventilatory support) may be required in some patients who do not respond adequately to lesser measures, particularly if the pH falls below 7.25.
3. Treat the underlying disorder.

Respiratory Alkalosis

Respiratory alkalosis is defined by alveolar hyperventilation and exists when PCO_2 is less than expected.

Clinical Features

Symptoms of hyperventilation include dizziness, carpal-pedal spasm, and, frequently, a chest pain described as tightness.

Diagnosis and Differential

It is caused by conditions that stimulate respiratory centers, including CNS tumors or stroke, infections, pregnancy, hypoxia, and toxins (e.g., salicylates). Anxiety, pain, and iatrogenic overventilation of patients on mechanical ventilators also cause respiratory alkalosis.

Emergency Department Care and Disposition

1. Identify and treat the underlying cause.
2. Rule out life-threatening causes of hyperventilation before diagnosing anxiety. The use of "paper-bag" rebreathing in the treatment of respiratory alkalosis should be avoided because it may lead to hypoxia, and patients respond to calm reassurance, which is more effective treatment.

FURTHER READING

For further reading in *Tintinalli's Emergency Medicine: A Comprehensive Study Guide*, 8th ed., see Chapter 15, "Acid-Base Disorders," by Gabor D. Kelen, David D. Nicolaou and David M. Cline; Chapter 17, "Fluids and Electrolytes," by Roberta Petrino and Roberta Marino.

Therapeutic Approach to The Hypotensive Patient

Saurin P. Bhatt

Shock is circulatory insufficiency that creates an imbalance between tissue oxygen supply (delivery) and oxygen demand (consumption). Such tissue hypoperfusion is associated with decreased venous oxygen content and metabolic acidosis (lactic acidosis). Shock is classified into four categories based on etiology: (a) hypovolemic, (b) cardiogenic, (c) distributive (e.g., neurogenic and anaphylactic), and (d) obstructive.

CLINICAL FEATURES

Factors that influence the clinical presentation of a patient in shock include the etiology, duration, and severity of the shock state and the underlying medical status of the patient. Often the precipitating cause of shock may be readily apparent (e.g., acute myocardial infarction, trauma, gastrointestinal [GI] bleeding, or anaphylaxis). It is not uncommon for the patient to present with nonspecific symptoms (e.g., generalized weakness, lethargy, or altered mental status). A targeted history of the presenting symptoms and previously existing conditions (e.g., cardiovascular disease, GI bleeding, adrenal insufficiency, or diabetes) will aid in identifying the cause and guide the initial treatment of shock. Drug use (prescribed and nonprescribed) is an essential element of the initial history. Medication use may be the cause or a contributing factor to the evolution of shock. For example, diuretics can lead to volume depletion and cardiovascular medications (e.g., β-blockers) can depress the pumping action of the heart. The possibility of drug toxicity and anaphylactic reactions to medications also should be considered.

Assessment of vital signs is a routine part of the physical examination; however, no single vital sign or value is diagnostic in the evaluation of the presence or absence of shock. The presence of hyperthermia or hypothermia may be a result of endogenous factors (e.g., infections or hypometabolic states) or exogenous causes (e.g., environmental exposures). The heart rate is typically elevated; however, bradycardia may be present with many conditions, such as excellent baseline physiologic status (young athletes), intraabdominal hemorrhage (secondary to vagal stimulation), cardiovascular medication use (e.g., β-blockers and digoxin), hypoglycemia, and preexisting cardiovascular disease.

The respiratory rate is frequently elevated early in shock. Increased minute ventilation, increased dead space, bronchospasm, and hypocapnia may be seen. As shock progresses, hypoventilation, respiratory failure, and respiratory distress syndrome may occur.

Shock is usually, but not always, associated with systemic arterial hypotension, defined as a systolic blood pressure (BP) below 90 mm Hg. The insensitivity of blood pressure to detect global tissue hypoperfusion has been repeatedly confirmed. Thus, shock may occur with a normal blood pressure, and hypotension may occur without shock. Early in shock, the systolic and diastolic BPs may initially be normal or elevated in response to a compensatory mechanism such as tachycardia and vasoconstriction.

As the body's compensatory mechanisms fail, BP typically falls. Postural changes in BP, commonly seen with hypovolemic states, will precede overt hypotension. The pulse pressure, the difference between systolic and diastolic BP measurements, may be a more sensitive indicator. The pulse pressure usually rises early in shock and then decreases before a change in the systolic BP is seen.

In addition to these vital sign abnormalities, physical examination findings in shock may include neck vein distention or flattening and cardiac dysrhythmias. A third heart sound (S3) may be auscultated in high-output states. Decreased coronary perfusion pressures can lead to myocardial ischemia, decreased ventricular compliance, increased left ventricular diastolic pressures, and pulmonary edema.

Decreased cerebral perfusion leads to mental status changes such as weakness, restlessness, confusion, disorientation, delirium, syncope, and coma. Patients with long-standing hypertension may exhibit these changes without severe hypotension. Cutaneous manifestations may include pallor, pale or dusky skin, sweating, bruising, petechiae, cyanosis (may not be evident if the hemoglobin level is less than 5 g/dL), altered temperature, and delayed capillary refill.

GI manifestations resulting from low flow states may include ileus, GI bleeding, pancreatitis, acalculous cholecystitis, and mesenteric ischemia. To conserve water and sodium, levels of aldosterone and antidiuretic hormone are increased. This results in a reduced glomerular filtration rate, redistribution of blood flow from the renal cortex to the renal medulla, and oliguria. In sepsis, a paradoxical polyuria may occur and be mistaken for adequate hydration.

Early in shock a common metabolic abnormality is a respiratory alkalosis. As the shock state continues and compensatory mechanisms begin to fail, anaerobic metabolism occurs, leading to the formation of lactic acid and resulting in a metabolic acidosis. Other metabolic abnormalities that may be seen are hyperglycemia, hypoglycemia, and hyperkalemia.

DIAGNOSIS AND DIFFERENTIAL

The clinical presentation and presumed etiology of shock will dictate the diagnostic studies, monitoring modalities, and interventions used. The approach to each patient must be individualized; however, frequently performed laboratory studies include complete blood count; platelet count; electrolytes, blood urea nitrogen, and creatinine determinations; prothrombin and partial thromboplastin times; and urinalysis. Other tests commonly used are arterial blood gas, lactic acid, fibrinogen, fibrin split products, D-dimer, and cortisol determinations; hepatic function panel; cerebrospinal fluid studies; and cultures of potential sources of infection. A pregnancy test should be performed on all females of childbearing potential. No single laboratory value is sensitive or specific for shock. Other common diagnostic tests include radiographs (chest and abdominal), electrocardiographs, computed tomography scans (chest, head, abdomen, and pelvis), and echocardiograms. Bedside ultrasound (US) may also help determine the etiology of shock. The following US views are helpful in this assessment: subcostal cardiac, parasternal long-axis cardiac, apical four-chamber cardiac inferior vena cava, right upper quadrant abdominal, pelvic, and abdominal aorta.

Continuous monitoring of vital signs should be instituted in all patients. Modalities such as pulse oximetry, end-tidal CO_2, central venous pressure, central venous O_2 saturation, cardiac output, and calculation of systemic vascular resistance and systemic oxygen delivery may be indicated.

A search to determine the etiology of the shock must be undertaken. Lack of response to appropriate stabilization measures should cause the clinician to evaluate the patient for a more occult cause. First, the physician must be certain that the basic steps of resuscitation have been carried out appropriately. Consider whether or not the patient has been adequately volume resuscitated. Early use of vasopressors may elevate the central venous pressure and mask the presence of continued hypovolemia. Ensure that all equipment is connected and functioning appropriately. Carefully expose and examine the patient for occult wounds. Consider less commonly seen diagnoses, such as cardiac tamponade, tension pneumothorax, adrenal insufficiency, toxic or allergic reactions, and occult bleeding (e.g., rupture ectopic pregnancy, or occult intraabdominal or pelvic bleeding) in the patient who is not responding as expected.

Please refer to other chapters in this book regarding the evaluation of the specific forms of shock.

EMERGENCY DEPARTMENT CARE AND DISPOSITION

The goal of intervention is to restore adequate tissue perfusion in concert with the identification and treatment of the underlying etiology.

1. **Airway:** Aggressive airway control, best obtained through endotracheal intubation, is indicated. Remember that associated interventions such as medications (i.e., sedatives can exacerbate hypotension) and positive pressure ventilation may reduce preload and cardiac output and may contribute to hemodynamic collapse.
2. **Breathing:** All patients should receive supplemental high-flow oxygen. If mechanical ventilation is used, neuromuscular blocking agents should be used to decrease lactic acidosis from muscle fatigue and increased oxygen consumption. Arterial oxygen saturation should be restored to >93% and ventilation controlled to maintain a $PaCO_2$ of 35 to 40 mm Hg.
3. **Circulation: Circulatory** hemodynamic stabilization begins with IV access through large-bore peripheral venous lines. Central venous access aids in assessing volume status (preload) and monitoring $ScvO_2$. US guidance has proven helpful with these procedures. Central venous access is the preferred route for the long-term administration of vasopressor therapy. The Trendelenburg position does not improve cardiopulmonary performance compared with the supine position, and it may worsen pulmonary gas exchange and predispose to aspiration. Passive leg raising above the level of the heart with the patient supine can be effective. Early surgical consultation is indicated for internal bleeding. Most external hemorrhage can be controlled by direct compression. Rarely will clamping or tying off of vessels be needed.
4. The type, amount, and rate of fluid replacement remain areas of controversy. There is no difference in survival comparing crystalloid with colloid resuscitation. Crystalloid solutions continue to be recommended because of the increased cost of colloid agents. Most practitioners use isotonic crystalloid intravenous fluids (0.9% NaCl, Ringer lactate) in the

initial resuscitation phase. Due to the increased cost, lack of proven benefit, and potential for disease transmission (with FFP), the routine use of colloids (5% albumin, purified protein fraction, fresh-frozen plasma [FFP], and synthetic colloid solutions [hydroxyethyl starch or dextran 70]) is questionable. Standard therapy in the hemodynamically unstable patient is 20 to 40 mL/kg given rapidly (over 10 to 20 minutes). Because only about 30% of infused isotonic crystalloids remain in the intravascular space, it is recommended to infuse approximately three times the estimated blood loss in acute hemorrhagic shock. However, the benefits of early and aggressive fluid replacement in these trauma patients remain unproven as do the benefits of permissive hypotension.

5. Blood remains the ideal resuscitative fluid. When possible, use fully cross-matched PRBCs. If the clinical situation dictates more rapid intervention, type-specific, type O (rhesus negative to be given to females of childbearing years) may be used. The decision to use platelets or FFP should be based on clinical evidence of impaired hemostasis and frequent monitoring of coagulation parameters. Platelets are generally given if there is ongoing hemorrhage and the platelet count is 50000/mm^3 or lower; administer 6 units initially. FFP is indicated if the prothrombin time is prolonged beyond 1.5 seconds; administer 2 units initially. Trauma patients requiring transfusion of multiple units of packed RBCs should receive FFP and platelets early in ratios that approach 1:1:1 in order to address the accompanying coagulopathy that will likely be present. The use of fresh whole blood has also been advocated and may be the most effective approach for such patients. The potential need for FFP and platelet transfusions should be considered early and reassessed frequently in an effort to detect and limit the adverse effects of trauma-induced coagulopathy.
6. Vasopressors are used after appropriate volume resuscitation has occurred and there is persistent hypotension. Possible choices include **dobutamine** 2.0 to 20.0 μg/kg/min, **dopamine** 5.0 to 20.0 μg/kg/min, **norepinephrine** 0.5 to 30.0 μg/min, and **epinephrine** 2.0 to 10.0 μg/min.
7. The goal of resuscitation is to maximize survival and minimize morbidity using objective hemodynamic and physiologic values to guide therapy. A goal-directed approach of urine output >0.5 mL/kg/h, CVP 8 to12 mm Hg, MAP 65 to 90 mm Hg, and $ScvO_2$ >70% during ED resuscitation of septic shock significantly decreases mortality.
8. Acidosis should be treated with adequate ventilation and fluid resuscitation. The use of **sodium bicarbonate** 1 mEq/kg use is controversial. Use only in the setting of severe acidosis refractory to above-mentioned methods. Correct only to arterial pH 7.25.
9. Early surgical or medical consultation for admission or transfer is indicated.

FURTHER READING

For further reading in *Tintinalli's Emergency Medicine: A Comprehensive Study Guide*, 8th ed., see Chapter 12, "Approach to Shock," by Bret A. Nicks and John Gaillard; Chapter 13, "Fluid and Blood Resuscitation in Traumatic Shock," by David M. Somand and Kevin R. Ward.

Anaphylaxis, Acute Allergic Reactions, and Angioedema

Alix L. Mitchell

Allergic reactions range from localized urticaria to life-threatening anaphylaxis. Anaphylaxis refers to the most severe form of immediate hypersensitivity reaction and encompasses both IgE-mediated reactions and anaphylactoid reactions, which do not require a previous sensitizing exposure.

CLINICAL FEATURES

Anaphylaxis may occur within seconds or be delayed over an hour after an exposure; rapid reactions are associated with higher mortality. Common exposures are foods, medications, insect stings, and allergen immunotherapy. Many cases are idiopathic. Criteria for anaphylaxis describe an acute progression of organ system involvement that may lead to cardiovascular collapse. Organ system involvement can include dermatologic (pruritus, flushing, urticaria, erythema multiforme, angioedema), respiratory tract (dyspnea, hypoxia, wheezing, cough, stridor), cardiovascular (dysrhythmias, collapse, arrest), gastrointestinal (cramping, vomiting, diarrhea), genitourinary (urgency, cramping), and eye (pruritus, tearing, redness). A biphasic response may occur causing recurrence of symptoms up to 11 hours after the initial exposure, but clinically important events are uncommon. Patients on β-blockers are susceptible to an exaggerated allergic response and may be refractory to first-line treatment.

Angioedema is caused by edema in the dermis, often of the face, neck, or extremities. Angioedema may accompany allergic reactions, or it may be triggered by angiotensin-converting enzyme inhibitors (ACEIs) or due to hereditary angioedema. **Urticaria** is a pruritic cutaneous reaction that may be associated with allergic reactions but may also be nonallergic. Many urticarial reactions are caused by viruses.

DIAGNOSIS AND DIFFERENTIAL

Anaphylaxis is a clinical diagnosis. A history of exposure to an allergen, such as a new drug, food, or sting may make the diagnosis obvious. There is no specific test to verify the diagnosis in real time. Anaphylaxis should be considered in any rapidly progressing multi-system illness. Workup is directed at ruling out other diagnoses while stabilizing the patient. The differential depends on the organ systems involved and may include myocardial ischemia, gastroenteritis, asthma, carcinoid, epiglottitis, hereditary angioedema, and vasovagal reactions.

EMERGENCY DEPARTMENT CARE AND DISPOSITION

Resuscitation must begin with airway, breathing, and circulation. Patients should be placed on a cardiac monitor with pulse oximetry and intravenous access obtained.

1. Administer oxygen as indicated by oximetry. Angioedema or respiratory distress should prompt early consideration for intubation.
2. Limit further exposure. This may be as simple as stopping an intravenous drug or removing a stinger. First-aid measures, ice, and elevation may be helpful for local symptoms. Gastric decontamination is not recommended for ingested allergens.
3. First-line therapy for anaphylaxis is **epinephrine**. In patients without cardiovascular collapse, administer 0.3 to 0.5 mg (0.3 to 0.5 mL of 1:1000; pediatric dose, 0.01 mg/kg) intramuscularly in the thigh. The dose may be repeated every 5 minutes as needed. Patients who are refractory to IM dosing or with cardiovascular compromise should receive intravenous epinephrine. A bolus of 100 μg (place 0.1 mL of 1:1000 in 10 mL normal saline) can be infused over 5 to 10 minutes. If needed, proceed to an infusion (start at 1 μg/min of mix of 1 mL 1:1000 dilution added to 500 mL NS infused at 0.5 mL/min, titrate as needed; pediatric dose, 0.1 to 0.3 μg/kg/min). Stop the infusion for chest pain or arrhythmias. For patients with refractory shock who do not tolerate IV epinephrine, another vasopressor should be chosen. There is no evidence for superiority of any specific agent.
4. Hypotensive patients require aggressive fluid resuscitation with **normal saline** 1 to 2 L (pediatric dose, 10 to 20 mL/kg).
5. Steroids are generally recommended in order to control persistent or delayed reactions, although supportive evidence is sparse. Severe cases can be treated with **methylprednisolone** 125 mg IV (pediatric dose, 2 mg/kg) or **hydrocortisone** 500 mg IV (pediatric dose, 10 mg/kg).
6. Antihistamines have theoretical benefit. **Diphenhydramine** 50 mg is typically given IV or IM (pediatric dose, 1 mg/kg). In addition, an H_2 blocker such as **ranitidine** 50 mg IV (pediatric dose, 0.5 mg/kg) is recommended in severe cases.
7. Bronchospasm should be treated with nebulized β-agonists such as **albuterol** 2.5 mg. If refractory, add nebulized **ipratropium bromide** 250 μg and intravenous **magnesium** 2 g (25 to 50 mg/kg in children) infused over 20 minutes.
8. For patients on β-blockers with hypotension refractory to epinephrine and fluids, use **glucagon** 1 mg IV every 5 minutes (pediatric dose, 50 μg/kg). An infusion of 5 to 15 μg/min should be started once blood pressure improves.
9. **Angioedema** is treated with supportive care and consideration for early intubation if the airway is compromised. Episodes may last hours to days. Patients with mild swelling without airway involvement can be observed for 12 to 24 hours and discharged if symptoms are improving. ACEI-induced angioedema can be treated with **icatibant** (30 mg SC). **C1 esterase inhibitor (human)** (1000 U IV) has been shown to be effective in case series. The ACEI must be discontinued.
10. Patients with hereditary angioedema can be treated with intravenous **C1 esterase inhibitor replacement** (C1 esterase inhibitor (human) 20 U/kg; C1 esterase inhibitor (recombinant) 50 U/kg to maximum 4200 units). Treatment with **fresh frozen plasma** has been used as an alternative when C1 esterase inhibitor replacement is not available (2 to 3 U IV). **Icatibant** (30 mg SC) and **ecallantide** (30 mg SC) are also effective in shortening attacks of hereditary angioedema.

11. Unstable or refractory patients merit admission to the intensive care unit. Patients with moderate to severe symptoms should be admitted for observation. Patient with mild allergic reactions should be observed in the ED and may be sent home if symptoms are stable or improving. Stable patients who received epinephrine are generally felt to be safe for discharge after 4 hours without symptoms. Consider longer observation for patients with a history of severe reactions, patients on β-blockers, and patients who live alone or might have difficulty returning.
12. Discharge patients on a 3-day course of antihistamines and prednisone; longer courses may be necessary for idiopathic anaphylaxis. Counsel all patients about the need to return to the ED for recurrence of symptoms. Instruct patients in avoiding future exposures to the allergen, if known. All patients who have experienced a severe allergic reaction or anaphylaxis should have and know how to use an **epinephrine autoinjector**. Consider Medic-Alert bracelets and referral to an allergist in these patients.

FURTHER READING

For further reading in *Tintinalli's Emergency Medicine: A Comprehensive Study Guide*, 8th ed., see Chapter 14, "Anaphylaxis, Allergies, and Angioedema," by Brian H. Rowe and Theodore J. Gaeta

SECTION 2

Analgesia, Anesthesia, and Sedation

Acute Pain Management and Procedural Sedation

Michael S. Mitchell

Acute pain is the chief complaint for 75% to 80% of all ED visits. Procedural sedation and analgesia often are needed for painful interventions or diagnostic studies.

CLINICAL FEATURES

Responses to pain vary and may include increased heart rate, blood pressure, respiratory rate, and behavioral changes, however these responses may only have a mild correlation, so they cannot be relied upon exclusively. Pain is most objectively assessed with the use of several validated pain scales, though these scales may not be as accurate in elderly patients or trauma patients. Pain scales are a mainstay of assessing pain in young children.

EMERGENCY DEPARTMENT CARE AND DISPOSITION

During the primary assessment, determine the patient's perception of the degree of pain and continue to reassess their pain after any intervention. Be aware that children are vulnerable to oligoanalgesia for several reasons including difficulty assessing their pain and provider discomfort as well as unfamiliarity with medication dosing regimens.

Pharmacologic and nonpharmacologic interventions may be helpful for treating anxiety and pain in the ED. Nonpharmacologic interventions include the application of heat or cold, immobilization and elevation of injured extremities, and distraction methods, such as feeding sucrose solution to infants. When pharmacologic intervention is needed, the selection of agent should be guided by the severity of pain necessitating analgesia, the route of delivery, and the desired duration of effects.

Acute Pain Control

Nonopioid Analgesics, such as **acetaminophen,** 650 to 1000 mg PO (15 mg/kg PO or PR in children) or nonsteroidal anti-inflammatory drugs (NSAIDS) such as **ibuprofen,** 400 to 800 mg PO (10 mg/kg PO in children) can be used to treat mild to moderate pain. Parenteral

NSAIDs are no more effective than oral medications. Adverse effects of NSAIDS include gastrointestinal irritation, renal dysfunction, platelet dysfunction, and impaired coagulation. Furthermore, NSAIDs increase the risk of cardiac death in patients with ischemic heart disease. Aspirin should be avoided in children because of an association with Reye syndrome.

Opiates, such as **morphine,** 0.1 mg/kg IV (0.1 to 0.2 mg/kg IV in children), **fentanyl,** 1 μg/kg IV (1 to 2 μg/kg in children), and **hydromorphone,** 0.2 to 1 mg IV (0.01 mg IV in children) are the agents of choice for moderate to severe pain. Children require more opiates proportionate to their weight than adults. The goal of therapy is to titrate the doses to effect. Side effects of opiates include respiratory depression, nausea and vomiting, confusion, pruritus, and urinary retention. Oral opioids may be tried as an alternative to parenteral administration, however they can have variable absorption and a slower effect.

Special caution should be given to the use of codeine and tramadol. Codeine is not a reliable analgesic as up to 10% of the US population lack the necessary enzyme to convert it to its active state. Tramadol can produce significant CNS toxicity.

Procedural Sedation and Analgesia (PSA)

Procedural sedation is the use of medication to induce a depressed level of consciousness while maintaining cardiorespiratory function so that a painful procedure can be performed. There are various levels of sedation achieved with different medications. See Table 7-1. Be aware that with increased depth of sedation, the risk of depressed breathing and potential loss of airway patency is increased.

Preparation

Recent oral intake is not a contraindication to procedural sedation in the emergency department. If concerned, however, waiting 3 hours after last oral intake is associated with a low risk of aspiration regardless of the level of sedation. The complication rate of PSA depends strongly on depth of sedation and patient's physiological reserve as determined by chronic or acute illness. Consider anesthesia consultation for patients with significantly limited physiologic reserve, especially cardiorespiratory conditions,

TABLE 7-1 Levels of Sedation and Analgesia

	Responsiveness	Airway	Breathing	Circulation
Minimal sedation (aka "anxiolysis")	Normal but slowed response to verbal stimulation	Unaffected	Unaffected	Unaffected
Moderate sedation (aka "conscious sedation")	Purposeful response to verbal or physical stimulation	Usually maintained	Usually adequate	Usually maintained
Deep sedation	Purposeful response after repeated or painful physical stimulation	May be impaired	May be suppressed	Usually maintained

those with severe systemic disease, at the extremes of age, and those with predicted difficult airway.

When PSA is performed, necessary equipment includes a continuous cardiac monitor with pulse oximetry, oxygen, suction, and immediate availability of appropriately sized resuscitation equipment. Informed consent should be obtained. The patient should be under constant observation by a provider trained in airway management. Blood pressure, heart rate, respiratory rate, and level of consciousness should be monitored. Some advocate routine use of capnography to monitor ventilation in sedated patients, as it has been shown to detect changes in ventilation before clinical observation allowing for earlier recognition of adverse events. The application of supplemental oxygen reduces hypoxemia and has no adverse clinical effects.

The analgesic or sedative agents chosen should be individualized to the patient and the planned procedure. The agents used for PSA often have a narrow therapeutic index. Therefore, these medications should be administered in small, incremental intravenous doses, with adequate time between doses to determine peak effect. All patients undergoing PSA should be reassessed continuously. Patients experiencing transient respiratory depression can usually be managed by bag-mask ventilation.

Sedation Management

Table 7-2 describes selected sedation agents for procedural sedation.

Nitrous Oxide is used for minimal sedation and is supplied in a 50:50 mixture with oxygen. It requires a special setup of a demand delivery system and a scavenging system to prevent exam room accumulation of nitrous oxide. It is contraindicated in pregnant women and those with pneumothorax, pneumocephalus, and vascular air embolus.

Fentanyl has a rapid onset of action and is easily titratable. Chest wall rigidity unresponsive to naloxone may occur at higher doses (5 to 15 mcg/kg) or when rapidly administered potentially necessitating neuromuscular blockade and mechanical ventilation. Slow administration (e.g., over 3 to 5 minutes) and careful flushing of the IV can prevent rigid chest syndrome.

Midazolam is commonly used as a sole agent for minimal sedation. Respiratory depression and hypotension may develop. Flumazenil quickly reverses sedation and respiratory depression due to benzodiazepines. Routine use to reverse sedation is not recommended.

Ketamine is a dissociative analgesic with sedative, analgesic, and amnestic properties that causes minimal respiratory depression and has a minimal effect on blood pressure. Ketamine may be administered IV or IM. In lower doses, it can produce analgesia. In higher doses (approximately 1mg/kg and above IV) a critical dosing threshold is exceeded and produces a dissociative state. Ketamine may cause increased intraocular pressure, hypersalivation, laryngospasm, and a hallucinatory emergence reaction in older children and adults. Ketamine can cause vomiting, especially in adolescents. Pretreatment with ondansetron can reduce the incidence of vomiting. There is conflicting data on whether ketamine causes increased intracranial pressure, thus there is no concluding evidence to restrict its use in head injury patients. Emergence reaction is best treated with **midazolam** (0.1 mg/kg IM or IV). Ketamine is contraindicated in children less than 3 months as well as those with increased intraocular pressure or obstructive

TABLE 7-2 Sedation Agents for Adult Procedural Sedation and Analgesia

Medication	Recommended Dosage	Route of Administration	Peak Effect	Approximate Duration	Use
Nitrous oxide	50:50 mixture with oxygen	Inhalational	1–2 min	3–5 min	Minimal sedation
Midazolam	0.05–0.1 mg/kg. May repeat 0.05 mg/kg every 2 min until adequately sedated 0.1 mg/kg	IV IM	2–3 min 15–30 min	20–30 min 1–2 h	Minimal or moderate sedation Minimal sedation
Fentanyl	1–3 μg/kg, can be titrated up to 5 μg/kg	IV	2–3 min	30–60 min	Minimal sedation
Fentanyl and midazolam	1–2 μg/kg fentanyl plus 0.1 mg/kg midazolam	IV	2–3 min	1 h	Moderate and deep sedation
Methohexital	1 mg/kg	IV	1 min	3–5 min	Moderate or deep sedation
Pentobarbital	2.5 mg/kg followed by 1.25 mg/kg, as needed, up to two times	IV rate should be <50 mg/min	3–5 min	15 min	Minimal and moderate sedation. Frequently used for radiologic procedures.
Ketamine	1 mg/kg 2–5 mg/kg	IV IM	1–3 min 5–20 min	15–30 min 30–60 min	Dissociative sedation Dissociative sedation
Ketamine and midazolam	Ketamine as above plus midazolam, 0.03–0.05 mg/kg	IV	1–3 min	30–60 min	Dissociative sedation
Etomidate	0.15 mg/kg, followed by 0.1 mg/kg every 2 min, if needed	IV	15–30 s	3–8 min	Moderate and deep sedation
Propofol	0.5–1.0 mg/kg, followed by 0.5 mg/kg every 3 min, if needed	IV	30–60 s	5–6 min	Moderate and deep sedation
Ketamine and propofol "ketofol"	Ketamine 0.125–0.5 mg/kg and Propofol 0.5 mg/kg	IV	30–60 s	15 min	Moderate and deep sedation

hydrocephalus and should be used in caution in patients with significant upper respiratory tract infectious symptoms or those undergoing a procedure involving major stimulation of the oropharynx (e.g., endoscopy).

Etomidate is a rapid onset sedative with short duration of effect. It causes temporary adrenal insufficiency which is associated with increased mortality in critically-ill patients; however, this effect has not been shown to cause adverse events when used in stable patients. Up to 20% of patients can have myoclonic jerking.

Propofol is an anesthetic agent administered by intravenous infusion that has a short duration of effect, which results in shorter recovery time and ED length of stay. The most common side effect is respiratory depression and apnea. Side effects include hypotension, therefore hypovolemia should be corrected before propofol administration. Adjunct analgesic is mandatory for painful procedures. Pain at the IV site is common during administration and can be blunted with adjunct use of lidocaine (e.g., 0.05 mg/kg IV). Propofol use is contraindicated in patients who are allergic to eggs or soy products.

Ketamine and Propofol can be used in combination and may have synergy with each other. Ketamine may blunt the hypotension and respiratory depression seen with propofol. Propofol may prevent the emergence reaction and vomiting seen with ketamine. Ketamine use precludes the use of an analgesic with propofol alone. The greatest advantage of using this combination is likely that sedation can be achieved with lower doses of either drug used alone.

Elderly

Procedural sedation in the elderly is associated with increased adverse events. The risk of respiratory depression is increased with all agents. Etomidate is a good choice owing to its minimal cardiovascular effects. When using propofol in this age group, the initial and subsequent doses should be 50% of those recommended for younger adults.

Children

Children of all ages feel pain, even neonates. Anxiety issues, pain control, and need for sedation must be addressed. Anxiety may be a significant barrier to a successful procedure performance, especially when patient's cooperation is needed. Parents can provide significant anxiety relief and should be allowed to stay with children. Age appropriate distraction techniques should also be employed. Benzodiazepines, such as midazolam, provide effective pharmacologic anxiety relief when needed. Oral sucrose is an effective analgesic in infants undergoing painful procedures such as IV catheter placement. Procedural sedation and analgesia should be used when performing painful procedures or when procedures require the patient to be still. Common medications used for pediatric procedural sedation are listed in Table 7-3.

Disposition

Patients are eligible for discharge only when fully recovered. When discharged, the patient must be accompanied by an adult and should not drive or operate machinery for 24 hours. Because many of the agents used for PSA produce anterograde amnesia, discharge instructions must be given to responsible accompanying adults.

TABLE 7-3 Medications for Procedural Sedation

Class	Drug	Route	Dose	Onset	Duration	Advantages	Disadvantages	Examples	Comments
Anxiolytic	Midazolam	PO, PR, IV, IM, IN	PO/PR 0.5 mg/kg IV/IM 0.05–0.1 mg/kg IN 0.2–0.4 mg/kg	PO/PR 20–30 min IV 3–5 min IM 10–20 min IN 5–10 min	1–4 h	Flexible route of administration	No analgesia, paradoxical reaction	Premedication for IV start, laceration repair using local anesthetic	Acidic, nasal administration stings, may cause increased secretions; oral/rectal slow onset, less predictable
Hypnotic/sedative	Propofol	IV	1–2 mg/kg, followed by 0.5 mg/kg repeat doses as needed	Seconds	Minutes	Rapid onset and short duration, motionlessness, muscle relaxant	No analgesia, respiratory and cardiovascular depressant	CT scan, LP with topical analgesic, laceration repair, reduction of dislocation	Non-analgesic, increased requirement for younger patients, painful injection
	Etomidate	IV	0.2–0.3 mg/kg	Seconds	Minutes	Rapid onset, short duration	No analgesia, myoclonus, respiratory depressant	CT scan, short procedures requiring motionlessness	Avoid in patients with increased tone (e.g., CP) due to myoclonic jerks, painful injection
	Pentobarbital	IV	1–2 mg/kg, repeated every 3–5 min as needed	<1 min	15–45 min	Well studied, motionlessness, neuroprotective	No analgesia, respiratory and cardiovascular depressant	CT scan, no reversal agent	Variable dosing, long recovery times
	Methohexital	IV	0.5–1 mg/kg	Seconds	10–60 min	Rapid onset	No analgesia, respiratory and cardiovascular depressant	CT scan, no reversal agent	—

Dissociative	Ketamine	IV, IM	IV 1–1.5 mg/kg IM 4–5 mg/kg	IV 1–2 min IM 3–5 min	IV 15 min IM 30–45 min	Analgesic, anesthetic, motionlessness, respiratory and cardiovascular stimulant, bronchodilator	Increased intraocular pressure, salivation; emetogenic; laryngospasm	Painful procedures requiring motionlessness (complex lacerations, fracture reductions, I & D), no reversal agent	Consider pretreatment with ondansetron; atropine and midazolam co-administration unnecessary
Combinations	Fentanyl + midazolam	IV	Fentanyl 1–2 μg/kg, midazolam 0.05–0.1 mg/kg	1–2 min	1–3 h	Analgesic and anxiolytic	Respiratory depressant	Fracture reduction, reduction of dislocation, laceration repair	Reversal with flumazenil and naloxone
	Propofol + ketamine	IV	Propofol 1 mg/kg, ketamine 0.5 mg/kg	1 min	Propofol (minutes); ketamine 15–45 min	Decreased dosing for both agents, complementary side effects (lessens respiratory and cardiovascular depression, emesis)	—	Fracture reduction, I & D, complex laceration	Consider ondansetron pretreatment
Other	Nitrous oxide	Inhaled	Titrate to effect	Minutes	Minutes	Self-dosing	Not readily available	Adjunct to anesthetics	—

Abbreviations: CP = cerebral palsy; I & D = incision and drainage; IN = intranasally.

Local and Regional Anesthesia

Local and regional anesthetics are essential tools for ED pain management. Agents can be administered topically, intravenously, by infiltration directly into the area to be anesthetized, or into the area of the peripheral nerves supplying the area. This discussion focuses on topical and infiltrative anesthetics.

The toxicity of local anesthetics (LAs) is related to the total dose and the rate of plasma concentration increase. The risk of toxicity is heightened in the setting of hypoxia, hypercarbia, and acidosis. Toxic effects include CNS effects progressing to coma and cardiovascular effects progressing to cardiovascular collapse. Allergic reactions to LAs are uncommon and are usually due to a preservative. If an allergy is suspected, the best approach is to use a preservative-free agent from the other class of LAs. Alternatively, diphenhydramine or benzyl alcohol may be used as an LA in the setting of a true allergy to conventional LAs.

LAs often cause pain during administration. Slow injection through a 27- or 30-gauge needle, injecting through the wound margin, using warm solution, and using buffered (with sodium bicarbonate) solution decrease injection pain.

Epinephrine (1:100 000) is often added to LAs before administration. Addition of epinephrine increases the duration of anesthesia, provides wound hemostasis, and slows systemic absorption. Epinephrine is safe for use in end-arterial fields, but should be avoided in those with suspected digital vascular injury or those with known peripheral vascular disease.

Lidocaine, which is the most commonly used LA in the ED, has a 2- to 5-minute onset of effect and a 1- to 2-hour duration of effect. The maximum dose of infiltrative lidocaine is 4.5 mg/kg without or 7 mg/kg with epinephrine. Lidocaine is buffered to decrease the pain of injection by adding 1 mL $NaHCO_3$ to 9 mL lidocaine, but for maximum effectiveness, it should only be added immediately before use.

Bupivacaine, which has an onset of effect of 3 to 7 minutes and duration of effect of 90 minutes to 6 hours, is preferred for prolonged procedures. The maximum dose of infiltrative **bupivacaine** is 2 mg/kg without or 3 mg/kg with epinephrine. Buffer bupivacaine with 1 mL $NaHCO_3$ to 29 mL bupivacaine.

Local Anesthetic Infiltration

LAs can provide anesthesia at a site by infiltrating directly into the site or by infiltrating around the peripheral nerves supplying the site. For some wounds, LA infiltration around the peripheral nerves is advantageous due to decreased total LA required and decreased pain at the site of injection. During administration, the syringe plunger must be drawn back to avoid intravascular injection of LA.

Topical Anesthetics

Topical anesthetics can eliminate the need for LA infiltration, are applied painlessly, do not distort wound edges, and may provide hemostasis. Common preparations include lidocaine, epinephrine, and tetracaine (LET), lidocaine and prilocaine (EMLA), and various preparations of lidocaine. LET is applied by placing a LET-saturated cotton ball or gauze pad onto an open wound for a minimum of 20 to 30 minutes. LET should not be used on mucus membranes or in end-arterial fields.

EMLA is a cream composed of lidocaine and prilocaine used only on intact skin to relieve the pain associated with venipuncture, arterial puncture, port access, and other superficial skin procedures. It has a 45- to 60-minute onset of effect and a 60-minute duration upon withdrawal. Because prilocaine may cause methemoglobinemia, EMLA should be used with caution in infants younger than 3 months and avoided in patients predisposed to methemoglobinemia.

Regional Blocks

Regional anesthesia is a technique that infiltrates local anesthetic agents adjacent to peripheral nerves ("nerve blocks") and is typically used for complicated lacerations, fractures, and dislocations. Distortion of the site is avoided. US guidance can be used. Care must be taken not to inject the anesthetic solution directly into the nerve. Prior to anesthetic use, distal neurovascular and neurologic status should be assessed. This chapter will discuss commonly used regional blocks in basic descriptions.

Digital Blocks

Purpose: Finger and toe blocks are advantageous because less anesthetic is needed, better anesthesia is obtained, and tissues are not distorted. The onset of anesthesia is delayed when compared with that of LA. Assess and document neurovascular status before the procedure.

Positioning: Place the hand in the prone (palm down) position. The nerves travel on the lateral aspect of the finger on both the dorsal and palmar sides.

Technique: Insert the needle on the dorsal surface of the proximal phalanx and advance toward the volar surface staying immediately adjacent to the phalanx. Aspirate to ensure no vascular puncture has occurred and inject 1 mL of anesthetic. Slowly retract the needle while injecting another 1 mL of anesthetic. Prior to withdrawing the needle, direct it across the dorsum to the other side of the digit and inject 1 mL while withdrawing slowly. Repeat the first injection on the other side of the digit. Toes can be blocked in the same manner.

Flexor Tendon Sheath Digital Nerve Block

Purpose: This is a one-injection alternative to the traditional digit block. Be aware that this technique may not provide adequate anesthesia to the distal fingertip.

Positioning: Place the hand in the supine (palm up) position. Have the patient flex the finger to identify the flexor tendon and its corresponding tendon sheath.

Technique: Inject the needle at the distal palmar crease into the flexor tendon sheath. Once the “pop” is felt, inject 2 to 3 mL of anesthetic.

Intercostal Nerve Block

Purpose: This block will provide anesthesia in a band-like fashion above and below the affected rib. These blocks are useful to ameliorate pain from a rib fracture or are useful in tube thoracostomy placement.

Positioning: The patient sits upright with the ipsilateral arm raised and resting on the head. The site of injection is either the mid-axillary line of the affected rib or the "rib angle," which is approximately 6 cm posterior of the mid-axillary line and immediately lateral to the paraspinous muscles. The "rib angle" site is preferred to ensure adequate analgesia to all branches of the intercostal nerve.

Technique: Palpate the inferior border of the rib to be blocked and retract the skin cephalad. Raise a wheal in the subcutaneous space and insert the needle bevel up and direct it toward the lower aspect of the bone with needle up and syringe down allowing a needle angle of approximately 10 degrees off perpendicular. Once bone is contacted, release the skin retraction and march the needle caudally until it drops off the bone. Aspirate before injection, and inject 2 to 5 mL of anesthetic. Note that pneumothorax can occur in up to 9% of patients, so close monitoring for respiratory symptoms is recommended for 30 minutes after procedure.

Femoral Nerve Block

Purpose: The femoral nerve block and a larger block involving the femoral, obturator, and lateral femoral cutaneous nerves ("three-in-one" block) are good for proximal femur fractures and hip fracture patients.

Positioning: The patient lies supine and the inguinal crease is exposed. The femoral nerve is 1 cm lateral to the femoral artery at the inguinal crease and is fairly superficial.

Technique: Ultrasound guidance is recommended. Locate the nerve location as described above and raise a wheal of anesthetic. With US guidance, direct the needle toward the femoral nerve. Correct positioning is confirmed when the patient reports anterior thigh parathesias. If this is not felt, the needle may need to be directed more laterally to find the nerve. Once found, retract the needle slightly and inject approximately 20 mL of anesthetic into the perineural space. To perform the "three-in-one" block, hold firm pressure distal to the injection site for 5 minutes to help promote cephalad distribution of the anesthetic.

Hematoma Block

Purpose: This block delivers anesthesia to a fracture site to aid in reduction.

Positioning: The patient is supine with the limb placed to access the fracture site.

Technique: A sterile approach is recommended. Direct the needle toward the fracture site. Aspiration of blood will confirm that the needle is likely within the confines of the hematoma. Inject 5 to 15 mL of anesthetic. Be careful not to exceed the maximum dose of anesthetic.

FURTHER READING

For further reading in *Tintinalli's Emergency Medicine: A Comprehensive Study Guide*, 8th ed., see Chapter 35, "Acute Pain Management," by James Ducharme; Chapter 113, "Pain Management and Procedural Sedation in Infants and Children," by Peter S. Auerbach; Chapter 36, "Local and Regional Anesthesia," by Douglas C. Dillon and Michael A. Gibbs; and Chapter 37, "Procedural Sedation," by Chris Weaver.

Chronic Pain

David M. Cline

MANAGEMENT OF PATIENTS WITH CHRONIC PAIN

Chronic pain is a painful condition that lasts longer than 3 months, pain that persists beyond the reasonable time for an injury to heal, or pain that persists 1 month beyond the usual course of an acute disease. Complete eradication of pain is not a reasonable endpoint in most cases. Rather, the goal of therapy is pain reduction and a return to functional status.

Clinical Features

Signs and symptoms of chronic pain syndromes are summarized in Table 8-1. Many of these syndromes will be familiar to emergency physicians.

Complex regional pain type I, previously known as *reflex sympathetic dystrophy,* and complex regional pain type II, previously known as *causalgia,* may be seen in the emergency department (ED) 2 weeks or more

TABLE 8-1 Signs and Symptoms of Selected Chronic Pain Syndromes

Disorder	Pain Symptoms	Signs
Transformed migraine	Initially migraine-like, becomes constant, dull, nausea, vomiting	Muscle tenderness and tension, normal neurologic examination
Fibromyalgia	Diffuse muscular pain, stiffness, fatigue, sleep disturbance	Diffuse muscle tenderness, >11 trigger points
Poststroke pain	Same side as weakness, throbbing, shooting pain, allodynia	Loss of hot and cold differentiation
Chronic back pain	Constant dull pain, occasionally shooting pain, pain does not follow nerve distribution	No trigger points, poor ROM in involved muscle
HIV-associated sensory neuropathy	Symmetric pain and paresthesia, most prominent in toes and feet	Sensory loss in areas of greatest pain symptoms
Complex regional pain types I and II	Burning persistent pain, allodynia, associated with immobilization/disuse (type I) or peripheral nerve injury (type II)	Early: edema, warmth, local sweating; late: the early signs alternate with cold, pale, cyanosis, eventually atrophic changes
Postherpetic neuralgia	Allodynia, shooting, lancinating pain	Sensory changes in the involved dermatome
Painful diabetic neuropathy	Symmetric numbness and burning or stabbing pain in lower extremities; allodynia may occur	Sensory loss in lower extremities
Phantom limb pain	Variable: aching, cramping, burning, squeezing, or tearing sensation	May have peri-incisional sensory loss

Abbreviations: HIV, human immunodeficiency virus; ROM, range of motion.

after an acute injury. These disorders should be suspected when a patient presents with classic symptoms: allodynia (pain provoked with gentle touch of the skin) and a persistent burning or shooting pain. Early associated signs during the disease include edema, warmth, and localized sweating.

Diagnosis and Differential

The most important task of the emergency physician is to distinguish chronic pain from acute pain that heralds a life- or limb-threatening condition. A complete history and physical examination should confirm the chronic condition or point to the need for further evaluation when unexpected signs or symptoms are elicited.

Rarely, a provisional diagnosis of a chronic pain condition is made for the first time in the ED. The exception is a form of post-nerve injury pain—complex regional pain. The sharp pain from acute injuries, including fractures, rarely continues beyond 2 weeks duration. Pain in an injured body part beyond this period should alert the clinician to the possibility of nerve injury.

Definitive diagnostic testing of chronic pain conditions is difficult, requires expert opinion and, often, expensive procedures such as magnetic resonance imaging, computed tomography, or thermography. Therefore, referral to the primary source of care and eventual specialist referral are warranted to confirm the diagnosis.

Emergency Department Care and Disposition

1. Opioids are not recommended for the primary treatment chronic pain in the ED. Patients who state their prescription opioids have been lost or stolen should be referred to their pain specialist or primary care doctor and the prescription should not be refilled by the emergency physician.
2. The evidence-based management of chronic pain conditions is listed in Table 8-2. The need for longstanding treatment of chronic pain conditions limits the safety of the nonsteroidal anti-inflammatory drugs. Doses of drugs are as follows. **Amitriptyline**—start 25 mg/d PO.

TABLE 8-2 Management of Selected Chronic Pain Syndromes

Disorder	Primary Treatment	Secondary Treatment
Transformed migraine	Stop prior medications	Celecoxib or prednisone taper
Fibromyalgia	Duloxetine	Pregabalin
Chronic back or neck pain	Duloxetine	Amitriptyline
Poststroke pain	Pregabalin	Gabapentin
HIV-associated sensory neuropathy	Optimize antiretroviral therapy	Lamotrigine
Complex regional pain types I and II	Acute: Prednisone taper	Ketamine by specialist
Postherpetic neuralgia	Pregabalin or gabapentin	Amitriptyline
Painful diabetic neuropathy	Duloxetine	Pregabalin or gabapentin
Phantom limb pain	Gabapentin	Amitriptyline

Gabapentin is started with an initial dose of 300 mg daily and is increased up to a maximum of 1200 mg three times daily according to response. **Pregabalin**—start 50 mg three times daily. **Duloxetine**—start 30 mg PO daily. **Lamotrigine**—begin with 25 mg daily.

3. Referral to the appropriate specialist is one of the most productive means to aid in the care of chronic pain patients who present to the ED. Possible outcomes of referral to pain specialists include optimization of medical therapy, trigger point injections, dedicated exercise programs, physical therapy, epidural steroid injections, or nerve blocks as indicated.

MANAGEMENT OF PATIENTS WITH ABERRANT DRUG-RELATED BEHAVIOR

The spectrum of patients with aberrant drug-related behavior includes those who have chronic pain and are now dependent on narcotics to "hustlers" who are obtaining prescription drugs to sell on the street.

Clinical Features

Because of the wide spectrum of patients with aberrant drug-related behavior, the history given may be factual or fraudulent. Patients with aberrant drug-related behavior may be demanding, intimidating, or flattering. In one ED study, the most common complaints of patients seeking drugs were (in decreasing order) back pain, headache, extremity pain, and dental pain. Many fraudulent techniques are used, including "lost" prescriptions, or doctor's note explaining need for opioids, "impending" surgery, fictitious hematuria with a complaint of kidney stones, self-mutilation, and fictitious injury.

Diagnosis and Differential

The diagnosis of aberrant drug-related behaviors may not be possible in the ED. The medical record can provide a wealth of information regarding the patient, including documentation proving that the patient is supplying false information. Most states now have controlled drug databases that can be queried. Aberrant drug-related behaviors are listed in Table 8-3. The predictive behaviors are illegal in many states and form a solid basis to refuse narcotics to the patient.

TABLE 8-3 Aberrant Drug-Related Behaviors
Forges/alters prescriptions*
Sells controlled/illicit drugs*
Uses aliases to receive opioids*
Current illicit drug use*
Fictitious illness, requests opioids
Conceals multiple ED visits for opioids
Conceals multiple physicians prescribing opioids
Abusive when refused

*Unlawful in many states.

Emergency Department Care and Disposition

The treatment of aberrant drug-related behavior is to refuse the controlled substance, consider the need for alternative medication or treatment, and consider referral for drug counseling.

FURTHER READING

For further reading in *Tintinalli's Emergency Medicine: A Comprehensive Study Guide*, 8th ed., see Chapter 38 "Chronic Pain," by David M. Cline.

Emergency Wound Management

SECTION 3

Evaluating and Preparing Wounds

CHAPTER 9

Timothy J. Reeder

CLINICAL FEATURES

Traumatic wounds are regularly encountered problems in the emergency department. It is important to document important historical information such as the mechanism, timing, location of injury, and the degree of contamination. Associated symptoms of pain, swelling, paresthesias, and loss of function should be identified. Determine factors that affect wound healing, such as patient age, location of injury, medications, chronic medical conditions, and previous keloid or scar formation. Adults with the sensation of a foreign body are much more likely to have retained a foreign body that should be removed. Review allergies, particularly to latex, and determine whether tetanus immunization is required (see Chapter 94). When caring for wounds, the ultimate goal is to restore the physical integrity and function of the injured tissue without infection.

When treating a wound, consider factors that impact risks for infection, such as time since injury, mechanism, and location. Shear forces are produced by sharp objects with relatively low energy, resulting in a wound with a straight edge and little contamination that can be expected to heal with a good result. Wounds caused by compression forces crush the skin against the underlying bone and often produce stellate lacerations. Tension forces may produce flap-type lacerations with surrounding devitalized tissue and may be more susceptible to infection. Other predictive factors for infection include location, depth, characteristics, contamination, and patient age. The risk of infection also relates to the interaction of bacterial contamination and blood supply. The density of bacteria is quite low over the trunk and proximal arms and legs, and thus these areas have lower risks for infection. Moist areas such as the axilla, perineum, and exposed hands and feet have a higher degree of colonization and may be at higher risk of infection. Wounds located on the face or scalp, both highly vascularized areas, are at lower risk for infection.

Wounds of the oral cavity are heavily contaminated with bacteria, although evidence supporting routine antibiotic use in simple intra-oral laceration is inconclusive. Wounds sustained from contaminated objects or environments and animal and human bites have an increased infection risk.

Wounds contaminated with feces have a high risk of infection even when treated with antibiotic therapy. Although there is no clearly defined relationship between time to closure and infection rate, consider time since injury when making decisions about wound repair. Delayed primary closure after 4 days of open wound management is recommended for wounds with a high risk for infection during the first care encounter.

DIAGNOSIS AND DIFFERENTIAL

Wound examination is greatly facilitated by a cooperative patient, good positioning, optimal lighting, and little or no bleeding. A thorough examination will minimize the risk of missed foreign bodies, tendon injuries, and nerve injuries. While performing wound assessment, repositioning the joint or extremity in the position assumed during injury may help identify underlying damaged structures.

Assess wound location, size, shape, margins, and depth. Pay particular attention to sensory and motor functions, tendon injury, vascular compromise, and injuries to specialized structures. Carefully palpate and inspect the wound and surrounding area to identify a retained foreign body or bone injury, and consider radiographic imaging when these complicating features are suspected. For wounds overlying joints, consider additional assessment to determine whether a violation of the joint space may have occurred.

EMERGENCY DEPARTMENT CARE AND DISPOSITION

Proper wound preparation is an important first step to restoring the integrity and function of the injured tissue, preventing infection, and maximizing cosmetic results.

Anesthesia

1. Control pain with local or regional anesthesia to enable better preparation and evaluation of the wound.
2. Perform a neurovascular examination of the involved and distal areas before anesthesia. Two-point discrimination (normal <6 mm) will help identify digital nerve injury.

Irrigation

1. Wound irrigation reduces the risk of infection.
2. Use low-pressure irrigation with a slow, gentle wash for simple uncontaminated wounds in highly vascular areas such as the face and scalp.
3. Use high-pressure irrigation with an appropriate 18-gauge catheter, syringe, and splash guard for contaminated wounds.
4. Consider anesthesia before irrigation.
5. Wound soaking is not effective in cleaning contaminated wounds and may increase wound bacterial counts.
6. Although sterile normal saline solution is commonly used, tap water is safe and effective. There is no added benefit of adding povidone iodine or hydrogen peroxide to irrigation fluid. Polyhexanide irrigation may have benefit in high-risk wounds.
7. Warmed fluids may be more comfortable for wound irrigation.

Skin Disinfection and Sterile Technique

1. Sterilizing the surrounding skin with a povidone iodine- or chlorhexidine-containing agent is common practice. Avoid contact with nonintact skin when these agents are used.
2. Full sterile technique has not been shown to reduce infection after repair of wounds in the acute setting. Clean, nonsterile gloves and attention to cleanliness may be used to improve efficiency and cost savings.

Hemostasis

1. Control of bleeding is necessary for proper wound evaluation and treatment.
2. Direct pressure is the preferred method and is usually effective.
3. Epinephrine-containing local anesthetics can be helpful in controlling bleeding associated with wounds and can be used for digital nerve blocks, nose, and ears except in patients with underlying small vessel disease.
4. Other means of hemostasis can be used, such as applying pressure with gelatin, cellulose, or collagen sponges placed directly into the wound.
5. Ligation of minor vessels may be necessary and can be achieved by ligating with an absorbable suture material after isolating and clamping the involved vessel.
6. Cautery, with a bipolar device for vessels <2 mm and battery-powered device for capillaries, can be used to control extensive bleeding.
7. Finger tourniquets or a blood pressure cuff placed proximal to the injury and inflated above the systolic blood pressure will control bleeding. The duration of tourniquet use should be minimized and not left in place for more than 20 to 30 min at a time.

Foreign Body and Hair Removal

1. Visually inspect the full depth and course of all wounds for foreign bodies. Carefully remove foreign debris with forceps.
2. Many opaque foreign bodies can be detected by routine radiographs. Foreign bodies with densities similar to those of soft tissue may require the use of computed tomography, magnetic resonance imaging, or ultrasound to visualize.
3. Routine hair removal does not appear to have an effect on infections, and shaving may increase the rate of postoperative skin and soft tissue infections.
4. When hair removal is required to adequately assess or repair a wound, clip with scissors 1 to 2 mm above the skin surface.

Debridement

1. Devitalized tissue may increase the risk of infection and delay healing. Debridement removes foreign matter, bacteria, and devitalized tissue and creates a clean wound edge.
2. Elliptical excision around the wound edges with a standard surgical blade is the easiest technique for excisional debridement.
3. Wounds with an extensive amount of nonviable tissue may require a large amount of tissue removal and will need more delayed wound closure or grafting. In general, a surgical specialist should be consulted to manage these wounds.

Prophylactic Antibiotics

Although there is no clear evidence that antibiotic prophylaxis prevents wound infection in most emergency department patients, it may have a role in selected higher-risk wounds and populations.

1. When used, antibiotic prophylaxis should be initiated before significant tissue manipulation, performed with agents that are effective against predicted pathogens, and administered through routes that rapidly achieve desired blood levels. Oral antibiotics may be as effective as intravenous if the agent has sufficient spectrum of coverage and rapid absorption.
2. Most non-bite infections are caused by staphylococci or streptococci, and coverage with a β-lactam antibiotics is typically adequate.
3. Prophylactic antibiotics are recommended for human bites, mammalian bites to the hand, and other high-risk bite wounds (see Chapter 15, Puncture Wounds and Bites).

FURTHER READING

For further reading in *Tintinalli's Emergency Medicine: A Comprehensive Study Guide*, 8th ed., see Chapter 37, "Wound Evaluation," by Adam J. Singer and Judd E. Hollander; and Chapter 40, "Wound Preparation," by Aleksandr M. Tichter, Wallace A. Carter, and Susan C. Stone.

CHAPTER 10 Methods for Wound Closure

Corey R. Heitz

Wound closure in the emergency department can reduce the risk of infection, provide for improved cosmetic outcome, and maintain the skin's protective functions. Methods for wound repair include primary closure (immediately after injury), secondary closure (allowing a wound to heal on its own, which may be useful for contaminated or infected wounds), and delayed closure (packing the wound and performing closure at a later date once infection is ruled out).

Clinicians should consider several factors when choosing a wound closure method: time since injury, wound tension, whether tension is static or dynamic, and risk of scar formation. The cosmetic outcome after wound closure is primarily a function of technique and not necessarily reflective of the specific closure method or device that is selected. Options for closure include sutures, staples, adhesive tape, tissue adhesives, and hair apposition.

SUTURES

Sutures are strong, reliable, and adaptable and allow good approximation of wounds that are under tension. Absorbable suture material loses its tensile strength in <60 days and thus does not require removal after healing. Nonabsorbable sutures maintain their tensile strength and will require removal after a suitable time period for tissue healing. For most emergency department applications, either choice is acceptable as both have similar rates of infection, cosmetic outcomes, and wound dehiscence risks. Absorbable sutures are suitable for deep tissue structures such as dermis and fascia or when avoiding the need for suture removal is desired. Often, monofilament nonabsorbable sutures are used due to ease of use, good tensile strength, and low rates of infection. Suture material is available in a wide variety of sizes, with higher gauge sizes (such as 5-0 and 6-0) being very thin with less tensile strength. Smaller gauge sizes (such as 3-0 and 4-0) are larger in diameter with greater strength. Large gauge (e.g., 6-0) is most often chosen for areas of low tension where minimizing scars is desired, such as on the face. Smaller gauge suture (e.g., 3-0) is often used for the scalp, extremities, or other areas where increased tension requires suture material with greater tensile strength. When placing sutures of any size, be sure to evert the skin edges and avoid applying excessive crushing force on the tissue that can further damage the area and impair healing. Direct pressure, topical vasoconstrictors, or local anesthetic with vasoconstrictor are all useful for achieving hemostasis when repairing a wound.

SUTURING TECHNIQUES

Simple Interrupted Percutaneous Sutures

Placing simple interrupted sutures is the easiest and most commonly used technique for wound repair. The needle is introduced on one side of the wound, through the deep tissues, and exits the other side of the wound

(Fig. 10-1). Be sure to keep the needle tip at 90 degrees to the skin and evert the wound edges for best results, and take care not to pucker the skin when tying the knot. Square knots are generally tied with the number of knots corresponding to the suture gauge (e.g.,four knots when using 4-0 suture material). Position the knots so that they all remain on the same side of the wound.

Continuous (Running) Percutaneous Sutures

A rapid method for closure of high-tension wounds, this method can be challenging to get cosmetically optimal results in irregularly shaped wounds and

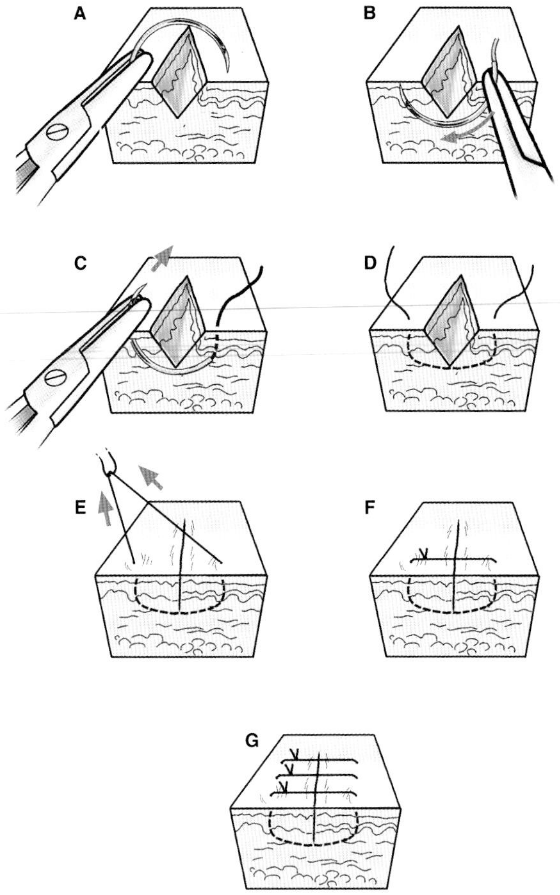

FIGURE 10-1. Placement of simple interrupted sutures. (A) Enter at 90 degrees. (B–D) Exit the same distance as the entrance. (E–G) Be consistent and tie knots on one side of wound.

Reproduced with permission from E. F. Reichman: *Emergency Medicine Procedures*. 2nd ed. New York: McGraw-Hill Education; 2013.

thus is most appropriate for long linear lacerations. Place a suture at one end of the wound, tie, but do not cut the suture material. Then sew back and forth down the wound at a 65 degree angle until the opposite end is reached, at which point the suture material is tied off and cut (Fig. 10-2).

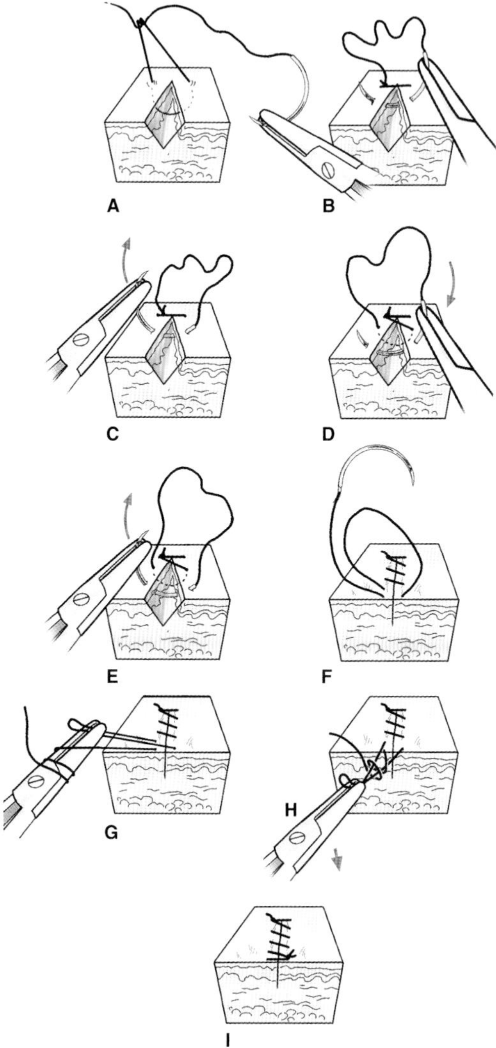

FIGURE 10-2. Continuous running. (A–C) Begin like a simple interrupted. (D–F) Be consistent, use a 65 degree angle. (G–I) Tie off at the end.

Reproduced with permission from E. F. Reichman: *Emergency Medicine Procedures*. 2nd ed. New York: McGraw-Hill Education; 2013.

Buried Dermal Sutures

These sutures are placed to reduce tension on the wound and close dead spaces by approximating underlying structures. Place these sutures by entering the deep tissues first and exiting in the subcutaneous layer, then entering the other side of the wound in the subcutaneous layer and exiting in the deep tissue (Fig. 10-3). This allows the knot to be buried deep within the tissue and thus should be completed with absorbable suture material. Closing adipose tissue with deep sutures is unnecessary as it does not

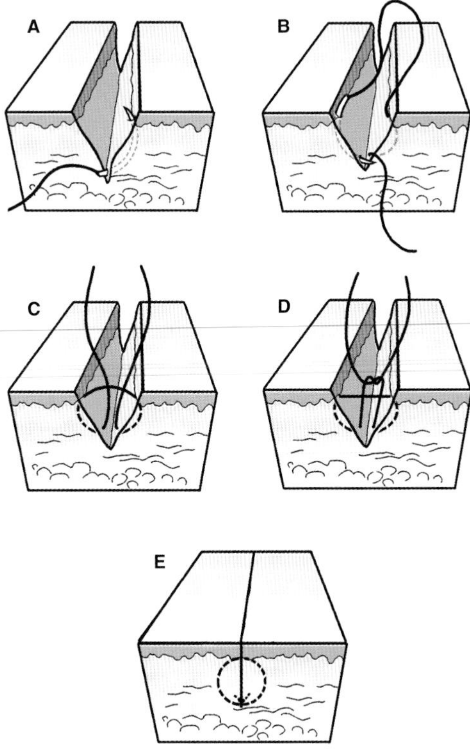

FIGURE 10-3. Buried (deep) dermal suture. Reverse of a simple interrupted, to bury the knot. (A) Insert the needle into one side of the base of the wound, and drive the needle from deep to superficial and exiting at the dermal–epidermal junction. (B) Insert the needle through the dermal–epidermal junction on the opposite side of the wound and drive it through the base of the wound. The suture should exit the base of the wound across from and level with the entrance site of the first throw. (C) Pull both free ends of the suture up and out through the laceration. (D) Tie a knot in the suture. (E) Pull both free ends of the suture to lower the knot to the base of the wound and oppose the tissue. Tie two additional knots to secure the suture. Cut off any excess suture.

Reproduced with permission from E. F. Reichman: *Emergency Medicine Procedures*. 2nd ed. New York: McGraw-Hill Education; 2013.

enhance cosmetic outcome or wound healing. Infection risks can be decreased when clinicians minimize the number of buried sutures used for wound repair.

Continuous Subcuticular Sutures

A more complex method, subcuticular sutures are performed with absorbable sutures and do not require removal. Begin by anchoring the suture at one end, and then weave horizontally in and out of the dermal–epidermal junction, subcutaneously (Fig. 10-4). This technique allows for excellent approximation of wound edges.

Vertical Mattress Sutures

Vertical mattress sutures allow for closure of deep and epidermal layers with a single suture placement, and allow for excellent wound edge eversion. Enter the wound on one side a few millimeters from the edge, take a

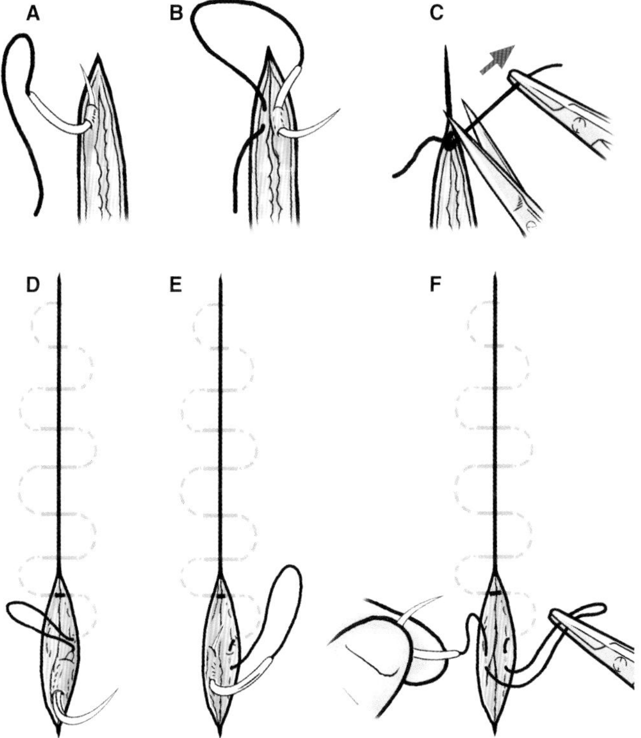

FIGURE 10-4. Continuous subcuticular suture. (A–C) Tie the anchor knot. (D, E) Use horizontal subcutaneous stitching. (F) Bury the knot at the end.

Reproduced with permission from E. F. Reichman: *Emergency Medicine Procedures*. 2nd ed. New York: McGraw-Hill Education; 2013.

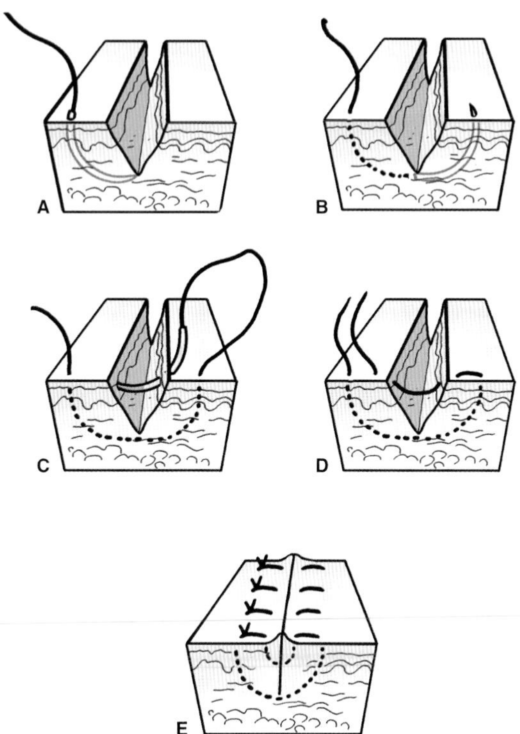

FIGURE 10-5. Vertical mattress suture. (A, B) Far-far. (C, D) Near-near. (E) Finished product, knots on one side.

Reproduced with permission from E. F. Reichman: *Emergency Medicine Procedures.* 2nd ed. New York: McGraw-Hill Education; 2013.

deep bite of tissue, and exit on the other side, similar to a simple interrupted suture technique. Then before tying the knot, reenter the same side of the wound that was just exited at a point closer to the wound edge and then exit in a similar position on the other side in a "far-far/near-near" fashion for each suture placement (Fig. 10-5).

Horizontal Mattress Sutures

For horizontal mattress sutures, begin similarly to a simple interrupted suture. Instead of tying the knot after the first suture throw, go several millimeters parallel to the wound and perform another throw, tying the knot on the original side of the wound (Fig 10-6). This technique is useful for wounds with poor circulation and other delicate areas as it distributes wound tension and prevents further skin disruption close to the wound edge.

Horizontal Half-Buried Mattress Sutures

This technique is useful for skin flaps and stellate lacerations because the suture passes through the dermis of the skin tip and not the epidermal layer.

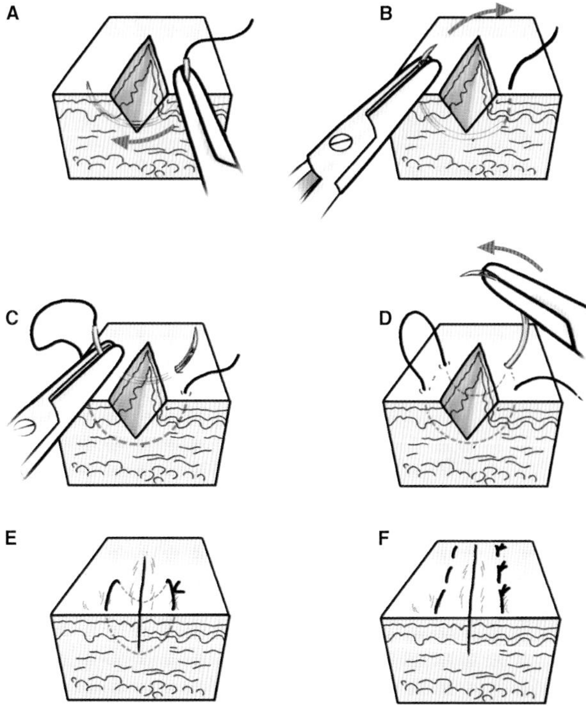

FIGURE 10-6. Horizontal mattress suture. (A, B) Start like a simple interrupted. (C) Enter on the same side as exit. (D–F) Exit and tie.

Reproduced with permission from E. F. Reichman: *Emergency Medicine Procedures*. 2nd ed. New York: McGraw-Hill Education; 2013.

Enter one side of the wound and run the suture in the dermal layer subcutaneously through the other edge(s), exiting near the original entrance point (Fig. 10-7).

NON-SUTURE TECHNIQUES

Staples

Staples are fast and easy to use but not as precise as other wound closure methods. Staples should not be used on the face as the cosmetic outcome is not as favorable as suture repairs. This wound closure method is excellent for scalp wound repair and other locations where cosmetic outcome is not as important. In some wounds, deep sutures may be needed to close dermal layers prior to staple application. Align the wound edges and keep the staple device perpendicular to and centered on the wound. Avoid firm downward pressure on the wound as this can cause depression of the wound edges. Instead, use gentle pressure to evert the wound edges at the time of each staple deployment (Fig. 10-8).

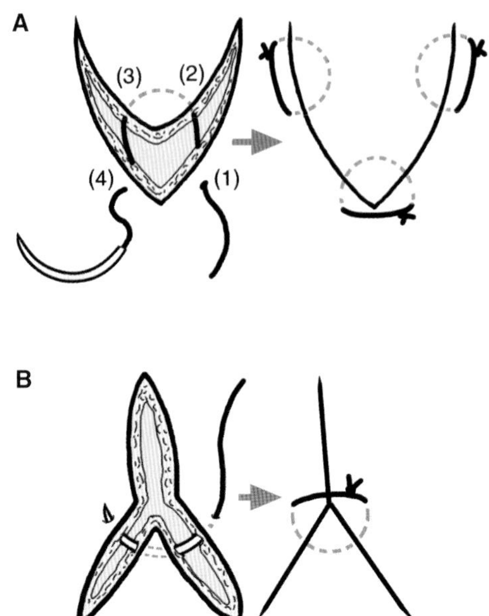

FIGURE 10-7. Horizontal half-buried suture. Enter and exit on the same side, keeping stitch buried under edges of flaps.

Reproduced with permission from E. F. Reichman: *Emergency Medicine Procedures*. 2nd ed. New York: McGraw-Hill Education; 2013.

Adhesive Tapes

Adhesive tapes are inexpensive, simple, painless, and rapid. They slough off when exposed to moisture and thus should only be used for low tension, fragile wounds such as skin tears. Use an adhesive adjunct such as tincture of benzoin and place the tape segments perpendicular to the wound about 3 mm apart. Reinforce with parallel strips, if needed.

Tissue Adhesives

Cyanoacrylate tissue adhesives are rapid, painless, and have similar tensile strength to 4-0 poliglecaprone subcuticular sutures. They provide a moisture and infection barrier, but can come off more easily when exposed to moisture. This wound repair does not require removal after healing, as the compound sloughs off spontaneously in 5 to 10 days. Do not use this wound repair material over joints or areas of high tension. Approximate the wound well, and place a thin coat of adhesive over the wound extending 5 to 10 mm on either side, repeating once dry (Fig. 10-9). Adhesive tape can be used as an adjunct for long or complex wounds.

Hair Apposition

Scalp wounds can be closed by hair apposition. After cleaning the wound thoroughly, twist several strands of hair together on either side. Then twist

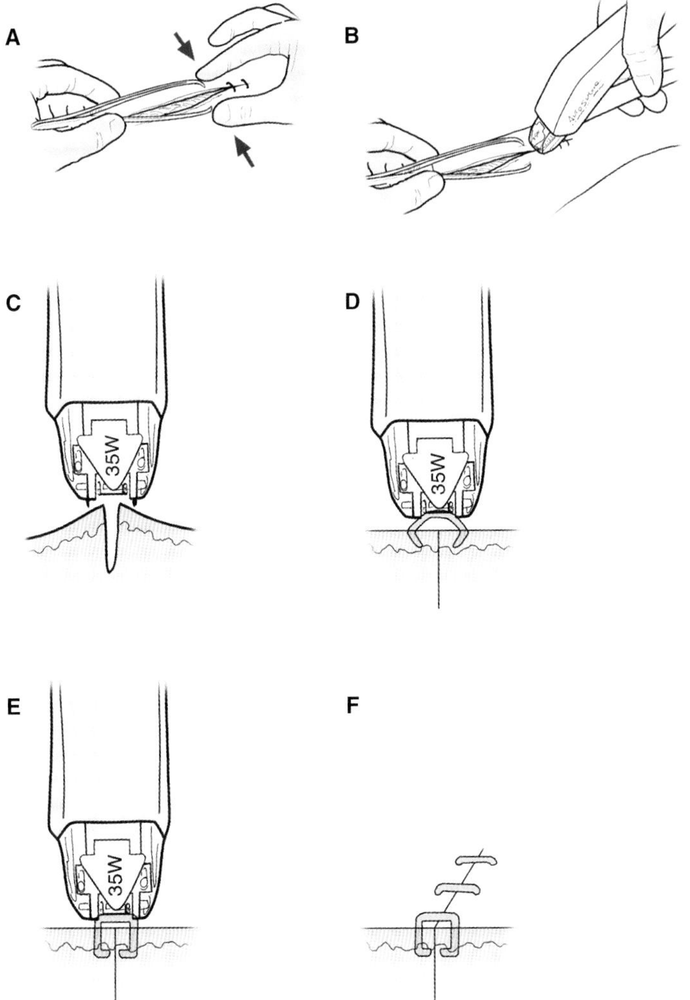

FIGURE 10-8. Laceration repair with staple closure. (A) The wound edges are opposed and everted. (B) The stapler is applied over the laceration. (C) The stapler is applied over the everted wound edges. (D) The plunger advances the staple into the wound margins. (E) The anvil bends the staple into shape. (F) The final result.

Reproduced with permission from E. F. Reichman: *Emergency Medicine Procedures*. 2nd ed. New York: McGraw-Hill Education; 2013.

these two bundles together and apply a drop of tissue adhesive to hold them together. This technique minimizes patient discomfort, but cannot be done for large lacerations (>10 cm), grossly contaminated wounds, uncontrolled bleeding, or gaping wounds with significant tension.

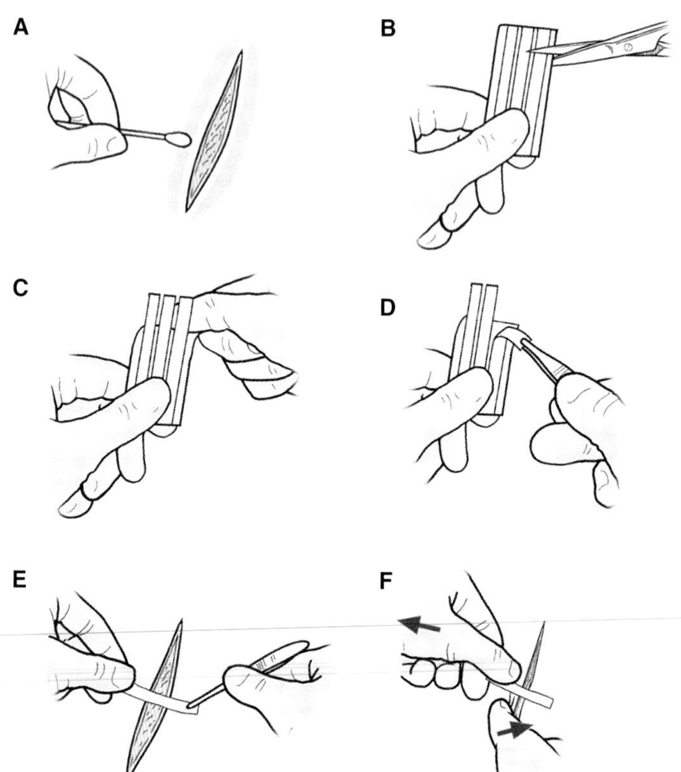

FIGURE 10-9. Laceration repair with adhesive tapes. (A) After the initial cleansing of the skin, clean the skin surface with acetone or alcohol to remove any surface oils. Allow the skin to dry. Apply benzoin solution to the skin on both sides of the wound with a cotton applicator. (B) Cut the skin closure tapes to the proper length. (C) Gently tear the end-tab off the back of the card to prevent the strips from deforming. (D) Remove a strip from the card. (E) Firmly secure the tape to one side of the wound. (F) Use the nondominant hand to oppose the wound edges as the tape is brought over and secured to the skin on the opposite wound edge. (Continued)

Reproduced with permission from E. F. Reichman: *Emergency Medicine Procedures*. 2nd ed. New York: McGraw-Hill Education; 2013.

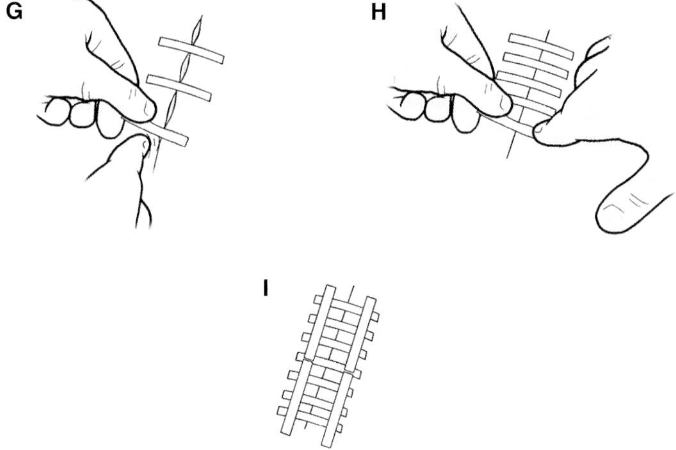

FIGURE 10-9. (G, H) Place additional tapes at 2 to 3 mm intervals until the wound edges are opposed. (I) Place pieces of tape across the tape edges to prevent premature removal and skin blistering from the tape ends.

FURTHER READING

For further reading in *Tintinalli's Emergency Medicine: A Comprehensive Study Guide*, 8th ed., see Chapter 41, "Wound Closure," by Adam J. Singer and Judd E. Hollander.

CHAPTER 11

Lacerations to The Face and Scalp

J. Hayes Calvert

SCALP AND FOREHEAD

The scalp and forehead have thick skin and little cushioning fat (Fig. 11-1). Wounds of the scalp and forehead can usually be repaired with primary closure when they are not visibly infected, regardless of the time since the injury and even if the injury was secondary to a bite. After performing wound cleansing and achieving hemostasis, palpate the base of the wound to assess for possible skull fracture. CT scan can be used to further evaluate an injury when an underlying fracture is suspected.

Examine the wound edges for signs of devitalized tissue that may require debridement. When hemostasis is not easily achieved, use direct pressure or vessel clamping to control bleeding at the wound edges. Irrigate the wound well to remove contamination and reduce the risk of wound infection. Close scalp lacerations with surgical staples or simple interrupted sutures using nonabsorbable monofilament or rapidly absorbable material.

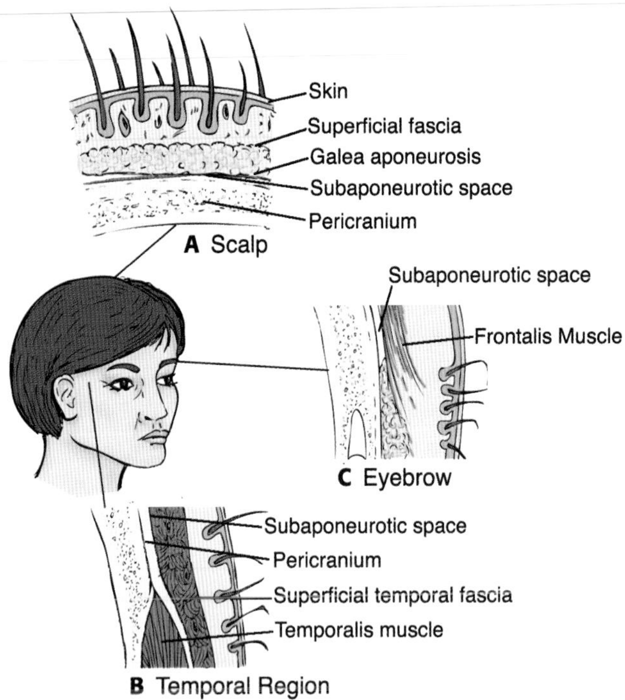

FIGURE 11-1. The layers of the scalp.

Consider a pressure dressing over deep scalp lacerations for the first 24 hours to reduce the chance of hematoma formation.

Superficial forehead lacerations are not associated with injury to the frontalis muscle, while deep lacerations do have damage to the frontalis muscle. Close superficial forehead lacerations with 6-0 nonabsorbable interrupted suture, rapidly absorbable suture, or tissue adhesive. Close the muscular layer of deep forehead lacerations with buried 5-0 absorbable suture, and then close the epidermal layer with 6-0 nonabsorbable suture, skin closure strips, or tissue adhesive. Eyebrows are important landmarks to assist with reapproximation of wound edges. When wounds involve the eyebrows, minimize skin debridement and leave suture tails long to facilitate removal. Remove scalp staples or sutures in 10 to 14 days, while forehead nonabsorbable sutures can be removed in 5 to 7 days.

EYELIDS

The eyelids are thin and offer limited protection from injuries to the globe and surrounding structures. Examine lid injuries for involvement of the canthi, the lacrimal system, or penetration through the tarsal plate or lid margin (Fig. 11-2). Eyelid injuries within 6 to 8 mm of the medial canthus are at risk for canalicular laceration, particularly when associated with medial wall blow-out fractures. Consider consultation with an ophthalmologist when ptosis is present or for complex eyelid wounds such as those involving the inner surface of the lid, lid margins, lacrimal duct, and tarsal plate. Close uncomplicated eyelid lacerations with nonabsorbable 6-0 or 7-0 simple interrupted percutaneous sutures. Avoid the use of tissue adhesive near the eye. Remove nonabsorbable sutures in 3 to 5 days.

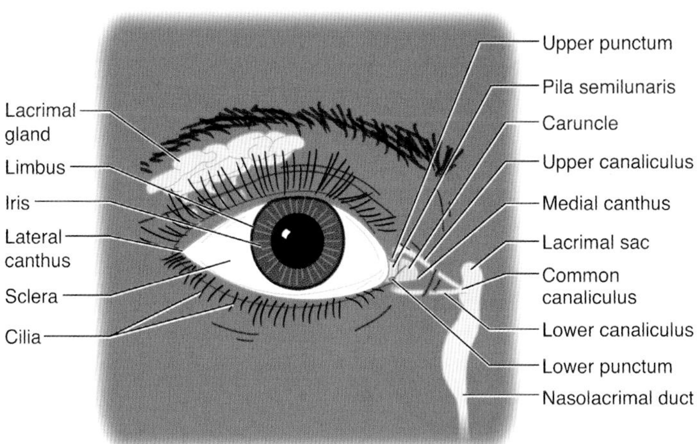

FIGURE 11-2. Periorbital anatomy.

NOSE

Examine nasal lacerations to determine depth and involvement of deep tissue layers. Exposed cartilage or deep involvement of the tissue layers increases the risk of infection. Topical lidocaine into the nasal cavity may provide sufficient anesthesia for some local wound repair, and injected intradermal lidocaine with or without epinephrine is appropriate when needed to facilitate wound evaluation, cleansing, and repair.

Close superficial nasal lacerations with 6-0 nonabsorbable monofilament simple interrupted sutures. When the laceration extends through all tissue layers, begin closure with a 5-0 nonabsorbable, monofilament suture that aligns the skin surrounding the entrances of the nasal canals to prevent malposition and notching of the alar rim. Gentle traction on the long, untied ends of this suture facilitates alignment of the mucosa and cartilage layers during subsequent suture placement. Close the mucosal layer with 5-0 rapidly absorbable interrupted sutures, and then irrigate the area gently from the outside before completing the repair. Avoid suture placement directly into the cartilage. Complete the repair with 6-0 nonabsorbable monofilament material close to the wound edges. Percutaneous nonabsorbable sutures should be removed in 3 to 5 days.

Drain small unilateral septal hematomas with an 18G needle, or incise the hematoma if it is larger. After the hematoma has been evacuated, place an anterior nasal packing to prevent reaccumulation. Consider a course of oral antibiotics to prevent infection while nasal packing is in place.

EAR

Close superficial lacerations of the ear with 6-0 nonabsorbable monofilament interrupted sutures, taking care to cover any exposed cartilage and minimize skin debridement. In most through-and-through lacerations of the ear, the skin can be approximated and the underlying cartilage will be supported adequately (Fig. 11-3). After laceration repair is complete,

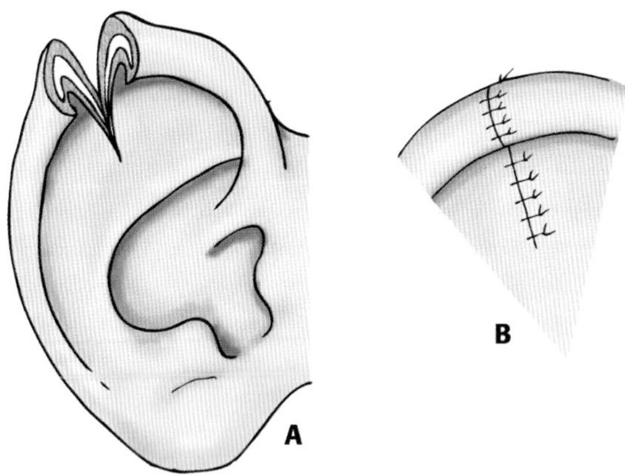

FIGURE 11-3. Repair of auricular laceration. **A.** Laceration through auricle. **B.** Interrupted 6-0 nonabsorbable sutures approximate the skin edges.

place a small piece of nonadherent gauze over the laceration and apply a pressure dressing to prevent development of a perichondral hematoma. To create a pressure dressing, place gauze squares behind the ear to apply pressure, and wrap the head circumferentially with gauze. Discontinue the pressure dressing after 24 hours when reevaluation demonstrates that no hematoma has accumulated. Consider consultation with an otolaryngologist or plastic surgeon for complex lacerations, ear avulsions, or auricular hematomas. Remove nonabsorbable percutaneous sutures in 5 to 7 days.

LIPS

The external surface of the lips has three distinct regions: the skin, the vermilion border (junction of the skin and red portion of the lips), and the oral mucosa. Isolated intraoral lesions of the lip often do not need to be sutured, especially if they are <1 cm in length. Repair large or gaping intraoral lip wounds with a rapidly absorbable 5-0 suture. Through-and-through lacerations of the lip that do not include the vermilion border can be closed in layers. Begin repair with 5-0 rapidly absorbable suture for the mucosal surface, then gently irrigate the wound from the outside before closing the orbicularis oris muscle with 4-0 or 5-0 absorbable suture. Finally, close the skin layer with 6-0 nonabsorbable monofilament sutures in a simple interrupted fashion.

Begin closure of a complicated lip laceration at the junction between the vermilion and the skin with a 6-0 nonabsorbable, monofilament suture to precisely align the edges of the vermilion border (Fig. 11-4). After placing that first stitch, continue to repair the vermilion and skin with the same 6-0 nonabsorbable monofilament suture and then use 5-0 rapidly absorbable suture for any needed mucosal surface repair. Consider oral antibiotics for contaminated wounds or through-and-through lacerations. Remove nonabsorbable percutaneous sutures in 5 to 7 days.

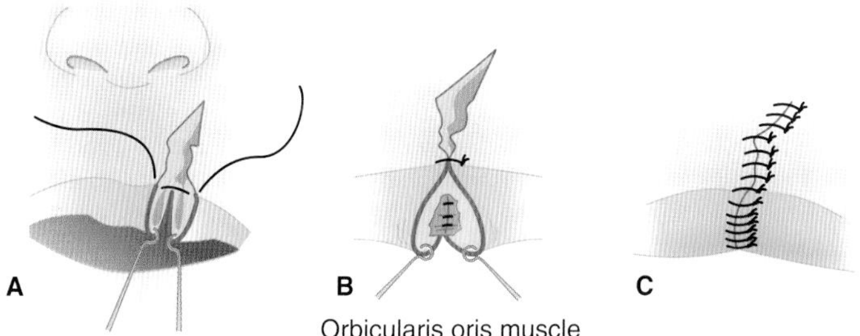

FIGURE 11-4. Lip laceration repair. **A.** The first suture is placed to align the vermilion skin junction. **B.** The orbicularis oris muscle is then repaired with 5-0 absorbable sutures. **C.** The irregular edges of the skin are then approximated with 6-0 nonabsorbable sutures.

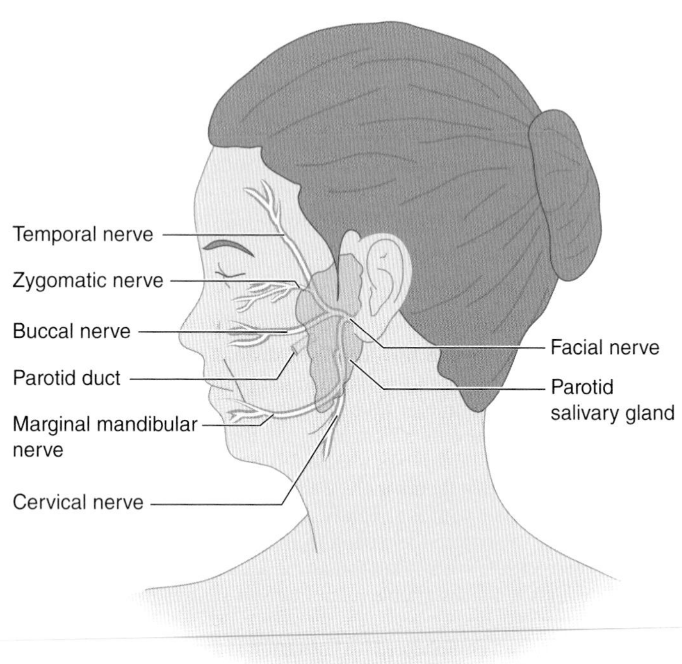

FIGURE 11-5. Cheek anatomy. The course of the parotid duct is within 1.5 cm of the midportion of a line drawn from the lower border of the tragus to the cheilion. The five branches of the facial nerve are the temporal, zygomatic, buccal, marginal mandibular, and cervical.

CHEEKS AND FACE

Evaluate cheek and other facial lacerations to determine wound depth and to assess for damage to the parotid gland, parotid duct, and facial nerve (Fig. 11-5), which would necessitate specialty consultation and operative repair. Repair superficial facial lacerations without underlying complications with 6-0 nonabsorbable monofilament, simple interrupted sutures. Tissue adhesive may also be used for wounds of appropriate size and location. Full-thickness cheek lacerations can be repaired in layers beginning with the intraoral mucosa using absorbable sutures. After irrigation of the external wound, close the subcutaneous and skin layers using 5-0 or 6-0 suture material. Remove nonabsorbable percutaneous sutures in 5 to 7 days.

FURTHER READING

For further reading in *Tintinalli's Emergency Medicine: A Comprehensive Study Guide*, 8th ed., see Chapter 42, "Face and Scalp Lacerations," by Wendy C. Coates.

CHAPTER 12

Injuries to the Arm, Hand, Fingertip, and Nail

John Pettey Sandifer

DIAGNOSIS AND DIFFERENTIAL

When taking a history, consider occupation, time and mechanism of injury, and hand dominance. Examination of all arm and hand injuries includes inspection at rest, evaluation of motor, nerve, and tendon functions, evaluation of sensory nerve function, and assessment of perfusion. Examine active motion and resistance to passive motion. (See Tables 12-1 and 12-2.) Examine all wounds for evidence of potential artery, nerve, tendon, or bone injuries, and the possible presence of foreign bodies, debris, or bacterial contamination.

Control bleeding to achieve adequate visualization and assessment of an injury. When necessary, a manual blood pressure cuff can be used as a temporary tourniquet for proximal injuries or a penrose drain can be used for distal finger injuries, taking care to apply for only limited time periods. Once adequate visualization is obtained, examine the wound for foreign bodies and tendon or joint capsule injuries. Examine the hand and arm throughout normal range of motion, including in the position of injury to avoid missing deep structure injuries that may have moved out of the field of view when examined in a neutral position. Obtain anteroposterior and lateral x-rays if bony injuries, retained radiopaque foreign bodies, or joint involvement are suspected.

EMERGENCY DEPARTMENT CARE AND DISPOSITION

1. Clean and irrigate all wounds after appropriate local anesthesia is provided.
2. Provide tetanus prophylaxis as indicated (see Chapter 16).

TABLE 12-1 Motor Testing of the Peripheral Nerves in the Upper Extremity

Nerve	Motor Exam
Radial	Dorsiflexion of wrist
Median	Thumb abduction away from the palm
	Thumb interphalangeal joint flexion
Ulnar	Adduction/abduction of digits

TABLE 12-2 Sensory Testing of Peripheral Nerves in the Upper Extremity

Nerve	Sensory Exam
Radial	First dorsal web space
Median	Volar tip of index finger
Ulnar	Volar tip of little finger

3. Consider consultation with a hand specialist for complex or extensive injuries, injuries that may require skin grafting, repairs requiring technically demanding skills, or injuries that may impact recovery of function.
4. Prophylactic antibiotics are not routinely needed for uncomplicated hand lacerations.
5. Consider antibiotics for complex wounds such as bites, injuries more than 12 hours old, contaminated wounds, exposed bone, or significant comorbidities.
6. See below for additional care instructions for specific injuries.

Dorsal Forearm, Wrist, and Hand Lacerations

1. Examine tendons and nerves distal to the wound to assess for potential injury.
2. Dorsal forearm and hand skin is often thin without underlying tissue. This can make wound edge approximation challenging.
3. For most lacerations, use 5-0 nonabsorbable sutures for closure. Consider subcuticular sutures with 5-0 absorbable material on the dorsum of the hand.

Clenched Fist Injuries

1. Clenched fist injuries, also known as "fight bites," occur when a patient throws a punch that impacts the front teeth of another individual and leads to lacerations over the dorsal metacarpophalangeal joint.
2. These lacerations often are accompanied with polymicrobial infections with pathogens such as *Staphylococcus aureus*, *Streptococcus* spp., *Corynebacterium* spp., and *Eikenella corrodens*.
3. Lacerations from clenched fist injuries are often not sutured, but instead allowed to heal by secondary intention. If signs of infection are already present, consider admission for IV antibiotics such as ampicillin–sulbactam or cefoxitin.
4. If outpatient treatment is recommended, splint the hand in a position of function with a 3- to 5-day course of prophylactic antibiotics such as amoxicillin–clavulanic acid. Arrange close follow-up in 24 to 48 hours with strict return instructions in the event of erythema, drainage, or increased pain.

Extensor Tendon Lacerations

1. Discuss tendon injuries with a hand specialist for preferred repair technique and to arrange follow-up. Experienced emergency physicians may repair simple extensor tendon injuries over the dorsum of the hand. Refer cases to a hand specialist when severe contamination or injuries to the tendons of the thumb are involved.
2. Small partial extensor tendon injuries (<50% transected) can be repaired with absorbable suture material, while larger injuries should be repaired with 4-0 or 5-0 colorless nonabsorbable suture. A figure-of-eight stitch with the knot at the edge of the tendon is recommended for repair of lacerated extensors. Splint the hand or digit in the position of function and recommend follow-up with a hand specialist within 7 days (Fig. 12-1).

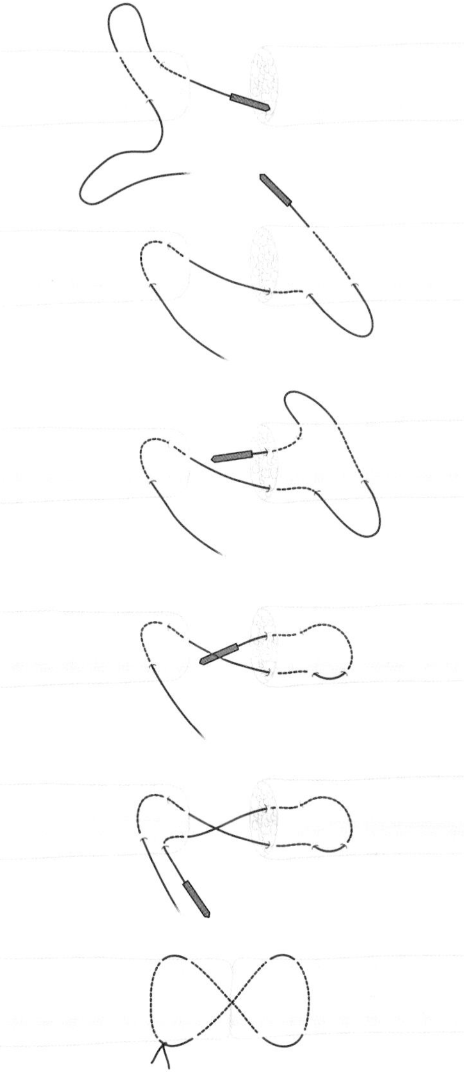

FIGURE 12-1. Extensor tendon laceration repair with a figure-of-eight stitch.

3. Lacerations to the extensor tendons over the distal interphalangeal (DIP) joint may produce a mallet deformity, and if not repaired may result in a swan neck deformity. Lacerations over the proximal interphalangeal joint may produce a boutonniere deformity. Open DIP tendon lacerations require operative repair by a hand surgeon; closed tendon injuries should be splinted in extension for up to 6 weeks or until operative repair. Refer these cases to a hand specialist.

Volar Forearm, Wrist, and Hand Lacerations

1. Linear lacerations over the volar aspect of the wrist or forearm may raise the possibility of self-inflicted injuries. In appropriate circumstances, question the patient about how the injury occurred and assess risks for possible self-injurious behavior.
2. Most simple lacerations to the volar surface of the forearm and wrist can be repaired with 4-0 or 5-0 nonabsorbable monofilament sutures.
3. Injuries that involve more than one parallel laceration, which may be seen with self-inflicted injuries, can sometimes be repaired with horizontal mattress sutures that cross adjacent lacerations. This can help to prevent compromising the vascular supply of any skin islands located between incisions (Fig. 12-2).
4. Examine the function of tendons and distal nerves individually to assess for possible damage. (See Tables 12-3 and 12-4.)

Palm Lacerations

1. Injuries to the palm can damage deep structures, even those with a benign superficial appearance. Regional anesthesia with a median or ulnar nerve block may be useful for exploring such wounds.

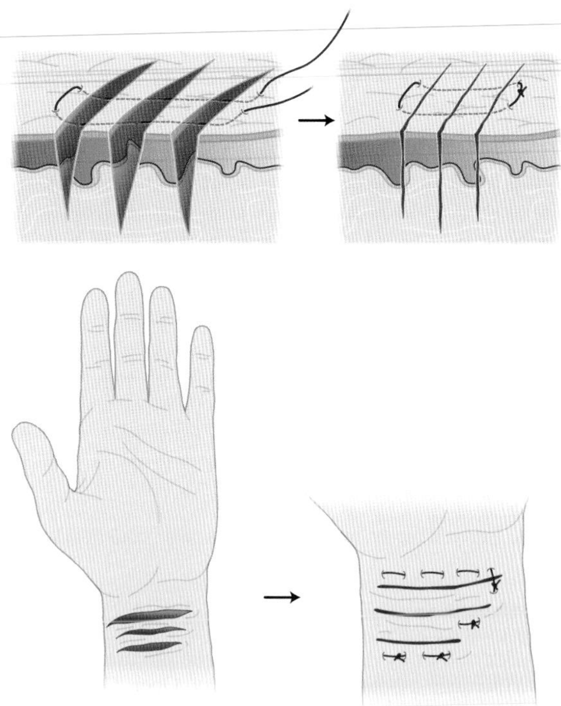

FIGURE 12-2. Horizontal mattress sutures for multiple parallel lacerations.

TABLE 12-3 Extensor Compartments in the Forearm Compartment

Compartment	Muscle	Function
First compartment	Abductor pollicis longus Extensor pollicis brevis	Abducts and extends thumb Extends thumb at MCP joint
Second compartment	Extensor carpi radialis longus Extensor carpi radialis brevis	Extends and radially deviates wrist Extends and radially deviates wrist
Third compartment	Extensor pollicis longus	Extends thumb at interphalangeal joint
Fourth compartment	Extensor digitorum communis Extensor indicis proprius	Splits into four tendons at level of the wrist; extends index, long, ring, and little digits Extends index finger
Fifth compartment	Extensor digiti minimi	Extends little finger at MCP joint
Sixth compartment	Extensor carpi ulnaris	Extends and radially deviates wrist

Abbreviation: MCP, metacarpophalangeal.

2. If no deep injury is identified, close the wound with sutures to re-oppose the skin creases accurately. Interrupted horizontal mattress sutures with 5-0 monofilament suture can be helpful to promote appropriate skin eversion.

Flexor Tendon Lacerations

1. Refer all flexor tendon injuries to a hand specialist. Many surgeons prefer to repair these injuries within 24 hours after injury.
2. Timely repair by a hand surgeon is important, as post-injury scarring and retraction make flexor tendon repairs more difficult after 10 to 14 days.

TABLE 12-4 Flexor Tendons in the Forearm

Flexor Tendon	Function
Flexor carpi radialis	Flexes and radially deviates wrist
Flexor carpi ulnaris	Flexes and ulnarly deviates wrist
Palmaris longus	Flexes wrist
Flexor pollicis longus	Flexes thumb at MCP and interphalangeal joints
Flexor digitorum superficialis	Flexes index, long, ring, and little digits at MCP and PIP joints
Flexor digitorum profundus	Flexes index, long, ring, and little digits at MCP, PIP, and DIP joints

Abbreviations: DIP, distal interphalangeal; MCP, metacarpophalangeal; PIP, proximal interphalangeal.

3. If operative repair is delayed, clean the wound and suture the overlying skin. Splint with the wrist and metacarpophalangeal joint flexed and the proximal interphalangeal and DIP joints in extension.

Finger Injuries

1. Many finger lacerations are straightforward and can be repaired by using 5-0 nonabsorbable suture materials.
2. Assess for underlying injuries, such as sensory nerve damage or extensor and flexor tendon injuries.
3. Partial or complete digit amputations should involve consultation with a hand surgeon to discuss whether implantation is a feasible option.
4. Digital nerve injuries are suspected when static two-point discrimination is >10 mm or distinctly greater on one side of the volar pad than the other.

Finger Tip Injuries

1. Successful repair of fingertip injuries requires knowledge of anatomy (Fig. 12-3) and an understanding of techniques of reconstruction.
2. Distal fingertip amputations with skin or pulp loss only are usually managed conservatively, with serial dressing changes.
3. For some distal fingertip amputations without exposed bone, a full-thickness skin graft using the severed tip itself may be considered. For larger injuries, skin can also be harvested from a distant site by a hand specialist with skin graft expertise.
4. Injuries with exposed bone are not amenable to skin grafting, and most of these injuries require specialist advice and management.

Injuries Involving the Nail and Nail Bed

1. Subungual hematomas of >50% of the nail bed are often decompressed by simple trephination of the nail plate. This produces good to excellent

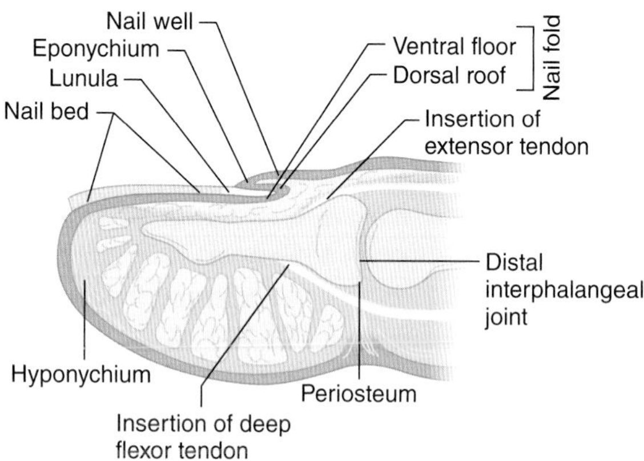

FIGURE 12-3. Anatomy of the perionychium.

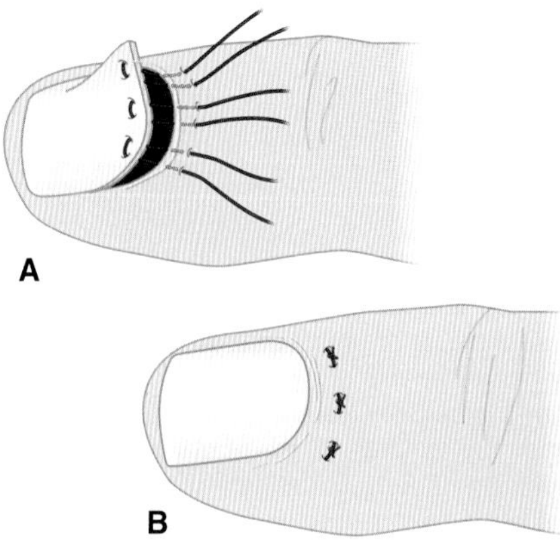

FIGURE 12-4. (A, B). Technique for repair of an avulsion of the germinal matrix using three horizontal mattress sutures.

outcomes in most patients regardless of subungual hematoma size, injury mechanism, or presence of fracture. Use of nail drill, electrocautery, scalpel, or 18 gauge needle is recommended for trephination.

2. Remove the nail only if there is an associated nail avulsion or surrounding nail fold disruption. Repair a nail bed laceration with 6-0 absorbable sutures to provide a smooth surface for nail regrowth. Clean and trephinate the removed nail and secure with sutures in its anatomic position.
3. Avulsion injuries to the nail bed have the poorest prognosis of any fingertip injury. Fragments of germinal matrix tissue left on the underside of the nail should be preserved and the nail anatomically reattached, if possible (Fig. 12-4). If there is extensive injury to the nail bed with avulsed tissue, consultation with a hand specialist is recommended.

Ring Tourniquet Syndrome

1. A tight ring encircling the proximal phalanx may become entrapped due to distal swelling. For this reason, rings should be removed from all injured fingers.
2. Ring removal techniques include lubrication, ring cutting, and the string or rubber band technique.

FURTHER READING

For further reading in *Tintinalli's Emergency Medicine: A Comprehensive Study Guide*, 8th ed., see Chapter 43, "Arm and Hand Lacerations," by Moira Davenport.

CHAPTER 13

Lacerations to the Leg and Foot

Moira Davenport

CLINICAL FEATURES

Lacerations to the leg and foot are commonly seen in the Emergency Department. The mechanism of injury determines the likelihood of disruption to underlying tissue, the risk of a retained foreign body, and the degree of potential contamination. See Chapter 9 for additional information about evaluating and preparing wounds for repair. As with other extremity injuries, evaluating limb positioning at the time of injury and replicating this during wound evaluation may help to uncover occult tendon injuries.

DIAGNOSIS AND DIFFERENTIAL

Assess lower extremity wounds for any associated nerve, vessel, or tendon injuries. Evaluate distal motor and sensory function and compare findings from the injured extremity to the contralateral side. Sensory function is best evaluated prior to providing anesthetic agents, but a full assessment of motor function and wound exploration may be easier to perform after the wound is anesthetized. Evaluate the superficial peroneal nerve (foot eversion), the deep peroneal nerve (foot inversion and ankle dorsiflexion), and the tibial nerve (ankle plantar flexion). Move the limb through its full range of motion to exclude tendon injury. Test each tendon function individually and visually inspect the wound at rest and in motion to rule out a partial laceration. Evaluate the extensor hallucis longus (great toe extension with ankle inversion), tibialis anterior (ankle dosiflexion and inversion), and achilles tendon (ankle plantar flexion and inversion).

Laboratory studies are not typically indicated for simple lacerations. Consider x-rays if there is suspicion for a fracture or radiopaque foreign body. Ultrasonography may also be useful to identify a foreign body, tendon injury, or bony abnormality.

EMERGENCY DEPARTMENT CARE AND DISPOSITION

General Recommendations

1. See Chapter 9 for discussion of wound preparation. Thorough wound exploration and irrigation of lower extremity wounds are important.
2. Wounds on the lower extremities may be under greater tension than those on an upper limb. Consider performing a layered closure with 4-0 absorbable material to close the fascia and interrupted 4-0 nonabsorbable sutures to close the skin, when appropriate. This type of layered closure is not typically required for wounds on the foot.
3. When possible, avoid placement of absorbable deep sutures in patients with diabetes, immunocompromise, or venous stasis changes due to an increased risk of infection.

4. Determine each patient's tetanus immunization status and update as necessary (see Chapter 94).
5. Cyanoacrylate glue is not used as often for wound repair on the lower extremities because of the greater wound tension associated with these injuries.
6. Once repaired, lacerations involving the joint or tendons should be splinted in a position of function.
7. Evidence does not support routine antibiotic prophylaxis in uncomplicated lacerations of the lower extremity. Antibiotics are recommended for open fractures, tendon or joint involvement, heavily contaminated wounds, bite wounds, patients with higher risks for infection, and wounds that exhibit early signs of infection.

Knee Injuries

1. Examine knee wounds throughout the range of movement of the joint. Assess patellar and quadriceps tendon function.
2. Evaluate these wounds to determine whether penetration of the joint capsule may have occurred. An x-ray may show air in the joint. Another approach to diagnose joint penetration is to inject 65 to 95 mL of sterile saline into the joint at a site separate from the laceration. Leakage of the solution from the wound indicates joint capsule injury.
3. Assess for potential injury to the popliteal artery, the popliteal nerve, and the tibial nerve.

Ankle Injuries

1. Move the ankle through its full range of motion and directly inspect the wound to ensure there are no tendon injuries. The Achilles tendon, the tibialis anterior, and the extensor hallucis longus in particular are at risk for injury and should be repaired if an injury is identified.
2. The Achilles tendon can rupture without a penetrating injury when a tensed gastrocnemius is suddenly contracted. The Thompson test can be used to assess the Achilles tendon. Have the patient kneel on a chair or lie supine with feet extending beyond the stretcher (see Fig. 13-1). Squeeze the patient's calf gently at the midpoint. Absent plantar flexion of the foot indicates complete Achilles tendon laceration.

Foot Injures

1. Explore lacerations on the sole of the foot to assess for tendon injury or retained foreign bodies. Place the patient in a prone position with the foot supported on a pillow or overhanging the bed.
2. Regional anesthesia can be helpful to facilitate exploration and repair of lacerations in this area.
3. Repair wounds as soon as possible after injury, ideally within 6 hours to minimize infection risks. Wounds presenting between 6 and 12 hours from the time of injury can often be repaired primarily. Evaluate each wound individually for infection risks.
4. When repairing foot wounds, a large needle is often required to penetrate the thick dermis of the sole. Use nonabsorbable 3-0 or 4-0 suture material to repair wounds located on the sole and 4-0 or 5-0 nonabsorbable sutures to repair the dorsal foot.

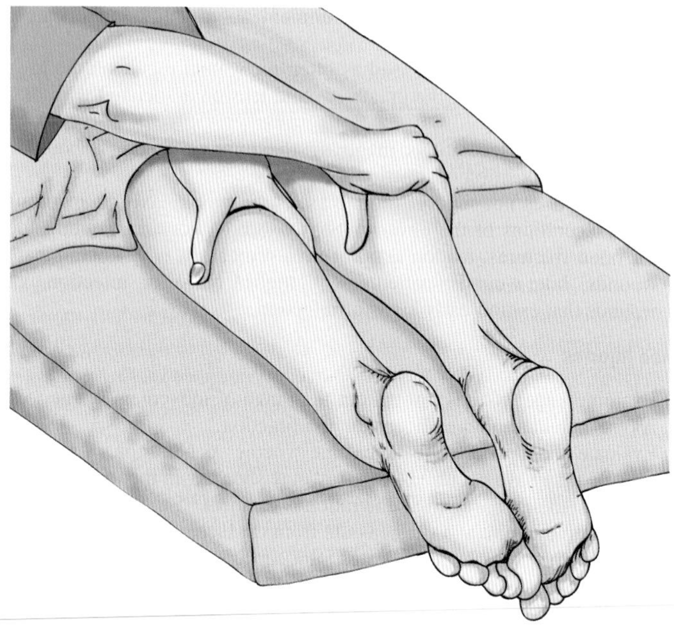

FIGURE 13-1. Thompson test. "With the patient's feet extending beyond the stretcher, squeeze both calfs at the midpoint. Normal response is shown on the patient's left, absent plantar flexion (abnormal) shown on patient's right."

5. Lacerations between the toes can be difficult to repair and may be facilitated by an assistant to hold the toes apart during repair. An interrupted mattress suture may be helpful to optimize adequate skin apposition.
6. Consider prescribing crutches and/or a walking boot after repair of a foot laceration.
7. Lawn mowers and bicycle spokes may cause extensive soft tissue injury along with underlying fractures and tendon lacerations. Severe injuries may require consultation with an orthopedic specialist.

Hair-Thread Tourniquet Syndrome

1. Hair-thread tourniquet syndrome is an unusual type of injury seen in infants. A long strand of hair or thread wraps around one of the toes and can lead to vascular compromise.
2. Remove the hair or thread completely to relieve neurovascular compromise by unwinding it, if possible. Otherwise, consider making a midline longitudinal incision along the extensor surface of the toe to cut the hair or thread.

DISPOSITION

1. Instruct patients to keep wounds clean and dry.
2. Recommend suture removal in 10 to 14 days for wounds of the lower limb and in 14 days for lacerations over joints.

3. Provide wound care instructions. Elevation of the affected limb can help to reduce edema and may aid healing.
4. Consider recommending a wound recheck after 48 hours for a heavily contaminated wound, when a complex repair is required, or if the patient is at higher risk for wound infections.
5. Crutches may be recommended for 7 to 10 days after a wound repair, as needed, to prevent additional tension on the wound during the initial healing process.

FURTHER READING

For further reading in *Tintinalli's Emergency Medicine: A Comprehensive Study Guide*, 8th ed., see Chapter 44, "Leg and Foot Lacerations," by Annabella Salvador-Kelly and Nancy Kwon.

CHAPTER 14

Soft Tissue Foreign Bodies

Michael T. Fitch

Emergency providers are often called upon to evaluate acute wounds that are at risk for embedded foreign bodies. Assessment of older wounds may also be complicated by retained foreign material that was initially unrecognized and can impact the healing process and risk of subsequent infection. Careful evaluation of wounds, radiographic imaging when indicated, and local exploration allow identification of most foreign bodies. Once identified, many foreign bodies can be removed in the emergency department, although some may be left in place or referred to appropriate specialists for delayed removal.

CLINICAL FEATURES

While only a small percentage of lacerations and puncture wounds contain foreign bodies, carefully assess all injuries to evaluate for potentially unrecognized retained material. The mechanism of injury, composition and shape of the wounding object, and the shape and location of the wound are all factors to consider. Objects that have broken, shattered, or splintered at the time of injury may increase the risk of an embedded foreign body. Brittle materials such as thorns, spikes, or branches may penetrate deeply into tissue before breaking. Wood splinters often fragment when pulled from a puncture wound.

Adult patients who complain of a foreign body sensation in an acute wound more than doubles the likelihood of one being present. Wounds that have healed but continue to be the source of sharp pain with movement or pressure over the site may represent a retained foreign object. Other potential signs of an unrecognized foreign body may include poor wound healing, recurrent infections, or the development of soft tissue masses.

Most foreign bodies can be identified through deliberate and careful exploration of wounds determined to be at risk. Use adequate lighting, appropriate anesthesia, and hemostasis techniques to optimize wound evaluation. Visually inspect all recesses of a wound, when possible, recognizing that wounds deeper than 5 mm or where the full depth cannot be visualized have a higher association with foreign bodies. Consider extending the wound margins with a scalpel to permit a more complete exploration when appropriate. Blind and gentle probing with a closed hemostat can be an effective method to identify some foreign bodies, such as glass fragments, when direct visualization is not possible.

DIAGNOSIS AND DIFFERENTIAL

When a foreign body is suspected but not identified and removed during visual inspection, consider radiographic imaging for further evaluation. Most foreign bodies can be seen on plain radiographs, although CT scan, ultrasound, or MRI may be indicated in some circumstances (Table 14-1). Use an underpenetrated soft tissue plain radiography technique or adjust

TABLE 14-1 Imaging Modalities for Detection of Soft Tissue Foreign Bodies

Material	Plain Radiographs	High-Resolution US	CT	MRI
Wood	Poor	Good	Moderate to good	Moderate
Metal	Excellent	Good	Excellent	Poor
Glass	Excellent	Good	Excellent	Good
Organic (e.g., plant thorns and cactus spines)	Poor	Good	Good	Good
Plastic	Moderate	Moderate to good	Good	Good
Palm thorn	Poor	Moderate	Good	Good

the contrast and brightness when using a digital system to increase the likelihood of identifying a foreign body. CT scan is capable of detecting more types of materials than plain film radiography, and may be useful for thorns, spines, wood splinters, or plastic foreign bodies. Ultrasound can be useful at the bedside for directing exploration and removal of foreign bodies. It is >90% sensitive for detecting foreign bodies larger than 4 to 5 mm taking into account the composition of the foreign body, proximity to echogenic structures, and operator experience. MRI is more accurate than the other modalities for identifying wood, plastic, spines, and thorns, but is often less available for emergency use.

EMERGENCY DEPARTMENT CARE AND DISPOSITION

1. Once a foreign body has been identified, consider the risks and benefits of immediate removal, delayed removal, or leaving in place. Consider the potential for infection, toxicity, functional problems, or persistent pain, recognizing that not all foreign bodies require removal. Objects that are small, inert, deeply embedded, and causing no symptoms can often be left in place. Thorns, wood splinters, spines, vegetative material, or contaminated objects are often best removed promptly to prevent subsequent inflammation, pain, or infection.
2. Techniques for soft tissue foreign body removal are based on clinical experience, as there are no systematic studies comparing different techniques. Many objects can be removed by the emergency provider when facilitated by adequate lighting, hemostasis, and anesthesia. Consider referral to a specialist for complicated or delayed foreign body removal. There is no proven benefit for prophylactic antibiotics for wounds that are not infected.
3. Provide tetanus immunization and appropriate wound care after foreign objects are removed. Primary closure of wounds can be considered after foreign contaminants are removed and the risks of infection are low. Consider delayed primary closure for wounds with higher risks of infection.
4. Superficially embedded metallic needles can be removed with a hemostat after a small incision over one end. Remove more deeply embedded

needles by making an incision at the midpoint of the needle, grasp it with a hemostat, and push it back out through the entrance wound. For needles perpendicular to the skin, extend an incision and use pressure on the wound edges to expose the needle and facilitate removal.

5. Wood splinters and organic spines can be removed using forceps when they are small and superficially located. Removal for deeper objects can be facilitated by an incision along the long axis of the foreign body when it is parallel to the skin surface. If the object is small and localization is difficult, a small elliptical block of tissue may be removed and the remaining wound closed primarily. Remove subungual splinters using traction or by excising a portion of nail over the splinter. Cactus spines embedded in the dermis may be removed individually or using an adhesive such as facial gel, rubber cement, or household glue applied to the skin and removed when dry.
6. Fishing hooks can be removed using one of several described techniques after providing adequate anesthesia to the skin around the site of entry. Superficial fishing hooks can be removed using a *retrograde technique* of gentle downward pressure on the shank while the hook is pulled back out the path of entry. The *string pull method* uses one hand to depress the shank of the hook to disengage the barb while the other hand gives a quick tug on a string that has been wrapped around the bend in the hook. When the *advance-and-cut technique* is used, the point and the barb of the fishhook are pushed through the skin and clipped with wire cutters, and the remaining part of the hook is threaded back through the original wound. The *incision technique* is nearly always successful, and involves enlarging the entrance wound to expose the bend in the hook and the barb until disengaged from the subcutaneous tissue. This technique allows for easier wound exploration and cleaning.

FURTHER READING

For further reading in *Tintinalli's Emergency Medicine: A Comprehensive Study Guide*, 8th ed., see Chapter 45, "Soft Tissue Foreign Bodies," by Richard L. Lammers.

CHAPTER 15 Puncture Wounds and Bites

Michael T. Fitch

PUNCTURE WOUNDS

Puncture wounds can be challenging to manage due to difficulty visualizing and cleaning the full depth of an injury. These injuries commonly occur to the extremities, such as on the plantar surface of the foot. Puncture wounds also include injuries caused by high-pressure injection equipment, health care associated needle-stick injuries, and some bite wounds from animals. Infections are reported in 6% to 11% of puncture wounds, with *Staphylococcus aureus* predominating (including methicillin-resistant *S. aureus*—MRSA). *Pseudomonas aeruginosa* is the most common pathogen in post-puncture wound osteomyelitis, particularly when penetration occurs through the sole of an athletic shoe. Post-puncture wound infections despite treatment with antibiotics suggest the possibility of a retained foreign body.

Clinical Features

Puncture wounds treated more than 6 hours after they occur have a greater risk of infection. Wood, glass, or plastic materials may break or splinter when an injury occurs, increasing the chance for retained fragments within the puncture track. Patient perception of a foreign body may be useful for predicting the presence of such a contaminant or fragment.

On physical examination, assess the wound and the likelihood of injury to structures beneath the skin by evaluating distal function of tendons, nerves, and blood vessels. Inspect the wound location, condition of surrounding skin, and the potential presence of foreign matter, debris, or devitalized tissue. Signs of infection include significant pain, swelling, erythema, warmth, fluctuance, decreased range of motion, or drainage from the site.

Diagnosis and Differential

Plain film radiographs should be obtained for any wound suspected of having a potential radiopaque retained foreign body (Table 15-1).

TABLE 15-1 Indications for Imaging in Puncture Wounds

Plain radiographs
Suspicion of fracture
Infected wound
Wound caused by materials prone to fragment (wood, glass, etc.)
Foreign body sensation reported by patient
CT or MRI
Suspected deep-space infection
Persistent pain after injury
Failure to respond to treatment

Organic substances, such as wood or plant matter, are not reliably detected by plan radiographs, but >90% of radiopaque foreign bodies that are >1 mm in diameter can be found this way. CT scan is the imaging modality to use when a retained foreign body continues to be suspected after negative plain film radiography.

Emergency Department Care and Disposition

Treatment recommendations for puncture wounds are based almost entirely on anecdotal evidence and uncontrolled case series.

1. Uncomplicated, clean puncture wounds less than 6 hours after injury and without foreign body should have superficial wound cleansing and tetanus prophylaxis as indicated. Soaking has no proven benefit. Debridement or coring of the wound tract does not reduce rates of infection. There is no proven benefit of prophylactic antibiotics for any type of puncture wound, and therefore routine use of antibiotics for healthy patients with clean puncture wounds is not recommended.
2. High-risk patients with plantar puncture wounds are recommended to receive prophylactic antibiotics along with superficial wound cleansing and tetanus prophylaxis. Consider antibiotics for diabetic patients or patients with other sources of impaired host defenses, forefoot puncture wound injuries, or punctures through athletic shoes. A first-generation cephalosporin, anti-staphylococcal penicillin, or macrolide are suitable antibiotics for most puncture wounds where antibiotics are prescribed. Consider an oral fluoroquinolone with anti-pseudomonal activity, such as **ciprofloxacin** 500 mg twice daily, for plantar puncture wounds through athletic shoes.
3. Cellulitis is a complication of puncture wounds that is most often localized without significant drainage and develops within the first 4 days after injury. This can usually be treated with a 7- to10-day course of a first-generation **cephalosporin, anti-staphylococcal penicillin, trimethoprim-sulfamethoxazole,** or **clindamycin**.
4. A local abscess may develop at the puncture site, especially if a foreign body remains. Treatment includes incision, drainage, and careful exploration for a retained foreign body. Antibiotics are typically only required if there is surrounding cellulitis.
5. Osteomyelitis is an uncommon but serious complication of puncture wounds and may have a greater prevalence in forefoot punctures through athletic shoes. Symptoms typically present more than 7 days after injury and diagnosis can be challenging as radiographs are normal in early stages. Elevations of erythrocyte sedimentation rate or C-reactive protein may support the diagnosis. MRI is the most commonly used imaging modality from the emergency department to help identify this complication. Surgical consultation with discussion of timing of IV antibiotics and admission for surgical treatment is important when osteomyelitis is diagnosed.

NEEDLE-STICK INJURIES

Needle-stick injuries in health care professionals create the most concerns about infection risk from potential exposure to hepatitis viruses or human immunodeficiency virus (HIV). The risk of infection after an inadvertent needle stick contaminated from an infectious source has been estimated to be negligible for hepatitis A, 6% for hepatitis B, 2% for hepatitis C, and 0.3% for HIV. Because recommendations in this area are complex and evolving, each hospital should have a predesigned protocol developed by infectious disease specialists for the evaluation, testing, and treatment of needle-stick injuries, including hepatitis B and HIV prophylaxis.

HIGH-PRESSURE-INJECTION INJURIES

High-pressure-injection injuries may present as puncture wounds, usually to the hand or foot. These are caused by industrial equipment that forces grease, paint, or other liquids through a small nozzle under high pressure. Patients initially may have pain with minimal swelling, but these injuries can still be severe as the injected liquid spreads along fascial planes and causes a delayed inflammatory response. Pain can be controlled with parenteral analgesics while avoiding digital blocks with local anesthesia as these can further increase tissue pressure. An appropriate hand specialist should be consulted for consideration of early surgical debridement of these injuries.

EPINEPHRINE AUTOINJECTOR INJURIES

These injuries typically occur when a patient inadvertently injects epinephrine into the hand or finger while attempting to treat an allergic reaction. Patients present with pain due to the needle stick, paresthesias, and epinephrine-induced vasospasm to the injected area. In the case of finger injections, the entire digit may be blanched and cold. There is no clear evidence that active treatment is better than observation alone, so many patients can be effectively treated with supportive care. Subcutaneous phentolamine injected into the original puncture site is the one treatment consistently described that rapidly reverses digital ischemia from accidental epinephrine injection. A mixture of 0.5 mL of standard phentolamine solution (5 mg/mL concentration) and 0.5 mL of 1% lidocaine solution will produce a 1 mL total volume containing 2.5 mg of phentolamine that can be subcutaneously injected directly through the site of an autoinjector puncture. Patients can be discharged home once ischemia is resolved, as relapse appears unlikely.

MAMMALIAN BITES

Clinical Features

Complications from bite wounds include tissue injury from the bite itself, local infections, or systemic illness. All wounds should be examined and cleaned well with irrigation and debridement as necessary. Evaluate for underlying injury to joints or tendons. Patient evaluation should also include assessment for the potential need for tetanus and/or rabies prophylaxis (see Chapter 94).

Diagnosis and Differential

Bite wounds with low risks for infection can often be repaired primarily. Face or scalp wounds without devitalized tissue that have no underlying fractures can be candidates for primary closure in patients with normal immune systems and wound healing properties. Delayed primary closure can be considered for wounds at higher risk of infection.

Emergency Department Care and Disposition

1. Consider primary closure for low-risk wounds after careful assessment, cleaning, and irrigation.
2. Avoid primary closure in patients with immunodeficiency or comorbidities that may impact successful wound healing.
3. High-risk wounds should be cleaned, debrided, and dressed to maintain a moist environment for healing. Recommend wound reevaluation for signs of infection in 24 to 48 hours.
4. Prophylactic antibiotics are recommended for human bites and for higher risk wounds, particularly if primary wound closure is required (Table 15-1).

INFECTIONS FROM CAT AND DOG BITES

Clinical Features

Most dog bite wounds are superficial and have a relatively low risk (5%) of infection. Cat bites tend to be deeper puncture wounds and are reported to become infected in up to 80% of patients who present for emergency care. However, the true rate of infection is likely much lower than this because most patients with cat bites do not present for care unless the bite appears severe or already has signs of infection.

Diagnosis and Differential

Despite a lack of evidence that antibiotics are effective for reducing the rates of infection after dog or cat bites, prophylactic antibiotics are often suggested for treatment of higher risk uninfected wounds. Many clinicians recommend antibiotics for cat bites, bites in immunocompromised patients, deep dog bite puncture wounds, hand wounds, or wounds needing debridement.

Emergency Department Care and Disposition

1. Common first-line antibiotics can be used when prophylactic antibiotics are desired (Table 15-2). **Amoxicillin-clavulanate**, 500 to 800 mg by mouth twice daily, is the antibiotic most commonly recommended for treatment of local infections after dog or cat bites.
2. **Penicillin** V 500 mg four times daily, or **ampicillin** 500 mg four times daily, may be adequate to cover *Pasteurella multocida* infections from cat bites and may be a lower cost alternative for prophylaxis of cat bites.
3. Cephalexin, dicloxacillin, erythromycin, or clindamycin alone are likely not sufficient for dog or cat bites, as they do not reliably provide coverage for *Pasteurella* species.
4. Serious systemic infections after dog or cat bites are rare, but can develop days after the injury. *Capnocytophaga canimorsus* produces a rare but fulminant bacteremic illness after a dog bite and is more common in alcoholics, post-splenectomy, or other immunosuppressed patients.

TABLE 15-2 Common Bites and First-Line Treatment

Animal	Organism	First-Line Antibiotic
Cat	*Pasteurella multocida* *Bartonella henselae* (cat-scratch fever)	Amoxicillin-clavulanate Azithromycin
Dog	*Pasteurella*, strepto-cocci, staphylococci, *Capnocytophaga canimorsus*	Amoxicillin-clavulanate
Human	*Eikenella*, staphylococci, streptococci Herpes simplex (herpetic whitlow)	Amoxicillin-clavulanate Acyclovir or valacyclovir
Rats, mice, squirrels, gerbils	*Streptobacillus moniliformis* (North America) or *Spirillum minus/minor* (Asia)	Amoxicillin-clavulanate
Livestock, large game animals	Multiple organisms *Brucella, Leptospira, Francisella tularensis*	Amoxicillin-clavulanate or specific agent for disease
Bats, monkeys, dogs, skunks, raccoons, foxes (all carnivores and omnivores)	Rabies	Rabies immune globulin, rabies vaccine
Monkeys	Herpes B virus (*Cercopithecine herpesvirus*)	Acyclovir or valacyclovir
Freshwater fish	*Aeromonas*, staphylococci, streptococci	Fluoroquinolone or trime-thoprim-sulfamethoxazole
Saltwater fish	*Vibrio*, staphylococci, streptococci	Fluoroquinolone

Broad-spectrum antibiotic coverage and appropriate resuscitative efforts are indicated with any such systemic infection.

5. Cat-scratch disease is characterized by regional lymphadenopathy 7 to 12 days after a cat bite or scratch, and is caused by *Bartonella henselae*. Antibiotics are not usually indicated as patients can be managed with pain relief and symptomatic care. Patients with severe painful lymphadenopathy may benefit from a 5-day course of **azithromycin**. Immunosuppressed patients can be treated with a 7- to 10-day course of **trimethoprim-sulfamethoxazole, ciprofloxacin,** or **rifampin**.

HUMAN BITES

Human bite wounds are at higher risk for polymicrobial infection with staphylococcal and streptococcal species or *Eikenella corrodens*. Treatment with prophylactic amoxicillin-clavulanate is recommended and typically suture repair is not advised with the possible exception of facial wounds. Infections requiring parenteral antibiotics can be treated with ampicillin-sulbactam, cefoxitin, or piperacillin-tazobactam. Patients with closed fist injuries, or "fight bite" wounds, to the knuckle caused by impact with another individual's teeth may require surgical treatment (see Chapter 12, Injuries to the Arm, Hand, Fingertip, and Nail).

RODENTS, LIVESTOCK, AND EXOTIC AND WILD ANIMALS

Rodent bites are typically trivial, rodents are not known to carry rabies, and these bites have a low risk for infection. Most patients can be treated conservatively with standard wound care. Livestock and large game animals can cause serious injury with a significant risk of infection and systemic illness caused by brucellosis, leptospirosis, or tularemia (see Chapters 97 and 98). Aggressive wound care and broad-spectrum prophylactic antibiotics are recommended.

FURTHER READING

For further reading in *Tintinalli's Emergency Medicine: A Comprehensive Study Guide*, 8th ed., see Chapter 46, "Puncture Wounds and Bites," by James Quinn

CHAPTER 16

Postrepair Wound Care

Eugenia B. Quackenbush

After an acute wound is repaired, focus subsequent wound care to optimize healing and prevent complications. Issues to consider include the appropriate use of dressings, efforts to minimize edema, prophylactic antibiotics, tetanus prophylaxis, cleansing, and use of packing or drains. Provide patients with appropriate pain control, follow-up instructions, and patient education.

USE OF DRESSINGS

Wound dressings provide a moist environment to promote epithelialization and speed healing. Cover appropriate sutured or stapled wounds with a protective, nonadherent dressing for 24 to 48 hours. Semipermeable films such as OpSite® are available as an alternative to conventional gauze dressings, although one of the disadvantages of these newer materials is their inability to absorb large amounts of fluid. As an alternative to traditional dressings, topical antibiotics may be used to facilitate a warm, moist environment to promote initial wound healing and may help to prevent scab formation. Wounds closed with tissue adhesives should not be treated with topical antibiotic ointment because it will loosen the adhesive and may result in wound dehiscence.

PATIENT POSITIONING AFTER WOUND REPAIR

Recommend elevation of the injured body part, if possible, to reduce edema around the wound and facilitate healing. Splints can be useful for extremity injuries as they decrease motion across the wound and may help limit movement-associated discomfort or the development of additional edema. Pressure dressings can be used in some circumstances to help minimize the accumulation of fluid and are useful for ear and scalp lacerations (see Chapter 11).

PROPHYLACTIC ANTIBIOTICS

Prophylactic antibiotics are not routinely recommended for all wounds, but instead should be reserved for selected special circumstances. When deciding whether or not to prescribe antibiotics, consider the mechanism of injury, location of the wound, degree of any bacterial or soil contamination, and host factors that may predispose to infection.

Prophylactic antibiotics are often recommended for human bites, dog or cat bites on the extremities (see Chapter 15), open fractures, and wounds with exposed joints or tendons (see Chapters 12 and 13). Patients with wounds in areas with lymphedema may also benefit from prophylactic antibiotics. When indicated, a 3- to 5-day course of antibiotics is adequate for nonbite injuries and a 5- to 7-day course is adequate for bite wounds. See Table 16-1 for recommended antibiotic regimens for those special circumstances when antibiotics may be indicated. Patients at high risk for infection should be advised to return for a wound check in 24 to 48 hours.

TABLE 16-1 Postrepair Oral Antibiotic Prophylaxis

Situation	Primary Recommendation	Alternative Recommendation
Uncomplicated patient	First-generation cephalosporin or antistaphylococcal penicillin	Macrolide Clindamycin
Grossly contaminated wounds and/or retained foreign body	Amoxicillin/clavulanate or second-generation cephalosporin	Clindamycin plus a fluoroquinolone
Bite wounds	Amoxicillin/clavulanate	Clindamycin plus either a fluoroquinolone or trimethoprim-sulfamethoxazole
Plantar puncture wounds	Ciprofloxacin	First-generation cephalosporin or antistaphylococcal penicillin
Underlying systemic immunodeficiency (AIDS, chronic steroid use, poorly controlled diabetes mellitus)	Amoxicillin/clavulanate or second-generation cephalosporin	Clindamycin plus a fluoroquinolone
Impaired local defenses (peripheral arterial disease, lymphedema)	Amoxicillin/clavulanate	Clindamycin or erythromycin

TETANUS PROPHYLAXIS

Evaluate patients to determine whether tetanus prophylaxis will be recommended. Inquire about the mechanism of injury, age of the wound, and the patient's tetanus immunization status. The only absolute contraindication to tetanus toxoid is a history of neurologic or severe systemic reaction after a previous dose (see Table 16-2 for a summary of recommendations for tetanus prophylaxis).

TABLE 16-2 Recommendations for Tetanus Prophylaxis

	Clean Minor Wounds		All Other Wounds*	
History of Tetanus Immunization	Administer Tetanus Toxoid†	Administer TIG‡	Administer Tetanus Toxoid	Administer TIG
<3 or uncertain doses	Yes	No	Yes	Yes
≥3 doses				
Last dose within 5 years	No	No	No	No
Last dose within 5–10 years	No	No	Yes	No
Last dose >10 years	Yes	No	Yes	No

*Especially if wound care delayed (>6 h), deep (>1 cm), grossly contaminated, exposed to saliva or feces, stellate, ischemic or infected, avulsions, punctures, or crush injuries.

†Tetanus toxoid: Tdap if adult and no prior record of administration; otherwise, tetanus-diphtheria toxoid if >7 years and diphtheria-tetanus toxoid if <7 years, preferably administered into the deltoid.

‡Tetanus immune globulin: adult dose, 250–500 IU administered into deltoid opposite the tetanus-diphtheria toxoid immunization site.

WOUND CLEANSING

Wounds that have been repaired with sutures or staples may be cleansed as early as 8 hours after closure without increasing the risk of wound infection. Clean the wound area with soap and water and examine for signs of infection daily. Application of topical antibiotics for the first 3 to 5 days may decrease scab formation and help to prevent wound edge separation. Patients with wounds closed with tissue adhesives may shower, but should not completely immerse the wound or apply topical antibiotics, as this will loosen the adhesive bond and cause earlier sloughing of the adhesive.

WOUND DRAINS

Drains or wound packing may be placed in healing wounds to remove interstitial fluid or blood, keep an open tract for drainage of infectious material, or to prevent an abscess from forming by allowing drainage from a contaminated area. Ribbon gauze packing is often used to pack an abscess cavity after incision and drainage, and can be changed regularly as long as the wound continues to drain. Closed drainage systems have largely replaced open wound drains placed after surgical procedures, as closed systems prevent secondary bacterial contamination into the wound. Provide appropriate follow-up instructions for patients with drains or packing in place.

PAIN CONTROL

Educate patients about the expected degree of pain associated with a wound and the measures they can take to reduce that pain. Splints may help to reduce pain and swelling in significant extremity lacerations. Analgesics may be needed for a short time period, although narcotic analgesia is rarely necessary after the first 48 hours of healing for most wounds.

FOLLOW-UP

Provide instructions for regular wound examination during the healing process and when to return for suture or staple removal. Recommend reevaluation in 24 to 48 hours for patients with high-risk wounds or comorbidities that may impair successful wound healing. Facial sutures are typically removed in 3 to 5 days, while sutures in most other areas of the body can be removed after 7 to 10 days of healing. Sutures in some locations such as the hands, feet, buttocks, or over joints should remain in place for 10 to 14 days to reduce the chance of wound dehiscence after suture removal.

When removing sutures or adhesive tapes, take care to avoid tension perpendicular to the wound that could cause dehiscence. When needed, gently debride scab or crusting over each suture with hydrogen peroxide–soaked gauze. Grasp the suture knot with forceps and use scissors or an appropriate scalpel blade to cut the suture. Remove skin staples with an appropriate device that deforms the center and extracts the legs from the skin. For wounds closed with tissue adhesive, advise patients to avoid rubbing, picking, scrubbing, or exposing the area to water for more than brief periods of time during the healing process. Tissue adhesive will slough off itself over time, typically within 5 to 10 days of application, as wound healing progresses.

PATIENT EDUCATION ABOUT LONG-TERM COSMETIC OUTCOME

Inform patients that all traumatic lacerations result in some degree of tissue scarring and that the short-term cosmetic appearance may not be predictive of the ultimate cosmetic outcome. Instruct patients to avoid sun exposure while wounds are healing, as wounds exposed to the sun can develop permanent hyperpigmentation. Patients should wear sunblock for at least 6 to 12 months after injury to optimize the cosmetic outcome.

FURTHER READING

For further reading in *Tintinalli's Emergency Medicine: A Comprehensive Study Guide*, 8th ed., see Chapter 47, "Postrepair Wound Care," by Adam J. Singer and Judd E. Hollander.

SECTION 4

Cardiovascular Diseases

Chest Pain: Cardiac or Not

Andrew Nyce

Millions of patients present to emergency departments (EDs) each year with acute nontraumatic chest pain. Varied clinical presentations coupled with a wide differential diagnosis make patients with chest pain some of the most challenging cared for by emergency care providers. An organized approach will assist clinicians when differentiating acute coronary syndrome (ACS) from other causes of chest pain.

CLINICAL FEATURES

Classically described cardiac chest pain is retrosternal in the left anterior chest with crushing, tightness, squeezing, or pressure that is often brought on by exertion and relieved with rest. Patients may also complain of dyspnea, diaphoresis, and nausea with pain radiating to the left shoulder, jaw, arm, or hand. Some patients, such as premenopausal and early menopausal women, racial minorities, diabetics, the elderly, and patients with psychiatric disease or altered mental status, may have nonclassic presentations of ACS that may or may not be associated with chest pain. Patients with acute myocardial infarction (AMI) who present without chest pain have diagnostic and treatment delays and a higher mortality rate compared to AMI patients who do have chest pain. The onset of symptoms attributed to cardiac disease may be sudden or gradual, and traditionally angina pain lasts 2 to 10 minutes, unstable angina lasts 10 to 30 minutes, and AMI pain often lasts longer than 30 minutes. Dyspnea at rest or with exertion, nausea, light-headedness, generalized weakness, acute changes in mental status, diaphoresis, or shoulder, arm, or jaw discomfort may be the only presenting symptoms for ACS for some patients.

Cardiac risk factors are useful in predicting coronary artery disease in patient populations but may be less useful when applied to an individual patient. Cocaine abuse and HIV infection can accelerate atherosclerosis. Classic symptoms such as radiation of pain to the arms, an exertional component, associated diaphoresis, nausea, and vomiting increase the likelihood that a patient is suffering from an AMI while other symptoms such as pain that is pleuritic in nature, positional, sharp and reproducible with palpation/positioning decrease the likelihood of disease. Unfortunately, there is no identifiable symptom complex that definitively rules in or out the disease without objective testing.

DIAGNOSIS AND DIFFERENTIAL

Patients with ACS often have a normal physical exam but may present with abnormal vital signs. Tachycardia may result from increased sympathetic tone and decreased left ventricular stroke volume. Bradycardia may result from ischemia to the conduction system. The degree of hemodynamic instability is dependent on the amount of myocardium at risk, associated dysrhythmias, or preexisting valvular or myocardial dysfunction. Patients with acute ischemia may have a third or fourth heart sound from changes in ventricular compliance, a new murmur from ruptured cordae tendineae or an aortic root dissection, or crackles on lung auscultation from congestive heart failure. Chest wall tenderness has been demonstrated in up to 15% of patients with AMI, making this physical examination finding unlikely to be useful by itself to completely exclude the possibility of ACS. Response to a particular treatment such as nitroglycerin or a "gastrointestinal (GI) cocktail" poorly discriminates between cardiac and noncardiac chest pain in isolation.

A detailed history and physical exam allows an emergency provider to risk stratify serious pathology in the differential diagnosis of a chest pain patient. Focused diagnostic testing should be performed based on the likelihood of serious pathology. When history and exam make ACS a likely potential cause, initial testing commonly includes an electrocardiogram (ECG), chest x-ray, and cardiac biomarkers.

Electrocardiography

Guidelines recommend ECG screening within 10 minutes of ED arrival for patients with chest pain of potential cardiac etiology. A normal ECG lacks the sensitivity to exclude ACS in isolation; notably patients with unstable angina or non-ST-segment elevation MI may have nonspecific or normal ECG tracings. ECGs demonstrating new ST-segment elevations ≥1 mm in two contiguous leads represent acute MI that will benefit from rapid reperfusion interventions. New ST-segment elevations, Q waves, left bundle branch block, and T-wave inversions or normalizations in symptomatic patients are suggestive of ischemia and should be further investigated. Misinterpretation of ECGs occurs in up to 40% of missed AMI cases, and the diagnostic value of an ECG can be improved by comparing it to a prior ECG and/or repeating it during the patient evaluation process.

Imaging

Chest radiography is commonly performed for patients with chest pain. Patients with ACS will most often have a normal chest x-ray, but images are useful to evaluate for other diagnostic possibilities such as thoracic aortic aneurysm, aortic dissection, pneumonia or pneumothorax. Chest CT may be useful to diagnose other possible conditions such as pulmonary embolism or aortic dissection.

Serum Markers

Due to its high sensitivity and nearly complete cardiac specificity, cardiac troponin (cTn) is the biomarker of choice for the detection of myocardial injury. Serum cTn should be obtained in patients with suspected ACS. While other clinical conditions such as aortic dissection, pulmonary embolism, acute CHF, aortic valve disease, and cardiac procedures can also be associated with an elevated troponin level, acute myocardial ischemia can be differentiated from nonischemic troponin elevations based on the pattern of elevation and the clinical context. With contemporary assays, cTn is detected as early as 2 hours after symptom onset in AMI patients but may not be reliably elevated until 6 hours after symptoms. Elevations peak at 48 hours from symptom onset and may remain elevated for 10 days. Patients with early presentation (within 6 hours of symptom onset) or those with intermittent symptoms should have serial measurements over time. A single cTn may be sufficient to exclude AMI for constant symptoms >8 to 12 hours. The measurement of cTn at short time intervals (delta cTn) is more sensitive for AMI than a single cTn. Patients with renal failure often have elevation of cTn and comparing baseline measures can assist the provider in risk stratifying the patient. Although almost obsolete, creatine kinase-MB testing may be useful in a subset of patients in whom the timing of infarction remains unclear.

Differential Diagnosis

Common causes of chest pain are listed in Table 17-1.

The classic symptoms of life-threatening causes of acute chest pain are listed in Table 17-2.

Pulmonary Embolism

Patients with pulmonary embolism often complain of sudden onset pleuritic chest pain associated with dyspnea, tachypnea, tachycardia, or hypoxemia. Risk factors include prolonged immobilization, active cancer, recent surgery or trauma, procoagulant syndromes, exogenous estrogen, or previous thromboembolic disease. Clinical decision aids such as the Wells and Revised Geneva Scores and the Pulmonary Embolism Rule-Out Criteria (PERC) can help risk stratify patients for diagnostic evaluation. Serum D-dimer may be a useful test in low-risk patients to help determine which patients need further

TABLE 17-1 Common Causes of Acute Chest Pain

Visceral Pain	Pleuritic Pain	Chest Wall Pain
Typical angina	**Pulmonary embolism**	Costosternal syndrome
Unstable angina	**Pneumonia**	Costochondritis (Tietze's syndrome)
Acute myocardial infarction	Spontaneous pneumothorax	Precordial catch syndrome
Aortic dissection	Pericarditis	Xiphodynia
Esophageal rupture	Pleurisy	Radicular syndromes
Esophageal reflux or spasm		Intercostal nerve syndromes
Mitral valve prolapse		Fibromyalgia

TABLE 17-2 Classic Symptoms of Potentially Life-Threatening Causes of Chest Pain*

Disorder	Pain Location	Pain Character	Radiation	Associated Signs and Symptoms
Acute coronary syndrome	Retrosternal, L chest, or epigastric	Crushing, tightness, squeezing, pressure	R or L shoulder, R or L arm/hand, jaw	Dyspnea, diaphoresis, nausea
Pulmonary embolism	Focal chest	Pleuritic	None	Tachycardia, tachypnea, hypoxia, may have hemoptysis
Aortic dissection	Midline, substernal	Ripping, tearing	Intrascapular area of back	Secondary arterial branch occlusion
Pneumonia	Focal chest	Sharp, pleuritic	None	Fever, hypoxia, may see signs of sepsis
Esophageal rupture	Substernal	Sudden, sharp, after forceful vomiting	Back	Dyspnea, diaphoresis, may see signs of sepsis
Pneumothorax	One side of chest	Sudden, sharp, lancinating, pleuritic	Shoulder, back	Dyspnea
Pericarditis	Substernal	Sharp, constant or pleuritic	Back, neck, shoulder	Fever, pericardial friction rub
Perforated peptic ulcer	Epigastric	Severe, sharp	Back, up into chest	Acute distress, diaphoresis

*A typical presentations are common.

Abbreviations: L, left; R, right.

testing with CT pulmonary angiography to identify pulmonary embolism. For more details, see Chapter 25, "Thromboembolism."

Aortic Dissection

Patients with aortic dissection classically describe a sudden onset of severe, tearing pain radiating to the intrascapular area of the back. Secondary symptoms result from arterial branch occlusions and may include ischemic stroke, AMI, or limb ischemia. Risk factors include male sex, age >50, uncontrolled hypertension, connective tissue disorders, cocaine use, bicuspid valve or aortic valve replacement, and pregnancy. Physical exam findings may include unilateral pulse deficits or focal neurologic deficits. If aortic dissection is suspected, obtain a CT aortogram or transesophageal echocardiogram. A normal chest x-ray and negative D-dimer lowers the probability but does not completely exclude the diagnosis of an aortic dissection. Additionally, this diagnosis can be associated with nonspecific ST segment or T-wave changes on ECG testing. For more details see Chapter 27, "Aortic Dissection and Aneurysms."

Esophageal Rupture (Boerhaave's Syndrome)

Patients with esophageal rupture often present with sudden-onset, sharp substernal chest pain that follows an episode of forceful vomiting. Patients are usually ill appearing with tachycardia, fever, dyspnea, and diaphoresis.

Physical examination may reveal crepitus in the neck or chest from subcutaneous emphysema, while audible crepitus on cardiac auscultation (Hamman's crunch) is a rare finding. A chest x-ray may be normal or demonstrate a pleural effusion (left more common), pneumothorax, pneumomediastinum, pneumoperitoneum, or subcutaneous air. Diagnosis is made via CT of chest with oral water-soluble contrast. For more details see Chapter 40, "Esophageal Emergencies."

Spontaneous Pneumothorax

A spontaneous pneumothorax causes sudden-onset, sharp, pleuritic chest pain with dyspnea. These classically occur in tall, slender male patients and risk factors include smoking, COPD, and asthma. Physical exam findings are inconsistent but auscultation may reveal decreased breath sounds on the affected side. The diagnosis is made by chest x-ray with only a small percentage of patients progressing to develop a tension pneumothorax. See more details in Chapter 32, "Spontaneous and Iatrogenic Pneumothorax."

Acute Pericarditis

Pain from acute pericarditis is typically sharp, severe, constant, and retrosternal that radiates to the back, neck, or jaw. Pain is classically worsened by lying supine and is relieved by sitting forward. The presence of a pericardial friction rub supports the diagnosis. ECG may show PR-segment depressions, diffuse ST-segment elevations, or T-wave inversions that are typically diffuse. See more details in Chapter 24, "The Cardiomyopathies, Myocarditis, and Pericardial Disease."

Musculoskeletal Causes

Chest pain due to irritation or inflammation of structures in the chest wall is commonly seen in the ED. Possible causes include costochondritis, xiphodynia (inflammation of the xiphoid process), precordial catch syndrome, intercostal strain due to coughing, and pectoralis muscle strain in the setting of recent physical exertion. Patients often complain of sharp pain that is worsened with movement of the chest wall and palpation. While chest wall tenderness is also present in some patients with ACS or other significant disease processes, a clear musculoskeletal etiology with completely reproducible pain in a patient without other symptoms or risk factors support this diagnosis.

Gastrointestinal Causes

Gastrointestinal disorders such as esophageal reflux, dyspepsia syndromes, and esophageal motility disorders often cannot be reliably differentiated from ACS by history and physical exam alone. Symptoms can range from a gnawing or burning pain in the lower chest with gastritis to postprandial dull, boring pain in the epigastric region with peptic ulcer disease. Esophageal spasm is often associated with reflux disease and is characterized by a sudden onset of dull or tight substernal chest pain. The pain is typically precipitated by drinking cold liquids and can be relieved by nitroglycerin. Clinicians should determine whether the symptoms are due to a GI disorder based on the clinical presentation and the absence of findings and/or risk factors suggesting an ischemic cause. Diagnostic decisions should not be made solely on the basis of a response to a therapeutic trial of antacids,

GI cocktails, or nitroglycerin. See more details in Chapter 40, "Esophageal Emergencies" and Chapter 41, "Peptic Ulcer Disease and Gastritis."

EMERGENCY DEPARTMENT CARE AND DISPOSITION

1. Patients with abnormal vital signs, concerning ECG findings, or clinical history concerning for an acute cardiac event should be promptly evaluated and treated according to immediate airway, breathing, or circulation needs.
2. Place patients with suspicious histories for serious pathology on cardiac monitors, establish IV access, and provide supplemental oxygen as necessary. Vital signs and pulse oximetry should be monitored at regular intervals.
3. Perform an ECG within 10 minutes in patients for whom there is a reasonable suspicion of myocardial ischemia.
4. Obtain a focused history to elicit potential features of life-threatening causes of chest pain such as ACS, aortic dissection, pulmonary embolism, severe pneumonia, and esophageal rupture. Ask about onset, timing, severity, radiation and character of the chest pain; alleviating and exacerbating factors; and presence of associated symptoms such as vomiting, diaphoresis, and dyspnea.
5. Perform physical examination of the thorax for prior surgical incisions, chest wall deformities, and symmetric rise and fall of the chest. Palpate for tenderness, masses, or crepitus. Auscultate to identify chest consolidation or pneumothorax, murmurs, gallops, or friction rubs.
6. Administer aspirin for patients at risk for AMI (see Chapter 18, "Acute Coronary Syndromes: Management of Myocardial Infarction and Unstable Angina," for details and additional medications).
7. Consider serum laboratory studies including cardiac troponin levels when concern for ACS remains after history and physical examination.
8. Consider chest radiography for patients with acute chest pain where the etiology remains uncertain after history and physical examination. Evaluate the radiograph for findings of pneumonia, pneumothorax, aortic dissection, pneumomediastinum, or other diagnoses.
9. ED treatment and disposition is contingent on the suspected etiology of the patient's chest pain. Patients in whom ACS cannot be reliably excluded after ED evaluation and diagnostic workup may require further diagnostic evaluation in the hospital.
10. The Thrombosis in Myocardial Infarction (TIMI) risk score or Global Registry of Acute Coronary Events score can aid clinicians when risk stratifying patients for ACS. However, a low-risk score is not sensitive enough to reliably exclude ACS or identify patients for early discharge without further evaluation.
11. If the etiology of chest pain remains unclear after the initial ED workup, clinicians should consider further testing and observation or admission as guided by clinical suspicion and findings.

FURTHER READING

For further reading in *Tintinalli's Emergency Medicine: A Comprehensive Study Guide*, 8th ed., see Chapter 48, "Chest Pain" by Simon A. Mahler.

Acute Coronary Syndromes: Myocardial Infarction and Unstable Angina

Maame Yaa A. B. Yiadom

Acute coronary syndromes (ACS) encompass a spectrum of cardiac disorders with myocardial ischemia and/or injury. These include ST-elevation myocardial infarction (STEMI), non-STEMI (NSTEMI), and unstable angina.

CLINICAL FEATURES

Chest pain is the most common symptom for patients with ACS. Important elements of the history include the timing of symptom onset, location, quality, severity, and duration. Also important is whether the pain is intermittent, constant, or waxing and waning. Twenty percent to 30% of all patients diagnosed with ACS report atypical symptoms, and their chief complaint may not include chest pain. These atypical symptoms can include shortness of breath, nausea, diaphoresis, back pain, abdominal pain, dizziness, or palpitations. Clinical features associated with chest pain that is diagnosed as ACS include substernal or left-sided chest pain, radiation of pain to one or both arms, and chest pain accompanied with nausea, vomiting, or diaphoresis.

Discuss risk factors for coronary artery disease (CAD) with patients to stratify the risk of ACS. These risk factors include older age, male gender, family history, smoking, hypertension, hypercholesterolemia, and diabetes. Patients with a long history of cocaine use may be at risk for accelerated CAD development, and recent use can cause acute ischemia from coronary vasospasm. The presence or absence of risk factors alone are poorly predictive of the likelihood of myocardial infarction in a patient presenting with acute symptoms. Physical examination can help identify signs of hemodynamic dysfunction from cardiac strain or acute heart failure such as pallor, diaphoresis, altered mental status, elevated jugular venous distension, peripheral edema, or rales on pulmonary exam.

DIAGNOSIS AND DIFFERENTIAL

Consider alternative diagnoses for patient symptoms based on clinical assessment, which may include diseases such as pulmonary embolism, congestive heart failure, gastroesophageal reflux disease, symptomatic hiatal hernia, chronic obstructive pulmonary disease, asthma, pneumonia, pneumothorax, pericarditis, myocarditis, aortic dissection, chest trauma, chest wall disorders, or mediastinal disorders.

Promptly obtain an ECG to assess for signs of cardiac ischemia. Findings diagnostic for STEMI include at least one of the four criteria listed in Table 18-1.

In the setting of symptoms suggestive of ischemia, ECG findings consistent with STEMI should be acted upon promptly to initiate appropriate

TABLE 18-1 Electrocardiographic ST-Segment-Based Criteria for Acute Myocardial Infarction

Location	Electrocardiographic Findings
Anteroseptal	ST-segment elevations in V1, V2, and possibly, V3
Anterior	ST-segment elevations in V_1, V_2, V_3, and V_4
Anterolateral	ST-segment elevations in V_1–V_6, I, and aVL
Lateral	ST-segment elevations in I and aVL
Inferior	ST-segment elevations in II, III, and aVF
Inferolateral	ST-segment elevations in II, III, aVF, and V_5 and V_6
True posterior*	Initial R waves in V_1 and V_2 > 0.04 s and R/S ratio ≥1
Right ventricular	ST-segment elevations in II, III, and aVF and ST elevation in right-side V_4

*Posterior wall infarction does not produce Q-wave abnormalities in conventional leads and is diagnosed in the presence of tall R waves in V_1 and V_2.

therapy. ECG findings that do not meet criteria for STEMI but raise concerns for NSTEMI or unstable angina may include ST or T wave changes in a coronary artery distribution (see Table 18-2).

For patients with suspected ACS, obtain serum troponin, chest radiograph, CBC, electrolytes, and PT/PTT. NSTEMI is diagnosed when an elevated serum troponin is identified in a patient with symptoms consistent with myocardial ischemia. Consider repeating troponin levels within 3 hours when diagnostic uncertainty remains. Over time, a patient may progress in disease severity, prompting consideration for serial ECGs to identify any dynamic ischemic changes, bedside echocardiography to assess for cardiac wall motion abnormalities, and/or additional serum troponin testing. Consult with cardiology to determine whether early cardiac catheterization may be appropriate for patients with NSTEMI who continue to have concerning symptoms or dynamic changes.

TABLE 18-2 Anatomic Distribution of Ischemic ECG Changes

Location	Location of ST or T Wave Changes	Coronary Artery Involvement
Inferior	II, III, AVF*	RCA in 80%; RCX in 20%
Lateral	I, AVL, V_{5-6}	LCX
Septal	V_{1-3}*	LAD septal branches
Anterior	V_{1-4}, loss of Q wave in V_{5-6}*	LAD
Right ventricular	V_1, right-sided V_4	RCA
Posterior	V_{7-9} (left-sided leads), R waves in V_1,	LCX
Atrial	V_{1-6}	RCA

*Can be accompanied with signs of dysrhythmia.

Abbreviations: RCA, right coronary artery; RCX, right circumflex artery; LCX, left circumflex artery; LAD, left anterior descending artery.

Unstable angina is a clinical diagnosis based on history, physical examination findings, and diagnostic testing that does not reveal a STEMI or NSTEMI. This may precede STEMI or NSTEMI or may be the presenting diagnosis that leads to a new diagnosis of CAD. Unstable angina characteristically presents with chest pain (or atypical ACS symptoms) associated with evidence of obstructive coronary artery disease and has one of the following three characteristics: (1) began within the past 2 months; (2) has increasing frequency, intensity, or duration of existing angina symptoms; or (3) existing angina begins to occur at rest. Additional diagnostic testing that may be helpful when unstable angina is considered includes coronary CT angiogram, exercise treadmill testing, cardiac nuclear perfusion imaging, or cardiac MRI.

EMERGENCY DEPARTMENT CARE AND DISPOSITION

1. STEMI treatment begins immediately upon recognition of diagnostic ECG findings. Goals include reperfusion by reducing thrombus, limiting thrombus extension, and relieving obstructive CAD. The effectiveness of interventions is time sensitive. Options include administering systemic thrombolytic therapy within 30 minutes of arrival or initiating percutaneous coronary intervention (PCI) within 90 minutes. PCI is the preferred therapy, when possible, based on greater benefits and fewer risks in patients without contraindications to thrombolysis (Table 18-3) who can achieve PCI within 120 minutes. See Table 18-3 for medications used in the treatment of STEMI.
2. For patients with a suspected ACS, begin cardiac monitoring, place an intravenous line, and provide supplemental oxygen if oxygen saturation is less than 95%. Administer **aspirin** 160 to 325 mg orally chewed. Consider oral, transdermal, or intravenous **nitroglycerin** to treat any ongoing angina. **Morphine sulfate** may be used as an adjunct if pain continues despite treatment with nitroglycerin.
3. **Clopidogrel** is recommended for use along with aspirin for patients with moderate to high-risk NSTEMI and STEMI, and in patients in whom PCI is planned. Use as an alternative to aspirin in patients allergic to aspirin. Clopidogrel increases risk of bleeding, and should be held at least 5 days before coronary artery bypass grafting (CABG).
4. Begin anticoagulation for patients with unstable angina or NSTEMI using **unfractionated heparin** or **low-molecular-weight heparins (LMWH).** These are also options for patients undergoing PCI revascularization, in consultation with your cardiology consultant. Unfractionated heparin is preferred for patients in whom CABG is planned.
5. Factor Xa inhibitors such as **fondaparinux** have similar efficacy to unfractionated heparin in patients with unstable angina or NSTEMI, and current guidelines consider it an option as an antithrombin. In STEMI patients lacking renal impairment, fondaparinux may be considered for those patients treated with thrombolytics that are not fibrin specific such as streptokinase.
6. Direct thrombin inhibitors, such as **bivalirudin**, bind directly to thrombin in clot and are resistant to agents that degrade heparin. Comparison of bivalirudin with unfractionated heparin found no outcomes benefit

TABLE 18-3 Drugs Used in the Emergency Treatment of STEMI

Antiplatelet Agents		
Aspirin	162–325 mg	
Clopidogrel	Loading dose of 600 mg PO followed by 75 mg/d. No loading dose is administered in patients > 75 years old receiving fibrinolytics	
Prasugrel	Loading dose of 60 mg promptly and no more than 1 h after PCI once coronary anatomy is defined and a decision is made to proceed with PCI	
Ticagrelor	Loading dose is 180 mg PO followed by 90 mg twice a day	
Antithrombins		
Unfractionated heparin	Bolus of 60 U/kg (maximum, 4000 U) followed by infusion of 12 U/kg/h (maximum, 1000 U/h) titrated to a partial thromboplastin time 1.5–2.5 × control	
Enoxaparin	30 mg IV bolus followed by 1 mg/kg SC every 12 h	
Fondaparinux	2.5 mg SC*	
Fibrinolytic Agents		
Streptokinase	1.5 MU over 60 min	
Anistreplase	30 U IV over 2–5 min	
Alteplase	Body weight > 67 kg: 15 mg initial IV bolus; 50 mg infused over next 30 min; 35 mg infused over next 60 min	
	Body weight < 67 kg: 15 mg initial IV bolus; 0.75 mg/kg infused over next 30 min; 0.5 mg/kg infused over next 60 min	
Reteplase	10 U IV over 2 min followed by 10 U IV bolus 30 min later	
Tenecteplase	Weight	Dose (total dose not to exceed 50 mg)
	<60 kg	30 mg
	≥60 but <70 kg	35 mg
	≥70 but <80 kg	40 mg
	≥80 but <90	45 mg
	≥90	50 mg
Glycoprotein IIb/IIIa Inhibitors†		
Abciximab	0.25 mg/kg bolus followed by infusion of 0.125 μg/kg/min (maximum, 10 μg/min) for 12–24 h	
Eptifibatide	180 μg/kg bolus followed by infusion of 2.0 μg/kg/min for 72–96 h	
Tirofiban	0.4 μg/kg/min for 30 min followed by infusion of 0.1 μg/kg/min for 48–96 h	
Other Anti-Ischemic Therapies		
Nitroglycerin	Sublingual: 0.4 mg every 5 min × 3 PRN pain IV: Start at 10 μg/min, titrate to 10% reduction in MAP if normotensive, 30% reduction in MAP if hypertensive	
Morphine	2–5 mg IV every 5–15 min PRN pain	

(Continued)

TABLE 18-3 Drugs Used in the Emergency Treatment of STEMI (Continued)

Metoprolol	50 mg PO every 12 h on first day, unless significant hypertension, may consider 5 mg IV over 2 min every 5 min up to 15 mg; withhold β-blockers initially if the patient is at risk for cardiogenic shock/adverse effects‡
Atenolol	25–50 mg PO, unless significant hypertension, may consider 5 mg IV over 5 min, repeat once 10 min later; withhold β-blockers initially if the patient is at risk for cardiogenic shock/adverse effects‡

*Fondaparinux should not be used as monotherapy for PCI; if used, addition of unfractionated heparin or bivalirudin is recommended before PCI.

†American College of Cardiology/American Heart Association 2009 focused update for STEMI patients recommended glycoprotein IIB/IIa inhibitors be given at the time of PCI; benefit prior to arrival in the cardiac catheterization laboratory is uncertain.

‡Risk factors for cardiogenic shock/adverse effects: (1) signs of heart failure; (2) evidence of a low cardiac output state; (3) increased risk for cardiogenic shock (cumulatively: age >70 years old, systolic blood pressure <120 mm Hg, sinus tachycardia >110 beats/min or bradycardia <60 beats/min, and longer duration of STEMI symptoms before diagnosis and treatment); or (4) standard relative contraindications to β-blockade (PR interval >0.24 s, second- or third-degree heart block, active asthma, or reactive airway disease).

Abbreviations: MAP, mean arterial pressure; PCI, percutaneous coronary intervention; PRN, as needed; STEMI, ST-segment elevation myocardial infarction.

in NSTEMI patients, but less bleeding occurred and no dosage adjustment is required in renal impairment. For patients with STEMI, bivalirudin may be considered as an alternative to unfractionated heparin and GP IIb/IIIa inhibitors.

7. In treatment settings without timely access to PCI, **fibrinolytics** are indicated for patients with STEMI if time to treatment is <6 to 12 hours from symptom onset, and the ECG has at least 1-mm ST-segment elevation in two or more contiguous leads. The dosages of individual fibrinolytic agents are listed in Table 18-3.
8. STEMI patients who have received fibrinolytics should receive full-dose anticoagulation started in the ED and maintained for a minimum of 48 hours. Similar efficacy and safety profiles have been demonstrated for tPA, rtPA, and TNK. Contraindications for fibrinolytics are listed in Table 18-4. Before administering thrombolytics, obtain informed consent. Arterial puncture should be avoided, as should venipuncture or central line placement in areas which are not readily compressible.
9. **Tissue plasminogen activator** (tPA) is a naturally occurring human protein and is not antigenic. tPA is fibrin-specific and has a half-life of 5 minutes. When compared with traditional dosing, front-loaded tPA has been shown to have superior 90-minute patency rates and reocclusion rates, with no increase in bleeding risk.
10. **Reteplase** (rPA) is a non-fibrin-specific deletion mutant of tPA with a prolonged half-life of 18 minutes and its use may have a faster time to perfusion. The main advantage of reteplase is that it is given as a double bolus rather than continuous infusion.

TABLE 18-4 Contraindications to Fibrinolytic Therapy in ST-Segment Elevation Myocardial Infarction

Absolute contraindications
Any prior intracranial hemorrhage
Known structural cerebral vascular lesion (e.g., arteriovenous malformation)
Known intracranial neoplasm
Ischemic stroke within 3 months
Active internal bleeding (excluding menses)
Suspected aortic dissection or pericarditis
Relative contraindications
Severe uncontrolled blood pressure (>180/100 mm Hg)
History of chronic, severe, poorly controlled hypertension
History of prior ischemic stroke >3 months or known intracranial pathology not covered in contraindications
Current use of anticoagulants with known INR >2–3
Known bleeding diathesis
Recent trauma (past 2 weeks)
Prolonged CPR (>10 min)
Major surgery (<3 weeks)
Noncompressible vascular punctures (including subclavian and internal jugular central lines)
Recent internal bleeding (within 2–4 weeks)
Patients treated previously with streptokinase should not receive streptokinase a second time
Pregnancy
Active peptic ulcer disease
Other medical conditions likely to increase risk of bleeding (e.g., diabetic retinopathy)

11. **Tenecteplase** (TNK) is a fibrin-specific substitution mutant of tPA that is given as a single weight-based bolus.
12. **Streptokinase** (SK) activates circulating plasminogen, is not fibrin-specific, and is capable of generating an allergic reaction (minor: 5% to 5.7%, anaphylaxis: <0.2% to 0.7%). Hypotension occurs in up to 15% of patients and is usually responsive to fluids and slowing of SK infusion. Contraindications include hypotension, prior SK administration within 6 months, and streptococcal infection within a year. SK's half-life is 23 minutes, but systemic fibrinolysis persists for 24 hours. Administer heparin within 4 hours of starting SK.
13. The most significant complication of systemic thrombolytics is bleeding, particularly intracranial hemorrhage. If significant bleeding occurs, discontinue thrombolytics, heparin, and aspirin. **Crystalloid** and **red blood cell** infusion may be necessary. **Cryoprecipitate** and **fresh frozen plasma (FFP)** may be used to reverse fibrinolysis by replenishing thrombotic factors. Begin with 10 units of cryoprecipitate and obtain fibrinogen levels. If the fibrinogen level is <1 g/L, administer a second 10 U of cryoprecipitate. If bleeding continues despite a fibrinogen >1 g/L, or if the fibrinogen level is <1 g/L after 20 U of cryoprecipitate, administer 2 U of FFP. If hemorrhage continues, administer platelets or antifibrinolytic agents such as aminocaproic acid or tranexamic acid.

14. Recent evidence shows no benefit to early IV administration of **β-blockers** on cardiac rhythm, infarct size, reinfarction, or mortality. Oral β-blocker therapy does not need to be initiated emergently unless there is a specific indication such as significant tachycardia or hypertension. β-blockers should be initiated within the first 24 hours of hospitalization for patients lacking contraindications.
15. **Glycoprotein IIb/IIIa (GP IIb/IIIa) antagonists** bind to platelets and inhibit their aggregation. Abciximab, eptifibatide, and tirofiban are currently available. There is no current evidence supporting the routine use of GP IIb/IIIa inhibitor therapy *prior* to angiography in patients with STEMI, and the use of these agents upstream is uncertain. Use of GP IIb/IIIa inhibitors should be guided by local interdisciplinary review of ongoing clinical trials, guidelines, and recommendations.
16. The disposition of ACS patients depends on their specific ischemic diagnosis and hemodynamic status. STEMI patients often are taken immediately to the catheterization laboratory for definitive treatment. Patients treated with thrombolytics who have continued hemodynamic instability and pain or have not reperfused may be candidates for rescue angioplasty. Emergent CABG may also be indicated for some patients. Patients in refractory cardiogenic shock should undergo emergent angioplasty. Intraaortic balloon pump or other LV-assisting devices may also be indicated for these patients. Admission to a critical care unit is appropriate.
17. NSTEMI or unstable angina patients who have ongoing chest pain, ECG changes, dysrhythmias, or hemodynamic compromise are also admitted for further care in a cardiac intensive care unit. Patients with symptoms of unstable angina but resolved chest pain, normal or nonspecific ECG changes, and no complications may often be admitted to a monitored inpatient bed.

FURTHER READING

For further reading in *Tintinalli's Emergency Medicine: A Comprehensive Study Guide*, 8th ed., see Chapter 49, "Acute Coronary Syndromes" by Judd E. Hollander and Deborah B. Diercks.

CHAPTER 19

Cardiogenic Shock

Brian Hiestand

Cardiogenic shock occurs when there is insufficient cardiac output to meet the metabolic demands of the tissues. It is most commonly caused by an acute myocardial infarction (AMI) with extensive cardiac tissue damage, impaired right ventricular cardiac contractility, or subsequent rupture of a papillary muscle. Other potential causes of cardiogenic shock include cardiotoxic drug effects, infection such as myopericarditis or endocarditis, and mechanical cardiac dysfunction caused by valvular disease, pulmonary embolism, cardiac tamponade, or myocardial contusion. Early treatment and stabilization of patients suffering from cardiogenic shock are important, as mortality approaches 50% for an AMI that is complicated by cardiogenic shock.

CLINICAL FEATURES

A hallmark of all types of shock is tissue hypoperfusion and the resulting end-organ manifestations of this lack of adequate blood supply. Cardiogenic shock generally presents with hypotension (systolic blood pressure [SBP] <90 mm Hg), although SBP may be greater than 90 mm Hg in some patients such as those with preexisting and uncontrolled hypertension. Sinus tachycardia is frequently seen, but may be absent particularly when patients are taking medications that can inhibit an appropriate tachycardic response, such as β-blockers. Evidence of end-organ tissue hypoperfusion in cardiogenic shock may include cool or mottled skin, oliguria, or altered mental status. Left ventricular failure can present with findings concerning for acute pulmonary edema, such as tachypnea, rales, wheezing, and frothy sputum. Patients with hypotension who have jugular venous distention without pulmonary edema may be suffering from right ventricular failure due to infarction, cardiac tamponade, or pulmonary embolism. The presence of a new heart murmur on cardiac auscultation may represent a ventricular septal defect or an acute valvular dysfunction from papillary muscle dysfunction or chordae tendineae rupture that can manifest clinically as cardiogenic shock.

DIAGNOSIS AND DIFFERENTIAL

Once the diagnosis of shock has been made, a key task for the clinician is to differentiate cardiogenic shock from shock that is caused by other disease processes, such as hypovolemia, overwhelming sepsis, or neurogenic shock. Evaluation of a hypotensive patient for signs of gastrointestinal bleeding, severe dehydration, potential sources of significant infection, or the presence of new neurologic deficits may help to establish an alternate diagnosis.

When cardiogenic shock is suspected, an electrocardiogram (ECG) is appropriate to assist in the detection of acute cardiac ischemia or infarction, arrhythmias, electrolyte abnormalities, or signs of drug toxicity with cardiac manifestations. ST-segment depression in the lateral leads of the ECG may be suggestive of a right ventricular infarction, which is associated with increased mortality and may not manifest itself with ST-segment elevation in a standard twelve lead ECG. Look for pulmonary edema, widened mediastinum, enlarged cardiac silhouette, or other alternative diagnoses such as pneumonia or pneumothorax on chest radiograph.

Bedside echocardiography, while not a substitute for emergent formal transthoracic echocardiography when clinically indicated, can rapidly exclude other causes of hypotension, identify some mechanical precipitants of shock, and help guide therapy. Visualization of the inferior cava can help to determine volume status when considering hypovolemic shock. A pericardial effusion can be diagnosed using limited bedside echocardiography and along with findings such as diastolic collapse of the right atrium and ventricle can be diagnostic for cardiac tamponade. Left ventricular function and cardiac contractility can also be evaluated with bedside testing and may support the clinician's impression of cardiogenic shock when decreased from normal cardiac function.

There is no single laboratory test that is diagnostic for cardiogenic shock. Obtain a complete blood count and chemistries (including liver function tests) to evaluate for anemia, potential signs of infection, and some components of end organ dysfunction. In the absence of ST-segment elevation that is diagnostic for an acute MI, elevations of cardiac markers such as troponin can establish the diagnosis of non-ST-segment elevation MI (NSTEMI). In addition, these markers may add prognostic value in patients with other causes of shock such as acute heart failure and sepsis. Given their high negative predictive value, natriuretic peptides, such as cardiac BNP or n-terminal pro-BNP, suggest a noncardiac etiology of patient condition if normal. In the setting of shock, serum lactate levels indicate the degree of hypoperfusion present and may be useful to follow during resuscitative efforts. Blood gas measurements will provide insight into acid-base status and CO_2 retention. Specialized laboratory testing, such as toxicology studies, should be guided by the specific clinical situation.

EMERGENCY DEPARTMENT CARE AND DISPOSITION

Airway management when necessary, circulatory stabilization, and arrangements for definitive cardiac care often occur simultaneously for patients in cardiogenic shock. Cardiology and/or cardiothoracic surgery should be consulted early when cardiogenic shock is diagnosed, as emergent coronary revascularization is an important intervention when ischemia is the underlying cause. Transfer to a facility with such specialized care should be arranged when indicated.

1. Supplemental oxygen should be provided. Noninvasive positive pressure ventilation may provide temporary support, but many patients in cardiogenic shock will require definitive airway management and thus endotracheal intubation should be considered as needed for respiratory support.

2. Intravenous access should be obtained. Cardiac rhythm and pulse oximetry monitoring should be initiated. Rhythm disturbances, hypoxia, hypovolemia, and electrolyte abnormalities should be identified and treated.
3. Early revascularization is required for cardiogenic shock due to acute cardiac ischemia. Percutaneous coronary intervention (PCI) is superior to fibrinolysis in the setting of cardiogenic shock. However, when PCI is not available (or prolonged transfer times are anticipated) fibrinolysis is superior to supportive measures alone.
4. In AMI, aspirin and heparin should be given unless there is an absolute contraindication present. Typical anti-anginal therapies may precipitate cardiovascular collapse, especially in patients with right ventricular ischemia. To treat acute chest pain in the setting of cardiogenic shock, consider cautious use of titrated intravenous **nitroglycerin** 5 to 100 μg/min or **morphine sulfate** given in 2 mg increments with close monitoring of blood pressure. Avoid the use of β-blockers in patients with cardiogenic shock as this may worsen cardiac function.
5. A small intravenous fluid challenge (250 to 500 mL bolus) with close monitoring for effectiveness may be considered for patients with mild hypotension and no pulmonary edema. Hypotension in the setting of right ventricular ischemia will warrant a more robust fluid resuscitation.
6. **Norepinephrine** may be considered for severe hypotension as a vasopressor and positive inotrope. An infusion should begin at 2 μg/min and titrated to the desired effect.
7. **Dobutamine** 2 to 20.0 μg/kg/min can be used to support blood pressure for hypotension due to cardiogenic shock in the absence of hypovolemia. Dobutamine may cause peripheral vasodilatation, and concomitant use of **dopamine** 2 to 20.0 μg/kg/min can be added and titrated to the desired effect with the lowest dose possible.
8. **Milrinone** may be considered as a positive inotrope and can be started with a loading dose of 50 μg/kg IV over 10 minutes followed by an infusion of 0.5 μg/kg/min.
9. In the setting of acute mitral regurgitation, afterload reduction via intravenous **sodium nitroprusside** 0.5 to 10.0 μg/kg/min should be combined with inotropic support via **dobutamine** 2 to 20.0 μg/kg/min.
10. Consider using intraaortic balloon pump counterpulsation (if available) as a temporizing measure to decrease afterload and to augment coronary perfusion. This is contraindicated in severe aortic regurgitation.
11. Consider more advanced mechanical circulatory support, such as percutaneous left ventricular assist devices or extracorporeal membrane oxygenation, in selected refractory cases.

FURTHER READING

For further reading in *Tintinalli's Emergency Medicine: A Comprehensive Study Guide*, 8th ed., see Chapter 50, "Cardiogenic Shock," by Casey Glass and David Manthey.

Low-Probability Acute Coronary Syndrome

David A. Wald

Patients presenting to the emergency department (ED) with chest pain or other symptoms suggesting possible coronary ischemia should be risk-stratified based on the probability of having an acute coronary syndrome (ACS). Patients with a low-probability ACS have no objective evidence of acute coronary ischemia or infarction. These patients do not have characteristic ST-segment elevation or depression on an electrocardiogram (ECG), and initial cardiac biomarkers are not elevated.

CLINICAL FEATURES

After performing an initial history and physical examination, an emergency provider needs to determine how much of a diagnostic evaluation to undertake for a patient presenting with chest pain. Approximately 3% to 6% of patients with an initial diagnosis of noncardiac chest pain or another alternative diagnosis may later develop a short-term adverse cardiac event, making risk stratification an important aspect of clinical decision making.

Among patients who are assessed as low-probability for ACS, aspects that have been shown to be associated with a low-risk profile include chest pain that is described as pleuritic, positional, sharp, stabbing, or that is found to be reproducible. High-risk historical features include chest pain that radiates to the arm or shoulders, is exertional, described as pressure, is accompanied by nausea or diaphoresis, or is similar to prior cardiac pain. However, even patients who present with atypical features may have some risk, and the absence of high-risk features alone cannot completely exclude the possibility of ACS. Significant coronary artery disease is rare in patients <30 years old, although age alone does not completely eliminate ACS as a cause of acute chest pain. In addition, treatment responsiveness to nitrates, antacids, or nonsteroidal anti-inflammatory medications cannot reliably confirm or exclude ACS. Focus the initial evaluation to identify potential alternative diagnoses and detect findings that may be consistent with heart failure or other underlying conditions.

The results and timing of previous cardiac testing, such as ECG, stress test, and cardiac catheterization, can be helpful to consider when determining the appropriate evaluation for possible ACS. For example, new ECG changes consistent with cardiac ischemia offer strong evidence of underlying cardiac disease. Conversely, a recent negative cardiac catheterization with no coronary luminal irregularities is associated with a very low incidence of myocardial infarction or ACS within a 2-year period. Previous stress test results can add evidence to the clinician's diagnostic decision making, but cannot confirm the presence or absence of disease.

DIAGNOSIS AND DIFFERENTIAL

The evaluation of patients presenting to the ED with possible ACS can be conceptualized into primary and secondary assessments (see Fig. 20-1). The goal of the primary evaluation is to identify patients with definite ACS

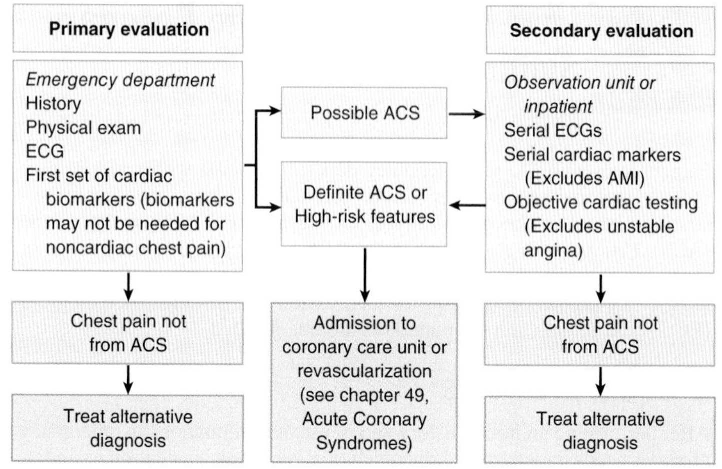

FIGURE 20-1. Evaluation process for patients with possible acute coronary syndrome (ACS). AMI, acute myocardial infarction.

and differentiate them from those with probable or possible ACS. Identifying patients with alternative causes of chest pain that are unlikely to be ACS should also be considered (see Chapter 17).

The primary evaluation for patients with suspected ACS includes a detailed history, physical examination, ECG, chest radiography as indicated, and cardiac biomarkers. Serial ECGs can be helpful in further evaluating patients with ongoing symptoms or changes in condition. Data obtained from this primary survey should be used to further risk-stratify patients presenting to the ED with possible ACS. Some experts have determined that when the pretest probability of ACS is ≤2% further testing is not indicated, whereas others have suggested a threshold of <1% to determine when additional testing is unnecessary.

Upon completion of the primary evaluation, classify patients into one of the following categories of the prognosis-based classification system: acute myocardial infarction (AMI), probable acute ischemia, possible acute ischemia, or definitely not ischemia (see Table 20-1). Patients with probable or possible acute ischemia can be further stratified based on their risk for adverse events using scoring systems such as the TIMI risk score or the HEART pathway based on clinical features, ECG findings, and initial diagnostic testing results. These scoring systems can assist clinicians in determining the extent of additional testing that is recommended.

The secondary assessment can be conducted in an ED, a hospital-based observation unit, or in the inpatient setting. The specific components of this secondary evaluation is informed by appropriate risk stratification. The goal of this assessment should be to exclude both components of ACS: myocardial infarction and unstable angina. In the absence of ST-segment elevation on the ECG, a myocardial infarction is excluded through the use of serial troponin measurements to detect myocardial necrosis. Serum troponin levels can take as long as 8 hours from the time of infarction to

TABLE 20-1 Prognosis-Based Classification System for ED Chest Pain Patients*

I. Acute myocardial infarction: immediate revascularization candidate
II. Probable acute ischemia: high risk for adverse events (any of the following): Evidence of clinical instability (i.e., pulmonary edema, hypotension, arrhythmia, transient mitral regurgitation murmur, diaphoresis) Ongoing pain thought to be ischemic (consider chest pain or discomfort as chief symptom, reproducing documented angina, or pain in setting of known coronary artery disease, including myocardial infarction) Pain at rest associated with ischemic ECG changes (consider new, or presumably new, transient, ST-segment deviation, 1 mm or greater, or T-wave inversion in multiple precordial leads) One or more positive myocardial marker measurements Positive perfusion imaging study
III. Possible acute ischemia: intermediate risk for adverse events. History suggestive of ischemia with absence of high-risk features, and any of the following: Rest pain, now resolved New onset of pain Crescendo pattern of pain Ischemic pattern on ECG not associated with pain (may include ST-segment depression <1 mm or T-wave inversion >1 mm)
IV. Possible acute ischemia: low risk for adverse events. History not strongly suggestive of ischemia and all of the following: ECG normal, unchanged from previous, or nonspecific changes Negative myocardial marker measurement *or (all of the following)* >2 weeks of unchanged symptom pattern or long-standing symptoms with only mild change in exertional pain threshold ECG normal, unchanged from previous, or nonspecific changes Negative initial myocardial marker measurement
V. Definitely not ischemia: very low risk for adverse events. All of the following: Clear evidence of nonischemic symptom etiology ECG normal, unchanged from previous, or nonspecific changes Negative initial myocardial marker measurement† *or* Unstructured clinician estimate of acute coronary syndrome ≤2%

*Authors' analyses from multiple sources.

†Literature not conclusive.

become elevated. Therefore, using cardiac biomarkers to diagnose a myocardial infarction in the absence of dynamic ECG changes should take into account the time from symptom onset and generally include multiple measurements. A modified approach in appropriate low-risk patients is to obtain two troponin measurements, at least 2 hours apart with one measurement at least 6 hours after the onset of pain.

Normal serial cardiac biomarker measurements reduce the likelihood of AMI but do not exclude unstable angina. Patients with a continued suspicion for ACS despite negative biomarkers often undergo some form of advanced cardiac testing. Common modalities of advanced cardiac testing include exercise or pharmacologically induced ECG stress test, stress echocardiography, nuclear imaging, cardiac magnetic resonance imaging

(MRI), computed tomography coronary angiography (CTCA), or cardiac catheterization. Based on risk stratification and institutional resources, some patients will undergo this type of testing during the initial hospitalization. However, additional testing as an outpatient is an option for low-risk patients in whom AMI has been excluded.

The use of advanced cardiac testing should be guided by general principles discussed below along with available resources and institutional practice patterns:

1. Cardiac imaging with CTCA may play a role in the evaluation of low-risk patients presenting with chest pain, as this approach can result in a more rapid and cost-effective diagnosis than stress myocardial perfusion imaging.
2. Noninvasive stress testing is often recommended for patients risk-stratified as low to intermediate risk. Treadmill exercise testing may be useful in patients who are able to exercise. In patients with physical limitations, pharmacologic stress testing may be necessary.
3. When stress testing is ordered, select a method of cardiac assessment such as electrocardiography, nuclear imaging, echocardiography, or magnetic resonance imaging. Selection from these options is often based on local practice, institutional expertise, and resource availability.
   a. ECG-based exercise treadmill testing is the least costly and most widely available but has the lowest sensitivity (68%) of the imaging options which may limit its use for high-risk patients. In addition, ECG-based exercise treadmill testing should not be used in patients with abnormal baseline ECGs due to difficulties in interpretation.
   b. Stress echocardiography has the advantages of no radiation exposure, improved sensitivity (80%), and wide availability.
   c. Nuclear imaging is also widely available, allows assessment of myocardial perfusion, and has high accuracy. However, there is associated radiation exposure and radioisotope-related delays.
   d. Cardiac MRI is also highly accurate and does not expose patients to radiation, but is less widely available.

EMERGENCY DEPARTMENT CARE AND DISPOSITION

The evaluation and treatment of patients with suspected ACS is typically initiated prior to either confirmation or exclusion of this condition. If an alternative diagnosis is confirmed and ACS is excluded, treatment should begin for the alternative diagnosis. Treat patients with suspected ACS as follows:

1. Provide supplemental **oxygen** via nasal cannula or as needed to maintain appropriate pulse oxygenation.
2. Administer **aspirin** 160 to 325 mg orally.
3. Provide **nitroglycerin** 0.4 mg spray or sublingual to treat suspected ischemic chest pain. Intravenous nitroglycerin may be used for patients with persistent ischemic chest pain unrelieved by other methods. Nitroglycerin paste applied to the skin is an alternative to intravenous nitroglycerin in patients without ongoing or recurrent ischemia.
4. Consider **morphine** 1 to 5 mg IV in patients with persistent ischemic chest pain.

5. Prescribe **metoprolol** 25 to 50 mg PO in the first 24 hours when ACS is suspected.
6. Antiplatelet and/or anticoagulant therapy may be appropriate for patients with definitive or likely ACS. The decision to administer these medications and specific doses may be institution-specific based on protocols or guidelines and are balanced with the patient's bleeding risk. These decisions may be determined through multidisciplinary discussions. These options include (a) dual antiplatelet therapy: a common regimen is **clopidogrel** 300 to 600 mg PO in addition to aspirin, (b) antithrombin therapy: common regimens are **heparin** 60 U/kg IV bolus (maximum bolus 4000 units) with 12 U/kg/h IV infusion (maximum infusion 1000 U/h) or **enoxaparin** 1 mg/kg SC every 12 hours.
7. Selected patients can be managed primarily in the ED or within a dedicated ED Observation Unit. Appropriately risk-stratified patients with negative serial cardiac markers, without diagnostic ECG changes, and who have normal advanced cardiac testing (when indicated) are unlikely to have ACS as a cause of their symptoms. Evaluate for alternative diagnoses and recommend appropriate close follow-up resources.
8. Patients with positive cardiac markers, diagnostic ECG changes, or positive diagnostic testing suggesting ACS should receive appropriate consultation and admission to the hospital for inpatient management.

FURTHER READING

For further reading in *Tintinalli's Emergency Medicine: A Comprehensive Study Guide*, 8th ed., see Chapter 51, "Low-Probability Acute Coronary Syndromes," by Kathleen A. Hosmer and Chadwick D. Miller.

CHAPTER 21

Syncope

Jo Anna Leuck

Syncope accounts for up to 2% of all emergency department (ED) visits and 6% of hospital admissions. Syncope is defined as a transient loss of consciousness accompanied by loss of postural tone, followed by complete resolution without intervention. Although syncope often is a benign vasovagal event, it may represent a life-threatening dysrhythmia or other condition, particularly in the elderly. Near-syncope, or feeling an impending loss of consciousness without syncope, may carry the same risk as syncope. In up to half of syncope cases presenting to the ED, there is no definite etiology established for the syncopal episode.

CLINICAL FEATURES

Cardiac-related syncope can be due to a structural cardiac lesion that limits the heart's ability to appropriately increase cardiac output. Examples of structural cardiac disease that can cause syncope include hypertrophic cardiomyopathy, aortic stenosis, pulmonary embolism, and myocardial infarction. Tachydysrhythmias such as ventricular tachycardia, torsades des pointes, and supraventricular tachycardia are common causes of syncope, but bradycardic syndromes may cause it as well. Syncope from a dysrhythmia is typically sudden and without prodrome. In young people, familial dysrhythmias such as Brugada or QT syndromes are uncommon but potentially serious causes of syncope.

Syncope is most commonly caused by vasovagal reflexes. Inappropriate vagal or sympathetic tone may lead to bradycardia, hypotension, or both. The hallmark of vasovagal syncope is a slow progressive prodrome of dizziness, nausea, pallor, diaphoresis, and diminished vision. The history should include a search for possible stimuli that are known to be associated with vasovagal syncope, such as phlebotomy, prolonged standing in a warm place, or fear. In situational syncope, the autonomic reflexive response results from a specific physical stimulus such as micturition, defecation, or extreme coughing. Carotid sinus hypersensitivity is another type of reflex-mediated syncope that is suggested by a history of presyncope when shaving, head-turning, or wearing of a constricting collar. This should be considered as a potential cause in elderly patients with recurrent syncope despite a negative cardiac workup.

Orthostatic syncope occurs when a sudden change in posture after recumbence is associated with inadequate compensatory increases in heart rate and peripheral vascular resistance. Orthostatic syncope can be due to decreased intravascular volume or poor vascular tone, which has a myriad of potential causes such as peripheral neuropathy, spinal cord injury, or medication side-effects. Since orthostatic changes can also be associated with other serious illnesses, alternative causes of syncope should still be considered even in the presence of orthostatic changes in blood pressure.

Neurologic syncope is rarely the primary cause of syncopal episodes, as patients with loss of consciousness with persistent neurological deficits or altered mental status do not meet the usual diagnostic criteria for syncope. When brainstem ischemia or vertebrobasilar insufficiency is the cause of syncope, patients will often report other posterior circulation deficits such as diplopia, vertigo, focal neurological deficits, or nausea associated with the syncopal episode. If patients report that upper extremity exercise preceded the event, there may be intermittent obstruction of the brachiocephalic or subclavian artery such as subclavian steal syndrome. Subarachnoid hemorrhage may also present with syncope, but it is usually accompanied by persistent symptoms such as headache. A traumatic subarachnoid hemorrhage can also occur as a result of injuries associated with syncope from another cause. Seizure is the most common disorder mistaken for syncope. Brief tonic-clonic movements are often seen with syncope, but the presence of a postictal state, tongue biting, incontinence, or an epileptic aura can point toward seizure as a more likely alternative diagnosis.

Medication-induced syncope can be a common complication of pharmacotherapy. Because of poor autonomic responses and multiple medications, the elderly are particularly prone to syncope as a side effect of medication use. Cardiovascular responses to orthostatic or vasodilatory challenges may be blunted by antihypertensive agents such as β-blockers and calcium channel antagonists. Cardiovascular medications may also cause conduction abnormalities or life-threatening dysrhythmias. Diuretics also contribute to the risk of orthostatic hypotension due to their volume-depleting effect.

DIAGNOSIS AND DIFFERENTIAL

Although an etiology for a syncopal episode may be difficult to establish, the most important components of the syncope workup are a comprehensive history, physical examination, and ECG. From there, risk stratification is a practical approach. The history should be directed to high-risk factors, including age, medications, and prodromal associations. Sudden events that occur without warning suggest dysrhythmias, while preceding exertion may imply a structural cardiopulmonary lesion. Associated symptoms such as palpitations or chest pains may suggest an underlying cardiac etiology, while vertigo or focal weakness can point toward a neurologic cause. Back or abdominal pain may suggest a leaking abdominal aortic aneurysm or ruptured ectopic pregnancy in the appropriate patient populations. Single-vehicle crashes or trauma in the absence of defensive injuries may prompt a consideration of syncope as a precipitating event. The medical history is useful in revealing likely cardiac or psychiatric causes for syncope. When present, a family history of cardiac disease or sudden death may also be informative.

Physical examination may occasionally reveal the cause of syncope. The cardiac examination may uncover a ventricular flow obstruction or a cardiac murmur suggestive of aortic stenosis or hypertrophic cardiomyopathy. Consider obtaining orthostatic vital sign measurements, as orthostatic hypotension with a systolic blood pressure drop of at least 20 mm Hg upon standing may support a diagnosis of vasovagal syncope. A significant blood pressure differential between upper extremities (>20 mm Hg) suggests subclavian steal syndrome as a possible etiology. In appropriate circumstances, a complete neurologic assessment or stool guaiac testing may yield information about secondary causes for syncope.

An ECG should be obtained for patients with syncope to assess for signs of ischemia or dysrhythmia. Suggestive ECG findings include prolonged QT interval, which may indicate a propensity for torsades des pointes, or PR interval shortening with a delta wave diagnostic for Wolf–Parkinson–White syndrome. Prolonged cardiac monitoring may show a transient recurrent dysrhythmia. Laboratory testing should be selective based on history and physical examination. An abnormal hemoglobin level in a patient with symptoms suggestive of anemia may explain orthostatic syncope and direct further workup. Women of childbearing age warrant a pregnancy test. Although not recommended routinely, serum electrolytes may be helpful in limited cases. If a patient is asymptomatic or does not have trauma, neuroimaging is not typically indicated in the routine workup of syncope.

EMERGENCY DEPARTMENT CARE AND DISPOSITION

By definition, syncope results in spontaneous recovery of consciousness. Therefore, the main goal of ED care is to identify those patients at risk for further medical problems.

1. Patients with an established medical condition leading to syncope, such as cardiac dysrhythmia, pulmonary embolism, or GI bleeding, can be appropriately managed by appropriately treating the underlying diagnosis. Patients for whom a life-threatening etiology is identified, including those with cardiac or neurologic causes, warrant admission.
2. Patients with unclear diagnoses who are at high-risk for morbidity and mortality are those for whom there is concern about sudden cardiac death or ventricular dysrhythmia. Per the San Francisco Syncope Rule and other studies, features that suggest a risk for adverse events include abnormal ECG, complaint of shortness of breath, systolic blood pressure of <90 mm Hg on arrival, hematocrit <30%, age older than 45 years, or a history of ventricular dysrhythmia or congestive heart failure. Consider admission for patients determined to be at higher risk to monitor for cardiac arrhythmias and to facilitate an expedited workup.
3. Patients with unclear diagnoses who are at low-risk are unlikely to have a cardiac etiology for their syncope. These patients lack the high-risk criteria noted above, tend to be young with few comorbidities, and have a normal physical examination and ECG. Low-risk patients can be safely discharged home with instructions for outpatient follow-up and to return for any recurrence of syncope or nearsyncopal symptoms.
4. Additional factors to consider when making inpatient versus outpatient decisions may include syncope while supine or during exercise, absence of prodromal symptoms, palpitations, or elderly patients.

FURTHER READING

For further reading in *Tintinalli's Emergency Medicine: A Comprehensive Study Guide*, 8th ed., see Chapter 52, "Syncope," by James Quinn.

CHAPTER 22 Acute Heart Failure

Lori J. Whelan

Acute heart failure covers a wide spectrum of illness, with symptoms ranging from a gradual increase in leg swelling, shortness of breath, or decreased exercise tolerance to the abrupt onset of pulmonary edema and respiratory distress. While the term congestive heart failure was historically used to describe volume overload, current terminology describes patients as having acute heart failure when they present with an acute exacerbation of chronic heart failure or when new-onset heart failure is diagnosed. Heart failure has a poor prognosis with an approximately 50% mortality rate within 5 years of initial diagnosis. The most common precipitating factors of acute heart failure are atrial fibrillation, acute myocardial infarction or ischemia, discontinuation of medications (diuretics), increased sodium load, drugs that impair myocardial function, and physical overexertion.

CLINICAL FEATURES

No single historical or physical finding is sensitive and specific enough to accurately diagnose acute heart failure in all patients. On physical examination, patients with acute heart failure may present with dyspnea, frothy pink sputum, or respiratory distress. Patients are frequently tachycardic and hypertensive, and a third heart sound (S3) may be identified on auscultation. Abdominojugular reflux and jugular venous distension may also be seen.

Acute heart failure can be further classified as follows:

1. **Hypertensive acute heart failure** is characterized by signs and symptoms of acute heart failure with relatively preserved left ventricular function, systolic blood pressure >140 mmHg, a chest radiograph compatible with pulmonary edema, and symptom onset less than 48 hours.
2. **Pulmonary edema** presents with respiratory distress, rales on chest auscultation, reduced oxygen saturation from baseline, and characteristic chest radiograph findings.
3. **Cardiogenic shock** is characterized by evidence of tissue hypoperfusion and systolic blood pressure <90 mmHg.
4. **Acute-on-chronic heart failure** has signs and symptoms of acute heart failure that are mild to moderate and do not meet criteria for hypertensive heart failure, pulmonary edema, or cardiogenic shock. Systolic blood pressure is typically <140 mmHg and >90 mmHg, associated with increased peripheral edema, and has symptom onset over several days.
5. **High-output failure** presents with high cardiac output, tachycardia, warm extremities, and pulmonary congestion.
6. **Right heart failure** is a low-output syndrome with jugular venous distention, hepatomegaly, and variable hypotension.

DIAGNOSIS AND DIFFERENTIAL

Commonly, patients with acute heart failure present with dyspnea and the differential diagnosis may include other conditions such as COPD, asthma, pneumonia, pneumothorax, pleural effusion, pulmonary embolus, and acute coronary syndrome. There is no single diagnostic test for heart failure; it is a clinical diagnosis based on the history, physical examination, and diagnostic testing. The most useful historical parameter is a history of acute heart failure. The symptom with the highest sensitivity for diagnosis is dyspnea on exertion (84%) and the most specific symptoms are paroxysmal nocturnal dyspnea, orthopnea, and edema (77% to 84%).

Chest radiographs showing pulmonary venous congestion, cardiomegaly, and interstitial edema are the most specific for a diagnosis of acute heart failure, although up to 20% of patients may have an initially negative CXR. ECG is not useful for diagnosis, although it may reveal an underlying cause or precipitant. BNP (B-type natriuretic peptide/*N*-terminal B-type natriuretic peptide) testing is useful to supplement provider assessment when diagnostic uncertainty exists. Bedside cardiac ultrasound may be useful to determine other causes for acute dyspnea, such as cardiac tamponade, and may also be useful to determine left ventricle function and volume status or identify signs of pulmonary congestion. These ancillary tests combined with an appropriate history and physical can help determine the likelihood of acute heart failure.

EMERGENCY DEPARTMENT CARE AND DISPOSITION

1. Provide supplemental **oxygen** to keep saturations above 95%.
2. Consider noninvasive ventilation with continuous positive airway pressure (CPAP) or bilevel positive airway pressure (BiPAP). Ensure adequate facemask seal, hemodynamic stability, and close monitoring for adequate tidal volumes, patient cooperation, and effectiveness.
3. While many patients with hypertensive acute heart failure present with severe hypertension, pulmonary edema can occur with systolic blood pressures as low as 150 mmHg. Prompt recognition of this condition and afterload reduction with vasodilators can improve symptoms and avoid the need for emergent intubation.
4. Administer **nitroglycerin** 0.4 mg sublingual up to one dose per minute or **nitroglycerin** 0.5 to 0.7 μg/kg/min IV up to 200 μg/min. Titrate dosages based on patient symptoms blood pressure levels.
5. **Nitroprusside** 0.3 μg/kg/min titrated upward every 5 to 10 minutes as needed to maximum 10 μg/kg/min may be initiated if elevated blood pressure is unresponsive to nitroglycerin.
6. When volume overload is suspected, consider loop diuretics such as **furosemide** 40 mg IV, **bumetanide** 1 to 3 mg IV, or **torsemide** 10 to 20 mg IV.
7. Shortness of breath, orthopnea, jugular venous distention, rales and possibly an S3 may be evident in patients with normotensive heart failure, even in the presence of normal vital signs, oxygen and ventilation. For these patients, treat with loop diuretics initially and then base additional treatment on responses to therapy.
8. Transient hypotension may develop after nitroglycerin is started. This may be due to marked clinical improvement, and should improve with decreasing the dose or discontinuing nitroglycerin. If hypotension persists, initiate an IV fluid bolus 250 to 1000 cc and consider causes such as right ventricular infarction, valvular pathology such as severe aortic stenosis, hypovolemia, or recent use of medications for erectile dysfunction

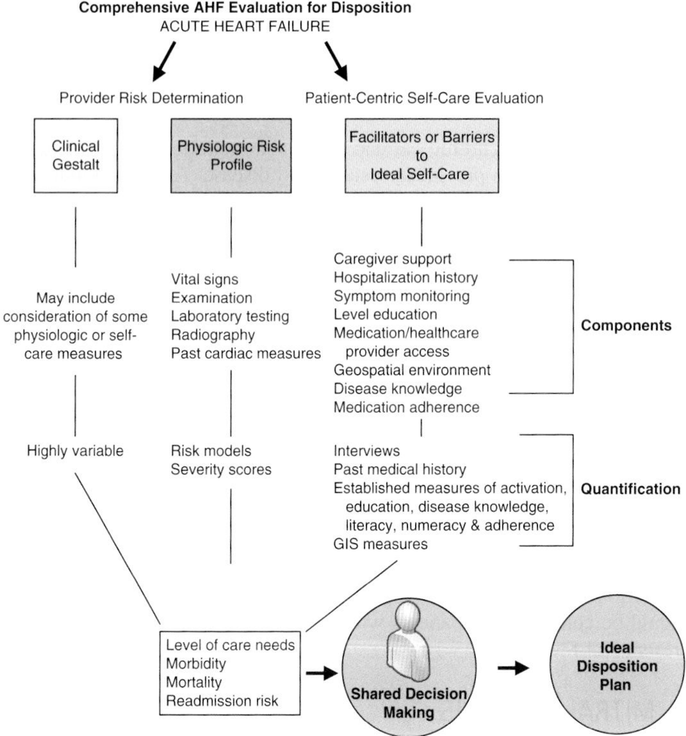

FIGURE 22-1. Factors impacting disposition decisions in ED patients with acute heart failure.

9. **Morphine** 2 to 5 mg IV can relieve congestion and anxiety but is associated with adverse events such as need for mechanical ventilation, prolonged hospitalization, ICU admission, and mortality.
10. For hypotensive patients or patients in need of additional inotropic support, see Chapter 19, "Cardiogenic Shock," for management recommendations.
11. Identify high-risk patient characteristics for severe illness that may require intensive care unit admission such as altered mental status, persistent hypoxia, hypotension, troponin elevation, ischemic ECG changes, BUN >43, creatinine >2.75, tachypnea, or inadequate urine output.
12. See Fig. 22-1 for some of the many factors to consider when making disposition decisions for outpatient management, observation care, inpatient admission, or need for intensive care for patients with acute heart failure.

FURTHER READING

For further reading in *Tintinalli's Emergency Medicine: A Comprehensive Study Guide*, 8th ed., see Chapter 53, "Acute Heart Failure," by Sean P. Collins and Alan B.Storrow.

CHAPTER 23

Valvular Emergencies

Boyd Burns

Many patients with chronic cardiac valve abnormalities who present for emergency care have previously established disease. Acute valvular dysfunction can present with significant symptoms, and emergency physicians must be alert to the presenting signs and symptoms to identify the undiagnosed patient. With bedside echocardiography becoming more commonly available, the initial diagnosis of valvular disease may become more common in the ED.

THE NEWLY DISCOVERED MURMUR

When an emergency provider identifies a new murmur on exam, the first step in the ED is to determine the potential clinical significance of this finding. Benign murmurs are not likely to cause symptoms and may be found incidentally. These are typically soft systolic ejection murmurs and occur after S_1 and end before S_2 and are not associated with specific symptoms. In contrast, a new diastolic murmur or a new systolic murmur with symptoms at rest warrants emergent echocardiographic imaging and further evaluation. In addition, risks for possible infections such as endocarditis should be considered in patients with a newly discovered murmur and the presence of fever (Fig. 23-1).

MITRAL STENOSIS

Clinical Features

Mitral stenosis prevents normal diastolic filling of the left ventricle, and dyspnea with exertion is the most common presenting symptom. In the past, hemoptysis was the second most common presenting symptom, but this is less common now that patients are typically diagnosed and treated earlier in the disease course. As the obstructive process progresses, left atrial pressures rise and lead to left atrial enlargement and symptoms of heart failure. Systemic emboli may develop, especially when accompanied by atrial fibrillation, and can result in myocardial, kidney, central nervous system, or peripheral infarction. Most patients with mitral stenosis eventually develop atrial fibrillation due to progressive dilatation of the atria. The classic murmur of mitral stenosis and associated signs are listed in Table 23-1.

Diagnosis and Differential

In the presence of mitral stenosis, the electrocardiogram (ECG) may demonstrate notched or diphasic P waves and right axis deviation. On the chest radiograph, straightening of the left heart border is a typical early radiographic finding suggestive of left atrial enlargement. Later in the illness, findings of pulmonary congestion develop, such as redistribution of flow to the upper lung fields, Kerley B lines, and an increase in vascular markings.

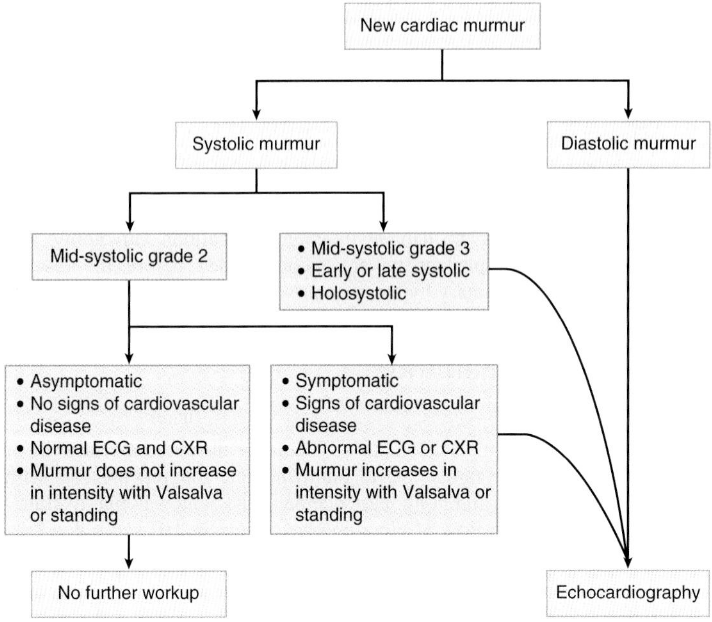

FIGURE 23-1. Algorithm for evaluation of newly discovered systolic murmur. CXR, chest x-ray.

The diagnosis of mitral stenosis is confirmed with echocardiography. The urgency for an accurate diagnosis and appropriate referral depends on the severity of symptoms and initial management will typically focus on symptom control.

TABLE 23-1 Comparison of Heart Murmurs, Sounds, and Signs

Mitral stenosis	Mid-diastolic rumble, crescendos into S_2	Loud snapping S_1, small apical impulse, tapping due to under-filled ventricle
Mitral regurgitation	Acute: harsh apical systolic murmur starts with S_1 and may end before S_2 Chronic: high-pitched apical holosystolic murmur radiating into S_2	S_3 and S_4 may be heard
Mitral valve prolapse	Click may be followed by a late systolic murmur that crescendos into S_2	Mid-systolic click; S_2 may be diminished by the late systolic murmur
Aortic stenosis	Harsh systolic ejection murmur	Paradoxical splitting of S_2, S_3, and S_4 may be present; pulse of small amplitude with a slow rise and sustained peak
Aortic regurgitation	High-pitched blowing diastolic murmur immediately after S_2	S_3 may be present; wide pulse pressure

Emergency Department Care and Disposition

1. Heart rate control is typically necessary for patients with persistent tachycardia and dyspnea who have atrial fibrillation with rapid ventricular response.
2. Anticoagulation is recommended for patients who have an atrial diameter greater than 55 mm, atrial fibrillation, left atrial thrombus, or a history of embolic disease.
3. Patients with asymptomatic mitral stenosis should be referred for outpatient evaluation, as mechanical intervention, balloon valvotomy, and valve repair or replacements are recommended before the disease progresses to pulmonary hypertension.

MITRAL REGURGITATION

Clinical Features

Acute mitral regurgitation secondary to rupture of the chordae tendineae or papillary muscles (or rarely due to blunt thoracic trauma) presents with dyspnea, tachycardia, and pulmonary edema as the acute valvular dysfunction allows retrograde flow of blood to occur from the left ventricle to the left atrium. These patients may quickly develop cardiogenic shock or cardiac arrest. Intermittent mitral regurgitation usually presents with acute episodes of respiratory distress due to pulmonary edema and may be asymptomatic between attacks. In contrast, chronic mitral regurgitation may be tolerated by patients for many years without specific treatment. In these cases, the first symptom is usually dyspnea with exertion that is sometimes precipitated by new-onset atrial fibrillation. If patients are not appropriately anticoagulated, systemic emboli may occur in up to 20% of patients and may initially be asymptomatic. The classic murmur and signs of mitral regurgitation are listed in Table 23-1.

Diagnosis and Differential

Consider mitral regurgitation in a patient without significant cardiomegaly who presents with new onset and marked pulmonary edema. In an acute valvular rupture, the ECG may show evidence of acute inferior wall infarction or ischemia. On chest radiography, acute mitral regurgitation from papillary muscle rupture may result in a minimally enlarged left atrium and pulmonary edema. In chronic disease, the ECG may demonstrate findings of left atrial and left ventricular hypertrophy associated with corresponding enlargement visible on chest radiography.

Echocardiography can confirm the diagnosis, and bedside testing may be needed in an acutely ill patient. While transthoracic echocardiography can help to make the diagnosis, this technique may underestimate lesion severity. Therefore, transesophageal echo should be used for definitive diagnostic purposes when a patient is stable and able to have this testing completed.

Emergency Department Care and Disposition

1. For acute mitral regurgitation due to papillary muscle rupture, emergent consultation for surgical repair is indicated.

2. **Nitrates** and noninvasive ventilation can be used to provide preload and afterload reduction and to decrease the work of breathing. **Dobutamine** may be used to provide inotropic support when necessary.
3. In severe cases, **aortic balloon counterpulsation** can be utilized to increase forward flow and mean arterial pressure while decreasing the severity of the regurgitation. This approach may be necessary to stabilize patients prior to emergent surgical repair.

MITRAL VALVE PROLAPSE

Clinical Features

Most patients with mitral valve prolapse are asymptomatic. When symptoms do occur, patients may report atypical chest pain, palpitations, fatigue, and dyspnea. The abnormal heart sounds are listed in Table 23-1. In patients with mitral valve prolapse who do not have mitral regurgitation at rest, exercise can provoke mitral regurgitation in about one-third of patients and is associated with a higher risk for morbid events.

Diagnosis and Differential

This diagnosis is unlikely to be made in the ED as the ECG and chest x-ray are usually normal. Echocardiography is recommended nonemergently to confirm the clinical diagnosis of mitral valve prolapse and to identify any associated mitral regurgitation. Echocardiography or consultation with a cardiologist can be performed on an outpatient basis and specific ED treatment for this conditionis rarely required.

Emergency Department Care and Disposition

1. Acute treatment for mitral valve prolapse is rarely required.
2. Patients with mitral valve prolapse who also have concomitant mitral regurgitation should receive recommendations for endocarditis prophylaxis.
3. Patients with palpitations attributed to mitral valve prolapse may be prescribed β-blocker therapy to provide symptomatic relief.

AORTIC STENOSIS

Clinical Features

Aortic stenosis presents an obstruction to left ventricular outflow. In the United Sates, the most common cause in adults is degenerative calcification associated with increasing age, hypertension, smoking, elevated cholesterol, and diabetes. The classic triad of symptoms is dyspnea, chest pain, and syncope. Dyspnea is usually the first symptom to appear, followed by paroxysmal nocturnal dyspnea, syncope on exertion, angina, and myocardial infarction. The classic murmur and associated signs of aortic stenosis are listed in Table 23-1. Blood pressure is typically normal or low, with a narrow pulse pressure.

Brachioradial delay is often present in aortic stenosis. To evaluate for this finding, the examiner palpates simultaneously the right brachial artery and the right radial artery of the patient, and any palpable delay is considered abnormal. Because patients with aortic stenosis are very preload dependent, the presence of atrial fibrillation may have significant consequences, as the absence of effective atrial contraction leads to a drop in cardiac output. This can lead to hypotension, especially when patients are treated with nitroglycerin for chest pain or dyspnea.

Diagnosis and Differential

Electrocardiogram and chest radiographic findings lack sensitivity and specificity for aortic stenosis. The ECG often demonstrates criteria for LVH and may have a left or right bundle branch block in up to 10% of patients. The chest radiograph is normal early, but eventually LVH and findings of congestive heart failure will develop if the patient does not have valve replacement. Transthoracic echocardiography can confirm the suspected diagnosis of aortic stenosis and determine disease severity.

Emergency Department Care and Disposition

1. Positive pressure ventilation and supplemental oxygen can be helpful in the treatment of pulmonary edema.
2. Negative inotropic drugs and vasodilators are often poorly tolerated and should be used with caution.
3. New-onset atrial fibrillation may require cardioversion to maintain cardiac output.
4. Patients discharged from the ED should avoid vigorous activity and be promptly seen in follow-up by a cardiologist.

AORTIC REGURGITATION

Clinical Features

Aortic regurgitation occurs when valve leaflets do not fully close and result in retrograde flow of blood from the aorta into the left ventricle during diastole. In acute disease, dyspnea from pulmonary edema is the most common presenting symptom. Patients may also complain of fever and chills when endocarditis is the underlying cause. Dissection of the ascending aorta that impacts the function of the aortic valve typically produces a "tearing" chest pain that may radiate between the shoulder blades. The classic murmur and signs of aortic regurgitation are listed in Table 23-1. Tachycardia develops in an attempt to maintain cardiac output in the setting of acute aortic regurgitation, although this may be inadequate and cardiogenic shock or arrest may occur.

Chronic aortic regurgitation typically presents with gradually worsening fatigue or dyspnea with exertion. Signs include a wide pulse pressure with a prominent ventricular impulse, and may be associated with head bobbing. A "water hammer pulse" characterized by a quick rise in peripheral pulse upstroke followed by a rapid collapse may also be present. Other classic findings may include an accentuated precordial apical thrust, pulsus bisferiens, a "to-and-fro" femoral murmur (Duroziez sign), and capillary pulsations visible at the proximal nailbed while pressure is applied at the tip (Quincke sign).

Diagnosis and Differential

In patients with acute aortic regurgitation, the chest radiograph demonstrates acute pulmonary edema with less cardiac enlargement than may be expected. When an aortic dissection is the underlying cause, a chest x-ray may demonstrate a widened mediastinum and prompt ordering of a CT of the chest with IV contrast. ECG changes that may be seen with aortic dissection include ischemia or findings of acute inferior myocardial infarction suggesting right coronary artery involvement.

In chronic aortic regurgitation, the ECG demonstrates LVH, and the chest radiograph may demonstrate LVH, aortic dilation, and/or evidence of congestive heart failure. Echocardiography is used to confirm the diagnosis and severity of valvular regurgitation. Bedside transthoracic echocardiography can be undertaken to further evaluate an unstable patient who may need emergency surgery. Otherwise, transesophageal echocardiography is recommended when aortic dissection is suspected to more completely evaluate the aorta and valvular function.

Emergency Department Care and Disposition

1. Patients with acute aortic regurgitation should have immediate surgical consultation for repair.
2. Treat pulmonary edema with oxygen and noninvasive ventilation, and prepare for intubation in the setting of respiratory failure. Diuretics and nitrates are typically ineffective.
3. **Nitroprusside** when used in combination with inotropic agents such as **dobutamine** or **dopamine** can reduce left ventricular end-diastolic pressure and augment forward flow.
4. Avoid β-blockers in the setting of acute aortic regurgitation as these can inhibit the reflex tachycardia that is necessary to maintain cardiac output.
5. Intraaortic balloon counterpulsation is contraindicated as it can worsen regurgitant flow.
6. Chronic aortic regurgitation is typically treated with vasodilators such as angiotensin-converting enzyme inhibitors or dihydropyridine calcium channel blockers.

RIGHT-SIDED VALVULAR HEART DISEASE

Pathologic tricuspid regurgitation is typically due to elevated right heart pressures or volume overload, which can be seen in conditions such as pulmonary hypertension, chronic lung disease, pulmonary embolism, and/or atrial septal defects. Acute tricuspid disease is most often found in the setting of acute endocarditis from organisms such as *Staphylococcus aureus*, which can lead to rapid valve destruction.

The pulmonic valve is least affected by acquired disease and most disease present here is congenital. Pulmonary hypertension, rheumatic heart disease, and carcinoid syndrome can all cause some degree of pulmonic valve disease.

Clinical Features

Clinically significant right-sided valvular disease leads to right heart failure symptoms such as jugular venous distension, peripheral edema, hepatomegaly, splenomegaly, and ascites. Dyspnea with exertion is often the first symptom in patients with right-sided valvular disease associated with pulmonary hypertension. Pulmonic stenosis often presents with dyspnea with exertion, syncope, chest pain, and findings consistent with right heart failure.

Diagnosis and Differential

Echocardiography is needed to confirm the diagnosis of right-sided valvular disease, and the transesophageal approach is more sensitive than transthoracic. Chest x-ray and ECG lack sensitivity and specificity, although chest radiography may demonstrate evidence of right atrial enlargement or right ventricular hypertrophy.

Emergency Department Care and Disposition

1. Target treatment of right-sided valvular disease based on the underlying causative disease process.
2. Patients with symptomatic pulmonic or tricuspid stenosis may be candidates for balloon valvotomy, while severe tricuspid regurgitation may require valve replacement.

PROSTHETIC VALVE DISEASE

Prosthetic valves are divided into two major groups: mechanical and bioprosthetic. Mechanical valves are more durable but require lifelong anticoagulation secondary to the thrombotic risk. Bioprosthetic valves, whether from bovine, porcine, or human sources, are less thrombogenic but more likely to fail and require repeat surgical repair.

Systemic thromboembolism is a common complication of mechanical heart valves, and therefore lifelong anticoagulation is recommended. Anticoagulation decreases the thrombotic risk from 8% to 1–2% per year. The risk for embolic complications is highest during the first three postoperative months, and prosthetic mitral valves are more likely than prosthetic aortic valves to produce emboli.

Malfunction of prosthetic valves can occur in many ways including thrombosis, dehiscence of sutures, gradual degeneration, or sudden fracture. Symptom progression is typically gradual except in acute failure, which can present with an acute onset of respiratory distress, pulmonary edema, and cardiogenic shock. Infectious complications of endocarditis carry a high mortality rate and occur in 6% of patients within 5 years of surgery.

Clinical Features

The replacement of a diseased or damaged valve relieves the obstruction or regurgitation that had developed, but any cardiac remodeling that occurred over time due to the abnormal valve will remain and can lead to chronic symptoms. Many patients will have continued dyspnea or other symptoms of heart failure because of the long-standing volume or pressure overload. These patients are also likely to have comorbid conditions such as coronary artery disease, systemic hypertension or atrial fibrillation.

Thromboembolism from a prosthetic valve source may cause transient neurologic symptoms, ischemic stroke, or ischemic episodes in an affected extremity or organ. Although anticoagulation can minimize the risks of thromboembolism, this is associated with its own potential complications from increased bleeding risks such as hemorrhagic stroke.

Acute failure of a prosthetic valve presents with acute respiratory distress, pulmonary edema, and cardiogenic shock and can be caused by mechanical valve failure, tearing of a bioprothesis, or presence of a large obstructive clot preventing proper closure of the valve. An acute valve failure often results in sudden death before emergent corrective surgery can be performed. A paravalvular leak may present with new congestive failure symptoms with severity based on the degree of the leak.

Diagnosis and Differential

Patients with prosthetic valves who present with new or increasing dyspnea on exertion, congestive heart failure, or chest pain are at risk for valvular malfunction. Patients with new neurologic symptoms may have thromboembolic disease or hemorrhagic stroke from excessive anticoagulation. The presence of a persistent fever or fever without a source should prompt concern for endocarditis, as patients with prosthetic valves are at increased risk for this infection.

Emergency Department Care and Disposition

1. The treatment and disposition of prosthetic valve dysfunction varies depending on the acuity, nature, and severity of the symptoms.
2. Emergent consulation with cardiology and cardiothoracic surgery experts is needed when acute prosthetic valve dysfunction is suspected. Emergency surgery or thrombolytic therapy may be required in severe cases.
3. **Aspirin** therapy is recommended for all patients with prosthetic valves. Anticoagulation for mechanical mitral valves requires an INR of 2.5–3.5 while mechanical aortic valves should be anticoagulated to an INR of 2.0–3.0.

FURTHER READING

For further reading in *Tintinalli's Emergency Medicine: A Comprehensive Study Guide*, 8th ed., see Chapter 54, "Valvular Emergencies," by William D. Alley and Simon A. Mahler.

The Cardiomyopathies, Myocarditis, and Pericardial Disease

Lorraine Thibodeau

Cardiomyopathies are the third most prevalent form of heart disease in the United States. Cardiomyopathies alter cardiac structure, myocardial function, and/or electrical conduction. Primary cardiomyopathies principally affect the myocardium and secondary cardiomyopathies are associated with other specific systemic disorders. Cardiomyopathies can be further categorized by systolic and/or diastolic dysfunction.

PRIMARY CARDIOMYOPATHIES WITH SYSTOLIC AND DIASTOLIC DYSFUNCTION

Dilated Cardiomyopathy

Dilated cardiomyopathy is the most common type of cardiomyopathy overall and is usually idiopathic, but may be familial or associated with specific associated causes. Peripartum cardiomyopathy is a form of dilated cardiomyopathy that affects pregnant women from 20 weeks gestation into the postpartum period. Idiopathic dilated cardiomyopathy is characterized by systolic and diastolic dysfunction and is the primary indication for cardiac transplant in the United States.

Clinical Features

Most patients with dilated cardiomyopathy present with signs and symptoms of acute heart failure from systolic pump dysfunction. Symptoms include dyspnea on exertion, orthopnea, and paroxysmal nocturnal dyspnea. Physical findings include rales, dependent edema, an enlarged liver, and a holosystolic murmur. Patients may also present with chest pain which may be a function of limited coronary vascular reserve.

Diagnosis and Differential

Typical chest radiograph and electrocardiogram (ECG) findings can be helpful, but the definitive diagnosis is typically made by echocardiogram. Chest radiographs usually show an enlarged cardiac silhouette, biventricular enlargement, and pulmonary vascular congestion. The ECG often shows left ventricular hypertrophy, left atrial enlargement, Q or QS waves, and poor R wave progression across the precordium. The diagnostic echocardiogram shows a decreased ejection fraction, ventricular enlargement, and increased systolic and diastolic volumes. The differential diagnosis includes acute myocardial infarction, restrictive pericarditis, acute valvular disruption, sepsis, or any other condition that results in a low cardiac output state.

Emergency Department Care and Disposition

Patients with symptomatic or newly diagnosed dilated cardiomyopathy typically require admission to a monitored bed or intensive care unit depending on severity of presentation. Patients with known dilated cardiomyopathy benefit from identification of an underlying cause for an exacerbation, including myocardial ischemia, anemia, infection, new-onset atrial fibrillation, bradydysrhythmia, valvular insufficiency, renal dysfunction, pulmonary embolism, or thyroid dysfunction.

1. Establish intravenous access, provide supplemental oxygen, and initiate cardiac monitoring.
2. Standard therapies for the treatment of acute heart failure should be employed. Guidelines from the American College of Cardiology that include issues important for the management of heart failure are available online at http://www.cardiosource.org/Science-And-Quality/Practice-Guidelines-and-Quality-Standards.aspx.
3. Complex ventricular ectopy can be treated with **amiodarone** 150 mg IV over 10 min and then 1 mg/min for 6 hours.
4. Chronic therapy includes diuretics and digoxin, which improve symptoms but have not been shown to impact survival. Angiotensin-converting enzyme (ACE) inhibitors and ß-blockers, such as carvedilol, are often used as they have been shown to improve patient survival.
5. A growing subset of advanced dilated cardiomyopathy patients are treated with Left Ventricular Assist Devices (LVADs) while awaiting heart transplant.

Myocarditis

Myocarditis is a common cause of dilated cardiomyopathy. Myocarditis is an inflammation of the myocardium and may be the result of a systemic disorder or an infectious agent including viral or bacterial etiologies. Pericarditis frequently accompanies myocarditis.

Clinical Features

Systemic signs and symptoms of myocarditis are nonspecific and can include myalgias, headache, rigors, and fever and tachycardia. Chest pain with a coexisting pericarditis is frequently present and may be accompanied by a pericardial friction rub. In severe cases, there may be symptoms of progressive heart failure with dyspnea on exertion, pulmonary rales, pedal edema, and/or cardiogenic shock.

Diagnosis and Differential

ECG may be normal or may demonstrate nonspecific changes such as atrioventricular block, prolonged QRS duration, or ST-segment elevation and PR depression if there is accompanying pericarditis. Chest radiography is typically normal, but may demonstrate pulmonary congestion if symptoms are severe. Cardiac enzymes may be elevated. Differential diagnosis includes cardiac ischemia or infarction, valvular disease, and sepsis.

Emergency Department Care and Disposition

1. Admission with supportive care is the mainstay of treatment for myocarditis.
2. Initiate appropriate antibiotics for patients with suspected bacterial myocarditis.
3. Patients with progressive heart failure symptoms associated with myocarditis may require admission to an ICU setting.

Left Ventricular Assist Devices

In patients with severe cardiomyopathy, LVADs may be used to augment left ventricular output. These devices consist of an implanted pump that transfers blood from the apex of the left ventricle to the proximal aorta. The pump receives its power from an external source (a battery or bedside power unit outside of the body) that is connected to a controller outside of the body. The controller drives the pump via a drive line that connects the pump to the outside battery and controller through a small abdominal wall incision.

Patients and their families usually have extensive training on the devices and should be involved in the evaluation of the LVAD patient. In addition, most patients will carry a card with their LVAD coordinator's contact information in the bag with their spare battery and controller. It is imperative to contact these coordinators as soon as possible to discuss diagnostic and management options.

Clinical Features

Most LVADs now employ pumps that create continuous blood flow to maintain a normal mean arterial pressure. However, because flow is continuous, many LVAD patients may not have a normal palpable pulse. Blood pressure readings can be obtained via Doppler or mechanical cuff. Auscultation reveals heart sounds associated with a whirr from the LVAD pump. The ECG should have discernible QRS complexes. The chest radiograph should show the LVAD components in place.

Emergency Department Care and Disposition

1. Many experts recommend to never perform CPR on an LVAD patient with hemodynamic instability, as chest compressions may dislodge the LVAD causing LV rupture with intractable hemorrhage.
2. Listen to the heart. If the whirr of the pump is heard, go on to step 3. If the whirr is not heard, enlist the patient and family to help search for a cause of mechanical failure and to change the battery and controller, but do not disconnect any of the equipment.
3. If the whirr of the pump is heard, obtain a blood pressure via Doppler or mechanical cuff, place the patient on the monitor, obtain IV access, and administer a bolus of normal saline.
4. Evaluate for the common complications (infection, anemia, bleeding, and thromboembolism). If identified, treat according to the following:
   a. Infection at the abdominal wall outlet for the drive site is treated with antibiotics.

b. Anemia secondary to red cell destruction from the pump or hemorrhage from anticoagulation is treated with blood transfusions as needed.
c. Thromboembolic events (such as pulmonary embolism, mesenteric ischemia, or stroke) are treated with heparin once bleeding has been ruled out.

5. If hypotension persists and/or if right ventricular failure is present, administer pressors to support appropriate hemodynamics.
6. Communication with the LVAD coordinator can be of considerable assistance to augment diagnostic and management strategies for any LVAD patient.

CARDIOMYOPATHIES WITH DIASTOLIC DYSFUNCTION

Hypertrophic Cardiomyopathy

Hypertrophic cardiomyopathy is characterized by asymmetric left ventricular and/or right ventricular hypertrophy primarily involving the intraventricular septum. The result is decreased compliance of the left ventricle leading to impaired diastolic relaxation and diastolic filling. Cardiac output and ejection fraction are usually normal. This condition is often hereditary.

Clinical Features

The type and severity of symptoms depend on age and tend to be more severe as patients get older. Dyspnea on exertion is the most common symptom, followed by chest pain, palpitations, and syncope. Patients may be aware of forceful ventricular contractions as well. Physical exam usually reveals a fourth heart sound and a systolic ejection murmur heard best at the lower left sternal boarder or apex that does not typically radiate to the neck. The examiner may enhance this murmur by having the patient Valsalva or stand, and a decrease in the murmur may be heard with maneuvers that increase LV filling such as squatting and passive leg elevation.

Diagnosis and Differential

The ECG in hypertrophic cardiomyopathy is nonspecific, but often demonstrates left ventricular hypertrophy and left atrial enlargement. Deep S waves may be seen with large septal Q waves (>0.3 mV) and upright T waves. In contrast, inverted T waves can suggest ischemia. Chest radiograph is usually normal. Echocardiography is the diagnostic study of choice and will demonstrate disproportionate septal hypertrophy.

Emergency Department Care and Disposition

Treatment is primarily supportive. Patients with suspected hypertrophic cardiomyopathy should be referred for echocardiographic evaluation.

1. Patients with suspected hypertrophic cardiomyopathy who have syncope should be hospitalized for cardiac monitoring and a thorough evaluation. This presentation can be a precursor to sudden cardiac death.
2. Following definitive diagnosis, ß-blockers, such as **atenolol** 25 to 50 mg orally every day, are the mainstay of treatment for patients with hypertrophic cardiomyopathy and chest pain.

Restrictive Cardiomyopathy

This type of cardiomyopathy is relatively uncommon and can be idiopathic or caused by a number of different etiologies such as sarcoidosis, scleroderma, and amyloidosis. In this disorder, ventricular filling is restricted leading to normal or diminished diastolic volume while systolic function is usually normal.

Clinical Features

The predominant symptoms are dyspnea, orthopnea, and pedal edema that occur without associated cardiomegaly or systolic dysfunction. Chest pain is uncommon. Physical examination is consistent with the degree of disease, and may show a third or fourth heart sound, cardiac gallop, pulmonary rales, jugular venous distension, inspiratory jugular venous distention (Kussmaul's sign), hepatomegaly, pedal edema, or ascites.

Diagnosis and Differential

The ECG is usually nonspecific, but may show conduction disturbances or low voltage in the setting of sarcoidosis or amyloidosis. The chest radiograph may show signs of acute heart failure without cardiomegaly. The differential diagnosis includes constrictive pericarditis and diastolic left ventricular dysfunction. Differentiating between restrictive cardiomyopathy and constrictive pericarditis is important as constrictive pericarditis can be treated surgically.

Emergency Department Care and Disposition

1. Most patients should be admitted for further diagnostic and therapeutic interventions.
2. Direct treatment towards symptom control by using diuretics and ACE inhibitors.
3. Some causes of restrictive cardiomyopathy may have specific treatment therapies, such as corticosteroids for sarcoidosis or chelation for the treatment of hemochromatosis.

Acute Pericarditis

Pericarditis involves inflammation of the layers covering the heart and may be idiopathic or due to infections such as a virus, bacteria, or fungus. Other etiologies include malignancy, drugs, radiation, connective tissue disease, uremia, myxedema, or postmyocardial infarction (Dressler's syndrome).

Clinical Features

The most common symptom of pericarditis is sharp or stabbing precordial or retrosternal chest pain that may radiate to the back, neck, shoulder, or arm. The classic description is pain that is made worse by lying supine, and lessened by sitting up and leaning slightly forward. Movement, swallowing, or inspiration may also aggravate the pain. Radiation to the left trapezial ridge is distinctive. Associated symptoms include recent or current infection, low-grade intermittent fever, dyspnea, and dysphagia. The physical exam is usually normal, but an intermittent friction rub heard best at the lower left sternal border or apex may be present.

Diagnosis and Differential

ECG changes of acute pericarditis and its convalescence have been divided into four stages. Stage 1 demonstrates diffuse ST-segment elevation, especially in leads I, V5, and V6, with PR-segment depression in leads II, aVF, and V4-6. As the disease begins to resolve (stage 2), the ST segments normalize and T-wave amplitudes decrease. In stage 3, T-wave inversion appears in leads previously showing ST elevations. Finally, stage 4 shows resolution of repolarization abnormalities and a return to a normal ECG.

When sequential ECGs are not available, it can be difficult to distinguish pericarditis from a normal variant with "early repolarization." In these cases, the finding of a ST-segment/T-wave amplitude ratio greater than 0.25 in leads I, V5, or V6 is suggestive of acute pericarditis.

Chest x-ray is usually normal but may show an enlarged cardiac silhouette if a large pericardial effusion is present. Echocardiography can be used to assess for the presence of an associated pericardial effusion. Routine laboratory testing may reveal additional abnormalities including an elevated creatine kinase or troponin in the setting of associated myocarditis.

Emergency Department Care and Disposition

1. Stable patients with idiopathic or presumed viral pericarditis can be treated as outpatients with nonsteroidal anti-inflammatory agents, such as **ibuprofen** 600 mg every 6 hours or 800 mg every 8 hours.
2. **Colchicine**, 0.5 mg orally twice a day, may be a beneficial adjuvant and may prevent recurrent episodes.
3. Patients with pericarditis who also have myocarditis, an enlarged cardiac silhouette on chest radiograph, an identified pericardial effusion by echo, uremic pericarditis, or hemodynamic compromise should be admitted into a monitored environment for further care.

Nontraumatic Cardiac Tamponade

When fluid accumulates in the pericardial space and eventually exceeds the filling pressure of the right ventricle, cardiac tamponade occurs resulting in restricted filling and decreased cardiac output. Potential etiologies include uremia, malignant effusion, hemorrhage associated with anticoagulation, bacterial or tubercular infection, chronic pericarditis, lupus, radiation, myxedema, or idiopathic.

Clinical Features

Patients with cardiac tamponade may present with mild to severe shock, and the most common chief complaint is dyspnea. Physical findings can include tachycardia, low systolic blood pressure, and a narrow pulse pressure. Pulsus paradoxus (a drop in systolic pressure greater than 10 mm Hg during normal inspiration), neck vein distention, distant heart sounds, and right upper quadrant pain (due to hepatic congestion) may be present. Pulmonary rales are usually absent.

Diagnosis and Differential

ECG may demonstrate low-voltage QRS complexes and ST elevations with PR depression as in pericarditis. Electrical alternans (beat-to-beat variability in the amplitude of the P and R waves unrelated to inspiratory cycle) is a classic but uncommon finding. Chest radiograph may or may not show an enlarged cardiac silhouette. Bedside ultrasound or echocardiogram is the diagnostic test of choice and demonstrates a large pericardial effusion with right atrium or ventricle diastolic collapse.

Emergency Department Care and Disposition

Cardiac tamponade is a rare and challenging diagnosis and when unrecognized can lead to hypotension and cardiac arrest with pulseless electrical activity (PEA).

1. Initiate resuscitative measures with large bore peripheral IVs, oxygen, and continuous cardiac monitoring.
2. An intravenous fluid bolus of 500 to 1000 mL normal saline can facilitate right heart filling and may temporarily improve patient hemodynamics.
3. When hemodynamics permit, perform pericardiocentesis in the cardiac catheterization lab or coronary care unit under echocardiographic guidance. Emergency pericardiocentesis in the ED may be required if patient is unstable.

Constrictive Pericarditis

Pericardial injury and inflammation can lead to abnormal diastolic filling of the cardiac chambers, which may lead to constrictive pericarditis. Potential causes include fungal or tuberculous pericarditis, uremic pericarditis, postcardiac trauma, and postsurgical changes after pericardiotomy.

Clinical Features

Typical presentations involve the gradual development of symptoms similar to heart failure and restrictive cardiomyopathy. Common signs and symptoms include exertional dyspnea, pedal edema, hepatomegaly, and ascites. Kussmaul's sign (inspiratory neck vein distention) is frequently seen in patients with constrictive pericarditis.

ECG findings are nonspecific, but may include low-voltage QRS complexes and inverted T waves. Chest radiography may demonstrate normal or slightly enlarged cardiac silhouette. Two-dimensional echocardiography is typically not useful, while CT scan, MRI, or Doppler echocardiography can be helpful for making this diagnosis.

Emergency Department Care and Disposition

1. Evaluate ventricular function when making the diagnosis of constrictive pericarditis.
2. Surgical pericardiectomy may be required when significant constriction and impaired ventricular filling are present.

FURTHER READING

For further reading in *Tintinalli's Emergency Medicine: A Comprehensive Study Guide*, 8th ed., see Chapter 55, "Cardiomyopathies and Pericardial Disease," by James T. Niemann.

CHAPTER 25 Venous Thromboembolism

Christopher Kabrhel

Venous thromboembolism (VTE) includes deep vein thrombosis (DVT) and pulmonary embolism (PE). DVT occurs when blood coagulates inside a deep vein such as those in the leg, arm, or pelvis. Most PEs occur when a portion of a venous clot breaks off, travels through the venous system through the right side of the heart, and subsequently enters a pulmonary artery. The clinical presentation of VTE is highly variable, thus clinicians must maintain a high index of suspicion for the diagnosis. Mortality from VTE is variable, with case fatality rates ranging from 1% to 45%, depending on the clinical presentation and comorbid conditions.

CLINICAL FEATURES

There are numerous factors that affect the risk of VTE and the clinical presentation. Factors that increase the risk of VTE include advanced age, obesity, pregnancy, prior VTE, malignancy, inherited thrombophilia, recent surgery or major trauma, immobility, an indwelling central venous catheter, smoking, long-distance travel, congestive heart failure, stroke, estrogen use, and inflammatory conditions.

Deep Vein Thrombosis

Patients with lower extremity DVT often present with calf or leg pain, redness, swelling, tenderness, and warmth. Patients with upper extremity DVT, which often occurs in the setting of an indwelling catheter, present with similar symptoms in an upper extremity. This classic constellation of findings is present in fewer than 50% of DVT patients, and while a 2-cm difference in lower leg circumference is predictive, pain in the calf with forced dorsiflexion of the foot (Homans' sign) is neither sensitive nor specific for DVT.

Uncommon but severe presentations of DVT include *phlegmasia cerulea dolens* and *phlegmasia alba dolens*. *Phlegmasia cerulea dolens* presents as an extremely swollen and cyanotic limb due to a high-grade obstruction that elevates compartment pressures and can compromise limb perfusion. *Phlegmasia alba dolens* has a similar pathophysiology but presents as a pale limb secondary to arterial spasm.

Pulmonary Embolism

The clinical presentation of PE is highly variable, ranging from sudden death to incidental diagnosis in patients who are completely asymptomatic. Consider the possibility of PE in a patient who experiences acute dyspnea, pleuritic chest pain, unexplained tachycardia, hypoxemia, syncope, or shock—especially in the absence of physical examination or radiographic findings for alternative diagnoses. The most common symptoms of an acute PE are dyspnea and pleuritic chest pain. Syncope occurs in 3% to 4% of patients with PE, which can be accompanied by convulsions or seizures. Physical findings that may accompany a PE include hypoxemia, tachypnea, tachycardia, hemoptysis, diaphoresis, and low-grade fever. Clinical signs of DVT occur in about 50% of patients with PE. Massive PE can cause hypotension, severe hypoxemia, or cardiopulmonary arrest. However, the clinical presentation of VTE can be insidious and there may be poor correlation between the size of a PE and the severity of symptoms.

DIAGNOSIS AND DIFFERENTIAL

The extremity pain and swelling associated with DVT are similar to other diagnoses such as cellulitis, congestive heart failure, musculoskeletal injuries, and venous stasis without thrombosis. The differential diagnosis for patients with symptoms concerning for PE may include many other pulmonary disorders, such as asthma, bronchitis, chronic obstructive pulmonary disease, pleural effusion, pneumonia, and pneumothorax. Cardiac disorders with symptoms similar to PE can include angina, myocardial infarction, congestive heart failure, pericarditis, and tachydysrhythmia. Muscle strain and costochondritis can mimic the pleuritic chest pain of PE. The presence of hypoxemia or dyspnea with clear lungs on physical exam and negative radiographic imaging prompt consideration for PE as a possible diagnosis.

Pretest Probability Assessment

Estimating the pretest probability for VTE is the first step for selecting a diagnostic pathway. Aggressive diagnostic testing can cause harm disproportionate to benefit, and therefore specific testing for PE is typically recommended for patients whose probability of disease is higher than 2.5%. Below this threshold, diagnostic testing is more likely to harm than help an individual patient. When a clinician's clinical gestalt after history and physical examination is that an individual patient is low risk for PE, the Pulmonary Embolism Rule-Out Criteria (PERC) rule can help to identify patients for whom specific diagnostic testing is not recommended (Table 25-1).

For patients that may need additional diagnostic testing, there are several clinical scoring systems that can be used to calculate a patient's pretest probability of VTE. The most robust systems are the Wells' Scores for PE and DVT (Tables 25-2 and 25-3).

TABLE 25-1 Pulmonary Embolism Rule-Out Criteria Rule (all nine factors must be present to exclude pulmonary embolism)

Clinical low probability (<15% probability of pulmonary embolism based on gestalt assessment)
Age <50 years
Pulse <100 beats/min during entire stay in ED
Pulse oximetry >94% at near sea level (>92% at altitudes near 5000 feet above sea level)
No hemoptysis
No prior venous thromboembolism history
No surgery or trauma requiring endotracheal or epidural anesthesia within the last 4 weeks
No estrogen use
No unilateral leg swelling, defined as asymmetrical calves on visual inspection with patient's heels raised off the bed

TABLE 25-2 Wells' Score for Pulmonary Embolism

Factors	Points*
Suspected deep venous thrombosis	3
Alternative diagnosis less likely than PE	3
Heart rate >100 beats/min	1.5
Prior venous thromboembolism	1.5
Immobilization within prior 4 weeks	1.5
Active malignancy	1
Hemoptysis	1

*Risk score interpretation (probability of PE): >6 points = high risk (78.4%); 2–6 points = moderate risk (27.8%); and <2 points = low risk (3.4%).

Source: Adapted with permission from Wells PS, Anderson DR, Rodger M, et al. Derivation of a simple clinical model to categorize patients probability of pulmonary embolism: increasing the models utility with the SimpliRED d-dimer. *Thromb Haemost.* 2000;83(3):416–420.

Diagnostic Testing

For patients who need additional testing and have low or intermediate pretest probability, serum D-dimer testing is the recommended initial test. The diagnostic sensitivity of automated quantitative D-dimer assays ranges from 94% to 98% and the specificity from 50% to 60% for PE and DVT. The D-dimer has a half-life of approximately 8 hours and can be elevated for at least 3 days after symptomatic VTE. Advanced age, pregnancy, active malignancy, recent surgery, liver disease, rheumatologic disease, infection, trauma, and sickle cell disease can all elevate D-dimer levels in the absence of VTE. D-dimer cutoffs for use in screening for VTE can be adjusted for age to maintain adequate exclusionary ability. The most commonly used formula

TABLE 25-3 Wells' Score for Deep Vein Thrombosis

Clinical Features	Points*
Active cancer (treatment within 6 months, or palliation)	1
Paralysis, paresis, or immobilization of lower extremity	1
Bedridden for >3 days because of surgery (within 12 weeks)	1
Localized tenderness along distribution of deep veins	1
Entire leg swollen	1
Unilateral calf swelling of >3 cm (below tibial tuberosity)	1
Unilateral pitting edema	1
Collateral superficial veins	1
Alternative diagnosis as likely as or more likely than deep venous thrombosis	–2
Prior history of DVT or PE†	1

*Risk score interpretation (probability of deep venous thrombosis) in original Wells' DVT model: ≥3 points: high risk (75%); 1 or 2 points: moderate risk (17%); <1 point: low risk (3%).

†Only awarded in the modified (dichotomized) Wells DVT model: ≤1 point DVT unlikely >1 point DVT likely.

Source: Adapted with permission from Geersing GJ, Zuithoff NP, Kearon C, et al: Exclusion of deep vein thrombosis using the Wells rule in clinically important subgroups: individual patient data meta-analysis. *BMJ.* March 10, 2014;348:g1340.

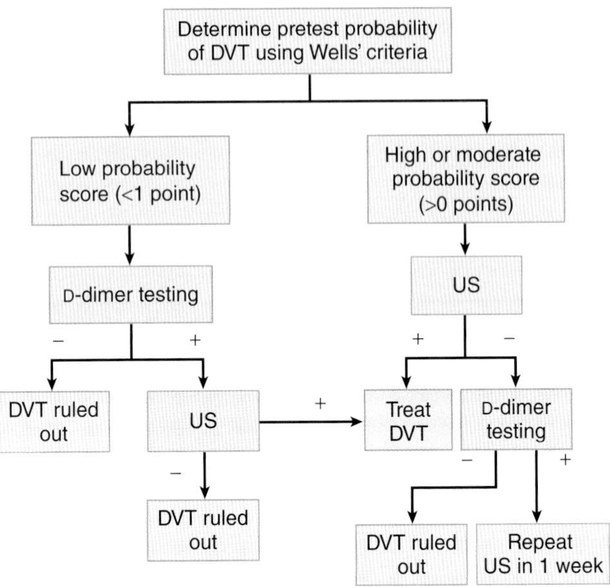

FIGURE 25-1. Diagnostic algorithm for deep vein thrombosis, applied in patients with leg symptoms compatible with DVT. +, positive test result; −, negative test result.

is age × 10 ng/mL to determine the upper limit of normal. For patients with high pretest probability of VTE, those with a positive D-dimer, or those in whom D-dimer testing is very likely to be positive, imaging is indicated.

Figure 25-1 illustrates a recommended diagnostic pathway for suspected DVT. Patients with a low pretest probability of DVT can be adequately evaluated with a serum D-dimer. Patients with a moderate or high pretest probability for DVT or those who have a positive D-dimer should undergo venous ultrasound (US). Venous US is nonionizing and has high sensitivity (90% to 95%) and specificity (95%) for lower extremity DVT. Sensitivity of venous US is lower for pelvic and isolated calf DVT and in obese patients. To rule out DVT in patients with high clinical probability, some diagnostic algorithms recommend both a negative initial ultrasound and a concurrent negative D-dimer or a follow-up ultrasound performed 1 week after the initial negative testing.

Figure 25-2 shows one recommended diagnostic algorithm for PE, though no singular diagnostic test or approach perfectly diagnoses or excludes PE. For patients who need radiographic imaging to evaluate for PE, a computed tomography (CT) pulmonary angiography of the chest is the test of choice (see Fig. 25-3) where a blood clot appears as a filling defect in a contrast-enhanced pulmonary artery. The sensitivity of a technically adequate CT for PE is about 90%, and specificity is 95%. Unfortunately, about 10% of scans are technically inadequate and should be interpreted with this limitation in mind. The negative likelihood ratio of a CT scan is 0.12, which is similar to that of a negative D-dimer. Therefore,

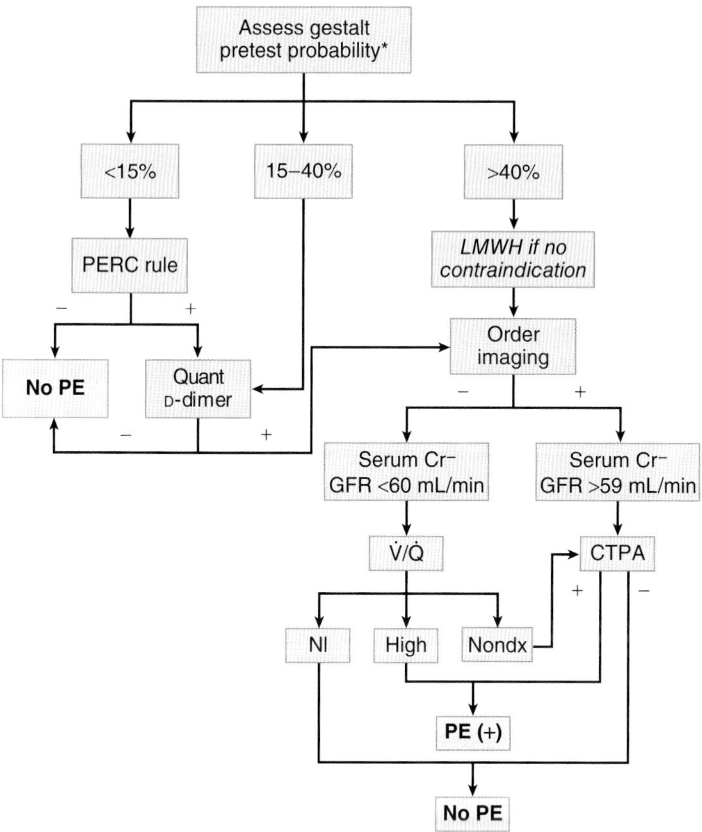

FIGURE 25-2. Pulmonary Embolism Rule-Out Criteria (PERC) rule—diagnostic algorithm for pulmonary embolism (PE). +, positive for PE; –, negative for PE; Cr, creatinine; High, high probability scan findings; LMWH, low-molecular-weight heparin; Nl, normal; Nondx, nondiagnostic (any reading other than normal or high probability); quant, quantitative.* Some physicians prefer to start with a clinical decision rule such as the Wells' score (where <2, 2 to 6, and >6 are used instead of <15%, 15% to 40%, and >40%, respectively). Note: Determine renal function by clinical picture (healthy, no risk factors for reduced glomerular filtration rate (GFR)) or calculated GFR. Nondiagnostic ventilation-perfusion ($\dot{V}/\dot{Q}$) scan findings require confirmation from results of another test, such as CT pulmonary angiography (CTPA), if benefits outweigh risks.

as with D-dimer testing, CT scan results should be interpreted in the appropriate context of pretest probability. Compared to other imaging modalities, CT scanning has the advantage of demonstrating important alternative diagnoses in 18% to 22% of patients.

Ventilation-perfusion ($\dot{V}/\dot{Q}$) scanning is another testing option to assess for possible PE. This is performed by comparing emission of radioisotope that has been injected into the pulmonary arteries to emission of radioisotope

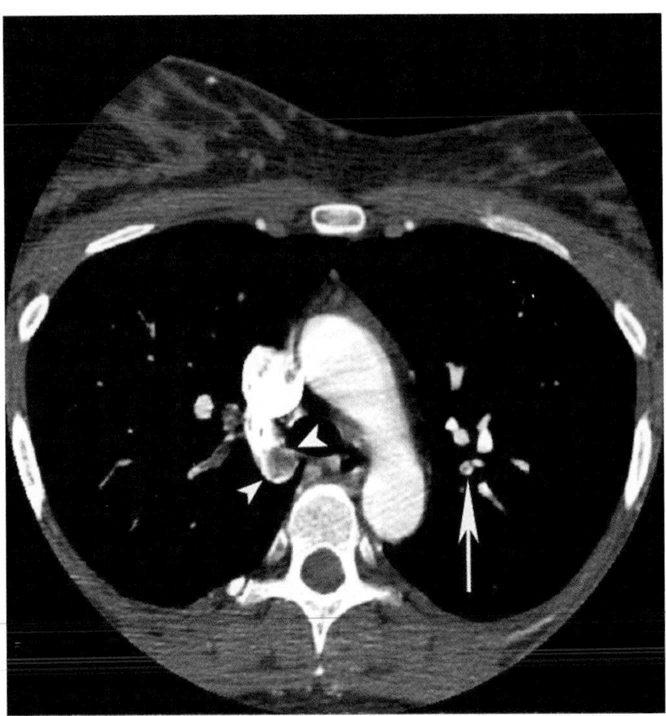

FIGURE 25-3. Axial image from a chest CT angiogram demonstrating a filling defect consistent with acute pulmonary embolism. Two *white arrowheads* outline a circular filling defect in the right middle lobar pulmonary artery. The *long white arrow* projecting in the left lung points to a filling defect in a segmental artery in the posterior medial segmental artery.

that has been inhaled into the alveoli. A $\dot{V}/\dot{Q}$ scan that demonstrates homogeneous scintillation throughout the lung in the perfusion portion rules out PE with 100% sensitivity. A $\dot{V}/\dot{Q}$ scan with two or more unmatched filling defects indicates 80% probability of PE. However, only about one-third of $\dot{V}/\dot{Q}$ scans demonstrate findings sufficient to diagnose or rule out PE with certainty.

EMERGENCY DEPARTMENT CARE AND DISPOSITION

The treatment of VTE consists of initial stabilization, anticoagulation, and thrombolytic or surgical therapy in severe cases. All patients suspected of having PE should have their cardiac rhythm, blood pressure, and pulse oxygenation measured.

1. Utilize supplemental oxygen when necessary to maintain adequate pulse oximetry readings.
2. Administer intravenous crystalloid fluids as needed to augment preload and correct hypotension.

3. Initial anticoagulation should be initiated as soon as possible to prevent further clot formation and allow endogenous fibrinolysis to proceed. Anticoagulation can be achieved by administering intravenous unfractionated heparin (**UFH**), subcutaneous low-molecular-weight heparin (**LMWH**), or a factor Xa inhibitor such as **rivaroxaban, apixaban,** or **fondaparinux. Dabigatran** (a direct thrombin inhibitor) and **edoxaban** (a factor Xa inhibitor) can also be used, but require initial anticoagulation with heparin for several days. (See Table 25-4.)
4. Current data favor the use of LMWH over UFH for treatment of PE or DVT, although the magnitude of benefit is small. LWMH can result in unpredictable anticoagulation in patients with severe renal insufficiency, so UFH is preferred in this setting. Potentially decreased absorption of LMWH in obese patients or high risk of bleeding in selected patients may also favor the use of UFH.
5. Systemic fibrinolytic therapy should be considered for selected patients with severe PE and no contraindications. Currently, the only patients with PE who have been shown to clearly benefit from thrombolytic

TABLE 25-4 Antithrombotic Therapy for Deep Venous Thrombosis and Pulmonary Embolism

	Dosage	Comments
Unfractionated heparin	80 U/kg bolus, then 18 U/kg/h infusion	Recommended if outpatient therapy not appropriate or in cases of severe renal failure
LMWHs		Outpatient treatment with LMWH preferred
Dalteparin	100 IU/kg SC every 12 h or 200 IU/kg SC every day	
Enoxaparin	1 mg/kg SC every 12 h or 1.5 mg/kg SC every day	
Tinzaparin	175 IU/kg SC every day	
Factor Xa inhibitors		
Fondaparinux	<50 kg, 5 mg SC every day; 50–100 kg, 7.5 mg SC every day; >100 kg, 10 mg SC every day	Do not use in renal failure
Target-specific anticoagulants		
Rivaroxaban (Xarelto®)	15 mg BID for 21 days, then 20 mg every day with food	No heparin requirement; good choice for outpatient treatment
Apixaban (Eliquis®)	10 mg BID for 7 days then 5 mg BID	No heparin requirement; good choice for outpatient treatment
Dabigatran (Pradaxa®)	150 mg BID	Requires run in of heparin for 5–10 days; renal excretion
Thrombolytic therapy	Tissue plasminogen activator or alteplase (Activase®), 10-mg IV bolus followed by 90 mg infused over 2 h	For PE with hemodynamic compromise; after infusion, begin unfractionated heparin or LMWH

Abbreviations: BID, twice a day; LMWH, low-molecular-weight heparin; VTE, venous thromboembolism.

therapy are those with a massive PE causing systolic blood pressure below 90 mm Hg or an observed decrease in blood pressure of 40 mm Hg. Fibrinolysis may also benefit patients with submassive PE that is associated with right heart strain on echocardiogram, elevated troponin or B-type natriuetric peptide, or severe hypoxemia and respiratory distress. In these patients fibrinolysis is associated with improved survival and quality of life, but with an increased risk of bleeding—especially among patients >65 years old. **Alteplase** (tPA) is the only fibrinolytic available in the United States that is Food and Drug Administration (FDA) approved for the treatment of PE and is administered as 100 mg infused over 2 hours. Heparin or LMWH is typically started after the thrombolytic infusion.

6. Severe DVT that causes *phlegmasia cerulea dolens* can lead to loss of limb and requires immediate treatment. The affected limb should be maintained at neutral level, constrictive clothing, casts, or dressings should be removed, and anticoagulation should be initiated. Catheter-based thrombectomy or thrombolysis should be discussed with an interventional radiologist, peripheral interventional cardiologist, or vascular surgeon. If this service is not available, consider intravenous thrombolysis.
7. Surgical and suction thromboembolectomy are options for patients with life-threatening PE and contraindications to fibrinolysis. The mortality associated with open surgical thromboembolectomy is high, but may be improved with early and appropriate patient selection.
8. An inferior vena cava filter should be considered when anticoagulation has failed, is contraindicated, or when submassive PE is associated with persistent large DVT.
9. Admit patients to an intensive care setting when signs of circulatory compromise are present or when thrombolytic therapy is given and close monitoring is needed. Patients with PE are typically admitted to a telemetry bed, but selected low-risk patients may be appropriate for outpatient management. Low-risk patients with DVT are often treated as outpatients. Appropriate follow-up must be assured when the eligibility for outpatient treatment is being evaluated, and practical limitations such as the ability to reliably comply with treatments at home should be considered.

FURTHER READING

For further reading in *Tintinalli's Emergency Medicine: A Comprehensive Study Guide*, 8th ed., see Chapter 56, "Venous Thromboembolism," by Jeffrey A. Kline.

CHAPTER 26 Systemic and Pulmonary Hypertension

Michael Cassara

Clinical presentations of acute systemic hypertension may be classified into following three categories:

1. **Hypertensive emergency** is characterized by elevated blood pressures with target organ dysfunction. Organ dysfunction is caused by persistent mechanical wall stress and endothelial injury leading to increased vascular permeability and fibrinoid necrosis within large arteries and arterioles of target organs such as brain, kidneys, heart, and lungs. Clinical manifestations of hypertensive emergency may include the following:

   - Chest pain associated with aortic dissection, acute pulmonary edema, or acute coronary syndrome.
   - Shortness of breath from acute pulmonary edema.
   - Acute neurologic symptoms such as altered mental status, focal motor or sensory deficits, headache, or visual disturbances. These can be associated with hypertensive encephalopathy, subarachnoid hemorrhage, intracranial hemorrhage, or acute ischemic stroke.
   - Peripheral edema secondary to acute renal failure or severe preeclampsia.
   - Sympathetic crisis due to sympathomimetic toxicity, adverse drug reactions and food–drug interactions, or pheochromocytoma.

2. **Hypertensive urgency** is accompanied by profound blood pressure elevations without acute target organ dysfunction. Some clinicians recommend acute pharmacologic treatment for blood pressures of 180/120 mm Hg or greater, although the clinical benefits of such acute interventions are unclear.
3. **Chronic systemic hypertension** is identified in patients with longstanding blood pressure elevations without obvious progression to acute target organ dysfunction. This diagnosis is defined by serial blood pressure measurements over several weeks. See Table 26-1.

TABLE 26-1 JNC7 Classification of Hypertension

Class	Systolic BP (mm Hg)		Diastolic BP (mm Hg)
Normal	<120	and	<80
Prehypertension	120–139	or	80–89
Stage 1	140–159	or	90–99
Stage 2	160 or greater	or	100 or greater

Abbreviations: BP, blood pressure; JNC7, *Seventh Report of the Joint National Committee on the Prevention, Detection, Evaluation, and Treatment of High Blood Pressure.*

CLINICAL FEATURES

Patients presenting with elevated blood pressure and accompanying acute symptoms often provide a history of hypertension. Many patients have coexisting medical conditions such as cardiovascular disease, renal dysfunction, cerebrovascular disease, diabetes, hyperlipidemia, chronic obstructive pulmonary disease, asthma, or renal artery stenosis. Secondary precipitants of acute hypertension may include pregnancy, sympathomimetic toxicity, adverse drug reactions, drug–drug interactions, or withdrawal from medications or recreational substances.

When a significantly elevated blood pressure is present, consider the possibility of hypertensive emergency in patients with any of the following signs and symptoms of target organ involvement:

- Nervous system signs and symptoms such as headaches, visual changes, papilledema, retinal exudates, seizures, encephalopathy, focal motor or sensory deficits, vomiting, seizures, or confusion
- Cardiovascular signs and symptoms such as chest pain, palpitations, dyspnea, rales, syncope, carotid bruits, new cardiac murmurs or gallops, asymmetric pulses, unequal blood pressures, pulsatile abdominal masses, or tearing pain radiating to the back or abdomen
- Renal system signs and symptoms such as anuria, peripheral edema, or hematuria

Consider preeclampsia in pregnant or recently postpartum patients with hypertension, hyperreflexia, and peripheral edema. Consider coarctation or aortic dissection in patients with hypertension, asymmetric peripheral pulses, and unequal blood pressures.

DIAGNOSIS AND DIFFERENTIAL

The primary goal of diagnostic testing is to reveal evidence of target organ injury when such injury is not otherwise clinically obvious. Urinalysis, pregnancy testing, and electrocardiograms are commonly ordered. When indicated in specific cases, additional testing such as metabolic profiles, toxicology screens, and radiographic imaging may provide additional supporting data. See Table 26-2.

Hematuria, proteinuria, and red cell casts on urinalysis, coupled with serum blood urea nitrogen, creatinine, and potassium elevations, suggest renal injury. Electrocardiographic abnormalities may reflect cardiac or renal dysfunction with findings such as tachycardia, altered QRS waveforms, and ST segment or T-wave changes. Chest radiographs may reveal findings of acute pulmonary edema or mediastinal widening suggestive of acute aortic dissection. Computed tomography or ultrasound may be necessary to confirm clinical suspicions when plain radiographs are nondiagnostic. Computed tomography of the head may reveal ischemic changes, edema, or hemorrhage.

EMERGENCY DEPARTMENT CARE AND DISPOSITION

Stabilize patients with hypertensive emergencies with an appropriate airway assessment, ventilatory support, supplemental oxygen administration, continuous cardiac monitoring, and intravenous catheter placement.

TABLE 26-2 Hypertensive Emergencies

Diagnostic Category	Evidence of Acute End-Organ Damage
Acute aortic dissection	Abnormal CT angiogram of chest and abdomen/pelvis or transesophageal echocardiogram of the aorta
Acute pulmonary edema	Interstitial edema on chest radiograph
Acute myocardial infarction	Changes on ECG or elevated levels of cardiac biomarkers
Acute coronary syndrome	Clinical diagnosis, changes on ECG, or elevated levels of cardiac biomarkers
Acute renal failure	Elevated serum creatinine level, proteinuria
Severe preeclampsia, HELLP syndrome, eclampsia	Proteinuria, hemolysis, elevated liver enzyme levels, low platelet counts
Hypertensive retinopathy	Retinal hemorrhages and cotton-wool spots, hard exudates, and sausage-shaped veins
Hypertensive encephalopathy	May see papilledema or arteriolar hemorrhage or exudates on funduscopic examination, may note cerebral edema with a predilection for the posterior white matter of the brain on MRI
Subarachnoid hemorrhage	Abnormal CT of the brain
Intracranial hemorrhage	Abnormal CT of the brain; RBC on lumbar puncture
Acute ischemic stroke	Abnormal MRI or CT of the brain
Acute perioperative hypertension	Clinical diagnosis; manifestations of other hypertensive emergencies
Sympathetic crisis	Clinical diagnosis in the setting of sympathomimetic drug use (i.e., cocaine or amphetamines) or pheochromocytoma (24-h urine assay for catecholamines and metanephrine or plasma fractionated metanephrines)

Abbreviation: HELLP, hemolysis, elevated liver enzymes, low platelets.

Formulate a problem-specific plan of care with a primary therapeutic goal of safely reducing arterial pressure while avoiding hypoperfusion.

1. **Aortic dissection.** Initiate treatments to reduce heart rate to 60 beats per minute or less and systolic blood pressure between 100 and 140 mm Hg, with an ideal target of less than 120 mm Hg. Initiate beta-adrenergic antagonists *before* starting vasodilator agents. Initial options include **esmolol** 250 to 500 μg/kg IV over 1 to 3 minutes followed by continuous infusion of 50 μg/kg/min, or **labetalol** 10 to 20 mg IV over 2 minutes followed by subsequent doses of 40 to 80 mg every 10 minutes as needed to a maximum dose of 300 mg. If beta-adrenergic antagonists are contraindicated, **diltiazem** 0.25 mg/kg over 2 minutes, alpha-adrenergic antagonists, benzodiazepines, or vasodilators may be necessary. When additional blood pressure control is needed, consider **nicardipine** 5 mg/h IV with incremental increases by 2.5 mg/h every 5 to 15 minutes to a maximum infusion rate of 15 mg/h. An alternative blood pressure control agent is **sodium nitroprusside** 0.3 to 0.5 μg/kg IV with incremental increases by 0.5 μg/kg/min.
2. **Acute hypertensive pulmonary edema.** The primary therapeutic goal is to reduce systemic afterload by 20% to 30%. There are no clear

evidence-based guidelines for the single best treatment for hypertensive pulmonary edema, although diuresis and vasodilation are commonly used. **Nitroglycerin** 0.4 mg sublingual up to three doses, topical 1 to 2 inches transdermal, or IV infusion starting at 5 μg/min with increases by 5 μg/min every 3 to 5 minutes up to 20 μg/min. Refractory cases can continue **nitroglycerin** IV infusion with incremental increases by 10 μg/min every 3 to 5 minutes to a maximum of 200 μg/min or add **nicardipine** (see dose above, #1). Consider **sodium nitroprusside** (see dose above, #1) when other agents are unsuccessful, keeping in mind its association with cyanide and thiocyanate toxicity in patients with prolonged therapy or renal failure. Intravenous **enalaprilat** 0.625 to 1.25 mg IV over 5 minutes every 4 to 6 hours, incrementally increased by 1.25 mg to a maximum of 5 mg every 6 hours is an additional adjunct, but may induce significant "first-dose" hypotension, and is pregnancy category D.

3. **Acute coronary syndromes.** The primary therapeutic goals are to limit ischemia and reduce the mean arterial pressure by no more than 25%. Sublingual or intravenous **nitroglycerin** (see dose above, #2) is preferred. Routine use of intravenous beta-adrenergic antagonists has fallen out of favor, and these agents are currently recommended only when patients have severe hypertension and should be avoided for those with risk for progression to cardiogenic shock. Oral beta-adrenergic antagonists may not provide sufficiently rapid blood pressure control in a hypertensive emergency.
4. **Acute sympathetic crisis.** The primary therapeutic goals are to decrease adrenergic stimulation and to relieve symptoms. **Benzodiazepines** are the recommended first intervention. **Nitroglycerin** (see dose above, #2), **phentolamine** 5 to 15 mg IV followed by continuous infusion of 0.2 to 0.5 mg/min, or **nicardipine** (see dose above, #1) are secondary adjuncts to consider.
5. **Acute renal failure.** The primary therapeutic goals are to reduce systemic vascular resistance with acute blood pressure reductions of less than 20% to help preserve renal blood flow. Recommended agents include **fenoldopam** 0.1 μg/kg/min IV titrated to desired effect every 15 minutes to a maximum of 1.6 μg/kg/min, **clevidipine** 1 to 2 mg/h IV, or **nicardipine** (see dose above, #1).
6. **Preeclampsia.** The primary therapeutic goals are to reduce significant elevations of blood pressure and prevent progression to eclampsia. **Labetalol** (see dose above, #1) and **hydralazine** 5 to 10 mg IV are commonly prescribed agents for blood pressure levels greater than 160/100 mm Hg.
7. **Hypertensive encephalopathy.** The primary therapeutic goal is to rapidly reduce significantly elevated mean arterial pressures by 20% to 25% once other neurologic emergencies are excluded. Recommended agents include **nicardipine** (see dose above, #1), **labetalol** (see dose above, #1), **fenoldopam** (see dose above, #5), or **clevidipine** (see dose above, #5).
8. **Subarachnoid hemorrhage.** The primary therapeutic goals for blood pressure control in subarachnoid hemorrhage are unclear, although reduction of systolic blood pressure to 160 mm Hg or lower is generally recommended. Recommended agents include **nicardipine** (see dose

above, #1), **labetalol** (see dose above, #1), **esmolol** (see dose above, #1), or **clevidipine** (see dose above, #5). Oral **nimodipine** may reduce vasospasm and subsequent cerebral infarction rate in patients with moderately increased blood pressure not requiring an intravenous agent.

9. **Intracranial hemorrhage.** The primary therapeutic goals for blood pressure control in intracranial hemorrhage are to reduce hemorrhage expansion and to lower systolic blood pressures to 120 to 160 mm Hg. Recommended agents include **nicardipine** (see dose above, #1), **labetalol** (see dose above, #1), or **esmolol** (see dose above, #1).
10. **Acute ischemic stroke:** The primary therapeutic goals for blood pressure control in acute ischemic stroke depend on the likelihood of fibrinolytic therapy, and should be balanced to avoid worsening ischemia from excessive blood pressure reduction. If fibrinolytic therapy is planned, blood pressure should be below 185/110 mm Hg, with a systolic blood pressure goal of 141 to 150 mm Hg. Recommended agents include **labetalol** (see dose above, #1), **nicardipine** (see dose above, #1), or **sodium nitroprusside** (see dose above, #1). If no fibrinolytic therapy is planned and significantly elevated blood pressures remain (e.g., 220/120 mm Hg), blood pressure should be lowered by no more than 10% to 15% in the first 24 hours.
11. For hypertensive urgency, useful agents include **labetalol** 200 to 400 mg orally, **captopril** 12.5 to 25 mg orally every 4 to 6 hours, **losartan** 50 mg orally per day, or **clonidine** 0.1 to 0.2 mg orally.
12. Consider starting an oral agent on an outpatient basis for asymptomatic patients with severe hypertension, such as those with systolic blood pressures above 180 to 200 mm Hg or diastolic blood pressures above 110 to 120 mm Hg. A diuretic agent such as **hydrochlorothiazide** 25 mg orally each day is an appropriate medication to consider starting in patients with uncomplicated asymptomatic severe hypertension. For patients with angina, postmyocardial infarction, migraines, or supraventricular arrhythmias, consider a beta-adrenergic antagonists such as **metoprolol** 50 mg orally once or twice daily. An angiotensin-converting enzyme inhibitor such as **lisinopril** 10 mg orally each day can be used in patients with a history of heart failure, renal disease, recurrent strokes, or diabetes mellitus.

CHILDHOOD HYPERTENSIVE EMERGENCIES

Hypertensive emergencies in children, as for adults, refer to profoundly elevated blood pressures associated with target organ damage. Neonates often present with nonspecific signs such as apnea, cyanosis, or poor feeding. Older children may present with symptoms and physical examination findings more typical of adults such as throbbing frontal headaches or blurred vision.

Renovascular lesions and pheochromocytoma are the most commonly identified etiologies for pediatric hypertensive emergencies. The decision to treat a hypertensive emergency in a child is based on the blood pressure and associated symptoms indicating target organ damage. Consider urgent treatment if the hypertensive blood pressure exceeds prior measurements by 30%, or if diastolic or systolic blood pressures exceed the 90th to 95th percentiles on a standardized table of blood pressure by age. The primary therapeutic goal for blood pressure control in an acutely symptomatic child with a hypertensive emergency is to lower the mean arterial pressure by 25% within 1 hour. Preferred medications include **labetalol** 0.2 to 1 mg/kg IV to a maximum of 40 mg per dose or a continuous infusion of 0.25 to 3 mg/kg/h or **nicardipine** 0.5 to 3 μg/kg/min IV.

The second-line agents include **hydralazine** 0.2 to 0.6 mg/kg IV to a maximum of 20 mg per dose, **esmolol** 100 to 500 μg/kg followed by an infusion of 50 to 150 μg/kg/min, or **clevidipine** 0.5 to 3.5 μg/kg/min IV. Refractory cases may be treated with **nitroprusside** 0.5 to 10 μg/kg/min IV. **Phentolamine** 0.1 mg/kg IV to a maximum of 5 mg is the drug of choice for significantly elevated blood pressure in the setting of a pheochromocytoma, while awaiting definitive surgical treatment.

PULMONARY HYPERTENSION

Pulmonary hypertension is characterized by an elevated pressure within the pulmonary vascular system compromising right ventricular function. Pulmonary hypertension is defined as a mean pulmonary artery pressure exceeding 25 mm Hg at rest or 30 mm Hg with exertion. Pulmonary hypertension can manifest with isolated pulmonary arterial pressure elevations or combined pulmonary arterial and venous pressure elevations. Definitive diagnosis requires right heart catheterization.

The most common symptom of pulmonary hypertension is dyspnea, either at rest or with exertion. Other symptoms include fatigue, syncope or near-syncope, and chest pain. Typically, this disorder will be seen in association with other cardiovascular or pulmonary disorders such as chronic obstructive pulmonary disease, left ventricular dysfunction, or disorders associated with hypoxemia.

When treating patients with suspected or known pulmonary hypertension:

- Provide supplemental oxygen to maintain saturation levels greater than 90% in patients presenting with hypoxia. Intubation in patients with severe pulmonary hypertension can cause rapid cardiovascular collapse due to increased intrathoracic pressure from positive pressure ventilation.
- Optimize intravascular volume to treat or prevent hypotension.
- Augment right ventricular function when necessary by using **dobutamine** 2 to 10 μg/kg/min IV or **milrinone** 0.375 μg/kg/min IV.
- Maintain coronary artery perfusion when necessary by using **norepinephrine** 0.05 to 0.75 μg/kg/min IV.
- Reduce right ventricular afterload with **prostanoids** (e.g., epoprostenol) and **phosphodiesterase-5 inhibitors** (e.g., sildenafil). Although these agents are rarely initiated in the emergency department, patients with previously diagnosed pulmonary hypertension may present already receiving continuous infusions of one of these agents. When assessing these patients in the acute setting, confirm catheter and pump function as one possible cause of clinical decompensation.

FURTHER READING

For further reading in *Tintinalli's Emergency Medicine: A Comprehensive Study Guide*, 8th ed., see Chapter 57, "Systemic Hypertension," by Brigitte M. Baumann; Chapter 58, "Pulmonary Hypertension," by Michael E. Winters.

CHAPTER 27

Aortic Aneurysms and Aortic Dissection

David E. Manthey

ABDOMINAL AORTIC ANEURYSMS

An abdominal aortic aneurysm (AAA) is commonly ≥3.0 cm in diameter and can be a significant cause of morbidity and mortality. Symptomatic aneurysms and those ≥5.0 cm in diameter frequently require prompt operative repair.

Clinical Features

An acute rupturing AAA is an emergent condition that will lead to death if not rapidly identified and repaired. The classically described presentation of a ruptured AAA is an older male smoker with atherosclerosis who presents with sudden severe back or abdominal pain, hypotension, and a pulsatile abdominal mass. Patients may also present with syncope or pain that localizes to the flank, groin, hip, or abdomen.

Half of patients with a rupturing aneurysm describe a ripping or tearing pain that is severe and abrupt in onset. On examination, patients may have a tender pulsatile abdominal mass, although this finding may be challenging to identify in obese patients. Patients with a ruptured AAA may present with persistent hypotension due to blood loss, although this may transiently improve due to compensatory mechanisms. Femoral pulsations are typically normal. Retroperitoneal hemorrhage may rarely present with external findings such as periumbilical ecchymosis (Cullen's sign), flank ecchymosis (Grey–Turner's sign), or a scrotal hematoma.

Aortoenteric fistulas, although rare, may present as gastrointestinal bleeding with either a small sentinel bleed or a massive life-threatening hemorrhage. Patients with prior aortic grafting are at an increased risk of this complication. The duodenum is a common site for fistula formation, and patients with this complication may present with hematemesis, melena, or hematochezia. Aortovenous fistulas can lead to high-output cardiac failure with decreased arterial blood flow distal to the fistula.

An uncommon presentation of AAA is rupture into the retroperitoneum, where significant fibrosis may lead to a chronic contained rupture. These patients can appear well and may complain of pain for an extended period of time before the diagnosis is made.

Clinicians may discover an asymptomatic AAA on physical examination or as an incidental finding on a radiologic study. Refer patients with a newly diagnosed AAA to a vascular surgeon for evaluation, keeping in mind that aneurysms larger than 5 cm in diameter are at a greater risk for rupture.

Diagnosis and Differential

Identifying a new AAA can be a challenging diagnosis. When the diagnosis is not initially identified, renal colic is the most common incorrect initial diagnosis. Consider this diagnosis in patients with symptoms of back pain, an intraabdominal process, testicular torsion, or gastrointestinal bleeding.

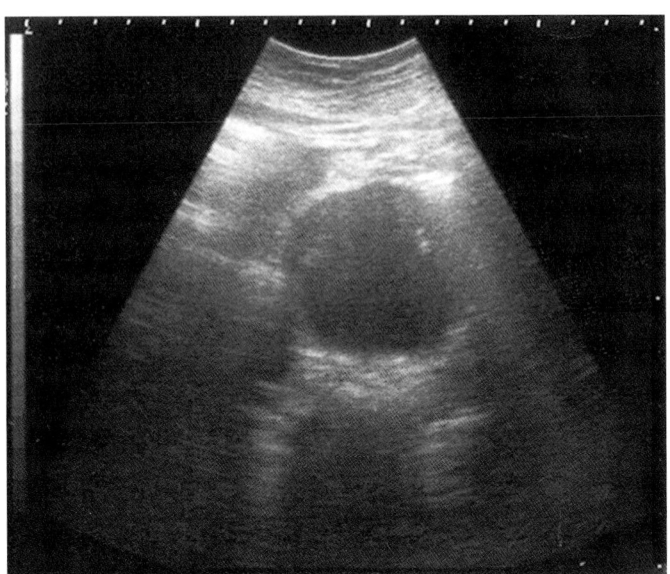

FIGURE 27-1. Ultrasound image of an abdominal aortic aneurysm in the transverse plane.

When the diagnosis is unclear, consider additional studies to further evaluate patients with symptoms concerning for an expanding or rupturing AAA. Bedside abdominal ultrasound has >90% sensitivity for identifying AAA and can be used to accurately measure the diameter of the aneurysm (see Fig. 27-1), although aortic rupture or retroperitoneal bleed cannot be reliably identified with this modality. Computed tomography (CT) can identify AAA and delineate the anatomic details of the aneurysm and any associated rupture. The role of plain radiography in the diagnosis of rupturing AAA is unclear, as a calcified, bulging aortic contour is present in only 65% of patients with a symptomatic AAA.

Emergency Department Care and Disposition

1. Consult emergently with a vascular surgeon when a rupturing AAA or aortoenteric fistula is suspected.
2. Stabilize hemodynamics by obtaining large-bore IV access and administering fluids judiciously to treat hypotension. Target a goal systolic blood pressure of 90 mm Hg, and transfuse packed red blood cells if needed. Provide pain control while avoiding hypotension.
3. When a small asymptomatic AAA (3.0 to 5.0 cm) is identified as an incidental finding, refer the patient to see a vascular surgeon. Large AAAs (>5.0 cm) are at higher risk for spontaneous rupture and may warrant close follow-up.
4. Nonaortic large-artery aneurysms can also cause symptoms from expansion and rupture (see Table 27-1). These can also be diagnosed and evaluated using ultrasound or CT scan.

TABLE 27-1 Nonaortic Large-Artery Aneurysms

Artery	Risk Factors	Clinical Presentation	Management
Popliteal (>2 cm or >150% of normal caliber)	Advanced age, male gender, trauma, congenital disorders	Most common peripheral aneurysm; discomfort behind knee with swelling with or without deep venous thrombosis	Thrombolysis, ligation, arterial bypass, endovascular repair
Subclavian	Arteriosclerosis, thoracic outlet obstruction	Pulsatile mass above or below clavicle, dysphagia, stridor, chest pain, hoarseness, upper extremity fatigue or numbness and tingling, limb ischemic symptoms	Surgical repair
Femoral	Advanced age, male gender, trauma, congenital disorders	Pulsatile mass with or without pain, limb ischemic symptoms, peripheral embolic symptoms	Thrombolysis, ligation, arterial bypass, endovascular repair
Femoral pseudoaneurysm	Prior femoral artery catheterization, trauma, infection	Pulsatile mass with or without pain	Surgical repair
Iliac	Pain in groin, scrotum, or lower abdomen; sciatica; vulvar or groin hematoma with rupture	Surgical repair	
Renal	Age 40–60 years, no gender preference, HTN, fibrodysplasia, arteriosclerosis	Flank pain, hematuria, collecting system obstruction, shock if ruptured	Surgical repair, nephrectomy
Splenic	Advanced age, female gender, HTN, congenital, arteriosclerosis, liver disease, multiparous, rupture increased in pregnancy	Rapid symptom onset; epigastric or left upper quadrant pain first, then diffuse abdominal pain with rupture, shock	Surgical repair, splenectomy, embolization if unruptured
Hepatic	Infection, arteriosclerosis, trauma, vasculitis	Obstructive jaundice, hemobilia from rupture into common bile duct, right upper quadrant pain, peritonitis, upper GI bleed	Surgical ligation, embolization

Abbreviation: HTN, hypertension.

AORTIC DISSECTION

Clinical Features

Aortic dissection occurs when blood dissects between the intimal and adventitial layers of the aorta, and classically presents with acute chest pain that is most severe at onset and radiates to the back. The location of the pain may indicate the area of the aorta that is involved. Sixty percent of patients with dissection of the ascending aorta have anterior chest pain, and involvement of the descending aorta may cause abdominal or back pain. The pain pattern may change as the dissection progresses from one anatomic area to another. The pain is most commonly described as sharp, ripping, or tearing pain. Syncope can occur in 10% of patients.

Most patients with aortic dissection are male (66%), older than 50 years, and have a history of hypertension. Chronic cocaine use and prior cardiac surgery are additional risk factors. Younger patients with identifiable risk factors such as connective tissue disorders, congenital heart disease, and pregnancy are also at risk. Up to 30% of patients with Marfan's syndrome will develop a dissection. Iatrogenic aortic dissection may occur after aortic catheterization or cardiac surgery.

The Stanford classification divides dissections into those that involve the ascending aorta (type A) and those that are restricted to the descending aorta (type B). The DeBakey classification divides dissections into three groups: involvement of the ascending and descending aortas (type I), involvement of only the ascending aorta (type II), or involvement of only the descending aorta (type III).

As an aortic dissection progresses, seemingly unrelated symptom complexes may present themselves. Presentations include aortic valve insufficiency, coronary artery occlusion with myocardial infarction, carotid involvement with stroke symptoms, occlusion of vertebral blood supply with paraplegia, cardiac tamponade with shock and jugular venous distention, compression of the recurrent laryngeal nerve with hoarseness of the voice, and compression of the superior cervical sympathetic ganglion with Horner's syndrome.

Findings on physical examination will depend on the location and progression of the dissection. A diastolic murmur of aortic insufficiency may be heard. Hypertension and tachycardia are common, but hypotension also may be present. Fifty percent of patients have decreased pulsation in the radial, femoral, or carotid arteries, although no specific threshold values have been defined for blood pressure differences in extremities. Forty percent of patients have neurologic sequelae.

Diagnosis and Differential

The differential diagnosis to be considered depends on the location and progression of the dissection, but may include myocardial infarction, pericardial disease, stroke, spinal cord disorders, and primary conditions causing abdominal, back, or chest pain.

D-dimer testing is one of several biomarkers that have been investigated for potential utility in identifying or excluding dissection. No current guideline endorses the use of D-dimer as the sole means for excluding aortic dissection, partially due to a false-negative rate as high as 18%.

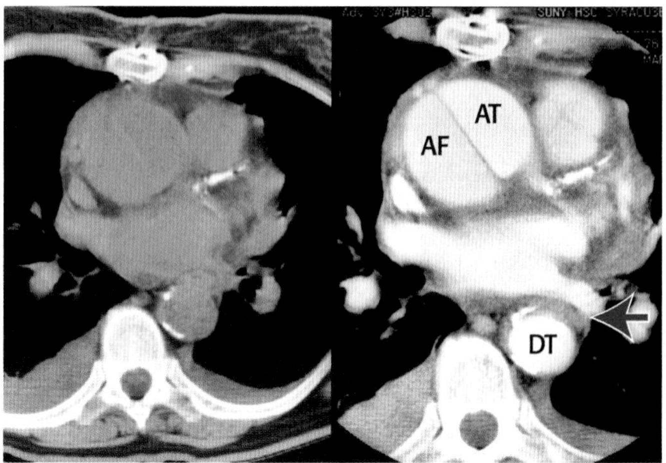

FIGURE 27-2. CT image of a type A aortic dissection. True and false lumens are present in the ascending aorta and descending aorta (descending false lumen at arrow) on noncontrast (*left*) and contrast (*right*) images. AF, ascending false lumen; AT, ascending true lumen; DT, descending true lumen.

The diagnosis of aortic dissection depends on radiographic confirmation. The most commonly found abnormalities on chest x-ray are an abnormal aortic contour and widening of the mediastinum, while other findings may include deviation of the trachea, mainstem bronchi, or esophagus, apical capping, pleural effusion, or displacement of aortic intimal calcifications. The chest x-ray is normal in 12% to 37% of patients with aortic dissection. CT scan with IV contrast is the imaging modality of choice and can reliably detect a false lumen as well as help to identify the extent of the dissection including extension into other vessels (see Fig. 27-2). Transesophageal echocardiograms are 97% to 100% sensitive and 97% to 99% specific. The preferential use of these studies may be institutionally dependent, and clinicians should coordinate diagnostic testing with the consulting vascular or thoracic surgeon.

Emergency Department Care and Disposition

1. Consult with a vascular or thoracic surgeon for patients with confirmed or strongly suspected aortic dissection to determine if operative intervention is indicated.
2. Stabilize hemodynamics with large-bore IV access, IV fluids for hypotension, and blood transfusion when required.
3. Manage hypertension with β-blockers such as **esmolol** 0.1 to 0.5 mg/kg IV bolus followed by a 0.025 to 0.2 mg/kg/min infusion, or **labetolol** 20 mg IV followed by subsequent doses of 20 to 40 mg IV every 10 minutes. Reduce the heart rate to a goal of between 60 and 70 beats per minute and the systolic blood pressure to a goal of 100 to 120 mm Hg.

4. Additional blood pressure reduction with agents such as **nitroprusside** or **nicardipine** should be used when needed after adequate inotropic blockade has been achieved and systolic blood pressures remain above 120 mm Hg.

FURTHER READING

For further reading in *Tintinalli's Emergency Medicine: A Comprehensive Study Guide*, 8th ed., see Chapter 59, "Aortic Dissection and Related Aortic Syndromes," by Gary A. Johnson and Louise A. Prince; and Chapter 60, "Aneurysmal Disease" by Louise A. Prince and Gary A. Johnson.

CHAPTER 28

Arterial Occlusion

Carolyn K. Synovitz

Peripheral arterial disease is defined as an ankle-brachial index (ABI) of <0.9 (see ABI definition below). The disease prevalence is 4.3% in Americans under age 40 years, and prevalence climbs to 15.5% in those over 70 years of age. High-risk individuals (such as those over 70 years, or those over 50 years with risk factors such as diabetes) should be evaluated carefully when complaints are indicative of possible occlusive arterial disease. Tobacco use significantly increases the risks that an individual will develop peripheral arterial disease. Limb ischemia from an acute arterial occlusion can lead to irreversible changes in peripheral nerves and skeletal muscle tissue in 4 to 6 hours. The most frequently diseased arteries leading to limb ischemia are the femoropopliteal, tibial, aortoiliac, and brachiocephalic. The common femoral and popliteal arteries are the most common sites of arterial embolism.

CLINICAL FEATURES

Patients with acute arterial limb ischemia typically present with one or more of the "six Ps": pain, pallor, poikilothermia (coldness), pulselessness, paresthesias, and paralysis. Pain is the earliest symptom and may increase with elevation of the limb. Changes in skin color with mottling, splotchiness, and cool temperature are common. Patients may present with muscle weakness as one early sign of limb ischemia, and the presence of acute anesthesia progressing to paralysis is concerning for acute ischemia that may negatively impact limb viability. A decreased pulse palpated distal to a vascular obstruction is an unreliable finding for early ischemia, especially in patients with chronic peripheral vascular disease and well-developed collateral circulation. Claudication is a cramping pain, ache, or tiredness in an ischemic limb that is brought on by exercise and relieved by rest. It is reproducible, resolves within 2 to 5 minutes of rest, and reoccurs at consistent walking distances. Claudication is a classically described symptom of peripheral vascular disease, but may only be present in 20% to 30% of patients with significant disease. These symptoms are contrasted with the pain of an acute episode of limb ischemia which is not well localized, is unrelieved by rest or gravity, and can present as a worsening of chronic pain when caused by an acute thrombotic event.

DIAGNOSIS AND DIFFERENTIAL

Although thromboembolic disease is the most common cause of acute arterial occlusion, the differential diagnosis for some of the presenting symptoms may include catheterization complications, vasculitis, Raynaud disease, thromboangiitis obliterans, blunt or penetrating trauma, or low-flow shock states such as sepsis. Vasospasm caused by intentional or accidental intraarterial drug injections may present as acute ischemic digits. Most commonly, a history of an abruptly ischemic limb in a patient with atrial fibrillation or recent myocardial infarction is strongly suggestive of an embolus. A history of chronic claudication suggests the presence of peripheral vascular disease, and an acute episode is likely caused by thrombosis and worsening limb ischemia. Examine the patient for differences in peripheral pulses, capillary refill, and skin findings on the extremities.

Objective bedside testing with a handheld Doppler can document the presence or absence of blood flow in an affected limb. Duplex ultrasonography can further be used to detect an obstruction to flow with sensitivity greater than 85%. In addition, the ABI can be easily measured in the emergency department using a blood pressure cuff and Doppler ultrasound to measure the systolic pressure of occlusion at the brachial artery and posterior tibial or dorsalis pedis arteries. The ABI is the leg occlusion pressure divided by the arm occlusion pressure and a normal ABI is >0.9. An abnormal ABI suggests peripheral vascular disease, and a ratio lower than 0.41:1 is concerning for critical limb ischemia. A CT angiogram is a diagnostic option that can be helpful in identifying the lesion location if the limb does not show signs of critical ischemia. The diagnostic gold standard is an arteriogram, which can define the anatomy of the obstruction and direct treatment of the limb.

EMERGENCY DEPARTMENT CARE AND DISPOSITION

1. Patients with acute arterial occlusion should be stabilized. Fluid resuscitation and pain medications should be administered as needed. Dependent positioning can increase perfusion pressure. Obtain an ECG and consider echocardiography to assess for conditions associated with embolism.
2. Staging of disease can be accomplished using the Rutherford Categories for acute limb ischemia (see Table 28-1). Patients that meet criteria I (Viable) to IIa (Marginally Threatened) may have diagnostic testing before definitive treatment. Patients with criteria IIb (Immediately Threatened) need immediate consultation and intervention. Patients that meet criteria III (Irreversible) may require limb amputation.
3. Initiate anticoagulation in patients with acute arterial occlusion using **unfractionated heparin** 80 U/kg intravenous bolus followed by IV infusion of 18 U/kg/h in collaboration with a consulting vascular surgeon.
4. Definitive treatment should be provided in consultation with a vascular surgeon and may include catheter-directed thrombolysis, percutaneous mechanical thrombectomy, revision of an occluded bypass graft, or revascularization.
5. All patients with an acute arterial occlusion should be admitted to a telemetry bed or to the intensive care unit, depending on the stability of the patient and the planned course of therapy.
6. Patients with chronic peripheral arterial disease who lack comorbidities and have no immediate limb threat can be discharged on **aspirin** 81 mg orally each day with an initial loading dose of 325 mg orally before discharge, with close vascular surgery or primary care follow-up for reassessment and further care.

TABLE 28-1 Rutherford Criteria for Acute Limb Ischemia

		Findings		Doppler Signals	
Category	Description/ Prognosis	Sensory Loss	Muscle Weakness	Arterial	Venous
I. Viable	Not immediately threatened	None	None	Audible	Audible
II. Threatened					
a. Marginally	Salvageable if promptly treated	Minimal (toes) or none	None	Inaudible	Audible
b. Immediately	Salvageable with immediate revascularization	More than toes, associated with rest pain	Mild, moderate	Inaudible	Audible
III. Irreversible	Major tissue loss or permanent nerve damage inevitable	Profound, anesthetic	Profound, paralysis (rigor)	Inaudible	Inaudible

Reproduced with permission from Rutherford RB, Baker JD, Ernst C, et al. Recommended standards for reports dealing with lower extremity ischemia: revised version. *J Vasc Surg.* September 1997;26(3): 517–538.

FURTHER READING

For further reading in *Tintinalli's Emergency Medicine: A Comprehensive Study Guide,* 8th ed., see Chapter 61, "Arterial Occlusion," by Anil Chopra and David Carr.

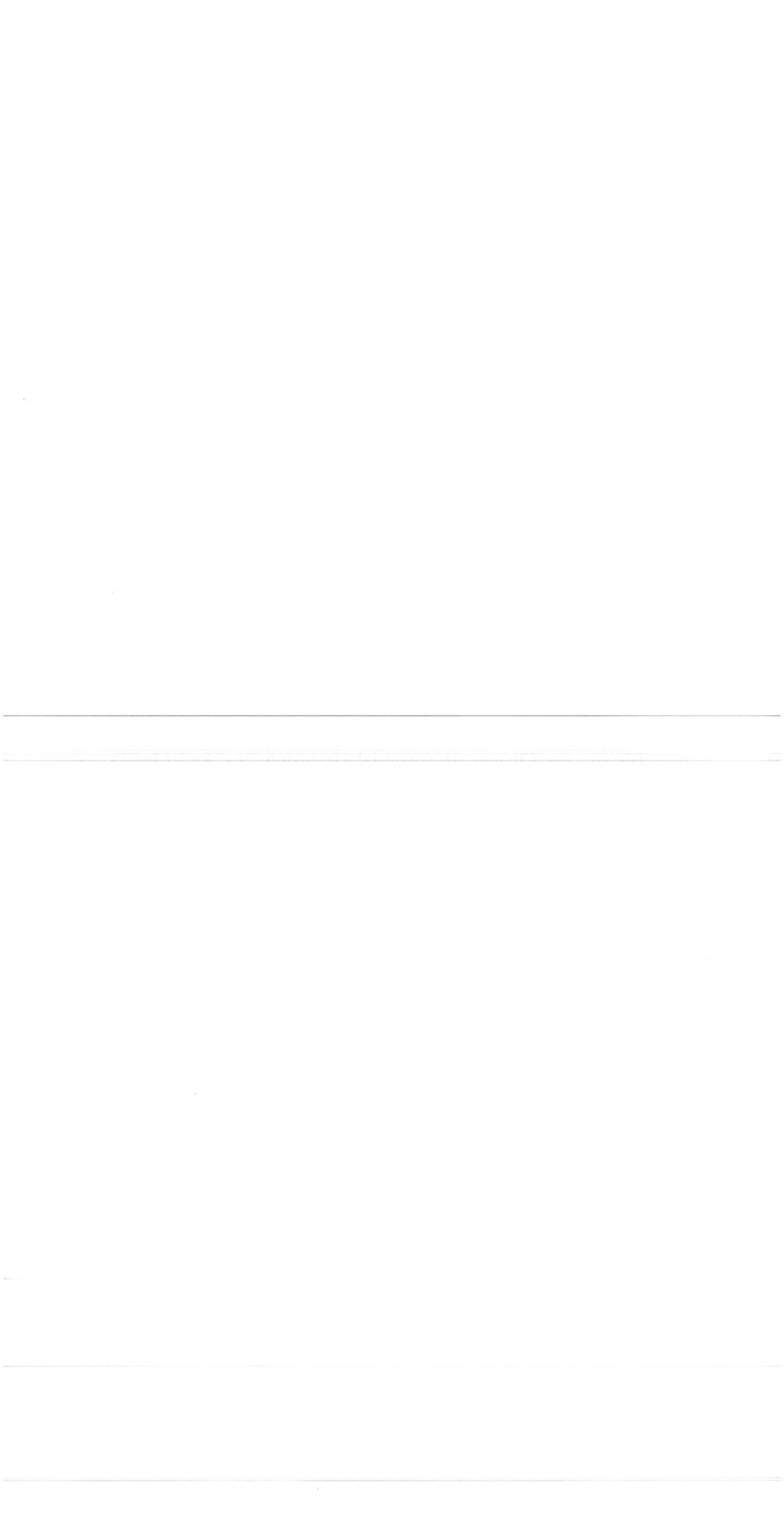

SECTION 5

Pulmonary Emergencies

Respiratory Distress

Baruch S. Fertel

The term respiratory distress includes both symptoms of dyspnea and signs indicating difficulty breathing. The cause of respiratory distress is often multifactorial and may include the findings of hypoxia, hypercapnia, and cyanosis.

DYSPNEA

Dyspnea is the subjective feeling of difficult, labored, or uncomfortable breathing. There is no single pathophysiologic mechanism that causes dyspnea and its etiology may be secondary to pulmonary, cardiac, or neurological dysfunction.

Clinical Features

The initial assessment of any patient with dyspnea should be directed toward identifying respiratory failure, which requires more immediate action. Dyspnea alone is a subjective complaint often difficult to quantify; therefore, objective findings are often needed to aid in diagnosis. Assess for signs of impending respiratory failure which include tachycardia, tachypnea, stridor, the use of accessory respiratory muscles (intercostals, sternocleidomastoid), stridor, lethargy, agitation, altered mental status, and inability to speak due to breathlessness. If present, oxygen should be administered immediately. Early use of noninvasive ventilation is often helpful in reversing the downward trajectory, although the need for aggressive airway management and mechanical ventilation should be anticipated. Lesser degrees of distress allow for a more detailed approach.

Diagnosis and Differential

The history and physical examination, together with ancillary testing, will help identify the etiology of dyspnea (Table 29-1).

It can be challenging to differentiate cardiac (CHF) and pulmonary causes. Signs such as an S_3 gallop, edema, jugular venous distention, a history of orthopnea, an elevated brain natriuretic peptide (BNP), or troponin and chest radiograph findings of edema and cardiomegaly may point to cardiac causes. Pulse oximetry is a rapid but insensitive screen for

TABLE 29-1 Common Causes of Dyspnea in the ED

Most Common Causes	Most Immediately Life-Threatening Causes
Obstructive airway disease: asthma, chronic obstructive pulmonary disease	Upper airway obstruction: foreign body, angioedema, hemorrhage
Decompensated heart failure/cardiogenic pulmonary edema	Tension pneumothorax
Ischemic heart disease: unstable angina and myocardial infarction	Pulmonary embolism
Pneumonia	Neuromuscular weakness: myasthenia gravis, Guillain-Barré syndrome, botulism
Psychogenic	Fat embolism

disorders of gas exchange as it may be falsely elevated as in methemoglobinemia. Arterial blood gas (ABG) analysis is more sensitive, detects both hypoxia and hypercarbia, and is useful for identifying metabolic causes, such as acidosis with compensatory tachypnea, but does not take into account work of breathing and fatigue. A peak expiratory flow rate may indicate reactive airway disease and a negative inspiratory force (NIF) may identify neurological causes of dyspnea. Additional ancillary tests that may prove helpful include a complete blood count to look for anemia, D-dimer assay when used with clinical decision rules to look for pulmonary embolus (PE), chest radiograph, electrocardiogram, and computed tomography of the chest. Bedside cardiopulmonary ultrasound is increasingly being used to look for pneumothorax, tamponade, pulmonary consolidation or effusion, right heart strain suggesting PE, and congestive heart failure.

Emergency Department Care and Disposition

1. The goal of oxygen therapy is to maintain the PaO_2 above 60 mm Hg or the oxygen saturation above 90%. Lower PaO_2 or saturation may be appropriate in those with longstanding lung disease such as chronic obstructive pulmonary disease (COPD).
2. After oxygenation has been ensured with an appropriate delivery device (nasal cannula, facemask, non-rebreather, BVM, NIV, or intubation) and the patient is stabilized, disorder-specific treatment and evaluation can be pursued.
3. The disposition of patients with dyspnea often depends on its etiology and acuity. Patients with hypoxia and an unclear cause of dyspnea will require hospital admission.

HYPOXIA AND HYPOXEMIA

Hypoxia is the insufficient delivery of oxygen to the tissues. Oxygen delivery is a function of cardiac output, hemoglobin concentration, and oxygen saturation. Hypoxemia is defined as a PaO_2 below 60 mm Hg. While hypoxia is often the result of hypoxemia, these two terms are not interchangeable and one can occur without the other. Hypoxemia results from a combination of five distinct mechanisms: (a) hypoventilation in which lack of ventilation increases $PaCO_2$, thereby displacing oxygen from the alveolus and lowering the amount delivered to the alveolar capillaries; (b) right-to-left shunt in which blood bypasses the lungs, thereby increasing the amount of unoxygenated blood entering the systemic circulation; (c) ventilation/perfusion mismatch in which areas of the lung are perfused but not ventilated; (d) diffusion impairment in which alveolar-blood barrier abnormality causes impairment of oxygenation; and (e) low inspired oxygen, such as that occurs at high altitude.

Clinical Features

Signs and symptoms of hypoxemia are nonspecific. Acute physiologic responses to hypoxemia include pulmonary arterial vasoconstriction and increases in minute ventilation and sympathetic tone manifesting as tachypnea, tachycardia, and an initial hyperdynamic cardiac state. The predominant features are often neurologic, and may include headache, somnolence, lethargy, anxiety, agitation, coma, or seizures. Chronic hypoxemia may result in polycythemia, digital clubbing, cor pulmonale, and changes in body habitus (e.g., pulmonary cachexia or barreled chest of COPD). Cyanosis may be present but is not a sensitive or specific indicator of hypoxemia.

Diagnosis and Differential

A formal diagnosis of hypoxemia requires ABG analysis; however, pulse oximetry may be useful for gross abnormalities or trends. Hypoxemia may be quantified, and clues to its etiology may be obtained, by calculation of the alveolar-arterial oxygen gradient ("A-a gradient," where the capital "A" represents alveolar oxygen tension and "a" indicates arterial oxygen level). The formula for calculating A-a gradient while breathing room air at sea level is

$$P(A - a)O_2 = 147 - (PaCO_2 \times 1.25) - PaCO_2$$

The A-a gradient is increased in cases of right-to-left shunts, ventilation-perfusion mismatch, and diffusion impairment. The normal value for a 20-year-old seated upright and healthy nonsmoker is 5 to 10; the upper limit of normal increases by 1 for each decade of life. Patients with shunt will often not respond to supplemental oxygen while those with VQ mismatch, diffusion impairment, low inspired oxygen will improve their $Pa0_2$.

Emergency Department Care and Disposition

Regardless of the specific cause of hypoxemia, the initial approach remains the same. The following are general treatment guidelines for hypoxia:

1. Supplemental oxygen is administered to achieve an O_2 saturation greater than 90%.
2. The airway is managed aggressively if there are signs of respiratory failure (see Chapter 1).
3. Cause-specific treatment and evaluation should be pursued.
4. All patients with new hypoxemia should be admitted and monitored until their condition is stabilized.

HYPERCAPNIA

Hypercapnia occurs exclusively due to alveolar hypoventilation (releasing of CO_2) and is defined as a $PaCO_2$ above 45 mm Hg. Factors that affect alveolar ventilation include respiratory rate, tidal volume, and dead space volume, all of which are controlled by the body to maintain $PaCO_2$ in a narrow range.

Clinical Features

The signs and symptoms of hypercapnia depend on the absolute value of the $PaCO_2$ and the rate of change. Acute elevations result in increased intracranial pressure, prompting patient complaints of headache, confusion, and lethargy. Coma, encephalopathy, and seizures may occur when the $PaCO_2$ acutely rises above 80 mm Hg; similar $PaCO_2$ levels may be well tolerated if elevations are chronic.

Diagnosis and Differential

The diagnosis of hypercapnia requires clinical suspicion and ABG analysis as pulse oximetry may be completely normal. In acute cases, the ABG will demonstrate an elevation in $PaCO_2$ with a respiratory acidosis and minimal metabolic compensation. Common causes of hypercapnia include COPD, respiratory center depression from drugs (e.g., opiates, sedatives, and anesthetics), neuromuscular impairment from disease (e.g., Guillain–Barré syndrome) or toxin (e.g., botulism), and finally thoracic cage disorders (e.g., morbid obesity, kyphoscoliosis).

Emergency Department Care and Disposition

Treatment of acute hypercapnia requires aggressive measures to increase minute ventilation.

1. Airway maintenance is crucial.
2. A trial of biphasic positive airway pressure or continuous positive airway pressure may prove helpful and improve minute ventilation; however, vigilance should be maintained in patients with depressed mental status as mechanical ventilation may be needed. Ensure that the respiratory rate is set to facilitate the removal of CO_2.
3. Where indicated, treatment should include condition-specific therapies, such as bronchodilators for COPD, or reversal agents for opiate overdose.
4. Disposition depends on acuity, but many patients with hypercapnia require hospital admission and monitoring.

WHEEZING

Wheezes are "musical" adventitious lung sounds produced by airflow through the central and distal airways. It is usually more prominent on exhalation, in contrast to upper airway stridor which is more prominent during inspiration, but it may be difficult to tell the two apart.

Wheezing is usually associated with lower airway disease such as asthma or other obstructive pulmonary diseases; however, the differential is broad and may also include pulmonary edema (commonly referred to as "cardiac asthma"), foreign body, bronchiolitis, and other pathologies.

COUGH

Cough is a protective reflex for clearing secretions and foreign debris from the tracheobronchial tree. Coughing is initiated by stimulation of irritant receptors located throughout the respiratory tract. Such irritants may include inflammation as in asthma, irritants such as mold or dust or pulmonary secretions.

Clinical Features

Acute cough (<3 weeks) is most often caused by infection of the respiratory tract, or allergic reactions. Common upper respiratory infections are associated with a combination of rhinorrhea, sinusitis, pharyngitis, and laryngitis, with the cough a result of drainage from the nasopharynx onto cough receptors in the pharynx and larynx. A productive cough is the hallmark of acute bronchitis. Pertussis may last 1 to 6 weeks. A subacute cough may last for 3 to 8 weeks and is often post-infectious and related to airway inflammation and secretions.

The most common cause of a chronic cough lasting more than 6 weeks is smoking. Features of smoking-related cough include peak severity in the morning and sputum production. Other causes of chronic cough include upper airway cough syndrome (formerly postnasal discharge) which is associated with mucus drainage from the nose, a history of "allergies or sinus problems," and frequent clearing of the throat or swallowing of mucus. Asthma-related chronic cough is often worse at night, exacerbated by irritants, and associated with episodic wheezing and dyspnea. Gastroesophageal reflux-related cough often has a history of heartburn, is worse when lying down, and improves with anti-acid therapy (e.g., antacids, H_2 blockers, or proton pump blockers). Angiotensin-converting enzyme (ACE) inhibitor or angiotensin II receptor blocker (ARB) therapy cough is highly variable in onset, severity, and variation during the day and can begin as early as 1 week to as late as 1 year after starting treatment. The cough is dry and typically resolves in 1 to 4 weeks after ACE or ARB therapy is stopped but may linger for up to 3 months.

Diagnosis and Differential

Obtain a chest radiograph in patients with purulent sputum and/or fever. Use spirometry to document the presence of airflow obstruction in patients with asthma. In both children and adults, acute coughing illnesses can last up to 3 weeks and appropriate guidance should be given.

In addition to disease-specific therapy, patients with acute cough may benefit from symptomatic treatment with antitussives, which block the cough reflex at various locations, or demulcents, which soothe the pharynx and somewhat suppress the cough reflex. For intractable coughing paroxysms in the ED, nebulized lidocaine may provide relief.

Figure 29-1 outlines a sequential approach for evaluation of subacute and chronic cough.

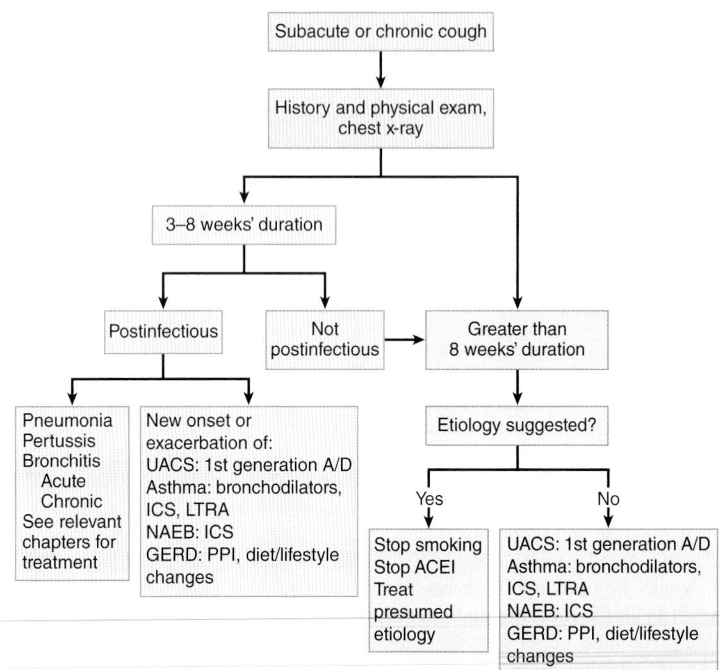

FIGURE 29-1. Evaluation of subacute and chronic cough for patients 15 years of age and older. ACEI, angiotensin-converting enzyme inhibitor; A/D, antihistamine/decongestant; GERD, gastroesophageal reflux disease; ICS, inhaled corticosteroids; LTRA, leukotriene receptor antagonist; NAEB, nonasthmatic eosinophilic bronchitis; PPI, proton pump inhibitor; UACS, upper airway cough syndrome.

HICCUPS

Hiccups are the involuntary spastic contraction of the inspiratory muscles.

Clinical Features

Benign hiccups are generally initiated by gastric distention from food or drink, especially carbonated beverages or alcohol. Persistent hiccups are usually the result of injury or irritation to a branch of the vagus or phrenic nerves.

Diagnosis and Differential

Determine whether a specific triggering event exists. Ask about the relationship with sleep; if there is resolution during sleep it suggests a psychogenic cause. Consider obtaining a chest radiograph to evaluate for intrathoracic pathology.

Emergency Department Care and Disposition

There are various physical maneuvers and drugs that can be used to terminate an acute episode.

Chlorpromazine is the only drug with FDA approval for hiccups though metoclopramide and haloperidol have also been used.

CYANOSIS

Cyanosis is a bluish color of the skin or mucous membranes, resulting from an increased amount of deoxyhemoglobin (reduced Hb). The detection of cyanosis is highly subjective and not a sensitive indicator of arterial oxygenation. It is usually visible when the deoxyhemoglobin level exceeds 5 mg/dL.

Clinical Features

The presence of cyanosis suggests tissue hypoxia. Cyanosis is divided into central and peripheral categories. Central cyanosis, which is most reliably observed under the tongue or on the buccal mucosa, is due to inadequate pulmonary oxygenation or abnormal hemoglobin such as methemoglobin and peripheral cyanosis of the fingers or extremities is due to diminished peripheral blood flow.

Diagnosis and Differential

The causes of cyanosis may be multifactorial (Table 29-2). In some cases, diagnosis is confounded by the coexistence of central and peripheral cyanosis. Pulse oximetry is easily available for continuous monitoring but may be inaccurate in the presence of a hemaglobinopathy. Obtain an ABG analysis *with* co-oximetry as ABG alone may also be misleading in the presence of a hemaglobinopathy. For example, methemoglobinemia and carboxyhemoglobinemia may cause cyanosis with a normal PaO_2. Methemoglobinemia is associated with blood that has been described as chocolate brown, and which does not change color with exposure to room air. An extremely elevated carboxyhemoglobin level may produce cherry-red mucous membrane discoloration. A hematocrit may demonstrate polycythemia vera or severe anemia, both of which may contribute to cyanosis.

TABLE 29-2 Differential Diagnosis of Cyanosis

Central Cyanosis	Peripheral Cyanosis
Hypoxemia	Reduced cardiac output
Decreased fraction of inspired oxygen: high altitude	Cold extremities
Hypoventilation	Maldistribution of blood flow: distributive forms of shock
Ventilation–perfusion mismatch	Arterial or venous obstruction
Right-to-left shunt: congenital heart disease, pulmonary arteriovenous fistulas, multiple intrapulmonary shunts	
Abnormal hemoglobin	
Methemoglobinemia: hereditary, acquired	
Sulfhemoglobinemia: acquired	
Carboxyhemoglobinemia	

PLEURAL EFFUSION

Pleural effusions result from fluid accumulating in the potential space between the visceral and parietal pleurae.

Clinical Features

A pleural effusion may be clinically silent or symptomatic, due to symptoms of an underlying disease, an increase in volume of the effusion with the production of dyspnea, or the development of inflammation and associated pain with respiration. Physical findings of a pleural effusion include percussion dullness and decreased breath sounds.

Diagnosis and Differential

The underlying etiologies of pleural effusion are numerous. In developed countries, the most common causes are heart failure, pneumonia, and cancer. The presence of pleural effusion on chest radiograph or ultrasound should prompt a search for the underlying cause.

Emergency Department Care and Disposition

Thoracentesis may be performed for diagnostic purposes to differentiate between an exudate and transudate or to identify infection. It may also be performed for therapeutic purposes if a patient has dyspnea at rest. Typically 1-1.5L are removed; more may precipitate re-expansion pulmonary edema.

The management of parapneumonic effusions and empyemas may include antibiotics to target the underlying infectious agent and the placement of a thoracostomy tube. The decision to admit should take into account the acuity and severity of symptoms.

FURTHER READING

For further reading in *Tintinalli's Emergency Medicine: A Comprehensive Study Guide*, 8th ed., see Chapter 62, "Respiratory Distress," by John Sarko, and J. Stephen Stapczynski.

Bronchitis, Pneumonia, and Novel Respiratory Infections

Jeffrey M. Goodloe

BRONCHITIS

Acute bronchitis is a commonly encountered, self-limited, infection producing inflammatory changes within the larger airways. Sharing the viral pathogens of upper respiratory infections, including those of the common cold, acute bronchitis is often caused by one of the following: influenza A or B virus, adenovirus, rhinovirus, parainfluenza virus, respiratory syncytial virus, or coronavirus. Far less frequent in etiology, the bacterial pathogens *Streptococcus pneumoniae*, *Haemophilus influenzae*, *Chlamydia pneumoniae*, *Mycoplasma pneumoniae*, and *Bordatella pertussis* may lead to more severe presentations in older populations, especially in those with increased comorbidities.

Clinical Features

The predominant cough of acute bronchitis may be productive and can easily last up to 3 weeks. Sputum purulence is usually indicative of sloughed inflammatory airway cells and, taken alone, does not indicate a bacterial etiology. Bronchitis most commonly lacks the suggestive symptoms and signs of pneumonia, specifically fever >38°C (100.4°F), adult heart rate >100 beats/min, and/or adult respiratory rate >24 breaths/min. Wheezing may be present.

Diagnosis and Differential

The diagnosis of acute bronchitis can be made clinically with the following criteria: (a) acute-onset cough (shorter than 3 weeks duration), (b) absence of chronic lung disease history, (c) normal vital signs, and (d) absence of auscultatory abnormalities that suggest pneumonia. Pulse oximetry is indicated if the patient describes dyspnea or appears short of breath. Bedside peak flow testing may reveal reductions in forced expiratory volume in 1 second. A chest radiograph is not required in non-elderly patients who appear nontoxic. Consider pertussis in adolescents and young adults whose coughs persist beyond 2 to 3 weeks, particularly if they exhibit coughing paroxysms with prominent post-tussive emesis or had exposure to pertussis.

Emergency Department Care and Disposition

1. The use of antibiotics for acute bronchitis, while commonly requested by patients and prescribed by practitioners, does NOT confer clinically relevant benefits in a viral illness, but produces side effects such as gastrointestinal distress, vaginitis, and future pathogen resistance.
2. If pertussis is strongly suspected, prescribe **azithromycin** 500 mg orally on day 1, followed by 250 mg orally on days 2 to 5. This treatment does not shorten the illness, but decreases coughing paroxysms and limits disease transmission.

3. Patients with evidence of airflow obstruction who are treated with bronchodilators experience faster cough resolution. **Albuterol** two puffs every 4 to 6 hours using a metered dose inhaler and spacer provides symptomatic relief in dyspnea and cough.
4. Consider additional agents for cough suppression, mucolysis, and other symptomatic relief on an individual basis factoring comorbidities, drug interactions, and potential side effects.
5. Discharge patients with instructions for timely follow-up with a primary care physician, smoking cessation when applicable, and when to return to the emergency department based upon clinical symptoms.

PNEUMONIA

Pneumonia is most commonly a bacterial infection of the alveolar lung. Pneumococcus (*Streptococcus pneumoniae*) is the classic bacterial etiology, although incidence from atypical and opportunistic agents, particularly if pneumonia is acquired in health care settings, is increasing. *Staphylococcus aureus*, *Klebsiella pneumoniae*, *Pseudomonas aeruginosa*, and *Haemophilus influenzae* are additional causative bacterial agents. *Legionella pneumophila*, *Mycoplasma pneumoniae*, *Chlamydia pneumoniae*, and a spectrum of respiratory viruses account for the bulk of atypical pneumonias. Anaerobes are less frequently encountered, but must be highly suspected if aspiration is suspected. Risk factors for pneumonia are multiple, and include diseases of the respiratory tract (e.g., chronic obstructive pulmonary disease or COPD) and immune system (e.g., cancer, AIDS), as well as chronic conditions associated with aspiration, bacteremia, and debilitation.

Clinical Features

Patients with undifferentiated bacterial pneumonia typically present with some combination of cough, fatigue, fever, dyspnea, sputum production, and pleuritic chest pain. Physical examination often reveals tachypnea, tachycardia, low pulse oximetry, and the auscultatory findings of bronchial breath sounds and rhonchi suggestive of consolidation. Impaired air passage may be indicated by wheezing. While historical features and associated symptoms and signs can prove helpful in predicting a likely causative organism, the treatment of pneumonia has shifted to empiric treatment based on the patient's environment. The clinician should differentiate between community acquired pneumonia (CAP) versus health care-associated pneumonia (HCAP) with HCAP's risk for organisms that require specific and/or broadened antibiotic coverage, such as *Pseudomonas aeruginosa* and/or methicillin-resistant *Staphylococcus aureus* (MRSA). Patients meeting criteria for HCAP include patients hospitalized over 48 hours within the prior 90 days, those receiving routine outpatient treatments of dialysis, chemotherapy, wound care, or home IV antibiotic therapy, and residents of a nursing facility.

Clinical features of aspiration pneumonitis depend on the volume and pH of the aspirate, the presence of particulate matter in the aspirate, and bacterial contamination. Although aspiration of acidic, larger volumes result in a relatively rapid onset of tachypnea, tachycardia, and respiratory distress that may progress to pulmonary failure, most cases of aspiration pneumonia progress insidiously. While aspiration pneumonias may occur anywhere in the lung, aspirated material has a predilection for the right lower lobe due to gravity and tracheobronchial tree anatomy. Untreated or partially treated aspiration pneumonia may progress to empyema, defined as pus in the pleural space, or a lung abscess.

Diagnosis and Differential

Uncomplicated presentations in otherwise healthy patients may not require use of radiology, laboratory, or pathology resources; however, chest radiography is most commonly used for diagnosis (see Fig. 30-1). Depending upon the anticipated etiology and disposition course, assessing white blood count with differential analysis, serum electrolytes, blood urea nitrogen, creatinine, glucose, blood gases, sputum Gram staining, and cultures of sputum and blood provide benefit, particularly in patients requiring intensive care unit (ICU) admission. Most patients do not require identification of a specific organism to make a diagnosis and begin treatment.

The differential diagnosis of nontrauma patients with respiratory complaints and radiographic abnormality is lengthy and partially includes noninfectious atelectasis; chronic pulmonary fibrosis; pleural effusion; chemical pneumonitis; inflammatory disorders, such as sarcoidosis; neoplasm; postsurgical changes; tuberculosis; bronchiolitis obliterans; pulmonary embolus;

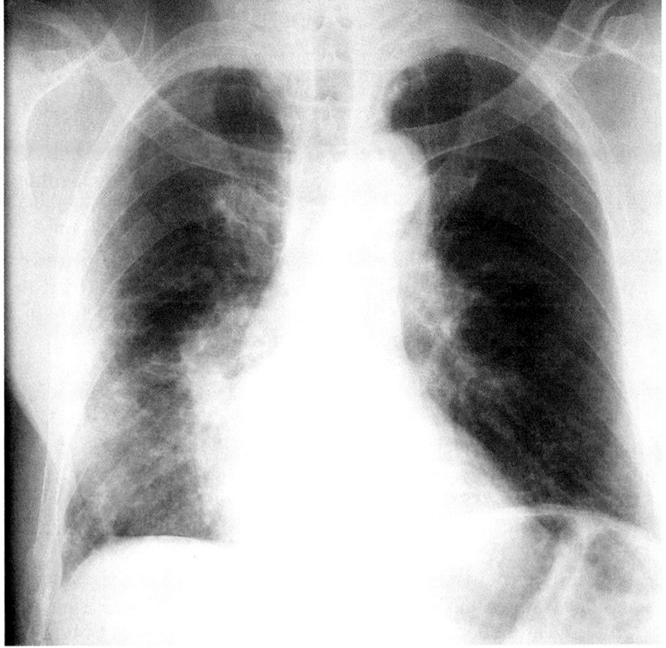

FIGURE 30-1. Lobar pneumonia.

congestive heart failure; and pulmonary vasculitides, such as Goodpasture disease or Wegener granulomatosis.

Emergency Department Care and Disposition

1. Support vital respiratory function (oxygenation, ventilation) as indicated, with rapidly impending or unresponsive respiratory failure managed via intubation and mechanical ventilation. Noninvasive positive pressure ventilation may prevent the need for intubation.
2. In general, progressive degrees of abnormal vital signs, comorbidities, and advancing age confer increased need for inpatient management. The complexity of pneumonia severity scoring as a means to determine discharge or admission prevents inclusion in this manual.
3. Begin antibiotic treatment in all cases of suspected bacterial pneumonia, with the specific choice(s) made considering the patient's recent environment, differentiating community acquired from HCAPs, comorbidities, drug allergies, drug–drug interactions, and local resistance patterns.
4. Specialty society guidelines and infectious disease consultation advice change with the advent of antimicrobials and resistance patterns. The antimicrobials listed here represent a summary of current and generally accepted antibiotic regimens for adults with the indicated clinical situations. Dosages may require adjustment for renal insufficiency.
5. Outpatient management of uncomplicated CAP in otherwise healthy patients: **azithromycin,** day 1 with 500 mg orally, followed by days 2 to 5 with 250 mg orally or **doxycycline** 100 mg orally twice daily for 10 days (this is a low-cost alternative). The Centers for Disease Control and Prevention (CDC) recommends reserving oral fluoroquinolones for those failing macrolide or tetracycline class therapy to minimize resistance.
6. Outpatient management of CAP in patients with significant comorbidities (and without health care–associated pneumonia suspected): **levofloxacin** 750 mg orally daily for 5 days OR **amoxicillin-clavulanate** 875/125 mg orally twice daily for 10 days PLUS **azithromycin,** day 1 with 500 mg orally, followed by days 2 to 5 with 250 mg orally.
7. Inpatient management of CAP in patients not requiring ICU admission: start antibiotic therapy with **levofloxacin** 750 mg IV OR **ceftriaxone** 1 g IV PLUS **azithromycin** 500 mg IV. Utilize antibiotics early in the course of any pneumonia requiring admission.
8. Inpatient management of CAP in patients requiring ICU admission: start antibiotic therapy with **ceftriaxone** 1 g IV PLUS **levofloxacin** 750 mg IV. If MRSA suspected, add **vancomycin** 10 to 15 mg/kg IV.
9. Inpatient management of suspected HCAP: start double coverage against *Pseudomonas* with (1) **levofloxacin** 750 mg IV PLUS (2) **cefepime** 1 to 2 g IV OR **piperacillin/tazobactam** 4.5 g IV. Also, cover suspected MRSA with **vancomycin** 10 to 15 mg/kg IV OR **linezolid** 600 mg IV.
10. Aspiration pneumonitis: prophylactic antibiotics are not recommended and their indiscriminate use may contribute to organism resistance. For witnessed aspirations, immediate tracheal suction followed by bronchoscopy, if needed, to remove large particles is indicated. In pneumonitis

that has already progressed to pneumonia prior to or shortly after emergency department presentation, start antibiotic therapy with **levofloxacin** 750 mg IV PLUS **clindamycin** 600 mg IV.

11. Empyema: **piperacillin/tazobactam** 4.5 g IV. If MRSA suspected, add **vancomycin** 10 to 15 mg/kg IV. Admit the patient and consult with a pulmonologist or thoracic surgeon early for further consideration of definitive diagnostic measures and treatment options to promote drainage.
12. Lung abscess: **clindamycin** 600 mg IV for anaerobic coverage plus **ceftriaxone** 1 g IV. A significant majority of lung abscesses are successfully treated with inpatient medical management and surgical consultation is required in only a minority of cases.
13. For patients with uncomplicated pneumonia, discharge instructions should, at a minimum, include timely follow-up with a primary care physician, smoking cessation (when applicable), and delineation of symptoms that should prompt a return visit to the emergency department.

NOVEL RESPIRATORY INFECTIONS

Severe acute respiratory syndrome (SARS) came to worldwide attention in the winter of 2003. Numerous deaths were reported in Asia, North America, and Europe. The etiologic agent is a coronavirus, SARS-CoV, spread by "droplet infection." In the event of SARS outbreak, up-to-date information can be found at the CDC website (http://www.cdc.gov/sars/who/clinicians.html) as well as at the World Health Organization (WHO) website (http://www.who.int/topics/sars/en/).

Middle East respiratory syndrome (MERS) was named in latter 2012 and became a more prominent global concern in the spring of 2014. A fatality rate approaching 50% was reported in the initial 100 diagnosed cases. Since these initial cases, mortality has decreased. The etiologic agent is a coronavirus. Respiratory symptoms predominate, though GI symptoms of abdominal pain and diarrhea may be present. Health care workers exposed via airborne transmission have become more common in case reports. Current, basic steps to reduce MERS coronavirus transmission to health care workers include wearing gloves, gown, eye protection and using a fit-tested N95 respirator facemask. Up-to-date information can be found at the CDC website (http://www.cdc.gov/coronavirus/mers/hcp.html) as well as at the WHO website (http://www.who.int/csr/disease/coronavirus_infections/en/).

FURTHER READING

For further reading in *Tintinalli's Emergency Medicine: A Comprehensive Study Guide*, 8th ed., see Chapter 64, "Acute Bronchitis and Upper Respiratory Tract Infections," by Cedric W. Lefebvre; Chapter 65, "Pneumonia and Pulmonary Infiltrates," by Gerald Maloney, Eric Anderson, and Donald M. Yealy, and Chapter 66, "Lung Empyema and Abscess," by Eric Anderson and Sharon E. Mace.

CHAPTER 31 Tuberculosis

Amy J. Behrman

Tuberculosis (TB) is the second most common cause of infectious disease deaths globally, with one-third of the world's population infected. Although active TB infection rates continue to decline in the United States, TB remains an important public health problem, particularly among immigrants, whose active TB case rate is 12 times higher than the US-born population. Other risk factors include HIV infection; living or working in prison, shelters, and long-term care facilities; and alcohol/drug abuse. Transmission occurs by inhalation of droplet nuclei and may lead to active primary infection or latent disease (which may reactivate later). Identifying and treating high-risk patients for active and latent TB is key to ongoing TB control.

CLINICAL FEATURES

Primary TB

Initial TB infection is usually asymptomatic in immune-competent adults, generally presenting with only a new positive reaction to TB skin testing (TST) or a new positive interferon gamma release assay (IGRA). These patients have normal chest radiographs (CXRs) and are presumed to have latent infections. When active primary TB does develop, symptoms often include fever, cough, weight loss, malaise, and chest pain. Some patients may present with active pneumonitis (which may be mistaken for community-acquired pneumonia) or extra-pulmonary disease.

Children are more likely to present with active early disease, although the presenting symptoms may be subtle even when CXRs are abnormal. Presenting symptoms may include fever, cough, wheezing, poor feeding, and fatigue. TB meningitis and miliary TB are more common in children than adults.

Immunocompromised patients are much more likely to develop rapidly progressive primary infections. All patients with active TB should be evaluated for immune-compromising conditions. Symptoms may be pulmonary (fever, cough, dyspnea, hemoptysis) or extrapulmonary, reflecting early hematogenous spread to the liver, bones, central nervous system, or other sites.

Reactivation TB

Latent TB infections will progress to active disease (i.e., reactivation TB) in 5% of cases within 2 years of primary infection; an additional 5% will reactivate over their lifetimes. Reactivation rates are higher in children, the elderly, persons with recent primary infection, those with immune compromise (in particular HIV), and those with chronic diseases such as diabetes and renal failure.

Most patients with reactivation TB present subacutely with fever, malaise, weight loss, fatigue, and night sweats. Most patients with active

TB will have pulmonary involvement and will develop productive coughs. Hemoptysis, pleuritic chest pain, and dyspnea may occur. Rales and rhonchi may be found, but the physical examination is not usually diagnostic.

Extrapulmonary TB develops in up to 20% of active TB cases. Lymphadenitis, with painless enlargement and possible draining sinuses, is a common presentation. Patients may also present with symptomatic pleural effusion, pericarditis, peritonitis, or meningitis. Additional sites of reactivation TB after hematogenous spread include bones, joints, adrenals, GI tract, and GU tract. Extrapulmonary reactivation TB is more common and often more severe in young children and immunocompromised patients as noted for primary TB infection above.

Miliary TB is a multisystem disease caused by massive hematogenous dissemination. It is also more common in immunocompromised patients and children. Symptoms are systemic with fever, weight loss, adenopathy, and malaise. Patients may present with multiorgan failure or Adult Respiratory Distress Syndrome (ARDS).

DIAGNOSIS AND DIFFERENTIAL

Variable presentations and limited testing options make TB diagnosis particularly challenging in the ED. Differential diagnoses may include other infectious causes of pulmonary and extrapulmonary lesions as well as malignancy. TB should always be considered in patients with prolonged febrile cough illnesses, particularly in known risk groups. TB should be considered in any HIV patient with respiratory symptoms, even if chest radiographs are normal (see Chapter 92 HIV Infections and AIDS).

Imaging

CXR remains the most useful ED diagnostic tool for TB. Active primary pulmonary TB usually presents with parenchymal infiltrates in any lung area. Hilar and/or mediastinal adenopathy may occur with or without infiltrates. Effusions, usually unilateral, may be seen with or without infiltrates.

Reactivation TB classically presents with lesions in the upper lobes or superior segments of the lower lobes (Fig. 31-1). Cavitation, calcification, scarring, atelectasis, hilar adenopathy, and effusions may be seen. Cavitation is associated with increased infectivity. Miliary TB may cause diffuse, small (1 to 3 mm) nodular infiltrates. Atypical CXRs are progressively more common with worsening immune compromise. Patients co-infected with HIV and TB are particularly likely to present with atypical imaging.

Stable scarring, volume loss, and calcified or noncalcified nodules may be found (often as incidental findings) in patients with asymptomatic latent TB infection; these patients are not infectious and do not require urgent treatment or isolation. Comparison with prior films is useful in determining the likelihood of active TB infection.

Laboratory Tests

Acid-fast staining of sputum can detect mycobacteria in many patients with pulmonary TB, although the yield is lower in HIV patients. Results may be available within several hours, with potential ED utility, but there

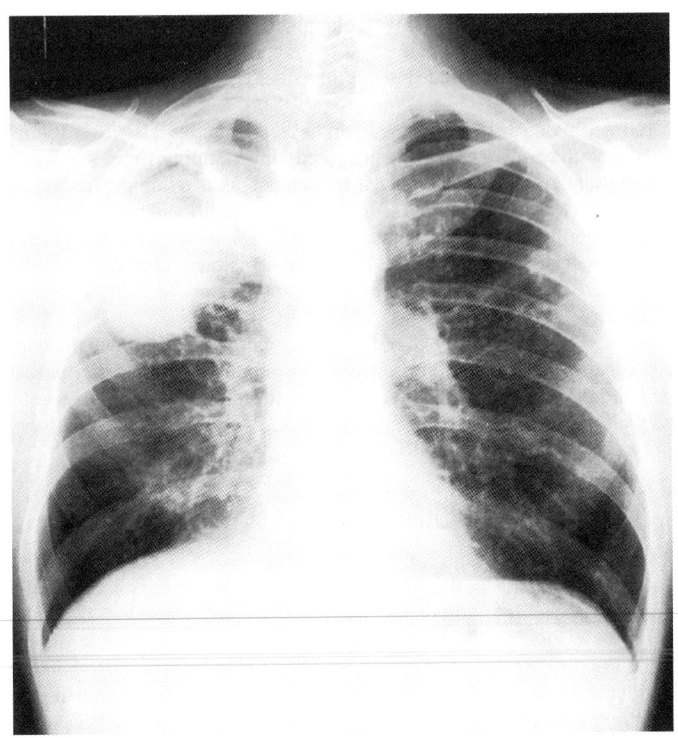

FIGURE 31-1. Cavitary tuberculosis of the right upper lobe.

are serious limitations. Many patients will have false negatives on a single sputum sample. Microscopy of nonsputum samples (e.g., pleural fluid, cerebrospinal fluid) is even less sensitive. Microscopy cannot differentiate between TB and nontuberculous mycobacteria. **Culture** of sputum (or other specimens) is the gold standard for diagnosing active TB. Unfortunately, definitive culture results take weeks. When available, newer technologies such as **TB-specific nucleic acid amplification tests (NAATs)** can produce results within 24 hours, a time frame potentially useful in ED management. These tests have poor negative predictive value, but a patient with positive microscopy and a positive NAAT should be treated for active TB unless subsequent cultures rule it out.

Tuberculin skin tests (TSTs) identify most patients with latent, prior, or active TB, but results are read 48 to 72 hours after placement, limiting the ED utility of this approach. Patients with disseminated TB, early active TB, or major immune compromise (especially HIV) may have false-negative TSTs. Immigrants who received BCG vaccine in childhood may have false-positive TSTs. **Interferon gamma release assays (IGRA)** of whole blood may become more useful than TST for ED evaluation of suspected TB, since these tests may be resulted within hours and may have better sensitivity and specificity in some situations. For instance, BCG alone should not cause a positive IGRA, making it useful for evaluating immigrants from high-prevalence countries.

EMERGENCY DEPARTMENT CARE AND DISPOSITION

1. Train ED and pre-hospital staff to identify patients at risk for active TB as early as possible during their care so that **airborne isolation and respiratory protection for staff** can be implemented as soon as possible to protect staff, visitors, and other patients. Consider the diagnosis of active TB in any patient with respiratory or systemic complaints, particularly if they are in higher risk groups, to facilitate treatment and reduce exposure risks.
2. Initial therapy for active TB should include at least four drugs until susceptibility profiles are available. The regimen usually includes **isoniazid** 5 mg/kg up to 300 mg PO daily in adults, **rifampin** 10 mg/kg up to 600 mg PO daily in adults, **pyrazinamide** 15 to 30 mg/kg up to 2 g PO daily in adults, and **ethambutol** 15 to 20 mg/kg up to 1.6 g PO daily in adults. Give **pyridoxine** 50 mg/day with INH to prevent neuropathy. Caution all patients to avoid alcohol and hepatotoxins during treatment. Directly observed therapy (DOT) may improve outpatient compliance with these complex regimens. (See http://www.cdc.gov/tb for DOT recommendations and long-term treatment options.)
3. Consider the possibility of multi-drug resistant **(MDR) TB** in patients with a prior history of TB, suboptimal prior treatment of TB, known or likely exposure to MDR TB, or persistently positive smears and symptoms after several months of treatment, and when there is known local drug resistance. Treatment of known or suspected MDR TB begins with four to six drugs judged likely to be effective by Infectious Disease consultation.
4. **Admission** is indicated for patients with clinical instability, hypoxia, dyspnea, diagnostic uncertainty, unreliable outpatient follow-up or compliance, and suspected or known MDR TB. ED physicians should know local laws and public health resources for case reporting, involuntary hospitalization, and treatment (including DOT). Patients with suspected TB should wear masks during all transport, and should be admitted to airborne-isolation single rooms.
5. Patients discharged from the ED with known or likely active TB infection must have urgent documented **referral to a physician or local public health department for long-term treatment and contact tracing**.
6. Persons with latent TB infection (defined as a positive TST and/or IGRA without active TB findings on imaging) should be referred to primary care or public health clinics for prophylaxis against reactivation TB.

FURTHER READING

For further reading in *Tintinalli's Emergency Medicine: A Comprehensive Study Guide*, 8th ed., see Chapter 67, "Tuberculosis," by Vu D. Phan and Janet M. Poponick.

CHAPTER 32 Spontaneous and Iatrogenic Pneumothorax

Mike Cadogan

Pneumothorax occurs when air or gas enters the pleural cavity, the potential space between the visceral and parietal pleura, leading to partial lung collapse. Smoking is the most common risk factor for spontaneous pneumothorax.

Primary pneumothorax occurs in patients without known lung disease and secondary pneumothorax occurs in the presence of known lung disease, such as chronic obstructive pulmonary disease, asthma, cystic fibrosis, interstitial lung disease, infection, connective tissue disease, and cancer. Latrogenic pneumothorax occurs secondary to invasive procedures such as needle biopsy of the lung, placement of a subclavian line, nasogastric tube placement or positive pressure ventilation, Tension pneumothorax results from positive pressure in the pleural space leading to decreased venous return, hypotension, and hypoxia. Hemopneumothorax occurs in 2% to 7% of patients with spontaneous pneumothorax. Treating the underlying disease may help decrease the risk of pneumothorax.

CLINICAL FEATURES

Sudden-onset dyspnea and ipsilateral, pleuritic chest pain are the most common presenting symptoms. The physical examination findings are often subtle. Sinus tachycardia is the most common physical finding. In spontaneous pneumothorax the classic examination findings of ipsilateral decreased breath sounds, reduced chest expansion, and hyperresonance to percussion are often absent. However, in traumatic pneumothorax, the positive predictive value of ipsilateral decreased breath sounds is 86% to 97%. Clinical hallmarks of tension pneumothorax include severe progressive dyspnea, tachycardia (>140 bpm), hypoxia, and ipsilateral decreased breath sounds. Tracheal deviations away from the affected side, distended neck veins, and cardiac apical displacement are late and infrequent signs of progressive tension.

DIAGNOSIS AND DIFFERENTIAL

Pneumothorax is an important differential consideration in patients with pleuritic chest pain, especially in those with underlying lung disease. Patients with pulmonary embolism, pneumonia, pericarditis, pleural effusions, or shingles can present with pain similar to those with pneumothorax. As clinical signs and symptoms are often subtle and variable, the definitive diagnosis is usually established with appropriate imaging. In stable patients with suspected pneumothorax, an erect posteroanterior (PA) chest radiograph is usually the primary investigation. Characteristically this demonstrates a displaced pleural line with absent lung markings extending from the visceral pleura (lung edge) to the chest wall (parietal pleura). Routine expiratory radiographs do not significantly enhance diagnostic yield. The presence of cardiophrenic recess hyperlucency and costophrenic angle enlargement (deep sulcus sign) on a supine anteroposterior radiograph is suggestive of pneumothorax.

Large emphysematous bullae may mimic pneumothorax. To prevent the potentially disastrous consequence of inserting a chest drain into a lung bulla mistaken for a pneumothorax, thoracic computed tomography (CT) should be used to clarify the diagnosis. Bedside ultrasound is a rapid, non-invasive method to diagnose pneumothorax in young, healthy patients with no underlying lung disease.

In normal lung, the visceral and parietal pleura are in direct contact and ultrasound can be used to demonstrate the lung moving back and forth beneath the ribs during respiration (lung sliding), and vertical reverberation artefacts (comet-tails). Features suggesting pneumothorax include absence of lung sliding, comet tail artefacts and a lung pulse in the presence of a distinct A lines and visualized lung point. Chest CT is effective at detecting pneumothorax, determining their size and volume, and detecting other lung pathology, and can differentiate large bullae from intrapleural air.

EMERGENCY DEPARTMENT CARE AND DISPOSITION

The ED treatment goal is the elimination of intrapleural air.

1. Tension pneumothorax should be diagnosed clinically—before a radiograph—and immediately treated by needle decompression followed by tube thoracostomy.
2. Administer **oxygen** >28% or 2 to 4 L by nasal cannula to increase pleural air resorption. Monitor for hypercapnia in patients with chronic obstructive pulmonary disease.
3. Observe patients with a small primary pneumothorax for at least 4 hours on supplemental oxygen, and then repeat the chest radiograph. If symptoms and chest radiograph have improved, the patient should return in 24 hours for repeat examination and then weekly until resolution. First-time spontaneous pneumothorax of <20% lung volume in a stable, healthy adult may be treated initially with oxygen therapy and observation.
4. Aspiration or tube thoracostomy is performed in order to rapidly reduce the volume of a closed pneumothorax and significantly shorten the time to pneumothorax resolution.
    a. For aspiration of a small primary or secondary spontaneous pneumothorax, insert a 14-G needle in adults (18-G needle in children) that is at least 2 in. (5 cm) long, followed by syringe aspiration and needle removal. Alternatively, a small catheter or pigtail catheter may be used and attached to a Heimlich valve or suction. Either of two locations may be used: anteriorly in the second intercostal space (ICS) at the midclavicular line (MCL) and laterally in the fourth or fifth ICS at the anterior axillary line (AAL). The fifth ICS AAL is the preferred location for needle thoracostomy decompression.
    b. Treat patients with a failed aspiration, large pneumothorax, recurrent pneumothorax, bilateral pneumothoraces, hemothorax, abnormal vital signs, or severe dyspnea using chest tube thoracostomy. Use a small 10- to 14-French chest tube for nontrauma, reserving larger 14- to 22-French chest tubes if a large air leak is probable, such as from mechanical ventilation or with underlying pulmonary disease.
5. Patients who require chest tube thoracostomy require admission to the hospital.

TREATMENT COMPLICATIONS

Intervention complications include intercostal vessel hemorrhage, lung parenchymal injury, empyema, and tube malfunction (development of an air leak or tension pneumothorax), and re-expansion lung injury. Re-expansion lung injury is uncommon and seen more often when there is collapse of the lung for greater than 72 hours, large pneumothoraces, rapid re-expansion, or negative pleural pressure suction of greater than 20 cm. Most patients with re-expansion injury require only observation and supplemental oxygen and rarely suffer adverse outcomes.

Iatrogenic Pneumothorax

Iatrogenic pneumothorax is a subset of traumatic pneumothorax and occurs more often than spontaneous pneumothorax. Transthoracic needle procedures (needle biopsy and thoracentesis) account for 50% of iatrogenic pneumothoraces with subclavian vein catheterization accounting for a further 25%. US guidance for central venous catheter insertion for thoracentesis reduces the pneumothorax complication rate. Factors associated with the increasing frequency of iatrogenic pneumothorax include underlying disease, body habitus, and experience of the operator. Although it is routine to obtain a chest radiograph after central line placement or transthoracic needle procedures, chest radiograph may not identify a pneumothorax if the patient is supine or if there is inadequate time for the pneumothorax to develop, with up to one-third detected later. Treatment for iatrogenic pneumothorax is generally the same as for spontaneous pneumothorax.

FURTHER READING

For further reading in *Tintinalli's Emergency Medicine: A Comprehensive Study Guide*, 8th ed., see Chapter 68, "Pneumothorax," by Bret A. Nicks and David Manthey.

CHAPTER 33 Hemoptysis

Nilesh Patel

Hemoptysis is the expectoration of blood from the lungs or tracheobronchial tree. *Massive hemoptysis* is defined as 100 mL of blood per 24 hours up to >1000 mL per 24 hours. Minor hemoptysis is defined as the production of smaller quantities of blood in a patient with no comorbid lung disease and stable vital signs. Hemoptysis results from the disruption of blood vessels within the bronchial circulation which supplies oxygenated blood to the bronchi, bronchioles, and lung parenchyma.

CLINICAL FEATURES

Hemoptysis may be the presenting symptom for many different diseases. Massive hemoptysis can often be life threatening. A careful history and physical can raise suspicion for the underlying diagnosis and guide the appropriate workup. The acute onset of fever, cough, and bloody sputum may indicate pneumonia or bronchitis. An indolent productive cough can indicate bronchitis or bronchiectasis. Dyspnea and pleuritic chest pain are potential indicators of pulmonary embolism, particularly in the presence of venous thromboembolic risk factors. Tuberculosis should be considered in the setting of fever, night sweats, and risk factors such as travel from endemic regions. Bronchogenic carcinoma may present with tobacco use, chronic weight loss, and a change in cough. Chronic dyspnea and minor hemoptysis may indicate mitral stenosis or alveolar hemorrhage syndromes (most commonly seen in patients with renal disease). Consider Goodpasture's syndrome in patients with hemoptysis, hematuria, and renal insufficiency.

The physical examination should begin with an assessment of airway, breathing, and circulation, with a focus on the vital signs. Common abnormal vital signs include fever and tachypnea. Tachypnea may be a sign of respiratory compromise with hypoxemia. Hypotension is an ominous sign, usually seen only in massive hemoptysis. The cardiac examination may reveal signs of valvular heart disease (e.g., the diastolic murmur of mitral stenosis). The nasal and oral cavities should be inspected carefully to help rule out an extrapulmonary source of bleeding (pseudohemoptysis).

DIAGNOSIS AND DIFFERENTIAL

A careful history and physical examination may suggest a diagnosis, although the cause of hemoptysis is undetermined in up to 30% of cases. Pulse oximetry and a chest x-ray (PA and lateral, if the patient's condition allows) are always indicated. Other tests that may be helpful include arterial blood gas, hemoglobin and hematocrit levels, platelet count, coagulation studies, urinalysis, and electrocardiogram. Chest CT should be considered if there is hemoptysis with an abnormal chest radiograph or if considering pulmonary embolism or carcinoma on the differential diagnosis. The long differential diagnosis list includes infectious, neoplastic, and cardiac etiologies. Infectious etiologies include bronchitis, bronchiectasis, bacterial pneumonia, tuberculosis, fungal pneumonia, and lung abscess.

Neoplastic etiologies include bronchogenic carcinoma and bronchial adenoma. Cardiogenic etiologies include mitral stenosis and left ventricular failure. Trauma, foreign body aspiration, pulmonary embolism (hemoptysis is one of the Wells criteria), primary pulmonary hypertension, pulmonary vasculitis, and bleeding diathesis, and coagulopathies secondary to medications are other potential causes.

EMERGENCY DEPARTMENT CARE AND DISPOSITION

1. Assess airway, breathing, and circulation in all patients who present with hemoptysis.
2. Administer supplemental oxygen as needed to maintain adequate oxygenation.
3. Administer normal saline or lactated Ringer's solution initially for resuscitation.
4. Type and cross-match blood if transfusion is necessary. Transfuse packed red blood cells as needed.
5. Administer fresh frozen plasma or prothrombin complex concentrates to patients with coagulopathies, including those taking warfarin; give platelets for thrombocytopenia (see Chapter 137, "Transfusion Therapy"). Other blood products can be considered as indicated.
6. Patients with ongoing massive hemoptysis may benefit from being placed in the decubitus position, with the bleeding lung in dependent position. This maneuver can also be performed after intubation in patients on mechanical ventilation.
7. Perform endotracheal intubation with a large diameter (8.0 mm) tube, which facilitates bronchoscopy, if there is respiratory failure or if the patient cannot clear blood or secretions from the airway. If bleeding is uncontrolled, consider preferentially intubating the mainstem bronchus of the unaffected lung (and using a tamponade device to stop bleeding in the alternate bronchus).
8. Admit any patient with moderate to severe hemoptysis to the hospital, and strongly consider placement in the intensive care unit. Patients with mild hemoptysis who have conditions that predispose them to severe bleeding also should be considered for admission. The advice of a pulmonologist or thoracic surgeon is required for decisions as to whether bronchoscopy, computed tomography, or angiography for bronchial artery embolization might be needed. For massive hemoptysis, emergent bronchoscopy may be indicated in the ED. If the appropriate specialists are not available, the patient should be stabilized and then transferred to another facility.
9. Treat patients who are discharged home for several days with cough suppressants, inhaled β-agonist bronchodilators as needed, and antibiotics if bacterial infection is thought to be the cause. Close follow-up is essential, particularly in those at high risk for neoplasm.
10. Most cases of mild hemoptysis are self-limited and patients can be discharged home with appropriate follow-up.

FURTHER READING

For further reading in *Tintinalli's Emergency Medicine: A Comprehensive Study Guide*, 8th ed., see Chapter 63, "Hemoptysis," by Troy Sims.

Asthma and Chronic Obstructive Pulmonary Disease

Stacey L. Poznanski

Although most asthmatic attacks are mild and reversible, severe attacks can be fatal and many patients develop chronic airflow limitation from permanent airway remodeling. Asthma is the most common chronic disease of childhood, while chronic obstructive pulmonary disease (COPD) is a leading cause of death in the world. COPD is the only major cause of death that is increasing in frequency, a phenomenon attributed to tobacco abuse. The prevalence has been stable in men, whereas the prevalence in women has doubled in the past few decades and women now account for >50% of COPD-related deaths.

CLINICAL FEATURES

Asthma is a chronic inflammatory disorder associated with hyperresponsiveness of the tracheobronchial tree and a continuum of acute bronchospasm and airway inflammation. COPD has two dominant forms: (a) pulmonary emphysema, defined in terms of anatomic pathology, characterized by destruction of bronchioles and alveoli and (b) chronic bronchitis, defined in clinical terms as a condition of excess mucous secretion in the bronchial tree, with a chronic productive cough for 3 months in each of two consecutive years. The World Health Organization's Global Institute for Chronic Obstructive Lung Disease definition of COPD encompasses both these forms as well as bronchiectasis, and asthma, and recognizes that most patients have a combination.

Acute exacerbations of asthma and COPD are usually associated with a trigger, such as smoking, respiratory infections, exposure to noxious stimuli (e.g., pollutants, cold, stress, antigens, or exercise), adverse response to medications (e.g., decongestants, β-blockers, nonsteroidal anti-inflammatory drugs), allergic reactions, hormonal changes during the normal menstrual cycle or pregnancy, and noncompliance with prescribed therapies. Although asthma exacerbations are due to expiratory airflow limitations, acute exacerbations of COPD are primarily due to ventilation–perfusion mismatch.

Classically, patients with exacerbations of asthma or COPD present with complaints of dyspnea, chest tightness, wheezing, and cough. Risk factors for death from asthma exacerbation include past history of severe exacerbation, ≥2 hospitalizations or >3 ED visits for asthma in the past year, >2 canisters per month of inhaled short-acting β_2 agonist (SABA), low socioeconomic status or history of illicit drug use, or psychiatric disease. Physical examination shows wheezing with prolonged expiration. Wheezing does not correlate with the degree of airflow obstruction; a "quiet chest" may indicate severe airflow restriction. Patients with severe attacks may be sitting upright with forward posturing, with pursed-lip exhalation, accessory muscle use, paradoxical respirations, and diaphoresis. Pulsus paradoxus of 20 mm Hg or higher may be seen. Severe airflow obstruction and ventilation/perfusion imbalance can cause hypoxia and hypercapnia. Hypoxia is characterized by tachypnea, cyanosis, agitation, apprehension, tachycardia, and hypertension. Signs of hypercapnia include confusion, tremor, plethora, stupor, hypopnea, and apnea. Impending respiratory failure may be signaled by alteration in mental status, lethargy, minimal or absent breath sounds, acidosis, worsening hypoxia, and hypercapnia.

DIAGNOSIS AND DIFFERENTIAL

Emergency department diagnosis of asthma or COPD usually is made clinically, although signs and symptoms do not always correlate well with severity of airflow obstruction. Severity can be measured more objectively by the forced expiratory volume in 1 second (FEV_1) and peak expiratory flow rate (PEFR) in cooperative patients. A FEV_1 or PEFR <40% of patients predicted in asthmatics indicates a severe exacerbation. Pulse oximetry is a fast, easy, and noninvasive means for assessing and monitoring oxygen saturation during treatment, but it does not aid in predicting clinical outcomes and cannot predict hypercapnia or acidosis. Arterial blood gas (ABG) is not needed in most patients with mild to moderate exacerbations and should be reserved for evaluation of hypercapnia and acidosis in severe cases. Compensated hypercapnia and hypoxia is common in COPD patients; comparison with previous ABG values is helpful. Normal or elevated $Paco_2$ in the setting of an acute, severe asthmatic attack is an ominous finding as it indicates respiratory fatigue.

Asthma and COPD can coexist or be mistaken for one another; this is especially true in females. The immediate diagnostic challenge is separating these diagnoses from other serious respiratory emergencies. Important asthma and COPD mimickers include acute heart failure, upper airway obstruction, pulmonary emboli, aspiration, endobronchial obstruction/mass, interstitial lung disease, and vocal cord dysfunction. Congestive heart failure (CHF) commonly coexists or mimics COPD and can also cause wheezing. Chest x-ray, brain natriuretic peptide (BNP), and signs of fluid overload (jugular venous distention or hepatojugular reflux) help differentiate COPD from CHF. Chest x-ray can be used to diagnose complications such as pneumonia and pneumothorax, but is not routinely indicated in mild to moderate asthma exacerbations. Electrocardiograms are useful to identify dysrhythmias or suspected ischemic injury in the appropriate patient population. A high index of suspicion is necessary to rule out pulmonary embolism.

EMERGENCY DEPARTMENT CARE AND DISPOSITION

Treatment may coincide with or precede history taking in acutely dyspneic patients, as patients can decompensate rapidly.

1. Administer supplemental **oxygen** to maintain Sao_2 above 90%. Caution is advised, as oxygen may exacerbate hypercapnia in the setting of COPD. Monitor closely with end-tidal CO_2 and oxygen saturation monitoring as well as venous blood gases, as indicated.
2. Short-acting β-adrenergic agonists (SABAs) are first-line agents used to treat acute bronchospasm in COPD and asthma. Aerosolized forms (by nebulizer or metered-dose inhaler with a spacer) minimize systemic toxicity and are preferred. **Albuterol sulfate** 2.5 to 5 mg is the most common agent used. Deliver doses every 20 minutes for three doses, then 2.5 to 10 mg every 1 to 4 hours as needed, or as continuous

nebulization (10 to 15 mg/h), titrating treatment to clinical response and signs of toxicity (tachycardia, hypertension, and palpitations). **Terbutaline** 0.25 mg or **epinephrine** 1:1000 0.3 to 0.5 mg) every 20 minutes for three doses SC may be administered to patients not tolerating aerosolized therapy. Epinephrine should be used with caution in the presence of underlying cardiovascular disease.

3. Anticholinergics are useful adjuvants for effect on the large, central airways. Nebulized **ipratropium** (0.5 mg = 2.5 mL) added to SABAs every 20 minutes for three doses, then as needed, may improve bronchodilation and decrease the need for hospitalization.
4. Give corticosteroids in the ED to patients with exacerbations of asthma and COPD. The initial dose is the equivalent of 40 to 60 mg of **prednisone**. Neither the choice of steroid nor the route of administration is critical. If the patient is unable to take oral medication, intravenous **methylprednisolone** 1 mg/kg may be used. Additional doses may be given every 4 to 6 hours. Inhaled steroids are not indicated for the treatment of acute symptoms.
5. Give antibiotics directed at *Streptococcus pneumoniae, Haemophilus influenzae,* and *Moraxella catarrhalis* to patients with COPD exacerbation who have a change in sputum volume or purulence. Commonly used agents include doxycycline, the macrolides (azithromycin), or amoxicillin with or without clavulanic acid. Antibiotic use in asthma should be reserved for concurrent bacterial infections such as pneumonia.
6. Administer intravenous **magnesium sulfate** (1 to 2 g over 30 minutes) to patients with severe asthma exacerbations (FEV_1 <25% predicted). Magnesium sulfate is not recommended for mild or moderate asthma exacerbations and should not be substituted for standard regimens. Current evidence does not support its use in COPD exacerbations.
7. Mechanical ventilation is necessary in patients with respiratory muscle fatigue, respiratory acidosis, altered mental status, or hypoxia refractory to standard therapies. **Noninvasive partial pressure ventilation (NPPV)** has become a useful alternative to intubation and invasive ventilation. NPPV lowers intubation rates, short-term mortality, and length of hospitalization in COPD. NPPV can be given by continuous positive airway pressure (CPAP) or bilevel positive airway pressure (BiPAP). BiPAP has the advantage of reducing the work of breathing. CPAP is titrated up to 15 cm H_2O, while BiPAP settings are between 8 and 20 cm H_2O for inspiration and 4 and 15 cm H_2O for expiration. NPPV is likely to fail when there is poor mask fit, or when the patient is unable to cooperate with (or tolerate) NPPV, is obtunded, cannot clear airway secretions, or is hemodynamically unstable.
8. When NPPV is not a viable option, **oral intubation** is indicated. Rapid inspiratory flow rates at a reduced respiratory frequency (12 to 14 breaths/min) plus adequate expiratory phase may help reduce air-trapping and subsequent barotrauma. Therapy is guided by pulse oximetry, capnography, and ABG results. Continue sedation and therapy for bronchospasm after the patient has been placed on mechanical ventilation as the purpose of mechanical ventilation is to eliminate the work of breathing and enable rest. Mechanical ventilation itself does not relieve the airflow obstruction.

9. **Ketamine** has been reported as therapy for refractory asthma, but controlled studies are lacking. An IV bolus dose of 0.2 mg/kg followed by an infusion of 0.5 mg/kg/h is sometimes used; ketamine is also a good agent if intubation is needed.
10. Admission criteria for patients with asthma include failure of outpatient treatment, persistent or worsening dyspnea, PEFR or FEV_1 <40% of predicted, hypoxia, hypercarbia, and altered mental status; presence of comorbidities increases likelihood of need for admission. As compared to asthmatics, patients with acute COPD exacerbations are more likely to require admission. Indications for COPD admission include therapeutic failure, frequent exacerbations or relapse after ED treatment, severe dyspnea, significant comorbidities, arrhythmias, older age, insufficient home support, worsening hypoxia and hypercapnia with acidosis, and impaired mental status.
11. Agents of uncertain or no benefit: In the absence of intubation, sedatives, hypnotics, and other medications that depress respiratory drive are generally contraindicated. The data supporting methylxanthines in acute asthma or COPD are conflicting; these medications have significant side effects, and they should be a third-line option at best.
12. Beta-blockers may exacerbate bronchospasm. Antihistamines and decongestants should be avoided as they diminish clearance of respiratory secretions. Mucolytics should also be withheld; they may exacerbate bronchospasm. Mast cell and leukotriene modifiers have no role in the treatment of acute exacerbations of asthma or COPD.
13. An 80%:20% mixture of helium and oxygen (Heliox) can lower airway resistance and aid in drug delivery in the patient with very severe asthma exacerbation; however, it does not reliably avert intubation, change admission rates, or decrease mortality. Care must be taken in the oxygen-dependent patient since Heliox administration may entail an FiO_2 less than 21%.
14. Administer a 5- to 10-day course of oral steroids (prednisone 40 to 60 mg/dose) to patients who improve enough to be discharged home. Consider adding inhaled corticosteroids for asthmatic patients with chronic symptoms. Close follow-up care must be arranged for discharged patients to ensure resolution of the exacerbation and review the management plan. Despite appropriate therapy, these patients have high relapse rates. Education of asthma and COPD patients before discharge (i.e., review of medications, inhaler techniques, use of PEFR measurements, avoidance of noxious stimuli, and need to follow-up) should be an integral part of ED care.

FURTHER READING

For further reading in *Tintinalli's Emergency Medicine: A Comprehensive Study Guide*, 8th ed., see Chapter 69, "Acute Asthma," by Rita K. Cydulka; Chapter 70, "Chronic Obstructive Pulmonary Disease," by Rita K. Cydulka and Craig G. Bates.

SECTION 6

Gastrointestinal Emergencies

CHAPTER 35 Acute Abdominal Pain

Bryan E. Baskin

Acute abdominal pain may be due to numerous etiologies including gastrointestinal, genitourinary, cardiovascular, pulmonary, musculoskeletal, dermatologic, neurogenic, and other sources creating visceral, parietal, or referred pain to the abdomen.

CLINICAL FEATURES

Consider immediate life threats that might require emergency intervention. Elicit time of pain onset; character, severity, location of pain and its referral (Fig. 35-1); aggravating and alleviating factors; and similar prior episodes. Cardiorespiratory symptoms, such as chest pain, dyspnea, and cough; genitourinary symptoms, such as urgency, dysuria, and vaginal discharge; and any history of trauma should be elicited. In older patients it is also important to obtain a history of myocardial infarction, dysrhythmias, coagulopathies, and vasculopathies. Past medical and surgical histories should be elicited, and a list of medications, particularly steroids, antibiotics, or nonsteroidal anti-inflammatory drugs (NSAIDs), should be noted. A thorough gynecologic history is indicated in female patients.

The physical examination should include the patient's general appearance. Patients with peritonitis tend to lie still. The skin should be evaluated for pallor, jaundice, or rash. The vital signs should be reviewed for signs of hypovolemia due to blood loss or volume depletion. Due to medications and/or the physiology of aging, elderly patients may not exhibit tachycardia in the face of hypovolemia or illness. A core temperature should be obtained; however, absence of fever does not rule out infection, particularly in the elderly. The abdomen should be inspected for contour, scars, peristalsis, masses, distention, and pulsation. The presence of hyperactive or high-pitched or tinkling bowel sounds increases the likelihood of small bowel obstruction.

Palpation is the most important aspect of the physical examination. The abdomen and genitals should be assessed for tenderness, guarding, masses,

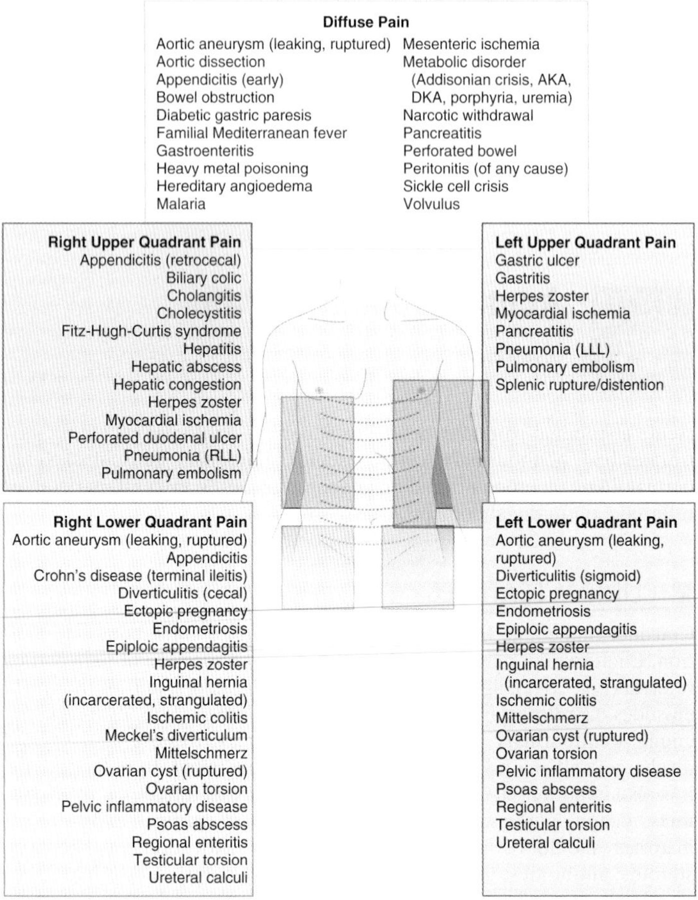

FIGURE 35-1. Differential diagnosis of acute abdominal pain by location. AKA, alcoholic ketoacidosis; DKA, diabetic ketoacidoisis; LLL, lower left lobe; RLL, right lower lobe.

organomegaly, and hernias. Rebound tenderness, often regarded as the clinical criterion standard of peritonitis, has several important limitations. In patients with peritonitis, the combination of rigidity, referred tenderness, and, especially, cough pain usually provides sufficient diagnostic confirmation; false-positive rebound tenderness occurs in about one patient out of four without peritonitis. This has led some investigators to conclude that rebound tenderness, in contrast to cough pain, is of no predictive value. A useful and underused test to diagnose abdominal wall pain is the sit-up test, also known as the *Carnett sign*. After identification of the site of maximum abdominal tenderness, the patient is asked to fold his or her arms across the chest and sit up halfway. The examiner maintains a finger on the tender area, and if palpation in the semisitting position produces the same or increased tenderness, the test is said to be positive for an abdominal wall syndrome.

Perform a pelvic examination in all postpubertal females. During the rectal examination, the lower pelvis should be assessed for tenderness, bleeding, and masses.

Elderly patients often fail to manifest the same signs and symptoms as younger patients, with decreased pain perception and decreased febrile or muscular response to infection or inflammation. This is similarly true of diabetics and immunocompromised patients. Due to this, morbidity and mortality of elderly patients presenting to EDs with abdominal pain are high. Biliary disease, bowel obstruction, diverticulitis, cancer, and hernia are more common causes of abdominal pain in patients over 50 years old. Hypotension from volume contraction, hemorrhage, or sepsis can be missed if a normally hypertensive patient appears normotensive. Conditions, somewhat less frequent but proportionately higher in occurrence, among the elderly include sigmoid volvulus, diverticulitis, acute mesenteric ischemia, and abdominal aortic aneurysm. Mesenteric ischemia should be considered in any patient older than 50 years with abdominal pain out of proportion to physical findings.

DIAGNOSIS AND DIFFERENTIAL

Suggested laboratory studies for goal-directed clinical testing are listed in Table 35-1. All women of child-bearing age with abdominal pain and/or abnormal vaginal bleeding should receive a qualitative pregnancy test. A complete blood count is neither sensitive nor specific to identify abdominal pathology; however, it remains the most commonly ordered test for ED patients with abdominal pain.

Plain abdominal radiographs can be helpful in patients with suspected obstruction, perforation (looking for free air), or to follow previously identified stones in renal colic patients; however, in general have low sensitivity. Ultrasonography is useful for the diagnosis of cholelithiasis, choledocholithiasis, cholecystitis, biliary duct dilatation, pancreatic masses, hydroureter or hydronephrosis, intrauterine or ectopic pregnancies, ovarian and tubal pathologies, free intraperitoneal fluid, suspected appendicitis (institution specific), and abdominal aortic aneurysm. Since ultrasound machines are portable, a bedside ultrasound can be performed quickly by an emergency provider. Computed tomography (CT) is currently the preferred imaging method for mesenteric ischemia, pancreatitis, aortic aneurysm, appendicitis, and urolithiasis and is superior for identifying virtually any abnormality that can be seen on plain films. Intravenous contrast is essential to identify vascular lesions, is helpful to identify inflammatory conditions (i.e., appendicitis), but is not needed for urolithiasis. Oral contrast aids in the diagnosis of bowel obstruction, but otherwise is less useful.

TABLE 35-1 Suggested Laboratory Studies for Goal-Directed Clinical Testing in Acute Abdominal Pain

Laboratory Test	Clinical Suspicion
Amylase	Pancreatitis (if lipase is not available)
Lipase	Pancreatitis
β-Human chorionic gonadotrophin	Pregnancy Ectopic or molar pregnancy
Coagulation studies (prothrombin time/ partial thromboplastin time)	GI bleeding End-stage liver disease Coagulopathy
Electrolytes	Dehydration Endocrine or metabolic disorder
Glucose	Diabetic ketoacidosis Pancreatitis
Gonococcal/chlamydia testing	Cervicitis/urethritis Pelvic inflammatory disease
Hemoglobin	GI bleeding
Lactate	Mesenteric ischemia
Liver function tests	Cholecystitis Cholelithiasis Hepatitis
Platelets	GI bleeding
Renal function tests	Dehydration Renal insufficiency Acute renal failure
Urinalysis	Urinary tract infection Pyelonephritis Nephrolithiasis
ECG	Myocardial ischemia or infarction

Source: Reproduced with permission from Fitch M. Utility and limitations of laboratory studies, in Cline DM, Stead LG (eds), *Abdominal Emergencies*. New York: McGraw-Hill Medical; 2008, p. 19.

EMERGENCY DEPARTMENT CARE AND DISPOSITION

Unstable patients should be resuscitated immediately, then diagnosed clinically with emergent surgical consultation.

1. The most common resuscitation need for abdominal pain patients is intravenous fluids with normal saline or lactated Ringer's (LR) solution. During the initial evaluation, the patient should have nothing by mouth.
2. The judicious use of analgesics is appropriate and may facilitate the ability to obtain a better history and more accurate physical examination. Consider **morphine** 0.1 mg/kg IV or hydromorphone 0.2 to 1 mg IV, which can be reversed by **naloxone** 0.4 to 2 mg SC/IV if necessary. NSAIDs such as ketorolac, 30 mg IV, or ibuprofen, (200 to 400 mg PO) are useful in patients with renal colic, but their use in other conditions is controversial and they can mask peritoneal inflammation.

3. Antiemetics, such as **ondansetron** 4 mg IM/IV, or **metoclopramide** 10 mg IM or slow IV, also increase the patient's comfort and facilitate assessment of the patient's signs and symptoms.
4. When appropriate, antibiotic treatment (i.e., **gentamicin** 1.5 mg/kg IV plus **metronidazole** 1 g IV; or **piperacillin-tazobactam**, 3.375 g IV) should be initiated, depending on the suspected source of infection. See specific chapters that follow in this section for additional antibiotics and guidelines.
5. Surgical or obstetric and gynecologic consultation should be obtained for patients with suspected acute abdominal or pelvic pathology requiring immediate intervention, including, but not limited to, abdominal aortic aneurysm, intraabdominal hemorrhage, perforated viscus, intestinal obstruction or infarction, ectopic pregnancy, or gynecologic emergencies. Historically, the "acute abdomen" or "surgical abdomen" has been identified by the presence of pain, guarding, and rebound as indicating a likely need for emergent surgery.
6. Indications for admission include toxic appearance, unclear diagnosis in elderly or immunocompromised patients, inability to reasonably exclude serious etiologies, intractable pain or vomiting, altered mental status, and inability to follow discharge or follow-up instructions. Continued observation with serial examinations is an alternative. Many patients with nonspecific abdominal pain can be discharged safely with 12 to 24 hours of follow-up and instructions to return immediately for increased pain, vomiting, fever, or failure of symptoms to resolve.

FURTHER READING

For further reading in *Tintinalli's Emergency Medicine: A Comprehensive Study Guide*, 8th ed., see Chapter 71, "Acute Abdominal Pain," by Mary Claire O'Brien.

CHAPTER 36 Nausea and Vomiting

Jonathan A. Maisel

Although nausea and vomiting are typically caused by gastrointestinal disorders, the clinician must consider systemic causes as well. Neurologic, infectious, cardiac, endocrine, renal, obstetric, pharmacologic, toxicologic, and psychiatric disorders may all be the cause of nausea and vomiting. A comprehensive history and physical examination, as well as the use of various diagnostic modalities, are needed to determine the cause and its complications.

CLINICAL FEATURES

History is essential in determining the cause of vomiting. Important features to elicit include the onset and duration of symptoms, the frequency and timing of episodes, the content of the vomitus (e.g., undigested food, bile-tinged, feculent), associated symptoms (e.g., fever, abdominal pain, diarrhea), exposure to foodborne pathogens, and the presence of sick contacts. A thorough past medical and surgical history (e.g., prior abdominal surgery) will also be valuable. Review the patient's medication list, as a variety of agents in therapeutic or toxic doses can trigger nausea and vomiting. The physical examination should initially focus on determining the presence or absence of a critical, life-threatening condition. Hypotension, tachycardia, lethargy, poor skin turgor, dry mucous membranes, and delayed capillary refill suggest significant dehydration. A careful abdominal examination will help clarify the presence or absence of a primary GI etiology. The extent to which the balance of the physical examination will be of value will be dictated by the history. In the event that a reliable history is not available (e.g., drug overdose, cognitive impairment), a comprehensive physical examination is warranted.

DIAGNOSIS AND DIFFERENTIAL

Vomiting with blood could represent gastritis, peptic ulcer disease, or carcinoma. However, aggressive nonbloody vomiting followed by hematemesis is more consistent with a Mallory-Weiss tear. The presence of bile rules out gastric outlet obstruction, such as from pyloric stenosis or strictures. The presence of abdominal distension, surgical scars, or an incarcerated hernia suggests a small bowel obstruction. The presence of fever would suggest an infectious (e.g., gastroenteritis, appendicitis, cholecystitis) or inflammatory cause. Vomiting with chest pain suggests myocardial infarction. Post-tussive vomiting suggests pneumonia. Vomiting with back or flank pain can be seen with aortic aneurysm or dissection, pancreatitis, pyelonephritis or renal colic. Headache with vomiting suggests increased intracranial pressure, such as with subarachnoid hemorrhage, tumor, or head injury. The presence of vertigo and nystagmus suggests either vestibular or CNS pathology. Vomiting in a pregnant patient is consistent with hyperemesis gravidarum in the first trimester; but in the third trimester, could represent preeclampsia if accompanied by hypertension. Associated medical conditions are also useful in discerning the cause of vomiting: diabetes mellitus suggests ketoacidosis, peripheral vascular disease suggests mesenteric ischemia, and medication use or overdose (e.g., lithium or digoxin) suggests toxicity.

All women of childbearing age warrant a pregnancy test. In vomiting associated with abdominal pain, liver function tests, urinalysis, and lipase or amylase determinations may be useful. Electrolyte determinations and renal function tests are usually of benefit only in patients with severe dehydration or prolonged vomiting. In addition, they may confirm the presence of adrenal insufficiency, with hyperkalemia and hyponatremia. Obtain specific drug levels for acetaminophen, salicylates, and digoxin when toxicity is suspected, and urine and/or serum toxicology screens when ethanol or illicit drug use is suspected. Urinalysis revealing ketones may suggest dehydration or diabetic ketoacidosis. The presence of nitrates, leukocyte esterase, bacteria and white blood cells is diagnostic of a urinary tract infection. The presence of red blood cells may suggest nephrolithiasis. The electrocardiogram and chest radiograph can be reserved for patients with suspected cardiac ischemia or pulmonary infection. Abdominal x-rays can be used to confirm the presence of intestinal obstruction. If plain x-rays are unrevealing, CT scan of the abdomen and pelvis with IV and PO contrast is not only helpful for revealing the location of a mechanical obstruction, but may also clarify alternative explanations for the patient's symptoms. CT scan of the brain will be helpful if a CNS lesion is suspected. Measuring intraocular pressure with a Tono-Pen® (Reichert, Inc., Depew, NY) is useful if glaucoma is suspected.

EMERGENCY DEPARTMENT CARE AND DISPOSITION

The treatment of nausea and vomiting consists of correcting fluid and electrolyte problems. In addition, one must initiate specific therapy for any life-threatening cause identified in the initial workup.

1. Resuscitation of seriously ill patients requires intravenous boluses of normal saline 20 mL/kg. Boluses may be repeated as necessary, targeting euvolemia. Caution should be used in the elderly, and those with compromised left ventricular function. Mildly dehydrated patients may tolerate an oral rehydration solution containing sodium as well as glucose to enhance fluid absorption. Many commercial products (e.g., Pedialyte®) are available.
2. Nutritional supplementation should be started as soon as nausea and vomiting subside. Patients can quickly advance from clear liquids to solids, such as rice and bread. Patients may benefit from avoiding raw fruit, caffeine, and lactose and sorbitol-containing products
3. Antiemetic agents are useful in actively vomiting patients with dehydration. **Ondansetron** 4 to 8 mg IV or ODT (children 0.15 mg/kg) is very effective and well tolerated, and can be administered to pregnant women (category B). **Promethazine** 25 mg (0.25 to 1 mg/kg in children over 2 years) IM or PR every 4 to 6 hours can be effective. **Prochlorperazine** 5 to 10 mg IM every 6 hours, or 25 mg PR every 12 hours is effective. **Metoclopramide** 10 mg (children 0.1 mg/kg) IV/IM every 6 to 8 hours is useful and can be administered to pregnant women (category B). **Meclizine** 25 mg PO every 6 hours is effective for vomiting associated with vertigo.

Patients with a life-threatening cause of vomiting require admission. In addition, toxic or severely dehydrated patients, particularly infants and the elderly, or those still intolerant of oral fluids after hydration, warrant admission. Patients with an unclear diagnosis, but favorable examination findings after hydration, can be discharged home safely with antiemetics. Work excuses are indicated for patients in the food, day care, and health care industries.

FURTHER READING

For further reading in *Tintinalli's Emergency Medicine: A Comprehensive Study Guide*, 8th ed., see Chapter 72, "Nausea and Vomiting," by Bophal Sarha Hang, Susan Bork, and Jeffrey Ditkoff.

Disorders Presenting Primarily with Diarrhea

Jonathan A. Maisel

Diarrhea is defined as three or more watery stools per day. There are four basic mechanisms: increased intestinal secretion (e.g., cholera), decreased intestinal absorption (e.g., enterotoxins, inflammation, or ischemia), increased osmotic load (e.g., laxatives, lactose intolerance), and abnormal intestinal motility (e.g., irritable bowel syndrome). Most cases are infectious in etiology.

DIARRHEA

Clinical Features

Determine if the diarrhea is acute (<3 weeks duration) or chronic (>3 weeks duration). Acute diarrhea is more likely to represent a serious problem, such as infection, ischemia, intoxication, or inflammation. Inquire about associated symptoms. Features such as fever, pain, presence of blood, or type of food ingested may help in the diagnosis of infectious gastroenteritis, food poisoning, diverticulitis, or inflammatory bowel disease. Neurological symptoms can be seen in certain diarrheal illnesses, such as seizure with shigellosis or hyponatremia, or paresthesias and reverse temperature sensation with ciguatoxin.

Details about the host can also better define the diagnosis. Malabsorption from pancreatic insufficiency or HIV-related bowel disorders need not be considered in a healthy host. Dietary practices, including frequent restaurant meals, exposure to day care centers, consumption of street vendor food or raw seafood, overseas travel, and camping with the ingestion of lake or stream water, may isolate the vector and narrow the differential diagnosis for infectious diarrhea (e.g., lakes or streams—*Giardia*; oysters suggest Vibrio; rice suggests *Bacillus cereus*; eggs suggest *Salmonella*; and meat suggests *Campylobacter*, *Staphylococcus*, *Yersinia*, *Escherichia coli*, or *Clostridium*). Certain medications, particularly antibiotics, colchicine, lithium, and laxatives, can all contribute to diarrhea. Travel may predispose the patient to enterotoxigenic *E. coli* or Giardia. Social history, such as sexual preference, drug use, and occupation, may suggest diagnosis such as HIV-related illness or organophosphate poisoning.

The physical examination begins with assessment of hydration status. Abdominal examination can narrow the differential diagnosis and reveal the need for surgical intervention. Even appendicitis can present with diarrhea in up to 20% of cases. Rectal examination can rule out impaction or presence of blood, the latter suggesting inflammation, infection, or mesenteric ischemia.

Diagnosis and Differential

The most specific tests in diarrheal illness all involve examination of the stool in the laboratory. Stool culture testing should be limited to severely dehydrated or toxic patients, those with blood or pus in their stool, immunocompromised patients, and those with diarrhea lasting longer than 3 days. Consider testing for *Salmonella*, *Shigella*, *Campylobacter*, Shiga toxin-producing *E. coli*, or amoebic infection. Make the laboratory aware of which pathogens you suspect. In patients with diarrhea >7 days, those who have traveled abroad, or consumed untreated water, an examination for ova and parasites may be useful to rule out *Giardia* or *Cryptosporidium*. Multiple samples may be required. Assay for *Clostridium difficile* toxin may be useful in ill patients with antibiotic-associated diarrhea or recent hospitalization.

Because most diarrheal illnesses are viral or self-limited, laboratory testing in routine cases is not indicated. However, in extremely dehydrated or toxic patients, electrolyte determinations and renal function tests may be useful. (Hemolytic-uremic syndrome, characterized by acute renal failure, thrombocytopenia, and hemolytic anemia, may complicate *E. coli* 0157:H7 infections in children and the elderly). If toxicity is suspected, tests for levels for theophylline, lithium, or heavy metals will aid in the diagnosis. Radiographs are reserved for ruling out intestinal obstruction or pneumonia, particularly *Legionella*. In addition, CT scanning or angiography may be indicated in acute mesenteric ischemia.

Emergency Department Care and Disposition

The treatment of diarrhea consists of correcting fluid and electrolyte problems. (Antibiotic-associated diarrhea often responds to withdrawal of the offending drug.) Initiate specific therapy for any life-threatening cause identified in the initial workup.

1. Replacement of fluids can be intravenous (boluses of 500 mL IV in adults, 20 mL/kg in children), with normal saline solution in seriously ill patients. Mildly dehydrated patients who are not vomiting may tolerate an oral rehydrating solution containing sodium (e.g., Pedialyte®, Gatorade®) and glucose to enhance fluid absorption (glucose transport unaffected by enterotoxins). The goal is 30 to 100 mL/kg over the first 4 hours.
2. Once patients tolerate oral fluids, introduce a "BRAT" diet (bananas, rice, apples, toast). Patients should avoid raw fruit, caffeine, lactose, and sorbitol-containing products.

Patients with an unclear diagnosis but favorable examination findings after hydration can be discharged home safely. Toxic or severely dehydrated patients, particularly infants and the elderly, warrant admission.

ACUTE INFECTIOUS AND TRAVELER'S DIARRHEA

Norovirus causes 50% to 80% of all infectious diarrheas in the United States, followed much less frequently by non-Shiga toxin-producing *E. coli*, *C. difficile*, invasive bacteria (*Campylobacter*, *Shigella*, *Salmonella*), Shiga toxin-producing *E. coli*, and protozoa. A history of foreign travel, with consumption of contaminated food or drink, is associated with an 80% probability of bacterial diarrhea, primarily toxin and nontoxin-producing strains of *E. coli*.

Diagnosis and Differential

Patients with severe abdominal pain, fever, and bloody stool should undergo stool studies for specific pathogens, including culture for *Salmonella*, *Shigella*, *Campylobacter*, and *E. coli* O157:H7; assay for Shiga toxin; and microscopy or antigen assay for *Entamoeba histolytica*. Exposure of a traveler or hiker to untreated water, and illness that persists for more than 7 days, should prompt an evaluation for a protozoal pathogen. Stool should be tested by enzyme immunoassay for *E. histolytica* antigen, *Giardia intestinalis* antigen, and *Cryptosporidium parvum* antigen.

Emergency Department Care and Disposition

Treatment of infectious diarrhea (including viral causes) includes antibiotics (see Table 37-1), antimotility agents, fluid resuscitation (oral or parenteral), and dietary modification. Probiotics are safe and may be beneficial.

Antimotility agents, such as **loperamide** 4 mg initially, then 2 mg following each unformed stool (16 mg/day maximum), will shorten the

TABLE 37-1 Antibiotic Recommendations for Infectious Diarrhea

Organism	Primary Treatment	Alternative Treatment
Empiric Tx – Traveler's Diarrhea	Ciprofloxacin 500 mg single dose or 500 mg BID × 3 days	Azithromycin 1000 mg single dose or trimethoprim/sulfamethoxazole 160 mg/800 mg single dose or BID × 3 days; or rifaximin 200 mg TID × 3 days
Empiric Tx – Infectious Diarrhea	Ciprofloxacin 500 mg BID × 5 days	Trimethoprim/sulfamethoxazole 160 mg/800 mg BID × 5 days
Clostridium difficile	Metronidazole 500 mg TID × 14 days	Vancomycin 125 mg QID × 14 days
Escherichia coli 0157:H7	No antibiotics	No antibiotics
Salmonella non-typhi	Ciprofloxacin 750 mg BID × 5 days	Azithromycin 500 mg daily × 7 days
Shigella	Ciprofloxacin 750 mg BID × 3 days	Azithromycin 500 mg daily × 3 days
Cyclospora	Trimethoprim/sulfamethoxazole 160 mg/800 mg BID × 10 days	
Giardia	Tinidazole 2 g single dose	Nitazoxanide 500 mg BID × 3 days
Vibrio cholerae	Doxycycline 500 mg single dose or azithromycin 1 g single dose	Trimethoprim/sulfamethoxazole 160 mg/800 mg BID × 3 days
Entamoeba histolytica	Metronidazole 750 mg TID × 10 days AND paromomycin 10 mg/kg TID × 7 days	Metronidazole AND iodoquinol 650 mg TID × 20 days
Listeria monocytogenes	No antibiotics	No antibiotics

duration of symptoms when combined with an antibiotic. Alternative agents include **bismuth subsalicylate** 30 mL or 2 tablets every 30 minutes for 8 doses, or **diphenoxylate and atropine** 4 mg four times daily. Avoid antimotility agents in the subset of patients with bloody or suspected inflammatory diarrhea because of the potential for prolonged fever, toxic megacolon in *C. difficile* patients, and hemolytic uremic syndrome in children infected with Shiga toxin-producing *E. coli*.

Most patients can be discharged home. Educate patients regarding the need for frequent hand washing to minimize transmission. Accordingly, patients employed in the food, day care, and health care industries should not return to work until diarrhea has resolved. Any toxic-appearing patient should be admitted. Consider admission for those at extremes of age as well.

Individuals should be counseled about the proper selection of food and beverages consumed when traveling abroad, as well as the use of bottled or boiled water for drinking, brushing teeth, and the preparation of food and infant formula.

CLOSTRIDIUM DIFFICILE-ASSOCIATED DIARRHEA AND COLITIS

Clostridium difficile is an anaerobic bacillus, which secretes two toxins that interact in a complex manner to cause illness ranging from diarrhea to pseudomembranous colitis. Pseudomembranous colitis is an inflammatory bowel disorder in which membrane-like yellowish plaques of exudate overlay and replace necrotic intestinal mucosa. Broad-spectrum antibiotics, most notably clindamycin, cephalosporins, ampicillin, amoxicillin, and fluoroquinolones, alter gut flora in such a way that *C. difficile* can flourish within the colon, causing enteropathy. Transmission of the organism can occur from contact with humans and fomites. *C. difficile* is the most common cause of infectious diarrhea in hospitalized patients and is now reported to affect healthy adults who were not exposed to a hospital setting.

Clinical Features

Onset is typically 7 to 10 days after initiating antibiotic treatment, but may occur up to several weeks following treatment. Clinical manifestations can vary from frequent, watery, mucoid stools to a toxic illness, characterized by profuse diarrhea, crampy abdominal pain, fever, leukocytosis, and dehydration.

Diagnosis and Differential

The diagnosis is confirmed by the demonstration of *C. difficile* toxin in stool. Colonoscopy is not routinely needed to confirm the diagnosis.

Emergency Department Care and Disposition

1. Ensure contact isolation, use of personal protective equipment, and appropriate hand hygiene with soap and water (alcohol-based rubs ineffective).
2. Mild *C. difficile* infection in an otherwise healthy patient can be treated with discontinuing the offending antibiotic, confirmation of infection, and clinical monitoring.

3. Oral **metronidazole** 500 mg three times daily for 14 days is the treatment of choice in patients with mild to moderate disease who do not respond to conservative measures.
4. Patients with severe diarrhea, those with a systemic response (e.g., fever, leukocytosis, or severe abdominal pain), and those whose symptoms persist despite appropriate outpatient management, must be hospitalized and should receive **vancomycin** 125 mg orally four times daily for 14 days.
5. Patients with pseudomembranous colitis complicated by toxic megacolon should receive **metronidazole** 500 mg IV every 6 hours AND **vancomycin** 500 mg orally every 6 hours. Toxic megacolon or intestinal perforation require immediate surgical consultation. Rarely, emergency colectomy may be required for fulminant colitis.

Use of antidiarrheal agents is controversial. Probiotic treatment is not a useful adjunct. Relapses occur in 20% to 30% of patients. A first relapse is treated with **metronidazole** 500 mg orally three times daily for 14 days. A second relapse is treated with **vancomycin** 125 mg orally four times daily for 14 days, followed by a four-week taper.

INFLAMMATORY BOWEL DISEASE/CROHN'S DISEASE

Crohn's disease is a chronic, idiopathic, granulomatous inflammatory disease, characterized by segmental ulceration of the GI tract anywhere from the mouth to the anus.

Clinical Features

The clinical course is variable and unpredictable, with multiple remissions and exacerbations. Patients commonly report a history of recurring fever, abdominal pain, and diarrhea over several years before a definitive diagnosis is made. Abdominal pain, anorexia, diarrhea, and weight loss occur in most patients. Patients may also present with complications of the disease, such as intestinal obstruction, intraabdominal abscess, or a variety of extraintestinal manifestations. Perianal fissures or fistulas, abscesses, and rectal prolapse can be seen in those with colonic involvement. Fistulas occur between the ileum and sigmoid colon; the cecum, another ileal segment, or the skin; or between the colon and the vagina. Abscesses can be intraperitoneal, retroperitoneal, interloop, or intramesenteric. Obstruction, hemorrhage, and toxic megacolon also occur. Toxic megacolon can be associated with massive GI bleeding.

Up to 40% of patients develop extraintestinal manifestations, including arthritis, uveitis, nephrolithiasis, and skin disease (e.g., erythema nodosum, pyoderma gangrenosum). Hepatobiliary disease, including gallstones, pericholangitis, and chronic active hepatitis, is commonly seen, as is pancreatitis. Some patients develop thromboembolic disease as a result of a hypercoaguable state. Malabsorption, malnutrition, and chronic anemia develop in longstanding disease. The recurrence rate for those with Crohn's disease is 25% to 50% when treated medically; higher for patients treated surgically.

Diagnosis and Differential

The definitive diagnosis of Crohn's disease is usually established months or years after the onset of symptoms. A careful and detailed history for previous bowel symptoms that preceded the acute presentation may provide clues to the correct diagnosis. Abdominal CT scanning is the most useful diagnostic test, potentially revealing bowel wall thickening, segmental narrowing, destruction of the normal mucosal pattern, mesenteric edema, abscess formation, and fistulas, as well as extraintestinal complications (e.g., gallstones, renal stones, sacroiliitis). Colonoscopy can detect early mucosal lesions, define the extent of colonic involvement, and identify colon cancer.

The differential diagnosis of Crohn's disease includes lymphoma, ileocecal amebiasis, sarcoidosis, chronic mycotic infections, tuberculosis, Kaposi sarcoma, *Campylobacter* enteritis, and *Yersinia* ileocolitis. Most of these conditions are uncommon, and the latter two can be differentiated by stool cultures. When confined to the colon, ischemic colitis, infectious colitis, pseudomembranous enterocolitis, irritable bowel syndrome, and ulcerative colitis should be considered.

Emergency Department Care and Disposition

Initial evaluation should determine the severity of the attack and identify significant complications. Laboratory evaluation includes complete blood count, chemistries, and type and cross match when indicated. Plain abdominal x-rays may identify obstruction, perforation, and toxic megacolon, which may appear as a long, continuous segment of air-filled colon greater than 6 cm in diameter. CT of the abdomen is the most useful test to confirm the diagnosis, and identify both intraintestinal and extraintestinal manifestations. Initial ED management includes intravenous fluid replacement, parenteral analgesia, bowel rest, correction of electrolyte abnormalities, and nasogastric suction if obstruction, ileus, or toxic megacolon is present. Additional treatment may include the following:

1. **Sulfasalazine** 3 to 5 g/day is effective for mild to moderate Crohn's disease, but has multiple toxic side effects, including GI and hypersensitivity reactions. **Mesalamine**, up to 4 g/day, is equally effective, with fewer side effects.
2. Intravenous **hydrocortisone** 300 mg/day is recommended for severe disease. Oral glucocorticoids (e.g., **prednisone** 40 to 60 mg/day) are often used as induction therapy.
3. Immunosuppressive drugs, **6-mercaptopurine** up to 1.5 mg/kg/day or **azathioprine** up to 2.5 mg/kg/day, are used as steroid-sparing agents, in healing fistulas, and in patients with serious surgical contraindications.
4. Oral antibiotics are first-line agents for perianal disease and can help induce remission. **Ciprofloxacin** 1 to 1.5 mg/kg/day, **metronidazole** 10 to 20 mg/kg/day, and **rifaximin** 800 mg twice daily are effective. Fulminant colitis should be treated intravenously with broad spectrum coverage, such as **piperacillin-tazobactam** 4.5 g four times daily.
5. Patients with medically resistant, moderate to severe Crohn's disease, may benefit from the antitumor necrosis factor antibody **infliximab** 5 mg/kg intravenously, or **adalimumab** 160 mg subcutaneously.
6. Diarrhea can be controlled by **loperamide** 4 to 16 mg/day, **diphenoxylate** 5 to 20 mg/day, or **cholestyramine** 4 g one to six times daily.

Hospital admission is recommended for those who demonstrate signs of fulminant colitis, peritonitis, obstruction, significant hemorrhage, severe dehydration, or electrolyte imbalance, or those with less severe disease who fail outpatient management. Surgical intervention is indicated in patients with intestinal obstruction or hemorrhage, perforation, abscess or fistula formation, toxic megacolon, or perianal disease, and in some patients who fail medical therapy. Alterations in therapy should be discussed with a gastroenterologist, and close follow-up must be ensured for patients discharged from the ED.

ULCERATIVE COLITIS

Ulcerative colitis is an idiopathic chronic inflammatory and ulcerative disease of the colon and rectum, characterized clinically by intermittent episodes of crampy abdominal pain, bloody diarrhea, and tenesmus, with complete remission between bouts.

Clinical Features

Patients with mild disease (60%), typically limited to the rectum, have fewer than four bowel movements per day, no systemic symptoms, and few extraintestinal manifestations. Patients with moderate disease (25%) have colitis extending to the splenic flexure. Severe disease (pancolitis) is associated with frequent daily bowel movements, weight loss, fever, tachycardia, anemia, and more frequent extraintestinal manifestations, including peripheral arthritis, ankylosing spondylitis, episcleritis, uveitis, pyoderma gangrenosum, erythema nodosum, hepatobiliary disease, thromboembolic disease, renal stones, and malnutrition.

Complications include GI hemorrhage (most common), perirectal abscess and fistula formation, obstruction secondary to stricture formation, and acute perforation. There is a 10- to 30-fold increase in the risk of developing colon carcinoma. The most feared complication is toxic megacolon, which presents with fever, tachycardia, dehydration, and a tender, distended abdomen. X-ray reveals a long, continuous segment of air-filled colon >6 cm in diameter. Perforation and peritonitis are life-threatening complications.

Diagnosis and Differential

The diagnosis of ulcerative colitis may be considered with a history of abdominal cramps, diarrhea, and mucoid stools. Laboratory findings are nonspecific and may include leukocytosis, anemia, thrombocytosis, decreased serum albumin levels, abnormal liver function test results, and negative stool studies for ova, parasites, and enteric pathogens. Abdominal CT scanning is important for the diagnosis of nonspecific abdominal pain or for suspected colitis. Colonoscopy can confirm the diagnosis and define the extent of colonic involvement. The differential diagnosis includes infectious, ischemic, radiation, antineoplastic agent induced, pseudomembranous, and Crohn's colitis. When the disease is limited to the rectum, consider sexually acquired diseases, such as rectal syphilis, gonococcal proctitis, lymphogranuloma venereum, and inflammation caused by herpes simplex virus, *Entamoeba histolytica*, *Shigella*, and *Campylobacter*.

Emergency Department Care and Disposition

Patients with severe disease should be admitted for intravenous fluid replacement, parenteral analgesia, bowel rest, correction of electrolyte abnormalities, and nasogastric suction if obstruction, ileus, or toxic megacolon is present. Consultation with both gastroenterology and surgery should be arranged for patients with significant GI hemorrhage, toxic megacolon, and bowel perforation. In addition, the following interventions should be considered:

1. Intravenous antibiotics, such as **piperacillin-tazobactam** 4.5 g every 6 hours, OR a combination of **ampicillin** 2 g every 6 hours + **metronidazole** 500 mg every 8 hours + **levofloxacin** 750 mg daily.
2. Parenteral steroid treatment with either **hydrocortisone** 100 mg every 8 hours, **methylprednisolone** 16 mg every 8 hours, or **prednisolone** 30 mg every 12 hours.
3. Intravenous **infliximab** 5 mg/kg can be effective in fulminant colitis unresponsive to intravenous corticosteroids.

The majority of patients with mild to moderate disease can be treated as outpatients. Therapy listed below should be discussed with a gastroenterologist, and close follow-up must be ensured.

1. For mild active proctitis and left-sided colitis, **mesalamine** suppositories (1000 mg at bedtime) or enemas (4 g at bedtime) are effective. However, topical steroid preparations (**beclomethasone**, **hydrocortisone**) may be better tolerated.
2. For patients who do not respond to or tolerate topical therapy, oral **mesalamine** 2.4 to 4 g/day is an effective alternative.
3. If topical therapy or oral mesalamine is unsuccessful, **prednisone** 40 to 60 mg/day orally can induce a remission. Once clinical remission is achieved, steroids should be slowly tapered and discontinued.
4. **Infliximab** 5 mg/kg intravenously may be considered for patients who are steroid dependent or refractory.

Supportive measures include a nutritious diet, physical and psychological rest, replenishment of iron stores, dietary elimination of lactose, and addition of bulking agents, such as **psyllium**. Antidiarrheal agents can precipitate toxic megacolon and should be avoided.

FURTHER READING

For further reading in *Tintinalli's Emergency Medicine: A Comprehensive Study Guide*, 8th ed., see Chapter 73, "Disorders Presenting Primarily with Diarrhea," by Nicholas E. Kman and Howard A. Werman.

CHAPTER 38

Acute and Chronic Constipation

Thomas E. Carter

Constipation is the most common digestive complaint in the United States. Gut motility is affected by diet, activity level, and multiple, often overlapping, causes.

CLINICAL FEATURES

Constipation is characterized by the presence of two or more of the following complaints straining, hard stools, incomplete evacuation, and fewer than three bowel movements per week. Constipation is chronic in patients with symptoms for 12 weeks consecutive or nonconsecutive of the preceding 12 months. Differentiating acute from chronic and functional from organic constipation can guide treatment. Functional constipation features include changes in medications or dietary supplements, a decrease in fluid or fiber intake, or a change in activity level including illness or injury. Organic constipation is suggested by acute onset, weight loss, rectal bleeding/melena, nausea/vomiting, inability to pass flatus, fever, rectal pain and change in stool caliber. Organic constipation has priority diagnosis of obstruction and carcinoma. A family history of colon, ovarian or uterine cancer plus an assessment of associated illnesses may elucidate other primary or comorbid diagnoses: cold intolerance (hypothyroidism), diverticulitis (inflammatory stricture), or nephrolithiasis (hyperparathyroidism). Diarrhea may occur with constipation/obstruction symptoms, as liquid stool can pass around an impaction or obstructive source.

Physical examination should focus on detection of hernias, abdominal masses, and ascites (carcinoma). Bowel sounds will be decreased in the setting of slow gut transit, but increased in the setting of obstruction. Visual and digital rectal examination will detect tone, masses, foreign bodies, hemorrhoids, abscesses, fecal impaction, anal fissures, or fecal blood. The latter, accompanied by weight loss or decreasing stool caliber, may confirm the presence of carcinoma. Fecal impaction may produce ulcers causing rectal bleeding.

DIAGNOSIS AND DIFFERENTIAL

The differential diagnosis for constipation is extensive, as noted in Table 38-1. Prioritize testing to evaluate organic constipation and complications of functional constipation based on suspicion; this may include a complete blood count (to rule out anemia), thyroid stimulating hormone (to rule out hypothyroidism), and electrolyte determinations (to rule out hypokalemia or hypercalcemia). Flat and erect abdominal films may be useful in confirming obstruction and pseudo-obstruction or assessing stool burden. computed tomography (CT) scan of the abdomen and pelvis with contrast may be necessary to identify organic causes of constipation including obstruction, carcinoma, or impaction.

Chronic constipation is usually a functional disorder that can be worked up on an outpatient basis. However, complications of chronic

TABLE 38-1 Differential Diagnosis of Constipation

Acute Causes
GI: quickly growing tumors, strictures, hernias, adhesions, inflammatory conditions, and volvulus
Medicinal: narcotic analgesic, antipsychotic, anticholinergic, antacid, antihistamine
Exercise and nutrition: decrease in level of exercise, fiber intake, fluid intake
Painful anal pathology: anal fissure, hemorrhoids, anorectal abscesses, proctitis
Chronic Causes
GI: slowly growing tumor, colonic dysmotility, chronic anal pathology
Medicinal: chronic laxative abuse, narcotic analgesic, antipsychotic, anticholinergic, antacid, antihistamine
Neurologic: neuropathies, Parkinson disease, cerebral palsy, paraplegia
Endocrine: hypothyroidism, hyperparathyroidism, diabetes
Electrolyte abnormalities: hypomagnesia, hypercalcemia, hypokalemia
Rheumatologic: amyloidosis, scleroderma
Toxicologic: lead, iron

constipation, such as fecal impaction and intestinal pseudo-obstruction, may become life-threatening and will require manual, colonoscopic, or surgical intervention.

EMERGENCY DEPARTMENT CARE AND DISPOSITION

Treatment of functional constipation is directed at severity, symptomatic relief, as well as addressing lifestyle issues. Occasionally, specific treatment is required for complications of constipation or for underlying disorders that can prevent organic constipation.

- The most important prescription for functional constipation is a dietary and exercise regimen that includes fluids (1.5 L/d), fiber (10 g/d), and exercise. Fiber in the form of bran (1 cup/d) or **psyllium** 1 tsp 3 times a day increases stool volume and gut motility. **Ducosate sodium** 100 mg daily/twice a day facilitates the mixture of stool fat and water improving symptoms of discomfort.
- Fecal impaction is unpleasant and uncomfortable stool should be removed manually with the aid of local anesthetic lubricant and parenteral analgesia or sedation as needed. In female patients, transvaginal pressure with the other hand may assist evacuation. The success of any other treatment regimen is often dependent on manual disimpaction. Following disimpaction, a regimen of diet, exercise, and medication should be prescribed to reestablish fecal flow.
- **Enemas of soapsuds** 1500 mL PR or **mineral oil** 100 to 150 mL PR are low-risk treatments, well tolerated, and should follow fecal disimpaction. Use care to avoid local trauma and rectal perforation.
- Medications alone may relieve mild cases of constipation. Stimulants can be either given by mouth, as with **docusate sodium/sennosides** 1 to 2 tablets PO daily or twice daily or per rectum, as with **bisacodyl** 10 mg PR three times daily in adults or children. In the absence of renal failure, saline laxatives such as **milk of magnesia** 15 to 30 mL PO once or twice a day or **magnesium citrate** 240 mL PO once are useful. Hyperosmolar agents such as **lactulose** or **sorbitol** 15 to 30 mL PO once or twice a day may be helpful, as is **polyethylene glycol** 17 g PO. In children, **glycerin rectal**

suppositories, or **mineral oil** (age 5 to 11 years: 5 to 15 mL PO daily; age >12 years: 15 to 45 mL PO daily) have been advocated.

- Management of constipation in palliative care, chronic opioid use, or abuse has no definitive regimen. When the above measures are unsuccessful, support is increasing for **methylnatrexone** 0.15 mg/kg subcutaneous a maximum dose of 12 mg.
- Many constipated patients can be safely discharged from the ED with established fecal flow or key aspects addressed (Tables 38-2 and 38-3). Early follow-up is indicated in patients with recent severe constipation;

TABLE 38-2 Suggested Laboratory Studies for Goal-Directed Clinical Testing in Acute Abdominal Pain

Laboratory Test	Clinical Suspicion
Amylase	Pancreatitis (if lipase is not available)
Lipase	Pancreatitis
β-Human chorionic gonadotrophin	Pregnancy Ectopic or molar pregnancy
Coagulation studies (prothrombin time/ partial thromboplastin time)	GI bleeding End-stage liver disease Coagulopathy
Electrolytes	Dehydration Endocrine or metabolic disorder
Glucose	Diabetic ketoacidosis Pancreatitis
Gonococcal/chlamydia testing	Cervicitis/urethritis Pelvic inflammatory disease
Hemoglobin	GI bleeding
Lactate	Mesenteric ischemia
Liver function tests	Cholecystitis Cholelithiasis Hepatitis
Platelets	GI bleeding
Renal function tests	Dehydration Renal insufficiency Acute renal failure
Urinalysis	Urinary tract infection Pyelonephritis Nephrolithiasis
ECG	Myocardial ischemia or infarction

Source: Reproduced with permission from Cline DM, Stead LG. *Abdominal Emergencies.* New York: McGraw-Hill Medical; 2008.

TABLE 38-3 Key Aspects to Address Before Discharging a Constipated Patient

Possible obstructing lesion
Systemic illness
Medication interaction/effect
Electrolyte imbalance
Potential for intestinal perforation with self-administered enemas

chronic constipation associated with systemic symptoms, such as weight loss, anemia, or change in stool caliber; refractory constipation; and constipation requiring chronic laxative use. Patients with organic constipation secondary to obstruction require hospitalization and surgical evaluation.

FURTHER READING

For further reading in *Tintinalli's Emergency Medicine: A Comprehensive Study Guide*, 8th ed., see Chapter 71, "Acute Abdominal Pain," by Mary Claire O'Brien.

CHAPTER 39 Gastrointestinal Bleeding

Mitchell C. Sokolosky

Gastrointestinal (GI) bleeding is a common problem in emergency medicine and should be considered life-threatening until proven otherwise. Acute upper GI bleeding is more common than lower GI bleeding. *Upper GI bleeding* is defined as that originating proximal to the ligament of Treitz. Upper GI bleeds can result from peptic ulcer disease, erosive gastritis and esophagitis, esophageal and gastric varices, and Mallory–Weiss syndrome. Lower GI bleeds most commonly result from diverticular disease, followed by colitis, adenomatous polyps, and malignancies. What may initially appear to be lower GI bleeding may be upper GI bleeding in disguise.

CLINICAL FEATURES

Most patients complain of hematemesis, coffee-ground emesis, hematochezia, or melena. Others will present with hypotension, tachycardia, angina, syncope, weakness, and confusion. Hematemesis or coffee-ground emesis suggests an upper GI source. Melena suggests a source proximal to the right colon. Hematochezia (bright red or maroon-colored) indicates a more distal colorectal lesion; however, approximately 10% of hematochezia may be associated with upper GI bleeding. Weight loss and changes in bowel habits are classic symptoms of malignancy. Vomiting and retching, followed by hematemesis, is suggestive of a Mallory–Weiss tear. A history of medication or alcohol use should be sought. This history may suggest peptic ulcer disease, gastritis, or esophageal varices. Spider angiomata, palmar erythema, jaundice, and gynecomastia suggest underlying liver disease. Ingestion of iron or bismuth can simulate melena, and certain foods, such as beets, can simulate hematochezia. However, stool heme (guaiac) testing will be negative.

DIAGNOSIS AND DIFFERENTIAL

The diagnosis may be obvious with the finding of hematemesis, coffee ground emesis, hematochezia, or melena. A careful ear, nose, and throat (ENT) examination can exclude swallowed blood as a source. Nasogastric (NG) tube placement and aspiration may detect occult upper GI bleeding. A negative NG aspirate does not conclusively exclude an upper GI source. Guaiac testing of NG aspirate can yield both false-negative and false-positive results. Most reliable is gross inspection of the aspirate for a bloody, maroon, or coffee-ground appearance. A rectal examination can detect the presence of blood, its appearance (bright red, maroon, or melanotic), and the presence of masses. All patients with significant GI bleeding require type and crossmatch for blood. Other important tests include a complete blood count, electrolytes, blood urea nitrogen, creatinine, glucose, coagulation studies, and liver function tests. The initial hematocrit level may not reflect the actual amount of blood loss. Upper GI bleeding may elevate the blood urea nitrogen level. Routine plain radiographs are of limited value. The initial diagnostic procedure of choice for lower GI bleeds—angiography, scintigraphy, or endoscopy—depends on resource ability and consultant preference. In one study, a cause for lower GI bleeding was found in <50% of cases.

EMERGENCY DEPARTMENT CARE AND DISPOSITION

1. Emergency stabilization (airway, breathing, and circulation) takes priority. Administer oxygen, insert large-bore intravenous catheters, and institute continuous monitoring.
2. Replace volume loss immediately with isotonic crystalloids (e.g., normal saline or Ringer lactate). The decision to transfuse blood is based on clinical factors (continued active bleeding and no improvement in perfusion after administration of 2 L of crystalloids) rather than initial hematocrit values. *The threshold for blood transfusion should be lower in the elderly.*
3. Replace coagulation factors, as needed.
4. A nasogastric tube is recommended in most patients with significant GI bleeding, regardless of the presumed source. If bright red blood or clots are found, perform *gentle* gastric lavage.
5. Consider early therapeutic endoscopy for significant upper GI bleeding. Timing of endoscopy for diagnosis and treatment of some lower GI bleeding sources can vary. *It is estimated that 80% of lower GI bleeding will resolve spontaneously.*
6. Proton pump inhibitors (e.g., **pantoprazole** 80 mg bolus followed by an infusion of 8 mg/h) are recommended for patients with nonvariceal bleeding from peptic ulcer disease.
7. Consider **octreotide** 25 to 50 μg bolus followed by 25 to 50 μg/h intravenously for patients with upper GI bleeding.
8. Balloon tamponade with the Sengstaken–Blakemore tube or its variants should only be considered an adjunctive or temporizing measure and is rarely used due to the high complication rate.
9. A surgical and gastroenterology consult should be obtained in patients with uncontrolled bleeding. Patients who do not respond to both pharmacologic and endoscopic treatments may require emergent surgery.
10. Most patients with GI bleeding will require hospital admission and early referral to an endoscopist.

FURTHER READING

For further reading in *Tintinalli's Emergency Medicine: A Comprehensive Study Guide*, 8th ed., see Chapter 75, "Upper Gastrointestinal Bleeding," by Christopher M. Ziebell, Andy Kitlowski, Janna M. Welch and Phillip A. Friesen; Chapter 76, "Lower Gastrointestinal Bleeding," by Bruce M. Lo.

CHAPTER 40 Esophageal Emergencies

Mitchell C. Sokolosky

Complaints of dysphagia, odynophagia, or ingested foreign body usually imply esophageal disease. Chest pain, upper gastrointestinal (GI) bleeding, malignancy, and mediastinitis may also be esophageal in nature. Many diseases of the esophagus can be evaluated over time in an outpatient setting, but several, such as esophageal foreign body and esophageal perforation, require emergent evaluation.

DYSPHAGIA

Dysphagia is difficulty with swallowing. Most patients with dysphagia have an identifiable organic cause. The two broad pathophysiologic groups of dysphagia are transfer dysphagia (oropharyngeal) and transport dysphagia (esophageal).

Clinical Features

A careful history is the key to the diagnosis of dysphagia. Determine whether solids, liquids, or both cause the symptoms and the time course and progression of symptoms. Dysphagia for solids that progresses to liquids suggests a mechanical or obstructive process. Dysphagia for both solids and liquids points to a motility disorder. A poorly chewed meat bolus may obstruct the esophagus and be the presenting sign for a variety of underlying esophageal pathologies. Esophageal filling proximal to the impacted bolus can cause inability to swallow secretions and can present an airway or aspiration risk. Physical examination of patients with dysphagia should focus on the head and neck and the neurologic examination, although the examination is often normal.

Diagnosis and Differential

The diagnosis of the underlying pathology of dysphagia is most often made outside the emergency department (ED). ED evaluation may include anteroposterior and lateral neck and chest x-rays. Direct laryngoscopy may identify lesions. Structural or obstructive causes of dysphagia include neoplasms (squamous cell is most common), esophageal strictures and webs, Schatzki ring, and diverticula. Motor lesions causing dysphagia include neuromuscular disorders (cerebrovascular accident is most common), achalasia, diffuse esophageal spasm, and esophageal dysmotility.

Emergency Department Care and Disposition

1. Aspiration is a major concern with most causes of dysphagia.
2. Most causes of dysphagia can be further evaluated and managed in the outpatient setting using a variety of tools including barium swallow (often first test), video esophagograpy, manometry, and esophagoscopy.
3. Many of the structural lesions ultimately will require dilatation as definitive therapy.

CHEST PAIN OF ESOPHAGEAL ORIGIN

Differentiating esophageal pain from ischemic chest pain is difficult at best and may be impossible in the ED. Patients with esophageal pain report symptoms that are also found in patients with coronary artery disease, and there is no historical feature that is sensitive or specific enough to differentiate the two. The best ED default assumption is that pain is cardiac in nature and not esophageal until proven otherwise.

Gastroesophageal Reflux Disease

Reflux of gastric contents into the esophagus causes a wide array of symptoms and long-term effects.

Clinical Features

Heartburn is the classic symptom of gastroesophageal reflux disease (GERD), although chest discomfort may be the only symptom. The association of pain with meals, postural changes, and relief of symptoms with antacids point to a diagnosis of GERD. Less obvious presentations of GERD include pulmonary symptoms, especially asthma exacerbations, and multiple ear, nose, and throat symptoms. GERD has also been implicated in the etiology of dental erosion, vocal cord ulcers and granulomas, laryngitis with hoarseness, chronic sinusitis, and chronic cough. Over time, GERD can cause complications such as strictures, inflammatory esophagitis, and Barrett esophagus (a premalignant condition).

Diagnosis and Differential

Diagnosis is suggested by history and favorable response to antacid treatment. However, some patients with symptoms due to cardiac ischemia also report improvement with the same therapy. Unfortunately, like cardiac pain, GERD pain may be squeezing or pressure-like and includes a history of onset with exertion or rest. Both types of pain may be accompanied by diaphoresis, pallor, radiation, and nausea and vomiting. An ECG and chest radiograph can be obtained in patients with ambiguous presentations. Given the serious outcome of unrecognized ischemic disease compared with the relatively benign nature of esophageal pain, a cautious approach is warranted.

Emergency Department Care and Disposition

1. Comprehensive treatment of reflux disease is done on an outpatient basis and involves decreasing acid production, enhancing upper tract motility, and eliminating risk factors for the disease.
2. Mild disease often is treated empirically with an H_2 blocker (e.g., **ranitidine** 150 mg PO twice daily) or proton pump inhibitor (e.g., **omeprazole** 20 to 40 mg PO daily).
3. Prokinetic drugs (e.g., **metoclopramide** 10 to 15 mg PO 30 minutes before meals and at bedtime) may reduce symptoms and decrease dose by 50% in elderly patients.
4. Patients should avoid agents that exacerbate GERD (ethanol, caffeine, nicotine, chocolate, or fatty foods), sleep with the head of the bed elevated (30°), and avoid eating within 3 hours of going to bed at night.

Esophagitis

Esophagitis can cause prolonged periods of chest pain and odynophagia. Esophagitis may be inflammatory (e.g., GERD, NSAIDs, potassium chloride, doxycycline, tetracycline, and clindamycin) or infectious if immunosuppressed (e.g., *Candida* most common, herpes simplex, cytomegalovirus (CMV), and aphthous ulceration). Withdrawal of offending agent is generally curative with medication-induced esophagitis. Patients with reflux-induced esophagitis require acid-suppressive medications. Infectious causes are established by endoscopy often with biopsy and specimen cultures.

Esophageal Perforation

Iatrogentic perforation is most common. Other causes include transient increase in intraesophageal pressure (*Boerhaave syndrome*), trauma, foreign body, infection, tumor, and aortic pathology. Perforation of the esophagus is associated with a high mortality rate.

Clinical Features

Pain is classically described as acute, severe, unrelenting, and diffuse and is reported in the chest, neck, and abdomen. Pain can radiate to the back and shoulders, or back pain may be the predominant symptom. Swallowing often exacerbates pain. Physical examination varies with the severity of the rupture and the elapsed time between the rupture and presentation. Abdominal rigidity with hypotension and fever often occur early. Tachycardia and tachypnea are common. Mediastinal emphysema takes time to develop. It is less commonly detected by examination or radiography in lower esophageal perforation and its absence does not rule out perforation. A Hammon crunch can sometimes be auscultated. Pleural effusions develop in 50% of patients with intrathoracic perforations and are uncommon in cervical perforations.

Diagnosis and Differential

Chest radiography can suggest the diagnosis. Given the limitations of CT, an esophagram or emergency endoscopy is most often used to confirm the diagnosis. Selection of the procedure depends upon the clinical setting and the resources available. Mistaking perforation for acute myocardial infarction, pulmonary embolism, or an acute abdomen can lead to delays in therapy.

Emergency Department Care and Disposition

1. Rapid, aggressive management is essential.
2. In the ED, initiate fluid resuscitation (see Chapter 5) and give broad-spectrum parental antibiotics to cover aerobic and anaerobic organisms. Examples include single drug coverage such as **piperacillin/tazobactam** 3.375 g intravenously (IV) or double drug coverage with **cefotaxime** 2 g IV or **ceftriaxone** 2 g IV plus **clindamycin** 600 mg IV or **metronidazole** 15 mg/kg IV once, then 7.5 mg/kg q6h (maximum 1 g/dose).
3. Obtain emergent surgical consultation.
4. All of these patients require hospitalization.

Swallowed Foreign Bodies

Children (18 to 48 months old) and those with mental illness account for most cases. Coins, toys, and crayons typically lodge in the anatomically narrow proximal esophagus. Adult candidates are those with esophageal disease, prisoners, and psychiatric patients. In adults, most impactions are distal. Complications include airway obstruction, stricture, and perforation. Once an object transverses the pylorus, it usually continues through the GI tract. Objects that become lodged distal to the pylorus are usually irregular, have sharp edges, and are wide (>2.5 cm) or long (>6 cm)

Clinical Features

Objects lodged in the esophagus can produce retrosternal pain, dysphagia, coughing, choking, vomiting, and aspiration, and the patient may be unable to swallow secretions. Adults with an esophageal foreign body generally provide unequivocal history. In the pediatric patient it may be necessary to rely on clues such as refusal or inability to eat, vomiting, gagging, choking, stridor, neck or throat pain, dysphagia, and drooling.

Diagnosis and Differential

Physical examination starts with an assessment of the airway. The nasopharynx, oropharynx, neck, and chest should also be examined. Occasionally, a foreign body can be directly visualized in the oropharynx. Plain films are used to screen for radiopaque objects. CT scanning has replaced the barium swallow test to evaluate for nonradiopaque objects.

Emergency Department Care and Disposition

1. Patients in extremis or with pending airway compromise are resuscitated in standard fashion and may require active airway management.
2. Emergent endoscopy is indicated for complete distal obstruction of the esophagus with pooling of secretions (often distal esophageal food impaction).
3. Hospital admission is generally not needed if the foreign body is easily removed by endoscopy without complications.
4. In stable patients, indirect or fiberoptic laryngoscopy may allow removal of very proximal objects.
5. Consult surgery for worrisome foreign bodies that are in the more distal GI tract.

Food Impaction

Meat is the most common cause of food impaction.

1. Complete esophageal obstruction requires emergency endoscopy.
2. Uncomplicated food impaction may be treated expectantly but should not be allowed to remain impacted for >12 to 24 hours.
3. The use of proteolytic enzymes (e.g., Adolph Meat Tenderizer, which contains papain) to dissolve a meat bolus is contraindicated.
4. **Glucagon** 1 to 2 mg for adults may be attempted but success rates are poor.

Coin Ingestion

1. Obtain radiographs on all children suspected of swallowing coins to determine the presence and location of the object. Coins in the esophagus present their circular face on anteroposterior films, as opposed to coins in the trachea, which show that face on lateral films.

2. Coins should be removed by endoscopy if lodged in the esophagus.
3. Removal of a coin with a Foley balloon catheter should be done under fluoroscopy by experienced hands. Complications include aspiration, airway compromise, and mucosal laceration.
4. Once in the stomach, coins almost always pass spontaneously.

Button Battery Ingestion

A button battery lodged in the esophagus is a true emergency requiring prompt removal because the battery may quickly induce mucosal injury and necrosis. Perforation may occur within 6 hours of ingestion.

1. Resuscitate the patient as needed.
2. Obtain radiographs to locate position of the battery.
3. Emergency endoscopy is indicated if battery is lodged in the esophagus. Foley balloon catheter technique may be considered if reliable history of ingestion ≤2 hours is obtained.
4. Batteries that have passed the esophagus can be managed expectantly with 24-hour follow-up examination. Repeat x-rays at 48 hour to ensure passage through pylorus. Most batteries pass through the body in 48 to 72 hours but may take longer.
5. Consult surgery if the patient develops symptoms or signs of GI tract injury.
6. The National Button Battery Ingestion Hotline at 202-625-3333 is a 24-hours, 7 days-a-week resource for help with management decisions.

Ingestion of Sharp Objects

1. Sharp objects in the esophagus, stomach, or duodenum require immediate removal by endoscopy in order to prevent complications such as perforation.
2. If the object is distal to the duodenum at presentation and the patient is asymptomatic, obtain daily plain films to document passage.
3. Consider surgical removal if 3 days elapse without passage.
4. Consult surgery immediately if the patient develops symptoms or signs of intestinal injury (e.g., pain, emesis, fever, and GI bleeding).

Narcotic Ingestion

1. The packets (condoms containing up to 5 g of narcotic) ingested by a narcotic courier (body packer) are often visible on plain x-ray.
2. Endoscopy is contraindicated because of the risk of iatrogenic packet rupture, which may be fatal.
3. Observation until the packet reaches the rectum is the favored treatment if the packets appear to be passing intact through the GI tract.
4. Whole-bowel irrigation may aid in the process of packet removal.

FURTHER READING

For further reading in *Tintinalli's Emergency Medicine: A Comprehensive Study Guide*, 8th ed., see Chapter 77, "Esophageal Emergencies" by Moss Mendelson.

Peptic Ulcer Disease and Gastritis

Teresa Bowen-Spinelli

Peptic ulcer disease (PUD) is a chronic illness manifested by recurrent ulcerations in the stomach and duodenum. Acid and pepsin are crucial for ulcer development, but the great majority of ulcers are directly related to infection with *Helicobacter pylori* or nonsteroidal anti-inflammatory drugs (NSAIDs) use. Gastritis is an acute or chronic gastric mucosal inflammation and has various causes. Dyspepsia is upper abdominal discomfort with or without other symptoms that can have various causes or be functional.

CLINICAL FEATURES

Peptic ulcer disease typically presents with burning epigastric pain, though it may be described as sharp, dull, and an ache, or an "empty" or "hungry" feeling. It may be relieved by the ingestion of food, milk, or antacids, presumably due to an acid buffering or a dilutional effect. The pain recurs as the gastric contents empty and the recurrent pain classically awakens the patient at night. Atypical presentations are common in the elderly and may include no pain, pain that is not relieved by food, nausea, vomiting, anorexia, weight loss, and/or bleeding.

A change in the character of the pain may herald the onset of a complication. Abrupt onset of severe pain is typical of perforation with spillage of gastric or duodenal contents into the peritoneal cavity. Back pain may represent pancreatitis from a posterior perforation. Nausea, vomiting, early satiety, and weight loss may occur with gastric outlet obstruction or cancer. Vomiting blood or passing melanotic stools with or without hemodynamic instability represents a bleeding complication.

DIAGNOSIS AND DIFFERENTIAL

Peptic ulcer disease cannot be definitively diagnosed on clinical grounds, but it can be strongly suspected in the presence of a "classic" history (as above) accompanied by "benign" physical examination findings and normal vital signs with or without mild epigastric tenderness. Examination findings that may be indicative of PUD complications include a rigid abdomen consistent with peritonitis in perforation, abdominal distension and succussion splash consistent with gastric outlet obstruction, occult or gross rectal blood, or blood in nasogastric aspirate consistent with bleeding.

The differential diagnosis of epigastric pain is extensive. Pain, radiating into the chest, and belching may point to gastroesophageal reflux disease; more severe pain in the right upper quadrant (RUQ) radiating around the right side of the abdomen with tenderness suggests cholelithiasis or biliary colic; pain radiating into the back is common with pancreatitis and/or a concomitant mass may represent a pseudocyst or if the mass is pulsatile may represent an abdominal aortic aneurysm. Chronic pain, anorexia, and weight loss with or without a mass may represent cancer. Myocardial ischemia may present as epigastric pain and should be strongly considered in the appropriate clinical setting, especially in the population of diabetics and the elderly.

Some ancillary tests may be helpful to exclude PUD complications and to narrow the differential. A normal CBC rules out chronic (but not acute) gastrointestinal (GI) bleeding. Elevated liver enzymes may indicate hepatitis. Elevated lipase may indicate pancreatitis. An upright xray may show free air in the setting a perforation and an abdominal US examination may show cholecystitis, cholelithiasis, or an abdominal arotic aneurysm. An ECG and troponin are indicated if myocardial ischemia is suspected.

The gold standard for diagnosis of PUD is visualization of an ulcer by upper GI endoscopy. Endoscopy is indicated in most patients with upper GI bleeding and in any patient with certain "alarm" features consistent with cancer: age >55 year, unexplained weight loss, early satiety or anorexia, persistent vomiting, dysphagia, anemia, abdominal mass, or jaundice. Because of the strong association of *H. pylori* infection with PUD, testing for the presence of *H. pylori* with PUD is usually indicated, but this is generally more appropriate at the time of follow-up with gastroenterologist.

EMERGENCY DEPARTMENT CARE AND DISPOSITION

After PUD is diagnosed, the goal of treatment is to heal the ulcer while relieving pain and preventing complications and avoiding recurrence. If the patient is infected with *H. pylori* then it must be eradicated in order to prevent ulcer recurrence. NSAIDs should be stopped whenever possible.

1. Proton pump inhibitors (PPIs) act to decrease acid production by blocking H+ ion secretion. They serve to heal ulcers faster than other therapies and also have an inhibitory effect on *H. pylori*. PPIs should be taken about 30 to 60 minutes prior to a meal. Include **omeprazole** 20 to 40 mg daily, **esomeprazole** 20 to 40 mg daily, 20 to 40 mg daily, **lansoprazole** 15 to 30 mg daily, **pantoprazole** 20 to 40 mg daily, or **rabeprazole** 20 mg daily.
2. Histamine-2 receptor antagonists (H_2RAs) inhibit acid secretion and are available over the counter. H_2RAs include **cimetidine** 200 to 400 mg twice a day, **famotidine** 10 to 20 mg twice a day; **nizatidine** 75 to 150 mg twice a day; and **ranitidine** 75 to 150 mg twice a day.
3. Liquid antacids relieve pain and heal ulcers by buffering gastric acid. Due to the minimal side effects of PPIs and H_2RAs, liquid antacids are generally used on an as needed basis for pain relief. Typical dosing is 15 mL, 1 hour after meals and at bedtime.
4. If present, *H. pylori* infection should be treated, though this would rarely be initiated in the ED. There are multiple therapies, but the most common is "triple therapy" formulation taken for 14 days which consists of a PPI, clarithromycin, and either amoxicillin or metronidazole.
5. Patients with complications always require consultation and most require admission for continued treatment. For the treatment of bleeding (see Chapter 39). For perforation provide resuscitation as needed, start broad-spectrum antibiotics, and obtain immediate surgical consultation. For gastric outlet obstruction provide resuscitation as needed, place a nasogastric tube, and admit for continued treatment.

6. When uncomplicated PUD is suspected in a stable patient, the great majority can be discharged home on a PPI or an H_2RA with a liquid antacid for breakthrough pain and with recommendations to follow-up with their primary care provider for further evaluation as indicated. Patients with "alarm" features who are stable enough for discharge should be referred for endoscopy.
7. Patients should be told that PUD is a presumptive diagnosis and that for definitive diagnosis gastroenterologists should perform an endoscopy. They should return for further evaluation or treatment if any of the following occur: worsening pain, increased vomiting, hematemesis or melena, weakness or syncope, fever, or chest pain.

FURTHER READING

For further reading in *Tintinalli's Emergency Medicine: A Comprehensive Study Guide*, 7th ed., see Chapter 78, "Peptic Ulcer Disease and Gastritis," by Matthew C. Gratton and Angela Bogle.

CHAPTER 42

Pancreatitis and Cholecystitis

Rita K. Cydulka

Acute pancreatitis (AP) is an inflammation of the pancreas. Disease severity ranges from mild local inflammation to multisystem organ failure secondary to a systemic inflammatory response. Cholelithiasis and alcohol abuse are the most common causes, but there are many potential etiologies. Patients without risk factors often develop pancreatitis secondary to medications or severe hyperlipidemia. Commonly used medications associated with pancreatitis include acetaminophen, carbamazepine, enalapril, estrogens, erythromycin, furosemide, hydrochlorothiazide, opiates, steroids, tetracycline, and trimethoprim-sulfamethoxazole.

PANCREATITIS

Clinical Features

The most common symptom is a midepigastric, constant, boring pain radiating to the back that is worse when the patient is supine and is often associated with nausea, vomiting, and abdominal distention. Low-grade fever, tachycardia, and hypotension may be present. Epigastric tenderness is common, whereas peritonitis is a late finding.

Physical findings are dependent on the severity of disease. Physical examination findings include epigastric tenderness, but tenderness may localize more to the right or left upper quadrant of the abdomen. Bowel sounds may be diminished and abdominal distention may be present secondary to ileus. Refractory hypotensive shock, renal failure, fever, altered mental status, and respiratory failure may accompany the most severe disease.

Diagnosis and Differential

The diagnosis should be suspected by the history and physical examination. The presence of two of the three following features makes the diagnosis more likely: (1) history and examination findings consistent with AP, (2) lipase or amylase levels at least two to three times the upper limit of normal, or (3) imaging findings consistent with pancreatic inflammation. Lipase is the preferred diagnostic test as it is more accurate. There are many sources of extrapancreatic amylase, making it relatively nonspecific. Normal serum amylase does not exclude the diagnosis of AP. There is no benefit to ordering both tests.

A CBC will identify leukocytosis or anemia. Liver studies can demonstrate associated biliary involvement. An elevated alkaline phosphatase level suggests biliary disease and gallstone pancreatitis. Persistent hypocalcemia (<7 mg/100 mL), hypoxia, increasing serum urea nitrogen, and metabolic acidosis are associated with a potentially complicated course.

Imaging can help confirm the diagnosis of pancreatitis, evaluate biliary involvement, and exclude causes of abdominal pain. Abdominal computed tomography (CT) scan is preferred over ultrasound as the latter is often limited by bowel gas overlying the pancreas. In the face of a typical clinical picture and laboratory results, emergency imaging may not be needed.

The differential diagnosis includes referred chest pain secondary to ischemic heart disease, pulmonary pathology such as pneumonia or empyema, hepatitis, cholecystitis or biliary colic, ascending cholangitis, renal colic, small bowel obstruction, peptic ulcer disease or gastritis, and acute aortic pathology such as aneurysm or dissection.

Emergency Department Care and Disposition

Care for the patient with pancreatitis includes fluid resuscitation; management of nausea, vomiting, and pain; and diligent monitoring of vital signs and pulse oximetry.

1. Initiate aggressive fluid resuscitation with crystalloid intravenous fluid. Pressors are indicated for hypotension not responsive to adequate fluid resuscitation.
2. All patients with nausea and vomiting should initially be NPO.
3. Administer antiemetics, such as **ondansetron** 4 mg or **prochlorperazine** 5 to 10 mg to reduce vomiting.
4. Administer parenteral analgesia for patient comfort. Intravenous opioids such as **morphine** 0.1 mg/kg are often required.
5. Administer oxygen to maintain a pulse oximetry reading of 95% oxygen saturation. Treat respiratory failure aggressively.
6. Treat patients with infected pseudocyst, abscess, or infected peripancreatic fluid with **imipenem-cilastatin** 500 mg IV, **meropenem** 1 g IV, or **ciprofloxacin** 400 mg IV and **metronidazole** 500 mg IV.
7. Patients with severe systemic disease will require intubation, intensive monitoring, bladder catheterization, and transfusion of blood and blood products as needed. Symptomatic hypocalcemia should be corrected. Laparotomy may be indicated for hemorrhage or abscess drainage.
8. Consult gastroenterology for patients with gallstone pancreatitis for endoscopic retrograde cholangiopancreatography (ERCP) and sphincterotomy.
9. Most patients will require hospitalization. Patients who demonstrate poor prognostic signs (dropping hemoglobin, poor urine output, persistent hypotension, hypoxia, acidosis, or hypocalcemia) despite aggressive early treatment should be admitted to the intensive care unit with surgical consultation.
10. Patients with mild disease, no biliary tract disease, and no evidence of systemic complications may be managed as outpatients with close follow-up if they tolerate clear liquids and oral analgesics in the ED. Instruct patients to increase their diet as tolerated once nausea is controlled.

CHOLECYSTITIS

Biliary tract emergencies most often result from obstruction of the gallbladder or biliary duct by gallstones. The four most common biliary tract emergencies caused by gallstones are biliary colic, cholecystitis, gallstone pancreatitis, and ascending cholangitis. Biliary disease affects all age groups, especially diabetics and the elderly. Gallstones, although common in the general population, remain asymptomatic in most patients. Common risk factors for gallstones and cholecystitis include advanced age, female sex and parity, obesity, rapid weight loss or prolonged fasting, familial tendency, use of some medications, Asian ancestry, chronic liver disease, and hemolytic disorders (e.g., sickle cell disease).

Clinical Features

Patients with biliary disease present with a wide range of symptoms. Biliary colic may present with epigastric or right upper quadrant pain, may range from mild to severe, and, although classically described as intermittent or colicky, is often constant. Nausea and vomiting are usually present. Pain may be referred to the right shoulder or left upper back. It may begin after eating but often bears no association to meals. Acute episodes of biliary colic typically last for 1 to 5 hours, followed by a gradual or sudden resolution of symptoms. Recurrent episodes are usually infrequent, generally at intervals longer than 1 week. Biliary colic seems to follow a circadian pattern, with highest incidence of symptoms between 9 PM and 4 AM.

Physical examination commonly demonstrates right upper quadrant or epigastric tenderness without findings of peritonitis.

Acute cholecystitis presents with pain similar to that of biliary colic that persists for longer than the typical 5 hours. Fever, chills, nausea, emesis, and anorexia are common. Past history of similar attacks or known gallstones may be reported. As the gallbladder becomes progressively inflamed, the initial poorly localized upper abdominal pain often becomes sharp and localized to the right upper quadrant. The patient may have moderate to severe distress and may appear toxic. Choledocholithiasis often presents with midline pain that radiates to the middle of the back.

Examination findings include tenderness in the right upper quadrant or epigastrum, and Murphy's sign (increased pain or inspiratory arrest during deep subcostal palpation of the right upper quadrant during deep inspiration). Murphy's sign is the most sensitive physical examination finding for the diagnosis of cholecystitis. Generalized abdominal rigidity suggests perforation and diffuse peritonitis. Volume depletion is common, but jaundice is unusual. Acalculous cholecystitis occurs in 5% to 10% of patients with cholecystitis, has a more rapid, aggressive clinical course, and occurs more frequently in patients with diabetes, the elderly, trauma or burn victims, after prolonged labor or major surgery, or with systemic vasculitides.

Ascending cholangitis, a life-threatening condition with high mortality, results from complete biliary obstruction (often a common bile duct stone; less commonly a tumor) with bacterial superinfection. Patients often present in extremis with jaundice, fever, confusion, and shock. Examination findings can be subtle. Patients commonly have focal right upper quadrant pain and nausea. Jaundice may or may not be present. The Charcot triad of fever, jaundice, and right upper quadrant pain is suggestive but all three components are usually not present at once.

Diagnosis and Differential

Suspicion of gallbladder or biliary tract disease must be maintained in any patient who presents with upper abdominal pain. The differential diagnosis is similar to that of AP (see Diagnosis and Differential section under the section Pancreatitis, earlier).

Patients with uncomplicated biliary colic usually have normal laboratory findings. The diagnosis is usually made based on the patient presentation, response to therapy, and examining the test results in aggregate.

Laboratory studies that may aid in diagnosis include a white blood cell count; leukocytosis with left shift suggests acute cholecystitis, pancreatitis, or cholangitis, but a normal white blood cell count does not exclude them. Serum bilirubin and alkaline phosphatase levels may be normal or mildly elevated in patients suffering from biliary colic or cholecystitis. Serum bilirubin and alkaline phosphatase levels are usually elevated in cases of choledocholithiasis and ascending cholangitis. Serum lipase or amylase levels should be checked to help exclude associated pancreatitis.

Ultrasound of the hepatobiliary tract is the initial diagnostic study of choice for patients with suspected biliary colic or cholecystitis (see Fig. 42-1). It can detect stones as small as 2 mm and signs of cholecystitis which include a thickened gallbladder wall (>3 to 5 mm), gallbladder distention (>4 cm in short-axis view), and pericholecystic fluid. A positive sonographic Murphy's sign is very sensitive for diagnosis of cholecystitis when it is elicited during the scan. Ultrasound has a strong positive predictive value (92%) when both a sonographic Murphy's sign and gallstones are present. Choledocholithiasis is suggested when the common bile duct diameter is greater than 5 to 7 mm.

Computed tomography of the abdomen is most useful when additional intraabdominal processes are suspected. Radionuclide cholescintigraphy (technetium-iminodiacetic acid [HIDA]) or diisopropyl iminodiacetic acid ([DISIDA] scans) offers a sensitivity of 97% and a specificity of 90% for cholecystitis. A reasonable emergency department (ED) approach to suspected cholecystitis would be to obtain an ultrasound scan and then a radionuclide scan if ultrasound fails to establish the diagnosis.

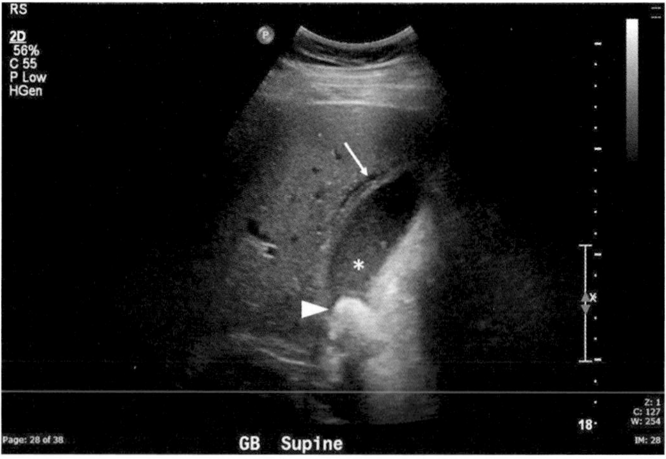

FIGURE 42-1. Abdominal US demonstrating acute cholecystitis with a gallstone (*arrow-head*), gallbladder sludge (*asterisk*), and pericholecystic fluid (*arrow*). Used with permission from Bart Besinger, MD, FAAEM.

Emergency Department Care and Disposition

Care for the patient with biliary disease includes fluid resuscitation and management of nausea, vomiting, and pain. Uncomplicated biliary colic can be managed without the aid of consultants. ED treatment includes the following measures:

1. Initiate aggressive fluid resuscitation with crystalloid intravenous fluid. Pressors are indicated for hypotension not responsive to adequate fluid resuscitation.
2. Patients should be made NPO.
3. Administer antiemetics, such as **ondansetron** 4 mg or **prochlorperazine** 5 to 10 mg to reduce vomiting.
4. Administer parenteral analgesia for patient comfort. Intravenous opioids such as **morphine** 0.1 mg/kg are often required. The intravenous nonsteroidal anti-inflammatory drug (NSAID) **ketorolac** 30 mg IV may also be helpful.
5. A nasogastric tube to low suction should be considered if the patient is distended or actively vomiting, or if vomiting is intractable to antiemetics.
6. Patients with acute biliary obstruction may require urgent decompression via endoscopic sphincterotomy of the ampulla of Vater.
7. Initiate early antibiotic therapy in any patient with suspected cholecystitis or cholangitis. Adequate therapy for uncomplicated cases of cholecystitis includes a parenteral third-generation cephalosporin (**cefotaxime** or **ceftriaxone** 1 g IV q12 to q24h) plus **metronidazole** 500 mg IV. Patients with ascending cholangitis, sepsis, or obvious peritonitis are best managed with triple coverage by using **ampicillin** (0.5 to 1.0 g IV q6h), **gentamicin** (1 to 2 mg/kg IV q8h), and **clindamycin** (600 mg IV q6h), or the equivalent substitutes (e.g., metronidazole for clindamycin, third-generation cephalosporins or piperacillin/tazobactam, or a fluoroquinolone for ampicillin).
8. Patients diagnosed with acute cholecystitis, gallstone pancreatitis, or ascending cholangitis require immediate surgical consultation with hospital admission. Patients with choledocholithiasis, gallstone pancreatitis, or ascending cholangitis may also require urgent gastroenterology consultation to facilitate ERCP and sphincterotomy. Signs of systemic toxicity or sepsis warrant admission to the intensive care unit pending surgical treatment.
9. Patients with uncomplicated biliary colic whose symptoms abate with supportive therapy within 4 to 6 hours of onset can be discharged home if they are able to maintain oral hydration. Oral opioid analgesics may be prescribed for the next 24 to 48 hours for the common residual abdominal aching. Arrange timely outpatient follow-up with a surgical consultant or the patient's primary care physician. Instruct patients to return to the ED if fever develops, abdominal pain worsens, for intractable vomiting, or if another significant attack occurs before follow-up.

FURTHER READING

For further reading in *Tintinalli's Emergency Medicine: A Comprehensive Study Guide*, 8th ed., see Chapter 79, "Pancreatitis and Cholecystitis," by Bart Besinger and Christine R. Stehman.

CHAPTER 43

Acute Appendicitis

Charles E. Stewart

Appendicitis is one of the most common surgical emergencies. Despite advances in laboratory testing and imaging, accurate diagnosis of appendicitis remains a challenge. Complications from misdiagnosis of appendicitis include intraabdominal abscess, wound infection, adhesion formation, bowel obstruction, and infertility.

CLINICAL FEATURES

The early signs and symptoms of appendicitis are quite nonspecific and progress with time. The most reliable symptom in appendicitis is abdominal pain. Pain commonly begins in the periumbilical or epigastric region. As peritoneal irritation occurs, the pain often localizes to the right lower quadrant. The final location of the pain depends on the location of the appendix. Other symptoms associated with appendicitis include anorexia, nausea, and vomiting, but these symptoms are neither sensitive nor specific. As the pain increases, irritation of the bladder and/or colon may cause dysuria, tenesmus, or other symptoms. Many patients have the "bump" sign, where the patient notes an increase in the abdominal pain associated with bumps in the ride to the hospital. Other physicians will have the patient jump up and down in the examining room to evoke the pain. (Such maneuvers illustrate peritoneal irritation, but are nonspecific for appendicitis.) If the pain suddenly decreases, the examiner should consider appendiceal perforation.

The classic point of maximal tenderness is in the right lower quadrant just below the middle of a line connecting the umbilicus and the right anterior superior iliac spine (McBurney's point). Patients may also have pain referred to the right lower quadrant when palpating the left lower quadrant (Rovsing's sign), pain elicited by extending the right leg to the hip while lying in the left lateral decubitus position (psoas sign), or pain elicited by passively flexing the right hip and knee and internally rotating the hip (obturator sign). Patients with a pelvic appendix may be quite tender on rectal examination, and patients with a retrocecal appendix may have more prominent flank pain than abdominal pain. No individual physical finding is sensitive or specific enough to rule in or rule out the diagnosis, and all physical findings and maneuvers depend on irritation of the peritoneum.

Fever is a relatively late finding in appendicitis and rarely exceeds 39°C (102.2°F), unless rupture or other complications occur. Meta-analysis of 42 studies found that fever was the single most useful sign, followed by rebound tenderness and migration of the pain to the right lower quadrant.

DIAGNOSIS AND DIFFERENTIAL

Even with that caveat, the diagnosis of acute appendicitis is primarily clinical. Symptoms with high sensitivity for appendicitis include fever, right lower quadrant pain, pain that occurs before vomiting, and absence of prior similar pain. Migration of the pain is thought to be a strong predictor for appendicitis. Physical signs with high specificity include right lower abdominal rigidity and positive psoas sign. In both children and adults, no single historical or physical examination finding is sufficient to make an unequivocal diagnosis of appendicitis. Consider appendicitis in any patient with atraumatic right-sided abdominal, periumbilical, or flank pain who has not previously undergone appendectomy.

Additional studies, such as complete blood count, C-reactive protein, urinalysis, and imaging studies, may be performed if the diagnosis is unclear, but lack the sensitivity to rule in or rule out the diagnosis. The combination of a normal WBC and C-reactive protein may have some utility as a negative screening test, as the likelihood of both being negative despite a pathologic diagnosis of appendicitis in a patient with a low pre-test probability is quite low. Unfortunately, these tests are often elevated in multiple conditions, so the reverse has almost no value. A pregnancy test must be performed in all females of reproductive age. A normal WBC does not rule out appendicitis. Urinalysis is useful to help rule out other diagnoses, but pyuria and hematuria can occur when an inflamed appendix irritates the ureter.

The differential diagnosis of right lower quadrant pain is wide and includes other gastrointestinal processes (e.g., inflammatory bowel disease, hernia, abscess, volvulus, diverticulitis), gynecologic or urological processes (e.g., ectopic pregnancy, ovarian torsion, renal colic, genitourinary (GU) infection or abscess), or musculoskeletal processes (e.g., muscular hematoma or abscess).

Scoring systems such as the Alvarado and Samuel scoring systems have been developed to aid in diagnosis. These scoring systems have uniformly had less sensitivity for diagnosis of appendicitis than the clinical judgment of an experienced examiner and should not replace this experienced-based decision.

The goal of imaging is to establish the diagnosis of appendicitis, avoid a negative appendectomy, and identify other potential causes of abdominal pain. Increased concerns about accumulated radiation exposure for children, potentially childbearing females, and pregnant patients have led to growing interest in alternatives to the CT scan. Unfortunately, imaging can also escalate the cost of the medical care.

Plain radiographs of the abdomen are not helpful.

Computed tomography (CT) is probably the imaging study of choice for most patients with an overall sensitivity of 96% and PPV of 96%. CT findings suggesting acute appendicitis include pericecal inflammation, abscess, and periappendiceal phlegmon or fluid collections (Fig. 43-1). CT has been shown to change management in women, decreasing unnecessary tests. CT may be conducted with or without contrast administered orally, intravenously, or rectally, depending on institutional experience and preference. Unenhanced CT scanning has 92% sensitivity and 96% specificity. Noncontrast CT should be considered an acceptable imaging modality in the workup of acute appendicitis. Clearly, no contrast should be used for patients with allergy to contrast or for patients with renal disease. CT findings of appendicitis may be obscured in the thin patient, as intraperitoneal fat serves as an intrinsic contrast medium in unenhanced CT.

Ultrasonography has a high sensitivity but is limited both by operator skill and in evaluating a ruptured appendix or an abnormally located (e.g., retrocecal) appendix. Reports of the effectiveness of ultrasound (US)

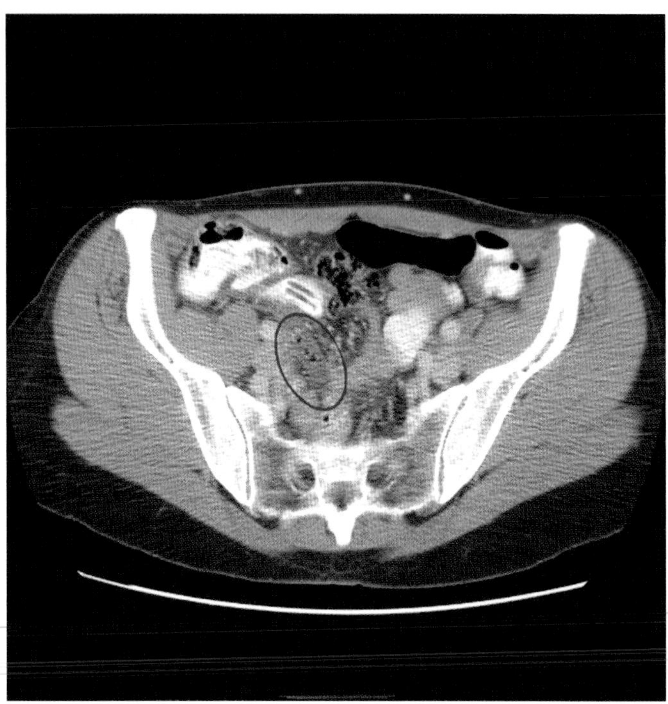

FIGURE 43-1. Acute appendicitis on contrast CT scan as evidenced by dilated and inflamed appendix.

diagnosis of appendicitis in pregnancy are conflicting, with some reporting US as useful and others reporting it as ineffective for diagnosis.

Graded compression ultrasonography is the initial modality of choice in both children and the pregnant patient to decrease radiation exposure. Overall sensitivity of US is 86% with positive predictive value (PPV) of 95%. Given the highly operator-dependent nature of ultrasonography, hospitals that frequently perform US for diagnosis of appendicitis may have greater reproducibility of high-quality studies. The diagnostic accuracy of abdominal US in children is better at ruling in acute appendicitis than excluding it.

Magnetic resonance imaging (MRI) for the diagnosis of appendicitis is accepted in many hospitals as a reliable technology that avoids completely the ionizing radiation risks. IV gadolinium contrast with MRI should be avoided in the pregnant patient as it crosses the placenta, given the teratogenic effects seen in animal studies. Gadolinium is not given to patients with renal disease as it may exacerbate the renal insufficiency.

The elderly patient is more likely to have preexisting comorbidities and may be taking medications that alter presentation, management, and outcomes. Elderly patients may have decreased perceptions of symptoms. Patients with communication difficulties and those with poor access to medical care may also have vague complaints, including diffuse pain, fever, or alteration in mental status. Such individuals commonly present later in the course of the disease and are more likely to have worse outcomes. In these patients, an atypical presentation is quite common and alternative or comorbid diagnoses are often found on imaging.

The pediatric patient who cannot verbalize symptoms also presents a significant challenge. Patients younger than 6 years have a high misdiagnosis rate due to poor communication skills and the association of many nonspecific symptoms. Careful history from the parent or guardian and equally careful physical examination are essential to accurate diagnosis. Coordinate imaging studies in these patients with your surgical consultant to ensure most accurate diagnosis with least radiation exposure.

Pregnant patients are at risk for misdiagnosis. Acute appendicitis is the most common surgical emergency in pregnancy, and delay in diagnosis is the greatest cause of increased morbidity in the pregnant woman with an acute abdomen. Ovarian torsion and ectopic or heterotopic pregnancy are additional considerations in the fertile female. If an abdominal US is nondiagnostic or not available, consider pelvic US, CT, or MRI.

EMERGENCY DEPARTMENT CARE AND DISPOSITION

1. Obtain surgical consultation before imaging when the diagnosis is thought to be clear. Patient should have nothing by mouth and should have intravenous (IV) access and fluids.
2. The treatment for acute appendicitis is appendectomy. If the local surgical services are inadequate or unavailable, transfer the patient to an appropriate facility.
3. Control pain with opioid analgesics, such as **fentanyl** 1 to 2 μg/kg IV every 1 to 4 hours or **morphine** 0.1 mg/kg.
4. Antibiotics given before surgery decrease the incidence of postoperative wound infection or, in cases of perforation, postoperative abscess formation. Several antibiotic regimens to cover anaerobes, enterococci, and gram-negative intestinal flora have been recommended, including **piperacillin/tazobactam** 3.375 g IV or **ampicillin/sulbactam** 3 g IV. Consult with the surgeon regarding the antibiotic regimen and timing.
5. In patients for whom the diagnosis is not clear, admit for observation, serial examinations, and surgical consultation. This is a safe option for high-risk patients (pediatric, geriatric, pregnant, or immunocompromised).
6. Stable, nontoxic-appearing patients with adequate pain control who can tolerate oral hydration have no significant comorbidities, and are able to return for reevaluation in 12 hours may be considered for discharge and 12-hour follow-up. These patients should be instructed to avoid strong analgesics, and should return if they develop increased pain, localization of the pain, fever, nausea, or other signs or symptoms of illness that are worsening or not resolving.

FURTHER READING

For further reading in *Tintinalli's Emergency Medicine: A Comprehensive Study Guide*, 8th ed., see Chapter 81, "Acute Appendicitis," by E. Paul DeKoning.

CHAPTER 44

Diverticulitis

James O'Neill

Diverticulitis is a common GI disorder that occurs when small herniations through the wall of the colon, or diverticula, become inflamed or infected.

CLINICAL FEATURES

Classically, diverticulitis presents with left lower abdominal pain, fever, and leukocytosis. The most common symptom is a steady, deep discomfort in the left lower quadrant of the abdomen. Pain may be constant or intermittent, with associated symptoms of change in bowel habits (constipation or diarrhea), nausea, vomiting, and anorexia. Urinary tract symptoms are less common. Patients with a redundant sigmoid colon, of Asian descent, or with right-sided disease may complain of pain in the suprapubic area or right lower quadrant. The presentation can mimic other diseases, such as appendicitis.

Patients have a low-grade fever, but the temperature may be higher in patients with generalized peritonitis and in those with an abscess. Physical findings range from mild abdominal tenderness to severe pain, obstruction, and peritonitis. Occult blood may be present in the stool.

DIAGNOSIS AND DIFFERENTIAL

The differential diagnosis includes acute appendicitis, colitis (ischemic or infectious), inflammatory bowel disease (Crohn's disease or ulcerative colitis), colon cancer, irritable bowel syndrome, pseudomembranous colitis, epiploic appendagitis, gallbladder disease, incarcerated hernia, mesenteric infarction, complicated ulcer disease, peritonitis, obstruction, ovarian torsion, ectopic pregnancy, ovarian cyst or mass, pelvic inflammatory disease, sarcoidosis, collagen vascular disease, cystitis, kidney stone, renal pathology, and pancreatic disease.

Diverticulitis can be diagnosed by clinical history and examination alone. In stable patients with past similar acute presentations, no further diagnostic evaluation is necessary unless the patient fails to improve with conservative medical treatment. If a patient does not have a prior diagnosis or the current episode is different from past episodes, diagnostic imaging should be performed to rule out other intraabdominal pathology and evaluate for complications. CT scan is the preferred imaging modality for its ability to evaluate the severity of disease and the presence of complications. CT with IV and oral contrast has documented sensitivities of 97% and specificities approaching 100%. Compression ultrasound is operator dependent and has been shown to have sensitivity and specificity greater than 80% with experienced operators. Laboratory tests, such as a CBC, liver function tests, and urinalysis, are not diagnostic but may help exclude other diagnoses.

EMERGENCY DEPARTMENT CARE AND DISPOSITION

ED care begins with fluid and electrolyte replacement, pain, and nausea control.

1. Ill-appearing patients, those with uncontrolled pain, vomiting, peritoneal signs, signs of systemic infection, comorbidities, or immunosuppression, and those with complicated diverticulitis (e.g., phlegmon, abscess, obstruction, fistula, or perforation), require admission and surgical consultation.
2. Uncomplicated diverticulitis is managed with oral antibiotics and a liquid diet, although recent data suggests that antibiotics may not be required in uncomplicated diverticulitis.
3. Outpatients should follow up with a gastroenterology specialist for an outpatient colonoscopy in 6 weeks if they show improvement. Patients with worsening of their condition during outpatient treatment will require admission to the hospital.

Please see Table 44-1 for antibiotic recommendations.

TABLE 44-1 Antibiotics for Diverticulitis

Outpatient 4–7 days	First line	Metronidazole 500 mg PO q6h PLUS Ciprofloxacin 750 mg PO BID OR Levofloxacin 750 mg PO q24h OR Trimethoprim-sulfamethoxazole (Bactrim) 1 tab PO BID
	Alternate	Amoxicillin-clavulanate extended release 1000/62.5 mg 2 tabs PO BID Moxifloxacin 400 mg PO q24h
Inpatient		
Moderate disease	First line	Metronidazole 500 mg IV TID PLUS Ciprofloxacin 400 mg IV BID OR Levofloxacin 750 mg IV q24h OR Aztreonam 2 g IV TID OR Ceftriaxone 1 g IV q24h
	Alternative	Ertapenem 1 g IV q24h Piperacillin-tazobactam 4.5 g IV q8h Moxifloxacin 400 mg IV q24h
Severe, life-threatening	First line	Imipenem 500 mg IV q6h Meropenem 1 g IV q8h Piperacillin-tazobactam 4.5 mg IV q8h
	Alternative	Ampicillin 2 g IV q6h PLUS Metronidazole 500 mg IV q6h PLUS Ciprofloxacin 400 mg IV q12h OR Amikacin, gentamicin, or tobramycin (Penicillin allergy: Aztreonam 2 g IV q6h PLUS metronidazole 500 mg IV q6h)

FURTHER READING

For further reading in *Tintinalli's Emergency Medicine: A Comprehensive Study Guide*, 8th ed., see Chapter 82, "Diverticulitis," by Graham Autumn.

CHAPTER 45

Intestinal Obstruction and Volvulus

Olumayowa U. Kolade

Intestinal obstruction results from mechanical blockage or the loss of normal peristalsis. Adynamic or paralytic ileus is more common and usually self-limiting. Common causes of mechanical small bowel obstruction (SBO) are adhesions due to previous surgery, incarcerated hernias, or inflammatory diseases. Other causes to consider are inflammatory bowel diseases, congenital anomalies, and foreign bodies. The most frequent causes of large bowel obstructions are cancer, diverticulitis with stricture, sigmoid volvulus, and fecal impaction. Consider intussusception in children. Sigmoid volvulus is more common in the elderly taking anticholinergic medications while cecal volvulus is more common in gravid patients. Intestinal pseudoobstruction (Ogilvie syndrome) may mimic large bowel obstruction. The elderly and bedridden and patients taking anticholinergic medications or tricyclic antidepressants are at increased risk for pseudoobstruction.

CLINICAL FEATURES

Crampy, intermittent, progressive abdominal pain and inability to have a bowel movement or to pass flatus are common presenting complaints. Vomiting, bilious in proximal obstructions and feculent in distal obstruction, is usually present. Patients with partial SBO can still pass flatus. Physical signs vary from abdominal distention, localized or general tenderness, to obvious signs of peritonitis. Localization of pain and the presence of abdominal surgical scars, hernia, or masses may provide clues to the site of obstruction. The abdomen may be tympanitic to percussion. Active, high-pitched bowel sounds can be heard in mechanical SBO. Bowel sounds may be diminished or absent if the obstruction has been present for many hours. Rectal examination may demonstrate fecal impaction, rectal carcinoma, or occult blood. Key features of ileus and mechanical bowel obstruction are described in Table 45-1. The presence of stool in the rectum does not exclude obstruction. Consider a pelvic examination in women. Systemic symptoms and signs depend on the extent of dehydration and the presence of bowel necrosis or infection.

TABLE 45-1 Key Features of Ileus and Mechanical Bowel Obstruction

	Ileus	Bowel Obstruction
Pain	Mild to moderate	Moderate to severe
Location	Diffuse	May localize
Physical examination	Mild distention, ± tenderness, decreased bowel sounds	Mild distention, tenderness, high-pitched bowel sounds
Laboratory	Possible dehydration	Leukocytosis
Imaging	May be normal	Abnormal
Treatment	Observation, hydration	Nasogastric tube, surgery

DIAGNOSIS AND DIFFERENTIAL

Suspect intestinal obstruction in any patient with abdominal pain, distention, and vomiting, especially in patients with previous abdominal surgery, abdominal/pelvic radiotherapy, or groin hernias.

Flat and upright abdominal radiographs and an upright chest x-ray can screen for obstruction (see Fig. 45-1), confirm severe constipation, or diagnose hollow viscous perforation with free air. The diagnostic procedure of choice in the ED is CT scanning using IV and oral contrast when possible. CT scanning can delineate partial versus complete bowel obstruction, partial SBO versus ileus, and strangulated versus simple SBO.

Laboratory tests may include a complete blood count, electrolytes, blood urea nitrogen, creatinine, lactate levels, coagulation profile, and type and cross-match. Suspect abscess, gangrene, or peritonitis if leukocytosis >20,000 or left shift is noted. An elevated hematocrit is consistent with dehydration.

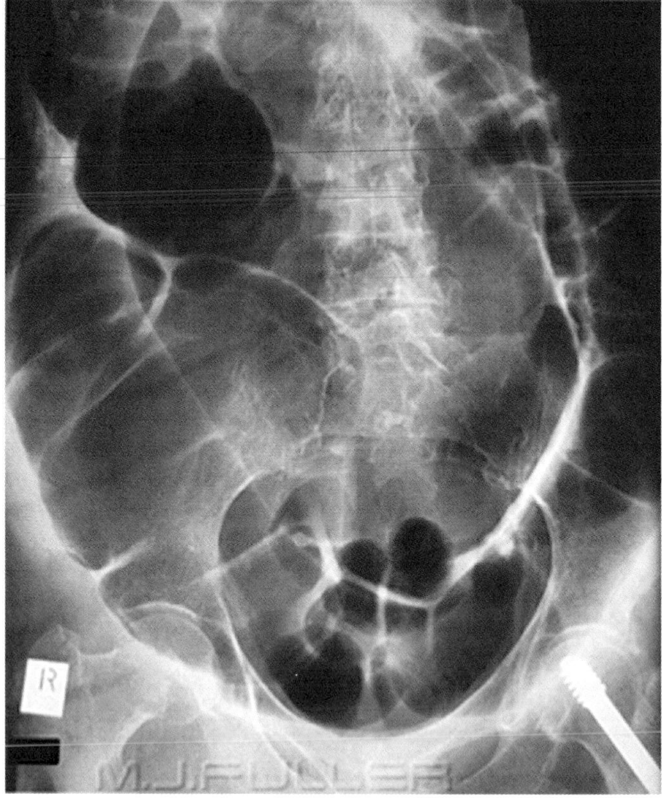

FIGURE 45-1. Sigmoid volvulus. Note that the open portion of the "C" formed by the twisted large bowel points toward the left side in the case of sigmoid volvulus. Reproduced with permission from Wikiradiography.com.

EMERGENCY DEPARTMENT CARE AND DISPOSITION

ED care is directed at vigorous fluid resuscitation with crystalloids, careful monitoring of response, and prompt surgical consultation. Surgical intervention is usually necessary to treat a mechanical obstruction.

1. Decompress the bowel with a nasogastric tube especially if vomiting or distension is present.
2. Administer preoperative broad-spectrum intravenous antibiotics coverage such as **piperacillin/tazobactam** 3.375 g IV every 6 hours, **tircarcillin-clavulanate** 3.1 g IV every 6 hours or **ampicillin/sulbactam** 3.0 g or double drug coverage with **cefotaxime** 2 g or **ceftriaxone** 2 g plus **clindamycin** 600 mg or **metronidazole** 1 g or a **carbapenem**, such as **meropenem** 1 g IV every 8 hours.
3. When the diagnosis is uncertain or if adynamic ileus is suspected, conservative measures, such as intravenous fluids and observation without surgical intervention, may be appropriate.
4. In patients with pseudoobstruction, colonoscopy is both diagnostic and therapeutic. Surgery is not indicated.

FURTHER READING

For further reading in *Tintinalli's Emergency Medicine: A Comprehensive Study Guide*, 8th ed., see Chapter 83, "Bowel Obstruction," by Timothy G. Price and Raymond J. Orthober.

CHAPTER 46

Hernia in Adults and Children

Louise Finnel

A hernia is a protrusion of any viscus from its normal cavity, for example, bowel bulging through the abdominal wall. Hernias are classified by anatomic location, hernia contents, and the status of those contents (e.g., reducible, incarcerated, or strangulated). The most common abdominal hernias are inguinal, ventral, and femoral hernias (Fig. 46-1).

Predisposing factors include family history, lack of developmental maturity, undescended testes, genitourinary abnormalities, conditions that increase intraabdominal pressure (e.g., ascites or pregnancy), chronic obstructive pulmonary disease, and surgical incision sites.

CLINICAL FEATURES

Most hernias are detected on routine physical examination or inadvertently by the patient. When the contents of a hernia can be easily returned to their original cavity by manipulation, the hernia is defined as *reducible*. A hernia becomes *incarcerated* when its contents are not reducible. Incarcerated hernias may lead to bowel obstruction and strangulation. *Strangulation* refers to vascular compromise of the incarcerated contents and is an acute surgical emergency. When not relieved, strangulation may lead to gangrene, perforation, peritonitis, and septic shock.

Symptoms other than an obvious protruding mass from the abdominal wall include localized pain, nausea, and vomiting. Signs of strangulation include severe pain and tenderness, induration, and erythema over the site. Children may exhibit irritability and poor feeding. Careful evaluation for obstruction is essential.

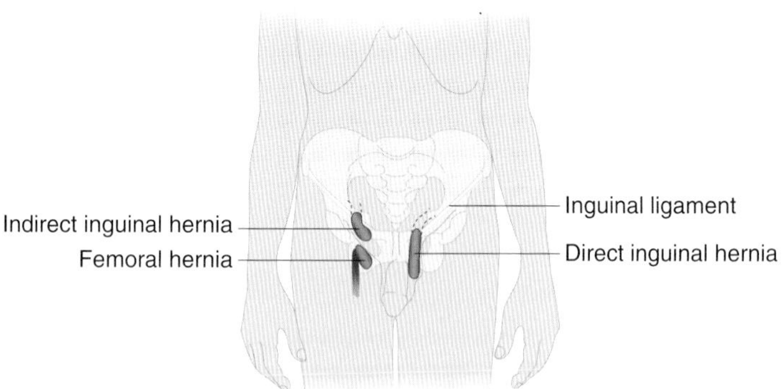

FIGURE 46-1. Groin hernias.

DIAGNOSIS AND DIFFERENTIAL

Physical examination is the predominant means of diagnosis. Laboratory testing is of minimal value. Ultrasonographic detection of hernias is operator and body habitus dependent but can be helpful in pediatric and pregnant patients where radiation exposure is a concern (Fig. 46-2). Computed tomography remains the best radiographic test for the evaluation of hernias and can more easily identify the less common hernia types such as Spigelian or obturator.

The differential diagnosis of a groin mass includes direct or indirect hernia, testicular torsion, tumor, groin abscess, hydrocele, varicocele, and hidradenitis. In children, retracted or undescended testes may be mistaken for inguinal hernias.

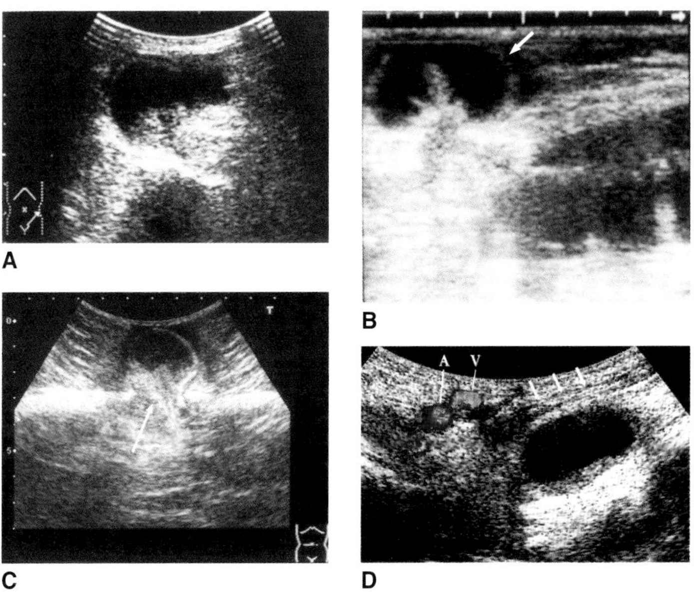

FIGURE 46-2. Ultrasonographic detection of incarcerated hernia. **A.** An incarcerated femoral hernia is demonstrated as a small - bowel segment herniated through the femoral canal. **B.** In an incarcerated incisional hernia, a small-bowel segment (arrow) is demonstrated as herniated through a small orifice in the abdominal wall. Dilated small-bowel loops are evident proximal to the incarceration. **C.** In an umbilical hernia, a herniated small - bowel segment is demonstrated within the fluid space in the hernia sac. The segment was softly strangulated at the femoral orifice (arrow) formed by a defect of the fascia and was easily reduced by manipulation in this case. **D.** An incarcerated obturator hernia is demonstrated deep in the femoral region. It locates posterior to the pectineus muscle (arrows) and medial to the femoral artery (A) and vein (V).Reproduced with permission from Ma OJ, Mateer JR, Reardon RF, et al: *Ma and Mateer's Emergency Ultrasound*, 3rd ed. New York: The McGraw-Hill Companies; 2014

TABLE 46-1 Steps for Hernia Reduction
1. NPO—in case reduction is unsuccessful
2. Adequate analgesia; children will require procedural sedation
3. Place patient in Trendelenberg position
4. Externally rotate and flex ipsilateral leg
5. Place a padded icepack to reduce swelling and blood flow to the area
6. Grasp and elongate the hernia neck with one hand
7. With the other hand apply firm steady pressure to proximal hernia at the site of the fascial defect

EMERGENCY DEPARTMENT CARE AND DISPOSITION

Do not attempt reduction if signs of strangulation exist, as dead bowel may then be introduced into the abdomen (Table 46-1).

Definitive Management

1. Adults with easily reducible hernias can be referred for outpatient surgical evaluation and repair. Patients should avoid heavy lifting and return to the ED if herniation recurs and cannot be reduced promptly. Discuss signs of obstruction with them prior to discharge.
2. Incarcerated hernias that can't be reduced with one or two attempts and strangulated hernias require emergent surgical consultation and intervention. Give nothing by mouth, initiate intravenous fluid resuscitation and administer intravenous opioid analgesia. Broad-spectrum antibiotics, such as **cefoxitin** 2 g IV or **piperacillin/tazobactam** 3.375 g IV, should be given if there is evidence of perforation or strangulation.
3. Infants with successfully reduced inguinal hernias should have surgical repair within 24 to 72 hours because one-third will redevelop incarceration.
4. Children with uncomplicated umbilical hernias may be discharged and followed longitudinally by their primary care providers. Refer children older than 4 years or those with hernias greater than 2 cm in diameter for surgical evaluation.

FURTHER READING

For further reading in *Tintinalli's Emergency Medicine: A Comprehensive Study Guide*, 8th ed., see Chapter 84, "Hernias in Adults," by Donald Byars and Turan Kayagil

CHAPTER 47

Anorectal Disorders

Chad E. Branecki

Anorectal disorders range from simple local disease processes to underlying serious systemic disorders. Most anorectal diseases originate in the anal crypts, glands, internal hemorrhoidal plexus, and external hemorrhoid veins. More serious life-threatening infections tend to lie in the deeper tissues such as the ischiorectal and pelvic-rectal spaces.

After a detailed history, a digital examination of the rectum should be performed, followed by anoscopy in the left lateral decubitus position. The supine or lithotomy position can be used for debilitated patients.

ANAL TAGS

Skin tags are usually asymptomatic minor projections of the skin at the anal verge, which may be from residual prior hemorrhoids. Most are asymptomatic but inflammation may cause itching or pain. Inflammatory bowel disease may be associated with sentinel tags; therefore, surgical referral is warranted.

HEMORRHOIDS

Engorgement, prolapse, or thrombosis of the internal or external hemorrhoidal vein(s) is termed hemorrhoids.

Clinical Features

Patients report painless, bright red rectal blood on the surface of the stool, toilet tissue, or dripping into the toilet bowl after defecation. Thrombosed hemorrhoids are usually painful and may appear as a bluish-purple mass protruding from the rectum. Large hemorrhoids may result in prolapse that may spontaneously reduce or require periodic manual reduction by patients or clinicians. They may become incarcerated and gangrenous, and require surgical intervention. Prolapse may cause mucous discharge and pruritus. If not reduced, severe bleeding, thrombosis, infarction, incarceration, urinary retention, or sepsis may occur.

Diagnosis and Differential

Internal hemorrhoids are not readily palpable and are best visualized through an anoscope. They are found at 2, 5, and 9 o'clock positions when patients are prone. Constipation, pregnancy, ascites, ovarian tumors, radiation fibrosis, and increased portal venous pressure are some of the common causes of hemorrhoids. Rectal and sigmoid colon tumors should be considered in patients older than 40 years.

Emergency Department Care and Disposition

Unless a complication is present, management is usually nonsurgical.

1. Hot sitz baths for at least 15 minutes, three times per day, and after each bowel movement will reduce pain and swelling. After the sitz baths, the anus should be gently but thoroughly dried.

2. Topical steroids and analgesics may provide temporary relief. Bulk laxatives, such as psyllium seed compounds or stool softeners, should be used after the acute phase has subsided. Laxatives causing liquid stool are contraindicated as they may result in cryptitis and sepsis.
3. Surgical treatment is indicated for severe, intractable pain, continued bleeding, incarceration, or strangulation.
4. Acute and recently thrombosed painful hemorrhoids (<48 hours) can be treated with clot excision. After analgesia, with a long acting local anesthetic such as 0.5% bupivacaine with epinephrine, an elliptical skin incision is made over the hemorrhoids and the thrombosed clot is evacuated (Fig. 47-1). Hemostasis is achieved by packing and pressure dressing. The pressure dressing may be removed after about 6 hours, when the patient takes the first sitz bath. Refer to a surgeon for definitive hemorrhoidectomy.

CRYPTITIS

Sphincter spasm, and superficial trauma from diarrhea, or repeated passage of large hard stools cause breakdown of the mucosa over the crypts. Infecting organisms enter the crypts and cause inflammation of anal glands, abscesses formation, fissures, and fistulae. Common symptoms include anal pain during bowel movements and itching, with or without rectal bleeding. Diagnosis is made by palpation of tender, swollen crypts with associated hypertrophied papillae. Anoscopy allows visualization of the inflamed crypts in posterior midline of the anal ring. Bulk laxatives, additional roughage, hot sitz baths, and warm rectal irrigations enhance healing. Surgical treatment may be needed in refractory cases.

ANAL FISSURES

Anal fissures are superficial linear tears of the anal canal usually caused by local trauma (e.g., passage of hard stool) and are the most common cause of painful rectal bleeding.

Clinical Features

Patients complain of sharp cutting pain with defecation that subsides between bowel movements. Bleeding is bright and in small quantities. Rectal examination is very painful and often not possible without application of topical anesthetic agents. Most fissures are located in the posterior midline. A sentinel pile may be noted in patients with chronic fissures. A non-posterior midline fissure should alert the physician to consider serious causes, such as Crohn's disease, ulcerative colitis, carcinomas, AIDS, tuberculosis, and sexually transmitted diseases.

Treatment is aimed at relieving sphincter spasm and pain, and preventing stricture formation. Hot sitz baths and the addition of bran (fiber) to the diet are helpful. Use of topical analgesics or steroids may be temporarily helpful. Surgical excision of the fissure may be required if the area does not heal in 6 weeks after adequate treatment.

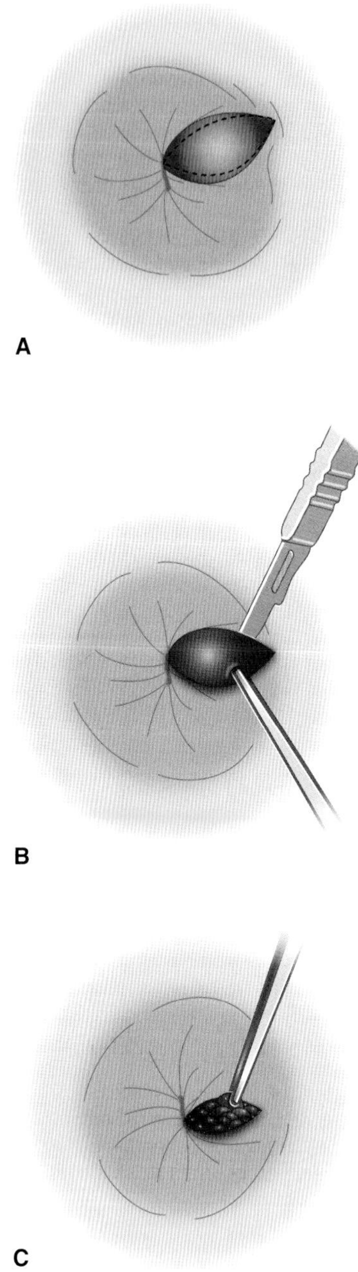

FIGURE 47-1. Elliptical incision of thrombosed external hemorrhoid. **A.** Elliptical incision. **B.** Unroofing of thrombosed external hemorrhoid. **C.** Evacuation of clot.

FISTULA IN ANO

An anal fistula is an abnormal inflammatory tract, originating from an infected anal gland. Fistulae commonly result from perianal or ischiorectal abscess. Crohn's disease, ulcerative colitis, tuberculosis, gonococcal proctitis, and carcinomas should also be considered in the etiology. Persistent bloody, malodorous discharge occurs as long as the fistula remains open. Blockage of the tract causes recurrent bouts of inflammation and abscess formation.

Ultrasonography with a 7 MHz endoprobe and enhanced with 3% hydrogen peroxide may aid in the diagnosis. Non-ill appearing patients can be treated with analgesics, antipyretics, and oral antibiotics such as ciprofloxacin 750 mg twice daily and metronidazole 500 mg four times daily for 7 days. Sitz baths and local cleaning will temporize the condition before surgery. Surgical excision is the definitive treatment and should not be delayed in ill-appearing patients.

ANORECTAL ABSCESSES

Abscesses start from the anal crypts and spread to involve the perianal, intersphincteric, ischiorectal, or deep perianal space. Perianal abscess is the most common and found at the anal verge (Fig. 47-2).

Clinical Features

Persistent dull, aching, throbbing pain that increases prior to defecation is typical. As the abscess progresses, pain and tenderness interfere with walking or sitting. Fever, leukocytosis, and a painful tender mass may be present upon digital rectal examination.

Emergency Department Care and Disposition

Simple isolated perianal abscess without systemic illness may be safely incised in the ED. Other perirectal abscesses, such as supralevator or ischiorectal abscesses, should be drained in the operating room. After adequate local and systemic analgesia, a cruciate incision is made over the abscess, and the "dog ears" are excised. Packing usually is not required. Sitz baths should be started the next day. Antibiotics usually are not necessary unless systemic infection or toxicity is present.

PROCTITIS

Proctitis is inflammation of the rectal mucosa. Common causes include prior radiation treatments, autoimmune disorders, vasculitis, ischemia, sexually transmitted infections (e.g., syphilis, gonorrhea, chlamydia, lymphogranuloma venereum, herpes simplex, chancroid, human papillomavirus), and other infectious diseases.

Clinical Features

Symptoms include anorectal pain, itching, discharge, diarrhea, bleeding, and lower abdominal cramping. Mucosal inflammation, erythema, bleeding, ulcers, or discharge may be noted during anoscopy.

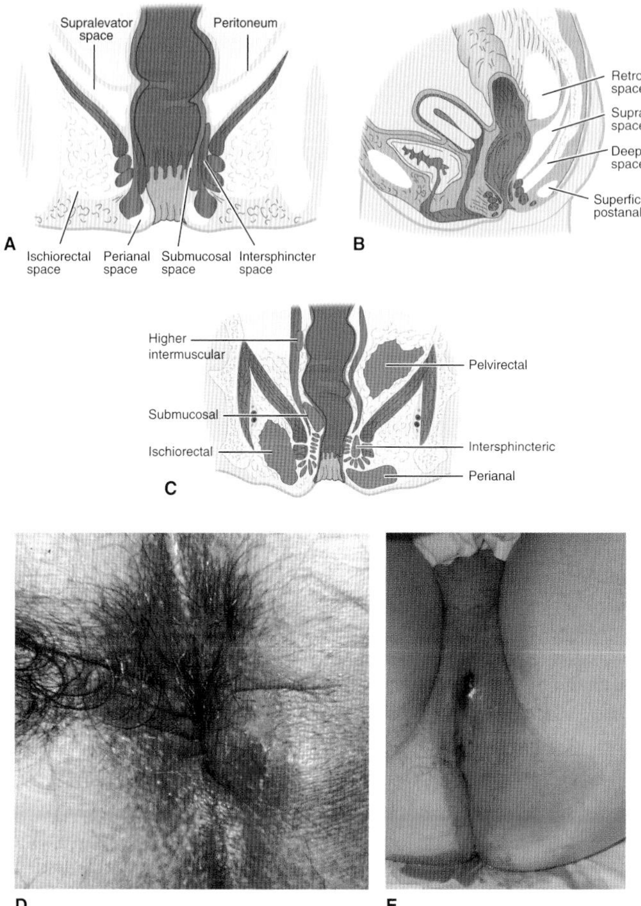

FIGURE 47-2. A, B. Anatomic classification of anorectal spaces. **C.** Anorectal abscesses. **D.** Perianal abscess. **E.** Complicated perirectal abscess.

A, B: Reproduced with permission from Reichman EF: *Emergency Medicine Procedures*. 2nd ed. New York: McGraw-Hill Education; 2013. **D:** Reproduced with permission from Knoop K, Stack L, Storrow A, et al: *Atlas of Emergency Medicine*, 3rd ed. New York: McGraw-Hill Education; 2010. Photo contributor: The American Society of Colon and Rectal Surgeons. **E:** Reproduced with permission from Knoop K, Stack L, Storrow A, et al: *Atlas of Emergency Medicine*, 3rd ed. New York: McGraw-Hill Education; 2010. Figure 9-35. Photo contributor: Lawrence B. Stack, MD.

Emergency Department Care and Disposition

Obtain cultures if an infectious cause is suspected. Stool softeners, sitz baths, good anal hygiene, and analgesics will provide some relief. Patient with enteric pathogens and sexually transmitted infections will require antibiotics directed at the suspected underlying pathogen. Arrange outpatient follow-up.

RECTAL PROLAPSE

Prolapse (procidentia) may involve the mucosa alone or all layers of the rectum. In addition, intussusception of the rectum may present as a prolapse.

Clinical Features

Most patients complain of protruding mass, mucous discharge, associated bleeding, and pruritus. Partial prolapse involves only the rectal mucosa and tends to protrude only a few centimeters from the dentate line. Complete prolapse involves all layers of the rectum, and appears like a red, ball-like mass and may extend up to 15 cm. Often, pain is not a significant feature.

Emergency Department Care and Disposition

In children, the prolapse can be gently reduced under proper analgesia and sedation. The child should then be referred to a specialist to ensure the prolapse is not due to an underlying condition. Every effort should be made to prevent the child from being constipated. In adults, reduction can be more difficult if the rectal walls have become edematous. Generous amounts of granulated sugar applied 15 minutes prior to the reduction may aid in the process with direct, continuous pressure. Lubricated gauze should be taped in place over the anal verge for a few hours after reduction. If the prolapse cannot be easily reduced, or there is evidence of ischemia, emergency surgical consultation and hospitalization are warranted.

ANORECTAL TUMORS

Factors such as smoking, anal intercourse, HIV, and genital warts are associated with anorectal cancer. Neoplasms that occur in this group include adenocarcinoma, malignant melanoma, and Kaposi's sarcoma. Patients present with nonspecific symptoms including sensation of a mass, pruritus, pain, and blood on the stool. Constipation, anorexia, weight loss, narrowing of the stool caliber, and tenesmus eventually develop. Anal margin neoplasms frequently present as an ulcer that fails to heal in a timely manner. Virtually all anorectal tumors can be detected by careful visual examination of the perianal area, digital palpation of the distal rectum and anal canal, and procto- or sigmoidoscopic examination. Complications of anorectal tumors include rectal prolapse, prolonged blood loss, perirectal abscesses, or fistulae. Refer all patients for proctoscopic or sigmoidoscopic examination and biopsy if the history or physical examination is suspicious for neoplasms.

RECTAL FOREIGN BODIES

Not all patients are forthcoming with accurate history of rectal foreign body insertion. Patients may instead complain of abdominal pain, anorectal bleeding, or discharge.

Clinical Features

Most foreign bodies are in the rectal ampulla and are palpable through digital and proctoscopic examination. Obtain abdominal and pelvis x-rays to demonstrate the position, shape, and number of foreign bodies. An upright film or CT scan may be useful to visualize a radiolucent foreign body and to detect free air, indicative of perforation.

Emergency Department Care and Disposition

Although some low-lying rectal foreign bodies can be removed in the ED, many require surgical consultation and intervention, especially if they are made of glass or contain sharp edges.

1. In the ED, procedural sedation accompanied by perianal and submucosal analgesia is used. Adequate sphincter relaxation is essential. Local infiltration anesthesia injected through a 30-gauge needle into the internal sphincter muscle circumferentially will provide good relaxation. Anal lubrication, the aid of obstetric forceps, a speculum or snares, and having the patient bear down may all be helpful in the extraction of the foreign body.
2. Large bulbar objects may create a vacuum-like effect proximally, making removal by simple traction impossible. In these cases, the vacuum can be overcome by passing a catheter around the foreign body into the ampulla and injecting air.
3. Occasionally, passing a Foley catheter proximal to the foreign body, inflating the balloon, and applying gentle traction may help maneuver the foreign body into a more desirable position for ease of removal.
4. Reevaluate the anus and rectum after foreign body removal for lacerations and perforation.

PRURITUS ANI

Pruritus ani can occur from a variety of anal and systemic problems. Common causes include diet, infectious agents, irritants, and tight-fitting undergarments. Pinworms (*Enterobius vermicularis*) are the most common cause of anal pruritus in children. The skin appears normal in early mild cases. In severe exacerbations the perianal area will appear reddened, excoriated, and moist. Increased fiber, sitz baths, antihistamines, zinc oxide ointment, or 1% hydrocortisone cream can be used to treat acute symptoms and enhance healing. Any underlying cause should also be treated. Consider referral to proctologist or dermatologist for resistant cases.

PILONIDAL SINUS

Pilonidal sinuses or cysts occur in the midline in the upper part of the natal cleft, which overlies the lower sacrum and coccyx. A pilonidal sinus is usually caused by foreign body granuloma reaction to ingrowing hair. Because of their proximity to the anus, infected pilonidal cysts (abscesses) are sometimes mistakenly diagnosed as perirectal abscesses.

Clinical Features

Pilonidal disease may present as a painless cyst, an infected abscess, or a chronic recurring cyst with drainage in the posterior midline over the sacrum and coccyx. Ultrasound can be used to determine the extent of the abscess before incision and drainage.

Emergency Department Care and Disposition

Acute infections may be drained in the ED and packed. The patient is placed prone and the buttocks are retracted. After appropriate sedation and local anesthesia, the abscess is drained and loculations are gently broken. The wound is packed loosely with gauze, and a bulky dressing is applied. The patient is advised to start sitz baths the following day. Antibiotics or cultures usually are not necessary, unless the patient is immunocompromised or there is evidence of surrounding cellulitis.

FURTHER READING

For further reading in *Tintinalli's Emergency Medicine: A Comprehensive Study Guide*, 8th ed., see Chapter 85, "Anorectal Disorders," by Brian E. Burgess

CHAPTER 48

Jaundice, Hepatic Disorders, and Hepatic Failure

Cem Oktay

JAUNDICE

Jaundice is a yellowish discoloration of skin, sclera, and mucous membranes resulting from the elevated levels of bilirubin in the circulation, usually presents at levels of >2.5 mg/dL. Hyperbilirubinemia occurs as a result of (1) overproduction (e.g., hemolysis), (2) inadequate cellular processing (e.g., infections, drugs, toxins), or (3) decreased excretion of bilirubin (e.g., pancreatic tumor, gallstone in the common bile duct). The causes of jaundice can also be classified as prehepatic, hepatic, and posthepatic.

Hyperbilirubinemia can be divided into two types: Unconjugated form results from the increased production of bilirubin or the impaired liver's ability to conjugate bilirubin. Conjugated form occurs as a result of impaired excretion of conjugated bilirubin in the setting of intrahepatic or extrahepatic cholestasis.

Clinical Features

Previously healthy young patients with acute hepatitis typically presents with a sudden onset of jaundice and a prodrome of fever, malaise, nausea, vomiting, and right upper quadrant abdominal pain resulting from the enlarged liver.

History of excessive alcohol consumption suggests alcoholic hepatitis. Jaundice usually develops gradually in the setting of alcoholic liver disease and cirrhosis.

Symptoms of anorexia, weight loss, and malaise associated with painless jaundice in older patients classically suggest hepatobiliary or pancreatic malignancy.

Liver metastases are suspected in patients with primary tumors and an enlarged, hard, tender, nodular liver accompanied by jaundice.

Inherited diseases such as Gilbert syndrome, glucose-6-phosphate dehydrogenase (G6PD) deficiency, can be the cause of jaundice when a family history of jaundice or a history of recurrent mild jaundice that spontaneously resolves or seen in response to a number of triggers such as certain foods, illness, or medication is present.

Jaundice can be seen in patients with the clinical signs and symptoms of cholecystitis in the setting of a retained gallstone in the common bile duct.

Patients with a history of biliary tract surgery, pancreatitis, cholangitis, or inflammatory bowel present with jaundice due to the development of biliary tract scaring or strictures.

Jaundice can be seen in patients with hepatomegaly, pedal edema, jugular venous distention, and a gallop rhythm due to the passive congestion of liver or acute ischemic hepatitis in patients with chronic heart failure.

Diagnosis and Differential

A detailed history, a carefully conducted physical examination, and routine laboratory tests lead to accurate diagnosis in 85% of patients with jaundice. Initial laboratory tests include serum bilirubin level (total and direct (conjugated) fractions; indirect (unconjugated) fraction can be calculated by subtraction), serum transaminases and alkaline phosphatase (ALP) levels, a complete blood count (CBC), and urinalysis to check for bilirubin and urobilinogen. Additional laboratory tests are ordered according to the clinical features to diagnose specific causes. These include serum lipase or amylase levels, prothrombin time (PT), electrolytes and glucose levels, blood urea nitrogen (BUN) and creatinine levels, γ-glutamyl transpeptidase (GGT), albumin, viral hepatitis panels, drug levels, and pregnancy test.

An increased total and indirect bilirubin signifies either an overproduction or an injury to hepatocytes themselves. Total and direct bilirubin is increased when there is some obstruction preventing the secretion of the conjugated bilirubin.

Transaminases (aspartate aminotransferase (AST) and alanine aminotransferase (ALT) are released into the circulation when there is hepatocyte injury or necrosis. The pattern of elevations in serum transaminases suggests the etiology of hepatocellular disease such as viral hepatitis, toxin- or drug-induced hepatitis, or cirrhosis. Enzyme levels may be near normal in the end-stage liver failure. Jaundice is more likely to be caused by sepsis or systemic infection, pregnancy, or inborn errors of metabolism, when transaminase levels are in normal range.

Hemolysis and hemoglobinopathy are considered when anemia is present in addition to normal liver transaminase levels; Coombs test and hemoglobin electrophoresis may be useful in diagnosis.

ALP elevation is associated with biliary obstruction and cholestasis. Serum GGT level is increased by alcohol consumption and drugs including hepatic microsomal enzyme activity.

Ultrasonogram of the liver, biliary tract, and pancreas is helpful in diagnosing an obstructive cause, or a mass or tumor in the liver, pancreas, and portal region. Computed tomography (CT) is superior to ultrasound (US) in detecting pancreatic or intraabdominal tumors. However, CT is more costly than and has similar sensitivity to US for detection of gallstones.

Emergency Department Care and Disposition

Treatment depends on the cause of the underlying condition leading to jaundice and any potential complications related to it.

Treatment is largely supportive; isotonic IV fluid therapy is administered if the patient is dehydrated. IV antibiotics are required since septic shock may develop expeditiously in patients with ascending cholangitis. Patients with extrahepatic obstructive jaundice without cholangitis should be admitted for drainage.

If the appropriate laboratory tests have been done in the emergency department (ED), further outpatient workup and treatment are appropriate when the patient is hemodynamically stable and has no evidence of hepatic failure or acute biliary obstruction. However, the patient should also be reliable to present the timely follow-up and has adequate social support.

HEPATIC DISORDERS

Specific entities addressed in this chapter include acute hepatitis, chronic liver disease, and complications of cirrhosis including ascites, spontaneous bacterial peritonitis (SBP), and hepatic encephalopathy.

ACUTE HEPATITIS

Hepatitis is an inflammation of the liver owing to infectious, toxic, or metabolic injury to hepatocytes. Patients can present to the ED anywhere along the spectrum of the disease from asymptomatic infection to an acute, or fulminant, liver failure to chronic cirrhosis. The most common causes are viral infection and toxic ingestion.

Clinical Features

Acute hepatitis typically presents with nausea, vomiting, and right upper quadrant abdominal pain. The patient with acute hepatitis can also have fever, diarrhea, jaundice, bilirubinuria, and an enlarged, tender liver. The presence of altered mental status, abnormal bleeding (bruising, bleeding gums, epistaxis, blood in the stool), ascites, and lower body edema suggests chronic disease or a fulminant liver failure.

Paying attention to the historical clues and risk factors is crucial in determining the etiology of hepatitis. Ingestion of acetaminophen (in one-time overdose or chronically high doses), mushrooms, raw oysters, and herbal remedies should be assessed in the history. Risk factors in the past medical history include chronic hepatitis, transfusion of blood products, positive human immunodeficiency virus status, frequent use of pain medications, or depression. A social history positive for injection drug use, chronic alcohol abuse, sexual promiscuity, or travel to countries with endemic parasitic liver diseases represents increased risk for liver disease.

Hepatitis A virus is transmitted by fecal-oral contamination that is associated with improper food handling. The most common transmission occurs from asymptomatic children to adults.

Hepatitis B virus (HBV) is transmitted sexually, by blood transfusion, by contaminated needles, and by perinatal transmission.

Hepatitis C virus (HCV) transmission occurs primarily through exposure to contaminated blood or blood products. HBV and HCV can lead to chronic infection, cirrhosis, and hepatocellular carcinoma.

Other hepatotropic viruses such as Hepatitis D and E viruses, cytomegalovirus, herpes simplex virus, coxsackievirus, and Epstein-Barr virus can cause acute hepatitis.

Toxic insults to the liver can cause acute hepatitis and fulminant liver failure. In addition to the most common toxic insult of acetaminophen, alcohol, a variety of prescription medications (e.g., certain antibiotics, statins, isoniazid), herbal remedies (e.g., black cohosh, chaparral, Echinacea, kava), and dietary supplements are associated with acute hepatitis and liver failure.

The clinical presentation of infectious hepatitis varies with the individual as well as with the specific causative virus. Asymptomatic incubation period is followed by a prodrome of nausea, vomiting, and malaise. Later on, patients may note dark urine (bilirubinuria) and clay-colored stools and jaundice.

Alcoholic liver disease can range from asymptomatic, reversible fatty liver to acute alcoholic hepatitis, cirrhosis, or a combination of acute and cirrhotic features. Acute alcoholic hepatitis develops in patients with asymptomatic liver disease (fatty liver can be seen on imaging) if they continue drinking. These patients may complain of gradual onset of anorexia, nausea, fever, dark urine, jaundice, weight loss, abdominal pain, and generalized weakness.

Fulminant hepatic failure is generally used to describe the development of encephalopathy within 8 weeks of the onset of symptoms in a patient with a previously healthy liver. Signs and symptoms of acute failure may include encephalopathy, cerebral edema, jaundice, ascites, right upper quadrant tenderness, and coagulopathy. Clinical features of hepatitis are listed in Table 48-1.

TABLE 48-1 Clinical Features of Hepatitis

	Acute Hepatitis	Chronic Disease/ Cirrhosis	Acute Liver Failure
Symptoms			
Nausea/vomiting/diarrhea	+	±	+
Fever	+	–	–
Pain	+	±	±
Altered mental status	–	±	+
Bruising/bleeding	–	±	+
Physical examination			
Jaundice	+	+	+
Hepatomegaly	+	–	±
Ascites	–	+	+
Edema	–	+	–
Skin findings (bruising, vascular malformations)	–	+	+
Lab abnormalities			
Elevated ALT/AST	+	+	±
AST/ALT > 2	+	±	±
Elevated PT/INR	–	±	+
Elevated ammonia	–	±	+
Low albumin	–	+	+
Direct bilirubinemia	–	+	±
Indirect bilirubinemia	+	+	±
Urobilinogen	+	+	+
Elevated blood urea nitrogen/creatinine	–	–	±
Radiologic findings			
Ascites	–	+	+
Fatty liver	+	–	–
Cirrhosis	–	+	+

Abbreviations: ALT, alanine aminotransferase; AST, aspartate aminotransferase; INR, International Normalized Ratio; PT, prothrombin time; +, typically present; –, typically absent; ±, variable.

Diagnosis and Differential

Traditional liver function panels include a mix of markers of hepatocyte injury, usually include AST, ALT, and ALP, as well as indicators of hepatocyte catabolic activity (direct and indirect bilirubin).

Elevations of transaminases in the hundreds of units per liter suggest mild injury, or smoldering inflammation. Levels in the thousands suggest extensive acute hepatic necrosis. Acute viral hepatitis may cause the levels of ALT to rise several thousand units per liter. Less significant elevations, less than five times normal, are typical of alcoholic liver disease. ALT is a more specific marker of hepatocyte injury than AST. Patients with acute alcoholic hepatitis have AST and ALT levels that rise to several hundred units per liter. A relative predominance of AST to ALT is expected in patients with alcoholic hepatitis.

ALP elevation is associated with biliary obstruction and cholestasis; elevations greater than four times normal strongly suggest cholestasis.

An elevated GGT in the setting of hepatitis suggests an alcoholic cause. It is also elevated by drugs such as phenobarbital and warfarin. It may rise in acute and chronic pancreatitis, acute myocardial infarction, uremia, COPD, rheumatoid arthritis, and diabetes mellitus.

Lactate dehydrogenase (LDH) is a nonspecific marker, which limits its utility.

Serum glucose level should immediately be checked in patients with altered mental status because severe hepatocellular injury can cause hypoglycemia. Hypoxia, sepsis, intoxication, intracranial lesions, or encephalopathy should also be considered in such a state.

Since nausea and vomiting may result in volume depletion and dehydration, serum electrolytes, BUN, and creatinine levels should be checked.

An elevated serum ammonia level is seen in patients with hepatic metabolic failure caused by acute and chronic liver diseases. Very high ammonia levels signify poor prognosis.

Prothrombin time serves as a true measure of liver function. Prolonged PT or elevated INR occurs in acute hepatitis and exacerbations of chronic compensated liver disease; however, it is a common complication of advancing cirrhosis and indicates significant liver dysfunction and a poor prognosis.

Albumin reflects the liver's synthetic function and may decrease in advancing cirrhosis or severe acute hepatitis. Low albumin suggests a poor short-term prognosis.

Serum bilirubin is somewhat insensitive for liver dysfunction. Hyperbilirubinemia in acute viral hepatitis varies in severity, and fractionation has no clinical value. However, the development of severe hyperbilirubinemia in primary biliary cirrhosis, alcoholic hepatitis, and acute liver failure suggests a poor prognosis.

Viral hepatitis serologies are often grouped into screening panels by hospital laboratories; however, these tests are rarely immediately available. Detection of immunoglobulin M anti-hepatitis A virus antibodies is standard for diagnosing acute infection with hepatitis A virus. Acute clinical illness in hepatitis B virus correlates with positive hepatitis B virus surface antigen (HBsAg). Hepatitis C virus is confirmed with positive anti-hepatitis C virus (anti-HCV) antibodies; however, this diagnosis may be masked by the 6- to 8-week delay between infection and antibody detection.

A CBC may be useful in detecting anemia, which suggests alcoholic hepatitis, decompensated cirrhosis, gastrointestinal bleeding, or a hemolytic process. Although white blood cell (WBC) count is not useful in diagnosis, a transient neutropenia followed by a relative lymphocytosis with atypical forms is seen with viral hepatitis.

The serum acetaminophen concentration is the basis for diagnosis and treatment in patients with the suspicion of toxic ingestion.

Differential diagnosis of acute hepatitis include viral hepatitis, drug- or toxin-induced hepatitis, alcoholic hepatitis, autoimmune hepatitis, cholecystitis and cholangitis, HELLP syndrome, hepatic, pancreatic, or biliary tumors, and metastatic liver diseases.

Emergency Department Care and Disposition

1. With the exception of acetaminophen toxicity (more completely discussed in Chapter 106), patients with acute hepatitis require supportive treatment with pain management, antiemetic medication, and fluid resuscitation.
2. Treat fluid and electrolyte imbalances secondary to poor oral intake, excessive diarrhea, or vomiting with intravenous crystalloids. Treat hypoglycemia with 1 ampule D50W IV. Administration of antiemetics may allow resumption of oral intake.
3. Admit high-risk patients, including the elderly and pregnant women, and patients with significant fluid and electrolyte imbalance or refractory vomiting. Other admission criteria include bilirubin ≥20 mg/dL, PT 50% above normal, hypoglycemia, low albumin, GI bleeding, encephalopathy, immunosupression, or suspected toxin-induced hepatitis.
4. Hospital admission is rarely required for patients with acute viral hepatitis. These patients can be managed as outpatients with the emphasis on rest, adequate oral intake, strict personal hygiene, and avoidance of hepatotoxins. Patients are recommended to return to the ED for poor oral intake, and worsening symptoms, particularly vomiting, jaundice, or abdominal pain. Follow-up visits should be arranged.
5. Management of alcoholic hepatitis is also supportive and can be managed as outpatients with emphasis on nutritional supplementations, including thiamine, magnesium, potassium, and folate, and adequate oral intake. All patients should be advised to avoid further alcohol ingestion and hepatotoxins. Patients and family members should be referred for detoxification or alcohol-dependency treatment. Prophylactic treatment for alcohol withdrawal is considered in patients who require hospital admission.
6. Patients with fulminant hepatic failure require critical care in the ED and admission to the intensive care unit. Aggressive support of circulation and respiration, monitoring and treatment of increased intracranial pressure if present, and correction of hypoglycemia and coagulopathy are warranted. Other treatments include oral lactulose, oral aminoglycoside antibiotics (neomycin, vancomycin), and diet modification for significant protein restriction. Early consultation with a hepatologist and liver transplant service is necessary.

CIRRHOSIS AND CHRONIC LIVER FAILURE

Cirrhosis is a chronic degenerative disease in which a critical amount of liver parenchyma is replaced by fibrotic tissue. Cirrhosis is often caused by alcoholic or chronic viral hepatitis; less common causes include drugs or toxins, hemochromatosis, Wilson's disease, and primary (idiopathic) biliary cirrhosis.

Clinical Features

Symptoms of cirrhosis develop gradually. Patients with cirrhosis may be asymptomatic or have nonspecific constitutional symptoms, such as fatigue, loss of appetite, general weakness, muscle wasting, nausea, vomiting, abdominal pain, and low-grade fever. Signs and symptoms of decompensation include abdominal distension due to ascites and hepatomegaly, altered mental status due to hepatic encephalopathy, pedal edema, jaundice, pruritus, splenomegaly, and spider angiomata.

Ascites, which is one of the hallmarks of cirrhosis, causes a protuberant abdomen. Intra-abdominal fluid can displace the diaphragm upward and produce pleural effusion with the possibility of respiratory compromise.

Hepatic encephalopathy causes a spectrum of illness ranging from chronic fatigue or mild confusion to acute lethargy. Hyperreflexia, spasticity, generalized seizure, and coma may also be present.

Patients with cirrhosis often present to the ED with worsening ascites and edema, altered mental status, abdominal pain resulting from complications such as SBP, gastrointestinal and variceal bleeding, and other concurrent infections including pneumonia and urinary tract infections.

Spontaneous bacterial peritonitis is a subtle crucial complication of ascites; however, it is difficult to diagnose because signs of abdominal pain and fever are not always present, and physical examination does not always demonstrate abdominal tenderness.

Hepatorenal syndrome is a complication of cirrhosis that often accompanies SBP. This syndrome is defined as functional renal failure in cirrhotic patients in the absence of intrinsic renal disease.

Hepatic encephalopathy may be worsened or precipitated by protein load from a large meal or from occult GI bleeding. Progressive liver disease, constipation, hypo- or hyperglycemia, electrolyte imbalances, alcohol withdrawal, hypoperfusion states such as sepsis, renal failure, medications such as antibiotics, and iatrogenic interventions can also compromise the liver's metabolic capacity and results in hepatic encephalopathy.

Diagnosis and Differential

Laboratory tests include transaminases (AST and ALT), ALP, total and direct bilirubin, LDH, albumin, ammonia, glucose, BUN and creatinine, electrolytes, PT/INR, and CBC. Transaminases may be near normal in the end-stage liver failure. PT and albumin reflects the liver's synthetic function. Prolonged PT is a common complication of advanced cirrhosis. Albumin may decrease in advanced cirrhosis. High ammonia is a sign of hepatic encephalopathy; however, levels of ammonia do not reliably correlate with mental status. Elevated serum ammonia levels do not obviate a thorough search for other multiple causes of altered mental status in patients with cirrhosis.

Patients who are diagnosed with ascites for the first time, or who have ascites and develop fever, abdominal pain, GI bleeding, or encephalopathy should undergo paracentesis to check for SBP. A 50 cc sample of ascitic fluid should be obtained for cell count, glucose and protein, Gram stain, and culture to identify bacterial peritonitis.

A total WBC count >1000/mm^3 or a neutrophil count >250/mm^3 is consistent with a diagnosis of SBP.

A 10 mL of ascitic fluid should be placed in a blood culture bottle at the bedside for best results. The most common isolates in SBP are Enterobacteriaceae (*Escherichia coli, Klebsiella pneumoniae*, etc.–63%) and *Streptococcus pneumoniae* (15%).

Bedside US can identify ascites and guide paracentesis (Fig. 48-1). US with duplex Doppler is the test of choice for identifying portal vein and hepatic vein thrombosis. Cancerous, vascular, or infectious lesions of the liver can be identified with US and abdominal CT. Consider obtaining a head CT to identify intracranial hemorrhage in patients with altered mental status.

Emergency Department Care and Disposition

1. Admit patients with ascites if they have significant respiratory compromise, abdominal pain, fever, acidosis, or leukocytosis for evaluation and treatment of SBP. Patients with new-onset or worsening hepatic encephalopathy, hepatorenal syndrome, coagulopathy with bleeding, severe hyponatremia, and severe hyper- or hypovolemia should also be managed in the hospital. Liver failure requires critical care in the ED and consultation with a gastroenterologist and a liver transplant center.

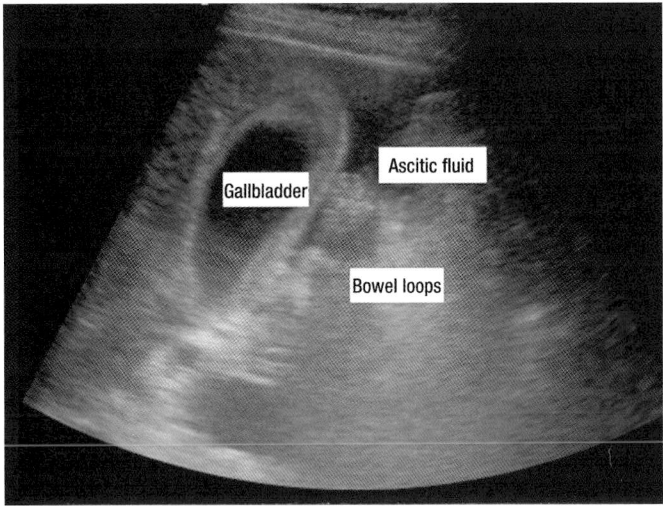

FIGURE 48-1. Sonographic image of ascitic fluid showing bowel loops and an edematous gallbladder wall, a common finding in patients with ascites. Used with permission from Michael S. Antonis, DO, sonographer.

2. Mild- to moderate-volume ascites can be managed with salt-restricted diet and diuretics as an outpatient basis in the absence of signs of infection and other complications. Recommended diuretics include spironolactone, 50 to 200 mg/d, and amiloride, 5 to 10 mg/d. Furosemide can be problematic because it can lead to overdiuresis. Fluid restriction is unnecessary unless serum sodium is less than 120 to 125 mEq/L.
3. Paracentesis is the recommended therapy for large-volume ascites. Removal of more than 1 L of ascitic fluid can cause hypotension so close monitoring is necessary for large-volume taps. For therapeutic paracentesis, it is recommended to administer albumin, 6 to 8 mg/L of fluid removed, for amounts greater than 4 L to prevent fluid shift and intravascular collapse.
4. Empiric antibiotic treatment is recommended in patients with SBP. Cefotaxime, 2 g IV in every 8 hours, is the first-line parenteral treatment. Administer IV fluoroquinolones except in patients who have received prophylactic quinolone treatment. Consider oral fluoroquinolones to treat very mild cases and assure close follow-up.
5. Lactulose is the mainstay of therapy for hepatic encephalopathy and is given PO or PR. The oral dose is 20 g diluted in a glass of water, fruit juice, or carbonated drink. 300 mL of diluted syrup with 700 mL of water or normal saline can be administered PR and the enema should be retained for 30 minutes.
6. Coagulopathy needs to be treated if the patient has uncontrolled bleeding or scheduled for a procedure. Give Vitamin K, 10 mg PO or IV . Consider fresh frozen plasma in doses appropriate for patient's PT level. Decreased or malfunctioning platelets should be replaced with pooled donor platelets.
7. Suspect gastroesophageal bleeding in patients with hematemesis, melena, or hematochezia. Specific treatments for variceal bleeding are addressed in Chapter 39.
8. Treat comorbidities such as electrolyte abnormalities, hypoglycemia, ventilatory and circulatory dysfunction, sepsis, and alcohol-related syndromes (withdrawal, ketoasidosis, Wernicke–Korsakoff syndrome) aggressively.
9. Choosing appropriate analgesics and sedatives in patients with compromised liver function is a complex decision. Avoid NSAIDs due to GI toxicity and possible potentiation of renal dysfunction. Acetaminophen may be used for short-term pain relief at a reduced dose of 2 g total per day, if needed. Opioids are contraindicated in patients with a history of encephalopathy or substance abuse. However, fentanyl and tramadol at reduced doses and increased dosing intervals are possible choices in select patients. Avoid benzodiazepine medication in patients with cirrhosis. Propofol is safe when short-term sedation is required.

FURTHER READING

For further reading in *Tintinalli's Emergency Medicine: A Comprehensive Study Guide*, 8th ed., see Chapter 80, "Hepatic Disorders," by Susan R. O'Mara and Kulleni Gebreyes.

Complications of General Surgical Procedures

Daniel J. Egan

As an increasing number of surgical procedures occur in outpatient settings and inpatient lengths of stay decrease, the emergency physician will encounter more postoperative patients and their complications. Common clinical situations presenting to the emergency department include: fever, respiratory complications, genitourinary complaints, wound infections, vascular problems, and complications of drug therapy. Specific problems not covered in other chapters of this book are discussed here.

CLINICAL FEATURES

Fever

The causes of postoperative fever are the 5 Ws: wind (respiratory), water (urinary tract infection [UTI]), wound, walking (deep venous thrombosis [DVT]), and wonder drugs (drug fever or pseudomembranous colitis [PMC]). Fever in the first 24 hours is usually due to atelectasis, but wound infections with necrotizing fasciitis, or clostridial infections must also be considered. In the first 72 hours, pneumonia, atelectasis, intravenous catheter-related thrombophlebitis, and infections are the major causes. UTIs are seen 1 to 5 days postoperatively. DVT does not typically occur until 5 days after the procedure, and wound infections generally manifest 7 to 10 days after surgery. Antibiotic-induced PMC is seen 6 weeks after surgery.

Respiratory Complications

Postoperative pain, splinting, and inadequate clearance of secretions lead to atelectasis. Fever, tachypnea, tachycardia, and mild hypoxia may be seen. Pneumonia may develop 24 to 96 hours later (see Chapter 30). Pulmonary embolism can occur any time postoperatively (see Chapter 25).

Genitourinary Complications

UTIs occur after any procedure, but more commonly after instrumentation of the GU tract or bladder catheterization. Elderly men, patients undergoing anorectal or prolonged operations, and those receiving spinal or epidural anesthesia are at increased risk for urinary retention presenting with lower abdominal pain and the inability to urinate (see Chapter 54). Decreased urine output should raise concerns for renal failure resulting from multiple causes, particularly volume depletion (see Chapter 50).

Wound Complications

Hematomas with pain and swelling at the surgical site result from inadequate hemostasis. A small portion of the wound may be opened to rule out infection. Seromas are collections of clear fluid under the wound. Wound infections present with pain, swelling, erythema drainage and tenderness. Risk factors include extremes of age, diabetes, poor nutrition, necrotic tissue, poor perfusion, foreign bodies, and hematomas. Necrotizing fasciitis should be considered in a systemically ill patient with rapidly expanding infection and pain out of proportion to examination (see Chapter 90). Superficial or deep fascial wound dehiscence can occur due to diabetes, poor nutrition, chronic steroid use, and inadequate or improper closure of the wound. Operative exploration may be required to determine the extent of dehiscence.

Vascular Complications

Superficial thrombophlebitis manifests with erythema, warmth, and fullness of the affected vein. It usually occurs in the upper extremities after intravenous catheter insertion or in the lower extremities due to stasis in varicosities. DVT most commonly occurs in the lower extremities postoperatively (see Chapter 25).

Drug Therapy Complications

Numerous medications cause fever without associated concomitant infection. Many antibiotics prescribed perioperatively can cause antibiotic-induced diarrhea. PMC, the most serious diarrheal complication, is caused by *Clostridium difficile* toxin. Watery or even bloody diarrhea, fever, and crampy abdominal pain are the usual complaints.

DIAGNOSIS AND DIFFERENTIAL

Postoperative patients with fever should have an evaluation focusing on the elements detailed above. Patients with suspected respiratory complications should have chest x-rays. Radiographs may demonstrate atelectasis, pneumonia, or pneumothorax. Additional imaging like CT or ultrasound may be indicated based on the operative procedure performed.

Patients with oliguria or anuria should be evaluated for signs of hypovolemia or urinary retention. Diagnosis of PMC is established by demonstrating *C difficile* cytotoxin in the stool. Nevertheless, in 27% of cases, the assay may be negative.

EMERGENCY DEPARTMENT CARE AND DISPOSITION

Contact the surgeon who performed the procedure to discuss patients who present with postoperative complications. Patients who are toxic appearing, have underlying debilitating conditions or elderly require hospitalization.

1. Patients with mild atelectasis and no evidence of hypoxemia may be managed as outpatients with pain control and increased deep breathing.
2. Postoperative pneumonia may be polymicrobial. Admission and antibiotic therapy to cover nosocomial infections such as *Pseudomonas* and methicillin-resistant *Staph aureus* are usually recommended (see Chapter 30).
3. Nontoxic patients with UTI can be managed as outpatients with oral antibiotic therapy geared toward appropriate organisms. Consider gram-positive flora when instrumentation has occurred. Ill-appearing patients require admission.
4. Wound hematomas may require removal of some sutures and evacuation. Consultation with the surgeon before treatment is appropriate.

Seromas can be confirmed and treated with needle aspiration. Admission may not be necessary for either of these processes.
5. Wound infections are often treated with oral antibiotics unless the patient shows signs of systemic toxicity or carries significant comorbidities. Perineal infections are often polymicrobial requiring parenteral antibiotics and admission. Necrotizing fasciitis needs immediate surgical debridement and broad-spectrum parenteral antibiotics (see Chapter 90).
6. Patients with superficial thrombophlebitis may be treated as outpatients with nonsteroidal anti-inflammatory drugs (NSAIDs), local heat application and elevation. Antibiotics may be indicated if surrounding cellulitis or lymphangitis are noted. Suppurative thrombophlebitis requires hospitalization and surgical excision.
7. Patients with suspected antibiotic-induced PMC will require fluid resuscitation and likely empiric therapy. Oral or intravenous **metronidazole** and oral **vancomycin** are treatments for this condition.

SPECIFIC CONSIDERATIONS

Complications of Breast Surgery

Although overall rates of complications are low following breast surgery, wound infections, hematomas, seromas, pneumothorax, and necrosis of the skin flaps may be seen. Lymphedema of the ipsilateral arm may occur after mastectomy.

Complications of Gastrointestinal Surgery

Stimulation of the splanchnic nerves during intraabdominal surgery may lead to dysmotility and a paralytic ileus. After gastrointestinal surgery, small bowel tone returns to normal within 24 hours and colonic function within 3 to 5 days.

Patients develop nausea, vomiting, constipation, and abdominal distention and pain. An adynamic ileus typically resolves after bowel rest, nasogastric suction and intravenous hydration. Prolonged ileus should prompt an investigation for nonneuronal causes like peritonitis, intra-abdominal abscesses, hemoperitoneum, pneumonia, sepsis, electrolyte imbalance, or medications. Abdominal imaging, complete blood cell count, basic metabolic panel, and urinalysis should be obtained. Occasionally, surgical intervention may be necessary for obstruction due to adhesions.

Intraabdominal abscesses are caused by preoperative contamination, intraoperative spillage of bowel contents or postoperative anastomotic leaks. Diagnosis is confirmed by computed tomography or ultrasonography. Antibiotic therapy as well as either percutaneous or surgical drainage will be required.

Pancreatitis occurs especially after direct manipulation of the pancreatic duct. The clinical spectrum extends from mild nausea and vomiting to severe abdominal pain and hemodynamic instability. Complications like pleural effusion and severe hemorrhage may occur. Serum amylase measurements are not specific and measurement of a lipase is more reliable.

Cholecystitis and biliary colic have been reported as postoperative complications. Elderly patients are more prone to develop acalculous cholecystitis. Characteristic lab findings of an obstructive process may be absent.

Fistulas, internal or external, may result from either technical complications or direct bowel injury. Fistulas can lead to electrolyte abnormalities and require surgical consultation and possible hospitalization. *Anastomotic leaks* occur primarily after esophageal, gastric and colonic procedures and can cause devastating consequences as a result of infection. Esophageal leaks occur within 10 days of the operation and carry very high morbidity and mortality rates.

Complications of bariatric surgery remain common, although mortality after the procedures is low. In the weeks after surgery, patients are at risk for leaks and bleeding. Dumping syndrome is seen in gastric bypass procedures due to the rapid influx of hyperosmolar chyme into the small intestine resulting in fluid sequestration and hypovolemia. Patients experience nausea, vomiting, epigastric discomfort, palpitations, dizziness, and sometimes syncope. Other complications include gastroesophageal reflux, vitamin and electrolyte deficiencies, ulcers, obstruction, gastric slippage, and band erosion.

Complications of laparoscopic procedures include problems related to pneumoperitoneum, traumatic injury from insertion of the needle and trocar, and retained stones after cholecystectomy.

Complications of transabdominal feeding tubes and *percutaneous endoscopic gastrostomy* tubes include infections, hemorrhage, peritonitis, aspiration, wound dehiscence, sepsis, and obstruction of the tube. Dislodged tubes should be replaced with the appropriately sized tube (same type if possible, or a temporary foley catheter).

Acute complications arising from stomas (ileostomy or colostomy) are usually due to technical errors of stoma placement. Later complications can be from the underlying disease, such as Crohn's disease or cancer. Ischemia, necrosis, skin maceration, bleeding, parastomal hernia, and prolapse may be seen.

The most common *complications of colonoscopy* are hemorrhage and perforation. Hemorrhage occurs typically due to polypectomy, biopsies, or mucosal lacerations or tearing. Perforation may be immediately apparent or symptoms may be delayed for several hours to days. Upright chest or abdominal radiographs may reveal free air but CT is most sensitive.

Rectal surgery complications include urinary retention (frequently after hemorrhoidectomy), constipation, prolapse, bleeding, and infections.

Tetanus has been known to occur in surgical wounds although, by far, this rare disease is more common after minor trauma.

FURTHER READING

For further reading in *Tintinalli's Emergency Medicine: A Comprehensive Study Guide*, 8th ed., see Chapter 87, "Complications of General Surgical Procedures," by Edmond A. Hooker

SECTION 7

Renal and Genitourinary Disorders

CHAPTER 50 Acute Kidney Injury

Sum Ambur

Patients with acute kidney injury (AKI) present with a wide variety of manifestations depending on the underlying etiology. AKI can be caused by hypovolemia, nephrotoxic medications, and anatomic problems of the genitourinary tract. Additional etiologies include cardiac, vascular, thrombotic, glomerular, and renal tubular disorders.

CLINICAL FEATURES

Deterioration in renal function leads to an excessive accumulation of nitrogenous waste products in the serum and significant electrolyte abnormalities. Patients usually have signs and symptoms of their underlying causative disorder but eventually develop stigmata of renal failure. Volume overload, hypertension, pulmonary edema, mental status changes or neurologic symptoms, nausea and vomiting, bone and joint problems, anemia, and increased susceptibility to infection (a leading cause of death) can occur as patients develop more chronic uremia.

DIAGNOSIS AND DIFFERENTIAL

History and physical examination usually provide clues to the etiology. Signs and symptoms of the underlying causative disorder should be vigorously sought. Physical examination should assess vital signs and volume status, establish urinary tract patency and output, and search for signs of chemical intoxication, drug usage, muscle damage, infection, or associated systemic disease. Diagnostic studies include urinalysis, blood urea nitrogen and creatinine levels, serum electrolytes, urinary sodium and creatinine, and urinary osmolality. Analysis of these tests allows most patients to be categorized as prerenal, renal, or postrenal. Fractional excretion of sodium can be calculated to help in this categorization (Table 50-1). Normal urinary sediment may be seen in prerenal and postrenal failure, hemolytic-uremic syndrome, and thrombotic thrombocytopenic purpura. The presence of albumin may indicate glomerulonephritis or malignant hypertension. Granular casts are seen in acute tubular necrosis. Albumin and red blood cell casts are found in glomerulonephritis, malignant hypertension, and autoimmune disease. White blood cell casts are seen in interstitial nephritis

TABLE 50-1 Laboratory Findings in Conditions That Cause Acute Renal Failure

Category	Dipstick Test	Sediment Analysis	Urine Osmolality (mOsm/kg)	Fractional Excretion of Sodium (%)
Prerenal	Trace to no proteinuria, SG >1.015	A few hyaline casts possible	>500	<1
Renal				
Ischemia	Mild to moderate proteinuria	Pigmented granular casts, renal tubular epithelial cells	<350	>1
Nephrotoxins	Mild to moderate proteinuria	Pigmented granular casts	<350	>1
Acute interstitial nephritis	Mild to moderate proteinuria, hemoglobin, leukocytes	White cells, eosinophils, casts, red cells	<350	>1
Acute glomerulonephritis	Moderate to severe proteinuria, hemoglobin	Red cells and red cell casts, red cells can be dysmorphic	>500	Depends on volume status
Postrenal	Trace to no proteinuria; hemoglobin and leukocytes possible	Crystals, red cells, white cells possible	<350	>1

Abbreviation: SG, specific gravity.

and pyelonephritis. Crystals can be present with renal calculi and certain drugs (sulfas, ethylene glycol, and radiocontrast agents). Renal ultrasound is the radiologic procedure of choice in most patients with renal failure when upper tract obstruction and hydronephrosis are suspected. Color-flow Doppler can assess renal perfusion and facilitate the diagnosis of large vessel causes of renal failure. Bedside sonography can quickly diagnose some treatable causes and give guidance for fluid resuscitation; inspiratory collapse of the intrahepatic inferior vena cava (IVC) can give a good measure of volume status and fluid responsiveness (Fig. 50-1).

Prerenal failure is produced by conditions that decrease renal perfusion and is the most common cause of community-acquired acute renal failure (70% of cases). It is also a common precursor to ischemic and nephrotoxic causes of intrinsic renal failure. Common causes of prerenal failure include hypovolemic states (vomiting/diarrhea, diuretics and other antihypertensives, reduced intake), fluid sequestration (cirrhosis, pancreatitis, burns, septic shock, others), blood loss, or decreased cardiac output from cardiac dysfunction. ***Intrinsic renal failure*** has vascular and ischemic etiologies; glomerular and tubulointerstitial diseases are also causative. Ischemic renal failure, traditionally known as acute tubular necrosis (ATN), is now called acute kidney injury (AKI). AKI, due to severe and prolonged prerenal etiologies, causes most cases of intrinsic renal failure. AKI is also the most common cause of hospital-acquired renal failure. Nephrotoxins (both physician prescribed and environmental) are the second most common cause of AKI. *Postrenal azotemia* occurs primarily in elderly men with high-grade prostatic obstruction. Lesions of the external genitalia (i.e., strictures) are also common causes. Significant permanent

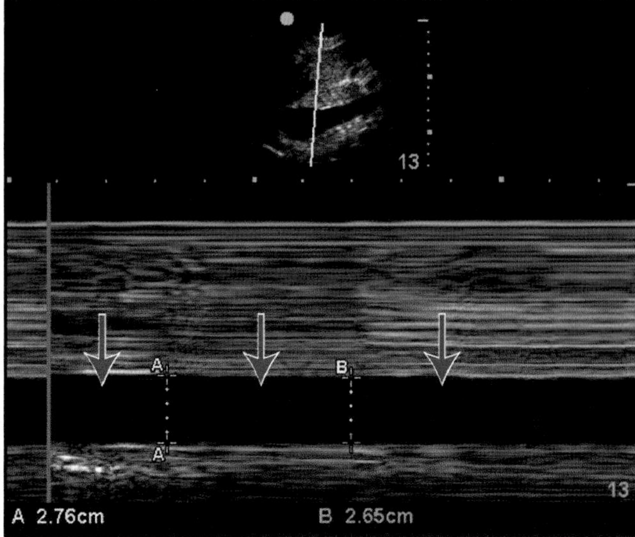

A

10

10

B

FIGURE 50-1. Ultrasound of the inferior vena cava. **A.** Dilated inferior vena cava (*arrows*) with little respiratory variation as might be expected in volume overload. **B.** An almost fully collapsed inferior vena cava at inspiration (*arrows*) and expiration (*arrowheads*) as might be expected in prerenal acute kidney injury. Used with permission from Michael B, Stone, MD, RDMS.

loss of renal function occurs over 10 to 14 days with complete obstruction, and worsens with associated UTI.

EMERGENCY DEPARTMENT CARE AND DISPOSITION

Emergency department goals in the initial care of patients with acute renal failure focus on treating the underlying cause with an emphasis on correcting fluid and electrolyte derangements. Efforts should be made to prevent further renal damage and provide supportive care while attempting to establish a diagnosis and facilitating further evaluation and treatment as appropriate. Urine output should be closely monitored and consideration should be given to placement of a Foley catheter. ECG should be performed to evaluate for hyperkalemia-associated changes. Appropriate labs including serum potassium, creatinine, and BUN should be obtained.

Prerenal Failure

1. Use isotonic fluids (normal saline or Lactated Ringer's solution) for volume resuscitation.
2. If cardiac failure is causing prerenal azotemia, optimize cardiac output to improve renal perfusion. Reducing intravascular volume (i.e., with diuretics) may be appropriate. Bedside echocardiography as well as sonographic assessment of the IVC may help guide this decision.

Renal Failure (Intrinsic)

Adequate circulating volume must be restored first; hypovolemia potentiates and exacerbates all forms of renal failure. Ischemia or nephrotoxic agents are the most common causes of intrinsic renal failure. History, physical examination, and baseline laboratory tests should provide clues to the diagnosis. Nephrotoxic medications and intravenous contrast should be avoided.

1. Vasopressor support with norepinephrine or dopamine may be needed as a temporizing measure to support mean arterial pressure and support renal perfusion in the setting of shock.
2. Use caution with renally excreted drugs (digoxin, magnesium, sedatives, and narcotics) and intravenous contrast because therapeutic doses may accumulate to excess and cause serious side effects. Fluid restriction may be required. Restoration of adequate intravascular volume with crystalloid infusion may be useful in the prevention of radiocontrast nephropathy.

Postrenal Failure

Establish appropriate urinary drainage; the exact procedure depends on the level of obstruction.

1. Place a Foley catheter to relieve obstruction caused by prostatic hypertrophy. However, there is no data to support the practice of intermittent catheter clamping to prevent hypotension and hematuria; urine should be completely and rapidly drained.

2. Percutaneous nephrostomy may be required for ureteral occlusion until definitive surgery to correct the obstruction can take place once the patient is stabilized.
3. For the acutely anuric patient, obstruction is the major consideration. If no urine is obtained on initial bladder catheterization and a bladder scan or bedside ultrasound reveals a full bladder, emergency urologic consultation may be necessary.
4. With chronic urinary retention, postobstructive diuresis may occur due to osmotic diuresis or tubular dysfunction. Patients may become suddenly hypovolemic and hypotensive. Urine output must be closely monitored, with appropriate fluid replacement as needed.

Dialysis

If treatment of the underlying cause fails to improve renal function, or in cases with severe hyperkalemia or hypervolemia, dialysis should be considered. It is prudent to consult with a nephrologist as soon as possible if urgent dialysis is a consideration.

1. The nephrologist usually makes decisions about dialysis. Dialysis is often initiated when the blood urea nitrogen is greater than 100 mg/dL or serum creatinine is greater than 10 mg/dL.
2. Patients with complications of acute renal failure such as cardiac instability (due to metabolic acidosis and hyperkalemia), intractable volume overload, hyperkalemia, and uremia (i.e., encephalopathy, pericarditis, and bleeding diathesis) not easily corrected by other measures should be considered for emergency dialysis.

Disposition

Patients with new-onset renal failure usually require hospital admission, often to an intensive care unit. Consider transferring patients to another institution if nephrology consultation and dialysis facilities are not available.

FURTHER READING

For further reading in *Tintinalli's Emergency Medicine: A Comprehensive Study Guide*, 8th ed., see Chapter 88, "Acute Kidney Injury," by Richard Sinert and Peter R. Peacock, Jr.

CHAPTER 51 Rhabdomyolysis

Annet Alenyo Ngabirano

Rhabdomyolysis is the destruction of skeletal muscle, caused by any mechanism that results in injury to myocytes and their membranes. Table 51-1 lists commonly recognized conditions associated with rhabdomyolysis. In general, the most common causes of rhabdomyolysis in adults are alcohol and drugs of abuse, followed by medications, muscle diseases, trauma, neuroleptic malignant syndrome, seizures, immobility, infection, strenuous physical activity, and heat-related illness. Multiple causes are present in more than half of patients. In children, rhabdomyolysis is less common and is thought to be more benign.

TABLE 51-1 Common Conditions Associated with Rhabdomyolysis in Adults

Trauma Crush injury Electrical or lightning injury **Drugs of abuse** Amphetamines (including ecstasy (3, 4-methylene-dioxymethamphetamine)) Caffeine Cocaine Ethanol Heroin Lysergic acid diethylamide Methamphetamines Opiates Phencyclidine **Environment and excessive muscular activity** Contact sports Delirium tremens Dystonia Psychosis Seizures Marathons, military basic training Heat stroke **Genetic disorders** Glycolysis and glycogenolysis disorders Fatty acid oxidation disorders Mitochondrial and respiratory chain metabolism disorders	**Immunologic diseases involving muscle** Dermatomyositis Polymyositis **Bacterial infection** *Clostridium* Group A β-hemolytic streptococci *Legionella* *Salmonella* *Shigella* *Staphylococcus aureus* *Streptococcus pneumoniae* **Viral infection** Coxsackievirus Cytomegalovirus Epstein–Barr virus Enterovirus Hepatitis virus Herpes simplex virus Human immunodeficiency virus Influenza virus (A and B) Rotavirus *Mycoplasma*	**Ischemic injury** Compartment syndrome Compression **Medications** Antipsychotics Barbiturates Benzodiazepines Clofibrate Colchicine Corticosteroids Diphenhydramine Isoniazid Lithium Monoamine oxidase inhibitors Narcotics Neuroleptic agents Phenothiazines Propofol Salicylates Selective serotonin reuptake inhibitors Statins Theophylline Tricyclic antidepressants Zidovudine Some novel cancer chemotherapeutic agents

CLINICAL FEATURES

Symptoms are usually acute in onset and include myalgias, stiffness, weakness, malaise, low-grade fever, and dark (usually brown) urine. Nausea, vomiting, abdominal pain, and tachycardia can occur in severe rhabdomyolysis. Muscle symptoms, however, may be present in only half of cases. Some patients may present with complications of rhabdomyolysis such as acute renal failure, metabolic derangements, disseminated intravascular coagulation, and mechanical complications (e.g., compartment syndrome or peripheral neuropathy) (Table 51-2).

Acute rhabdomyolysis may be present without any of these signs or symptoms and with normal findings on physical examination. For this reason, diagnosis is often made from a significant history, an elevated serum creatine kinase level or the presence of dark urine on routine laboratory testing.

DIAGNOSIS AND DIFFERENTIAL

An elevated serum creatine kinase is the most sensitive and reliable indicator of muscle injury. Diagnosis requires a fivefold or greater increase above the upper threshold of normal serum creatine kinase level in the absence of cardiac or brain injury. Persistently elevated levels despite treatment suggest ongoing muscle necrosis.

Myoglobinuria develops once skeletal muscle injury is >100 gram. Because myoglobin contains heme, qualitative tests such as the dipstick test do not differentiate among hemoglobin, myoglobin, and red blood cells. Therefore, suspect myoglobinuria when the urine dipstick test is positive for blood but no red blood cells are present on microscopic examination. Absence of an elevated serum myoglobin level or of myoglobinuria does not exclude the diagnosis as levels may return to normal within 1 to 6 hours after the onset of muscle necrosis.

Other laboratory studies are useful in identifying the common complications of rhabdomyolysis and the underlying cause. Urinalysis should be obtained for all patients. Serum electrolyte, calcium, phosphorus, and uric acid levels help detect hyperkalemia, abnormal calcium and phosphorus levels, and hyperuricemia. Serum creatinine and BUN levels are needed to identify acute renal failure. Because disseminated

TABLE 51-2 Complications of Rhabdomyolysis

- Acute renal failure
- Metabolic derangements
  - Hypercalcemia (late)
  - Hyperkalemia
  - Hyperphosphatemia
  - Hyperuricemia
  - Hypocalcemia
  - Hypophosphatemia (late)
- Disseminated intravascular coagulation
- Mechanical complications
  - Compartment syndrome
  - Peripheral neuropathy

intravascular coagulation is a potential complication, a baseline CBC should be obtained and a coagulopathic screen considered (e.g., prothrombin time, partial thromboplastin time, fibrin split products, and fibrinogen level). Other common laboratory findings in rhabdomyolysis include elevated levels of aldolase, lactate dehydrogenase, urea, creatine, and aminotransferases. Further laboratory testing should be guided by the medical history and clinical presentation.

Other causes of muscle pain and weakness besides rhabdomyolysis should be considered in the appropriate clinical setting. These include acute myopathies, periodic paralysis, polymyositis or dermatomyositis, and Guillain–Barré syndrome. Rhabdomyolysis associated with strenuous exercise, fasting, or repeat episodes of rhabdomyolysis suggests an inherited metabolic myopathy.

EMERGENCY DEPARTMENT CARE AND DISPOSITION

1. **Provide aggressive IV rehydration for 24 to 72 hours.** One method of rehydration is rapid correction of the fluid deficit with IV crystalloids followed by infusion of 2.5 mL/kg/h, with the goal of maintaining a minimum urine output of 2 mL/kg/h. Another method titrates infusion rates to a goal of 200 to 300 mL of urine output per hour.
2. **No prospective controlled studies have demonstrated benefit from alkalinization of the urine with sodium bicarbonate or forced diuresis with mannitol or loop diuretics.** Bicarbonate is widely recommended but without an evidence base. If bicarbonate is given, maintain an isotonic solution and avoid metabolic alkalosis or hypokalemia. Mannitol may be harmful because it may cause osmotic diuresis in hypovolemic patients.
3. Place a urinary catheter in patients in critical condition and those with acute renal failure to monitor urine output. Institute cardiac monitoring as electrolyte and metabolic complications can cause dysrhythmias. For patients with heart disease, comorbid conditions, or preexisting renal disease or for elderly patients, hemodynamic monitoring may be necessary to avoid fluid overload. Serial measurements of urine pH, electrolytes, creatine kinase, calcium, phosphorus, BUN, and creatinine are needed.
4. Monitor electrolytes. Hypocalcemia observed early in rhabdomyolysis usually requires no treatment. Give calcium, if needed, to treat hyperkalemia-induced cardiotoxicity or profound signs and symptoms of hypocalcemia. If hypercalcemia is symptomatic, continue saline diuresis. Treat hyperphosphatemia with oral phosphate binders when serum levels are >7 mg/dL. Treat hypophosphatemia when the serum level is <1 mg/dL. Hyperkalemia, which is usually most severe in the first 12 to 36 hours after muscle injury, can be significant and prolonged. Traditional insulin and glucose therapy, although recommended, may not be as effective in rhabdomyolysis-induced hyperkalemia. The use of ion-exchange resins (e.g., sodium polystyrene sulfonate) is effective. Dialysis may be needed (see Chapter 17, Fluids and Electrolytes, *Tintinalli's Emergency Medicine: A Comprehensive Study Guide*, 8th ed.).
5. Avoid prostaglandin inhibitors such as nonsteroidal anti-inflammatory drugs (NSAIDs) because of their vasoconstrictive effects on the kidney.

6. Finally, treat the underlying cause.
7. The majority of healthy patients with *exertional rhabdomyolysis* and *without comorbidities* (i.e., heat stress, dehydration, trauma) can be treated with oral or IV rehydration, observed in the ED, and then released. Otherwise, patients should be admitted for IV hydration, diuresis, management of complications, and treatment of the underlying cause. Admit to a monitored bed to identify dysrhythmias if they occur. Consult the nephrology service to evaluate the need for dialysis, especially for patients with hyperkalemia unresponsive to therapy.

FURTHER READING

For further reading in *Tintinalli's Emergency Medicine: A Comprehensive Study Guide*, 8th ed., see Chapter 89, "Rhabdomyolysis," by Francis L. Counselman and Bruce M. Lo.

Emergencies in Renal Failure and Dialysis Patients

Jonathan A. Maisel

Patients with end-stage renal disease (ESRD) may sustain multiple complications of their disease process and treatment. Emergent dialysis is most commonly required for hyperkalemia, severe metabolic acidosis, and pulmonary edema resistant to alternative therapy. See the appropriate chapters for discussion of the management of hypertension, heart failure, bleeding disorders, and electrolyte disorders.

CARDIOVASCULAR COMPLICATIONS

Elevated levels of troponin I and T are common, even in those who are asymptomatic, and are associated with increased long-term risk of ischemic heart disease. Myocardial infarction may be defined by a 20% or greater rise in the troponin value, with at least one value above the 99th percentile. Hypertension occurs in most patients starting dialysis. Management includes control of blood volume, followed by use of adrenergic-blocking drugs, angiotensin-converting enzyme inhibitors, or vasodilating agents. Congestive heart failure (CHF) may be caused by hypertension, coronary ischemia, and valvular disease, as well as uremic cardiomyopathy, fluid overload, and arteriovenous (AV) fistulas (high output failure). Treatment includes supplemental oxygen, bilevel positive airway pressure, nitrates, angiotensin converting enzyme inhibitors, and possibly **furosemide** 60 to 100 mg IV, as its pulmonary vasodilator effect may provide relief, even in oliguric patients. Preload can be further reduced by inducing diarrhea with **sorbitol** and with phlebotomy (minimum 150 mL). Blood should be collected in a transfusion bag so that it may be transfused back to the patient during subsequent dialysis. Hemodialysis (HD) is the definitive treatment. Pericarditis in ESRD patients is usually due to worsening uremia. Electrocardiographic (ECG) changes typical of acute pericarditis are not always seen. Pericardial friction rubs are louder than in most other forms of pericarditis, often palpable, and frequently persist after the metabolic abnormalities have been corrected. Uremic pericarditis is treated with intensive dialysis. Cardiac tamponade is the most serious complication of uremic pericarditis. It presents with changes in mental status, hypotension, or dyspnea. An enlarged heart on chest x-ray may suggest the diagnosis, which can be confirmed with echocardiography. Hemodynamically significant pericardial effusions require pericardiocentesis under fluoroscopic or ultrasonographic guidance.

NEUROLOGIC COMPLICATIONS

Uremic encephalopathy presents with altered mental status, cognitive defects, memory loss, slurred speech, and asterixis. The progressive neurologic symptoms of uremia are the most common indications for initiating HD. It should remain a diagnosis of exclusion until structural, vascular, infectious, toxic, and metabolic causes of neurologic dysfunction have been ruled out. Peripheral neuropathy, manifested by paresthesias, diminished deep tendon reflexes, impaired vibration sense, muscle wasting, and weakness, occurs in 60% to 100% of patients with ESRD. Autonomic dysfunction, characterized by postural dizziness, gastric fullness, bowel dysfunction, reduced sweating, reduced heart rate variability, and baroreceptor control impairment, is common in ESRD patients. Stroke is seen in 6% of HD patients, with half of cases being hemorrhagic, typically subdural hematomas. Stroke may be caused by cerebrovascular disease, head trauma, bleeding dyscrasias, anticoagulation, excessive ultrafiltration, or hypertension. Stroke should be considered in any ESRD patient presenting with a change in mental status.

HEMATOLOGIC COMPLICATIONS

Anemia is caused by decreased erythropoietin, blood loss from dialysis, frequent phlebotomy, and decreased red cell survival. Factitious anemia reflects changes in plasma volume related to dialysis. Abnormal hemostasis in ESRD is multifactorial in origin, resulting in an increased risk of gastrointestinal (GI) tract bleeding, subcapsular liver hematomas, subdural hematomas, and intraocular bleeding. Benefit may be seen following the infusion of **desmopressin** 0.3 μg/kg or **cryoprecipitate**. Immunologic compromise, caused by impaired leukocyte chemotaxis and phagocytosis, leads to high mortality rates from infection. Dialysis does not appear to improve immune system function.

GASTROINTESTINAL COMPLICATIONS

Anorexia, nausea, and vomiting are common symptoms of uremia, and are used as an indication to initiate dialysis, and assess its efficacy. Chronic constipation is common, due to decreased fluid intake and the use of phosphate-binding gels.

COMPLICATIONS OF HEMODIALYSIS

Hypotension is the most frequent complication of HD. Excessive ultrafiltration due to underestimation of the patient's ideal blood volume (dry weight) is the most common cause of intradialytic hypotension. Cardiac compensation for fluid loss may be compromised by diastolic dysfunction common in ESRD patients. Other causes of intradialytic hypotension include myocardial dysfunction from ischemia, hypoxia, arrhythmias, and pericardial tamponade, abnormalities of vascular tone secondary to sepsis or antihypertensive medications, and volume loss from inadequate oral intake, vomiting, diarrhea, GI bleeding, or blood tubing or filter leaks. Treatment consists of Trendelenberg positioning, oral salt solution, or infusion of normal saline solution. If these interventions fail, excessive ultrafiltration is unlikely, and further evaluation will be required.

Dialysis disequilibrium, caused by cerebral edema following large solute clearances, is characterized by nausea, vomiting, and hypertension, which can progress to seizures, coma, and death. Treatment consists of terminating dialysis, and administering mannitol intravenously to increase serum osmolality.

COMPLICATIONS OF VASCULAR ACCESS

Complications of vascular access account for more inpatient hospital days than any other complication of HD. Thrombosis or stenosis present with loss of the bruit and thrill over the access. These need to be treated within

24 hours with angiographic clot removal, angioplasty, or direct injection of thrombolytic into the access. Vascular access infections often present with signs of systemic sepsis, including fever, hypotension, and an elevated white blood cell count. Classic signs of pain, erythema, swelling, and discharge are often missing. Obtain both peripheral and catheter blood cultures simultaneously. A fourfold higher colony count in the catheter culture suggests it is the source. *Staphylococcus aureus* is the most common infecting organism, followed by gram-negative bacteria. Patients usually require hospitalization along with treatment with **vancomycin** 15 mg/kg IV and an aminoglycoside, such as **gentamycin** 100 mg IV. Potential life-threatening hemorrhage from a vascular access may result from a ruptured aneurysm or anastomosis, or overanticoagulation. Bleeding can often be controlled with 5 to 10 minutes of pressure at the puncture site. If this fails, the addition of an adsorbable gelatin sponge soaked in reconstituted **thrombin**, or a prothrombotic gauze, followed by 10 minutes of direct pressure may be effective. Life-threatening hemorrhage may require placement of a tourniquet proximal to the access, and vascular surgery consultation. If the etiology is excessive anticoagulation, the effects of heparin can be reversed with **protamine** 0.01 mg per unit heparin dispensed during dialysis or 10 to 20 mg **protamine** if the heparin dose is unknown. If a newly inserted vascular access continues to bleed, **desmopressin** 0.3 μg/kg IV can be given as an adjunct to direct pressure.

COMPLICATIONS OF PERITONEAL DIALYSIS

Peritonitis is the most common complication of peritoneal dialysis (PD). Signs and symptoms are similar to those seen in other patients with peritonitis, and include fever, abdominal pain, and rebound tenderness. A cloudy effluent supports the diagnosis. Peritoneal fluid should be sent to the laboratory for cell count, Gram stain, culture, and sensitivity. With peritonitis, cell counts usually reveal >100 leukocytes/mm^3, with >50% neutrophils. Gram stain is positive in only 10% to 40% of culture-proven peritonitis. Organisms isolated include *Staphylococcus epidermidis, S. aureus, Streptococcus* species, and gram-negative bacteria. Empiric therapy begins with a few rapid exchanges of dialysate to decrease the number of inflammatory cells within the peritoneum. The addition of **heparin** (500 to 1000 U/L dialysate) decreases fibrin clot formation. Empiric antibiotics, covering gram-positive organisms (e.g., **cephalothin** or **vancomycin** 500 mg/L dialysate) and gram-negative organisms (e.g., **gentamycin** 100 mg/L dialysate), are added to the dialysate. Inpatient versus outpatient treatment of PD-related peritonitis should be based on clinical presentation.

Infections around the PD catheter are characterized by pain, erythema, swelling, and discharge. Causative organisms are *S. aureus* and *Pseudomonas aeruginosa*. Outpatient treatment consists of a first-generation cephalosporin or **ciprofloxacin**.

FURTHER READING

For further reading in *Tintinalli's Emergency Medicine: A Comprehensive Study Guide*, 8th ed., see Chapter 90, "End-Stage Renal Disease," by Mathew Foley, Ninfa Mehta and Richard Sinert.

CHAPTER 53

Urinary Tract Infections and Hematuria

David R. Lane

URINARY TRACT INFECTIONS

Urinary tract infections (UTIs) are the most common bacterial infections treated in the outpatient setting. More than 50% of women experience one in their lifetimes, and approximately 12% of women have a UTI annually. UTIs are divided into two major categories: lower tract infections and upper tract infections. Lower UTIs include *urethritis*, typically caused by sexually transmitted diseases and differentiated by the presence of discharge, and *cystitis*, an acute bacterial infection of the urinary bladder. *Pyelonephritis* is an infection of the upper urinary tract structures including the ureters and kidneys. Differentiation of upper and lower UTIs is based on history and physical exam.

Uncomplicated UTI occurs in young, healthy, nonpregnant women with structurally and functionally normal urinary tracts.

Complicated UTI occurs in patients who are older, healthy, nonpregnant women with normal urinary tracts: that is, all men, and women who have a structural or functional genitourinary abnormality or an underlying predisposing medical condition that increases the risk of infection and recurrence or reduces the effectiveness of antimicrobial therapy.

Asymptomatic bacteriuria (ABU) is the presence of significant bacteria in urine without signs or symptoms that are referable to a urinary tract infection; the usual cutoff is a single organism isolated in a quantity of at least 100,000 colony forming U/mL. Screening and treatment is not generally recommended, with the exception of women who are pregnant or men who are going to undergo a transurethral prostate resection.

More than 80% of UTIs are caused by *Escherichia coli*. Other causative organisms include *Klebsiella*, *Proteus*, *Enterobacter*, *Pseudomonas*, *Chlamydia*, and *Staphylococcus saprophyticus*.

Clinical Features

Typical symptoms of cystitis include frequency, urgency, hesitancy, and suprapubic pain. Pyelonephritis is characterized by the addition of flank pain or costovertebral angle tenderness, particularly in conjunction with fever, chills, or nausea and vomiting. If vaginal or urethral discharge is present, urethritis, vaginitis, cervicitis, or PID are more likely than UTI. As in many diseases, diabetics and the elderly have a predilection for presenting atypically, and weakness, malaise, generalized abdominal pain, or altered mental status may be the only signs or symptoms noted.

Diagnosis and Differential

Diagnosis of UTI can be inferred from history and physical, and confirmed by *urine dipstick* or *urinalysis* and culture. Clean-catch midstream collection of urine is as accurate as urine obtained by catheterization if the patient follows instructions carefully. Catheterization should only be used in a patient that cannot void spontaneously, is too ill or immobilized, or is extremely obese. Note that 1% to 2% of patients develop a UTI after a single catheter insertion.

The two tests of interest on *urine dipstick* are nitrite reaction, a measure of bacteriuria, and leukocyte esterase, a measure of pyuria. Nitrite has a very high specificity (>90%), but a low sensitivity (50%); several organisms are not detected by this test (*Enterococcus*, *Pseudomonas*, and *Acinetobacter*). Leukocyte esterase sensitivity (77%) is affected by high levels of protein or glucose in the urine. In addition it may be falsely positive in vaginitis or cervicitis. If either nitrite or leukocyte esterase is positive, the sensitivity is 75% and specificity is 82%. If both are positive, the specificity is 98% to 100%. A positive urine dipstick nitrite or leukocyte test result supports the diagnosis of UTI; a negative test result does not exclude it.

Urinalysis also evaluates bacteriuria and pyuria, the urine white blood cell count. Bacteriuria is defined as any bacteria on a Gram-stained specimen of uncentrifuged urine, and has a sensitivity of 95% and specificity of over 60%. False-negative results may occur in patients with low-colony-count UTI or *Chlamydia* infections. False-positive results can occur with vaginal or fecal contamination. Pyuria is defined as greater than 2 to 5 white blood cells per high power field in women and 1 to 2 white blood cells per high power field in men. False-negative results may occur in symptomatic patients with dilute urine, incompletely treated UTI, an obstructed, infected kidney, or systemic leukopenia.

Urine culture should only be performed for the following patients: those with complicated UTI (including men and pregnant women), those with relapse or reinfection, children, and those who are septic. Finally, imaging (CT or ultrasound) should be limited to patients with severe or nonresponsive pyelonephritis, or if there is a significant concern for a renal stone.

No single test or combination of testing can effectively rule out UTI in women presenting to the ED with symptoms of cystitis, and if test results are equivocal, consider initiating empiric treatment.

The differential diagnosis for patients presenting with dysuria includes vaginitis and cervicitis in women and urethritis, prostatitis, and epididymitis in men. Intraabdominal pathology, bladder or urethral structural abnormalities or cancer, chemical irritation or allergies to hygienic products, and trauma are also considerations.

Emergency Department Care and Disposition

Appropriate antimicrobial treatment should rapidly improve symptoms in all UTIs and also minimize growing community antibiotic resistance. Consider using **nitrofurantoin** 100 mg extended release twice a day PO for 5 days as a first-line agent in uncomplicated UTI. Alternatives in uncomplicated UTI include **TMP-SMX DS** 160/800 mg twice a day for 3 days or **fosfomycin** 3 g in a single dose. Avoid flouroquinolones in uncomplicated UTI to reduce antibiotic resistance.

For complicated UTI or pyelonephritis, **ciprofloxacin** 500 mg twice a day for 7 days is considered the first-line agent. Alternatives include **levofloxacin** 750 mg daily for 5 days or **cefpodoxime** 400 mg twice a day for 7 to 14 days. If local resistance is less than 20%, **TMP-SMX DS**

160/800 mg twice a day for 7 to 14 days or **amoxicillin-clavulanate** 875/125 mg twice a day for 14 days are acceptable.

For pregnant patients, ABU should be treated with 3 days of **nitrofurantoin** and UTI should be treated with 7 days of **nitrofurantoin**. Fluoroquinolones and tetracyclines are teratogenic and should be avoided, and TMP-SMX should be used with caution in the first and third trimesters.

If there is suspicion for concomitant infection with gonorrhea or *Chlamydia*, antibiotic choice is more complex (see Chapter 87, "Sexually Transmitted Infections").

In addition to the antibiotic, prescribe a 2-day course of a bladder analgesic such as **phenazopyridine** 200 mg three times a day. Discharge instructions must include return precautions for uncontrolled pain, fever, vomiting, and also should encourage adequate hydration, completion of the entire antibiotic course, and outpatient follow-up with a primary care doctor.

Admit patients with pyelonephritis who exhibit intractable vomiting. Consider admission for pregnant females (20% will develop sepsis) and patients with inadequate outpatient follow-up. Parenteral antibiotic options for inpatient management of pyelonephritis include **ceftriaxone** 1 g IV daily, **ciprofloxacin** 400 mg IV every 12 hours, and **piperacillin-tazobactam**, 3.375 g IV every 6 hours.

HEMATURIA

Gross hematuria, visible to the eye, suggests a lower urinary tract source; however, other pigments such as myoglobin can simulate hematuria. Microscopic hematuria (>3 RBCs/HPF) suggests a renal source, though it can also be present in UTI.

Diagnosis and Differential

A urine dipstick is positive with approximately 5 to 20 red blood cells per milliliter of urine. A positive dipstick should be followed by microscopy. Urethral catheterization induces hematuria in 15% of patients. False-positives may also result from myoglobin, free hemoglobin due to hemolysis, and porphyrins. False-negative results may occur if the urine has a high specific gravity.

Any process that results in infection, inflammation, or injury to the kidneys, ureters, bladder, prostate, male genitalia, or urethra may result in hematuria. UTI is the most common cause of hematuria associated with urgency, dysuria, and nocturia, whereas painless hematuria is largely due to neoplastic, hyperplastic, or vascular causes. The most common causes of hematuria in patients <40 years are infections and inflammatory conditions, including UTI, prostatitis, urethritis, sexually transmitted diseases, epididymo-orchitis, nephrolithiasis, and tuberculosis. In older patients, consider renal and bladder cancer, as well as prostate tumors and benign prostatic hypertrophy in men. Consider strenuous exercise or poststreptococcal infection (in younger patients), as well as trauma, malignant hypertension, eroding abdominal aortic aneurysm, coagulopathy, foreign body, Henoch–Schonlein purpura, pulmonary-renal syndromes, sickle cell disease complications, and renal vein thrombosis. Hematuria in a patient taking oral anticoagulants should not be attributed to the anticoagulant alone, as the incidence of underlying disease is up to 80% in patients referred to urology. Imaging in the ED for hematuria should be limited to patients with trauma, symptoms of nephrolithiasis, or high concern for abdominal aortic aneurysm.

Emergency Department Care and Disposition

Treatment of hematuria is directed at the cause. ED management consists of the minimization of complications and appropriate referral or admission for further evaluation. All patients with hematuria should be promptly followed up by either primary care or urology.

Admit patients with infection associated with an obstructive stone, intractable pain or vomiting, hemodynamic instability, newly diagnosed glomerulonephritis, significant anemia, renal insufficiency, bladder outlet obstruction, preeclampsia, or any other potentially life-threatening cause of hematuria.

FURTHER READING

For further reading in *Tintinalli's Emergency Medicine: A Comprehensive Study Guide*, 8th ed., see Chapter 91, "Urinary Tract Infections and Hematuria," by Kim Askew.

CHAPTER 54

Acute Urinary Retention

Casey Glass

CLINICAL FEATURES

Urinary retention can be either acute or chronic. The most common cause of retention is outlet obstruction secondary to benign prostatic hyperplasia (BPH) in men, although medication use, acute neurologic dysfunction, urinary tract bleeding or calculi, and other anatomic obstruction are also common causes in both men and women. Acute syndromes typically present with rapid onset of lower abdominal pain occasionally radiating to the lower back. Patients typically complain of difficulty voiding but some may not volunteer this information. There is a 20% chance of a recurrence in the following 6 months after an episode of acute obstruction. Chronic obstruction usually presents with lower abdominal discomfort and the patient may note incomplete voiding or the need to void frequently. Overflow incontinence is often present.

The history should address previous episodes of obstruction, recent medication changes, and over-the-counter medicine use. Assess for any history of trauma or neurologic disability or symptoms of infection. It is critical to know if any recent urologic procedures or urinary catheterizations have been performed. The duration of symptoms is also important as it is associated with the development of postobstructive diuresis and renal dysfunction.

DIAGNOSIS AND DIFFERENTIAL

Causes of urinary retention may include anatomic obstruction, neurologic dysfunction, medication side effect, trauma to the genitourinary tract, infection, and psychological stress. Fever may indicate infection as either the cause or as a result of urinary outlet obstruction. Tachycardia and hypotension may resolve after the obstruction is relieved. The physical examination should address the functional and anatomic assessment of the lower urinary tract. Palpate the abdomen for a suprapubic mass corresponding to the distended urinary bladder. The penis should be examined for stricture at the meatus or palpable abnormalities of the penile urethra. In men the prostate should be assessed for size, texture, and tenderness. The female lower urinary tract should be evaluated for bladder prolapse or stricture of the urethral meatus. A pelvic exam is generally indicated to screen for infection or mass as a cause of obstruction. A comprehensive neurologic examination should be performed in all patients and perineal sensation and anal sphincter tone should be documented.

Bedside ultrasound can be very helpful both in distinguishing the degree of obstruction and in discriminating obstruction from the sensation of fullness associated with bladder spasm in conditions such as inflammatory or infectious cystitis. The patient should first be encouraged to attempt to void. After a voiding attempt the bladder is imaged with a low-frequency sector

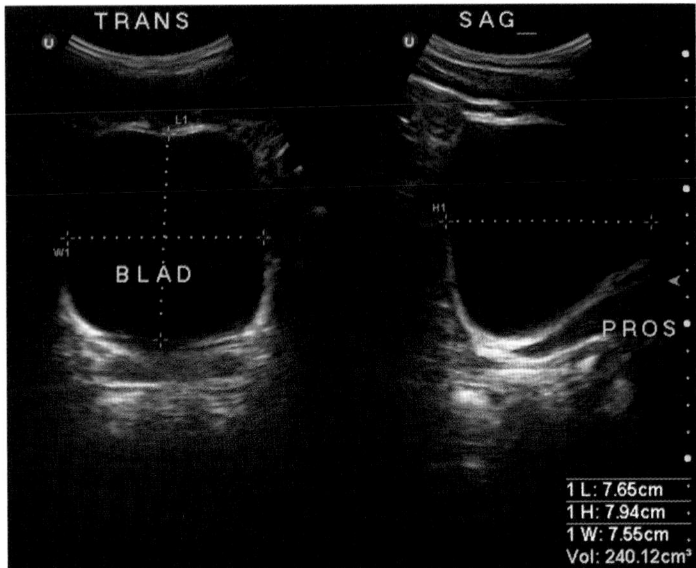

FIGURE 54-1. Transverse and sagittal views of the urinary bladder. The prostate is visualized as a medium echogenicity structure posterior and caudal to the bladder. Anterior-posterior, cradio-caudal, and transverse measurements of the bladder are obtained for calculation of the bladder volume. Reproduced with permission from Casey Glass, MD.

format probe in both the transverse and sagittal views (Figure 54-1). Many manufacturers have a calculation package available to estimate the retained urine volume. Residual volumes >50 to 150 cc are consistent with urinary retention; however, volumes in the setting of retention are typically greater than 300 cc.

EMERGENCY DEPARTMENT CARE AND DISPOSITION

The goals of emergency department care are relieving the discomfort of retention, assessing for any secondary injury to the renal system, and treatment of the primary cause of retention.

1. Most patients with bladder outlet obstruction are in distress, and passage of a urethral catheter alleviates their pain and urinary retention. Copious intraurethral lubrication including a topical anesthetic (2% lidocaine jelly) should be used. A 16-French Coudé catheter is recommended if straight catheters fail. The catheter should be passed to its fullest extent to obtain free urine flow before inflating the balloon. A catheter should not be placed if there is suspicion of trauma to the urethra, either secondary to a traumatic event or recent instrumentation. In most cases a catheter should be left indwelling and connected to a leg drainage bag. For cases of postanesthesia-related retention it is appropriate to remove the catheter after bladder drainage and then attempt a trial of spontaneous voiding.

2. The patient with obstruction from hematuria represents a special case. A 3-port Foley catheter should be placed and the bladder irrigated until returning fluid is free of blood. These patients are likely to need admission for continued irrigation as the catheter often becomes blocked with clot following placement.
3. Failure to pass a urethral Foley catheter, or recent urologic procedure or instrumentation requires the involvement of a urologist for catheter placement and consultation should not be delayed. Urgent urologic consultation is also indicated for obstruction secondary to stricture, prostatitis, or urethral trauma. Physicians familiar with the procedure may choose to place a suprapubic urinary catheter.
4. Send urine for routine analysis as well as culture. Assess electrolytes, blood urea nitrogen (BUN), and creatinine for postobstructive renal failure. Urine output should be monitored quantitatively.
5. Oxybutynin can be prescribed for control of bladder spasms. This anticholinergic medicine can itself cause a functional obstruction. Patients may also require pain medication for control of discomfort from bladder spasms. Treat male patients in whom BPH is the suspected etiology of their obstruction with an α-blocker.
6. Antibiotics are not indicated unless there is evidence of cystitis or other infection.
7. If urinary retention has been chronic, postobstructive diuresis may occur even in the presence of normal blood urea nitrogen and creatinine levels. In such patients, closely monitor urinary output, for 4 to 6 hours after catheterization. Hourly output of greater than 200 mL for more than 4 to 6 hours is an indication for admission and fluid replacement.
8. Address precipitating causes of retention. Discontinue offending medications. Infectious or neurologic causes must be completely evaluated; urgency of workup depends on patient acuity and comorbidities.
9. In all cases of urinary retention, urologic follow-up in 3 to 7 days is indicated for a complete genitourinary evaluation. Patients should usually expect to have the catheter removed at that visit.

FURTHER READING

For further reading in *Tintinalli's Emergency Medicine: A Comprehensive Study Guide*, 8th ed., see Chapter 92, "Acute Urinary Retention," by David Hung-Tsang Yen and Chen-Hsen Lee.

CHAPTER 55

Male Genital Problems

Gavin R. Budhram

TESTICULAR TORSION

Testicular torsion results from abnormal fixation of the testis within the tunica vaginalis, allowing the testis to twist. It exhibits a bimodal age distribution, peaking in the perinatal period and during puberty but may occur at any age. Although sometimes associated with trauma, torsion usually occurs in the absence of any preceding event.

Clinical Features

Because of the potential for infarction and infertility, testicular torsion must be the primary consideration in any male complaining of testicular pain. Pain usually occurs suddenly, is severe, and is felt in the lower abdominal quadrant, the inguinal canal, or the testis. The pain may be constant or intermittent but is not positional because torsion is primarily an ischemic event. Although symptom onset tends to occur after exertion, the testicle also may twist from unilateral cremasteric muscle contraction during sleep. Early in presentation, the affected testicle is firm, tender, elevated, and in a transverse lie compared to the contralateral testicle. The unilateral absence of the cremasteric reflex is a sensitive but nonspecific finding.

Diagnosis and Differential

Color-flow duplex ultrasound is the most commonly used confirmatory study, but sensitivity ranges from 69% to 90%. In addition, urinalysis is typically ordered, but pyuria does not rule out testicular torsion.

Torsion of the appendages is more common than testicular torsion but is not dangerous because the appendix testis and appendix epididymis have no known function. The diagnosis is supported by pain that is most intense near the head of the epididymis or testis, an isolated tender nodule, or the pathognomonic blue dot appearance of a cyanotic appendage with illumination through thin prepubertal scrotal skin. If normal intratesticular blood flow can be demonstrated with color Doppler, surgical exploration is not necessary because most appendages calcify or degenerate over 10 to 14 days and cause no harm. The differential for testicular torsion also includes epididymitis, inguinal hernia, hydrocele, and scrotal hematoma.

Emergency Department Care and Disposition

1. When the diagnosis of testicular torsion is obvious, immediate urologic consultation is indicated for exploration because imaging tests can be too time consuming. Testicular salvage rates are excellent with surgical detorsion within 6 hours of symptom onset, but decline rapidly thereafter.
2. The emergency physician can attempt manual detorsion. Most testes twist in a lateral to medial direction, so detorsion is performed in a

medial to lateral direction, similar to the opening of a book. The endpoint for successful detorsion is pain relief; urologic referral is still indicated.

3. Urology should be consulted early in the patient's course even if confirmatory testing is planned. When the diagnosis of testicular torsion cannot be ruled out by diagnostic studies or examination, urologic consultation is still indicated if suspicion is high.

EPIDIDYMITIS AND ORCHITIS

Clinical Features

Epididymitis is characterized by gradual onset of pain due to inflammation. Bacterial infection is the most common cause, with infecting agents dependent on the patient's age. In patients <35 years, epididymitis is due primarily to sexually transmitted diseases; culture or DNA probe for gonococcus and *Chlamydia* is indicated in males <35 years even in the absence of urethral discharge. Common urinary pathogens such as *Escherichia coli* and *Klebsiella* predominate in older men. Epididymitis causes lower abdominal, inguinal canal, scrotal, or testicular pain alone or in combination. Due to the inflammatory nature of the pain, patients with epididymitis may note transient pain relief when elevating the scrotal contents while recumbent (positive Prehn's sign).

Diagnosis and Differential

Initially, when tenderness is well localized to the epididymis, the clinical diagnosis is clear. However, progression of inflammation results in the physical examination finding of a single, large testicular mass (epididymo-orchitis), which is difficult to differentiate from testicular torsion or carcinoma. Testicular malignancy should be suspected in patients presenting with asymptomatic testicular mass, firmness, or induration. Ten percent of tumors present with pain due to hemorrhage within the tumor. Orchitis in isolation is rare; it usually occurs in conjunction with other systemic infections, such as mumps or other viral illnesses.

Emergency Department Care and Disposition

1. If the patient appears toxic, admission is indicated for intravenous antibiotics (e.g., **ceftriaxone** 1 to 2 g every 12 hours IV or **trimethoprim/sulfamethoxazole** 5 mg/kg IV of trimethoprim component every 6 hours).
2. Outpatient treatment is the norm in patients who do not appear toxic; urologic follow-up within 1 week is indicated. Age <35: Treat gonorrhea and *Chlamydia* with **ceftriaxone** 250 mg IM single dose plus **doxycycline** 100 mg PO twice daily for 10 days. Age >35: Treat gram-negative bacilli with **levofloxacin** 500 mg PO daily for 10 days or **ofloxacin** 300 mg PO twice daily for 10 days.
3. In addition, scrotal elevation, ice application, nonsteroidal anti-inflammatory drugs, opioids for analgesia, and stool softeners are indicated.
4. Orchitis is treated with disease-specific therapy, symptomatic support, and urologic follow-up.

ACUTE PROSTATITIS

Acute prostatitis is a bacterial inflammation of the prostate presenting with varying complaints of suprapubic or genital pain, back pain, perineal pain, voiding difficulties, frequency, dysuria, pain with ejaculation, and fever and chills. Patients at risk include those with anatomic or neurophysiologic lower urinary tract obstruction, acute epididymitis or urethritis, unprotected rectal intercourse, phimosis, and an indwelling urethral catheter. The causative organism is *E. coli* in most cases, with *Pseudomonas*, *Klebsiella*, *Enterobacter*, *Serratia*, or *Staphylococcus* causing the remainder. Physical examination usually reveals perineal, rectal, and prostate tenderness. The diagnosis is clinical as urinalysis and culture are often negative even after prostate massage. Treatment is **ciprofloxacin** 500 mg twice daily, or **levofloxacin** 500 mg PO daily, or **ofloxacin** 300 mg PO twice daily. All treatments should be for 2 to 4 weeks. Pain medicine may be required. Admission is not necessary unless the patient is septic, immunocompromised, has significant comorbidities, or has worsened on outpatient therapy. In this case, IV treatment with **piperacillin-tazobactam** 3.375 to 4.5 g or cefotaxime with an aminoglycoside may be initiated. Consider testing and treatment for gonorrhea and chlamydia in patients with risk factors for sexually transmitted disease.

SCROTUM

Scrotal abscesses may be localized to the scrotal wall or may arise from extensions of infections of intrascrotal contents (i.e., testis, epididymis, and bulbous urethra). A simple hair follicle scrotal wall abscess can be managed by incision and drainage; no antibiotics are required in immunocompetent patients. When a scrotal abscess is suspected to arise from an intrascrotal infection, ultrasound may demonstrate pathology in the testis and/or epididymis. Retrograde urethrography may be needed to identify a source in the urethra. Definitive care of any complex abscess calls for a urology consultation.

Fournier gangrene is a polymicrobial infection of the perineal subcutaneous tissues. Diabetic males are at highest risk, but any immunocompromised state can be associated with the disease. Prompt diagnosis is essential to prevent extensive tissue loss. Early surgical consultation is recommended for at-risk patients who present with scrotal, rectal, or genital pain. Treatment mainstays include aggressive fluid resuscitation with normal saline solution and broad-spectrum antibiotics to cover gram-positive, gram-negative, and anaerobic organisms: **imipenem** 1 g IV every 8 hours or **meropenem** 500 mg to 1 g IV every 8 hours plus **vancomycin** 1 g IV every 12 hours if methicillin-resistant *Staphylococcus aureus* is suspected. Care usually includes hyperbaric oxygen therapy (if readily available) and surgical debridement.

PENIS

Balanoposthitis is inflammation of the glans (balanitis) and foreskin (posthitis). Upon foreskin retraction, the glans and prepuce appear purulent, excoriated, malodorous, and tender. Treatment consists of cleaning with mild soap, ensuring adequate dryness, applying antifungal creams (**nystatin** 100,000 U/g, four times daily or **clotrimazole** 1% cream bid), and using an

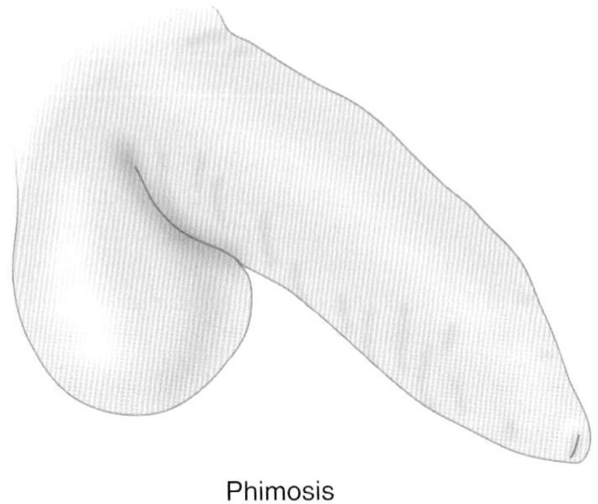

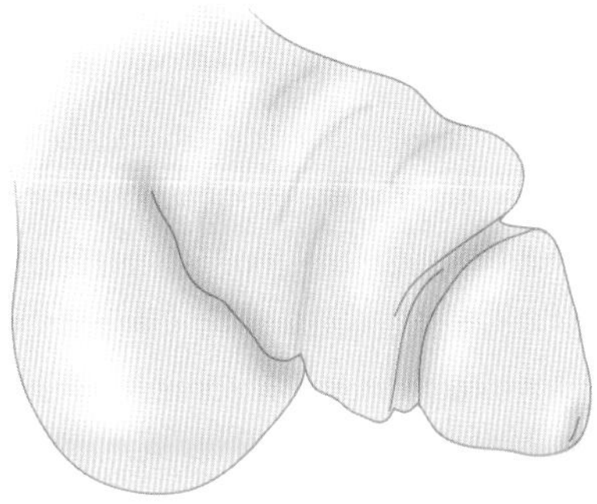

FIGURE 55-1. Phimosis and paraphimosis.

oral azole (**fluconazole** 150 mg single dose, reevaluate at 7 days for repeat dosing). Urologic referral is needed for reassessment and possible circumcision in recurrent cases. An oral cephalosporin (e.g., **cephalexin** 500 mg, times daily) should be prescribed in cases of secondary bacterial infection. Balanoposthitis can be the sole presenting sign of diabetes.

Phimosis is the inability to retract the foreskin proximally (Fig. 55-1). Physiologic phimosis is common in boys but less than 10% of foreskins remain nonretractile at age 3 with nearly all resolving by adolescence. Pathologic phimosis occurs as a result of infection, poor hygiene, or previous injury with scarring. Hemostatic dilation of the preputial ostium relieves urinary retention until definitive dorsal slit or circumcision can be performed. Topical steroid therapy, such as **hydrocortisone** 1% cream for 4 to 6 weeks, along with daily preputial retraction, reduces the rate of required circumcision.

Paraphimosis is the inability to reduce the proximal edematous foreskin distally over the glans (see Fig. 55-1). Paraphimosis is a true urologic emergency because the resulting glans edema and venous engorgement can progress to arterial compromise and gangrene. If surrounding tissue edema can be successfully compressed, as by wrapping the glans with 2 × 2-in. elastic bandages for 5 minutes, the foreskin may be reduced. Making several puncture wounds with a small (22- to 25-gauge) needle may help with expression of glans edema fluid. Local anesthetic block of the penis is helpful if patients cannot tolerate the discomfort associated with edema compression and removal. If arterial compromise is suspected or has occurred, local infiltration of the constricting band with 1% plain **lidocaine** followed by superficial vertical incision of the band will decompress the glans and allow foreskin reduction.

Penile entrapment injuries occur when various objects are wrapped around the penis potentially occluding vascular supply. Objects may be removed by a variety of techniques including compression, cutting, cooling the penis, and possibly even urologic surgical removal. Retrograde urethrogram and Doppler studies may be employed if indicated to assess urethral injury and distal penile arterial blood supply, respectively.

Penile fracture occurs when there is an acute tear of the penile tunica albuginea. The penis is acutely swollen, discolored, and tender in a patient with history of intercourse-associated trauma accompanied by a snapping sound and sudden loss of erection. Retrograde urethrography may be indicated for assurance of urethral integrity. Urologic consultation is indicated.

Peyronie disease produces progressive penile deformity, typically curvature with erections, that is painful and may result in erectile dysfunction or preclude successful vaginal intercourse. Examination shows a thickened plaque on the dorsal penile shaft. Assurance and urologic follow-up are indicated.

Priapism is a painful pathologic erection that may be associated with urinary retention. Infection and impotence are other complications. Corporal aspiration and instillation of an α-adrenergic antagonist (i.e., phenylephrine) is the next step and may need to be performed by the emergency physician when urologic consultation is not available. Even when emergency physicians provide stabilizing care, urologic consultation is indicated in all cases.

URETHRA

Urethritis is characterized by purulent urethral discharge. Diagnosis is clinical but is often confirmed with a first-void urine specimen. Causative agents are usually *Chlamydia trachomatis* or *Neisseria gonorrhoeae*, though *Trichomonas*, *Ureaplasma urealyticum*, and herpes simplex virus may also occasionally cause urethritis. Treatment is **ceftriaxone** 250 mg IM and **azithromycin** 1 g PO.

Urethral stricture is becoming more common due to the high incidence of sexually transmitted diseases and may result in urinary retention. A normal post-void residual volume should be less than 100 mL and can be estimated with bedside ultrasonography. If a patient's bladder cannot be cannulated, the differential diagnosis includes urethral stricture, voluntary external sphincter spasm, bladder-neck contracture, or benign prostatic hypertrophy. If a 14- or 16-Fr Foley cannot be passed, a Coudé catheter may be used to navigate a stricture. Retrograde urethrography can be performed to delineate the location and extent of a urethral stricture. Endoscopy is necessary to confirm bladder neck contracture or define the extent of an obstructing prostate gland. Suspected voluntary external sphincter spasm can be overcome by holding the patient's penis upright and encouraging him to relax the perineum and breathe slowly during the procedure. After no more than three gentle attempts to pass a 12-Fr Coudé catheter into a urethra prepared with anesthetic lubricant, urologic consultation should be obtained. In an emergency situation, suprapubic cystotomy can be performed using the Seldinger technique. Urologic follow-up should occur within 48 hours.

Urethral foreign bodies are associated with bloody urine and slow, painful urination. Radiography of the bladder and urethral areas may disclose a foreign body. Removal of the foreign body often requires urologic consultation for endoscopy or open cystotomy, though a gentle milking action of the proximal end of a urethral foreign body may be attempted. Retrograde urethrography or endoscopy is often required to confirm an intact urethra.

FURTHER READING

For further reading in *Tintinalli's Emergency Medicine: A Comprehensive Study Guide*, 8th ed., see Chapter 93, "Male Genital Problems," by Jonathan E. Davis.

CHAPTER 56

Urologic Stone Disease

Geetika Gupta

The acute phenomenon of renal stones migrating down the ureter is referred to as *renal colic*. Adults and children can develop kidney stones. In adults, the condition is more common in males than in females; kidney stones usually occur in the third to fifth decade of life. There is a reoccurrence rate of 37% within the first year of having a stone. Children under the age of 16 years constitute 7% of cases seen, with the distribution being equal between the sexes.

CLINICAL FEATURES

Patients usually present with an acute onset of severe pain, which may be associated with nausea, vomiting, and diaphoresis. Patients are frequently anxious, pacing, or writhing and are unable to hold still or converse. The pain is sharp and episodic in nature due to the intermittent obstruction of the ureter and is relieved after the stone passes. The pain typically originates in either flank with subsequent radiation around the abdomen toward the groin. However, as the stone passes into the distal ureter, where 75% of stones are diagnosed, the pain may be located in the anterior abdominal or suprapubic area. Vesicular stones may present with intermittent dysuria and terminal hematuria. Children may present in a similar fashion, but up to 30% have only painless hematuria. Vital signs may demonstrate tachycardia and an elevated blood pressure, which are secondary to pain. Fever may be present if there is a concomitant urinary tract infection. Examination may show costovertebral tenderness or abdominal tenderness, guarding, or rigidity. Hematuria may be present in 85% of patients with renal colic.

DIAGNOSIS AND DIFFERENTIAL

The consideration of urologic stones and renal colic is based on clinical judgment. The differential diagnosis includes abdominal aortic aneurysm and aortic dissection. Other concerning possibilities include appendicitis, mesenteric ischemia, cholecystitis, ectopic pregnancy, gonadal torsion, renal infarction, incarcerated hernia, epididymitis, salpingitis, pyelonephritis, herpes zoster, drug-seeking behavior, musculoskeletal strain, and papillary necrosis. Papillary necrosis may be present in patients with sickle cell disease, diabetes, nonsteroidal analgesic abuse, or infection. Patients receiving outpatient extracorporeal shock wave lithotripsy for urolithiasis may present to the emergency department (ED) with renal colic because the resulting "sludge" is passed in the urine.

Obtain a urinalysis to assess for hematuria and infection. Check serum renal function, as a majority of patients who are stone formers have decreased creatinine clearance. Get a pregnancy test in females of childbearing age.

The recommendation for the ideal modality of imaging is evolving. Imaging helps diagnose a ureteral stone, rules out other diagnoses, identifies complications, establishes the location of the stone, and/or assists with the management if the stone fails to pass spontaneously. Noncontrast helical computed tomography (CT) has the overall highest sensitivity and specificity. Positive findings include changes in the ureteral caliber, suspicious calcifications, stranding of perinephric fat, and dilation of the collecting system. It has a PPV of 96% and a NPV of 93% to 97%. It can be performed quickly and can rule in or rule out other diagnoses. The disadvantage of CT is radiation exposure; therefore, many facilities have adopted a low-dose CT protocol. It has similar sensitivities as regular dose radiation CT for stones >3 mm and individuals with a BMI >30 (Table 56-1).

The use of plain kidney-ureter-bladder film (KUB) is limited as only 90% of ureteral stones are radiopaque. A KUB cannot rule in or rule out a ureteral stone. The KUB is useful in following the progression of a stone, once visualized on CT, in the outpatient setting.

The IV pyelogram (IVP) is rarely used anymore in the ED. It provides information on renal function and anatomy and is used as an adjunct to CT.

Ultrasound (US), an anatomic rather than a functional test, is useful in patients for whom CT is not advised such as pregnant women and children. It detects hydronephrosis and larger stones but is not sensitive for midureteral or small, less than 5-mm stones. Sensitivity increases to 90% for stones >6 mm. A false-positive diagnosis of hydronephrosis may be related to a full bladder, renal cysts, and anatomic variation. A rapid bolus of crystalloid can result in a false-positive diagnosis of hydroureter. Bedside US by ED physicians may also decrease length of stay for selected patients.

TABLE 56-1 Ancillary Tests in Urologic Stone Disease

Test	Sensitivity (%)	Specificity (%)	LR+	LR–	Comments
Noncontrast CT	94–97	96–99	24–∞	0.02–0.04	Advantages: speed, no RCM, detects other diagnoses Disadvantages: radiation, no evaluation of renal function
IV urogram	64–90	94–100	15–∞	0.11–0.15	Advantage: evaluates renal function Disadvantage: RCM (allergy, nephrotoxicity, metformin related acidosis)
Ultrasound	63–85	79–100	10–∞	0.10–0.34	Advantages: safe in pregnancy, no RCM, no radiation, no known side effects Disadvantages: insensitive in middle third of the ureter, may miss smaller stones (<5 mm)
Plain abdominal radiograph	29–58	69–74	1.9–2.0	0.58–0.64	Advantage: may be used to follow stones Disadvantage: poor sensitivity and specificity

Abbreviations: LR = likelihood ratio; RCM = radiocontrast media.

EMERGENCY DEPARTMENT CARE AND DISPOSITION

Medications

1. Analgesia: Nonsteroidal anti-inflammatory drugs administered parenterally are considered the analgesics of choice. The prostaglandins promote dilation of the ureter and thus aid in the alleviation of the source of the pain. **Ketorolac** 30 mg IVP is the recommended starting dose. Caution should be used in the elderly, those with bleeding tendencies, and those with renal impairment. Opioids, in titrated doses such as **morphine** 5 mg IV or **hydromorphone** 1 mg IV, may also be used to assist in pain control. Care must be used when utilizing these medications in senior, pediatric, and pregnant populations.
2. Intravenous crystalloid: It is recommended to correct any volume deficits from vomiting or decreased oral intake. Studies have not shown it to be effective in pain control or stone passage.
3. Antiemetics: **Metoclopramide**, 10 mg IV, the only antiemetic drug specifically studied for the treatment of renal colic, has been shown to be effective in providing relief from nausea and pain. Other antiemetics may also be used.
4. Medical expulsion therapy: The use of α-blockers results in a 2- to 6-day improvement in rate and time to expulsion and decreased pain. Options include **tamsulosin** 0.4 mg daily up to 4 weeks, **terazosin** 5 to 10 mg daily, and **doxazosin** 4 mg daily. Steroids and calcium channel blockers are not recommended.
5. Antibiotics: If the urinalysis shows evidence for an infection, the choice of antibiotic is dictated by the local resistance patterns to gram-negative rods. Patients with an infected ureteral stone without significant obstruction, fever, or systemic illness may be discharged with a fluoroquinolone such as **ciprofloxacin** 500 mg twice a day for 10 to 14 days or **levofloxacin** 500 mg daily for 10 to 14 days, a third-generation cephalosporin such as **cefpodoxime** 200 mg twice a day for 10 to 14 days or other drugs with good local sensitivities. Close follow-up is essential.

Patients with a more complicated clinical situation should be admitted. Intravenous antibiotic selections to consider include **gentamicin** or **tobramycin** 1 mg/kg/dose every 8 hours *and* **ampicillin** 1 to 2 g every 4 hours; **piperacillin-tazobactam** 3.375 g every 6 hours; **cefepime** 2 g every 8 hours; **ticarcillin-clavulanic acid** 3.1 g every 6 hours, or **ciprofloxacin** 400 mg every 12 hours.

Disposition

If the stone is passed in the ED, no treatment is necessary other than elective urologic follow-up. Patients with small unilateral stones less than 5 mm, no complicated infection, and pain controlled by oral analgesics may be discharged with a urine strainer, prescriptions for oral analgesics and medical expulsive therapy, and urologic or primary care physician follow-up within 7 days. The rate of stone passage depends on its size and location. A stone measuring 5–6 mm in diameter takes 7 to 30 days to pass. Instruct patients to return if they develop fever, persistent vomiting, or uncontrolled pain.

TABLE 56-2 Indications for Admission in Patients with Nephrolithiasis

Absolute Indications for Admission	Relative Indications for Admission
Intractable pain or vomiting	Fever
Urosepsis*	Solitary kidney or transplanted kidney without obstruction
Single or transplanted kidney with obstruction*	Obstructing stone with signs of urinary infection
Acute renal failure	Urinary extravasation
Hypercalcemic crisis	Significant medical comorbidities
Severe medical comorbidities/advanced age	Stone unlikely to pass—large stone above the pelvic brim

*Indication for urgent decompression.

Urologic consultation on an emergent basis is needed in patients with a complete obstruction complicated by fever and/or urosepsis and in patients with a solitary or transplanted kidney. Discuss disposition with a urologist in patients with a stone larger than 5 mm, renal insufficiency, severe underlying disease, extravasation or complete obstruction, sloughed renal papillae, UTI, or failed outpatient management.

Hospitalization is indicated for patients who have a solitary or transplanted kidney with obstruction, uncontrolled severe pain, intractable emesis, acute renal failure, hypercalcemic crisis, severe medical comorbidities, and urosepsis. Consider admission for patients with a fever, solitary or transplanted kidney without obstruction, obstructing stone with infection, urinary extravasation, significant medical comorbitidies, or large proximal ureteral stone. (Table 56-2).

FURTHER READING

For further reading in *Tintinalli's Emergency Medicine: A Comprehensive Study Guide*, 8th ed., see Chapter 94, "Urologic Stone Disease," by David E. Manthey and Bret A. Nicks.

Complications of Urologic Procedures and Devices

Steven Go

COMPLICATIONS OF URINARY CATHETERS

Complications related to the use of urinary catheters are not infrequent and therefore the catheters **should be used only when absolutely necessary.** Silicone catheters are available for patients with latex allergies.

Catheter-Associated Urinary Tract Infection

Catheter-associated urinary tract infections (CA-UTIs) are a very common cause of nosocomial infections. Signs and symptoms of CA-UTI include fever, rigors, altered mental status, malaise, or lethargy, flank pain, costovertebral angle tenderness, acute hematuria, and pelvic discomfort. In those whose catheters have been removed, dysuria, urgent or frequent urination, or suprapubic pain or tenderness may indicate CA-UTI. Do not treat asymptomatic bacteriuria in a patient with a short-term catheterization, except in pregnancy or immediately posturologic procedure. CA-UTI in spinal cord injury patients may also present with increased spasticity, autonomic dysreflexia, and a sense of unease. Pyelonephritis is the most common complication of CA-UTI and should be suspected when fever is present. Other related infections include prostatitis, epididymitis, and scrotal abscess.

Diagnosis of CA-UTI in the ED is made clinically with urine microscopy. Send urine for culture. Add blood cultures if the patient is septic or immunocompromised. An ultrasound may be useful to identify urinary obstruction. Remember that pyuria is universal for patients with long-term (>1 month) indwelling catheters and in the absence of symptoms, pyuria should not be used in the diagnosis of infection. Hematuria is a better indicator of infection. Remove the urinary catheter if clinically feasible or replace the catheter if it is >7 days old. In patients with mild symptoms, empirically treat with **ciprofloxacin** 500 mg twice a day, **levofloxacin** 500 mg once a day, or **cefpodoxime** 200 mg twice a day. Tailor specific antibiotic choice to local bacterial sensitivities. Seven days is the recommended duration of antimicrobial treatment for patients with CA-UTI who have prompt resolution of symptoms, and 10 to 14 days of treatment is recommended for those with a delayed response. In patients with catheter-associated pyelonephritis, admission is frequently required. Check urine cultures and blood cultures if there is concern for sepsis.

Nondeflation of Foley Retention Balloon

Nondeflation of the Foley retention balloon prevents the removal of the catheter. Cut the plastic catheter valve just proximal to the inflation port and insert a flexible guide wire to expand the channel and deflate the balloon. If this is not successful, insert a 22-G central venous catheter (CVC) over the guide wire. Once the tip of the catheter enters the balloon, remove the guide wire and deflate the balloon. If the inflated balloon persists, instill 10cc of mineral oil through the CVC and wait 15 minutes to dissolve the balloon (this step may be repeated). If these methods fail, consult a urologist to remove the catheter.

COMPLICATIONS OF PERCUTANEOUS NEPHROSTOMY

Percutaneous nephrostomy is a urinary drainage procedure used for supravesical or ureteral obstruction. Bleeding may occur. Check hemoglobin, hematocrit, and renal function studies. Check platelet count and coagulation studies if a coagulopathy is suspected. Treat mild bleeding by irrigating the nephrostomy tube to clear the blood clots. If bleeding fails to resolve, a vascular injury may be present and emergent urology consult is indicated. Initiate fluid resuscitation and blood transfusion in severe cases.

Infectious complications from nephrostomy tubes include bacteriuria, pyelonephritis, renal abscess, and urosepsis. Culture the urine and wound drainage (if any) and administer antibiotics after consulting a urologist.

Catheter dislodgment, tube blockage, and residual stone fragments can occur. Obtain a CT scan and consult urology to treat these mechanical issues.

LITHOTRIPSY

Common post-lithotripsy complications include abdominal and flank pain, gross hematuria, skin ecchymosis, and ureteral obstruction from stone fragments. However, ruptured or perforated organs, infections (pyelonephritis, urosepsis, psoas abscess), vascular injury, and pancreatitis may also occur. The presence of hypotension, syncope, flank hematoma, drop in hemoglobin, and severe pain are all harbingers of serious complications (e.g., perinephric and renal hematomas). Administer supportive therapy with IV fluids, antiemetics, and analgesics. Check blood counts, creatinine, and urinalysis. Obtain cultures and administer antibiotics if indicated. If simple obstruction is suspected, obtain a renal ultrasound. Obtain a CT scan if a more severe injury is suspected. Consult urology early in the process as surgical intervention may be indicated in these cases.

COMPLICATIONS OF URETERAL STENTS

A range of infectious complications can occur from ureteral stents. Therefore, order a urinalysis and culture for urinary symptoms, incontinence, flank pain, or change in the baseline discomfort. Treat simple infections with outpatient antibiotics in consultation with a urologist, as stent removal is not always necessary. However, if pyelonephritis or urosepsis is suspected, obtain appropriate cultures, administer IV antibiotics, order imaging (abdominal series, ultrasound, and CT) to verify stent placement, and consult urology.

Late complications with long-term stent placement may be seen. New-onset abdominal pain, severe flank pain, fever, irritative bladder symptoms, or gross hematuria may be indicative of stent migration, obstruction, or infection. Obtain a urinalysis to evaluate for infection, imaging to evaluate stent position, and urologic consultation. However, new anemia without hematuria may be indicative of a retroperitoneal hematoma and is diagnosed with CT. Assume vascular fistulization from an eroding stent in the presence of severe gross hematuria, syncope, or hypotension. Resuscitate these patients, order lab studies, irrigate the bladder, and transfuse appropriately. Obtain urology consultation immediately.

COMPLICATIONS OF ARTIFICIAL URINARY SPHINCTERS

The artificial sphincter is a device used for urinary incontinence from various causes. Skin flora cause early infections, while later infections are usually due to gram-negative pathogens. **Never introduce a urinary drainage catheter through an artificial urinary sphincter**. Obtain urinalysis, appropriate labs, cultures, and imaging, and administer IV antibiotics as indicated. Consult a urologist for further evaluation and management.

COMPLICATIONS OF ERECTILE DYSFUNCTION DEVICES

Injections for erectile dysfunction can result in priapism, which requires emergent urologic consultation. The most common complication of vacuum devices is pain from improper use, but skin necrosis and infections can occur. Infection of implanted penile prostheses (both early and late), erosion of the prosthesis into the penile tissue, and prosthesis migration can occur. Administer broad-spectrum IV antibiotics if infection is present and consult a urologist for device removal.

FURTHER READING

For further reading in *Tintinalli's Emergency Medicine: A Comprehensive Study Guide*, 8th ed., see Chapter 95, "Complications of Urologic Procedures and Devices," by Elaine B. Josephson.

SECTION 8

Gynecology and Obstetrics

CHAPTER 58 Vaginal Bleeding and Pelvic Pain in the Nonpregnant Patient

Joelle Borhart

VAGINAL BLEEDING

Abnormal vaginal bleeding is a common complaint in females presenting to the ED. Determination of pregnancy status in patients of reproductive age is critical to formulate the appropriate differential diagnosis and to guide subsequent testing and decision making.

Clinical Features

All patients should be asked about the amount and duration of bleeding. Reproductive and sexual history, history of sexually transmitted infections, trauma, medications, and the possibility of foreign bodies should be elicited. Symptoms of a possible bleeding disorder (history of bruising, epistaxis, other abnormal bleeding), endocrine disorder, or liver disease should be noted. A complete abdominal and pelvic examination, including speculum and bimanual exam, should be performed on nonvirginal patients to look for structural or traumatic causes of bleeding. Skin or conjunctiva pallor, abnormal vital signs, or a report of dizziness, syncope, or weakness can indicate significant blood loss.

Diagnosis and Differential

In prepubertal girls, causes of vaginal bleeding include genital trauma and/or sexual abuse, vaginitis, tumors, and foreign bodies. Bleeding coupled with vaginal discharge raises concerns for retained foreign bodies. Up to 20% of adolescents with abnormal uterine bleeding may have a primary coagulation disorder such as von Willebrand disease. Anovulatory cycles are also common during the teenage years. In women of reproductive age and perimenopausal women, bleeding can arise from the uterus or cervix and is most commonly due to anovulation, pregnancy, exogenous hormone use, coagulopathy, uterine leiomyomas, cervical and endometrial polyps, pelvic infections, and thyroid dysfunction. In postmenopausal women, the most common causes of vaginal bleeding are exogenous estrogens, atrophic vaginitis, endometrial lesions including cancer, and other tumors.

The new term *abnormal uterine bleeding (AUB)* encompasses all causes of abnormal bleeding in nonpregnant women and divides etiologies of AUB into structural and nonstructural causes. The use of the term *dysfunctional uterine bleeding* is no longer recommended. AUB may be ovulatory or anovulatory. Anovulatory cycles are common at the extremes of reproductive age. Patients with anovulatory cycles may present with prolonged menses, irregular cycles, or intermenstrual bleeding. Usually the bleeding is painless and minimal, but severe bleeding can occur, resulting in anemia and iron depletion.

A pregnancy test must be obtained on all women of reproductive age to rule out pregnancy as a cause of bleeding. Other laboratory evaluation is guided by the history and physical examination. A CBC should be checked if signs of excessive bleeding or anemia are present. A prolonged PT or elevated INR may identify a coagulopathy. Obtain thyroid function tests in patients with symptoms and signs of thyroid dysfunction. Ultrasonography is an important imaging modality to determine uterine size, characteristics of the endometrium, and to detect structural abnormalities. Ultrasound may be deferred for outpatient evaluation in stable, nonpregnant patients as the results will rarely change ED management.

Emergency Department Care and Disposition

Most patients with vaginal bleeding are hemodynamically stable and need no acute intervention. Patients who are unstable with persistent bleeding require aggressive resuscitation: IV crystalloids, blood products, and gynecologic consultation for urgent D and C.

1. For unstable patients with severe bleeding high-dose IV estrogen is considered first-line treatment. Give **conjugated estrogen** (e.g., Premarin®) 25 mg IV every 2 to 6 hours until bleeding slows followed by an oral contraceptive. These patients should be admitted to a gynecologic service for further management.
2. In stable patients short-term hormonal therapy may be prescribed to temporize an acute bleeding episode. Choices include the following:
   a. Oral contraceptive regimen: **ethinyl estradiol** 35 μg and **norethindrone** 1 mg (e.g., Ortho-Novum 1/35®) three tablets daily for 7 days. Alternatively, a taper may be given: four tablets for 2 days, three tablets for 2 days, two tablets for 2 days, and one tablet for 3 days.
   b. **Medroxyprogesterone** 20 mg three times per day for 7 days or 10 mg per day for 10 days.
   c. **Tranexamic acid** (e.g., Lysteda®), an antifibrinolytic agent, 600 to 1300 mg every 8 hours for 3 days. Withdrawal bleeding may be heavy and typically occurs 3 to 10 days after the hormonal therapy has stopped. Obtain gynecologic consultation if administration is considered.
3. If there is any concern for malignancy, hormonal therapy is best deferred until the patient is evaluated by gynecology and a decision about a biopsy is made.
4. Nonsteroidal anti-inlammatory drugs (NSAIDs), such as **naproxen** 500 mg twice daily PO or **ibuprofen** 400 mg every 6 hours PO, may reduce bleeding.
5. Stable patients may be discharged home and instructed to follow-up with their gynecologic provider.

PELVIC PAIN

Pelvic pain generally arises from gynecologic pathology but referred pain from extrapelvic conditions, such as inflammatory bowel disease, urinary tract infections or stones, diverticulitis, leaking abdominal aneurysm, or appendicitis, need to be considered. Pregnancy should be excluded in all women of reproductive age. Pelvic inflammatory disease is a common cause of pelvic pain and is discussed in Chapter 64.

Clinical Features

Pelvic pain may be acute or chronic, intermittent or continuous. Attention to the characteristics of the pain will aid in determining etiologies. Sudden onset of unilateral pain suggests an ovarian cyst, ovarian torsion, obstruction, or renal lithiasis. Gradual onset suggests an infectious process or slowly enlarging mass. Other attributes, such as the relationship of the pain with the menstrual cycle, aggravating and relieving factors, and associated urinary, GI, and systemic symptoms assist in developing the differential diagnosis.

A complete abdominal and pelvic examination, including speculum and bimanual exams should be performed. A pregnancy test should be done to rule out pregnancy in women of reproductive age. Other testings, such as urinalysis, CBC, and ultrasound, are guided by the history and physical examination.

Diagnosis and Differential

Ovarian Cysts

Symptomatic ovarian cysts typically cause sudden-onset unilateral pain. Cysts can be complicated by bleeding from the cyst wall (hemorrhagic cyst) or by cyst rupture. A ruptured cyst can causes abnormal vital signs and an acute abdomen. Cysts that are >8 cm, multiloculated, or solid are concerning for malignancy, dermoid cysts, or endometriomas ("chocolate cysts"). In women who are postmenopausal, an ovarian mass is malignant until proven otherwise. All patients with cysts should follow-up with their gynecologic provider for further evaluation.

Ovarian Torsion

Ovarian torsion results in the sudden onset of severe adnexal pain from ischemia of the ovary. Torsion is a surgical emergency and rapid intervention is necessary to preserve ovarian function. A history of acute onset of severe unilateral pain may be obtained, though atypical presentations are common. Pain may develop after exertion. Risk factors for torsion include pregnancy (enlarged corpus luteum), large ovarian cysts or tumors, and chemical induction of ovulation (ovarian hyperstimulation syndrome). Ultrasound with Doppler flow imaging is the diagnostic procedure of choice but is not 100% sensitive. Imaging early in the process may show congestion from venous outflow obstruction with preserved arterial flow and images obtained during a transient period of detorsion may appear normal. Analgesia, gynecologic consultation, and preparation for surgery are warranted if the diagnosis is suspected.

Endometriosis

Endometriosis results from endometrium-like tissue implanted outside of the uterus causing chronic inflammation. Symptoms include recurrent pelvic pain associated with menstrual cycles, dyspareunia, and infertility. The definitive diagnosis is usually not made in the ED. Treatment consists of analgesics and gynecologic referral.

Leiomyomas

Leiomyomas (uterine fibroids) are benign smooth muscle tumors, often multiple, seen most commonly in women in middle and later reproductive years. About 30% of women with leiomyomas will develop symptoms such as abnormal vaginal bleeding, dysmenorrhea, bloating, backache, urinary symptoms, and dyspareunia. Severe pain can result with torsion of a pedunculated fibroid, or ischemia and infarction of a fibroid. Bimanual examination may demonstrate a mass or an enlarged uterus. Pelvic ultrasound is confirmatory. Treatment consists of NSAIDs or other analgesics for pain, hormonal manipulation for excessive bleeding, and referral to a gynecologist for definitive therapy.

Emergency Department Care and Disposition

Most patients are ultimately discharged from the ED even though there may not be a specific diagnosis. It is common and appropriate to discharge patients with a diagnosis of undifferentiated abdominal pain. Patients should receive detailed discharge instructions with strict return precautions outlined. Follow-up instructions should also be very specific. Reevaluation in 12 to 24 hours can be scheduled if any concern persists. Analgesics, such as **NSAIDs**, provide effective pain control for most outpatients, although some patients will require opioids, such as **oxycodone/acetaminophen** (5/325) one to two tablets every 4 to 6 hours PO for a few days.

FURTHER READING

For further reading in *Tintinalli's Emergency Medicine: A Comprehensive Study Guide*, 8th ed., see Chapter 96, "Abnormal Uterine Bleeding," by Bophal Sarha Hang; Chapter 97, "Abdominal and Pelvic Pain in the Nonpregnant Female," by Melanie Heniff and Heather R.B. Fleming.

CHAPTER 59

Ectopic Pregnancy and Emergencies in The First 20 Weeks of Pregnancy

Robert Jones

ECTOPIC PREGNANCY

Ectopic pregnancy (EP) is the leading cause of maternal death in the first trimester. Major risk factors include history of pelvic inflammatory disease, surgical procedures on the fallopian tubes including tubal ligation, previous EP, diethylstilbestrol exposure, intrauterine device use, and assisted reproduction techniques. The most common extrauterine location is the fallopian tube. This diagnosis must be considered in every woman of childbearing age presenting with abdominal pain and/or vaginal bleeding.

Clinical Features

The classic triad of abdominal pain, vaginal bleeding, and amenorrhea used to describe EP may be present, but many cases occur with more subtle findings. Presenting signs and symptoms may be different in ruptured versus nonruptured EP. Location of the EP will also determine the clinical features. The vast majority of EPs implant in the ampullary portion of the fallopian tube but additional implantation locations include the cervix, abdomen, and cesarean scar. Ninety percent of women with EP complain of abdominal pain; 50% to 80% have vaginal bleeding; and 70% give a history of amenorrhea. The pain described may be sudden, lateralized, extreme, or relatively minor and diffuse. The presence of hemoperitoneum with diaphragmatic irritation may cause the pain to be referred to the shoulder or upper abdomen. Presenting vital signs may be entirely normal even with a ruptured EP. There is poor correlation with the volume of hemoperitoneum and vital signs in EP. Relative bradycardia, as a consequence of vagal stimulation, may be present even in cases with rupture and hemoperitoneum. Physical examination findings are highly variable. The abdominal examination may show signs of localizing or diffuse tenderness with or without peritoneal signs. The pelvic examination findings may be normal but more often show cervical motion tenderness, adnexal tenderness with or without a mass, and possibly an enlarged uterus. Vaginal bleeding, ranging from spotting to heavy, is often present. Fetal heart tones may be heard in cases of EP beyond 12 weeks of gestation.

Diagnosis and Differential

The definitive diagnosis of EP is made either by ultrasound (US) or by direct visualization during surgery. The diagnosis of pregnancy is central to the diagnosis of possible EP and needs to be confirmed first. Urine pregnancy testing (for urinary β-human chorionic gonadotropin [β-hCG]) is a qualitative screening test with a threshold for detection of >20 mIU/mL of β-hCG. Urine qualitative testing is 95% to 100% sensitive and specific as compared with serum testing. Dilute urine, particularly when β-hCG levels are <50 mIU/mL, may result in a false-negative result. Quantitative serum testing for the diagnosis of pregnancy is virtually 100% sensitive for detecting β-hCG levels >5 mIU/mL and should be performed when the diagnosis of EP is considered but urine results are negative.

The primary goal of US in suspected EP is to determine if an intrauterine pregnancy (IUP) is present, since US cannot rule out the presence of EP. The transabdominal examination is usually performed first due to its wider field of view; the transvaginal examination is performed if the transabdominal examination is not diagnostic. When US reveals an unequivocal IUP and no other abnormalities, EP is effectively excluded unless the patient is at high risk for heterotopic pregnancy. Actual visualization of an EP with US occurs in a minority of cases. Sonographic findings of an empty uterus without an adnexal mass or free fluid in a woman with a positive pregnancy test result are considered indeterminate. In such situations, the findings must be evaluated in context with the patient's quantitative β-hCG level. A high β-hCG level (>6000 mIU/mL for transabdominal US or >1500 mIU/mL for transvaginal US) with an empty uterus is suggestive of EP. If the β-hCG is low (<1500 mIU/mL transvaginal), then the pregnancy may indeed be intrauterine or ectopic but often too small to be visualized on US or the patient may have already had a miscarriage. In this situation, repeat quantitative β-hCG testing in 2 days must be performed. β-hCG should increase at least 66% in that period; EP has a slower rate of increase. Since many EPs will have β-hCG levels <1500 mIU/mL, quantitative β-hCG levels should not be used to determine the need for US imaging.

Differential diagnosis in the patient presenting with abdominal pain, vaginal bleeding, and early pregnancy includes threatened, incomplete, or missed abortion, recent elective abortion, implantation bleeding, molar pregnancy, heterotopic pregnancy, or corpus luteum cyst.

Emergency Department Care and Disposition

Treatment of patients with suspected EP depends on the patient's vital signs, physical signs, and symptoms. Close communication with the obstetric-gynecologic consultant is essential.

1. For unstable patients, insert two large-bore intravenous lines and begin rapid infusion of crystalloid and/or packed red blood cells to maintain blood pressure.
2. Perform a bedside urine pregnancy test.
3. Notify the obstetric-gynecologic consultant immediately if the patient is unstable, even before laboratory and diagnostic tests are complete.
4. Draw blood for blood typing, and rhesus (Rh) factor determination (or cross-matching for the unstable patients), quantitative β-hCG determination (if indicated), and serum electrolyte determination, as required. Rh-negative women with EP should receive 50 μg of **anti-Rho (D) immunoglobulin.**
5. Reliable, stable patients with indeterminate US results and a β-hCG level below 1000 mIU/mL can be discharged with ectopic precautions and follow-up in 2 days for repeat β-hCG determination and obstetric-gynecologic reevaluation.

6. Definitive treatment, as determined by the obstetric-gynecologic consultant, may involve laparoscopy, dilation and curettage, or medical management with methotrexate. Methotrexate therapy, even when used in properly selected patients with EP, has a treatment failure rate of up to 36%, so proper selection is essential.

THREATENED ABORTION AND ABORTION

According to the World Health Organization, between 20% and 40% of pregnancies will spontaneously abort. Approximately 75% of these spontaneous abortions will occur before 8 weeks of gestation.

Clinical Features

Vaginal bleeding in the first 20 weeks, with a closed cervical os, benign examination, and no passage of tissue, is termed *threatened abortion.* A dilated cervix increases the likelihood of abortion (*inevitable abortion*). *Incomplete abortion* is defined as partial passage of the conceptus and is more likely between 6 and 14 weeks of pregnancy. The patient may report passage of grayish white products of conception (POC), or the POC may be evident on pelvic examination. *Complete abortion* is passage of all fetal tissue before 20 weeks gestation. All recovered POC should be sent for pathologic examination. *Missed abortion* is fetal death at less than 20 weeks without passage of any fetal tissue for 4 weeks after fetal death. *Septic abortion* implies evidence of infection during any stage of abortion, with signs and symptoms of pelvic pain, fever, cervical motion or uterine tenderness, or purulent or foul-smelling drainage.

Diagnosis and Differential

Perform a pelvic examination and obtain a complete blood count (CBC), blood typing (and cross-matching for unstable patients) and rhesus (Rh) factor determination, urine pregnancy test, quantitative β-hCG, and urinalysis. The differential diagnosis includes EP, implantation bleeding, and gestational trophoblastic disease (GTD). Implantation bleeding, which is usually scant and painless, is a diagnosis of exclusion. GTD is a proliferative disease of the trophoblast that includes complete hydatidiform mole, partial mole, trophoblastic tumor, and choriocarcinoma. Patients with GTD present with bleeding, an enlarged uterus out of proportion to menstrual age, and a significantly elevated β-hCG level. Also consider the possibility of a molar pregnancy in patients with hyperemesis gravidarum or pregnancy-induced hypertension before 24 weeks of gestation.

Emergency Department Care and Disposition

Treatment of patients with suspected threatened abortion and abortion depends on the patient's vital signs, physical signs, and symptoms. Close communication with the obstetric-gynecologic consultant is essential.

1. Patients who are symptomatic or demonstrate signs of hemodynamic instability should receive supplemental oxygen, be placed on a cardiac monitor, and have two large-bore intravenous (IV) lines established. The obstetric-gynecologic consultant is consulted emergently in the unstable patient.

2. Initiate aggressive IV crystalloid and/or packed red blood cell infusion, when appropriate, to help correct hypovolemia.
3. Rh-negative women with threatened abortion or abortion should receive **anti-Rho (D) immunoglobulin**. There is no uniform agreement on dosing. Dosing recommendations range from 50 to 300 μg in these patients.
4. US imaging should be performed when the patient is stable.
5. Incomplete abortion or GTD requires dilation and curettage. The decision to proceed with medical treatment, such as **misoprostol**, or surgical treatment, such as dilation and curettage, should be made in conjunction with the consulting obstetrician. GTD patients must receive close follow-up until quantitative β-hCG has returned to zero. Failure of the β-hCG to return to normal may indicate choriocarcinoma.
6. Septic abortion requires gynecologic consultation and broad-spectrum antibiotics such as **ampicillin/sulbactam** 3 g IV or **clindamycin** 600 mg plus **gentamicin** 1 to 2 mg/kg IV.
7. Patients with threatened abortion or complete abortion may be discharged with close follow-up arranged. Discharge instructions include pelvic rest (no intercourse or tampons) and instructions to return for heavy bleeding, fever, or pain.

NAUSEA AND VOMITING OF PREGNANCY

Nausea and vomiting of pregnancy generally are seen in the first 12 weeks and affect 60% to 80% of pregnant women. Cases can range from mild symptoms to hyperemesis gravidarum.

Clinical Features

Findings on physical examination are usually normal except for signs of volume depletion. The presence of abdominal pain in nausea and vomiting of pregnancy or hyperemesis gravidarum is highly unusual and should suggest another diagnosis.

Diagnosis and Differential

Diagnostic workup may include CBC, serum electrolytes, blood urea nitrogen, creatinine, and urinalysis. Differential diagnosis includes ruptured EP, cholelithiasis, cholecystitis, gastroenteritis, pancreatitis, appendicitis, hepatitis, peptic ulcer disease, pyelonephritis, fatty liver of pregnancy, and hemolysis with elevated liver enzymes and low platelets (known as HELLP syndrome).

Emergency Department Care and Disposition

1. Rehydration should begin with IV fluid such as 5% dextrose in normal saline or 5% dextrose in Lactated Ringer's solution. Failure to include dextrose may result in prolonged ketosis.
2. Frequently used antiemetics are **metoclopramide** 10 mg IV every 6 to 8 hours, **promethazine** 12 to 25 mg IV every 4 hours (pregnancy class C, but widely used), and **ondansetron** 4 to 8 mg IV every 4 to 8 hours.
3. If the patient improves in the emergency department (urine ketones clearing and tolerating oral liquids), she may be discharged with a prescription for an antiemetic. **Doxylamine with pyridoxine** 50 mg PO

every evening may be added as maintenance therapy for nausea and vomiting.

4. Admission is indicated for intractable vomiting, persistent ketonuria, electrolyte abnormalities, or weight loss greater than 10% of prepregnancy weight. Systemic steroids, such as **methylprednisolone,** 16 mg PO or IV every 8 hours for 3 days and tapered over 2 weeks to the lowest effective dose can be initiated in consultation with an obstetrician.

FURTHER READING

For further reading in *Tintinalli's Emergency Medicine: A Comprehensive Study Guide*, 8th ed., see Chapter 98, "Ectopic Pregnancy and Emergencies in the First 20 Weeks of Pregnancy," by Heather A. Heaton.

Comorbid Diseases in Pregnancy

Abigail D. Hankin

Many medical conditions can present in the context of pregnancy, either as a preexisting condition or arising during pregnancy. This chapter focuses on conditions that require different management when encountered in the pregnant patient. Some disorders are covered in other chapters within this text, including hypertension (Chapters 26 and 61), HIV infection (Chapter 92), and cardiac rhythm disturbances (Chapter 2).

DIABETES

Diabetics are at increased risk for complications of pregnancy and acute complications of diabetes. Many patients with gestational diabetes are managed with diet alone, though some patients require oral hypoglycemics such as metformin or glyburide. Insulin therapy is necessary for some patients with gestational diabetes and nearly all patients with type I or II diabetes. Insulin requirements increase as a pregnancy progresses, from 0.7 U/kg/d during the first trimester to 1.0 U/kg/d at term.

Pregnant patients are at increased risk of diabetic ketoacidosis (DKA), and DKA can occur more rapidly, and at lower glucose levels, than in nonpregnant patients. DKA should be considered for any pregnant diabetic patient who is ill appearing and/or has a blood glucose level ≥180 mg/dL. Treatment of DKA includes supplemental oxygen, left lateral decubitus positioning, and usual DKA care: isotonic fluid resuscitation to correct volume deficits, administration of continuous insulin, correction of electrolyte abnormalities, and treatment of the underlying cause (see Chapter 129).

Mild hypoglycemia (glucose <70 mg/dL and able to follow commands) is treated with a snack of milk and crackers. Severe hypoglycemia (glucose <70 mg/dL and unable to follow commands) should be treated with 50 mL of **50% dextrose in water** IV, with 1 to 2 mg of **glucagon** given IM or subcutaneous if IV access is delayed. Subsequently, the patient should be given 5% dextrose solution IV at 50 to 100 mL/h.

HYPERTHYROIDISM

Hyperthyroidism in pregnancy increases the risk of preeclampsia, congenital anomalies, and neonatal morbidity. Clinical features may be subtle and may mimic normal pregnancy. Treatment is with **propylthiouracil** (PTU). Patients on PTU are at risk for purpuric rash and agranulocytosis.

Thyroid storm presents with fever, volume depletion, or cardiac decompensation manifesting as high-output heart failure. Management is similar to nonpregnant patients (see Table 60-1).

HYPERTENSION

Treatment is often considered for chronic hypertension, defined as blood pressure >140/90 mm Hg measured on two occasions before 20 weeks gestation or sustained beyond 12 weeks gestation. Chronic hypertension is

TABLE 60-1 Principles of Treatment of Thyroid Storm during Pregnancy

Principle	Comment
Inhibit thyroid hormone release with thionamides (PTU is preferred over methimazole; also blocks conversion of T_4 to T_3)	**Propylthiouracil** (PTU) 600–1000 mg PO loading dose followed by 200–250 mg PO every 4 h (first trimester) or **Methimazole** 40 mg PO loading dose followed by 25 mg PO every 4 h (second and third trimesters)
Inhibit new thyroid hormone production (give at least 1 h after above step)	**Lugol solution** 8–10 drops every 6–8 h or **Potassium iodine** 5 drops PO every 6 h or **Iopanoic acid** 1 g IV every 8 h **Do not use radioactive iodine because the fetus will concentrate iodine-131 after the 10th to 12th week of gestation, resulting in congenital hypothyroidism**
Block peripheral thyroid hormone effects	**Propranolol** 1–2 mg IV every 10–15 min and start **Propranolol** 40 mg PO every 6 h or **Esmolol** 500 μg/kg IV bolus, then 50 μg/kg/min maintenance Hold if evidence of heart failure is present
Prevent conversion of T_4 to T_3	**Hydrocortisone** 100 mg IV every 8 h or **Dexamethasone** 2 mg IV every 6 h
Supportive care	Left lateral decubitus position Oxygen Cooling blankets IV fluids Acetaminophen 650 mg PO every 4 h

typically treated with **labetalol**, **nifedipine**, or **methyldopa** while angiotensin receptor blockers and angiotensin-converting enzyme inhibitors are avoided in pregnancy.

Acute hypertensive crisis in pregnancy is treated with labetalol or hydralazine (see Table 60-2).

While blood pressure is being managed, fetal well-being should be closely monitored, and clinicians should consider superimposed preeclampsia.

DYSRHYTHMIAS

Dysrhythmias may be precipitated by pregnancy and labor/delivery. Supraventricular tachycardias are treated with vagal maneuvers, β-blockers, adenosine, verapamil, and diltiazem at usual dosages. Patients with atrial fibrillation who require anticoagulation should be managed with unfractionated or low-molecular-weight heparin (LMWH). Electrical cardioversion may be used to treat dysrhythmias when indicated and have not been shown to be harmful to the fetus. Amiodarone should only be used to treat resistant, life-threatening dysrhythmias, as its use has been linked to fetal neurotoxicity.

TABLE 60-2 Treatment of Hypertension in Pregnancy

Agent	For Existing Hypertension	Adjunct to Existing Treatment	Urgent Control of Acute Hypertension	Potential Adverse Effects (Maternal)
Hydralazine	N/A	50–300 mg daily in 2–4 divided doses; use with methyldopa or labetalol to prevent reflex tachycardia*	Loading dose of 5 mg IV or IM, maintenance dose there after of 5–10 mg every 20–40 min up to 300 mg; *or* constant infusion of 0.5–10 mg/h	Delayed hypotension
Hydrochlorothiazide	N/A	12.5–50 mg daily	N/A	Volume depletion and electrolyte disorders
Labetalol	200–2400 mg daily in 2–3 divided doses	N/A	Loading dose of 20 mg IV; maintenance dose of 20–80 mg up to 300 mg; *or* constant infusion of 1–2 mg/min	Headache
Nifedipine	30–120 mg daily as slow-release preparation	N/A	10–30 mg orally, repeated after 45 min if needed	Headache, interference with labor
Methyldopa	0.5–3.0 g daily in 2–3 divided doses	N/A	N/A	Sedation, elevated liver function tests, depression

*Risk of fetal bradycardia and neonatal thrombocytopenia.

Abbreviation: N/A, not applicable.

THROMBOEMBOLISM

Deep venous thrombosis (DVT) and pulmonary embolism (PE) are the most common causes of maternal morbidity and mortality in industrialized nations. Factors associated with increased risk of thromboembolism include advanced maternal age, increasing parity, multiple gestations, operative delivery, bed rest, and obesity. Symptoms of DVT and PE may be mistaken for symptoms of normal pregnancy. Table 60-3 shows the various imaging modalities to consider for the diagnosis of PE in pregnancy. DVT and PE are treated with unfractionated or low-molecular-weight heparin at usual doses. Warfarin is contraindicated (see Chapter 25).

TABLE 60-3 Imaging Modalities for Diagnosis of Pulmonary Embolism in Pregnancy

	Radiation	Limitations	Disadvantages	Advantages	Lactation
Chest radiograph	Minimal	Nonspecific and nonsensitive	Results determine next imaging study, requiring more time to diagnosis	May identify another cause of pulmonary symptoms	No change
CT-PA	High maternal breast radiation; lower fetal radiation than V/Q scan	Contrast allergy and renal insufficiency	Hyperdynamic state in pregnancy can affect interpretation	High sensitivity and specificity; needed if abnormal chest radiograph	No need to discard breast milk
V/Q scan	Low breast radiation but higher fetal radiation than CT-PA	Not useful if abnormal chest radiograph, asthma, COPD, underlying pulmonary disease	If negative or inconclusive and suspicion for PE remains, will need a CT-PA; limited availability and time for isotope preparation, which delays diagnosis	Negative perfusion study effectively rules out PE	Discard breast milk for 12 h
MRI/MRV	No radiation	Gadolinium safety for fetus is unknown; do not use in maternal renal insufficiency	Limited availability	Can detect pelvic and iliac thrombosis	No need to discard breast milk

Abbreviations: COPD, chronic obstructive pulmonary disease; CT-PA, chest CT–pulmonary angiography; V/Q scan, ventilation-perfusion scan; MRV, magnetic resonance venography.

ASTHMA

Symptoms of acute asthma exacerbation include cough, wheezing, and dyspnea. Acute therapy includes maintenance of oxygen saturation >95%, administration of inhaled β_2-agonists, systemic corticosteroids, and fetal monitoring. Aerosolized **ipratropium** may be added in severely obstructed patients. **Terbutaline sulfate**, 0.25 mg SC every 20 minutes, may also be used. Subcutaneous epinephrine should be avoided, if possible. Peak expiratory flow rate (PEFR) is not altered in pregnancy, with goal PEFR between 380 and 550 L/min. Patients who are discharged home should receive oral **prednisone** 40 to 60 mg/d for 5 to 10 days in addition to a rescue β-agonist.

CYSTITIS AND PYELONEPHRITIS

Clinical features of cystitis and pyelonephritis are similar in pregnant and nonpregnant women, as are the causative microbes. Cystitis may be treated with **nitrofurantoin**, 100 mg PO twice daily for 3 to 7 days, while trimethoprim-sulfamethoxazole should be avoided due to concerns of fetal kernicterus during the third trimester. Fluoroquinolones and tetracyclines should also be avoided in pregnancy. Pregnant patients with pyelonephritis are treated aggressively because of increased risk of preterm labor and sepsis, and should be admitted for IV hydration and a second- or third-generation cephalosporin. Many providers continue antibiotic suppression for the remainder of the pregnancy.

SICKLE CELL DISEASE

Pregnant women with sickle cell disease are at higher risk of miscarriage, preterm labor, and vasoocclusive crises. Clinical features, evaluation, and treatment are similar to nonpregnant patients. Management of vasoocclusive crisis includes aggressive hydration, analgesia, identification and treatment of the underlying cause, and fetal monitoring. Opiates can be used, while NSAIDs should be avoided, particularly after 32 weeks gestation. Blood transfusion should be considered when conservative measures have failed, or with severe anemia, preeclampsia, hypoxemia, acute chest syndrome, or a new-onset neurological event.

HEADACHES

Headaches can be a presenting symptom of a wide variety of benign and life-threatening disorders, including intracranial hemorrhage, central vein thrombosis, mass, infection, and preeclampsia/eclampsia. Warning symptoms of potentially life-threatening disease include acute onset, postpartum headaches, neurological deficits, fever, and papilledema or retinal hemorrhages. If indicated, CT scan of the brain should be performed with appropriate shielding of the uterus. Migraine headaches should be treated with acetaminophen, antiemetics and, if necessary, narcotics. Ergot alkaloids and triptans should not be used.

SEIZURE DISORDERS

Seizure frequency may increase in patients with epilepsy due to altered drug pharmacokinetics. Acute seizure management is similar to that in nonpregnant patients, with emphasis on supplemental oxygen and left lateral decubitus positioning (see Chapter 145). Status epilepticus with prolonged maternal hypoxia and acidosis has a high mortality rate for the mother and infant, and should be treated aggressively with early intubation and ventilation.

SUBSTANCE ABUSE

Cocaine use is associated with increased incidence of fetal death in utero, placental abruption, preterm labor, premature rupture of membranes, spontaneous abortion, intrauterine growth restriction, and fetal cerebral infarcts. Treatment of acute cocaine intoxication is unchanged in pregnancy. Acute opiate withdrawal in pregnant women can be treated with clonidine, 0.1 to 0.2 mg SL every hour as needed for symptoms, not to exceed 0.8 mg. Patients should be referred to addiction specialists for methadone or buprenorphine/naloxone therapy. Alcohol use contributes to increased rates of spontaneous abortion, low birthweight, preterm deliveries, and fetal alcohol syndrome. Treatment of severe alcohol withdrawal does not differ from treatment in nonpregnant patients.

MEDICATIONS IN PREGNANCY AND LACTATION

Table 60-4 lists common emergency department medications that are known to be unsafe in pregnancy. For any drug not listed in the table, the National Library of Medicine provides detailed information online in the Drugs and Lactation Database (LactMed).

TABLE 60-4 Drugs Used in Emergency Settings with Known Adverse Effects in Human Pregnancy

Drug	Effect
Angiotensin-converting enzyme inhibitors and angiotensin receptor blockers	Renal failure, oligohydramnios
Aminoglycosides	Ototoxicity (gentamicin class D, Black Box Warning)
Androgenic steroids	Masculinize female fetus
Anticonvulsants (carbamazepine, hydantoins, valproate)	Dysmorphic syndrome, anomalies, neural tube defects
Antithyroid agents	Fetal goiter
Aspirin (high doses)	Bleeding, antepartum and postpartum
Cytotoxic agents (e.g., methotrexate)	Multiple anomalies
Erythromycin estolate	Maternal hepatotoxicity
Fluoroquinolones	Fetal cartilage abnormality

(Continued)

TABLE 60-4 Drugs Used in Emergency Settings with Known Adverse Effects in Human Pregnancy (Continued)

Drug	Effect
Isotretinoin	Hydrocephalus, deafness, anomalies
Lithium	Congenital heart disease (Ebstein's anomaly)
Nonsteroidal anti-inflammatory drugs (prolonged use after 32 weeks)	Oligohydramnios, constriction of fetal ductus arteriosus
Streptomycin	Fetal cranial nerve VIII damage
Sulfonamides	Fetal hemolysis, neonatal kernicterus (near term)
Tetracyclines	Fetal teeth and bone abnormalities
Trimethoprim, methotrexate	Folate antagonist (first trimester)
Thalidomide	Phocomelia
Warfarin	Embryopathy—nasal hypoplasia, optic atrophy

DIAGNOSTIC IMAGING IN PREGNANCY

The threshold for teratogenesis from ionizing radiation is 10 rads, with the first trimester being the most vulnerable period. The effects of radiation exposure change with gestational age. No single test exceeds the teratogenic threshold, but teratogenic effects of multiple imaging should be considered cumulatively. Ultrasound and magnetic resonance imaging have not been associated with teratogenic effects.

FURTHER READING

For further reading in *Tintinalli's Emergency Medicine: A Comprehensive Study Guide*, 8th ed., see Chapter 99, "Comorbid Disorders in Pregnancy," by Lori J. Whelan.

Emergencies After 20 Weeks of Pregnancy and The Postpartum Period

Kathleen Kerrigan

THROMBOEMBOLIC DISEASE OF PREGNANCY

Deep vein thrombosis (DVT) and pulmonary embolism (PE) are the leading causes of maternal morbidity and mortality in industrialized nations. Symptoms are similar to those seen in nonpregnant women. Evaluation for DVT should begin with ultrasound of the lower extremities. If there is a concern for PE initiate the evaluation with a chest radiograph. D-dimer may not be helpful to diagnose or exclude thromboembolic disease as levels increase throughout pregnancy. Consensus guidelines recommend obtaining a V/Q scan or CT pulmonary angiography next if the chest radiograph is nondiagnostic. DVT and PE are treated with unfractionated heparin or low-molecular-weight heparin. Do not use warfarin in pregnancy as it crosses the placenta, potentially causing fetal CNS abnormalities and embryopathies such as bone and cartilage abnormalities as well as nasal and limb hypoplasia.

CHEST PAIN

The underlying causes of chest pain in pregnancy are similar to those of nonpregnant women. Some disorders, such as aortic dissection and cardiomyopathy, may be associated with pregnancy. Treat pregnant women with acute myocardial infarction with aspirin, heparin, and percutaneous intervention rather than thrombolytics. Treat congestive heart failure and pulmonary edema with standard modalities except for sodium nitroprusside. It should be avoided as it can cause thiocyanate and cyanide accumulation in the fetus.

Chronic Hypertension

Chronic hypertension is defined as blood pressure at or above 140/90 mmHg prior to pregnancy, prior to 20 weeks' gestation or lasting more than 12 weeks after delivery. These patients are at risk for abruption, preeclampsia, low birth weight, cesarean delivery, premature birth, and fetal demise.

Gestational Hypertension

Gestational hypertension is defined as blood pressure at or above 140/90 mmHg after 20 weeks or in the immediate postpartum period but without proteinuria.

Hypertension in pregnancy is defined as a systolic blood pressure ≥140 mmHg or diastolic ≥90 mmHg on two occasions at least 4 hours apart in a woman who was normotensive prior to 20 weeks' gestation.

Preeclampsia

Preeclampsia is characterized by hypertension, greater than 140/90 mmHg, on two occasions at least 4 hours apart and proteinuria ≥300 mg in 24 hours in patients at 20 weeks' gestation until 4 to 6 weeks after delivery. In the absence of proteinuria, thrombocytopenia with platelet count less than 100,000, elevation of liver enzymes twice normal, new renal insufficiency with a creatinine of 1.1 or a doubling of serum creatinine, pulmonary edema, or new-onset mental status disturbances or visual disturbances can be used to make the diagnosis of preeclampsia. Edema may or may not be present. Symptoms of severe preeclampsia reflect end-organ involvement and may include headache, visual disturbances, mental status changes, edema, oliguria, dyspnea due to pulmonary edema, and abdominal pain. Blood pressure in severe preeclampsia is typically elevated to 160/110 mmHg or more.

HELLP Syndrome

HELLP syndrome is probably a clinical variant of preeclampsia. It is characterized by hemolysis, elevated liver enzymes, and low platelets. Patients usually complain of abdominal pain, especially epigastric and right upper quadrant pain. Because the blood pressure is not always elevated, HELLP syndrome should be considered in the evaluation of all pregnant women greater than 20 weeks' gestation with abdominal pain.

Eclampsia

Eclampsia is preeclampsia with seizures.

Diagnosis and Differential

Preeclampsia is a clinical diagnosis. The following laboratory abnormalities may be seen in severe preeclampsia: anemia, thrombocytopenia, elevated creatinine, elevated liver enzymes, elevated LDH. The HELLP variant is diagnosed by laboratory tests: schistocytes on peripheral smear, platelet count lower than 150,000/mL, and elevated aspartate aminotransferase and alanine aminotransferase levels. The differential diagnosis of preeclampsia includes worsening of preexisting hypertension, transient hypertension, renal disease, fatty liver disease of pregnancy, and coagulation disorders. Focused ultrasonography or a CT scan of the pelvis and abdomen should be done if concerns for subcapsular hematoma exist as this has a high risk of maternal and fetal mortality if ruptured.

Emergency Department Care and Disposition

1. Treat severe preeclampsia and eclampsia with **magnesium sulfate** loading dose of 4 to 6 g IV over 20 minutes, followed by a maintenance infusion of 1 to 2 g/h to prevent seizure. Monitor serum magnesium levels and reflexes.
2. Treat severe hypertension, greater than 160/110 mm Hg, with **labetalol** 20 mg IV initial bolus, followed by repeat boluses of 40 to 80 mg, if needed, to a maximum of 300 mg for blood pressure control or **hydralazine** 5.0 mg IV initially, followed by 5 to 10 mg every 10 minutes.
3. Consult an obstetrician emergently for severe preeclampsia or eclampsia.

4. Hospitalize all patients with a sustained systolic blood pressure ≥140 mmHg or diastolic ≥90 mmHg plus any symptoms of preeclampsia.
5. Definitive treatment requires delivery of the fetus.
6. In patients with mild preeclampsia, outpatient management may be appropriate after consultation with an obstetrician. Arrangements must be made for frequent laboratory evaluation and close fetal surveillance.

VAGINAL BLEEDING DURING THE SECOND HALF OF PREGNANCY

Placental abruption, placenta previa, and preterm labor are the most common causes of vaginal bleeding during the second half of pregnancy.

Clinical Features

Placental Abruption

Placental abruption, the premature separation of the placenta from the uterine wall, must be considered in all pregnant females near term who present with painful vaginal bleeding. Clinical features include vaginal bleeding, abdominal pain, uterine tenderness, hypertonic contractions, increased uterine tone, fetal distress, and, in severe cases, disseminated intravascular coagulation (DIC), and fetal and/or maternal death. Vaginal bleeding may be mild or severe, depending on whether the area of abruption communicates to the cervical os. Abruption of greater than 50% of the placenta usually results in fetal demise. Be aware of the possibility of abruption after trauma, even minor trauma.

Placenta Previa

Placenta previa is the implantation of the placenta over the cervical os. Clinical features include painless, bright red vaginal bleeding. The amount of bleeding is frequently large as opposed to normal "bloody show," when a small amount of bright red blood and mucous are passed.

Diagnosis and Differential

Transabdominal ultrasound should be obtained prior to performing speculum or digital pelvic examination to differentiate abruption placenta from placenta previa as it is contraindicated in previa. If transabdominal ultrasound is nondiagnostic, transvaginal ultrasound should be considered. The transvaginal ultrasound must be performed by someone experienced in transvaginal ultrasound, as positioning is extremely important. Ultrasound is very sensitive in detecting placenta previa but has limited sensitivity in diagnosing placental abruption.

Emergency Department Care and Disposition

1. Hemodynamic instability is managed with IV normal saline or packed red blood cells.
2. Obtain emergent obstetric consultation, complete blood count (CBC), type and cross, baseline coagulation studies, and electrolyte studies on all patients.
3. Obtain a DIC profile on patients with suspected placental abruption.

4. Give **Rh (D) immune globulin** 300 μg IM to Rh-negative patients.
5. Patients with placental abruption or placenta previa may need emergent cesarean delivery.
6. Do not use tocolytics in patients with suspected abruption.

Premature Rupture of Membranes

Premature rupture of membranes (PROM) is rupture of membranes before the onset of labor. Clinical presentation includes a rush of fluid or continuous leakage of fluid from the vagina. Diagnosis is confirmed by finding a pool of fluid in the posterior fornix with pH greater than 7.0 and a ferning pattern on smear. Sterile speculum examination may be done; however, **digital pelvic examination should be avoided because it increases the rate of infection and decreases the latent period from rupture until delivery.** Tests for chlamydia, gonorrhea, bacterial vaginosis, and group B *Streptococcus* should be performed. Management of PROM depends on gestational age and maturity of the fetus, condition of the fetus, concern for infection, and presence of other complicating factors. Antibiotics and steroids may be appropriate. An obstetrics consultation should be obtained to assist with treatment and admission decisions.

PRETERM LABOR

Clinical Features and Diagnosis

Preterm labor is defined as labor before 37 weeks' gestation. Clinical features include regular uterine contractions with effacement and dilatation of the cervix. Cervical fluid should be examined for possible PROM. Only after premature rupture of membranes and placenta previa have been excluded should digital examination be performed; use sterile gloves. Obtain tests for chlamydia, gonorrhea, bacterial vaginosis, and group B *Streptococcus*. Perform an ultrasound for fetal age, weight, anatomy, and amniotic fluid level if possible but obstetric consultation should not be delayed awaiting results.

Emergency Department Care and Disposition

1. Monitor mother and fetus.
2. Consult an obstetrician for admission and decision making regarding tocolytics.
3. If tocolytics are initiated, administer glucocorticoids to the mother to hasten fetal lung maturity if the gestational age is less than 34 weeks. **Dexamethasone** 6 mg IM is commonly used.
4. Do not use tocolytics if placental abruption is suspected.
5. Gestational age younger than 34 weeks is associated with poorer outcomes; if possible, the patient should be transferred to a tertiary care center with a high-risk intensive care unit.

POSTPARTUM HEMORRHAGE

The differential diagnosis of hemorrhage in the first postpartum day includes uterine atony, uterine rupture, laceration of the lower genital tract, retained placental tissue, uterine inversion, and coagulopathy. After the first 24 hours, retained products of conception, uterine polyps, or coagulopathy such as von

Willebrand disease are more likely causes. An enlarged and "doughy" uterus suggests uterine atony; a vaginal mass suggests an inverted uterus. Bleeding despite good uterine tone and size may indicate retained products of conception or uterine rupture. The vagina and cervix must be inspected for lacerations. The first priority of ED management is stabilization of the patient with crystalloid IV fluids and/or packed red blood cells, if needed. CBC, clotting studies, and type and cross must be obtained. Uterine atony is treated with uterine massage and **oxytocin** 20 units in one liter of normal saline IV at 200 mL/h. Minor lacerations may be repaired in the ED. Extensive lacerations, retained products of conception, uterine inversion, or uterine rupture require emergency operative treatment by the obstetrician.

POSTPARTUM ENDOMETRITIS

Postpartum endometritis is a polymicrobial infection with symptoms that usually begin several days after delivery. Clinical features include fever, lower abdominal pain, and foul-smelling lochia. Physical examination reveals uterine or cervical motion tenderness and discharge. CBC, urinalysis, and cervical cultures should be obtained. Admission for antibiotic treatment is indicated for patients who appear ill, have had a cesarean section, or who have underlying comorbidities. Antibiotic regimens for outpatients may include clindamycin or doxycycline. Do not use doxycycline in patients who are breastfeeding. Inpatient regimens include **clindamycin** 450 to 900 mg IV every 8 hours plus **gentamicin** 1.5 mg/kg IV every 8 hours or **cefoxitin** 1 to 2 g IV every 6 hours.

MASTITIS

Mastitis is cellulitis of the periglandular breast tissue. Clinical features include swelling, redness, and tender engorgement of the involved portion of the breast, with or without fever and chills. Milk stasis presents similarly, except it lacks erythema, fever, or chills. For cellulitis, initiate treatment with **dicloxacillin** 500 mg orally four times daily or **cephalexin** 500 mg orally four times daily. **Clindamycin** 300 mg PO every 6 hours may be used in patients with penicillin allergy or if concerns about MRSA exist. Oral analgesics may be needed. Patients should continue nursing on the affected breast. However, in cases of purulent discharge, the mother should pump and discard the milk rather than nurse. Differentiate mastitis from breast abscess using bedside ultrasound.

AMNIOTIC FLUID EMBOLISM

Amniotic fluid embolism is a sudden, catastrophic illness with mortality rates of 60% to 80%. Clinical features include sudden cardiovascular collapse with hypoxemia, pulmonary edema, altered mental status, seizures, and DIC along with sudden onset of fetal distress. Death can occur rapidly. Treatment is supportive; treat hypoxia, hypotension, and hypoperfusion.

FURTHER READING

For further reading in *Tintinalli's Emergency Medicine: A Comprehensive Study Guide*, 8th ed., see Chapter 100, "Maternal Emergencies After 20 Weeks of Pregnancy and in the Postpartum Period," by Janet Simmons Young.

CHAPTER 62

Emergency Delivery

Stacie Zelman

Precipitous delivery in an emergency setting can be a source of significant anxiety for an emergency physician. While emergency delivery is a relatively uncommon occurrence, careful preparation and education can help in avoiding serious complications, and result in a positive outcome for the mother and child.

CLINICAL FEATURES

Any pregnant woman who is beyond 20 weeks' gestation and appears to be in active labor should be evaluated expeditiously. Initial evaluation should include complete maternal vital signs and fetal heart monitoring. A persistently slow or fast fetal heart rate (less than 110 beats/min or greater than 160 beats/min) is an indicator of fetal distress. History includes frequency and time of onset of contractions, leakage of fluid, vaginal bleeding, estimated gestational age, and prenatal care. A focused physical examination should include an abdominal examination evaluating fundal height, abdominal or uterine tenderness, and fetal position. A bimanual or sterile speculum examination should be performed if no contraindications exist such as active vaginal bleeding. After the exam, place the patient in the left lateral decubitus position to prevent maternal hypotension.

False labor is characterized by irregular, brief contractions usually confined to the lower abdomen. These typically painless contractions, commonly called Braxton–Hicks contractions, are irregular in intensity and duration. True labor is characterized by painful, regular contractions of steadily increasing intensity and duration leading to progressive cervical dilatation. True labor typically begins in the fundal region and upper abdomen and radiates into the pelvis and lower back.

DIAGNOSIS AND DIFFERENTIAL

Patients without vaginal bleeding should be assessed with sterile speculum and bimanual examinations to evaluate the progression of labor, cervical dilation, and rupture of membranes. Patients with active vaginal bleeding require initial evaluation with ultrasound to rule out placenta previa. Spontaneous rupture of membranes typically occurs with a gush of clear or blood-tinged fluid. If ruptured membranes are suspected, a sterile speculum examination should be performed and amniotic fluid obtained from the fornix or vaginal vault. Amniotic fluid is alkaline, will stain Nitrazine paper dark blue and will "fern" if dried on a slide. The presence of meconium in amniotic fluid should be noted. Avoid digital examinations in the preterm patient in whom prolongation of gestation is desired as even one examination increases the chance of infection.

EMERGENCY DEPARTMENT CARE AND DISPOSITION

If the cervix is dilated in a woman experiencing active contractions, further transport, even short distances, may be hazardous. Preparations should be made for emergency delivery. Assess fetal position by physical examination, and confirm by ultrasound, if possible. Place the patient in the dorsal lithotomy position. Notify an obstetrician, if one is available.

Emergency Delivery Procedure (Fig. 62-1)

1. **Control of the delivery** of the neonate is the major challenge.
   a. As the **infant's head** emerges from the introitus, support the perineum with a sterile towel placed along the inferior portion of the perineum with one hand while supporting the fetal head with the other.
   b. Exert mild counter-pressure to prevent the rapid expulsion of the fetal head, which may lead to third- or fourth-degree perineal tears.
   c. As the infant's head presents, use the inferior hand to control the fetal chin while keeping the superior hand on the crown of the head, supporting the delivery.
   d. Ask the mother to breathe through contractions rather than bearing down and attempting to push the baby out rapidly.
2. After delivery of the head, palpate the neck for the presence of a **nuchal cord** (may be present in up to 35% of deliveries).
   a. If the cord is loose, reduce it over the infant's head; delivery may then proceed as usual.
   b. If the cord is tightly wound, clamp it in the most accessible area using two clamps in close proximity and cut to allow delivery of the infant.
3. After delivery of the head, the head will restitute or turn to one side or the other.
   a. As the head rotates, hands are placed on either side, providing gentle downward traction to deliver the anterior shoulder.
   b. Guide the shoulders upward, delivering the posterior shoulder and allowing the remainder of the infant to be delivered.
4. Place the posterior (left) hand underneath the infant's axilla before delivering the rest of the body. Use the anterior hand to grasp the infant's ankles and ensure a firm grip.
5. Wrap the infant in a towel and stimulate him or her while drying.
6. Double clamp the umbilical cord and cut with sterile scissors.
7. Place the infant in a warm incubator, where postnatal care may be provided and calculate **Apgar scores** at 1 and 5 minutes after delivery. Scoring includes general color, tone, heart rate, respiratory effort, and reflexes.
8. If an **episiotomy** is necessary (e.g., with a breech presentation), it may be performed as follows:
   a. Inject a solution of 5 to 10 mL of 1% **lidocaine** with a small-gauge needle into the posterior fourchette and perineum.
   b. While protecting the infant's head, make a 2- to 3-cm cut with scissors to extend the vaginal opening at the midline or 45 degrees from midline.
   c. Support the incision with manual pressure from below, taking care not to allow the incision to extend into the rectum (less likely with the mediolateral incision).

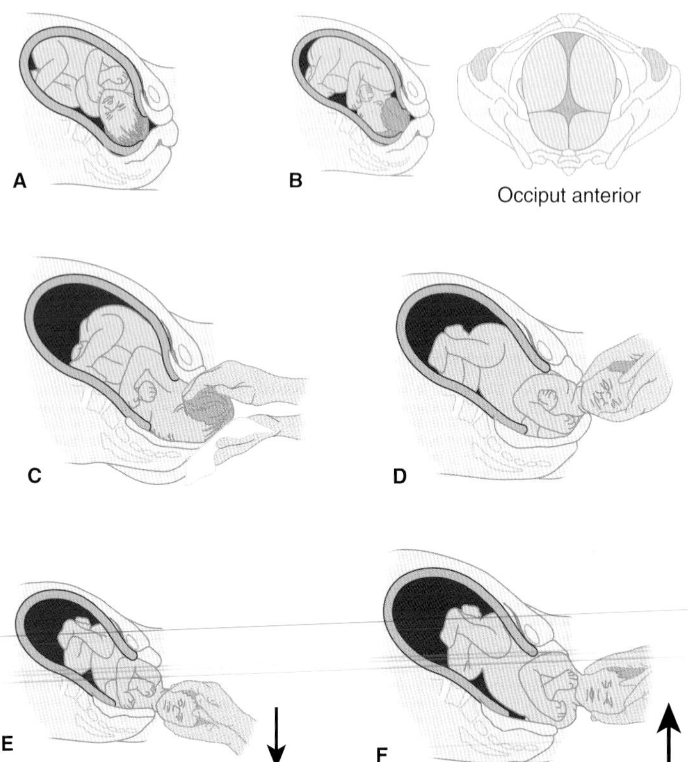

FIGURE 62-1. Movements of normal delivery. Mechanism of labor and delivery for vertex presentations. **A.** Engagement, flexion, and descent. **B.** Internal rotation. **C.** Extension and delivery of the head. After delivery of the head, the neck is checked for encirclement by the umbilical cord. **D.** External rotation, bringing the thorax into the anteroposterior diameter of the pelvis. **E.** Delivery of the anterior shoulder. **F.** Delivery of the posterior shoulder. Note that after delivery, the head is supported and used to gently guide delivery of the shoulder. Traction should be minimized.

CORD PROLAPSE

If bimanual examination shows a **palpable, pulsating cord:**

a. Do not remove the examining hand; use the hand to elevate the presenting fetal part to reduce compression of the cord.
b. Immediate obstetric assistance is necessary, as a **cesarean section is indicated**.
c. Keep the examining hand in the vagina while the patient is transported and prepped for surgery to prevent further compression of the cord by the fetal head. Do not attempt to reduce cord.

SHOULDER DYSTOCIA

Initially recognized after the delivery of the fetal head, when routine downward traction is insufficient to deliver the anterior shoulder. The anterior shoulder is trapped behind the pubic symphysis.

a. After delivery of the infant's head, the head retracts tightly against the perineum ("Turtle sign").
b. Upon recognizing shoulder dystocia, suction the infant's nose and mouth and call for assistance to position the mother in the extreme lithotomy position, with legs sharply flexed up to the abdomen (**McRoberts maneuver**) and held by the mother or an assistant.
c. Next, an assistant should apply downward suprapubic pressure to disimpact the anterior shoulder from the pubic symphysis.
d. Do not apply fundal pressure because this will further force the shoulder against the pelvic rim.
e. A **Woods Corkscrewmaneuver** may be attempted—place fingertips behind the anterior shoulder and in back of the posterior shoulder of the infant, and rotate the shoulder girdle 180°.

BREECH PRESENTATION

The primary concern with breech presentation is head entrapment.

a. Breech presentations may be classified as **frank, complete, incomplete, or footling**.
b. In any breech delivery, immediate obstetric consultation should be requested.
c. **Frank and complete breech presentations:**
    - Serve as a dilating wedge nearly as well as the fetal head, and delivery may proceed in an uncomplicated fashion.
    - Main point is to allow the delivery to progress spontaneously. This lets the presenting portion of the fetus to dilate the cervix maximally.
d. Consult obstetrical texts for a detailed description of maneuvers for breech delivery.
e. **Footling and incomplete breech positions** are not considered safe for vaginal delivery because of the possibility of cord prolapse or incomplete dilatation of the cervix.

POSTPARTUM CARE

The placenta should be allowed to separate spontaneously and assisted with gentle traction. Aggressive traction on the cord risks uterine inversion, tearing of the cord, or disruption of the placenta, which can result in severe vaginal bleeding. After removal of the placenta, gently massage the uterus to promote contraction. Infuse **oxytocin** 10 to 40 U/1000 mL NS at a moderate rate to maintain uterine contraction. Oxytocin may also be given as 10 U IM. Episiotomy or laceration repair may be delayed until an experienced obstetrician is able to close the laceration and inspect the patient for fourth-degree (rectovaginal) tears.

FURTHER READING

For further reading in *Tintinalli's Emergency Medicine: A Comprehensive Study Guide*, 8th ed., see Chapter 101, "Emergency Delivery," by Sarah Elisabeth Frasure.

CHAPTER 63

Vulvovaginitis

Robert R. Cooney

Causes of vulvovaginitis include infections, irritants, allergies, reaction to foreign bodies, and atrophy. The normal vaginal flora help maintain an acidic pH between 3.8 and 4.5, which decreases pathogen growth.

BACTERIAL VAGINOSIS

Bacterial vaginosis (BV) is the most common cause of malodorous vaginal discharge. However, up to 50% of infected women are asymptomatic. BV occurs when vaginal lactobacilli are replaced by anaerobes such as *Gardnerella vaginalis*, *Mycoplasma*, and *Ureaplasma*.

Clinical Features

The most common symptom is malodorous or "fishy smelling" vaginal discharge. Vaginal irritation, excoriation, fissures, and edema are uncommon. A combination of history, vaginal examination, and point-of-care testing confirm the diagnosis.

Diagnosis and Differential

The diagnosis can be made if three of the following four criteria are present: (1) vaginal discharge, (2) vaginal pH greater than 4.5, (3) positive amine test (fishy odor when 10% KOH is added to the discharge), and (4) clue cells seen on saline wet preparation.

Emergency Department Care and Disposition

Treat with **metronidazole** 500 mg PO twice daily for 7 days. **Clindamycin 2%** intravaginal cream at night for 7 days or **metronidazole 0.75%** intravaginal gel daily for 5 days are alternatives. Treatment is not recommended for male partners or asymptomatic women. To avoid a disulfram-like reaction, patients treated with metronidazole should refrain from alcohol use during treatment and for 24 hours after ending treatment.

All symptomatic pregnant women should be treated, and women at high risk of preterm labor should be considered for treatment. Preferred treatment in pregnancy is **metronidazole** 250 mg PO twice daily for 7 days.

CANDIDA VAGINITIS

Candida albicans is the second most common cause of infectious vaginitis. Conditions that promote *Candida* vaginitis include systemic antibiotics, diabetes, pregnancy, hormone replacement therapy, and birth control pills. Incidence is decreased in postmenopausal patients. Candidiasis is not typically considered a sexually transmitted disease, though it can be transmitted sexually.

Clinical Features

The most common symptom of *Candida* vaginitis is pruritus. Other symptoms include vaginal discharge, external dysuria, and dyspareunia. Exam may reveal vulvar and vaginal edema, erythema, and a thick "cottage cheese" discharge.

Diagnosis and Differential

Diagnosis is confirmed if vaginal pH is 4 to 4.5 and budding yeast or pseudohyphae are present on microscopy. Ten percent KOH dissolves vaginal epithelial cells, leaving yeast buds and pseudohyphae intact and easier to see. Use of KOH increases the sensitivity to 80%, with a specificity approaching 100%.

Emergency Department Care and Disposition

Single-dose treatment with **fluconazole**, 150 mg PO, is as effective as topical treatments. Almost all topically applied azoles are equally efficacious and available over-the-counter. Treatment options include **clotrimazole**, **butoconazole**, **miconazole**, **terconazole**, and **tioconazole** in several strengths and formulations. Pregnant patients should avoid oral fluconazole and instead use intravaginal agents for 7 days. For nonpregnant patients with complicated candidiasis, **fluconazole** 150 mg PO is given on days 1 and 3.

TRICHOMONAS VAGINITIS

Trichomoniasis is a common sexually transmitted disease caused by the protozoan *Trichomonas vaginalis*.

Clinical Features

Presenting symptoms include a frothy, malodorous vaginal discharge, pruritus, and vaginal irritation. However, up to 50% of women harboring the organism are asymptomatic.

Diagnosis and Differential

Saline wet prep shows motile, pear-shaped, flagellated trichomonads. Microscopy should be performed immediately after obtaining the sample or the organisms may lose motility. The sensitivity of microscopy is 60% to 70%. The sensitivity of culture is 95% but results are not readily available in the ED. New point-of-care PCR-based tests are now available as well.

Emergency Department Care and Disposition

The treatment of choice for trichomoniasis is **metronidazole** 2 g single oral dose or **tinidazole** 2 g single oral dose. **Metronidazole** 500 mg twice daily for 7 days is recommended for patients who fail single-dose therapy. Metronidazole gel is much less efficacious and thus not recommended for use. Sexual partners should be treated to avoid retransmission of disease. Patients should also be counseled to abstain from sexual activity until treatment course is completed and they are asymptomatic.

CONTACT VULVOVAGINITIS

Common causes of contact vulvovaginitis include douches, soaps, bubble baths, deodorants, perfumes, feminine hygiene products, topical antibiotics, and tight undergarments. Patients complain of perineal burning, itching, and local swelling. Examination findings may include redness, edema, and ulceration. Vaginal pH changes may promote overgrowth of *Candida*, obscuring the primary problem.

Try to identify the precipitating agent and rule out infectious causes. Most cases resolve spontaneously when the precipitant is withdrawn. For more severe reactions, cool sitz baths, compresses with Burow's solution, and topical corticosteroids may help. Oral antihistamines are drying but may be helpful if a true allergy is identified. Concomitant *Candida* infections should be treated as previously discussed.

VAGINAL FOREIGN BODIES

Patients with a vaginal foreign body present with chronic, foul-smelling or bloody discharge. In younger girls, common items include toilet paper, toys, and small household objects. Items seen in adults include a forgotten or irretrievable tampon, packets of illegal drugs, or items used for sexual stimulation. Removal of the object is usually curative.

ATROPHIC VAGINITIS

After menopause, the lack of estrogen stimulation leads to vaginal mucosal atrophy with a subsequent loss of resistance to minor trauma or infection. Bleeding can occur. The vaginal pH also increases, and subsequent changes in the vaginal flora can predispose to bacterial infection with purulent discharge. Treatment consists primarily of topical estrogen creams. Estrogen creams should not be prescribed in the emergency department for women with prior reproductive tract cancer or postmenopausal bleeding.

BARTHOLIN GLAND CYST AND ABSCESS

Bartholin glands are located in the labia minora at the 4 and 8 o'clock position. Obstruction of the gland may result in cyst or abscess formation. Patients present with pain and swelling that develops over several days. Exam will reveal pain, induration, and fluctuance. Patients without an abscess may be treated with broad-spectrum antibiotics, analgesics, and sitz baths. In addition, patients with an abscess require an incision and drainage with the placement of a Word catheter and referral for definitive surgical management.

FURTHER READING

For further reading in *Tintinalli's Emergency Medicine: A Comprehensive Study Guide*, 8th ed., see Chapter 102, "Vulvovaginitis," by Ciara J. Barclay-Buchanan and Melissa A. Barton.

CHAPTER 64

Pelvic Inflammatory Disease

Abigail D. Hankin

Pelvic inflammatory disease (PID) comprises a spectrum of infections of the female upper reproductive tract, including endometritis, salpingitis, tubo-ovarian abscess, and pelvic peritonitis. *Neisseria gonorrhoeae* and *Chlamydiatrachomatis* are frequently isolated pathogens; however, many other microorganisms have been associated with PID, including vaginal flora, gram-negative rods, streptococci, and mycoplasmas. Risk factors for PID include age (teenagers are at greatest risk), multiple sexual partners, a new sexual partner within the past 30 days, presence of other sexually transmitted diseases, and intrauterine device insertion within the prior 3 weeks. PID occurs less commonly in pregnancy, but is associated with increased maternal morbidity and preterm labor. Complications of PID include significantly increased risk for ectopic pregnancy, infertility, and chronic pain, even after only a single episode of PID.

CLINICAL FEATURES

Clinical diagnosis of PID is complicated due to the wide variation in symptoms and clinical findings. Common presenting complaints include lower abdominal pain (seen in >90%), vaginal discharge (75%), vaginal bleeding, urinary discomfort, fever, nausea, and vomiting. Many women with PID may have nonspecific or very subtle symptoms. Physical exam may show lower abdominal tenderness, cervical motion tenderness, or uterine/adnexal tenderness. Mucopurulent cervicitis is a common finding, and its absence should prompt consideration of alternative causes of the patient's symptoms.

DIAGNOSIS AND DIFFERENTIAL

Given the clinical variability in the diagnosis of PID and the potential sequelae of delayed treatment, the United States Centers for Disease Control and Prevention recommends empiric treatment for PID based on the minimal criteria listed in Table 64-1. No single laboratory test is highly sensitive or specific for PID. Laboratory evaluation should include a pregnancy test, wet preparation of vaginal secretions, and DNA probe or culture for *N. gonorroheae* and *Chlamydia trachomatis*. Treatment, when indicated, should not be delayed pending test results.

The differential diagnosis includes gastroenteritis, diverticulitis, ectopic pregnancy, spontaneous or septic abortion, ovarian cyst, pyelonephritis, and renal colic.

EMERGENCY DEPARTMENT CARE AND DISPOSITION

1. Treatment guidelines from the Centers for Disease Control and Prevention are outlined in Tables 64-2 and 64-3. Patients with mild to moderate symptoms may be treated with oral therapy as outpatients with appropriate oral antibiotics and adequate analgesia .

TABLE 64-1 Diagnostic Criteria for Pelvic Inflammatory Disease

Group 1: Minimum criteria. Empiric treatment if no other cause to explain findings.
Uterine or adnexal tenderness
Cervical motion tenderness
Group 2: Additional criteria improving diagnostic specificity.
Oral temperature >101°F (38.3°C)
Abnormal cervical or vaginal mucopurulent secretions
Elevated erythrocyte sedimentation rate
Elevated C-reactive protein level
Laboratory evidence of cervical infection with *Neisseria gonorrhoeae* or *Chlamydia trachomatis* (i.e., culture or DNA probe techniques)
Group 3: Specific criteria for PID based on procedures that may be appropriate for some patients.
Laparoscopic confirmation
Transvaginal US (or MRI) showing thickened, fluid-filled tubes with or without free pelvic fluid or tubo-ovarian complex
Endometrial biopsy results showing endometritis

Source: Reproduced with permission from Centers for Disease Control and Prevention; Workowski KA, Berman SM. Sexually transmitted diseases treatment guidelines, 2010. *MMWR Recommend Rep.* 2010;59(RR-12):12.

2. Suggested criteria for admission include toxic appearance, inability to tolerate oral medication, nausea and vomiting, inability to exclude alternative diagnoses or surgical emergency, failure to respond to outpatient management, pregnancy, immunosuppression, concern for noncompliance, and tubo-ovarian abscess.
3. Outpatients should be reevaluated in the emergency department or by their gynecologist within 72 hours of emergency department discharge.
4. Provide preventative counseling and test or refer for HIV testing. The patient and their sexual partner(s) must complete the full treatment course before resuming sexual activity to prevent reinfection.

TABLE 64-2 Parenteral Treatment Regimens for Pelvic Inflammatory Disease

Cefotetan, 2 g IV every 12 h, or cefoxitin, 2 g IV every 6 h
plus
Doxycycline, 100 mg PO or IV every 12 h*
or
Clindamycin, 900 mg IV every 8 h
plus
Gentamicin, 2 mg/kg IV or IM loading dose, followed by gentamicin, 1.5 mg/kg every 8 h maintenance dose†
Alternative Parenteral Regimen (limited data on effectiveness)
Ampicillin/sulbactam, 3 g IV every 6 h
plus
Doxycycline, 100 mg PO or IV every 12 h*

*PO doxycycline has the same bioavailability as IV doxycycline and avoids painful infusion.

†Gentamicin dosing may be 3 to 5 mg/kg every 24 h.

Source: Reproduced with permission from Centers for Disease Control and Prevention; Workowski KA, Berman SM. Sexually transmitted diseases treatment guidelines, 2010. *MMWR Recomm Rep.* 2010;59(RR-12):12.

TABLE 64-3 Oral and Outpatient Treatment Regimens for Pelvic Inflammatory Disease

Ceftriaxone, 250 mg IM once, *or* cefoxitin, 2 g IM once, *and* probenecid, 1 g PO once administered concurrently *or* Other parenteral third-generation cephalosporin (e.g., ceftizoxime or cefotaxime) *plus* Doxycycline, 100 mg PO twice a day for 14 days *with or without* Metronidazole, 500 mg PO twice a day for 14 days
If parenteral cephalosporin therapy is not feasible and community prevalence of fluoroquinolone resistance is low: Levofloxacin, 500 mg PO, *or* ofloxacin, 400 mg twice daily every day for 14 days *with or without* Metronidazole, 500 mg PO twice a day for 14 days

Note: Other parenteral third-generation cephalosporins can be substituted for ceftriaxone or cefoxitin. Since the Centers for Disease Control and Prevention guidelines were published in 2006, clinically significant resistance to the fluoroquinolones (6.7% of infections in heterosexual men, an 11-fold increase from 0.6% in 2001) has emerged in the United States. Fluoroquinolone antibiotics are no longer recommended to treat gonorrhea in the United States. Fluoroquinolones may be an alternative treatment option for disseminated gonococcal infection if antimicrobial susceptibility can be documented.

FURTHER READING

For further reading in *Tintinalli's Emergency Medicine: A Comprehensive Study Guide*, 8th edition, see Chapter 103, "Pelvic Inflamatory Disease," by Suzanne M. Shepherd, Brian Weiss, and William H. Shoff.

Complications of Gynecologic Procedures

Robert R. Cooney

The most common reasons for emergency department visits during the postoperative period after gynecologic procedures are pain, fever, and vaginal bleeding. A focused but thorough evaluation should be performed, including sterile speculum and bimanual examination. Consultation with the gynecologist who performed the procedure is indicated.

COMPLICATIONS OF ENDOSCOPIC PROCEDURES

Laparoscopy

The major complications associated with laparoscopy are thermal injury of the bowel, viscus perforation, hemorrhage, vascular injury, ureteral or bladder injuries, incisional hernia, and wound dehiscence. Bowel injury should be suspected if pain is greater than expected after laparoscopy. Thermal injury is easily missed due to delayed development of symptoms for several days to weeks postoperatively. Patients with the above typically present with bilateral lower abdominal pain, fever, elevated white blood cell count, and peritonitis. X-rays can show an ileus or free air under the diaphragm. Early gynecology consultation should be obtained.

Hysteroscopy

Complications of hysteroscopy are rare but include uterine perforation, postoperative bleeding, fluid overload from absorption of distention media, gas embolism, and infection. Bleeding may originate from the uterus after resection or the cervix due to lacerations or tears. Management includes packing of the vaginal vault and consultation with a gynecologist.

OTHER COMPLICATIONS OF GYNECOLOGIC PROCEDURES

Vaginal Cuff Cellulitis

Cuff cellulitis, a common early complication after hysterectomy, is an infection of the contiguous retroperitoneal space immediately above the vaginal apex and the surrounding soft tissue. Patients typically present with fever, abdominal pain, pelvic pain, back pain, and purulent vaginal discharge. Cuff tenderness and induration plus purulent discharge are prominent during the gynecologic exam. Abscesses are rare, but will present as a fluctuant mass near the cuff approximately 10 to 14 days postoperatively. Treat with broad-spectrum antibiotics. Recommended regimens include **imipenem-cilastatin**, **gentamicin and clindamycin**, or **ciprofloxacin** plus **metronidazole**. Admit for continuation of antibiotics and consideration of drainage by interventional radiology.

Postoperative Wound Infection

Patients with wound infections generally present with fever and increasing pain at the surgical site. Onset is typically within 2 weeks of surgery. Exam will reveal erythema, tenderness, induration, and possibly incisional drainage. Treatment includes drainage and antibiotic treatment directed at methicillin-resistant *Staphylococcus aureus* and streptococci. Patients with invasive infections should be admitted.

Ureteral Injury

Ureteral injury can occur during abdominal hysterectomy, resulting from crushing, transecting, or ligating trauma. These patients present soon after surgery with flank pain. They may also complain of fever, costovertebral angle tenderness, and hematuria. The workup includes a urinalysis and a CT scan with IV contrast or an intravenous pyelogram to evaluate for obstruction. These patients should be admitted for ureteral catheterization and possible repair, although delayed repair after percutaneous nephrostomy is also acceptable.

Vesicovaginal Fistula

Vesicovaginal fistulas can occur after abdominal hysterectomy. Patients typically present 10 to 14 days following surgery with a watery vaginal discharge. Placing a cotton tampon in the vagina and instilling methylene blue through a urinary catheter can confirm the diagnosis. The tampon should stain within 20 minutes. Management includes placement of a Foley catheter and prompt gynecologic consultation.

Postconization Bleeding

The most common complication associated with loop electrocautery, laser ablation, and cold-knife conization of the cervix is bleeding, which can be rapid and excessive. Delayed hemorrhage can occur 1 to 2 weeks postoperatively. Direct visualization of the bleeding site is required. Applying Monsel's solution, direct pressure for 5 minutes with a large cotton swab, or cauterization with silver nitrate is a reasonable first step. If unsuccessful, the bleeding site may be better visualized and treated in the OR.

Septic Pelvic Thrombophlebitis

Septic pelvic thrombophlebitis is a rare complication that may follow cesarean delivery or hysterectomy. The presenting complaint is typically abdominal pain and fever. CT and MRI aid in the diagnosis but do not exclude the disease if negative. Patients are admitted for anticoagulation and IV antibiotics.

Induced Abortion

Complications associated with induced abortion may be characterized by time of occurence. These include uterine perforation, cervical lacerations, retained products of conception, and postabortal endometritis (Table 65-1). Patients with retained products of conception usually present with excessive bleeding and abdominal pain. Pelvic examination reveals an enlarged and tender uterus with an open cervical os. A pelvic ultrasound should be

TABLE 65-1 Complications Associated with Induced Abortion

Timing	Complication	Possible Etiologies
Immediate complications: within 24 h postprocedure	Bleeding, pain	Uterine perforation, cervical lacerations
Delayed complications: between 24 h and 4 weeks postprocedure	Bleeding	Retained products of conception, postabortive endometritis
Late complications: >4 weeks postprocedure	Amenorrhea, psychological problems, Rh isoimmunization	—

done to confirm the diagnosis. Treatment is dilatation and curettage or medical management with misoprostol. Endometritis can occur with or without retained products of conception and is treated with antibiotics. Women who are Rh negative require **$\mathbf{Rh_0}$ immunoglobulin**, 300 μg IM, after spontaneous or induced abortion.

Assisted Reproductive Technology

Complications related to ultrasound-guided aspiration of oocytes include ovarian hyperstimulation syndrome, pelvic infection, intraperitoneal bleeding, and adnexal torsion. Ovarian hyperstimulation syndrome can be a life-threatening complication of assisted reproduction. Mild cases present with abdominal distention, ovarian enlargement, and weight gain. In severe cases, patients have rapid weight gain, tense ascites from third spacing of fluid into the abdomen, pleural effusions, hemodynamic instability, oliguria or electrolyte abnormalities. Renal impairment and increased coagulability may also be noted. Avoid bimanual pelvic exam to prevent rupturing the ovaries. Workup includes CBC, electrolytes, liver enzymes, coagulation studies, and type and crossmatch. Initiate IV volume replacement and consult with gynecology for admission.

Postembolization Syndrome

Postembolization syndrome consists of postprocedure pelvic pain, fever, and leukocytosis lasting up to 7 days caused by myometrial and fibroid ischemia and necrosis after uterine fibroid embolization. Exam may reveal vaginal discharge of fibroid expulsion. Evaluate patients for other causes of fever and provide pain control. Patients with inadequate pain control or those in whom an infection is present may require admission.

FURTHER READING

For further reading in *Tintinalli's Emergency Medicine: A Comprehensive Study Guide*, 8th ed., see Chapter 105, "Complications of Gynecologic Procedures," by Nikki Waller.

SECTION 9

Pediatrics

CHAPTER 66 Fever and Serious Bacterial Illness in Children

Todd P. Chang

FEVER AND SERIOUS BACTERIAL ILLNESS (SBI)

Fever is the most common pediatric chief complaint presenting to an emergency department (ED) and accounts for 30% of outpatient visits. Infants and children are at relatively high risk for serious bacterial illness (SBI), which includes urinary tract infection (UTI), pneumonia, bacteremia or sepsis, and meningitis—in decreasing prevalence. Neonates are at the highest risk due to their immature immune response, while infants from 1 to 3 months of age gradually transition to the lower risk profile of older infants and children. The incidence of UTI is 5% overall in children 2 months to 2 years, with a prevalence of 3% to 8% in all febrile children visiting an ED. Widespread vaccination has dropped the incidence of occult bacteremia for children 3 to 36 months of age to 0.5% to 0.7%, with further decreases expected with the 13-valent pneumococcal conjugate vaccine. Meningitis risk decreases from about 1% in the first month of life to <0.1% later in infancy and childhood.

Clinical Features

In the neonate or infant <3 months of age, the threshold for concerning fever is 38°C (100.4°F); in infants and children 3 to 36 months old, the threshold is 39°C (102.2°F). In general, higher temperatures are associated with a higher incidence of SBI. Immature development may make reliable examination of younger infants difficult. Persistent crying, inability to console, poor feeding, or temperature instability may be the only findings suggestive of an SBI. In the neonate, there may not be any findings other than fever.

Diagnosis and Differential

Infants <3 months

An ill-appearing infant should be managed aggressively for SBI, with full sepsis evaluation, parenteral antibiotics, and admission, but a well-appearing febrile infant less than 3 months of age presents a challenge because history and physical examination are rarely helpful in diagnosing or excluding SBI in this age group. Meningismus is rarely present; rales may not be appreciated without strong negative inspiratory forces; and bacteremia occurs even in the well-appearing infant. A history of cough, tachypnea, or hypoxemia (by pulse oximetry), however, should alert the examiner to a possible lower respiratory tract infection and consideration of the diagnosis of pneumonia.

All febrile infants 0 to 28 days of age should receive full SBI evaluations, admission, and empiric antibiotic treatment. Antibiotic coverage in this age group includes **ampicillin** 50 mg/kg IV for *Listeria monocytogenes* and either **gentamicin** 2.5 mg/kg IV or **cefotaxime** 50 mg/kg IV for other common organisms. Avoid using ceftriaxone in this age group. Sepsis testing includes complete blood count (CBC), blood culture, urinalysis and urine culture, and lumbar puncture for CSF indices and culture. Obtain a chest radiograph if any respiratory signs described above are present, and order stool studies if the infant has diarrhea.

Febrile infants 29 to 90 days old without a focal source may be stratified to low or high risk of SBI using one of three classic criteria: Rochester Criteria, Boston Criteria, or Philadelphia Protocol. To meet low-risk SBI status, the infant must be well-appearing with a normal urinalysis and normal White Blood Cell (WBC) count, between 5,000/mm^3 and 15,000/mm^3 for the Rochester and Philadelphia, and 5,000/mm^3 and 20,000/mm^3 for Boston. A negative CSF (WBC $<$ 10 per hpf in Boston and WBC $<$ 8 per hpf in Philadelphia) is also required for Boston and Philadelphia, and each criteria set has other parameters to complete a low-risk status (Table 66-1). Obtain a chest radiograph for infants with a suggestion of lower respiratory tract disease. Although there is evidence to support the use of any of these three criteria, the overall incidence of bacteremia is dropping due to two factors: empiric antibiotic treatment of women testing positive for Group B streptococcus during the third trimester and the effects from herd immunity from *Haemophilus* and pneumococcal vaccines.

All ill-appearing infants should receive parenteral antibiotic therapy (Table 66-2) and be admitted to the hospital. Infants older than 28 days at low risk for SBI may be managed conservatively as inpatients with **ceftriaxone** 50 mg/kg IM/IV pending cultures; as inpatients without antibiotics; as outpatients with ceftriaxone; or as outpatients without antibiotics. The key deciding factor should be the physician's comfort level and the ability for close follow-up, typically within 12 to 24 hours. If antibiotics are administered (inpatient or outpatient), obtain CSF and urine and blood cultures prior to administration of antibiotics.

Well-appearing febrile infants between the ages of 29 and 90 days with an identifiable viral source of infection (e.g., respiratory syncytial virus [RSV] or influenza) should have urinary tract infection (UTI) and bacteremia ruled out before being discharged from the ED. Chest radiographs should be obtained at the discretion of the clinician, but are not indicated for well-appearing infants over 29 days with RSV. Consider deferring lumbar puncture if a virus is identified as the cause of the symptoms.

Some evidence supports the use of serum biomarkers such as C-reactive protein and procalcitonin to differentiate SBI from viral illness.

TABLE 66-1 Comparison of Low-Risk Rochester Criteria, Philadelphia Protocol, and Boston Criteria for Assessment of Fever in Well-Appearing Neonates and Infants*

Low-Risk Criteria for Serious Bacterial Infection*	Rochester Criteria	Philadelphia Protocol	Boston Criteria
Fever	T ≥ 38°C (100.4°F)	T ≥ 38.2°C (100.8°F)	T ≥ 38°C (100.4°F)
Age	≤ 60 days	29–56 days	28–89 days
Past medical history	Term infant ≥ 37 weeks gestation No perinatal or postnatal antibiotics No treatment for jaundice No chronic illnesses or admissions Not hospitalized longer than mother	No immunodeficiency syndrome	No immunizations within 48 h No recent antibiotics
Physical examination	Well appearing Unremarkable examination	Same	Same
Laboratory values			
Blood count	WBC ≥ 5000, ≤ 15,000/mm^3 Absolute band count ≤ 1500/mm^3	WBC ≤ 15,000/mm^3 Band-to-neutrophil ratio ≤ 0.2	WBC ≤ 20,000/mm^3
Urinalysis	WBC ≤ 10 per high-power field	WBC ≤ 10 per high-power field	WBC ≤ 10 per high-power field
Stool	WBC ≤ 5 per high-power field	–	–
Lumbar puncture and cerebrospinal fluid findings	None	WBC ≤ 8 per high-power field	WBC ≤ 10 per high-power field Negative Gram stain
Chest radiograph	None	Negative	Negative if obtained
Comments	Excluded lumbar puncture, so number of missed meningitis cases is unknown. UTIs missed in those with negative urinalysis. The least sensitive of the low-risk criteria.	Sensitivity of low-risk criteria for SBI 98%; specificity 44%; PPV 14%; NPV 99.7%	5% of low-risk neonates and infants had SBI (8 bacteremia, 8 UTI, 10 bacterial gastroenteritis); 96% sensitive to ceftriaxone

Abbreviations: NPV, negative predictive value; PPV, positive predictive value; SBI, serious bacterial illness; T, temperature; UTI, urinary tract infection.

*Any single deviation from the criteria is interpreted as failure of low-risk criteria.

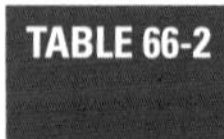

TABLE 66-2 Suggested Guidelines for the Evaluation and Management of Neonates, Infants, and Children with Fever Who Are Well Appearing, Have Had All Relevant Immunizations, and Have No Clinical Source for Fever

Age Group	Evaluation	Treatment
Neonate, 0–28 days* of age, ≥ 38°C (100.4°F) SBI incidence of ill appearing: 13%–21%; if not ill appearing: < 5%	CBC and blood culture *and* Urinalysis and urine culture *and* CSF cell count, Gram stain, and culture Chest x-ray is optional, if no respiratory symptoms Stool culture if diarrhea is present	*Admit and treat with:* Parenteral antibiotic therapy with ampicillin, 50 mg/kg, and either cefotaxime, 50 mg/kg, or gentamicin, 2.5 mg/kg

Abbreviations: CSF, cerebrospinal fluid; SBI, serious bacterial illness; UTI, urinary tract infection.

*For preterm infants, count age by estimated postconception date and not by actual delivery date for the first 90 days of life.

Infants 3 to 36 Months

Physical examination findings become more reliable with increasing age, though meningeal signs remain unreliable up to 2 years old. Viral illnesses account for most febrile illnesses in this age group. Diagnostic testing should be guided by clinical findings, including ill appearance; however, UTIs are still prevalent in this age group, even with no focal symptoms besides fever. Females prior to toilet training, circumcised boys younger than 6 months of age, and uncircumcised boys under 1 year of age are at risk for occult UTI. Obtain both a urinalysis and urine culture (by catheterization or suprapubic tap) if a source for the fever is not otherwise identified. Consider CBC and blood culture for bacteremia/sepsis and CSF studies for meningitis, although these are much less common.

Older Febrile Children

The risk for bacteremia in children older than 3 years is <0.2%. CBC and blood cultures are not routinely recommended in immunized older children with fever. Etiologies to consider in older febrile children include viral infections, streptococcal pharyngitis, pneumonia, and sinusitis. Testing is directed by clinical presentation.

Emergency Department Care and Disposition

For the management of pneumonia, see Chapter **71**; for the management of UTI, see Chapter **75**; and infections of the ears, nose, and throat are covered in Chapter **68**. Fever is not typically harmful to children, although it makes children uncomfortable and may potentiate seizures. Counsel parents against "fever phobia." To reduce a fever:

1. Remove excessive clothing and blankets to increase heat loss through radiation.
2. Administer **acetaminophen** 15 mg/kg PO/PR every 4 hours (up to 5 times a day).
3. Consider **ibuprofen** 10 mg/kg PO in children older than 1 year of age; the dose can be repeated every 6 to 8 hours (maximum of 40 mg/kg in 24 hours), and can be given concurrently with acetaminophen.

Patients who are called to return to the ED for evaluation of positive blood cultures require repeat evaluation. Patients with positive blood cultures without contaminants should be hospitalized and treated with parenteral antibiotics. Well-appearing afebrile children already on antibiotics should complete the course of therapy. If the patient is afebrile, clinically well, without a focus of infection, and not currently on antibiotics, repeat testing or treatment is not usually necessary. If the child with a positive blood culture remains febrile or continues to appear ill, a full sepsis workup (CBC, repeat blood culture, lumbar puncture, urinalysis, and urine culture) should be performed. The patient should be hospitalized and given parenteral antibiotics (Table 66-3).

TABLE 66-3 Suggested Guidelines for the Evaluation and Management of Neonates, Infants, and Children with Fever Who Are Well Appearing, Have Had All Relevant Immunizations, and Have No Clinical Source for Fever

Age Group	Evaluation	Treatment
Infants 57 days* to 6 months*of age, ≥ 38°C (100.4°F) Non-UTI SBI incidence is estimated to be negligible; UTI is 3%–8%	Urinalysis and urine culture alone *or* For conservative management, treat infants 57–90 days using Philadelphia Protocol or Boston Criteria above	*Discharge if negative* *Treat for UTI* with cefixime, 8 mg/kg/dose daily, or cefpodoxime, 5 mg/kg/dose twice a day, or cefdinir, 7 mg/kg/dose twice daily for 10 days as outpatient *Admit and treat* with parenteral ceftriaxone if fails conservative criteria for discharge
Infants 57 days to 6 months*of age ≥ 39°C (102.2°F) SBI incidence is estimated as < 1%; non-UTI SBI incidence is estimated to be negligible; UTI is 3%–8%	Urinalysis and urine culture alone *or* Urinalysis and urine culture in addition to CBC and blood culture	*Discharge if negative* *Treat for UTI as above* If WBC ≥ 15,000/mm^3, consider treatment with ceftriaxone, 50 mg/kg IV/IM, and follow-up in 24 h If WBC ≥ 20,000/mm^3, consider chest x-ray and CSF testing†
Infants/children 6 to 36 months of age Non-UTI SBI incidence is < 0.4% UTI in girls ≤ 8% UTI in boys (<12 months) ≤ 2% Uncircumcised boys (1–2 years) remains 2%	Consider Urinalysis and urine culture, based on the following: Girls 6–24 months Boys 6–12 months Uncircumcised boys 12–24 months	*Discharge if negative* *Treat for UTI* as above as outpatient

Abbreviations: CSF, cerebrospinal fluid; SBI, serious bacterial illness; UTI, urinary tract infection.

*For preterm infants, count age by estimated postconception date and not by actual delivery date for the first 90 days of life.

†Meningismus is difficult to discern in infants < 6 months of age, and especially in infants < 2 months of age. Therefore, we recommend routine CSF testing in infants < 2 months of age, but selective CSF testing in infants 2–6 months of age. There is no absolute cutoff point for prediction of meningitis with a peripheral WBC count.

SEPSIS

Sepsis (bacteremia with clinical evidence of systemic infection) can rapidly progress to multiorgan failure and death. Risk factors include prematurity, immunocompromised state, recent invasive procedures, and indwelling foreign objects such as catheters.

Clinical Features

Clinical signs may be vague and subtle in the young infant, including lethargy, poor feeding, irritability, or hypotonia. Fever is common; however, very young infants may be hypothermic. Tachypnea and tachycardia are usually present as a result of fever but also may be secondary to hypoxia and metabolic acidosis. Sepsis can rapidly progress to shock, manifest as prolonged capillary refill, decreased peripheral pulses, altered mental status, and decreased urinary output. Hypotension is usually a late sign of septic shock in infants and children; sustained tachycardia for age is often the only sign available to the clinician of impending shock.

Diagnosis and Differential

Diagnosis is based on clinical findings and confirmed by positive blood culture results. Though international criteria for sepsis have been published, all infants who appear toxic should be considered septic. The laboratory evaluation of a child with presumed sepsis includes CBC, blood culture, complete metabolic panel, blood lactate, catheterized urinalysis with culture and sensitivities, chest radiograph, lumbar puncture, and stool studies in the presence of diarrhea. Infants are at particular risk for hypoglycemia with SBI and sepsis, and a glucose level should always be checked.

Emergency Department Care and Disposition

1. ABCs. Administer high-flow oxygen, institute cardiac monitoring, and secure IV or IO access immediately. Perform endotracheal intubation in the presence of respiratory failure or severe respiratory distress.
2. Treat shock with **20 mL/kg boluses** of **0.9% normal saline** solution; preferably 60 mL/kg within 15 minutes. For infants, push actual volumes using multiple saline flushes. Repeat boluses until vital signs, perfusion, mental status, and urine output improve, up to 100 mL/kg total volume.
3. Treat hypoglycemia with **5 mL/kg 10% dextrose**.
4. Initiate antibiotic therapy promptly, as soon as IV access is achieved. Do not delay due to difficulty with procedures such as lumbar puncture. Empiric antibiotic choices include **cefotaxime** 50 mg/kg IV **or piperacillin-tazobactam** 100 mg/kg IV; because of ceftriaxone-resistant *S. pneumoniae*, add **vancomycin** 15 mg/kg IV for ill-appearing infants.
5. Treat volume-refractory shock with **dopamine** 5 to 20 μg/kg/min or **norepinephrine** 0.1 to 0.2 μg/kg/min.
6. Consider the presence of drug-resistant organisms, immune-incompetence, or infection with unusual or opportunistic organisms.

MENINGITIS

Meningitis is usually a complication of a primary bacteremia and has a peak incidence in children between birth and 2 years of age. Prematurity and immature immunity put children at higher risk.

Clinical Features

Meningitis may present with the subtle signs that accompany less serious infections, such as otitis media or sinusitis. Irritability, inconsolability, hypotonia, and lethargy are most common in infants. Older children may complain of headache, photophobia, nausea, and vomiting and exhibit the classic signs of meningismus with complaints of neck pain. Occasionally, meningitis presents as a rapidly progressive, fulminant disease characterized by shock, seizures, or coma, or with febrile status epilepticus.

Diagnosis and Differential

Diagnosis is made by lumbar puncture and analysis of the cerebrospinal fluid (CSF). The CSF should be examined for white blood cells, glucose and protein, Gram stain, and culture. Consider herpes simplex virus (HSV) PCR in the seizing neonate and any child with CSF pleocytosis or xanthochromia. In the presence of known immunocompromised state, consider infections with opportunistic or unusual organisms. Perform cranial computed tomography before lumbar puncture in the presence of focal neurologic signs or increased intracranial pressure.

Emergency Department Care and Disposition

1. Treatment should always begin with the ABCs and restoration of oxygenation and perfusion (see specific treatment recommendations under the section "Sepsis").
2. Empiric antibiotic therapy is based on the patient's age and listed in Table 66-4. Do not defer or delay antibiotics when meningitis is strongly suspected. Administer **acyclovir** 20 mg/kg IV for any suspicion of herpes encephalitis.

TABLE 66-4 Suggested Guidelines for the Evaluation and Management of Neonates, Infants, and Children with Fever Who Are Well Appearing, Have Had All Relevant Immunizations, and Have No Clinical Source for Fever

Age Group	Treatment
Neonate, 0–28 days*of age, ≥ 38°C (100.4°F) SBI incidence of ill appearing: 13%–21% ; if not ill appearing: < 5%	*Admit and treat with:* Parenteral antibiotic therapy with ampicillin, 50 mg/kg, and either cefotaxime, 50 mg/kg, or gentamicin, 2.5 mg/kg
Infant 29–56 days* of age, ≥ 38.2°C (100.8°F) (Philadelphia Protocol) SBI incidence of ill appearing: 13%–21%; if not ill appearing: < 5%	*Discharge if:* WBC ≤15,000/mm³ and ≥ 5000/mm³ and < 20% band forms Urinalysis negative CSF WBC <10 cells/mm³ Negative chest x-ray or fecal leukocytes if applicable *Admit if:* Any of above criteria are not met and treat with parenteral ceftriaxone, 50 mg/kg with normal CSF, 100 mg/kg with signs of meningitis

(Continued)

TABLE 66-4 Suggested Guidelines for the Evaluation and Management of Neonates, Infants, and Children with Fever Who Are Well Appearing, Have Had All Relevant Immunizations, and Have No Clinical Source for Fever (Continued)

Age Group	Treatment
Infants 57 days*to 6 months*of age, ≥ 38°C (100.4°F) Non-UTI SBI incidence is estimated to be negligible. UTI is 3%–8%	*Discharge if negative* *Treat for UTI* with cefixime, 8 mg/kg/dose daily, or cefpodoxime, 5 mg/kg/dose twice a day, or cefdinir, 7 mg/kg/ dose twice daily for 10 days as outpatient *Admit and treat* with parenteral ceftriaxone if fails conservative criteria for discharge
Infants 57 days to 6 months*of age ≥ 39°C (102.2°F) SBI incidence is estimated as < 1%; non-UTI SBI incidence is estimated to be negligible. UTI is 3%–8%	*Discharge if negative* *Treat for UTI as above* If WBC ≥ 15,000/mm^3, consider treatment with ceftriaxone, 50 mg/kg IV/IM, and follow-up in 24 h If WBC ≥ 20,000/mm^3, consider chest x-ray and CSF testing†
Infants/children 6–36 months of age Non-UTI SBI incidence is < 0.4% UTI in girls ≤ 8% UTI in boys (< 12 months) ≤ 2% Uncircumcised boys (1–2 years) remains 2%	*Discharge if negative* *Treat for UTI* as above as outpatient
Children > 36 months and older	*Discharge and treat with antipyretics:* acetaminophen, 15 mg/kg PO/PR every 4 h, or ibuprofen, 10 mg/kg PO every 6 h as needed

Abbreviations: CSF, cerebrospinal fluid; SBI, serious bacterial illness; UTI, urinary tract infection.

*For preterm infants, count age by estimated postconception date and not by actual delivery date for the first 90 days of life.

†Meningismus is difficult to discern in infants < 6 months of age, and especially in infants < 2 months of age. Therefore, we recommend routine CSF testing in infants < 2 months of age, but selective CSF testing in infants 2–6 months of age. There is no absolute cutoff point for prediction of meningitis with a peripheral WBC count.

3. The role of steroids in the management of meningitis is highly controversial, but only exert possible benefit when given prior to antibiotics.
4. Admit, hydrate, and give meningitis doses of antibiotic for any patient suspected of having meningitis for whom efforts at lumbar puncture fail. Obtain blood and urine cultures. Lumbar puncture may be successful after hydration.

FURTHER READING

For further reading in *Tintinalli's Emergency Medicine: A Comprehensive Study Guide*, 8th ed., see Chapter 116, "Fever and Serious Bacterial Illness in Infants and Children," by Vincent J. Wang.

CHAPTER 67 Common Neonatal Problems

Lance Brown

In general, the signs and symptoms of illness are vague and nonspecific in neonates making the identification of specific diagnoses challenging. The survival of premature infants has produced a population of children whose corrected gestational age (chronological age since birth in weeks minus the number of weeks of prematurity) makes them, in many ways, similar to neonates. Neonates present to the emergency department (ED) with conditions ranging from normal to critical.

WEIGHT GAIN, FEEDING, AND STOOLING

Bottle-fed infants generally take 6 to 9 feedings (2 to 4 oz) in a 24-hour period, with a relatively stable pattern developing by the end of the first month of life. Breast-fed infants generally prefer feedings every 1 to 3 hours. Infants may lose up to 12% of their birth weight during the first 3 to 7 days of life. After this time, infants are expected to gain about 1 oz/d (20 to 30 g/d) during the first 3 months of life. Parental perception that an infant's food intake is inadequate may prompt an ED visit. If the patient's weight gain is adequate and the infant appears satisfied after feeding, parental reassurance is appropriate.

Regurgitation occurs when gastric contents are effortlessly expelled, typically within 30 minutes of feeding, and, though potentially large in volume, are never projectile or bilious. Regurgitation is typically a self-limited condition and if an infant is thriving and gaining weight appropriately, reassurance is appropriate.

Vomiting is differentiated from regurgitation by forceful contraction of the diaphragm and abdominal muscles. Vomiting has a variety of causes and is rarely an isolated symptom. Etiologies are diverse and include increased intracranial pressure (e.g., nonaccidental trauma), infections (e.g., urinary tract infections, sepsis, or gastroenteritis), hepatobiliary disease (usually accompanied by jaundice), and inborn errors of metabolism (usually accompanied by hypoglycemia and metabolic acidosis). Bilious vomiting in a neonate or infant should be considered a surgical emergency with particular concern for malrotation with midgut volvulus.

The number, color, and consistency of stool in the same infant changes from day to day and differs among infants. Normal breast-fed infants may go 5 to 7 days without stooling or have six to seven stools per day. Color has no significance unless blood is present, or the stool is acholic (i.e., white).

Infants without normal stooling in the first 2 days of life may have anatomic anomalies (e.g., intestinal stenosis or atresias), cystic fibrosis, Hirschsprung disease, or meconium ileus or plug. Constipation that develops later in the first month of life suggests Hirschsprung disease, hypothyroidism, anal stenosis, or anterior anus. Although bacterial infection may cause bloody diarrhea, this is rare in neonates. The most common cause of blood in the stool in neonates is anal fissures. Breast-fed infants may have heme-positive stool from swallowed maternal blood due to bleeding nipples. Necrotizing enterocolitis may present as bloody diarrhea and usually presents with other signs of sepsis (e.g., jaundice, lethargy, fever, poor feeding, or abdominal distention). Abdominal radiography may demonstrate pneumatosis intestinalis or free air. Dehydrated neonates should be admitted for parenteral rehydration.

Abdominal distention can be normal in the neonate and is usually due to lax abdominal muscles, relatively large intraabdominal organs, and swallowed air. In general, if the neonate appears comfortable, is feeding well, and the abdomen is soft, there is no need for concern.

BREATHING AND CRYING

A normal respiratory rate for a neonate is from 30 to 60 breaths/min. Periodic breathing manifests as alternating episodes of rapid breathing with brief (<5 to 10 seconds) pauses in respiration. Periodic breathing is usually normal in neonates. Apnea is formally defined as a cessation of respiration for longer than 10 to 20 seconds with or without accompanying bradycardia and cyanosis. Apnea generally signifies critical illness including infection, CNS injury, and metabolic disease, and prompt investigation and admission for monitoring and treatment should be initiated. Apnea may be the first sign of bronchiolitis with respiratory syncytial virus in neonates and can occur before wheezing. Chlamydia and pertussis can also cause apnea in the young infant.

Noisy breathing in a neonate is usually benign. Infectious causes of stridor seen commonly in older infants and young children (e.g., croup) are rare in neonates. Stridor in a neonate is often due to a congenital anomaly, most commonly, laryngomalacia. Other causes include webs, cysts, atresias, stenoses, clefts, and airway hemangiomas. Nasal congestion from a mild upper respiratory tract infection may cause significant respiratory problems in a neonate. Neonates are obligate nasal breathers and feed for relatively prolonged periods while breathing only through their noses. The use of saline drops and nasal suctioning is typically effective.

There are benign to life-threatening causes of prolonged crying in infants. True inconsolability represents a serious condition in most infants and requires investigation for injury (accidental or inflicted), infection, supraventricular tachycardia (SVT), corneal abrasion, hair tourniquet, hernia or testicular torsion, or an abdominal emergency. If, after a thorough ED evaluation, a cause for excessive crying has not been identified and the child continues to be inconsolable, admission to the hospital for further evaluation is warranted.

Intestinal colic is a common cause of crying in infants. The cause is unknown. The incidence is about 13% in neonates. The formal definition includes crying for at least 3 hours per day for at least 3 days per week over a 3-week period. Intestinal colic seldom lasts beyond 3 months of age. No effective treatment has been identified. In general, the initial diagnosis of colic is not made in the ED and it is a diagnosis of exclusion.

SLEEPING, SEIZURES, AND SEEMINGLY ABNORMAL MOVEMENTS

Normal newborns awaken at variable intervals that can range from about 20 minutes to 6 hours. Neonates and young infants tend to have no differentiation between day and night until approximately 3 months of age. Seizures in neonates may present with subtle signs and symptoms including eye deviation, tongue thrusting, eyelid fluttering, periods of apnea, pedaling movements or arching. All seizures in neonates, unlike some in older infants and young children, require an extensive workup including testing of serum calcium level and admission to the hospital. Seizures need to be differentiated from benign conditions such as a Moro reflex or benign neonatal sleep myoclonus. Benign neonatal sleep myoclonus was first described in 1982 and consists of lightning-like rhythmic jerks of the extremities when the infant is sleeping, is stopped when the neonate is touched or awakened, occurs only during sleep, requires no workup, and is best handled with reassurance.

FEVER AND SEPSIS

Fever in the neonate (age 28 days or younger) is defined as the history of documented fever by a parent or presence of a rectal temperature of 38°C (100.4°F) or higher in the ED. Fever in the neonate must be taken seriously, and at this point in time the proper management includes a complete sepsis workup, administration of parenteral antibiotics (e.g., cefotaxime and ampicillin), and admission to the hospital. For further detailed discussion, see Chapter 66.

ALTE/BRUE

An apparent life-threatening event (ALTE), recently renamed brief resolved unexplained event (BRUE) by the American Academy of Pediatrics, is defined as an event occurring in an infant younger than 12 months involving a brief, but now resolved episode of one or more of the following: (1) cyanosis or pallor; (2) irregular, decreased, or absent breathing; (3) hyper- or hypotonia; or (4) altered responsiveness. According to the definition of BRUE, these infants appear well on presentation to the ED and there is no explanation of the qualifying event. The new guidelines emphasize categorization into lower risk and higher risk, with lower risk criteria being: (1) age > 60 days; (2) prematurity ≥ 32 weeks, and postconceptional age ≥ 45 weeks; (3) first BRUE; (4) duration of event < 1 minute; (5) no CPR by a healthcare provider; 6) no concerning historical or physical examination features. If not considered lower risk, they are categorized as higher risk. Recommendations for further evaluation of lower risk patients show limited benefit, but the strength of the evidence to support these recommendations is only moderate to poor. Evaluation for higher risk patients may include a complete blood count; electrolytes, calcium, phosphorous, magnesium, and ammonia levels; urine toxicological screen; chest radiograph; electrocardiogram; testing for respiratory syncytial virus or pertussis; and a sepsis workup, including blood, urine, and cerebrospinal fluid. A brain CT may be included in cases of suspected nonaccidental trauma. There is no relation between ALTE/BRUE and sudden infant death syndrome, which are now considered distinct entities.

JAUNDICE

There are multiple causes of jaundice, and the likelihood of any specific cause is based on the age of onset. Jaundice that occurs within the first 24 hours of life tends to be serious in nature and usually is addressed while the patient is in the newborn nursery. Jaundice that develops during the second or third day of life is usually physiologic; if the neonate is gaining weight, feeding and stooling well, is not anemic, does not have an elevated direct (conjugated) bilirubin level greater than one-third the total, and does not have a total bilirubin level indicating the need for phototherapy (check www.bilitool.org) reassurance and close follow-up are appropriate. Jaundice that develops after the third day of life is generally serious. Causes include sepsis, UTI, congenital TORCH infections, hemolytic anemia, biliary atresia, breast milk jaundice, and hypothyroidism. Workup of these infants usually includes a complete sepsis evaluation, including a lumbar puncture, a peripheral blood smear, complete blood count, total and direct bilirubin levels, liver function tests, reticulocyte count, and a Coombs test. Empiric antibiotics are generally administered when sepsis is suspected.

ORAL THRUSH AND DIAPER RASH

Intraoral lesions due to *Candida* are typically white and pasty and cover the tongue, lips, gingiva, and buccal mucosa. Treatment consists of topical application of oral nystatin suspension four times a day.

Two main types of diaper rash are common in neonates: contact dermatitis and candidal diaper dermatitis. Contact dermatitis is macular, erythematous, and has sharply demarcated edges. Treatment consists of frequent diaper changes, air drying, and application of a barrier cream containing zinc oxide. Candidal dermatitis presents with erythematous plaques with a scalloped border and satellite lesions. Treatment consists of frequent diaper changes and application of nystatin cream at least four times a day.

EYE COMPLAINTS

Red eyes in neonates run the spectrum from benign to sight threatening. A common benign finding is a corneal abrasion from uncoordinated hand movements and untrimmed fingernails in neonates. Fluorescein staining is diagnostic. Cloudy corneas suggest acute glaucoma. Prompt pediatric ophthalmologic consultation is indicated. Conjunctivitis in the neonatal period may be related to sexually transmitted infections. Gonococcal conjunctivitis typically occurs in the first few days of life and presents with copious discharge. In these cases, a sepsis workup, ocular irrigation, parenteral antibiotics, prompt ophthalmology consultation, and admission to the hospital are indicated. After the first week of life, chlamydial conjunctivitis is more common and may range from mild to severe. Topical drops are inadequate treatment for chlamydial conjunctivitis. Oral erythromycin is indicated.

ABDOMINAL CATASTROPHES

Surgically correctable abdominal emergencies in neonates are uncommon, may present with nonspecific symptomatology, and, when suspected, require prompt consultation with an experienced pediatric surgeon. Common signs and symptoms include irritability and crying, poor feeding, vomiting, constipation, and abdominal distention. Bilious vomiting is suggestive of malrotation with midgut volvulus and requires emergent surgical consultation and radiologic evaluation (upper gastrointestinal series with small bowel follow through). Projectile vomiting following feeds suggests pyloric stenosis, which is evaluated with ultrasound. A groin mass may represent an incarcerated hernia; inguinal hernias are common among premature infants.

INBORN ERRORS OF METABOLISM

Typical presentations of inborn errors of metabolism include lethargy or cardiorespiratory arrest. Most neonates will have inborn errors of metabolism diagnosed after successful resuscitation. Adding a properly obtained serum ammonia level to the usual laboratories obtained during resuscitation may assist in facilitating the diagnosis of some inborn errors of metabolism.

CONGENITAL ADRENAL HYPERPLASIA

These neonates present with virilization, ambiguous genitalia, and hyperpigmentation and may be in shock on presentation. Laboratory values include hyponatremia and hyperkalemia. In addition to usual resuscitation measures, hydrocortisone administered intravenously, intramuscularly, or intraosseously at a dose of 12.5 to 25 mg is indicated.

CONGENITAL HEART DISEASE AND CYANOSIS

Many disorders can present with cyanosis, and differentiating among them can be a diagnostic challenge. However, symptom patterns may help differentiate various causes and assist in suggesting the correct diagnosis and course of action. Rapid, unlabored respirations and cyanosis that does not respond to oxygen therapy suggest cyanotic heart disease with right-to-left shunting. Irregular or shallow breathing and cyanosis suggest sepsis, CNS disease, or metabolic disorders. Labored breathing with grunting and retractions is suggestive of pulmonary disease such as pneumonia or bronchiolitis. All cyanotic neonates should be admitted to the hospital for monitoring, therapy, and further investigation.

NONACCIDENTAL TRAUMA

A battered child may present with unexplained bruises at different ages, skull fractures, intracranial injuries identifiable on computed tomography of the head, extremity fractures, cigarette burns, retinal hemorrhages, unexplained irritability, lethargy, or coma.

FURTHER READING

For further reading in *Tintinalli's Emergency Medicine: A Comprehensive Study Guide*, 8th ed., see Chapter 114, "Neonatal Emergencies and Common Neonatal Problems," by Quynh H. Doan and Niranjan Kissoon; Chapter 115, "Sudden Infant Death Syndrome and Apparent Life-Threatening Event," by Claudius Ilene and Joel S. Tieder.

Common Infections of the Ears, Nose, Neck, and Throat

Yu-Tsun Cheng

This chapter is limited to infections of the ears, nose, neck, and throat. Further information can be found in Chapter 69 "Upper Respiratory Emergencies—Stridor and Drooling," as well as Chapter 151 "Ear, Nose and Sinus Emergencies" and Chapter 153 "Neck and Upper Airway Disorders."

ACUTE OTITIS MEDIA

Acute otitis media (AOM) accounts for 7.4% of all visits to emergency departments in the United States. AOM is an infection of the middle ear space that commonly affects young children because of relative immaturity of the upper respiratory tract, especially the eustachian tube. The most common pathogens in the post-pneumococcal vaccine era are *Streptococcus pneumoniae* (49%) and nontypeable *Haemophilus influenzae* (29%).

Clinical Features

Peak age is 6 to 18 months. Symptoms include fever, poor feeding, irritability, vomiting, ear pulling, and earache. Signs include bulging, pus behind the tympanic membrane (Fig. 68-1), an immobile tympanic membrane (TM), loss of visualization of bony landmarks within the middle ear, and bullae on the TM (bullous myringitis). Mastoiditis is the most common suppurative complication of AOM. The primary symptoms of mastoiditis include fever, protrusion of the auricle, and tenderness over the mastoid area.

Diagnosis and Differential

Making an accurate diagnosis is the most important first step. The definition of AOM requires three equally important components: (a) acute onset (<48 hours) of signs and symptoms, (b) middle-ear effusion (see Fig. 68-1), and (c) signs and symptoms of middle ear inflammation. A red TM alone does not indicate the presence of an ear infection. Fever and prolonged crying can cause hyperemia of the TM alone. Pneumatic otoscopy can be a helpful diagnostic tool; however, a retracted drum for whatever reason will demonstrate decreased mobility. Other common causes of acute otalgia are a foreign body in the external ear canal or otitis externa.

Emergency Department Care and Disposition

1. *Treatment of pain is essential for all children diagnosed with AOM.* Topical analgesics such as benzocaine-antipyrene are recommended for routine use, unless there is a known perforation of the TM. **Acetaminophen** 15 mg/kg or **ibuprofen** 10 mg/kg can be used.
2. Consider the use of a wait-and-see prescription for the treatment of uncomplicated AOM. Parents are given a prescription, and if the child is not better or becomes worse within 48 to 72 hours, the parents are advised to fill the prescription. Contraindications to the use of a wait-and-see prescription are as follows: age <6 months, an immunocompromised

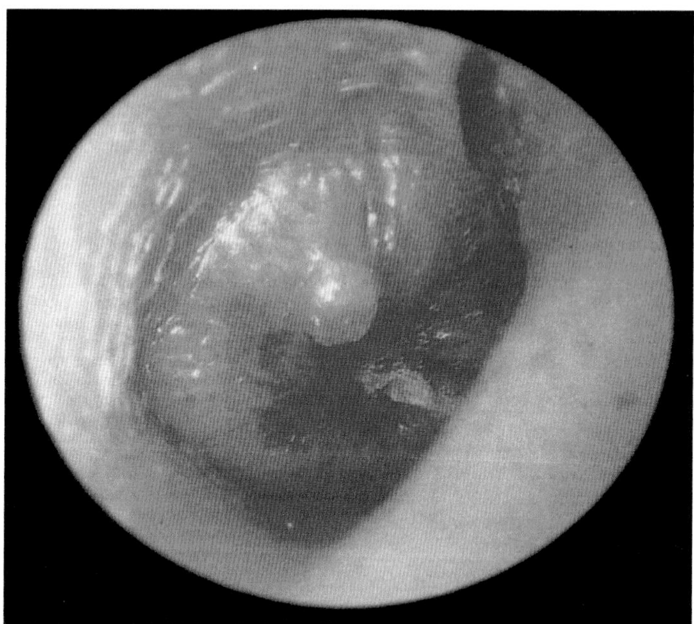

FIGURE 68-1. Acute otitis media in a 3-year-old child with an outward bulge of the tympanic membrane and an exudative process in the middle ear space. Used with permission from Dr. Shelagh Cofer, Department of Otolaryngology, Mayo Clinic.

state, ill-appearance, recent use of antibiotics, or the diagnosis of another bacterial infection. If any of these conditions are met, the child should be prescribed an immediate antibiotic.

3. **Amoxicillin** 40 to 45 mg/kg/dose PO given twice daily remains the first drug of choice for uncomplicated AOM.
4. Second-line antibiotics include **amoxicillin/clavulanate** 40 to 45 mg/kg/dose (based on the amoxicillin component) given twice daily. **Cefpodoxime** 5 mg/kg/dose twice daily, **cefuroxime** 15 mg/kg/dose twice daily, **cefdinir** 7 mg/kg/dose twice daily, and **ceftriaxone** 50 mg/kg/dose IM for one to three daily doses are alternatives. For patients allergic to the previously mentioned antibiotics, **azithromycin** 10 mg/kg/dose PO on the first day followed by 5 mg/kg/dose PO for four more days can be used.
5. Infants younger than 60 days with AOM are at risk of infection with group B *Streptococcus*, *Staphylococcus aureus*, and gram-negative bacilli and should undergo evaluation and treatment for presumed sepsis.
6. In uncomplicated AOM, symptoms resolve within 48 to 72 hours; however, the middle-ear effusion may persist as long as 8 to 12 weeks. Routine follow-up is not necessary unless the symptoms persist or worsen.
7. If mastoiditis is suspected, obtain a CT scan of the mastoid. If the diagnosis is confirmed, obtain consultation with an otorhinolaryngologist and start parenteral antibiotics.

Uncomplicated AOM is treated as an outpatient, whereas mastoiditis typically requires inpatient treatment.

OTITIS EXTERNA

Otitis externa (OE) is an inflammatory process involving the auricle, external auditory canal (EAC), and surface of the TM. It is commonly caused by *Pseudomonas aeruginosa* and *S. aureus*, which often coexist.

Clinical Features

Peak seasons for OE are spring and summer, and the peak age is 7 to 12 years. Symptoms include earache, itching, and, less commonly, fever. Signs include erythema, edema of the EAC, white exudate on the EAC and TM, pain with motion of the tragus or auricle, and periauricular or cervical adenopathy.

Diagnosis and Differential

Diagnosis for OE is based on clinical signs and symptoms. A foreign body within the external canal should be excluded by carefully removing any debris that may be present.

Emergency Department Care and Disposition

1. Cleaning the ear canal with a small tuft of cotton attached to a wire applicator is the first step. Place a wick in the canal if significant edema obstructs the EAC.
2. Consider oral analgesics, such as **ibuprofen** at 10 mg/kg/dose every 6 hours.
3. **Fluoroquinolone**-otic drops are now considered the preferred agents over neomycin containing drops. **Ciprofloxacin with hydrocortisone**, 0.2% and 1% suspension (Cipro HC), 3 drops twice daily or **ofloxacin** 0.3% solution 5 to 10 drops twice daily can be used. Ofloxacin is used when TM rupture is found or suspected.
4. Oral antibiotics are indicated if auricular cellulitis is present.

Follow-up should be advised if improvement does not occur within 48 hours; otherwise routine follow-up is not necessary. Malignant OE is characterized by systemic symptoms and auricular cellulitis. This condition can result in serious complications and requires hospitalization with parenteral antibiotics.

ACUTE BACTERIAL SINUSITIS

Sinusitis is an inflammation of the paranasal sinuses that may be secondary to infection or allergy, and may be acute, subacute, or chronic. Acute bacterial sinusitis is defined as an infection of the paranasal sinuses with complete resolution in <30 days. The major pathogens in childhood are *Streptococcus pneumoniae*, *Moraxella catarrhalis*, and nontypeable *Haemophilus influenzae*.

Clinical Features

Two major types of sinusitis may be differentiated on clinical grounds: acute severe sinusitis and mild subacute sinusitis. Acute severe sinusitis is associated with elevated temperature, headaches, and localized swelling and tenderness or erythema in the facial area corresponding to the sinuses. Such localized findings are seen most often in older adolescents. Mild subacute sinusitis is manifest in childhood as a protracted upper respiratory infection associated with purulent nasal discharge persisting in excess of two weeks. Fever is infrequent. Chronic sinusitis may be confused with allergies or upper respiratory infections.

Diagnosis and Differential

The diagnosis is made on clinical grounds without laboratory or radiographic studies. Transillumination of the maxillary or frontal sinuses is seldom helpful. Nasal congestion lasting 3 to 7 days often accompanies viral upper respiratory infections and should not be diagnosed as acute sinusitis, nor treated with antibiotics. *Similarly, colored drainage from the nose as a solitary symptom does not suggest a diagnosis of sinusitis and should not be treated with antibiotics.* Imaging studies are not needed to confirm a diagnosis of acute bacterial sinusitis in children <6 years of age with persistent symptoms.

Emergency Department Care and Disposition

Patients with mild symptoms suggestive of a viral infection can be observed for 7 to 10 days, with no antibiotics prescribed. Suspect acute bacterial sinusitis if symptoms persist or are severe: fever >39°C, purulent nasal drainage for >3 days and ill-appearance.

1. For children with mild to moderate sinusitis, treat with **amoxicillin** 40 to 45 mg/kg/dose PO twice daily for 10 to 14 days.
2. For children who present with severe symptoms, are in day care, or have recently been treated with antibiotics, prescribe **amoxicillin/clavulanate** 40 to 45 mg/kg/dose twice a day (based on the amoxicillin component), or oral second- and third-generation cephalosporins such as **cefuroxime** 15 mg/kg PO twice a day or **cefpodoxime** 5 mg/kg PO twice a day.

STOMATITIS AND PHARYNGITIS

Herpangina, hand, foot, and mouth disease (HFMD), and herpes simplex gingivostomatitis are the primary infections that cause stomatitis in children and are all viral. The vast majority of pharyngitis is caused by viral infections; however, group A β-hemolytic *Streptococcus* (GABHS) and *Neisseria gonorrhoeae* are bacterial infections that require accurate diagnoses. The identification and treatment of GABHS pharyngitis is important to prevent the suppurative complications and the sequelae of acute rheumatic fever.

Clinical Features

Herpangina causes a vesicular enanthem of the tonsils and soft palate, affecting children 6 months to 10 years of age during late summer and early fall. The vesicles are painful and can be associated with fever and dysphagia. HFMD usually begins as macules which progress to vesicles of the palate, buccal mucosa, gingiva, and tongue. Similar lesions may present on the palms of hands, soles of feet, and buttocks. Herpes simplex gingivostomatitis often presents with abrupt onset of fever, irritability, and decreased oral intake with edematous and friable gingiva. Vesicular lesions often with ulcerations are seen in the anterior oral cavity.

Peak seasons for GABHS are late winter or early spring, the peak age is 5 to 15 years, and it is *rare before the age of 2 years*. Symptoms include sore throat, fever, headache, abdominal pain, enlarged anterior cervical nodes, palatal petechiae, and hypertrophy of the tonsils. With GABHS there is usually the absence of cough, coryza, laryngitis, stridor, conjunctivitis, and diarrhea. A scarlatinaform rash associated with pharyngitis may indicate GABHS and is commonly referred to as *scarlet fever*.

Epstein-Barr Virus (EBV) is a herpes virus and often presents much like streptococcal pharyngitis. Common symptoms are fever, sore throat, and malaise. Cervical adenopathy may be prominent and often is posterior. Hepatosplenomegaly and splenomegaly may be present. EBV should be suspected in the child with pharyngitis nonresponsive to antibiotics in the presence of a negative throat culture.

Gonococcal pharyngitis in children and nonsexually active adolescents should alert one to the possibility of sexual abuse. Gonococcal pharyngitis may be associated with infection elsewhere including proctitis, vaginitis, urethritis, or arthritis.

Diagnosis and Differential

The diagnoses of herpangina, HFMD, and herpes simplex gingivostomatitis are based on clinical findings. To diagnose GABHS, current guidelines recommend the use of **Centor criteria** to determine which patients require testing: (a) tonsillar exudates, (b) tender anterior cervical lymphadenopathy, (c) absence of cough, and (d) history of fever. With two or more criteria, testing should be performed with a rapid antigen detection test and/or culture. If the rapid antigen test is negative, a confirmatory throat culture is recommended.

Diagnosis of EBV is often clinical. A heterophile antibody (monospot) can aid in the diagnosis. The monospot may be insensitive in children <2 years of age and is often negative in the first week of illness. If obtained, the white blood cell count may show a lymphocytosis with a preponderance of atypical lymphocytes. Diagnosis of gonococcal pharyngitis is made by culture on Thayer-Martin medium. Vaginal, cervical, urethral, and rectal cultures also should be obtained if gonococcal pharyngitis is suspected.

Emergency Department Care and Disposition

1. Treatment of herpangina, HFMD, and herpes simplex gingivostomatitis is primarily supportive. Systemic analgesics such as a combination of **ibuprofen** and **acetaminophen** should be considered. Parenteral hydration may be necessary if the child cannot tolerate oral fluids. Occasionally oral narcotics may be required.
2. Antibiotics for the treatment of GABHS pharyngitis should be reserved for patients with a positive rapid antigen test or culture. Antibiotic choices for GABHS include **penicillin V** (children 250 mg PO twice daily, adolescent/adult 500 mg PO twice daily) for 7 to 10 days; **benzathine penicillin G** 1.2 million units IM (600,000 units IM for patients weighing less than 27 kg) once; or **amoxicillin 50 mg/kg once daily** for 7 to 10 days.

3. Treat gonococcal pharyngitis with **ceftriaxone** 250 mg IM. When gonococcal pharyngitis is suspected, empiric treatment of chlamydia is recommended with **azithromycin** 1 g PO given in the emergency department. Appropriate follow-up should be encouraged for treatment failure and symptomatic contacts. Follow-up for suspected gonococcal pharyngitis should include local reporting agencies and social service investigations.
4. EBV is usually self-limited and requires only supportive treatment including antipyretics, fluids, and rest.

CERVICAL LYMPHADENITIS

Acute, unilateral cervical lymphadenitis is commonly caused by *S. aureus* or group A *Streptococcus*. Bilateral cervical lymphadenitis is often caused by viral entities such as EBV and adenovirus. Chronic cervical lymphadenitis is less common but may be caused by *Bartonella henselae* or *Mycobacterium* species.

Clinical Features

Acute cervical lymphadenitis presents with tender, >1 cm nodes often with overlying erythema. Bilateral cervical lymphadenitis presents with small, rubbery lymph nodes and usually self-resolves. *Bartonella* results from the scratch of a kitten with ipsilateral cervical lymphadenitis.

Diagnosis and Differential

Most cases are diagnosed clinically, although culture may guide effective antimicrobial treatment. Differential may also include sialadenitis (infection of the salivary glands), which is usually caused by *S. aureus*, as well as gram-negative and anaerobic bacteria.

Emergency Department Care and Disposition

1. **Either amoxicillin plus clavulanic acid** 20 mg/kg/dose given twice daily or **clindamycin** 10 mg/kg/dose given three times daily for 7 to 10 days is recommended first-line antibiotics for the treatment of acute cervical lymphadenitis.
2. The presence of a fluctuant mass may require incision and drainage in addition to antimicrobial therapy.

Most cases of acute bilateral cervical lymphadenitis resolve without antibiotics, as they often represent viral infection or reactive enlargement. Chronic cases of lymphadenitis are often treated surgically, with directed antimicrobial therapy in some cases depending on clinical diagnosis.

FURTHER READING

For further reading in *Tintinalli's Emergency Medicine: A Comprehensive Study Guide*, 8th ed., see Chapter 118 "Ear and Mastoid Disorders in Infants and Children by Carmen Coombs; Chapter 120, "Nose and Sinus Disorders in Infants and Children" by Joanna S. Cohen and Dewesh Agrawal; Chapter 121 "Mouth and Throat Disorders in Infants and Children" by Derya Caglar, Richard Kwun, and Abigail Schuh; and Chapter 122 "Neck Masses in Infants and Children" by Charles E.A. Stringer and Vikram. Sabhaney

Upper Respiratory Emergencies—Stridor and Drooling

Christopher S. Cavagnaro

The physical sign common to all causes of upper respiratory tract obstruction is stridor. Laryngomalacia, due to a developmentally weak larynx, accounts for 60% of stridor in the neonatal period, but is self-limited and rarely requires treatment. Common causes of stridor in children >6 months of age discussed here include viral croup, epiglottitis, bacterial tracheitis, airway foreign body, retropharyngeal abscess, and peritonsillar abscess.

VIRAL CROUP (LARYNGOTRACHEOBRONCHITIS)

Viral croup is responsible for most cases of stridor after the neonatal period. It is usually a benign, self-limited disease caused by edema and inflammation of the subglottic area. Croup is most prevalent in the fall and early winter, and children ages 6 months to 3 years are most commonly affected, with a peak at an age of 12 to 24 months.

Clinical Features

Croup typically begins with a 1- to 3-day prodrome of cough, coryza, and low-grade fever, followed by a 3- to 4-day period of classic barking cough, though cough and stridor may be abrupt in onset. Symptoms peak on days 3 to 4 and are often more severe at night. Physical examination classically shows stridor, with a greater inspiratory component. Severe cases may have stridor at rest, tachypnea, nasal flaring, and retractions.

Diagnosis and Differential

The diagnosis of croup is clinical: a barking, seal-like cough and history or finding of stridor in the appropriate setting is diagnostic. The differential diagnosis includes epiglottitis, bacterial tracheitis, or foreign body aspiration. Radiographs are not necessary, unless other causes are being considered. Neck or chest radiographs may demonstrate subglottic narrowing or the "steeple sign," though this sign is neither sensitive nor specific for croup.

Emergency Department Care and Disposition

1. Patients with significant stridor should be kept in a position of comfort with minimal disturbance; monitor pulse oximetry and provide oxygen as needed.
2. Administer **dexamethasone** 0.15 to 0.6 mg/kg (10 mg maximum) PO or IM (may use the IV formulation orally). Nebulized **budesonide** (2 mg) may also be clinically useful, if unable to tolerate oral treatment. Even patients with mild croup symptoms benefit from steroids; therefore, most ED patients diagnosed with croup should be treated with a single dose of corticosteroids.
3. Nebulized **racemic epinephrine** (2.25%), 0.05 mL/kg/dose up to 0.5 mL, should be used to treat moderate to severe cases (significant stridor at rest). Alternatively **L-epinephrine** (1:1000), 0.5 mL/kg/dose up to

5 mL, can be used. Children with stridor associated only with agitation do not need epinephrine.

4. Although intubation should be performed when clinically indicated, aggressive treatment with epinephrine usually prevents intubation. When necessary, consider a smaller endotracheal tube than estimated by age to avoid trauma to the inflamed mucosa.
5. **Heliox** (70% helium/30% oxygen mixture) has theoretical benefits for severe refractory croup given its decreased airway resistance, though studies have shown no definitive advantage and it is limited by the low fractional concentration of oxygen.
6. Children with persistent stridor at rest, tachypnea, retractions, or hypoxia, or those who require more than two treatments of epinephrine should be admitted to the hospital.
7. Discharge criteria include the following: at least 3 hours since the last dose of epinephrine, nontoxic appearance, no clinical signs of dehydration, room air oxygen saturation greater than 90%, parental ability to recognize changes in the patient's condition, and no social concerns with access to telephone and a relatively short transit time to the hospital.

EPIGLOTTITIS

Epiglottitis, or supraglottitis, is life threatening and can occur at any age. Historically caused by *Haemophilus influenzae* type b, vaccination has decreased the occurrence of epiglottitis. In immunized children, most cases are caused by *Streptococcus* and *Staphylococcus* species. *Candida* may be a cause in immunocompromised patients.

Clinical Features

Classically, there is abrupt onset of high fever, sore throat, and drooling. Symptoms may progress rapidly to stridor and respiratory distress. Cough may be absent and the voice muffled. The patient is toxic in appearance and may assume a tripod or sniffing position to maintain the airway. The presentation in older children and adults can be subtler. The only complaint may be severe sore throat, with or without stridor. The diagnosis is suggested by severe sore throat, a normal-appearing oropharynx, and a striking tenderness with gentle movement of the hyoid.

Diagnosis and Differential

Radiographs are usually unnecessary to make the diagnosis in patients with a classic presentation. If the diagnosis is uncertain, then lateral neck films should be taken at the bedside in extension and during inspiration with a minimum of disturbance. If it is necessary for the patient to be moved to the radiology suite, a physician trained in airway management should be present at all times. The epiglottis is normally tall and thin, but in epiglottitis, it is very swollen and appears squat and fat like a thumbprint (called the "thumb sign") at the base of the hypopharynx (Fig. 69-1). False-negative radiographic evaluations do occur, and, if suspicion remains, gentle direct visualization of the epiglottis is necessary to exclude the diagnosis. Blood cultures are positive in up to 90% of patients, whereas cultures from the epiglottis are less sensitive.

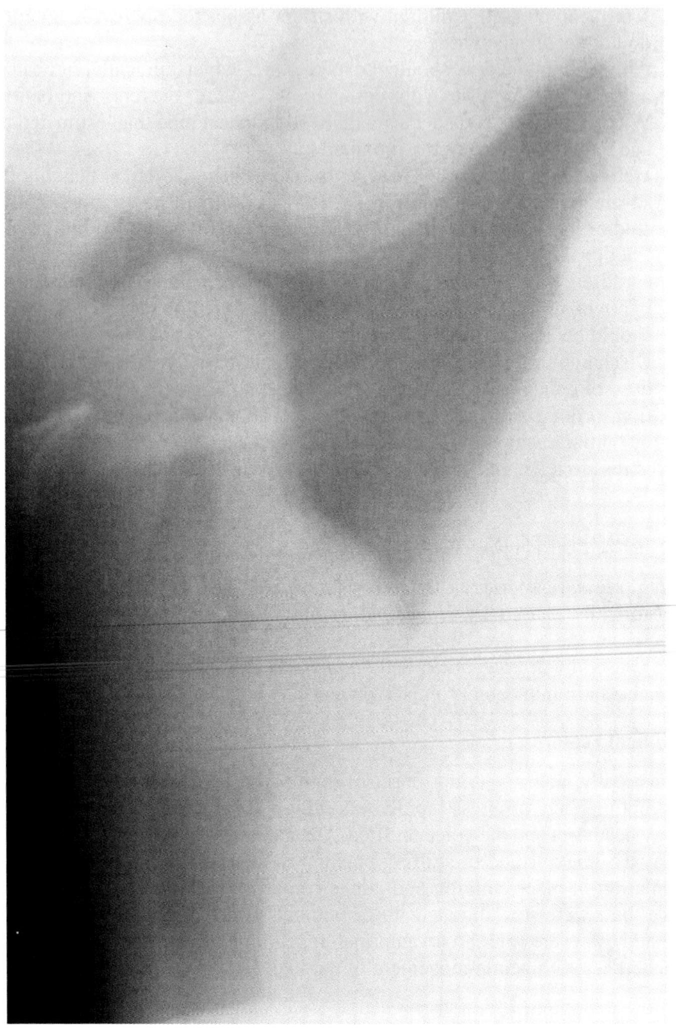

FIGURE 69-1. Lateral neck view of a child with epiglottitis. Courtesy of W. McAlister, MD, Washington University School of Medicine, St. Louis, MO.

Emergency Department Care and Disposition

1. Keep the patient seated and upright. Provide oxygen and administer nebulized **racemic or L-epinephrine**. Heliox also can be attempted.
2. In the event of total airway loss, attempt bag-valve-mask ventilation.
3. Alert a referral center or pediatric otolaryngologist or anesthesiologist to coordinate decisions regarding definitive airway management.
4. The most experienced individual should perform intubation as soon as the diagnosis is made. Use sedation, paralytics, and vagolytics as

indicated. Multiple endotracheal tube sizes must be immediately available. For the patient who is able to maintain their airway, use of paralytics must be accompanied by the certainty that intubation will be successful or that a surgical airway can immediately be performed if unsuccessful.

5. Steroids may be employed to decrease mucosal edema of the epiglottis. Use **methylprednisolone** 2 mg/kg IV or **dexamethasone** 0.15 to 0.6 mg/kg IV.
6. Administer antibiotics: **cefuroxime** 50 mg/kg/dose IV, **cefotaxime** 50 mg/kg/dose IV, or **ceftriaxone** 50 mg/kg/dose IV are appropriate empiric options. In regions with increased cephalosporin resistance, **vancomycin** 10 mg/kg/dose IV should be added.

BACTERIAL TRACHEITIS

Bacterial tracheitis (membranous laryngotracheobronchitis or "bacterial croup") is uncommon and can present as either a primary or secondary infection. The mean age of presentation is between 5 and 8 years of age, compared with younger ages as had been previously described. It is usually caused by *Staphylococcus aureus*, *Streptococcus pneumoniae*, or β-lactamase–producing gram-negative organisms (*H. influenzae* and *Moraxella catarrhalis*).

Clinical Features

Patients with bacterial tracheitis appear toxic and have more respiratory distress than do patients with croup. They commonly present with sudden worsening of an upper respiratory infection with fever, sore throat, stridor, and cough occasionally productive of thick sputum.

Diagnosis and Differential

If obtained, radiographs of the lateral neck and chest usually demonstrate subglottic narrowing of the trachea with irregular densities and ragged and indistinct borders. Bronchoscopy, however, is most diagnostic.

Emergency Department Care and Disposition

1. Manage patients' airways as above for epiglottitis; patients frequently require intubation. Ideally, perform intubation and bronchoscopy in the operating room where cultures and Gram stain may be obtained to guide antibiotic therapy.
2. Administer empiric parenteral antibiotics: **ampicillin/sulbactam** 50 mg/kg/dose IV or **ceftriaxone** 50 mg/kg/dose IV **plus clindamycin** 10 mg/kg/dose IV. In areas with increasing *S. aureus* resistance, consider the addition of **vancomycin** 10 mg/kg/dose IV.

AIRWAY FOREIGN BODY

Foreign body (FB) aspirations cause more than 3000 deaths each year and have a peak incidence between ages 1 and 3 years. In children younger than 6 months, the cause is usually secondary to a feeding by a well-meaning sibling. The most common FB aspirations fall into two groups: food and toys. Commonly aspirated foods include peanuts, sunflower seeds, raisins, grapes, and hot dogs, but almost any object may be aspirated. Unlike small round metal objects, aspirated vegetable matter commonly causes intense pneumonitis and subsequent pneumonia and suppurative bronchitis. A FB aspiration should be suspected if there is a history of sudden onset of coughing or choking and should be considered in all children with unilateral wheezing.

Clinical Features

At presentation many patients are asymptomatic. There may or may not be a witnessed aspiration. The primary symptom is cough, which is classically abrupt in onset, and may be associated with gagging, choking, stridor, or cyanosis. Signs depend upon the location of the FB and the degree of obstruction: stridor and hoarseness with a FB in the laryngotracheal area; unilateral wheezing and decreased breath sounds with a bronchial FB. Symptoms, however, are unreliable in localizing the level of FB. Wheeze may be present in 30% of laryngotracheal FB aspirations and stridor in up to 10% of bronchial aspirations. Eighty to 90% of FBs are located in the bronchi. Patients with immediate onset of severe stridor and cardiac arrest usually have laryngotracheal aspirations.

Diagnosis and Differential

FB aspiration is easily confused with more common causes of respiratory diseases because patients may have fever, wheezing, or rales. While plain chest radiographs may be helpful to confirm a diagnosis, they can be normal in >50% of tracheal FB and 25% of bronchial FB. More than 75% of FB in children <3 years of age are radiolucent. In cases of complete obstruction, atelectasis may be found. In partial obstructions, a ball valve effect occurs, with air trapping caused by the FB leading to hyperinflation of the obstructed lung apparent during expiration. Thus, in a stable cooperative child, inspiratory and expiratory posteroanterior chest radiographs may be helpful. In a stable but noncooperative child, decubitus films may be used, but are less sensitive than fluoroscopy. FB aspiration is definitively diagnosed preoperatively in only one-third of cases; thus, if clinically suspected, bronchoscopy is indicated.

Upper esophageal FBs are usually radiopaque and can impinge on the posterior aspect of the trachea. Patients may present with stridor, and typically have dysphagia. Radiographically, flat FBs such as coins are usually oriented in the sagittal plane when located in the trachea and in the coronal plane when in the esophagus.

Emergency Department Care and Disposition

1. If FB aspiration or airway obstruction is clearly present, perform basic life support (BLS) procedures to relieve airway obstruction (see Chapter 3).
2. If BLS maneuvers fail, perform direct laryngoscopy and extraction of the FB with Magill forceps. If the FB cannot be seen, orotracheal intubation with dislodgement of the FB distally may be lifesaving.
3. If an obstructive laryngotracheal FB cannot be removed or dislodged, an emergent surgical airway may be required.

4. Definitive treatment of partial airway obstruction usually requires rigid bronchoscopy in the operating room under general anesthesia.

RETROPHARYNGEAL ABSCESS

Retropharyngeal abscesses form within a potential space present only in young children and usually occur in children younger than 4 years of age.

Clinical Features

Patients classically present with fever, drooling, and dysphagia, and may have inspiratory stridor. Patients may hold their neck in an unusual position with torticollis, hyperextension, or stiffness. Reported complications include rapidly fatal airway obstruction from sudden rupture of the abscess pocket, aspiration pneumonia, empyema, mediastinitis, and erosion into the jugular vein and carotid artery.

Diagnosis and Differential

Physical examination of the pharynx may show a retropharyngeal mass. Although palpation commonly will demonstrate fluctuance, this could lead to rupture of the abscess. Lateral neck radiograph performed during inspiration may show a widened retropharyngeal space. The diagnosis is suggested when the retropharyngeal space at C2 is twice the diameter of the vertebral body or greater than one half the width of C4. CT of the neck with IV contrast is very helpful for diagnosis and defining extent of the infection and may help differentiate between cellulitis and abscess.

Emergency Department Care and Disposition

1. Immediate airway stabilization is the first priority. Intubate unstable patients before performing CT.
2. Antibiotic choice is controversial because most retropharyngeal abscesses contain mixed flora. Consider **ampicillin/sulbactam** 50 mg/kg/dose IV or **clindamycin** 10 mg/kg/dose IV. Substitute **ceftriaxone** 50 mg/kg/dose IV for ampicillin/sulbactam in the penicillin-allergic patient.
3. Consider adjunctive treatment with parenteral steroids (e.g., **dexamethasone** 0.15 to 0.6 mg/kg IV to a maximum of 10 mg) to reduce inflammation and edema.
4. Retropharyngeal cellulitis and some very small abscesses may improve with antibiotics alone. Most abscesses, however, will require otolaryngology consult for operative incision and drainage.

PERITONSILLAR ABSCESS

A peritonsillar abscess is a typically unilateral, deep, oropharyngeal polymicrobial infection, most commonly seen in adolescents and young adults.

Clinical Features

Patients usually appear acutely ill with sore throat, fevers, chills, dysphagia/odynophagia, trismus, drooling, and a muffled "hot potato" voice. The uvula is displaced away from the affected side. As a rule, the affected tonsil is anteriorly and medially displaced.

Diagnosis and Differential

The diagnosis and differentiation from aperitonsillar cellulitis can typically be made through careful visualization of the oral cavity. Classic findings include uvular deviation away from the abscess, soft palate displacement, trismus, and localized fluctuance; airway compromise may occur. In typical cases, imaging studies are unnecessary, though in patients with toxic appearance or atypical exam findings, computed tomography (CT) with contrast or ultrasound is indicated.

Emergency Department Care and Disposition

1. Treat most cases with needle aspiration, antibiotics, and pain control. Administer topical (e.g., benzocaine or endocaine spray), oral (e.g., oxycodone or vicodin), or parenteral (e.g., fentanyl, morphine) analgesics, then aspirate the abscess using a large gauge needle. Avoid deep penetration, which could injure adjacent vascular structures and result in significant bleeding. The last centimeter of the tip of a needle guard can be cut off, and carefully reattached to the aspirating syringe, covering all but the end of the needle, to limit the depth of penetration.
2. Consider **clindamycin** 10 mg/kg/dose IV or **ampicillin/sulbactam** 50 mg/kg/dose IV. Definitive follow-up is essential in all cases. Oral antibiotics for outpatient treatment include **amoxicillin/clavulanate** 45 mg/kg/dose given twice daily or **clindamycin** 10 mg/kg/dose every eight hours.
3. Formal incision and drainage in the operating room is sometimes necessary, especially in young or uncooperative patients. Most patients can be discharged safely on oral antibiotics following drainage.
4. Consider empiric IV fluid boluses, as patients may be dehydrated on presentation, and/or may not drink as well after incision and drainage.

FURTHER READING

For further reading in *Tintinalli's Emergency Medicine: A Comprehensive Study Guide*, 8th ed., see Chapter 123, "Stridor and Drooling" by Elisa Mapelli and Vikram Sabhaney.

CHAPTER 70 Wheezing in Infants and Children

Richard J. Scarfone

ASTHMA

Asthma is the most common chronic disease of childhood and the most frequent reason for hospitalization of children. The primary pathologic event is airway inflammation causing recurrent episodes of wheezing, dyspnea, and cough associated with airflow obstruction that is variably reversible. The most common triggers are viral infections, allergens, exercise, and environmental irritants including cigarette smoke and cold air.

Clinical Features

Wheezing, a high-pitched sound that occurs when there is an elevation of airway resistance, is the hallmark of an acute asthma exacerbation. Associated findings may include cough, shortness of breath, and chest tightness or pain. To optimize medical management, clinical features are used to classify severity as mild, moderate, or severe. In addition to degree of wheezing, the other important clinical features used to define illness severity include respiratory rate, work of breathing as indicated by retractions and/or nasal flaring, aeration quality, and inspiratory/expiratory ratio. Serial assessments are key to emergency department (ED) management because changes in clinical status and response to treatment are usually more relevant to outcome and need for admission than the level of severity at presentation.

Hypoxemia, while frequent, is usually mild (SpO_2 >92%) and due to V/Q mismatch, which may worsen during initial treatment with bronchodilators for a period of 1 to 2 hours. If available, end-tidal CO_2 ($ETCO_2$) by capnometry should be monitored during severe exacerbations. Hypocapnia is expected early in the course of an asthma exacerbation, thus a normal or minimally elevated $ETCO_2$ may be a sign of impending ventilatory failure.

Diagnosis and Differential

The differential diagnosis of wheezing in infants and children is extensive—asthma and bronchiolitis being the most common causes. Consideration of patient age, presenting signs and symptoms, response to therapy, and time of year helps differentiate the two diseases. For children >2 years old who do not have a prior history of asthma, a provisional diagnosis of asthma is made when there are signs and symptoms of wheezing, shortness of breath, cough, dyspnea, diminished air entry, or retractions **and** demonstration of reversibility with an inhaled β_2-agonist (e.g., albuterol). On the other hand, children <2 years old without a prior history or family history of wheezing and presenting during a respiratory viral epidemic with a preceding upper respiratory infection should be treated as having bronchiolitis.

Chest radiography should be considered if the patient fails to improve as expected, fever is present, there is concern for possible pneumothorax (pain or significant hypoxia) or foreign body (unilateral wheezing), or for patients with focal lung findings.

Emergency Department Care and Disposition

An inhaled β_2-agonist, most often albuterol, is the mainstay of acute asthma therapy and its frequency of administration should be titrated to the child's degree of illness.

1. Administer **oxygen** for saturations below 92%.
2. Deliver **albuterol** by metered-dose inhaler with spacer 4 to 8 puffs every 20 minutes up to three doses or nebulization 2.5 to 5 mg every 20 minutes up to three doses. These routes are equally effective and either is indicated for the initial treatment of mild to moderately ill patients. Continuously nebulized albuterol 0.5 mg/kg/h is used for those who are more severely ill. **Ipratropium** plus albuterol is superior to albuterol alone in the treatment of acute severe asthma. Ipratropium should be given concurrently with nebulized or meter-dosed albuterol 0.25 to 0.5 mg Q 20 minutes × 3 doses. Levalbuterol is not any more effective or safer than albuterol and is more expensive.
3. Administer **systemic corticosteroids** in all but the most mildly ill patients who respond immediately to albuterol. Early administration, even at the time of triage, decreases hospital admission rates. **Prednisone or prednisolone** 2 mg/kg/dose, maximum 60 mg/dose or **dexamethasone** 0.6 mg/kg to a maximum of 10 to16 mg may be used. Dexamethasone's long half-life allows for shorter duration of therapy for discharged patients. Severely ill children should be treated with IV methylprednisolone 1 mg/kg/dose.
4. **Systemic β-agonists** have no advantage over inhaled albuterol except for children with poor ventilation and impaired delivery of inhaled albuterol. **Terbutaline** has selective β_2 activity and can be administered SQ or IM 0.01 mg/kg, maximum 0.4 mg, Q 20 minutes × 3 doses to those without IV access. **Epinephrine** continues to be used by some clinicians for its α-agonist activity that may shrink edematous mucosa. It is given SQ or IM 0.01 mg/kg, maximum 0.5 mg, Q 15 minutes.
5. Consider **magnesium sulfate** 50 to 75 mg/kg, maximum 2 g, IV over 10 to 20 minutes in the patient with poor ventilation. An IV fluid bolus of 20 cc/kg should precede magnesium administration to avoid a clinically significant decline in blood pressure.
6. Other interventions, such as the use of **ketamine** 2 mg/kg IV followed by 2 to 3 mg/kg/h or **helium-oxygen** (in a 60:40 or 70:30 ratio) may be considered in a critically ill patient not responding to other measures who is otherwise approaching the need for intubation and mechanical ventilation.
7. **Helium-oxygen (Heliox)** as a 60:40 or 70:30 (helium:oxygen) mix may restore laminar airflow and improve alveolar ventilation. Nebulized albuterol may be administered with this treatment. A maximum FiO_2 of 40% can be administered with helium, so patients requiring high concentrations of oxygen are not candidates for this therapy.
8. Administer **IV fluids** (normal saline) to patients in status asthmaticus who have decreased oral intake or are nil per os (NPO) due to the severity of the episode.

9. Admit children to the hospital who do not respond adequately to treatment (e.g., persistent hypoxemia or continuing to require albuterol therapy at least every 2 hours) or whose caretaker may not be able to provide necessary ongoing care.
10. An extremely small number of children will require intubation and mechanical ventilation despite aggressive management. It is best to try to avoid this due to challenges in ventilatory management and the potential for barotrauma; additionally, laryngoscopy during intubation may precipitate laryngospasm. In this setting, **noninvasive ventilation** strategies such as bilevel positive airway pressure (BiPAP) may prevent the need for mechanical ventilation. Should a patient progress to this stage, the most experienced operator available should perform the procedure, and a carefully considered sequence of rapid-sequence intubation medications chosen. These often include premedication with atropine 0.02 mg/kg (minimum 0.5 mg, maximum 1 mg) and lidocaine 1.5 mg/kg and sedation with ketamine 2 mg/kg, followed by paralysis using succinylcholine 2 mg/kg or rocuronium 1 mg/kg to provide optimal intubating conditions. Permissive hypercapnia is a strategy that may minimize barotrauma.
11. Following initial therapy, most children will improve and may be observed off of albuterol therapy. The duration of observation will vary; in general, those who were sicker on arrival should be observed at least 2 to 3 hours post-albuterol before making a decision to discharge home. **Admit** children to the hospital who either do not respond adequately to initial treatment or don't maintain that response (e.g., hypoxemia, work of breathing, significant tachypnea, and/or failure to normalize aeration).
12. **Discharge planning** should include an "action plan" (available at http://www.nhlbi.nih.gov/health/public/lung/asthma/actionplan_text.htm), albuterol as MDI or nebulizer, oral corticosteroids, and follow-up with the primary care provider.

BRONCHIOLITIS

Bronchiolitis is the most frequent lower respiratory infection in the first 2 years of life and is most commonly caused by *respiratory syncytial virus* (RSV). Infection causes acute airway inflammation and edema, small airway epithelial cell necrosis and sloughing, increased mucus production and mucus plugs, and bronchospasm, all of which can vary considerably between patients and during the course of the illness.

Clinical Features

Most patients have wheezing and rhinorrhea typical of an upper respiratory infection (URI) in addition to some combination of fever, tachypnea, cough, rales, use of accessory muscles, and nasal flaring. Apnea and dehydration are of great concern and may be more common in infants younger than 3 months or those born prematurely. Hypoxemia, cyanosis, altered mental status, and fatigue are ominous signs and may portend respiratory failure. Disposition decisions should be made with consideration of signs of severity as well as the typical time course for illness: severity increases over the first 3 to 5 days with total duration of illness 7 to 14 days.

Diagnosis and Differential

Bronchiolitis, like asthma, typically has wheezing as its most prominent clinical sign. In contrast to asthma, however, most infants with bronchiolitis are unresponsive to both **β-agonists** and corticosteroids. Thus, it is important to differentiate the two conditions. In general, patients with bronchiolitis are <2 years old (peaking presentation is 6 to12 months of age), do not have a past history or family history of wheezing or atopic disease, have a URI, and present during a RSV or other respiratory viral pathogen outbreak. Diagnosis is clinical and does not require laboratory or radiologic studies.

Routine testing for RSV or other pathogens is expensive and is rarely helpful; it may be indicated only if the information is necessary for infection control measures for hospitalized patients. Routine performance of radiographs increases inappropriate antibiotic use and does not change time to recovery. Radiographs are indicated only if other diseases or foreign body aspiration are suspected, or if the patient has severe disease.

Emergency Department Care and Disposition

1. **Nasal suctioning and saline drops:** Deep suctioning of the nasal passages after saline instillation may substantially decrease work of breathing, correct hypoxemia, and enable the patient to feed normally. Nasal vasoconstrictors are not indicated and have resulted in tachydysrhythmias. Mildly ill, well-hydrated patients need to be treated with suctioning only.
2. Provide **oxygen** to maintain saturations >90%. The use of heated, humidified, **high-flow nasal cannula (HFNC) therapy** provides delivery of an air/oxygen blend, up to 12 L/min in infants. Its use approximates continuous positive airway pressure to improve ventilation in a minimally invasive manner and should be considered for all moderately to severely ill infants.
3. **Nebulized α- and β-agonists** should not be routinely used. However, use of a β_2-agonist (albuterol) might be considered for a moderately ill infant, particularly if there is a personal or family history of asthma or atopic disease. **Nebulized epinephrine** 0.5 mL of 1:1000 in 2.5 mL saline is not routinely effective but may be reserved for those ill enough to require hospitalization and who had a suboptimal response to β_2-agonists. If these medications are used, an objective measure (e.g., respiratory rate or bronchiolitis score) should be used to assess response; lack of response should lead to a discontinuation of that therapy.
4. As with epinephrine, consider **nebulized hypertonic saline** 3% or 5%, 3 to 5 mL by nebulizer to decrease mucus production and viscidity for hospitalized infants unresponsive to other interventions.
5. Provide **isotonic IV fluids (normal saline)** if necessary. Patients with bronchiolitis may not be able to feed normally, and when respiratory rates exceed 60 to 70 breaths/min there is increased risk of aspiration of feedings.
6. **Corticosteroids** should not be used routinely for patients with bronchiolitis. A large multicenter study found no benefit of dexamethasone over placebo, whereas a second study found that the combination of dexamethasone and epinephrine was beneficial. However, the benefit was

marginal and the doses of dexamethasone were large. Potential adverse effects of these medications and lack of sufficient evidence for benefit preclude their routine use.

7. **Ventilatory support:** Noninvasive measures (CPAP or BiPAP) may improve oxygenation and ventilation, decrease work of breathing, and delay or obviate the need for endotracheal intubation. Additionally, application of CPAP may prevent further apnea in affected infants.
8. **Decision for hospitalization:** Caution should be the rule when making disposition decisions about very young infants in respiratory distress due to an illness without effective outpatient therapies. Careful and serial observations (including pulse oximetry) and reassessment are keys to determining disposition. Persistent hypoxia, significant tachypnea or work of breathing, and inability to feed or maintain hydration are all indications for hospitalization. Decision-makers must also consider where in the clinical course of illness the patient resides (severity increases over the first 3 to 5 days of illness), the ability of caretakers to manage the illness, and the availability of follow-up. In addition, patients with risk factors for apnea and/or severe disease with possible respiratory failure should be identified early, including (a) young developmental age (< 6 to12 weeks) or prematurity (< 37 weeks); (b) witnessed apnea; (c) hemodynamically significant congenital heart disease: on medication for CHF; moderate to severe pulmonary hypertension; cyanotic CHD; (d) chronic lung disease: bronchopulmonary dysplasia; congenital malformations; cystic fibrosis; and (e) immunocompromised state (Table 70–1).

TABLE 70-1 Dosages of Medications for Asthma Exacerbations

Medication	American Pediatric Dosages	Alternate Pediatric Dosages
Bronchodilators		
Salbutamol/ albuterol (aerosol or nebulized)	• MDI (90 μg/puff); *delivered via valved holding chamber:* • ≤ 1 year: 2 puffs/dose • 1–3 years: 4 puffs/dose • ≥ 4 years: 8 puffs/dose	• MDI (100 μg/puff); *delivered via valved holding chamber:* • ≤ 1 year: 2 puffs/dose • 1–3 years: 4 puffs/dose • 4–6 years: 6 puffs/dose • ≥ 7 years: 8 puffs/dose
	• Nebulization (unit dose nebule or 5 mg/mL solution): • 0.15–0.3 mg/kg/dose (minimum 2.5 mg)	• Nebulization (unit dose nebule or 5 mg/mL solution): • < 10 kg: 1.25-mg nebule or 0.25 mL of 5-mg/mL solution* • 10–20 kg: 2.5-mg nebule or 0.5 mL of 5-mg/mL solution* • > 20 kg: 5-mg nebule or 1 mL of 5-mg/mL solution*
	• IV: • *Not available*	• IV: • 0.5–3 mg/kg/h continuous infusion (maximum 15 mg/h)
	• PO: • *Not recommended*	• PO: • *Not recommended*

(Continued)

TABLE 70-1 Dosages of Medications for Asthma Exacerbations (Continued)

Medication	American Pediatric Dosages	Alternate Pediatric Dosages
Ipratropium bromide (aerosol or nebulized)	• MDI (20 μg/puff); *delivered via valved holding chamber:* • 4–8 puffs/dose PRN, alternated with salbutamol	• MDI (20 μg/puff); *delivered via valved holding chamber:* • 3 puffs/dose for all patients, alternated with salbutamol
	• Nebulization: • 250–500 μg for all patients, mixed with salbutamol	• Nebulization: • 250 μg for all patients, mixed with salbutamol
Systemic corticosteroids		
Prednisone (PO)	1–2 mg/kg/dose (maximum 60 mg) for 3–10 days	2 mg/kg (maximum 60 mg) in ED, then 2 mg/kg/d bid for 4 days
Methylprednisolone (IV, IM)	2 mg/kg/dose load, then 0.5–1 mg/kg/dose every 6 h	1 mg/kg/dose (maximum 125 mg/dose), repeated every 6 h or change to oral regimen
Dexamethasone (PO, IV, IM)	0.6 mg/kg/dose (maximum 16 mg) for 1–2 days	• Multiple dosing regimens: • 0.6 mg/kg/d for 1–2 days • 0.3 mg/kg/d for 3–5 days
Other medications		
Magnesium sulfate (IV)	25–75 mg/kg/dose (maximum 2 g) × 1	50 mg/kg/dose × 1 *(monitor blood pressure)*
Ketamine (IV)[†]	1–2 mg/kg/dose × 1	2 mg/kg/dose × 1 *(may alleviate need for intubation, given as induction agent for intubation)*

[*]Mixed in 3 mL of normal saline solution.

[†]Consider only if standard therapies have failed in order to prevent intubation.

Abbreviation: MDI = metered-dose inhaler.

FURTHER READING

For further reading in *Tintinalli's Emergency Medicine: A Comprehensive Study Guide*, 8th ed., see Chapter 124, "Wheezing in Infants and Children," by Allan Shefrin, Alia Busuttil and Roger Zemek.

CHAPTER 71

Pneumonia in Infants and Children

Ameer P. Mody

Pneumonia, infection of the lower respiratory tract, is one of the leading causes of pediatric morbidity and mortality throughout the world. The etiologic agent, clinical presentation, and severity of illness vary greatly based on the age of the child. In neonates (age 0 to 30 days), group B streptococci and other gram-negative enteric bacteria are common pathogens. Pneumonia caused by *Chlamydia trachomatis* has largely been eliminated in developed countries, but should be considered when the mother had little or no prenatal care. In infants and toddlers (1 month to 2 years), respiratory syncytial virus (RSV), influenza virus, parainfluenza virus, and human metapneumovirus are some of the common viral pathogens. *Streptococcus pneumoniae* and *Haemophilus influenzae* are the most common bacterial pathogens. Pneumonia in children aged 2 to 5 years is most likely caused by respiratory viruses, followed by *S. pneumoniae, H. influenzae*, and *Staphylococcus aureus*. In children 5 to 13 years of age, *Mycoplasma pneumoniae* is the most likely etiology of community-acquired pneumonia followed by *S. pneumoniae and Chlamydophila pneumoniae*. Adolescents typically follow the same seasonal and epidemiologic patterns of healthy adults with community-acquired pneumonia.

CLINICAL FEATURES

The clinical presentation of pneumonia varies with the age of the patient, although most pediatric patients will have some combination of fever, preceding viral illness, tachypnea, respiratory distress, rales, and diminished breath sounds. Tachypnea is the most sensitive finding in pediatric patients with pneumonia (see Table 71-1). Symptoms of pneumonia may be subtle in neonates and infants, but these patients may be more severely ill. Fever or hypothermia, apnea, tachypnea, poor oral intake, vomiting, lethargy, grunting, or shock may be present in these patients. In older children and teens, community-acquired pneumonia presents more similarly to adult patients with a viral prodrome, fever, cough, abnormal lung sounds, vomiting, pleuritic chest pain, tachypnea, or hypoxemia. In younger children, particularly with lower lobe pneumonias, abdominal pain may be a

TABLE 71-1 Tachypnea as an Indicator for Pneumonia

Age	Tachypnea	Comments
0–60 days	> 60 breaths/min	> 70 breaths/min indicates severe disease
2–12 months	> 50 breaths/min	> 60 breaths/min indicates severe disease
1–5 years	> 40 breaths/min	> 50 breaths/min indicates severe disease
> 5 years	> 20 breaths/min	> 50 breaths/min indicates severe disease

predominant complaint. The clinical manifestations of bacterial and viral pneumonias overlap in all age groups, making the clinical distinction very challenging.

DIAGNOSIS AND DIFFERENTIAL

For most pneumonias, the etiologic agent is never determined. The diagnosis of pneumonia should primarily be made on clinical grounds; chest radiography is not required and not considered the gold standard for diagnosis. Chest radiography is not 100% sensitive, nor specific for the diagnosis of pneumonia, and does not distinguish between bacterial or viral etiologies. The presence of fever plus tachypnea, decreased breath sounds, or fine crackles predicts pneumonia with 93% to 96% sensitivity. If all four variables are present, the sensitivity is 98%. Chest radiography should be reserved for patients in which the differential diagnosis is in question (aspirated foreign body, congestive heart failure, mediastinal mass) or a complication of pneumonia is suspected (failure of outpatient therapy, pleural effusion, cavitary pneumonia, significant patient comorbidities, age <3 months). Routine laboratory testing is not required for well-appearing children with mild community-acquired pneumonia. For neonates or older patients with significant respiratory distress or toxic appearance, a blood culture, complete blood count, and serum electrolytes should be obtained. Rapid viral antigen testing (if available) for RSV, influenza, and human metapneumovirus can be valuable if they are quick and specific, as results may negate the need for imaging, invasive testing, and antibiotic therapy.

EMERGENCY DEPARTMENT CARE AND DISPOSITION

The ED care of pediatric pneumonia is age-dependent but follows the principles of supportive care of respiratory distress, hypoxemia, dehydration, and fever. Oxygen should be given for respiratory distress or oxygen saturations less than 92% on room air. Antipyretics should be administered for febrile patients and may resolve tachypnea associated with fever. Patients with wheezing should be given bronchodilators. Dehydration (caused by respiratory distress, increased insensible losses, and diminished oral intake associated with pneumonia) should be corrected with boluses of 20mL/kg of normal saline. Antibiotic therapy should be initiated for patients based on suspicion of bacterial pathogen, age of patient, and severity of illness (see Table 71-2).

Neonates with pneumonia have a significant risk for respiratory decompensation and should be admitted and monitored closely. Most healthy infants (>3 months) and children with pneumonia can be treated as outpatients. Criteria utilized to determine need for admission include work of breathing (presence of significant tachypnea, retractions, grunting), hypoxemia, poor oral intake, persistent vomiting, dehydration, and social factors (access to follow-up medical care, inadequate family resources, inability to follow treatment plan). Pediatric intensive care consultation and admission should be considered for infants with severe respiratory distress, impending respiratory failure, or shock.

TABLE 71-2 Empiric antibiotic therapy for Pneumonia

Age	Bacterial Pathogens	Outpatient Treatment	Inpatient Treatment
Neonates	Group B *Streptococcus* Gram-negative enterics *Listeria monocytogenes*	Initial outpatient treatment not indicated	Ampicillin + gentamycin or cefotaxime
1–3 months	*Streptococcus pneumonia* *Chlamydia trachomatis* *Haemophilus influenza* *Bortadella pertussis* *Staphylococcus aureus*	Initial outpatient treatment not indicated	Ampicillin or Ceftriaxone or Cefotaxime or Vancomycin. Macrolide should be utilized if *C. trachomatis* or *B. pertussis* is suspected
3 months–5 years	*S. pneumonia* *H. influenzae type b* Nontypeable *H. influenza* *S. aureus*	Amoxicillin +/− clavulanic acid or cefuroxime axetil	Ampicillin or Ceftriaxone or Cefotaxime or Vancomycin +/− macrolide
5–18 years	*Mycoplasma pneumonia* *S. pneumonia* *Chlamydophila pneumonia* *H. influenzae type b* *S. aureus*	Azithromycin (if *M. pneumoniae* suspected) or Amoxicillin +/− clavulanic acid or cefuroxime axetil	Ampicillin or Ceftriaxone or Cefotaxime or Vancomycin +/− macrolide

FURTHER READING

For further reading in *Tintinalli's Emergency Medicine: A Comprehensive Study Guide*, 8th ed, see Chapter 125, "Pneumonia in Infants and Children," by Joseph E. Copeland.

CHAPTER 72 Pediatric Heart Disease

Garth D. Meckler

There are six common clinical presentations of pediatric heart disease: cyanosis, shock, congestive heart failure (CHF), pathologic murmur, hypertension, and syncope. Table 72-1 lists the most common lesions in each category. While cyanosis and shock typically appear in the first weeks of life and are often dramatic in their presentation, the symptoms of CHF may be subtle and include respiratory distress or feeding intolerance, which may be misdiagnosed as viral upper respiratory tract illness, especially in winter months. A high index of suspicion must therefore be maintained in order to make the correct diagnosis. This chapter focuses on conditions producing cardiovascular symptoms seen in the emergency department (ED) that require immediate recognition, therapeutic intervention, and prompt referral to a pediatric cardiologist.

The evaluation of an asymptomatic murmur is a nonemergent diagnostic workup that can be done on an outpatient basis. Innocent murmurs, often described as flow murmurs, are of low intensity, are brief, and occur during systole. In general, common pathologic murmurs in children are typically harsh, holosystolic, continuous, or diastolic in timing, and often radiate.

TABLE 72-1 Clinical Presentations of Congenital Heart Disease

Clinical Presentation	Causative Conditions in Neonates	Causative Conditions in Infants and Children
Cyanosis	Transposition of the great arteries, TOF, tricuspid atresia, truncus arteriosus, total anomalous pulmonary venous return	TOF, Eisenmenger's complex
Cardiovascular shock	Critical AS, coarctation of the aorta, HLHS	Coarctation of the aorta (infants)
Congestive heart failure	Rare: PDA, HLHS	PDA, VSD, ASD, atrioventricular canal
Murmur	PDA, valvular defects (AS, PS)	VSD, ASD, PDA, outflow obstructions, valvular defects (AS, PS)
Syncope	–	AS, PS, Eisenmenger's complex
Hypertension	–	Coarctation of the aorta
Dysrhythmias	–	ASD, Ebstein's anomaly, postsurgical complication after repair of congenital heart defect

Abbreviations: AS = aortic stenosis; ASD = atrial septal defect; HLHS = hypoplastic left heart syndrome; PDA = patent ductus arteriosus; PS = pulmonic stenosis; TOF = tetralogy of Fallot; VSD = ventricular septal defect.

They may be associated with abnormal pulses or symptoms such as syncope or CHF.

The treatment of dysrhythmias is discussed in Chapter 3, pediatric hypertension is discussed in Chapter 26, and syncope is discussed in Chapter 78. Chest pain is usually of benign etiology in children, though may occasionally represent congenital (e.g., Anomalous Left Coronary Artery arising from Pulmonary Artery, ALCAPA) or acquired (e.g., Kawasaki disease, myocarditis, pericarditis, cardiomyopathy) heart disease. Myocarditis and cardiomyopathy are covered in Chapter 24, chest pain and acute coronary syndrome in Chapters 17 and 18, and Kawasaki disease in Chapter 83.

CYANOSIS AND SHOCK

Cardiac causes of cyanosis and shock typically present in the first 2 weeks of life and present in the critically ill neonate. The differential diagnosis, however, is broad at this age, and, in addition to congenital heart disease, the clinician should consider infection (sepsis, pneumonia), metabolic disease (see Chapter 79), and nonaccidental trauma. For the neonate presenting with cyanosis, the hyperoxia test helps differentiate respiratory disease from cyanotic congenital heart disease (although imperfectly). When placed on 100% oxygen, the infant with cyanotic congenital heart disease will fail to demonstrate an increase in Pao_2 or pulse oximetry, while those with respiratory causes will often respond with an improvement in Pao_2 or pulse oximetry.

Clinical Features

Acral cyanosis (blue discoloration of the distal extremities) can be normal in the neonate, but central cyanosis (including the mucus membranes of the mouth) is the cardinal feature of cyanotic congenital heart disease. Appreciation of cyanosis in dark-skinned neonates may be difficult, and an accurate set of vital signs including preductal and postductal pulse oximetry (i.e., right upper extremity and either lower extremity) and four-extremity blood pressures are essential. Cyanosis associated with a heart murmur strongly suggests congenital heart disease, but the absence of a murmur does not exclude a structural heart lesion. The cyanotic infant may be tachypneic, as well, though the increased respiratory rate in cyanotic heart disease is often effortless and shallow unless associated with congestive heart failure, which is rare in the first week of life.

Shock with or without cyanosis, especially during the first 2 weeks of life, should alert the clinician to the possibility of ductal-dependent congenital heart disease in which systemic (shock) or pulmonary (cyanosis) blood flow depends on patency of the fetal ductus arteriosis. Shock in the neonate is recognized by inspection of the patient's skin for pallor (or, more often, an "ashen grey" appearance), mottling, cyanosis, and assessment of the mental status appropriate for age. Mental status changes include apathy, irritability, or frank lethargy. Tachycardia and tachypnea may be the initial signs of impending cardiovascular collapse. Distal pulses should be assessed for quality, amplitude, and duration, and a differential between preductal (right brachial) and postductal (femoral) pulses or blood pressure is classic for ductal-dependent lesions such as coarctation of the aorta.

Diagnosis and Differential

The workup for congenital heart disease begins with chest radiograph and electrocardiogram (ECG) with pediatric analysis. Chest radiographs are assessed for heart size, shape, and pulmonary blood flow. An abnormal right position of the aortic arch may be a clue to the diagnosis of congenital cardiac lesion. Increased pulmonary vascularity may be seen with significant left-to-right shunting or left-sided failure. Decreased pulmonary blood flow is seen with right-sided outflow lesions such as pulmonic stenosis. Cyanotic heart lesions often demonstrate right axis deviation and right ventricular hypertrophy on ECG while left outflow obstruction (e.g., coarctation of the aorta) may show left ventricular hypertrophy. Echocardiography is generally required to define the diagnosis.

The differential diagnosis for cyanosis or shock due to congenital heart disease typically includes cyanotic lesions: transposition of the great vessels, tetralogy of Fallot, and other forms of right ventricular outflow tract obstruction or abnormalities of right heart formation. Acyanotic lesions that can present with shock include severe coarctation of the aorta, critical aortic stenosis, and hypoplastic left ventricle. It should be noted that cyanosis may accompany shock of any cause.

Transposition of the great vessels represents the most common cyanotic defect presenting in the first week of life. This entity is easily missed due to the absence of cardiomegaly or murmur, unless there is a coexistent ventricular septal defect (VSD). Symptoms (before shock) include central cyanosis, increased respiratory rate, and/or feeding difficulty. There is usually a loud and single S2. Chest radiographs may show an "egg on a string" shaped heart with a narrow mediastinum and increased pulmonary vascular markings. ECG may show right-axis deviation and right ventricular hypertrophy.

Tetralogy of Fallot is the most common cyanotic congenital heart disease overall, and can present with cyanosis later in infancy or childhood. Physical examination reveals a holosystolic murmur of VSD, a diamond-shape murmur of pulmonary stenosis, and cyanosis. Cyanotic spells in the toddler may be relieved by squatting. Chest radiograph may show a boot-shape heart with decreased pulmonary vascular markings or a right-sided aortic arch. The ECG often demonstrates right ventricular hypertrophy and right axis deviation.

Hypercyanotic episodes, or "tet spells," may bring children with tetralogy of Fallot to the ED in dramatic fashion. Symptoms include paroxysmal dyspnea, labored respirations, increased cyanosis, and syncope. Episodes frequently follow exertion due to feeding, crying, or straining with stools and last from minutes to hours.

Left ventricular outflow obstruction syndromes may present with shock, with or without cyanosis. Several congenital lesions fall into this category, but in all these disorders, systemic blood flow is dependent on a large contribution of shunted blood through a patent ductus arteriosus. When the ductus closes, infants present with decreased or absent perfusion, pallor or an ashen appearance, hypotension, tachypnea, and severe lactic acidosis. Diminished lower extremity pulses and BP, particularly compared to right brachial pulse and BP, are classic for coarctation of the aorta.

Emergency Department Care and Disposition

1. Cyanosis and respiratory distress are first managed with high-flow oxygen, cardiac and oxygen monitoring, and a stable intravenous or intraosseous line. Caveats: neonates tolerate low oxygen saturations well due to oxygen-avid fetal hemoglobin; oxygen is a potent pulmonary vasodilator and may lead to "pulmonary steal" of systemic blood flow, worsening systemic shock in ductal-dependent systemic blood flow such as coarctation of the aorta. Treatment with prostaglandins (see below) is critical in these cases.
2. For severe shock in infants suspected of having shunt-dependent lesions, give **prostaglandin E1** (PGE1) in an attempt to reopen the ductus. Treatment begins with 0.05 μg/kg/min and should be tapered to the lowest effective dose; the rate may be increased to 0.2 μg/kg/min if there is no improvement. Side effects include fever, skin flushing, diarrhea, and periodic apnea.
3. Obtain immediate consultation with a pediatric cardiologist and, if the patient is in shock, a pediatric intensivist.
4. Management of hypercyanotic spells consists of positioning the patient in the knee-to-chest position and administration of **morphine sulfate** 0.2 mg/kg SC, IM, or IO. Resistant cases should prompt immediate consultation with a pediatric cardiologist for consideration of phenylephrine for hypotension or propranolol for tachycardia.
5. Consider and treat noncardiac causes of symptoms; administer a fluid challenge of 10 to 20 mL/kg of normal saline solution and empiric administration of antibiotics as indicated. Fluids should be administered more judiciously to neonates with congenital heart disease, typically using10 mL/kg boluses.
6. **Epinephrine** is the initial drug of choice for hypotension. An infusion is started at 0.05 to 0.5 μg/kg/min and titrated to the desired blood pressure.

By definition, these children are critically ill and require admission, usually to the neonatal or pediatric intensive care unit.

CONGESTIVE HEART FAILURE

Clinical Features

Congestive heart failure from congenital or acquired heart disease typically presents after the neonatal period, usually in the second or third month of life (congenital) or later in childhood (acquired causes). The distinction between pneumonia and CHF in infants requires a high index of clinical suspicion and is often difficult. Pneumonia can cause a previously stable cardiac condition to decompensate; thus, both problems can present simultaneously. Presenting symptoms include poor feeding, diaphoresis, irritability or lethargy with feeding, weak cry, and, in severe cases, grunting, nasal flaring, and respiratory distress. Note that the early tachypnea of CHF in infants is typically "effortless" and is the first manifestation of decompensation, followed by increased work of breathing and rales on examination.

Diagnosis and Differential

Cardiomegaly evident on chest radiograph is universally present except in constrictive pericarditis. A cardiothoracic index greater than 0.6 on the PA chest radiograph is abnormal. The primary radiographic signs of cardiomegaly on the lateral chest radiograph are an abnormal cardiothoracic index and lack of retrosternal air space due to the direct abutment of the heart against the sternum.

Once CHF is recognized, age-related categories simplify further differential diagnosis (Table 72-2). Congenital cardiac causes of CHF are best categorized by age of onset. Early-onset CHF is associated with ductal-dependent lesions such as coarctation of the aorta and may be abrupt in onset; persistent patent ductus arteriosis (PDA) may also present in the neonatal period with CHF. Rarely, sustained tachyarrhythmias may present with CHF in the neonatal period. By contrast, lesions that result in pulmonary overcirculation such as VSD or atrial septal defect (ASD) present with gradual development of failure in the second or third month of life. Onset of CHF after age 3 months usually signifies acquired heart disease such as cardiomyopathy or myocarditis. The exception is when pneumonia, endocarditis, or another complication causes a congenital lesion to decompensate.

Cardiomyopathy presents with respiratory distress and feeding difficulties and is easily confused with upper respiratory tract infection. A pathologic gallop (S3 and or S4) is key to recognition. Rales and organomegaly are often present, and cardiomegaly and pulmonary vascular congestion are noted on chest radiography.

Myocarditis is often preceded by a viral respiratory illness, presents with nonspecific symptoms, and is more common in school age children. Presenting symptoms include shortness of breath, vomiting, poor feeding, lethargy, and fever. Signs of poor perfusion, organomegaly, and

TABLE 72-2 Differential Diagnosis of Congestive Heart Failure Based on Age at Presentation

Cardiac Lesion	Chest Radiograph	Electrocardiogram
Tetralogy of Fallot	Boot-shaped heart, normal-sized heart, decreased pulmonary vascular markings	Right axis deviation, right ventricular hypertrophy
Transposition of the great arteries	Egg-shaped heart, narrow mediastinum, increased pulmonary vascular marking	Right axis deviation, right ventricular hypertrophy
Total anomalous pulmonary venous return	Snowman sign, significant cardiomegaly, increased pulmonary vascular markings	Right axis deviation, right ventricular hypertrophy, right atrial enlargement
Tricuspid atresia	Heart of normal to slightly increased size, decreased pulmonary vascular markings	Superior QRS axis with right atrial hypertrophy, left atrial hypertrophy, left ventricular hypertrophy
Truncus arteriosus	Cardiomegaly, increased pulmonary vascular markings	Biventricular hypertrophy

tachypnea and tachycardia are common. ECG may show diffuse ST changes, dysrhythmias, or ectopy, which is associated with an increased risk of sudden death; a prolonged QRS duration of >120 ms is associated with poor clinical outcome. Chest radiograph shows cloudy lung fields from inflammation or pulmonary edema. Cardiomegaly with poor distal pulses and prolonged capillary refill, however, distinguish it from common pneumonia. Cardiac Troponin T is a highly sensitive, though nonspecific, test for myocarditis and levels <0.01 ng/mL reliably exclude myocarditis.

Usually pericarditis presents with pleuritic and positional chest pain. Muffled heart sounds and a friction rub may be present on physical examination. Cardiomegaly is seen on a chest radiograph. An echocardiogram is performed urgently to distinguish a pericardial effusion from dilated or hypertrophic cardiomyopathy, and to determine the need for pericardiocentesis.

If an infant presents in pure right-sided CHF, the primary problem is most likely to be pulmonary, such as cor pulmonale. In early stages, periorbital edema is often the first noticeable sign. This may progress to hepatomegaly, jugular venous distention, peripheral edema, and anasarca.

Emergency Department Care and Disposition

1. The infant who presents with mild tachypnea, hepatomegaly, and cardiomegaly should be seated upright in a comfortable position, oxygen should be given, and the child should be kept in a neutral thermal environment to avoid metabolic stresses imposed by hypothermia or hyperthermia.
2. If the work of breathing is increased or CHF is apparent on chest radiograph, **furosemide,** 1 to 2 mg/kg, should be administered parenterally.
3. Hypoxemia is usually corrected by administration of oxygen, fluid restriction, and diuresis, although continuous positive airway pressure (CPAP or BIPAP) is sometimes necessary.
4. Stabilization and improvement of left ventricular function is often first accomplished with inotropic agents. **Digoxin** is used in milder forms of CHF. The appropriate first digitalizing dose to be given in the ED is 20 to 30 μg/kg in neonates and 30 to 50 μg/kg in infants and children between 1 month and 2 years of age.
5. When CHF progresses to cardiogenic shock (absent distal pulses and decreased end-organ perfusion), continuous infusions of inotropic agents, such as dopamine or dobutamine, are indicated instead of digoxin. The initial starting range for **dopamine** is 5 to 15 μg/kg/min and **dobutamine** 2.5 to 15 μg/kg/min but may result in significant tachycardia in infants. **Milrinone** is another inotrope that improves diastolic relaxation and vasodilation without increasing myocardial oxygen demand and is given as 50 μg/kg IV over 10 to 60 minutes followed by continuous infusion of 0.25 to 0.75 μg/kg/min.
6. Aggressive management of secondary derangements, including respiratory insufficiency, acute renal failure, lactic acidosis, disseminated intravascular coagulation, hypoglycemia, and hypocalcaemia, and fever should be implemented.

7. Definitive diagnosis and treatment of congenital defects presenting with CHF often requires cardiac catheterization followed by surgical repair. See the previous section for recommendations regarding administration of prostaglandin E1 as a temporizing measure before surgery.

FURTHER READING

For further reading in *Tintinalli's Emergency Medicine: A Comprehensive Study Guide*, 8th ed., see Chapter 126, "Congenital and Acquired Pediatric Heart Disease" by Esther L.Yue and Garth D. Meckler.

CHAPTER 73 Vomiting and Diarrhea in Infants and Children

Stephen B. Freedman

Gastroenteritis is a major public health problem, accounting for up to 20% of all acute care outpatient visits to hospitals. Most children who come to the emergency department because of vomiting and/or diarrhea have a self-limited viral disorder. Nevertheless, loss of water and electrolytes can lead to clinical dehydration and may result in hypovolemic shock or life-threatening electrolyte disturbances.

CLINICAL FEATURES

The evaluation of the child's hydration status is the cornerstone to clinical management, regardless of whether the presenting complaint is vomiting or diarrhea (Table 73-1). Viral, bacterial, and other infectious organisms can cause gastroenteritis, and spread most commonly occurs by the fecal-to-oral route. Viral pathogens cause disease by invading tissue and altering the intestine's ability to absorb water and electrolytes. Bacterial pathogens cause diarrhea by producing enterotoxins and cytotoxins and by invading the intestine's mucosal absorptive surface. Dysentery occurs when bacteria invade the mucosa of the terminal ileum and colon, producing diarrhea with blood, mucus, or pus. Table 73-2 lists common infectious agents, clinical features, and treatments of diarrhea in children. Infants are at greater risk for rapid dehydration and hypoglycemia, as they are with chronic illnesses, high-risk social situations, or malnutrition.

DIAGNOSIS AND DIFFERENTIAL

Acute gastroenteritis is a clinical diagnosis that is characterized by the presence of three or more diarrheal stools in a 24-hour period, and may be accompanied by vomiting, poorly localized abdominal pain, and fever. Because gastroenteritis-induced dehydration is usually isotonic, serum electrolytes are not routinely helpful unless signs of severe dehydration are present or intravenous rehydration fluids will be administered. The

TABLE 73-1 Clinical Dehydration Score

Score	General Appearance	Eyes	Oral Mucosa (Tongue)	Tears
0	Normal	Normal	Moist	Normal
1	Thirsty, restless, lethargic but irritable	Mildly sunken	Sticky	Decreased
2	Drowsy/nonresponsive, limp, cold, diaphoretic	Very sunken	Dry	None

Score >0 = some dehydration; score >5 = moderate-severe dehydration.

TABLE 73-2 Clinical Features and Treatment of Bacterial Gastroenteritis

Organism	Typical Clinical Features	Risk Factors	Complications	Antimicrobial Therapy
Shigella	• Ranges from watery stools without constitutional symptoms to fever, abdominal pain, tenesmus, mucoid stools, hematochezia; *Shigella dysenteriae* serotype 1 causes more severe symptoms	• Contact with infected host or fomite, poor sanitation, crowded living conditions, day care	• Pseudomembranous colitis, toxic megacolon, intestinal perforation, bacteremia, • Reiter's syndrome, hemolytic-uremic syndrome, encephalopathy, seizures, hemolysis	• Typically self-limited • Treat if: immunocompromised, severe disease, dysentery or systemic symptoms • If susceptibility unknown: azithromycin, ceftriaxone, ciprofloxacin; if susceptible, ampicillin or trimethoprim-sulfamethoxazole
Salmonella	• Nontyphoidal: May be asymptomatic or cause watery diarrhea, mild fever, abdominal cramps • Enterica serotypes: "enteric fever" may include high fever, constitutional symptoms, headache, abdominal pain, dactylitis, hepatosplenomegaly, rose spots, altered mental status	• Direct contact with animals: poultry, livestock, reptiles, pets; consuming food contaminated by human carrier: beef, poultry, eggs, dairy, water	• Meningitis, brain abscess, osteomyelitis, bacteremia, dehydration, endocarditis, enteric (typhoid or paratyphoid) fever	• Typically self-limited • Treat if: < 3 months of age, hemoglobinopathy, immunodeficiency, chronic GI tract disease, malignancy, severe colitis, bacteremia, sepsis • Options: ampicillin, amoxicillin, trimethoprim-sulfamethoxazole; if resistant, azithromycin, fluoroquinolone • Invasive disease: cefotaxime, ceftriaxone
Campylobacter	• Diarrhea, hematochezia, abdominal pain, fever, malaise	• Contamination from poultry feces or undercooked poultry, untreated water, unpasteurized milk, pets (dogs, cats, hamsters, birds); person-to-person transmission possible	• Acute: dehydration, bacteremia, focal infections, febrile seizures • Convalescence: reactive arthritis, Reiter's syndrome, erythema nodosum, acute idiopathic polyneuritis, Miller Fisher syndrome, myocarditis, pericarditis	• Often self-limited; 20% have relapse or prolonged symptoms • Treat if: moderate-severe symptoms, relapse, immunocompromised, day care and institutions • Options: erythromycin, azithromycin, ciprofloxacin

Escherichia coli–Shiga toxin producing	• Initially nonbloody diarrhea, often becoming bloody; severe abdominal pain	• Food or water contaminated with human or cattle feces, undercooked beef, unpasteurized milk	• Hemorrhagic colitis, hemolytic-uremic syndrome	• None indicated; debated risk of increased incidence of hemolytic-uremic syndrome with treatment
E. coli–enteropathogenic	• Severe watery diarrhea, usually children <2 years in resource-limited countries	• Food or water contaminated with feces	• Dehydration	• Treat if severe • Options: trimethoprim-sulfamethoxazole, azithromycin, ciprofloxacin
E. coli–enterotoxigenic	• Moderate watery diarrhea, abdominal cramps; traveler's diarrhea	• Food or water contaminated with feces	• Dehydration	• Treat if severe • Options: trimethoprim-sulfamethoxazole, azithromycin, ciprofloxacin
E. coli–enteroinvasive	• Fever, bloody or nonbloody diarrhea, dysentery	• Food or water contaminated with feces	• Dehydration	• Treat if severe • Options: trimethoprim-sulfamethoxazole, azithromycin, ciprofloxacin
E. coli–enteroaggregative	• Watery diarrhea, may be prolonged	• Food or water contaminated with feces	• Dehydration	• Treat if severe • Options: trimethoprim-sulfamethoxazole, azithromycin, ciprofloxacin
Yersinia	• Bloody diarrhea with mucus, fever, abdominal pain; pseudoappendicitis syndrome: fever, right lower quadrant pain, leukocytosis; *Yersinia* pseudotuberculosis causes fever, scarlatiniform rash, abdominal pain	• Contaminated food: improperly cooked pork, unpasteurized milk, untreated water; contact with animals (ungulates, rodents, rabbits, birds)	• Acute: bacteremia, pharyngitis, meningitis, osteomyelitis, pyomyositis, conjunctivitis, pneumonia, empyema, endocarditis, acute peritonitis, liver/spleen abscess; convalescence: erythema nodosum, glomerulonephritis, reactive arthritis	• Typically self-limited; if severe, treat with trimethoprim-sulfamethoxazole, aminoglycosides, cefotaxime, fluoroquinolones, tetracycline, doxycycline, chloramphenicol
Vibrio cholerae	• Voluminous watery diarrhea, usually without cramps or fever, classically described as "rice water" stools	• Travel to affected areas, consumption of contaminated water or food (particularly undercooked seafood)	• May rapidly lead to hypovolemic shock, hypoglycemia, hypokalemia, metabolic acidosis, seizures	• Treat if moderate or severe: azithromycin, doxycycline; ciprofloxacin or trimethoprim-sulfamethoxazole if resistant

exception is infants in the first 6 months of life, in whom significant sodium abnormalities may develop. Bedside glucose should be checked in all patients with altered mental status; hypoglycemia can develop rapidly in the setting of protracted vomiting or diarrhea in infants and toddlers. Stool cultures are reserved for cases in which the child has traveled to a high-risk country, is highly or persistently febrile, has had more than 10 stools in the previous 24 hours, or has blood in the stool. In the setting of a known outbreak of *Escherichia coli* O157:H7, consider stool cultures and blood tests to check for evidence of hemolysis, thrombocytopenia, and acute kidney injury.

Although diarrhea is the most prominent symptom of acute gastroenteritis in infants and children, other etiologies of diarrhea that may result in significant morbidity must be considered: bacterial colitis, Hirschsprung disease, partial obstruction, inflammatory bowel disease, and hemolytic uremic syndrome. Acute appendicitis typically manifests with abdominal pain followed by vomiting associated with constipation; however, it may also cause diarrhea, particularly once the appendix has perforated (see Chapter 74, "Pediatric Abdominal Emergencies").

Vomiting is also a common and nonspecific presentation for other disease processes, such as otitis media, urinary tract infection, sepsis, malrotation, intussusception, increased intracranial pressure, metabolic acidosis, and drug or toxin ingestions. Consequently, *isolated vomiting*, though most often of viral origin, requires a careful and thoughtful evaluation before being diagnosed as acute gastroenteritis. Specific clinical findings, such as bilious or bloody vomitus, hematochezia, or abdominal pain, should trigger concerns for a disease process other than simple viral gastroenteritis.

EMERGENCY DEPARTMENT CARE AND DISPOSITION

Dehydration (Vomiting and/or Diarrhea)

1. Because most cases are self-limited, oral rehydration is generally all that is necessary. Vomiting is not a contraindication to oral rehydration; the key is to give small amounts of the solution frequently. Use of a commercially available **oral rehydration solution** (ORS) containing 45 to 60 mmol/L of sodium is recommended. Many other beverages traditionally suggested for children with vomiting and diarrhea, such as tea, juice, or sports drinks, are deficient in sodium and may provide excessive sugar, resulting in amplified fluid losses. Give **ORS** 50 to 100 mL/kg of body weight, plus additional ORS to compensate for ongoing losses. Aim for about 30 mL (1 ounce) of ORS per kilogram of body weight per hour. Consider nasogastric administration of fluids if oral challenge fails.
2. Administer intravenous or intraosseous isotonic crystalloid to children with severe dehydration, hemodynamic compromise, or when altered mental status precludes safe oral administration of fluid. Give **normal saline** or Ringer's lactate as a 20-mL/kg bolus every 20 minutes until perfusion improves and urine output is adequate.
3. Treat hypoglycemia with 10% dextrose 5 mL/kg in infants or 25% dextrose 2 mL/kg in toddlers and older children.

Vomiting

1. Treat dehydration, hypoglycemia, and electrolyte abnormalities as mentioned earlier.
2. **Ondansetron** 0.15 mg/kg/dose should be administered (or 2 mg for 8 to <15 kg; 4 mg for 15 to <30 kg; 8 mg if ≥30 kg) as an adjunct to oral rehydration therapy in children with persistent vomiting. Oral dosing is preferred as the main objective is to support the success of oral rehydration; intravenous ondansetron administration results in greater QT prolongation and its use should be avoided.
3. Most children can be discharged if they are tolerating oral rehydration, have adequate urine output, and ongoing fluid losses have been minimized. Continuation of a normal diet (including lactose-containing milk or formula) is recommended. Patients who cannot tolerate oral fluids, have significant ongoing losses, severe electrolyte abnormalities, or surgical abdominal processes, require admission to the hospital.

Diarrhea

1. Treat dehydration and hypoglycemia as above.
2. Children with mild diarrhea who are not dehydrated may continue routine feedings. Do not withhold feedings >4 hours in a dehydrated child or for any length of time in a child who is not dehydrated. There is no need to dilute formula because more than 80% of children with acute diarrhea can tolerate full-strength milk safely.
3. Antidiarrheal and antimotility agents such as loperamide are not recommended in children and are contraindicated in young children.
4. Antibiotics are unnecessary for the vast majority of children with acute gastroenteritis and may be associated with increased risk for hemolytic uremic syndrome. See Table 73-2 for specific treatment recommendations by pathogen.
5. All infants and children who appear toxic or have high-risk social situations, significant dehydration, significant ongoing fluid losses, altered mental status, inability to drink, or laboratory evidence of hemolytic anemia, thrombocytopenia, azotemia, or a significant sodium abnormality should be admitted.
6. Children who respond to oral or intravenous hydration can be discharged. Instructions should be given to return to the emergency department or seek care with the primary care provider if the child becomes unable to tolerate oral hydration, develops bilious vomiting, becomes less alert, or exhibits signs of dehydration, such as no longer wetting diapers. Dietary recommendations include a diet high in complex carbohydrates, lean meats, vegetables, fruits, and yogurt. Fatty foods and foods high in simple sugars should be avoided. The BRAT diet is discouraged because it does not provide adequate energy sources.

FURTHER READING

For further reading in *Tintinalli's Emergency Medicine: A Comprehensive Study Guide*, 8th edition, see Chap. 128, "Vomiting, Diarrhea, and Dehydration in Infants and Children," by Stephen B. Freedman and Jennifer D. Thull-Freedman.

CHAPTER 74

Pediatric Abdominal Emergencies

Janet Semple-Hess

ABDOMINAL PAIN

The assessment of acute abdominal pain can be challenging given the preverbal state of young children, the varied number of diagnoses that present similarly, and increasing appreciation of risks associated with pediatric diagnostic imaging.

Clinical Features

Presenting signs and symptoms differ by age. The key gastrointestinal (GI) signs and symptoms include pain, vomiting, diarrhea, constipation, fever, jaundice, and masses. Abdominal pain in children younger than 2 years typically manifests as fussiness, irritability, lethargy, or grunting. Toddlers and school-age children often localize pain poorly and point to their umbilicus, or may present as refusal to ambulate. Pain may be peritoneal and exacerbated by motion, or spasmodic, and associated with restlessness. Abdominal pain may originate from non-GI sources, and associated symptoms may help localize extra-abdominal causes such as cough with pneumonia or sore throat in streptococcal pharyngitis.

Vomiting and diarrhea are common in children. These symptoms may be the result of a benign process or indicate the presence of a life-threatening condition. Bilious vomiting is almost always indicative of a serious process, especially in the neonate. Upper GI bleeding in children presents with hematemesis, which is often frightening to caretakers, but rarely serious in an otherwise healthy infant or child. Lower GI bleeding presents with melena or hematochezia, and the distinction between painless and painful rectal bleeding can help differentiate likely etiologies. Jaundice can be an ominous sign, and sepsis, congenital infections, hepatitis, anatomic problems, and enzyme deficiencies should be considered in the evaluation of these patients. Abdominal masses may be asymptomatic (e.g., Wilms tumor) or associated with painless vomiting (e.g., pyloric stenosis) or colicky abdominal pain (e.g., intussusception).

Diagnosis and Differential

Obtain a thorough history from parent and child (if possible), including the quality and location of pain, chronology of events, feedings, bowel habits, fever, weight changes, and other systemic signs and symptoms. Begin the physical examination with an assessment of the child's overall appearance, vital signs, and hydration status. Observation should precede auscultation and palpation. Extra-abdominal areas including the chest, pharynx, testes, scrotum, inguinal area, and neck should also be evaluated. Adolescent females who are sexually active with lower abdominal pain may require a bimanual exam. The likely etiologies of abdominal pain vary with age. Table 74-1 classifies emergent and nonemergent conditions by age group.

TABLE 74-1 Causes of Abdominal Pain by Age Group

Age	Emergent	Nonemergent
0–3 months	Necrotizing enterocolitis Volvulus Incarcerated hernia Testicular torsion Nonaccidental trauma Hirschsprung's enterocolitis	Constipation Acute gastroenteritis Colic
3 months to 3 years	Intussusception Volvulus Testicular torsion Appendicitis Vaso-occlusive crisis Tumor Pneumonia Urinary tract infections	Urinary tract infections Constipation Henoch–Schönlein purpura Acute gastroenteritis
3 years through ado lescence	Appendicitis Diabetic ketoacidosis Vaso-occlusive crisis Ectopic pregnancy Ovarian torsion Testicular torsion Cholecystitis Pancreatitis Urinary tract infections Tumor Pneumonia	*Streptococcus* pharyngitis Inflammatory bowel disease Pregnancy Renal stones Peptic ulcer disease/gastritis Ovarian cysts Henoch–Schönlein purpura Constipation Acute gastroenteritis Nonspecific viral syndromes

Neonates and Young Infants (0 to 3 Months)

Life-threatening abdominal conditions in young infants include necrotizing enterocolitis, malrotation with midgut volvulus, incarcerated hernias, and nonaccidental trauma. Other urgent conditions include pyloric stenosis and testicular torsion. Inconsolability, lethargy, and poor feeding may be the only indication of serious underlying disease. Bilious vomiting in an infant indicates intestinal obstruction and should be considered a surgical emergency until proven otherwise. Common non-life-threatening causes of abdominal pain in young infants include colic (see Chapter 67) milk-protein allergy or gastroesophageal reflux. Fever requires thorough investigation for a source (see Chapter 66). Other causes of irritability in infants should be considered, including hair or thread tourniquets of the digits and genitalia, and corneal abrasions (see Chapter 67).

Helpful studies in this age group include abdominal two-view radiographs to identify obstruction, pneumatosis intestinalis, or free air; abdominal ultrasound to diagnose pyloric stenosis, testicular torsion, and hernias; and upper GI contrast studies to identify malrotation. Useful laboratory studies include serum electrolytes to identify abnormalities resulting from vomiting and dehydration and a CBC, coagulation panel, and type and screen if concern is for a surgical abdomen with perforation.

Malrotation of the intestine can present with life-threatening *volvulus*. Symptoms include bilious vomiting, abdominal distention, and obstipation, or, occasionally, streaks of blood in the stool. The vast majority of cases present within the first month of life. Patients are ill-appearing and may present in compensated or decompensated shock. A "bird's beak" appearance on an upper GI series is suggestive of this diagnosis. Immediate surgical consultation and aggressive fluid resuscitation are critical to improve outcomes.

Pyloric stenosis usually presents with progressive nonbilious, projectile vomiting occurring just after feeding. Pyloric stenosis occurs most commonly in the third or fourth week of life, but may be seen anywhere from 1 to 12 weeks of age. A left upper quadrant pyloric mass, or "olive," may be present, but is usually difficult to detect, and peristaltic waves may be noted following a feeding trial in the ED. Ultrasound is the imaging modality of choice. Electrolytes may demonstrate a characteristic hypochloremic metabolic alkalosis, which must be corrected prior to definitive surgical care. While pyloric stenosis is not a surgical emergency, the resultant dehydration from persistent vomiting requires immediate medical treatment.

Necrotizing enterocolitis, although rare outside of the neonatal unit, should be considered in any infant younger than 3 weeks of age, especially if premature. Vomiting, poor feeding, and abdominal distention may be present, and abdominal films may show pneumatosis intestinalis, as well as portal vein gas. Immediate surgical/neonatology consultation, NPO, IVF hydration, and broad-spectrum antibiotics for intestinal flora should be instituted if suspected.

Hirschsprung's disease is a pathologic cause of constipation in this age group, as true constipation is unusual. Key history for Hirschprung's disease is delayed passage of meconium at birth (more than 24 hours). Symptoms include infrequent and often explosive bowel movements, poor feeding and growth, and progressive abdominal distension. Toxic megacolon may occur as a complication and if suspected, emergent surgical consultation is warranted.

Older Infants and Toddlers (3 Months to 3 Years)

The differential diagnosis of acute abdominal pain in this age group includes intussusception, gastroenteritis (see Chapter 73), constipation, urinary tract disease (see Chapter 75), and nonaccidental trauma. Though less common in this age group, acute appendicitis, diabetic ketoacidosis or other metabolic diseases, tumors such as Wilm's, neuroblastoma or hepatoblastoma and malrotation with midgut volvulus must be considered.

Imaging studies are guided by the differential diagnosis: radiographs can help rule out free air or obstruction, and confirm suspected constipation; ultrasound can help identify intussusception, abdominal or renal mass, or appendicitis, and air-contrast enema is both diagnostic and potentially therapeutic for intussusception. A CBC and electrolytes may be helpful in evaluating complications of vomiting and diarrhea, and urinalysis will identify pyelonephritis as a potential cause of abdominal pain in this age group. A bedside glucose is helpful in the lethargic child or in cases with persistent or prolonged vomiting.

Intussusception occurs when one portion of the bowel telescopes into another, which can result in a partial or complete obstruction, bowel-wall edema, and eventually bowel ischemia. The greatest incidence occurs between 6 to 18 months of age, and it is the most common cause of

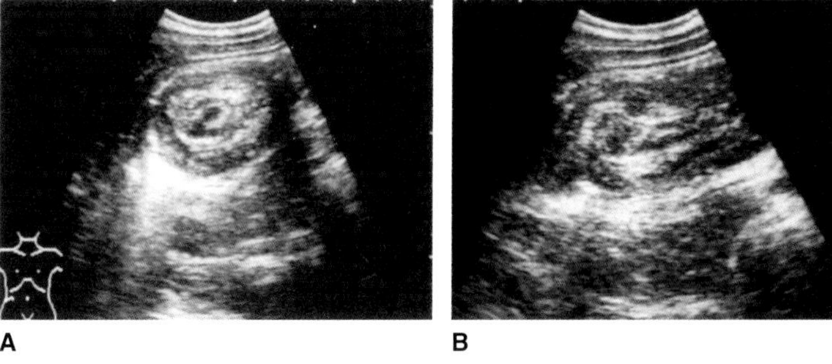

FIGURE 74-1. A and B. Ultrasound image of intussusception showing the classic target appearance of bowel-within-bowel. Reproduced with permission from Ma OJ, Mateer JR, Blaivas M: Emergency Ultrasound, 2nd ed. New York: McGraw-Hill; 2008.

intestinal obstruction in children under 2 years of age. The classic presentation of intermittent paroxysms of abdominal pain with pain-free intervals (or lethargy), vomiting (may be bilious), and "currant jelly stool" are not present in all patients, and bloody stools is a late sign. Stool testing may reveal occult blood in 70% of intussusception cases. Providers must have a high index of suspicion for intussusception in patients presenting with nonspecific changes in mental status or who are ill-appearing without any apparent etiology. Ultrasound should be performed if the diagnosis is ambiguous, and may demonstrate the classic "target sign" (see Fig. 74-1). In more classic cases, air or barium enema should be performed, and can be both diagnostic and therapeutic. Radiologic reduction requires a readily available pediatric surgeon for irreducible cases or perforation during the procedure. Uncomplicated cases of intussusception successfully reduced by enema may be discharged after observation if tolerating oral fluids and has reliable follow-up, as there is a 10% recurrence risk.

Constipation, defined as infrequent, hard stools, is a common cause of abdominal pain in children and may be a sign of either a pathologic (e.g., Hirschsprung disease, cystic fibrosis, spinal cord abnormality, or infant botulism) or functional process. History is key to the diagnosis. For neonates, verify passage of meconium in the first 24 hours of life. A rectal examination is recommended to assess presence of stool, rectal tone, sensation, and size of the anal vault. A careful neurologic examination should be completed to assess for neuromuscular causes. A single upright abdominal radiograph may be helpful to visualize fecal retention or impaction, and to help rule out the concern for obstruction. Treatment in the ED with suppositories or enemas may be necessary, and outpatient maintenance therapy such as with polyethylene glycol for older children (older than 12 months) is essential to prevent recurrence. Admission is indicated for patients with impaction associated with vomiting, dehydration, and failure of outpatient treatment.

Children (3 to 15 Years Old)

Acute abdominal pain in children 3 to 15 years old includes a range of diagnoses, including appendicitis (Chapter 43), constipation, gastroenteritis, urinary tract infection, streptococcal pharyngitis (Chapter 68), pneumonia (Chapter 71), pancreatitis (Chapter 42), and functional abdominal pain. In adolescents, gall bladder disease (cholelithiasis, biliary colic, or cholecystitis), renal stones, ovarian pathology (cysts or torsion), and testicular torsion should be considered. Diabetes and diabetic ketoacidosis are more prevalent in this age group and commonly present as vague abdominal pain. The presence of a parent and allowing the child to sit on the parents' lap are helpful in examining younger children. Older children may not readily offer important history surrounding embarrassing topics such as constipation and genital pain. Adolescents should be interviewed alone to provide confidentiality and facilitate discussion of potentially important information surrounding sexual activity and other sensitive subjects.

Henoch–Schönlein purpura (HSP) is an idiopathic vasculitis of children between 2 and 11 years of age. HSP classically presents with palpable purpura, acute abdominal pain, and arthritis. A urinalysis should be obtained to identify hematuria, with subsequent renal function tests when blood is present, as up to 30% of children with HSP will develop renal involvement, sometimes months later. Abdominal pain in HSP is caused by bowel wall edema and GI vasculitis, and may occur before typical rash of HSP appears. Microscopic and even gross GI bleeding is not uncommon, though rarely life-threatening. Intussusception (ileo-ileo as compared to the classic ileo-colic in idiopathic intussception) occurs in 3.5%, and must be considered in patients with significant abdominal pain. Treatment of HSP is primarily supportive: joint pain responds well to nonsteroidal anti-inflammatory medications; severe abdominal pain may improve with corticosteroids. Consultation and follow-up with a pediatric rheumatologist or nephrologist may be necessary for more severe symptoms or renal involvement with hypertension.

GASTROINTESTINAL BLEEDING

Upper GI (UGI) bleeding is distinguished from lower GI (LGI) bleeding anatomically at the ligament of Treitz. The presentation of GI bleeding in children varies, and includes bright red blood in small strands or clots in emesis or stool, vomiting of gross blood (hematemesis), black tarry stools (melena), or profuse bright red blood per rectum. Occult bleeding may present with pallor, fatigue, or anemia.

The first step in management is to evaluate the need for acute resuscitation, and distinguish the bleed as UGI or LGI. Confirmation through gastric or fecal occult blood testing is useful to distinguish substances that grossly mimic blood. Foods such as beets, cranberries, and red food dyes can appear like blood in stool. A thorough history and physical examination is important to determine the location, amount, and etiology of the bleed. Examination for extra-GI sources is also important (e.g., epistaxis is a common cause of hematemesis in children). Ask about recent dental surgery or gingival bleeding. Post-tonsillectomy bleeding is an important and potentially serious cause of hematemesis. A common cause of hematemesis in the newborn is swallowed maternal blood (either post-delivery or from fissures in mother's nipples).

The differential diagnosis of UGI and LGI bleeding by age group is summarized in Table 74-2. In general, UGI bleeding in children without

TABLE 74-2 Age-Based Causes of Upper and Lower GI Bleeding

Upper GI Bleeding

Neonate	Infant/Toddler	Child/Adolescent
Common	*Common*	*Common*
Swallowed maternal blood/ maternal "sore nipples"	Non-GI source (e.g., epistaxis)	Mallory–Weiss tear
	Mallory–Weiss tear	Gastritis (especially *Helicobacter pylori* gastritis)
Trauma (nasogastric tube in NICU)	Esophagitis	Esophagitis
Uncommon	Gastritis	Peptic ulcer disease
Stress ulcer/gastritis	*Uncommon*	*Uncommon*
Esophagitis/GERD	Stress gastritis or ulcer	Esophageal varices
Vascular malformation	Peptic ulcer disease	Toxic/caustic ingestion
Hemorrhagic disease of newborn (vitamin K deficiency)	Vascular malformation	Foreign body
Coagulopathy/bleeding diathesis	GI duplication	Vasculitis
Coagulopathy associated with infection	Gastric/esophageal varices Bowel obstruction Toxic/caustic ingestion Coagulopathy/bleeding diathesis Foreign body	Vascular malformation Bowel obstruction Crohn's disease Coagulopathy/bleeding diathesis GI stromal tumors Dieulafoy's lesion

Lower GI Bleeding

Neonate	Infant/Toddler	Child/Adolescent
Common	*Common*	*Common*
Swallowed maternal blood	Anal fissure	Anal fissure
Anal fissure	Milk/soy protein allergy	Infectious gastroenteritis
Milk/soy protein allergy	Infectious gastroenteritis	Polyps; benign, familial
Infectious gastroenteritis	*Uncommon*	*Uncommon*
Uncommon	Intussusception	Henoch–Schönlein purpura
Meckel's diverticulum*	Meckel's diverticulum*	Hemorrhoids
Necrotizing enterocolitis	GI duplication	Inflammatory bowel disease
Vascular malformation	Hemolytic-uremic syndrome	Meckel's diverticulum*
Hemorrhagic disease of newborn (vitamin K deficiency)	Henoch–Schönlein purpura	Hemolytic-uremic syndrome
Intussusception	Malrotation with volvulus	Vascular malformation
Malrotation with volvulus	Polyps; benign, familial	Celiac disease
Hirschsprung-associated enterocolitis (toxic megacolon)	Coagulopathy/bleeding diathesis	
GI duplication	Vascular malformation	

*Most common cause of severe LGI bleeding in all ages.

Abbreviation: NICU, neonatal intensive care unit.

underlying portal hypertension is rarely life-threatening. While most causes of LGI bleeding in children are also benign, potential emergent causes include vascular malformations, Meckel diverticula, hemolytic uremic syndrome, and intussusception. In cases of melena, evaluate for causes of UGI bleeding and HSP. In cases of bright red blood per rectum, evaluate for anal fissure. For painless hematochezia, consider Meckel diverticulum, or arteriovenous malformation. For hematochezia in the setting of abdominal pain, the differential is larger including HSP, hemolytic uremic syndrome, infectious gastroenteritis, inflammatory bowel disease, milk-protein allergy in infants, intussusception, and necrotizing enterocolitis (neonates).

Laboratory studies and imaging should be completed as dictated by other associated signs and symptoms. Mild bleeding can typically be managed by a consultant on an outpatient basis. Stool studies for infectious causes should be sent if suspected. Moderate and severe bleeding requires acute resuscitation with isotonic crystalloid and, potentially, blood products. While acute shock should be treated immediately, overexpansion of intravascular volume should be avoided, particularly for variceal bleeding or more chronic conditions. Consultation with a pediatric surgeon, gastroenterologist, or critical care physician may be necessary, depending on the etiology.

FURTHER READING

For further reading in *Tintinalli's Emergency Medicine: A Comprehensive Study Guide*, 8th ed., see Chapter 130, "Acute Abdominal Pain in Infants and Children" by Ross J. Fleischman; Chapter 131, "Gastrointestinal Bleeding in Infants and Children" by Sarah M. Reid.

CHAPTER 75

Pediatric Urinary Tract Infections

Marie Waterhouse

Urinary tract infections (UTIs) are relatively common in children, from infancy through adolescence. The incidence and clinical presentation of pediatric UTI vary by age and gender.

CLINICAL FEATURES

There are several age-specific clinical presentations for pediatric UTI. Neonates present with a clinical syndrome indistinguishable from sepsis, and may often have nonspecific symptoms such as fever, jaundice, poor feeding, vomiting, irritability, or lethargy. Older infants and young children typically present with gastrointestinal symptoms such as abdominal pain, vomiting, or decreased appetite. School-age children and adolescents present similarly to adults, and often, but not always, complain of specific urinary symptoms such as dysuria, frequency, urgency, or hesitancy. Infants and young children are more likely to have fever and upper tract disease, necessitating longer courses of antibiotic treatment. Adolescents without fever, flank pain, or vomiting may be treated similarly to adults with shorter course antibiotic regimens.

DIAGNOSIS AND DIFFERENTIAL

The gold standard for the diagnosis of pediatric UTI is the growth of a single urinary pathogen from a properly obtained urine culture. For infants and children in diapers, urine obtained by sterile transurethral catheterization is preferred. Ultrasound-guided suprapubic bladder aspiration is an acceptable alternative, but is more invasive and rarely performed. For toilet-trained children who can void on command (usually ascertained by asking a parent, but generally at around 3 years old), urine may be collected as a clean catch specimen. Bagged urine specimens have virtually no role in diagnosis of pediatric UTI, and are never appropriate for urine culture.

Urine microscopy and chemical test strips (dipstick) have similar test characteristics in terms of sensitivity and specificity; however, dipstick is usually faster and more convenient, and a finding of positive nitrites is highly specific for the presence of gram-negative bacteriuria, obviating the need for urine microscopy. In cases where dipstick is indeterminate (i.e., "trace" leukocyte esterase), subsequent urine microscopy may be helpful in increasing diagnostic certainty. Microscopy is typically considered positive if more than five white blood cells per high-power field or bacteria are seen. Because young infants void frequently, and often do not store urine in the bladder long enough to accumulate leukocytes or nitrites, urinalysis is less sensitive in this age group, and culture should be sent regardless of negative urinalysis result.

Young children may also experience urinary symptoms from urethritis secondary to irritant soaps, clothing, or poor hygiene. Physical exam should assess for vaginitis in girls, or meatitis or balanitis in boys. Adolescents may have urinary symptoms as a manifestation of a sexually transmitted disease such as *Chlamydia trachomatis*. An appropriate sexual history should be obtained in teenagers, and a pelvic examination may be indicated for sexually active females (for a discussion of sexually transmitted diseases, see Chapter 87).

EMERGENCY DEPARTMENT CARE AND DISPOSITION

The treatment and disposition of infants and children with UTI depend on age and clinical severity. In general, antibiotics should not be given until after urine culture has been obtained. However, timely antibiotic administration takes precedence in the septic patient.

1. Treat neonates for sepsis and obtain cultures of blood and CSF in addition to urine. Administer parenteral antibiotics and admit to the hospital: **ampicillin** 50 mg/kg/dose plus **gentamicin** 3 to 5 mg/kg/dose; or **ampicillin** 50 mg/kg/dose plus **cefotaxime** 50 mg/kg/dose are appropriate empiric choices.
2. Treat infants from 1 month to 2 years of age with an intravenous third-generation cephalosporin such as **ceftriaxone, cefotaxime**, or **cefepime** (all are dosed at 50 mg/kg/dose). Ceftriaxone has the advantage of maintaining efficacy for 12 to 24 hours per dose. After an initial dose of IV antibiotics, well-appearing infants in this age group may be treated with a course of oral antibiotics, which is equally effective to parenteral treatment. Young infants must have close follow-up with their primary care providers, and be urged to return if they cannot tolerate oral therapy or are worsening. Children who are dehydrated, ill-appearing, have persistent vomiting, or are medically complex may require inpatient parenteral treatment. Antibiotic choices in all cases are guided by local susceptibility patterns. In communities where cephalexin, amoxicillin, or trimethoprim-sulfamethoxazole resistance has emerged, a third-generation oral cephalosporin such as **cefixime** 4 mg/kg/dose given twice daily or **cefdinir** 7 mg/kg/dose given twice daily should be considered. If *Enterococcus faecalis* has been found on prior urine cultures, add **amoxicillin** 25 mg/kg/dose given twice daily or **ampicillin** IV 50 mg/kg/dose to standard therapy. Treat for 7 to 14 days, as short-course therapy is not effective in young children.
3. Children older than 2 years who are not ill-appearing and who can tolerate oral fluids may be treated exclusively with oral antibiotics for a course of 7 to 14 days, as described above. Again, local antibiotic susceptibility patterns should guide antibiotic choice.
4. Well-appearing adolescent females older than 13 years with simple cystitis may be treated similarly to adults with a short course of oral antibiotics (see Chapter 53).

FURTHER READING

For further reading in *Tintinalli's Emergency Medicine: A Comprehensive Study Guide*, 8th ed., see Chapter 132, "Urinary Tract Infection in Infants and Children," by Justin W. Sales.

Seizures and Status Epilepticus in Children

Ara Festekjian

The causes and manifestations of seizures are numerous, ranging from benign to life threatening. Seizure precipitants include fever, CNS infections, head injury, structural brain abnormalities, hypoglycemia, electrolyte abnormalities, hypoxemia, toxin exposure, dysrhythmias, metabolic disorders, congenital infections, and neurocutaneous syndromes.

CLINICAL FEATURES

The clinical features of seizure activity depend on the affected area of the brain and can range from classic tonic-clonic movements to subtle behavioral changes; they may be generalized (with loss of consciousness) or partial (with focal motor or behavioral features). Rhythmic repetitive movements, bowel or bladder incontinence, a postictal state, and tongue biting are highly suggestive of seizures.

Motor changes (tonic or clonic) may be focal or generalized, and seizures may present with atony (sudden loss of tone or "drop attack") in some age groups. Additional seizure manifestations include staring spells ("absence") or changes in mental status or behavior, which can be complex, such as automatisms (blinking, bicycling, or lip smacking in infants), vocalizations, or hallucinations.

Associated clinical signs include alteration in autonomic dysfunction, such as mydriasis, diaphoresis, tachypnea or apnea, tachycardia, hypertension and salivation, and postictal somnolence. Transient focal deficits may represent Todd's paralysis following a seizure.

DIAGNOSIS AND DIFFERENTIAL

The diagnosis of seizure disorder is based primarily on history and physical examination. Bedside glucose testing should be performed on all children who are seizing or postictal, but the clinical scenario should direct additional laboratory and imaging tests. Screening tests for electrolytes are not indicated in most cases of childhood seizures including simple febrile seizures or first time afebrile seizures, unless otherwise indicated by the specific history. The suggested ED evaluation of differing clinical scenarios presenting with seizures is listed in Table 76-1.

Status epilepticus is defined as seizure activity lasting >30 minutes or multiple seizures without a return to normal mental status between seizures. Five minutes have been suggested as an operational definition because seizures lasting longer than 5 minutes usually do not resolve without treatment. Status epilepticus is a medical emergency, and is more responsive to medications when treated early and aggressively.

Seizures must be distinguished from other events that masquerade as seizures in children such as syncope, breath-holding spells, gastroesophageal reflux (Sandifer's syndrome), chorea (acute rheumatic fever), myoclonic jerks, rigors, startle reflex, tics, pseudo-seizures, migraine

TABLE 76-1 Suggested ED Evaluation of Pediatric Seizures
Age of child
Seizure duration and description of seizure activity prior to arrival
History of trauma
History of possible ingestion
History of fever
History of associated illness (vomiting or diarrhea)
Feeding problems (especially in an infant)
Changes in behavior
History of seizures and type of seizures
History of developmental delay
Other medical history
Medications
• Anticonvulsants with milligrams per kilogram dose and recent changes or missed doses • Recent new medications (may alter metabolism of antiepileptic drugs) • Allergies
Developmental history
Family history of seizures

variants, and night terrors. Primary seizures should be distinguished from seizures secondary to treatable or life-threatening causes such as trauma, infection, hypoglycemia, metabolic abnormalities, or electrolyte abnormalities.

EMERGENCY DEPARTMENT CARE AND DISPOSITION

1. The management of the seizing child requires immediate supportive care, termination of the seizure with anticonvulsant medication, and correction of reversible causes such as hypoglycemia or metabolic abnormalities.
2. Ensure a patent airway, apply oxygen to all seizing patients, and assist ventilation as indicated. If rapid-sequence intubation is required, continuous EEG monitoring should be arranged alongside anticonvulsant administration as neuromuscular blockade obscures the ability to clinically assess for ongoing seizures.
3. Treat hypoglycemia with 4 to 5 mL/kg **10% dextrose** in infants or 2 mL/kg **25% dextrose** in older children IV/IO.
4. Administer **lorazepam**, 0.1 mg/kg or **midazolam** 0.1 to 0.2 mg/kg IV/IO. If vascular access is not available, administer midazolam 0.2 mg/kg IN (maximum dose 10 mg). Repeat benzodiazepine dose in 5 minutes if seizure persists and prepare to support breathing and blood pressure with repeated dosing.
5. Administer second-line or third-line antiepileptic drugs if more than 2 doses of benzodiazepine are required. Consider using 2 of the following 4 medications, and moving on to fourth-line treatments if seizures are refractory to treatment. For infants, use **phenobarbital** 20 mg/kg IV/IO (maximum 800 mg). For older children: **fosphenytoin** 20 PE/kg IV/IO

over 20 minutes; **valproic acid** 20 mg/kg IV/IO; and **levetiracetam** 20 to 30 mg/kg IV/IO.

6. Fourth-line treatment strategies include continuous infusions in the ICU setting of propofol, midazolam, or pentobarbital, or induction of general inhaled anesthesia. **Propofol** dose is 0.5 to 2 mg/kg or 1.5 to 4 mg/kg/hr IV/IO; or **midazolam** continuous infusion: 0.05 to 0.4 mg/kg/hr IV/IO.
7. Treat electrolyte abnormalities as follows: for hyponatremia < 120 mEq/L, **3% NaCl** 4 to 6 mL/kg, for hypocalcemia, < 7 mg/dL of calcium and < 0.8 mmol/L of ionized calcium, 0.3 mL/kg of **10% calcium gluconate**, over 10 minutes, and for hypomagnesemia < 1.5 mEq/L, 50 mg/kg of **magnesium sulfate** over 20 minutes.
8. Children who present to the ED following a brief seizure and who regain a normal mental status without focal neurologic deficits are candidates for discharge and outpatient follow-up. Patients presenting to the ED with ongoing seizures meet the definition for status epilepticus and even when seizure termination is achieved in the ED, it is suggested that they be admitted for further observation. All infants with true seizures should be admitted to the hospital. Patients with refractory seizures, those with seizures from acute traumatic brain injury, CNS infection, or serious metabolic or electrolyte abnormalities typically require treatment in the ICU setting.

Febrile Seizure

Seizures in the setting of fever are common in children and are usually benign. Simple febrile seizures (SFS) occur between 6 months and 6 years of life, are brief (<15 minutes), and generalized. Patients with SFS require no specific ED evaluation or medication for their seizure, though evaluation for a treatable source of fever such as a urinary tract infection, and antipyretics may be indicated. Children experiencing SFS have the same 1% risk of developing epilepsy as the general population. Complex febrile seizures (>15 minutes in duration, focal, or recurrent) carry a slightly higher risk for epilepsy, but also do not routinely require ED evaluation or treatment. Febrile status epilepticus is treated as above with the addition of neuroimaging, CSF analysis and culture, and potential antibiotics and acyclovir as indicated.

First Seizure

The overall risk of recurrence after a single afebrile seizure is about 40%. Emergent neuroimaging is not necessary in the ED in the patient with a normal neurologic exam, though outpatient MRI and EEG may be of benefit. Most neurologists do not recommend starting anticonvulsant medication after a first seizure.

FURTHER READING

For further reading in *Tintinalli's Emergency Medicine: A Comprehensive Study Guide*, 8th ed., see Chapter 135, "Seizures in Infants and Children," by Maija Holsti.

Altered Mental Status and Headache in Children

Carlo Reyes

HEADACHE

Pediatric headache accounts for 1% of emergency department visits. The vast majority of headaches in children have a benign etiology. Factors associated with serious or dangerous causes of headache include preschool age, occipital location, recent onset of headache, and inability of the child to describe the quality of the head pain.

Clinical Features

Headaches can be classified as primary or secondary. Primary headaches are associated with normal physical exam findings, are self-limited, and may be recurrent. Examples of primary headache include physiologic or functional (migraine, tension, cluster). Secondary headaches are usually anatomic (vascular malformation, tumor) or infectious (sinusitis, dental abscess), and have higher morbidity and mortality if left untreated. A careful history and physical examination should focus on identifying or excluding secondary headaches. Historical findings that suggest secondary headache include acute onset; associated fever or stiff neck; morning vomiting; behavioral changes; altered mental status; "worst ever" headache; sleep disturbance; associated trauma or toxic exposure; or aggravation by coughing, Valsalva, or lying down. Physical findings suggestive of secondary headaches include blood pressure abnormalities, nuchal rigidity, head tilt, ptosis, retinal hemorrhage or papilledema, visual field defects, and neurologic findings (altered mental status, ataxia, and hemiparesis).

Diagnosis and Differential

Pertinent historical features of pediatric headache include severity and quality of pain, age of first occurrence, precipitants, rapidity of onset, location, duration, and associated symptoms. Physical examination should include a thorough general examination with careful attention to the neurologic examination, including cranial nerves, gait, strength, and mental status. The history and physical exam should guide the work up. For instance, CT is indicated to rule out suspected intracranial hemorrhage. Magnetic resonance imaging better visualizes the posterior fossa, the most common location of pediatric brain tumors, and either modality may be used for space-occupying lesions elsewhere. *Importantly, neuroimaging in children is usually not indicated unless there is an abnormal neurologic exam, altered mental status, concurrent seizures, a recent "worst headache of life" complaint, or change in type of headache.*

Emergency Department Care and Disposition

1. For secondary headaches, evaluate and treat underlying cause and pain.
2. For primary headaches, narcotics are not recommended. Most primary headaches respond to **ibuprofen** 10 mg/kg or **acetaminophen** 15 mg/kg.
3. For migraines: **prochlorperazine** 0.15 mg/kg, **metoclopramide** 0.1 mg/kg, or **ketorolac** 0.5 mg/kg are widely used for abortive migraine therapy. **Metoclopramide** and **prochlorperazine** are often given with **diphenhydramine** 1 mg/kg to prevent extrapyramidal side effects. "Migraine cocktails" that include **ketorolac, prochlorperazine** or **metoclopramide,** and **diphenhydramine** appear effective and safe. **Sumatriptan** 5 to 10 mg (in children weighing 20 to 39 kg) or 20 mg (>40 kg children) nasal spray or 0.1 mg/kg subcutaneously is commonly used.
4. Cluster and tension headaches are managed much the same way as migraines. **Sumatriptan** as dosed above and **high-flow oxygen** (7 L/min non-rebreather mask) can be used for cluster headaches. Tension headaches usually respond to first-line oral therapy such as **ibuprofen** 10 mg/kg.
5. For headaches that disrupt activities of daily living or school performance, refer to their primary care provider or pediatric neurologist to consider prophylactic regimens.
6. In general, most patients may be discharged after relief of symptoms. Patients with life-threatening causes of headache require admission for definitive care. Patients with intractable pain also may need admission.

ALTERED MENTAL STATUS

Altered mental status (AMS) in a child is defined as the failure to respond to the external environment in a manner consistent with the child's developmental level. In treating children with AMS, aggressive resuscitation, stabilization, diagnosis, and treatment must occur simultaneously to prevent morbidity and death.

Clinical Features

The spectrum of AMS ranges from confusion to lethargy, stupor, and coma indicative of depression of the cerebral cortex or localized abnormalities of the reticular activating system. Important historical elements to consider include prodromal events (recent illnesses, exposures, trauma), risk factors (medications, social or family history, potential for abuse), and other associated symptoms. A head-to-toe exam should be performed to identify occult infection, trauma, toxicity, or metabolic disease. A child's mental status can be assessed by the Glasgow coma scale, or the simpler AVPU scale, where A means "alert," V means "responsive to verbal stimuli," P means "responsive to painful stimuli," and U means "unresponsive," corresponding to a GCS of 15, 13, 8, and 3, respectively.

Pathologic causes of altered mental status can be divided into supratentorial lesions, subtentorial lesions, and metabolic encephalopathy. Supratentorial lesions are due to compression of the brainstem, resulting in altered level of consciousness and focal motor abnormalities with a rostral-to-caudal progression of dysfunction, and fast component of nystagmus away from the stimulus during cold caloric testing. Subtentorial lesions produce rapid loss of consciousness, cranial nerve abnormalities, abnormal breathing patterns, asymmetric or fixed pupils, and no eye movement during cold caloric testing. Metabolic encephalopathy produces decreased level of consciousness before exhibiting motor signs, which are symmetrical when present. Pupillary reflexes are intact in metabolic encephalopathy except with profound anoxia, opiates, barbiturates, and anticholinergics.

Diagnosis and Differential

A thorough history and physical examination are paramount to determining the diagnosis. The familiar mnemonic AEIOU TIPS (alcohol, encephalopathy, insulin, opiates, uremia, trauma, infection, poisoning, and seizure) is helpful in organizing diagnostic possibilities (Table 77-1).

TABLE 77-1 AEIOU TIPS: A Mnemonic for Pediatric Altered Mental Status

A	**Alcohol.** Ethanol. Isopropyl alcohol. Methanol. Concurrent hypoglycemia is common. **Acid-base and metabolic.** Hypotonic and hypertonic dehydration. Hepatic dysfunction, inborn errors of metabolism. **Arrhythmia/cardiogenic.** Stokes–Adams, supraventricular tachycardia, aortic stenosis, heart block, pericardial tamponade, hypertensive encephalopathy.
E	**Encephalopathy.** Reye's syndrome. Parainfectious encephalomyelitis. Autoimmune encephalitis. **Endocrinopathy.** Addison's disease can present with AMS or psychosis. Thyrotoxicosis can present with ventricular dysrhythmias. Pheochromocytoma can present with hypertensive encephalopathy. **Electrolytes.** Hypo-/hypernatremia and disorders of calcium, magnesium, and phosphorus can produce AMS.
I	**Insulin.** AMS from hyperglycemia is rare in children, but diabetic ketoacidosis is the most common cause. Hypoglycemia can be the result of many disorders. Irritability, confusion, seizures, and coma can occur with blood glucose levels < 40 mg/dL. **Intussusception.** AMS may be the initial presenting symptom.
O	**Opiates.** Common household exposures are to Lomotil, Imodium, diphenoxylate, and dextromethorphan. Clonidine, an α-agonist, can also produce similar symptoms. **Oxygen.** Disorders of airway, breathing, or circulation may adversely affect oxygen delivery to the brain; hypercapnia from primary lung disease or neurologic dysfunction also may result in altered mental status.
U	**Uremia.** Encephalopathy occurs in over one-third of patients with chronic renal failure. Hemolytic-uremic syndrome can produce AMS in addition to abdominal pain. Thrombocytopenic purpura and hemolytic anemia also can cause AMS. In children with chronic renal failure, neurologic dysfunction may develop secondary to stroke, hypertension, or metabolic derangements.

(Continued)

TABLE 77-1 AEIOU TIPS: A Mnemonic for Pediatric Altered Mental Status (Continued)

T	**Trauma.** Hypovolemia or hemorrhage from multisystem trauma may lead to insufficient cerebral perfusion and result in altered mental status. Consider concussion, hemorrhage or contusion, or epidural or subdural hematoma. Remember to look for signs of child abuse, particularly shaken baby syndrome with retinal hemorrhages. **Tumor.** Primary, metastatic, or meningeal leukemic infiltration. Intracerebral tumors commonly produce focal neurologic signs, and posterior fossa tumors typically block the ventricular system and create signs and symptoms suggestive of hydrocephalus. Supratentorial and infratentorial tumors may present abruptly with altered mental status, fever, or meningismus after an intratumor hemorrhage. **Thermal.** Hypo- or hyperthermia. Progressive hypothermia leads to insidious altered mental status. Temperatures > 41°C (105.8°F) result in headache, weakness, and dizziness followed by confusion, euphoria, combativeness, and altered mental status.
I	**Infection.** Bacterial meningitis, encephalitis, and brain abscess are the most important causes of AMS in children, especially AMS with fever. Brain abscess is characterized by fever and headache before AMS changes. Presenting symptoms also include generalized or focal seizures. Any systemic infection associated with vasculitis or shock may lead to altered mental status secondary to cerebral hypoperfusion. **Intracerebral vascular disorders.** Subarachnoid, intracerebral, or intraventricular hemorrhages can be seen with trauma, ruptured aneurysm, or arteriovenous malformations. Venous thrombosis can follow severe dehydration or pyogenic infection of the mastoid, orbit, middle ear, or sinuses. Arterial thrombosis is uncommon in children, except in those with homocystinuria. Intracerebral and intraventricular hemorrhages may follow birth asphyxia or trauma in neonates, but in older children, they may signify a congenital or acquired coagulopathy. Cerebral emboli from bacterial endocarditis may cause altered mental status. Acute confusional migraine may be associated with profound alterations in consciousness. Children with sickle cell anemia can develop cerebral thrombosis, status epilepticus, and coma.
P	**Psychogenic.** Rare in children, characterized by decreased responsiveness with normal neurologic examination including oculovestibular reflexes. Psychogenic unresponsiveness may be a conversion reaction, an adjustment reaction, a panic state, or malingering. **Poisoning/ingestion.** Drugs, toxins, or illicit substances can be ingested by accident, through neglect or abuse, or in a suicidal gesture.
S	**Seizure.** Generalized motor seizures and absence status epilepticus are often associated with prolonged unresponsiveness in children. In a child with a history of seizures who presents with AMS, consider nonconvulsive status epilepticus. Seizures in a febrile child suggest intracranial infection. Shunt malfunction should be considered among patients with a ventriculoperitoneal shunt for hydrocephalus.

Abbreviation: AMS, altered mental status.

Diagnostic adjuncts largely depend on the clinical situation and must be determined immediately after the primary and secondary survey. Rapid bedside glucose determination can immediately confirm either hypoglycemia, or hyperglycemia due to diabetic ketoacidosis. Toxicity due to poisoning or ingestion may require a reversal agent. If meningitis or encephalitis is suspected, lumbar puncture should be done immediately after initial resuscitation and stabilization. Neuroimaging may be indicated in the setting of trauma or suspicion of space-occupying lesion.

Emergency Department Care and Disposition

Treatment priorities should concentrate on stabilization and reversal of life-threatening conditions.

1. Ensure airway, breathing, and circulation. Immobilize the cervical spine if trauma is suspected and obtain appropriate imaging studies when the patient is stabilized.
2. Provide continuous pulse oximetry and supplemental **oxygen** as needed to correct hypoxia, including bag-valve-mask and intubation when appropriate. Consider capnometry for intubated patients.
3. Administer fluid resuscitation with 20 mL/kg fluid boluses of **isotonic crystalloid** for hypotension. Fluid boluses may be repeated up to 60 mL/kg. Intravenous pressors are indicated if hypotension persists.
4. Treat hypoglycemia with **10% dextrose 5 mL/kg** in infants or **25% dextrose 2 mL/kg** in older children.
5. Control core body temperature to minimize metabolic demands. Prevent hypothermia with warming lamps and treat hyperthermia when present.
6. Treat seizures with benzodiazepines (see Chapter 76).
7. For suspected opiate or clonidine overdose, administer **naloxone** 0.01 to 0.1 mg/kg IV every 2 minutes. For iatrogenic benzodiazepine overdose, consider **flumazenil** 0.01 mg/kg IV in the setting of known, isolated benzodiazepine ingestion.
8. Administer empiric antibiotics, **ceftriaxone** or **cefotaxime** 50 mg/kg/dose, and consider additional **vancomycin** 10 mg/kg/dose for suspected meningitis.
9. Patients with AMS will require admission and neurologic observation. Only those with a transient, rapidly reversible, and benign cause of AMS may be discharged from the emergency department after a period of observation with follow-up scheduled within 24 hours of discharge.

FURTHER READING

For further reading in *Tintinalli's Emergency Medicine: A Comprehensive Study Guide*, 8th ed., see Chapter 136, "Headache in Children," by David C. Sheridan and Garth Meckler; Chapter 137 "Altered Mental Status in Children" by Sarah Mellion and Kathleen Adelgais.

Syncope and Sudden Death in Children and Adolescents

Derya Caglar

Syncope is a presenting symptom for 1% to 3% of all pediatric emergency visits. It is more common in adolescents than younger children. Up to 50% of adolescents experience at least one syncopal episode which is usually transient and self-limited, but can be a symptom of serious cardiac disease.

Sudden, unexpected death in children comprises 2.3% of all pediatric deaths, of which sudden cardiac death makes up about one-third. The risk of sudden cardiac death is greater in patients with congenital or acquired heart disease, even those that have undergone corrective surgery. Except for trauma, sudden cardiac death is the most common cause of sports-related deaths. Hypertrophic cardiomyopathy and congenital artery anomalies are the most common cause of sudden cardiac death in adolescents without known cardiac disease. Other causes of sudden cardiac death in children include myocarditis, congenital heart disease, and conduction disturbances.

CLINICAL FEATURES

Syncope is the sudden onset of falling accompanied by a brief episode of loss of consciousness. Involuntary motor movements may occur with all types of syncopal episodes but are most common with seizures. Table 78-1 lists the most common causes of syncope by category.

Neurally mediated syncope is the most common cause in children. This type of syncope typically lasts <1 minute and is preceded by sensations of nausea, warmth, or light-headedness with a gradual visual grayout. Cardiac syncope occurs when there is an interruption of cardiac output from an intrinsic problem such as tachydysrhythmia, bradydysrhythmia, outflow obstruction, and myocardial dysfunction. Syncope resulting from cardiac causes usually begins and ends abruptly and may be associated with chest pain, palpitations, or shortness of breath. Risk factors associated with serious causes of syncope are presented in Table 78-2. Events easily mistaken for syncope are presented in Table 78-3 in addition to common associated symptoms.

DIAGNOSIS AND DIFFERENTIAL

No specific historical or clinical features reliably distinguish between vasovagal syncope and other causes. A thorough history and physical examination can help to arouse or allay suspicion of serious causes. The most important step in evaluation of children with syncope is a detailed history, including a thorough description of the event, associated symptoms, circumstances, personal or family history of cardiac disease, medications, drugs, intake, and intercurrent illness. Syncope during exercise suggests a more serious cause. Approximately 25% of children who suffer sudden death have a history of syncope. If witnesses note that the patient appeared lifeless or cardiopulmonary resuscitation was performed, a search for serious pathologic conditions must be undertaken.

TABLE 78-1 Causes of Syncope in Children and Adolescents
Neurally mediated: most common cause of syncope in children (80%)
Vasovagal: $<$ 1 min duration, prolonged standing, emotional upset, warning signs
Orthostatic: light-headedness with standing may precede; due to hypovolemia
Situational: urination, defecation, coughing, and swallowing may precipitate familial dysautonomia
Breath-holding: 6-18 months old, crying leads to breath-holding, syncope, short-lived
Cardiac dysrhythmias: events that usually start and end abruptly
Prolonged Q-T syndrome
Supraventricular tachycardia / Wolff-Parkinson-White syndrome
Sick sinus syndrome: associated with prior heart surgery
Atrioventricular block: most common in children with congenital heart disease; acquired cardiac disease (myocarditis, muscular dystrophy, Lyme)
Pacemaker malfunction
Structural cardiac disease:
Hypertrophic cardiomyopathy: commonly exertional syncope; infants present with congestive heart failure and cyanosis
Dilated cardiomyopathy: idiopathic, postmyocarditis, or congenital
Congenital heart disease
Valvular diseases: aortic stenosis often congenital; Ebstein malformation; mitral valve prolapse (associated with syncope but NOT increased risk of sudden death)
Arrhythmogenic right ventricular dysplasia: congestive heart failure, cardiomegaly
Pulmonary hypertension: dyspnea on exertion, exercise intolerance, shortness of breath
Coronary artery abnormalities: aberrant left main artery causing external compression during physical exercise
Medications and drugs: antihypertensives, tricyclic antidepressants, cocaine, diuretics, antidysrhythmics

The physical examination includes complete cardiovascular (heart sounds, murmurs, rhythm, and the character of pulses), neurologic, and pulmonary examinations. Strongly consider obtaining an ECG on all patients with syncope. Routine bloodwork is not indicated in children with clear vasovagal syncope. Tests should be directed by the history and exam: a classic story for vasovagal syncope with a normal physical examination requires no further testing. Palpitations or exertional syncope require ECG evaluation for potential dysrhythmias. Sudden collapse, especially during exercise, suggests structural abnormalities, particularly when associated with a murmur on physical examination. ECG,

TABLE 78-2 Risk Factors for a Serious Cause of Syncope
Exertion preceding the event
Age $<$ 6 years
History of cardiac disease or heart murmur in the patient
Family history of sudden death, long QT syndrome, sensorineural hearing loss, or cardiac disease
Recurrent episodes
Recumbent episode
Prolonged loss of consciousness
Associated chest pain or palpitations
Absence of premonitory symptoms or physical precipitating factors
Use of medications that can alter cardiac conduction

TABLE 78-3 Events Easily Mistaken for Cardiovascular Syncope

Condition	Distinguishing Characteristics
Basilar migraine	Headache, rarely loss of consciousness, other neurologic symptoms
Seizure	Loss of consciousness simultaneous with motor event, prolonged postictal phase
Vertigo	Rotation or spinning sensation, no loss of consciousness
Hyperventilation	Inciting event, paresthesias or carpopedal spasm, tachypnea
Hysteria	No loss of conciousness, indifference to event
Hypoglycemia	Confusion progressing to loss of consciousness, requires glucose administration to terminate

chest x-ray, and echocardiography should be considered in this setting. Syncope associated with chest pain may require cardiac troponins as part of the evaluation to rule out ischemic heart disease (e.g., aberrant left coronary artery). Electrolytes, thyroid studies, chest x-ray, and urine pregnancy testing or drug screen should be considered in the appropriate clinical setting.

EMERGENCY DEPARTMENT CARE AND DISPOSITION

1. Strongly consider obtaining an electrocardiogram (ECG) in all patients.
2. If vasovagal syncope is likely, patients may be discharged home with reassurance and advised to increase water and salt intake.
3. Consider an echocardiogram for patients with known or suspected cardiac disease. If an echocardiogram is not immediately available, the urgency for obtaining the study should be determined in consultation with a cardiologist.
4. If no clear cause is found, the child may be discharged to be further evaluated and followed by the primary care provider unless there are cardiac risk factors or exercise-induced symptoms for which referral to a cardiologist is warranted.
5. Patients with a normal ECG but a history suggesting a dysrhythmia are candidates for outpatient monitoring and cardiac workup.
6. Children with documented dysrhythmias should be admitted. All children admitted for syncope should undergo cardiac monitoring. Children who are survivors of sudden cardiac arrest should be admitted to a pediatric intensive care unit.

FURTHER READING

For further reading in *Tintinalli's Emergency Medicine: A Comprehensive Study Guide*, 8th ed., see Chapter 127, "Syncope, Dysrhythmias, and ECG Interpretation," by Andrew C. Dixon.

Hypoglycemia and Metabolic Emergencies in Infants and Children

Teresa J. Riech

HYPOGLYCEMIA

Hypoglycemia in children may be due to inadequate oral intake, excess insulin, low levels of hyperglycemic hormones (e.g., cortisol or growth hormone), inborn errors of metabolism, or systemic infection. Prompt recognition and treatment of hypoglycemia are essential to avoid potentially severe and permanent neurologic injury, and bedside glucose testing should be considered in any neonate, infant, or child with altered mental status.

Clinical Features

Hypoglycemic children may manifest symptoms related to adrenergic hormone release including tachycardia, diaphoresis, tremors, anxiety, irritability, and tachypnea. Severe hypoglycemia may result in apnea or seizures, particularly in neonates and infants, who may not manifest typical signs and symptoms of older children and adults. Neonates and infants with hypoglycemia may also present with altered mental status and nonspecific symptoms such as poor feeding, an abnormal or high-pitched cry, temperature instability, and irritability or lethargy. Hypoglycemia often accompanies critical illness (sepsis) and the features of that illness may dominate the clinical picture, thereby masking the signs of hypoglycemia.

Diagnosis and Differential

Hypoglycemia is defined as a plasma glucose concentration less than 45 mg/dL in symptomatic children and less than 35 mg/dL in asymptomatic neonates. Bedside glucose testing is the most important diagnostic test in any neonate or infant who is critically ill or has altered mental status. Abnormal results should be confirmed with a venous sample, but treatment should not be delayed for confirmatory results. Urine testing for ketones is important, as ketonuria is associated with ketotic hypoglycemia, adrenal insufficiency, and other inborn errors of metabolism. Absent urine ketones are associated with hyperinsulinemic states, infants of a diabetic mother, as well as disorders of fatty acid oxidation and mitochondria.

Emergency Department Care and Disposition

1. For neonates administer **10% dextrose** 5 mL/kg IV/IO/PO/NG. Treat infants with the same dose of 10% dextrose, or **25% dextrose** 2 mL/kg IV/IO/PO/NG. Give older children 2 mL/kg of **25% dextrose** IV/IO/PO/NG.
2. Administer maintenance dextrose for persistent hypoglycemia using **10% dextrose** at 1.5 times maintenance.
3. When intravenous access is not immediately available, consider **glucagon** 0.03 mg/kg IM or subcutaneous (maximum 0.5 mg).

4. If adrenal insufficiency is suspected, give **hydrocortisone** 25 mg IV/IM for neonates and infants, 50 mg for toddlers and school-age children, and 100 mg for everyone else. Steroids should be given early in patients with hypopituitarism and adrenal insufficiency.
5. Consider empiric antibiotics for suspected sepsis.

INBORN ERRORS OF METABOLISM

Inborn errors of metabolism are challenging childhood disorders representing a broad spectrum of diseases with nonspecific signs and symptoms. Delay in accurate diagnosis and treatment can lead to significant morbidity and mortality. Despite the myriad etiologies, the principles of initial emergency department (ED) diagnosis and management are relatively simple. The sudden acute deterioration of a healthy neonate should always prompt consideration of metabolic disease, and making a definitive diagnosis is less important than having a high index of suspicion and implementing supportive care.

Clinical Features

Vomiting, altered mental status, and poor feeding are the most common features of metabolic emergencies. Seizures may accompany some metabolic crises. Tachypnea due to metabolic acidosis and tachycardia from dehydration, as well as hypotension due to hypovolemia or adrenal insufficiency, may be noted. Rarely, some metabolic disorders may be associated with characteristic body or urine odors or other phenotypic stigmata (e.g., ambiguous genitalia and hyperpigmentation in congenital adrenal hyperplasia, as discussed separately below). Most metabolic toxins cross the placenta and are cleared by maternal enzymes; therefore, newborns are asymptomatic, and symptoms present after feeding begins.

Diagnosis and Differential

Screening laboratory tests for suspected inborn errors of metabolism include a bedside glucose, urine for ketones, a blood gas analysis for metabolic acidosis, serum ammonia, basic metabolic panel, and lactate level. Figure 79-1 details the diagnostic evaluation recommended in the ED. Additional laboratory tests for definitive diagnosis that should be considered based on initial screening results include liver function tests, CBC, lactate dehydrogenase, creatine kinase, serum amino acids and acylcarnitine profile, urine organic acids, and reducing substances. The differential diagnosis of shock in the neonate includes sepsis, congenital heart defects, and abdominal catastrophes.

Emergency Department Care and Disposition

Despite the diverse etiology and complexity of inborn errors of metabolism, ED resuscitation and stabilization of patients with these disorders are relatively simple. Neonates, infants, and children presenting in metabolic crisis, regardless of cause, show some combination of dehydration, metabolic acidosis, and encephalopathy, which must be immediately addressed. The goals of treatment are to improve circulatory status by restoring circulatory volume, provide energy substrate to halt catabolism, remove the

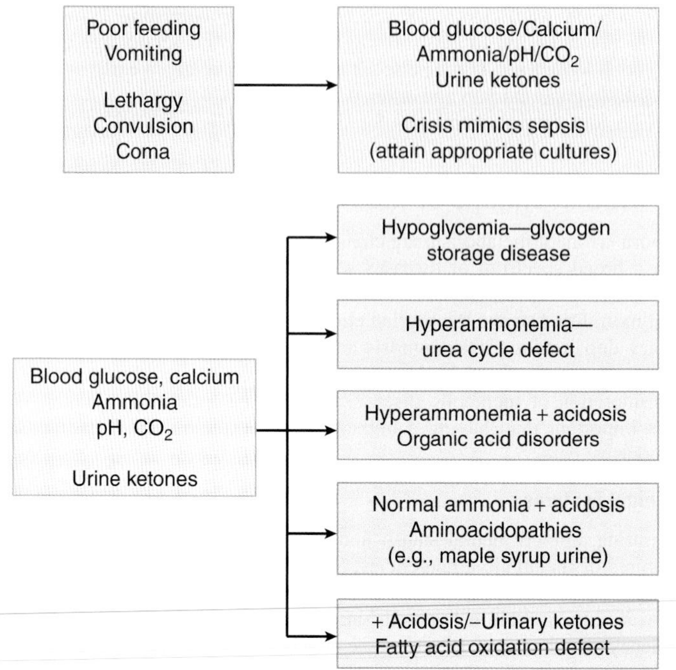

FIGURE 79-1. Approach to suspected metabolic disorders.

inciting metabolic substrate (formula or breast milk), and help eliminate toxic metabolites.

1. Attend to Airway, Breathing, Circulation, and Disability (ABCD). If apnea, hypoventilation, or hypoxemia necessitates endotracheal intubation, avoid prolonged use of paralytics because metabolic acidosis can be worsened by respiratory acidosis if insufficient ventilation is provided.
2. Restore circulation with **0.9% saline boluses** of 20 mL/kg, reassessing after each bolus.
3. Make patients NPO, and correct hypoglycemia as above with D10 in neonates and infants or D25 in children.
4. Begin **10% dextrose infusion** at twice maintenance rate.
5. Consider broad-spectrum antibiotics.
6. Specific metabolic treatments are guided by the underlying defect and should be determined in consultation with a metabolic specialist. Substrates to facilitate shunting of metabolic pathways or hemodialysis may be needed.
7. Reflexive use of bicarbonate should be avoided; however, in select cases of severe acidosis (pH < 7.0), treatment with 0.5 mEq/kg/h of sodium bicarbonate may be considered.

Patients with a newly diagnosed or suspected metabolic disorder and those who are dehydrated or otherwise decompensated require admission

TABLE 79-1 Conditions Associated with Hypoglycemia in Infants and Children

Neonates	Infancy and Childhood
Infant of a diabetic mother	Idiopathic ketotic hypoglycemia/starvation
Congenital heart disease	Diabetes mellitus/endocrine disorder
Infection/sepsis	Infection/sepsis
Adrenal hemorrhage	Inborn errors of metabolism
Hypothermia	Hypothermia
Hypoglycemia-inducing drug use by mother	Drug induced (salicylates, etc.) Hyperinsulinism
Maternal eclampsia	Idiopathic
Fetal alcohol syndrome	
Hypopituitarism	

for dextrose and specific treatment. Transfer to a pediatric hospital may be required (Table 79-1).

CONGENITAL ADRENAL HYPERPLASIA

Congenital adrenal hyperplasia results from deficiency in one of the enzymes involved in the production of cortisol, which leads to decreased cortisol levels sometimes accompanied by mineralocorticoid deficiency ("salt wasting syndrome"). Steroid precursors may be shunted to androgen production with virilization of females.

Clinical Features

Patients with salt-wasting adrenal hyperplasia typically present in the second to fifth week of life with nonspecific symptoms including shock, vomiting, lethargy, irritability, and poor feeding. On examination, females may have clitoromegaly and males may have a small penis or hypospadias. Hyperpigmentation may be noted on axillae and around the nipples.

Diagnosis and Differential

The most important laboratory tests include bedside glucose and electrolytes, as hyponatremia and hyperkalemia are often present and suggest the diagnosis. Serum potassium levels of 6 to 12 mEq/kg are not unusual but are rarely associated with ECG abnormalities. Definitive diagnosis depends on analysis of blood hormone levels. If possible, blood should be obtained for analysis before treatment with exogenous steroids; however, treatment should not be delayed in the critically ill neonate. The differential diagnosis includes sepsis, congenital heart disease, and other inborn errors of metabolism.

Emergency Department Care and Disposition

1. Administer **0.9% saline boluses** of 20 mL/kg IV/IO.
2. Treat hypoglycemia as above.
3. Administer **hydrocortisone** IV/IO/IM: 25 mg for neonates, 50 mg for toddlers and school-age children, and 100 mg for adolescents.

TABLE 79-2 Management of Hypoglycemia in the ED

Patient Age	Dextrose Bolus Dose	Dextrose Maintenance Dosage	Other Treatments to Consider
Neonate	D10 5 mL/kg PO/NG/IV/IO	6 mL/Kg/h D10	Glucagon, 0.03 mg/ kg IM/IV Hydrocortisone, 25 g PO/IM/IV/IO
Infant	D10 5 mL/kg PO/NG/IV/IO *or* D25 2 mL/kg	6 mL/Kg/h D10	Glucagon, 0.03 mg/ kg IM/IV Hydrocortisone, 25 g PO/IM/IV/IO
Child	D25 2 mL/kg PO/NG/IV/IO	6 mL/kg/h D10 for the first 10 kg + 3 mL/kg/h for 11–20 kg + 1.5 mL/kg/h for each additional kg >20 kg	Glucagon, 0.03 mg/kg/ IM/IV, Hydrocortisone, 50 g PO/IM/IV/IO
Adolescent	—	6 mL/kg/h D10 for the first 10 kg + 3 mL/kg/h for 11–20 kg + 1.5 mL/kg/h for each additional kg >20 kg	Glucagon, 0.03 mg/ kg IM/IV Hydrocortisone,100 g PO/IM/IV/IO

Abbreviations: D10, 10% dextrose; D25, 25% dextrose; NG, (Via) nasogastric tube.

4. Treat hyperkalemia with **calcium gluconate** 100 mg/kg IV (1 mL/kg) and **bicarbonate** 1 mEq/kg IV. Insulin should be avoided as it may cause profound hypoglycemia.

Neonates with adrenal crisis from adrenal hyperplasia require hospitalization. Infants with shock or severe hyperkalemia should be admitted to the ICU with endocrine consultation. Those with a known diagnosis of adrenal hyperplasia who have normal vital signs and are able to tolerate oral intake may be discharged home after administration of hydrocortisone as above with instructions to triple their usual home dose of steroid until fever, vomiting, or diarrhea resolve and when next-day follow-up can be assured) (Table 79-2).

FURTHER READING

For further reading in *Tintinalli's Emergency Medicine: A Comprehensive Study Guide*, 8th ed., see Chapter 144, "Metabolic Emergencies in Infants and Children," by Garth Meckler, Nadeemuddin Qureshi, Mohammed Al-Mogbil, and Osama Y. Kentab.

CHAPTER 80

Diabetes in Children

Adam Vella

Type 1 diabetes, an autoimmune disease, is characterized by an abrupt and frequently complete decline in insulin production. Type 2 diabetes is marked by increasing insulin resistance and occurs in overweight adolescents with a strong genetic predisposition. Diabetic ketoacidosis (DKA) is the leading cause of mortality in patients with diabetes <24 years of age, and cerebral edema is the leading cause of mortality in DKA.

DKA is much more common in patients with type 1 diabetes than in those with type 2, but patients with type 2 diabetes may develop hyperglycemic hyperosmolar nonketotic syndrome (HHNS) with acidosis, which can result in severe total body water, potassium, and phosphorus deficits. About 4% of children with newly diagnosed type 2 diabetes present with HHNS, which has a case fatality rate of 12%.

CLINICAL FEATURES

Polyuria, polydipsia, and polyphagia are the classic triad leading to the diagnosis of type 1 diabetes. Other common symptoms include weight loss, secondary enuresis, anorexia, vague abdominal discomfort, visual changes, and genital candidiasis in a toilet-trained child. Symptoms of DKA include excessive thirst, weakness, vomiting, loss of appetite, confusion, abdominal pain, shortness of breath, and a generally ill-appearance. Occasionally, children with DKA present to the ED complaining primarily of abdominal pain, which may mimic acute appendicitis; Kussmaul breathing (hyperpnea from acidosis) may be mistaken for hyperventilation from anxiety or respiratory distress from pulmonary disease.

Premonitory symptoms of cerebral edema occur in 50% of patients and include severe headache, declining mental status, and seizures. Cerebral edema is rare (0.5% to 1% of all children presenting with DKA) but typically occurs 6 to 12 hours after initiating therapy. Although the etiology of this complication is unknown, it is felt that several factors may contribute, including young age, severe hyperosmolality, severe acidosis, and failure of the serum sodium level to rise commensurately with the fall in glucose level during therapy.

DIAGNOSIS AND DIFFERENTIAL

The diagnosis of diabetes is established by demonstrating hyperglycemia and glucosuria in the absence of other causes such as steroid therapy, Cushing syndrome, pheochromocytoma, hyperthyroidism, or other rare disorders. DKA is generally defined as a metabolic acidosis (pH <7.30 or serum bicarbonate level of <15 mEq/L) with hyperglycemia (serum glucose level of >200 mg/dL) in the presence of ketonemia or ketonuria. In adolescent patients without known diabetes, consider toxic ingestions of ethylene glycol, isopropyl alcohol, or salicylates.

Cerebral edema in DKA is a clinical diagnosis based on altered mental status not attributed to hypovolemia. Treatment should begin prior to obtaining head CT when suspected. CT imaging can confirm the diagnosis, and intracranial pressure monitoring may be indicated.

EMERGENCY DEPARTMENT CARE AND DISPOSITION

The treatment of DKA consists of judicious fluid resuscitation, insulin therapy, correction of electrolyte abnormalities, and close monitoring. Patients should be placed on a cardiac monitor, noninvasive blood pressure device, and pulse oximetry, and intravenous lines should be established.

1. Administer 10 mL/kg normal saline (NS) bolus over 1 hour if the child is hemodynamically stable. If shock is suspected or hypotension is present give an initial 20 mL/kg NS bolus and repeat as needed until the blood pressure normalizes. Once vital signs have stabilized, resist the desire to correct the fluid deficit too rapidly, especially if there is a high calculated osmolality (i.e., >340 mOsm/L).
2. Follow the initial bolus with NS at 1.5 times the calculated maintenance rate.
3. If [K^+] is 3.5 to 5.5 mEq/L and patient is urinating, add 30 mEq [K^+]/L (1/2 as KCl and 1/2 as potassium phosphate). If initial [K^+] is 2.5 to 3.5 mEq/L, add 40 mEq [K^+]/L; consider adding more if the [K^+] is <2.5 mEq/L.
4. Begin regular insulin infusion at 0.1 U/kg/h after IV fluid bolus (if given) is complete. Adjust dose to maintain glucose decline at 50 to 100 mg/dL/h. Do not decrease insulin infusion below 0.05 U/kg/h until ketonuria has resolved. High-dose insulin therapy and insulin boluses increase the risk of complications and should not be given.
5. Add dextrose to IV fluids when blood glucose is <200 to 250 mg/dL. Glucose levels correct faster than ketoacidosis, so supplement with dextrose and continue the insulin drip until ketoacidosis has resolved.
6. Measure serum electrolyte levels every 2 hours; measure serum glucose level every hour.
7. **The use of bicarbonate in the treatment of DKA is not recommended**, as it does not improve outcomes and has been associated with a fourfold increase in the development of cerebral edema. Bicarbonate administration should be limited to critically ill patients with a pH of <7.0 and hemodynamic compromise unresponsive to fluid resuscitation.
8. **Management of cerebral edema**. Treat patients with altered mental status suggestive of cerebral edema with **mannitol** 0.25 to 1 g/kg. Consider 3% hypertonic saline, 10 mL/kg over 30 minutes. Restrict additional IV fluids to minimum required to maintain IV access. Use caution if endotracheal intubation is required and avoid eucapnea as severe metabolic acidosis requires a compensatory respiratory alkalosis, and a rise in CO_2 may worsen systemic and intracellular acidosis, leading to hyperemia and worsening of cerebral edema.
9. Most patients with DKA require admission to the intensive care unit, even when in stable condition, because of intensive monitoring needs. Furthermore, many hospitals restrict the use of insulin infusions to

intensive care settings. Patients with cerebral edema require ICU admission and possible intracranial pressure monitoring. Consultation with the patient's primary care physician and a pediatric endocrinologist should be made early in the course of therapy.

FURTHER READING

For further reading in *Tintinalli's Emergency Medicine: A Comprehensive Study Guide*, 8th ed., see Chapter 145, "Diabetes in Children," by Adam Vella.

CHAPTER 81 Fluid and Electrolyte Therapy in Infants and Children

Ron L. Kaplan

The most common disorder of fluid balance in children requiring emergency care is dehydration. Dehydration is the result of a negative fluid balance that can result from decreased fluid intake, increased output (renal, GI, or insensible losses from the skin or respiratory tract), or conditions such as sepsis, burns, and diabetes.

CLINICAL FEATURES

The presence of fluid and electrolyte disturbances is often suggested by a thorough history. Children with chronic underlying disease are at particular risk. The clinical appearance depends on the degree of dehydration, the rate at which the fluid was lost, and the age of the patient.

Though the gold standard for assessing dehydration is comparison of pre-illness weight with weight on presentation to the emergency department (ED), a reliable and recent pre-illness weight is rarely available in the ED. Physical examination can provide an estimation of the degree of dehydration, which is typically classified as mild, moderate, or severe. Clinical signs and symptoms of dehydration are listed in Table 81-1. An important exception to the reliability of signs and symptoms to predict degree of dehydration occurs in hypernatremic dehydration, when fluid

TABLE 81-1 Clinical Guidelines for Assessing Dehydration in Children

	None to Mild (<3% Body Weight Loss)	Mild to Moderate (3% to 9% Body Weight Loss)	Severe (>9% Body Weight Loss)
Mental status	Well, alert	Fatigued, restless, irritable	Apathetic, lethargic, unconscious
Thirst	Normal, slight increase, or refusing fluids	Increased, eager to drink	Very thirsty or too lethargic to drink
Heart rate	Normal	Normal to increased	Tachycardia or bradycardia in critically ill children
Pulse quality	Normal	Normal to reduced	Weak, thready
Eyes	Normal	Slightly sunken	Sunken
Tears	Present	Decreased	Absent
Mucous membranes	Moist	Dry	Parched
Anterior fontanelle	Normal	Sunken	Sunken
Capillary Refill	Normal	3 to 4 s	>4 s
Extremities	Warm	Warm to cool	Cold, mottled, cyanotic
Urine output	Normal	Decreased	Minimal

Source: Used with permission from Stephen Freedman, MD and Jennifer Thull-Freedman.

loss occurs primarily from the interstitial and intracellular spaces and clinical signs of intravascular volume depletion may be minimal. In this setting, however, the skin may have a characteristic doughy feel.

DIAGNOSIS AND DIFFERENTIAL

If available, the absolute and relative fluid deficit can be calculated from a pre-illness weight: 1 kg of weight loss is equivalent to 1 L of fluid deficit. In the absence of a reliable pre-illness comparison weight, the diagnosis of dehydration is based primarily on historical data and physical examination findings (Table 81-1).

Routine laboratory testing is not required in mild to moderate dehydration, but serum electrolytes and other studies may be indicated in the setting of severe dehydration, signs and symptoms of electrolyte abnormalities, or certain underlying medical conditions. A rapid bedside glucose test should be done on any child presenting with altered sensorium. Infants are at particular risk of hypoglycemia.

EMERGENCY DEPARTMENT CARE AND DISPOSITION

The management of fluid and electrolyte disturbances in infants and young children revolves around a few basic principles: (a) identification and treatment of shock; (b) administration of appropriate fluids to replace fluid deficits, ongoing losses, and maintenance fluid requirements; (c) identification and treatment of causes that have specific therapies (e.g., diabetic ketoacidosis, sepsis, and inborn errors of metabolism). The most common approaches to rehydration include oral rehydration therapy and parenteral therapy, though rehydration through nasogastric tube is also effective, simple, and well tolerated.

1. Treat hypovolemic shock with an initial bolus of 20 mL/kg of isotonic crystalloid: normal saline (NS) or lactated Ringer (LR) solution IV/IO. Repeat boluses every 10 to 20 minutes until mental status, vital signs, and peripheral perfusion improve. Up to 60 mL/kg or more may be needed in the first hour; care must be taken to monitor for signs of volume overload or myocardial dysfunction.
2. Oral rehydration is as effective as intravenous therapy and is recommended by the World Health Organization (WHO) for mild to moderate dehydration. Administer frequent small sips of oral rehydration solution containing glucose and electrolytes (e.g., Rehydralyte®) by mouth or nasogastric tube. Give 50 mL/kg orally over 4 hours for mild dehydration and 100 mL/kg for moderate dehydration. Vomiting is not a contraindication to attempting oral rehydration. Ondansetron may be used to facilitate oral rehydration if nausea or vomiting persists. Give 0.1 mg/kg IV or 0.15 mg/kg PO or by oral disintegrating tablet with a maximum dose of 8 mg.
3. Treat patients who cannot tolerate oral or enteral rehydration with IV or IO administration of NS or LR. If shock is not present, administer 20 mL/kg over 1 hour and repeat as needed. After initial volume replacement, 5% dextrose in 0.9% saline may be started at one to two times maintenance while determining disposition.

4. For maintenance treatment, use the following formula to determine fluid rate:
   For the first 10 kg: 100 mL/kg/d or 4 mL/kg/h
   For the second 10 kg: 50 mL/kg/d or 2 mL/kg/h
   For each kg >20 kg: 20 mL/kg/d or 1 mL/kg/h

   Isotonic fluids such as 5% dextrose in 0.9% saline should be used for maintenance treatment after the first week of life in order to avoid iatrogenic hyponatremia. 10% dextrose with no electrolytes should be used on day 1 of life and 5% dextrose in 0.45% saline can be used on days 2 to 7 of life.
5. Treat specific electrolyte disturbances, as listed in Table 81-2. Of note, overly rapid correction of hypo- or hypernatremia may lead to severe CNS sequelae. If neurologic symptoms such as seizures or altered mental status accompany hyponatremia, administer 2 to 3 mL/kg of 3% saline until symptoms resolve or the serum sodium is >120 mEq/L. Otherwise, correct the hyponatremia slowly over 48 hours to avoid CNS osmotic demyelination. Hypernatremia must be corrected slowly as well, in order to prevent cerebral edema and central pontine myelinolysis.

TABLE 81-2 Electrolyte Disorders in Infants and Children and Initial Management

Electrolyte Disorder	Common Causes	Symptoms and Signs	Initial Treatment Recommendations
Hyponatremia	Vomiting, diarrhea, excess free water intake	Mental status changes, seizures, hyporeflexia	IV normal saline starting with a 20 mL/kg bolus For seizures: 4 mL/kg of 3% saline over 30 min Further correction slowly over 48 h
Hypernatremia	Vomiting, diarrhea, insensible losses, diabetes insipidus, renal disease	Diarrhea, mental status changes, ataxia, doughy skin, seizures, hyperreflexia	IV normal saline starting with a 20 mL/kg bolus Further correction to take place slowly over 48 h
Hypokalemia	Vomiting, DKA	Muscle weakness, ileus	Generally tolerated well, replace orally over several days If severe: IV 0.2 to 0.3 mEq/kg/h of KCl
Hyperkalemia*	Cortical adrenal hyperplasia (neonates), renal failure. May be due to hemolysis of blood sample	ECG changes: peaked T waves, prolonged PR interval, widening of QRS	Insulin 0.1 unit/kg *plus* 25% glucose, 0.5 g/kg IV Calcium gluconate 10%, 1 mL/kg IV, no faster than 1 mL/min Albuterol, 0.5% solution, 2.5 mg via nebulization For other treatments, see Chapter 4.

(Continued)

TABLE 81-2 Electrolyte Disorders in Infants and Children and Initial Management (Continued)

Electrolyte Disorder	Common Causes	Symptoms and Signs	Initial Treatment Recommendations
Hypocalcemia	Dietary or vitamin D deficiency, hypoparathyroid and chronic renal failure	Vomiting, irritability, muscle weakness, tetany, seizures	Calcium gluconate 10%, 1 mL/kg IV, no faster than 1 mL/min
Hypercalcemia	Malignancy, hypervitaminosis D or A	Fatigue, irritability, anorexia, vomiting, constipation	IV normal saline starting at 20 mL/kg Consider furosemide 1-2 mg/kg IV, maximum dose 40 mg
Hypomagnesemia	Diarrhea, short gut, diuretics, chemotherapy	Muscle spasms, weakness, ataxia, nystagmus, seizures ECG changes: prolonged PR and QTc, torsades de pointes	For seizures or dysrhythmia: IV magnesium sulfate 1 mEq/kg slowly over 4 h Asymptomatic patients can be treated with oral supplements
Hypermagnesemia	Ingestion of antacids or renal dysfunction	Hypotension, respiratory failure, loss of deep tendon reflexes ECG changes: widening of QRS, PR, QTc	Remove exogenous source of magnesium If severe: calcium gluconate 10% 1 mL/kg IV no faster than 1 mL/min

*Mild hyperkalemia usually well tolerated in neonates.

Most children with mild to moderate dehydration can be managed as outpatients without any laboratory evaluation in the emergency department. Admission criteria include young infants with ongoing significant fluid losses; severe dehydration; significant electrolyte or metabolic derangements; persistent vomiting and failed attempts at oral rehydration; or an underlying diagnosis requiring ongoing inpatient treatment (e.g., DKA or inborn errors of metabolism).

FURTHER READING

For further reading in *Tintinalli's Emergency Medicine: A Comprehensive Study Guide*, 8th ed., see Chapter 129, "Fluid and Electrolyte Therapy in Infants and Children," by Chan Melissa and Enarson Paul.

CHAPTER 82

Musculoskeletal Disorders in Children

Mark X. Cicero

CHILDHOOD PATTERNS OF INJURY

The growth plate (physis) is the weakest point in children's long bones and the frequent site of fractures. The ligaments and periosteum are stronger than the physis; therefore, they tolerate mechanical forces at the expense of physeal injury. The blood supply to the physis arises from the epiphysis, so separation of the physis from the epiphysis may result in growth arrest. The Salter–Harris classification is used to describe fractures involving the growth plate (Figs. 82-1 and 82-2).

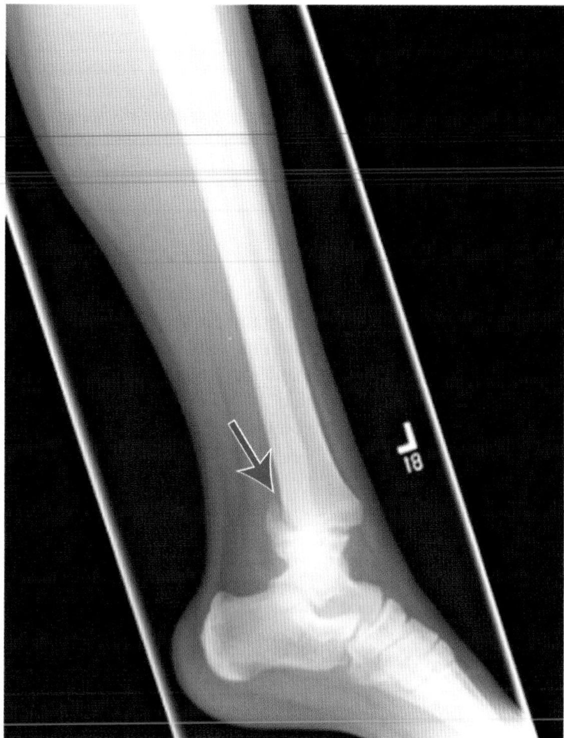

FIGURE 82-1. Salter–Harris type II fracture of distal tibia. Lateral radiograph illustrating fracture extending through physeal growth plate and metaphysis with dorsal displacement of epiphysis requiring reduction. Used with permission from Wake Medical Center, Raleigh, NC.

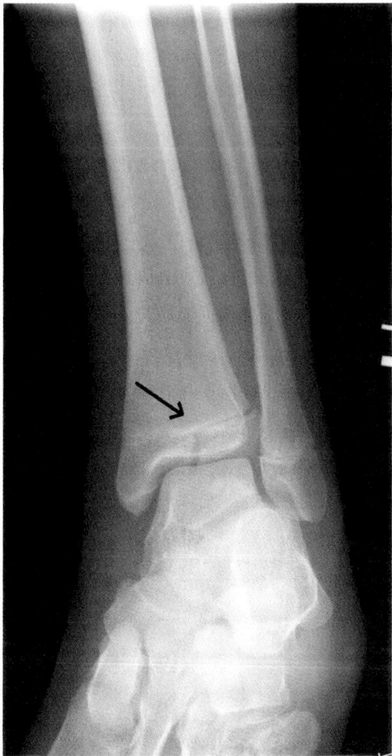

FIGURE 82-2. An x-ray of a Salter–Harris type III fracture of the distal tibia, also known as Tillaux's fracture. Note the intra-articular component extending through the growth plate and the medial epiphysis of the tibia. Reproduced with permission from Schafermeyer RW, Tenebein M, Macias CG: *Strange and Schafermeyer's Pediatric Emergency Medicine*, 4th ed. New York: McGraw-Hill, Inc; 2015.

Salter–Harris Type I Fracture

In type I physeal fracture, the epiphysis separates from the metaphysis. The reproductive cells of the physis stay with the epiphysis. There are no bony fragments, and these injuries have a low incidence of growth disturbance. Diagnosis is suspected clinically in children with point tenderness over a physis. On radiograph, there may be no abnormality; there may be an associated joint effusion; or there may be epiphyseal displacement from the metaphysis. In the absence of epiphyseal displacement, the diagnosis is clinical. Treatment consists of splint immobilization, ice, elevation, and referral to orthopedics. Type I fractures of the distal fibula are not associated with growth arrest and can be followed by a primary care physician (PCP) or by orthopedics after splinting.

Salter–Harris Type II Fracture

A type II physeal fracture goes through the physis and out through the metaphysis. Growth is preserved because the physis remains with the epiphysis. Diagnosis is made by noting a metaphyseal triangular-shaped fragment without epiphyseal involvement on radiograph. Treatment is closed reduction (if necessary) with analgesia and sedation followed by splint or cast immobilization, and follow-up with orthopedics.

Salter–Harris Type III Fracture

The hallmark of type III physeal fracture is an intra-articular fracture of the epiphysis with the cleavage plane continuing along the physis. The prognosis for bone growth depends on the circulation to the epiphyseal bone fragment and is usually favorable. Diagnosis is made radiographically with an epiphyseal fragment without a metaphyseal fracture. Reduction of the unstable fragment with anatomic alignment of the articular surface is critical. Open reduction is sometimes required.

Salter–Harris Type IV Fracture

The fracture line of type IV physeal fractures begins at the articular surface and extends through the epiphysis, physis, and metaphysis. Diagnosis is made radiographically with both epiphyseal and metaphyseal fractures. Especially when there is displacement of the bony fragments, open reduction is usually required to reduce the risk of premature bone growth arrest.

Salter–Harris Type V Fracture

In type V physeal fracture, severe compressive forces essentially crush the physis. There is usually no epiphyseal displacement. The diagnosis is often difficult. An initial diagnosis of sprain or type I injury may prove incorrect when later growth arrest occurs. Radiographs may look normal or demonstrate focal narrowing of the epiphyseal plate. There is usually an associated joint effusion. Treatment consists of casting, nonweight bearing, and close orthopedic follow-up in anticipation of bone growth arrest.

Torus Fractures, Greenstick Fractures, and Plastic Deformities

Children's long bones are more compliant than those of adults and tend to bow and bend under forces where an adult's might fracture. Torus (*buckle*) fractures involve a bulging or buckling of the bony cortex, usually of the metaphysis. Patients have point tenderness over the fracture site and soft tissue swelling. Radiographs may be subtle but show cortical disruption. Torus fractures are not typically angulated, rotated, or displaced, so reduction is not necessary. Splinting in a position of function for 3 to 4 weeks is often preferred over casting. Orthopedic follow-up is usually recommended.

In greenstick fractures, the cortex and periosteum are disrupted on one side of the bone but intact on the other. If the degree of angulation is significant, treatment is closed reduction and immobilization.

Plastic deformities, also known as bowing or bending fractures, are seen in the forearm and lower leg in combination with a completed fracture in the companion bone. The diaphyseal cortex is deformed, but the periosteum is intact. Treatment requires prompt orthopedic consultation for closed reduction and realignment.

FRACTURES ASSOCIATED WITH CHILD ABUSE

Certain injury patterns are consistently seen in abused children, particularly multiple fractures in various stages of healing. Please see Chapter 187 for details.

SELECTED PEDIATRIC INJURIES

Clavicle Fracture

Clavicles are commonly fractured in children, and may occur in newborns during difficult deliveries, presenting in neonates with nonuse of the arm. If the fracture was not initially appreciated, parents may notice a bony callus at age 2 to 3 weeks. In older infants and children, the usual mechanism is a fall onto the outstretched arm or shoulder. Care of the patient with a clavicle fracture is directed toward pain control. Even displaced fractures usually heal well, although patients may have a residual bump at the fracture site. A simple sling is effective and less painful than other methods of clavicle immobilization. Newborns require no specific treatment. Orthopedic consultation in the emergency department (ED) is required for an open fracture (which also requires antibiotics), displacement of the medial clavicle, or a skin-tenting fracture fragment that has the potential to convert to an open fracture. Otherwise, routine follow-up with the PCP is usually adequate.

Supracondylar and Condylar Fractures

The most common elbow fracture in childhood is the supracondylar fracture of the distal humerus. The mechanism is commonly a fall onto the outstretched arm. Children complain of pain on passive elbow flexion and hold the forearm pronated. The close proximity of the brachial artery to the fracture predisposes the artery to injury. Subsequent arterial spasm or compression by casts may further compromise distal circulation. A forearm compartment syndrome (resulting in Volkmann ischemic contracture) may occur.

Radiographs show the injury, but the findings may be subtle. Type I fractures have no displacement or angulation, or may have a posterior fat pad as the only radiographic manifestation of a fracture. Confirmation of a fracture may be seen on an x-ray taken 2 to 4 weeks later, when a periosteal reaction is visible. Type II fractures are angulated, but the posterior cortex is intact, while type III fractures are completely displaced with no cortical contact.

In cases of neurovascular compromise, immediate fracture reduction is indicated. If an ischemic forearm compartment is suspected after reduction, surgical decompression or arterial exploration may be indicated. Outpatient treatment is acceptable for type I fractures after appropriate immobilization. Such children need orthopedic reassessment within 2 to 7 days. Orthopedic consultation and admission is recommended for patients with type II or III fractures. Open reduction with operative pinning is usually required.

Lateral and medial condylar fractures and intercondylar and transcondylar fractures carry risks of neurovascular compromise, especially to the ulnar nerve. These patients have soft tissue swelling and tenderness while maintaining the arm in flexion. Depending on the displacement visualized on x-ray, patients may require open reduction.

Radial Head Subluxation ("Nursemaid's Elbow")

Radial head subluxation is a very common injury seen most often in children 1 to 4 years of age. The typical history is that the child was lifted or pulled by the hand or wrist, though 50% have no such history and parents may report a fall or simply that their child refuses to use the arm. The arm is held in adduction, flexed at the elbow, with the forearm pronated. Gentle examination demonstrates no tenderness to direct palpation, but attempts to supinate the forearm or move the elbow cause pain. If the history and examination are strongly suggestive, radiographs are not needed. However, if the history is atypical or there is point tenderness or signs of trauma, radiographs should be obtained.

There are two maneuvers for reduction. The first, the supination/flexion technique, is performed by holding the patient's elbow at 90° with one hand and then firmly supinating the wrist and simultaneously flexing the elbow so that the wrist is directed to the ipsilateral shoulder. There may be a "click" with reduction, and the child may transiently cry and resist. The second, the hyperpronation technique, is reported to be more successful. The hyperpronation technique is performed by holding the child's elbow at 90° in one hand and then firmly pronating the wrist while extending the elbow. Usually the child will resume normal activity in 5 to 10 minutes if reduction is achieved. If the child is not better after a second reduction attempt, alternate diagnoses and radiographs should be considered. No specific therapy is needed after successful reduction. Parents should be reminded to avoid linear traction on the arm because there is a risk of recurrence.

Forearm Injuries

Torus Fractures

Torus fractures, also called buckle fractures, are among the most common pediatric bony injuries and may occur in the radius or ulna. Treatment consists of pain management with NSAIDs, application of a volar splint, and follow-up with the PCP or orthopedics in 1 to 3 weeks.

Fractures of the Radial and Ulnar Shafts

Metaphyseal Fractures

Any metaphyseal fracture with rotational deformity or more than 10 degrees of angulation in children above 8 years of age, or more than 15 to 20 degrees in younger children, requires consultation with an orthopedist to determine the need for reduction. Otherwise, immobilization in a splint with follow-up with orthopedics within 1 week is adequate treatment.

Diaphyseal Fractures

Most diaphyseal forearm fractures warrant urgent orthopedic consultation. Transverse fractures of one or both bones may remain unstable despite attempts at closed reduction. Two fracture-dislocation injuries with especially guarded prognoses are an ulnar fracture with a radial head dislocation (Monteggia's fracture) and a radial shaft fracture with distal radioulnar joint dislocation (Galeazzi's fracture).

Wrist Fractures

Carpal bone injuries are rare in young children, and gain frequency in older children and adolescents, when athletic pursuits generate greater force. The scaphoid fracture requires a high index of suspicion. Snuffbox tenderness and tenderness of the lateral wrist with axial compression of the thumb warrant application of a thumb spica splint and follow-up with an orthopedist, even when radiographs show no scaphoid fracture.

Lower Extremity Injuries

Slipped Capital Femoral Epiphysis

Slipped capital femoral epiphysis (SCFE) is more common in obese children, with a peak incidence between ages 14 and 16 years (11 and 13 years in girls). Clinically, the child presents with pain at the hip or referred to the thigh or knee. With a chronic SCFE, children complain of dull pain in the groin, anteromedial thigh, and knee, which becomes worse with activity. With walking, the leg is externally rotated and the gait is antalgic. Hip flexion is restricted and accompanied by external rotation of the thigh. Acute SCFE is due to trauma or may occur in a patient with preexisting chronic SCFE.

The differential includes septic arthritis, toxic synovitis, Legg–Calvé–Perthes disease, and other hip fractures. Children with SCFE are not febrile or toxic and have normal white blood cell counts and erythrocyte sedimentation rates. Obtain bilateral hip radiographs in any adolescent with hip pain. Bilateral anteroposterior and frog-leg lateral radiographs of the hips are preferred. Medial slips of the femoral epiphysis will be seen on anteroposterior views, whereas frog-leg views detect posterior slips. In the anteroposterior view, a line along the superior femoral neck should transect the lateral quarter of the femoral epiphysis, and will not if the epiphysis is slipped.

The management of SCFE is operative. Immediate non-weight-bearing upon diagnosis is important and admission for surgical pinning is typical. The main long-term complication is avascular necrosis of the femoral head and premature closure of the physis.

Femoral Fracture

All femoral shaft fractures should prompt emergent orthopedic consultation. In infants and nonambulatory children with femoral fractures, evaluation for nonaccidental trauma is warranted. In young children who are injured, femur fractures rarely cause hypotension. When hypotension is present, searching for another serious hemorrhagic injury is key.

Knee Injuries

Fractures of the Distal Femoral Physis

Fractures through the distal femoral physis are uncommon yet carry a significant complication rate. The popliteal artery lies close to the distal femoral metaphysis and may be injured along with the peroneal nerve. In these cases, immediate orthopedic evaluation is needed.

Patellar Dislocation

Often, there is a history of the kneecap "popping" out of place. Reduction is performed by extending the affected knee while gently "lifting" the patella medially into place. After reduction, radiographs are obtained to evaluate for fracture. A knee immobilizer and crutches are provided, and follow-up is with orthopedics.

Tibia Fractures

Toddler's Fracture

The toddler's fracture is an isolated spiral fracture of the distal tibia in a toddler. The typical mechanism is external rotation of the foot with the knee flexed. Clinically, there is often refusal to bear weight, and usually pain with palpation and rotation of the distal tibia, although swelling may be minimal or absent and occasionally there is no tenderness. Obtain radiographs with standard and oblique views of the leg in the limping toddler, even in the absence of physical examination findings. Radiographically, a fracture line may be noticed at the distal third of the tibial shaft. If a toddler's fracture is clinically suspected and initial radiographs are negative, immobilization and no immobilization are both management options with follow-up in 1 week for repeat x-rays and/or bone scan or MRI. The leg should not be in a circumferential cast if the diagnosis is not clear. For fractures evident on radiograph, immobilize the leg in a long leg splint or above knee cast with adequate flexion for car seat use and provide orthopedic follow-up within 72 hours for definitive casting if not done in the ED.

Distal tibial Salter–Harris types I and II fractures are the most common tibial fractures in children. If any significant displacement is evident, closed reduction and immobilization are usually sufficient ED management. The Salter–Harris type III fracture of the distal tibia typically requires open reduction when there is displacement. The Tillaux fracture is a Salter–Harris type III fracture through the anterolateral physis: it is usually managed surgically. The triplane fracture is a Salter–Harris type IV fracture. A computed tomography scan is warranted, and management is usually surgical.

Foot and Ankle Injuries

Most nondisplaced fractures of the metatarsals and phalanges can be managed by immobilization in a posterior short-leg splint and follow-up with an orthopedist. Significantly displaced fractures of the metatarsals and phalanges, as well as those of the great toe, that have intra-articular involvement may require fixation, although this can typically be done on an outpatient basis. Fractures of the base of the fifth metatarsal are common with inversion injuries of the ankle as in adults. The evaluation of ankle injuries should therefore include radiographs of the foot when there is tenderness over the fifth metatarsal bone.

SELECTED NONTRAUMATIC MUSCULOSKELETAL DISORDERS OF CHILDHOOD

Kawasaki's disease is discussed in Chapter 83.

Acute Septic Arthritis

Septic arthritis occurs in all ages, but especially in children younger than 3 years. The hip is most often affected, followed by the knee and elbow. If left untreated, purulent joint infection leads to total joint destruction. Please see Chapter 180, "Acute Disorders of the Joints and Bursae" for additional information.

Radiographs may show joint effusion, but this is nonspecific. The differential includes osteomyelitis, transient synovitis, cellulitis, septic bursitis, acute pauciarticular juvenile idiopathic arthritis (JIA), acute rheumatic fever, hemarthrosis, and SCFE. Distinguishing septic arthritis from osteomyelitis may be quite difficult. Osteomyelitis is more tender over the metaphysis, whereas septic arthritis is more tender over the joint line. Joint motion is much more limited in septic arthritis. Prompt arthrocentesis is the key to diagnosis at the bedside or, in the case of the hip, via ultrasound guidance. Synovial fluid shows WBCs and organisms.

Prompt open joint drainage and washout in the operating room is critical in the case of the hip, or arthroscopically or via arthrocentesis in more superficial joints. In all pediatric patients, when the organism is unknown, initial treatment is **vancomycin** 10 mg/kg IV every 6 hours or **clindamycin** 10 mg/kg IV every 6 hours *and* **cefotaxime** 50 mg/kg. The prognosis depends on the duration between symptoms and treatment, which joint is involved (worse for the hip), presence of associated osteomyelitis (worse), and the patient's age (worse for the youngest children).

Henoch–Schönlein Purpura

Henoch–Schönlein purpura (HSP) is a small-vessel vasculitis characterized by purpura, arthritis, abdominal pain, and hematuria. See Chapter 74, "Pediatric Abdominal Emergencies," for a discussion of HSP.

SELECTED PEDIATRIC RHEUMATOLOGIC DISORDERS

Transient Synovitis of the Hip

Transient or toxic synovitis is the most common cause of hip pain in children younger than 10 years. The peak age is 3 to 6 years, and the cause is unknown. Symptoms may be acute or gradual. Patients have pain in the hip, thigh, and knee, and an antalgic gait. Pain limits range of motion of the hip, but in contrast to septic arthritis, passive range of motion remains possible. There may be a low-grade fever, but patients do not appear toxic. The WBC and ESR are usually normal or mildly elevated. Radiographs of the hip are normal or show a mild to moderate effusion. The main concern is differentiation from septic arthritis, particularly if the patients are febrile, with elevation of WBC or ESR and effusion. Diagnostic arthrocentesis is required when the diagnosis is in doubt with fluoroscopic or ultrasound guidance. The fluid in transient synovitis is a sterile clear transudate.

Once septic arthritis and hip fracture have been ruled out, patients can be treated with weight-bearing as tolerated, no strenuous activity for 1 to 2 weeks, anti-inflammatory agents such as **ibuprofen** 10 mg/kg every 6 hours, and close follow-up.

Legg–Calvé–Perthes Disease

Legg–Calvé–Perthes disease is avascular necrosis of the femoral head, complicated by a subchondral stress fracture. Collapse and flattening of the femoral head ensues, with a potential for subluxation. The result is a painful hip with limited range of motion, muscle spasm, and soft tissue contractures. Children have a limp and chronic dull pain in the groin, thigh, and knee, which becomes worse with activity. Systemic symptoms are absent. Hip motion is restricted; there may be flexion and abduction contracture and thigh muscle atrophy. Initial radiographs in the first 1 to 3 months show widening of the cartilage space in the affected hip and diminished ossific nucleus of the femoral head. The second sign is subchondral stress fracture of the femoral head. The third finding is increased femoral head opacification. Deformity of the femoral head then occurs, with subluxation and protrusion of the femoral head from the acetabulum.

Bone scan and magnetic resonance imaging are very helpful in making this diagnosis by showing bone abnormalities well before plain films. The differential diagnosis includes transient synovitis, tuberculous arthritis, tumors, and bone dyscrasias.

In the ED, it is key to consider this chronic and potentially crippling condition. Initial management is non-weight-bearing and referral to a pediatric orthopedist for definitive care.

Osgood–Schlatter Disease

Osgood–Schlatter disease is common, and affects boys more than girls, usually between the ages of 10 and 15 years. The cause is repetitive stress on the tibial tuberosity by the quadriceps muscle, leading to inflammation. Prolonged basketball play is a frequent culprit. Children have pain and tenderness over the tuberosity, and symptoms are usually bilateral. The patellar tendon is thick and tender, with the tibial tuberosity enlarged and indurated.

Radiographs show soft tissue swelling over the tuberosity and patellar tendon thickening without knee effusion. Normally, the ossification site at the tubercle at this age will be irregular, but the prominence of the tubercle is characteristic of Osgood–Schlatter disease.

The disorder is self-limited. Acute symptoms improve after temporary avoidance of the offending activity. Crutches may be necessary, with a knee immobilizer or cylinder cast rarely needed. Exercises to stretch taut and hypertrophied quadriceps muscles are helpful.

Acute Rheumatic Fever

Acute rheumatic fever (ARF) is an acute inflammatory multisystem illness primarily affecting school-age children. It is not common in the United States, but there have been recent epidemics. ARF is preceded by infection with certain strains of group A β-hemolytic *Streptococcus*, which stimulates antibody production to host tissues. Children develop ARF 2 to 6 weeks after symptomatic or asymptomatic streptococcal pharyngitis. Arthritis, which occurs in most initial attacks, is migratory and polyarticular, primarily affecting the large joints. Carditis occurs in 33% of patients. Sydenham chorea occurs in 10% of patients and may occur months after the initial infection. The rash, erythema marginatum, is fleeting, faint, and serpiginous, usually accompanying carditis. Subcutaneous nodules, found on the extensor surfaces of extremities, are quite rare. Carditis confers greatest mortality and morbidity.

Various tests are used to confirm prior streptococcal infection (throat culture and streptococcal serology) or to assess carditis (electrocardiogram, chest radiograph, and echocardiogram). The differential includes JIA, septic arthritis, Kawasaki's disease, leukemia, and other cardiomyopathies and vasculitides. In the ED, carditis is the main management issue. Most patients are admitted.

Significant carditis is managed initially with **prednisone** 1 to 2 mg/kg/d. Arthritis is treated with high-dose **aspirin** 75 to 100 mg/kg/d to start. All children with ARF are treated with **penicillin** (or **erythromycin**, if allergic): **benzathine penicillin** 600,000 to 1.2 million U IM is given based on weight or oral **penicillin VK** 250 mg for young children and 500 mg for older children given twice daily for 10 days. Long-term prophylaxis is indicated for patients with ARF, and lifelong prophylaxis is recommended for patients with carditis.

Post-Infectious Reactive Arthritis

Because of increased group A β-hemolytic streptococcal infections, post-infectious reactive arthritis (PIRA) is also increasing. PIRA is a sterile, inflammatory, nonmigratory mono- or oligoarthritis occurring with infection at a distant site with β-hemolytic *Streptococcus*, or less commonly with *Staphylococcus* or *Salmonella*. Unlike ARF, PIRA is not associated with carditis and in general is a milder illness. However, the arthritis in PIRA is more severe and prolonged as compared with ARF.

To make the diagnosis of PIRA, antecedent infection with group A *Streptococcus* must be determined with throat culture or fourfold rise in ASO or anti-DNase B titer. PIRA is responsive to nonsteroidal anti-inflammatory drugs. If group A *Streptococcus* is recovered from the throat, treatment with penicillin or erythromycin should be instituted.

Juvenile Idiopathic Arthritis

The group of diseases comprised by juvenile idiopathic arthritis (JIA) share the findings of chronic noninfectious synovitis and arthritis, but with systemic manifestations. Pauciarticular disease is the most common form, usually involving a single large joint such as the knee. Permanent joint damage occurs infrequently. Polyarticular disease occurs in one-third of cases. Large and small joints are affected, and there may be progressive joint damage. Systemic JIA occurs in 20% of patients. This form is associated with high fevers and chills. Extra-articular manifestations are common, including a red macular coalescent rash, hepatosplenomegaly, and serositis. The arthritis in this form may progress to permanent joint damage.

In the ED, laboratory tests focus mostly on excluding other diagnoses. Complete blood count, ESR, and C-reactive protein may be normal. Arthrocentesis may be necessary to exclude septic arthritis, particularly in pauciarticular disease. Radiographs initially show joint effusions but are nonspecific. The diagnosis of JIA is not likely to be made in the ED.

Initial therapy for patients with an established diagnosis includes nonsteroidal anti-inflammatory drugs. Glucocorticoids are occasionally used, for example, for unresponsive uveitis or decompensated pericarditis or myocarditis.

FURTHER READING

For further reading in *Tintinalli's Emergency Medicine: A Comprehensive Study Guide*, 8th ed., see Chapter 140, "Musculoskeletal Disorders in Children," by Karen J.L. Black, Catherine Duffy, Courtney Hopkins-Mann, Demilola Ogunnaiki-Joseph, and Donna Moro-Sutherland.

CHAPTER 83 Rashes in Children

Lance Brown

Though rarely life-threatening, rashes are a common reason for emergency department (ED) visits in children. Helpful clues to the specific diagnosis of rash in a child include signs and symptoms that preceded or presented with the exanthem, whether mucous membranes are involved, immunization history, human and animal contacts, and environmental exposures. Identifying outbreaks among multiple children may be useful. Pediatric exanthems can be broadly classified by etiologic agent. With few exceptions, outpatient management is appropriate for most of these conditions.

VIRAL INFECTIONS

Enterovirus

Enteroviruses include **coxsackie viruses**, **echoviruses**, and **polioviruses** with a diverse range of clinical presentations. Enterovirus infections typically occur in epidemics in the summer and early fall. Many enteroviral infections lack specific clinical syndromes and presentation may include fever, upper and lower respiratory tract symptoms, gastrointestinal symptoms, meningitis, and myocarditis. The rashes of enteroviral infections also have a variety of appearances, including diffuse macular eruptions, morbilliform erythema, vesicular lesions, petechial and purpural eruptions, rubelliform rash, roseola-like rash, and scarlatiniform eruptions.

One distinctive enteroviral infection is **hand-foot-and-mouth disease**. Initially, patients typically present with fever, anorexia, malaise, and a sore mouth. Oral lesions appear on days 2 or 3 of illness followed by skin lesions. The oral lesions start as very painful 4- to 8-mm vesicles on an erythematous base that then ulcerate. The typical location of the oral lesions is on the buccal mucosa, tongue, soft palate, and gingiva. Skin lesions start as red papules that change to gray—3- to 7-mm vesicles that ultimately heal in 7 to 10 days. Typical locations of skin lesions include the palms, soles, and buttocks. A similar enanthum without involvement of the hands and feet is caused by a different viral subtype and is known as **herpangina** (most commonly caused by coxsackievirus A).

Management of presumed enteroviral infections typically involves symptomatic therapy ensuring adequate hydration, antipyretics/analgesics, or a combined suspension of diphenhydramine liquid and Maalox® applied in small quantities to the lesions (or swish and spit) three times daily and before feeding. Occasional narcotics may be required to facilitate adequate outpatient hydration.

Measles

Due to immunizations, measles is no longer common, but recent outbreaks have occurred among unimmunized groups. Infection typically occurs in the winter and spring. The incubation period is 10 days, followed by a 3-day prodrome of upper respiratory symptoms and then malaise, fever, coryza, conjunctivitis, photophobia, and cough. Ill appearance is expected. Just before the development of a rash, Koplik spots, tiny white lesions on the buccal mucosa, may be seen with a "grains of sand" appearance that is pathognomonic for measles. The exanthem develops 14 days after exposure. Initially, a red, blanching, maculopapular rash develops. The rash progresses from the head to the feet and rapidly coalesces on the face, and lasts about a week. As the rash resolves, a coppery brown discoloration may be seen and desquamation can occur. Measles is self-limited and treatment is supportive.

Rubella

Now quite rare due to immunizations, rubella (German measles) can be seen in teenagers, typically in the spring. The incubation period is 12 to 25 days and prodromal symptoms are similar to measles. The rash develops as fine, irregular pink macules and papules on the face that spread to the neck, trunk, and arms in a centrifugal distribution. The rash coalesces on the face as the eruption reaches the lower extremities and then clears in the same order as it appeared. Lymphadenopathy typically involves the suboccipital and posterior auricular nodes. Treatment is supportive.

Erythema Infectiosum

Erythema infectiosum (also known as *fifth disease*) is a febrile illness caused by parvovirus B19, typically occurring in the spring, and most commonly affecting children ages 5 to 15 years. The rash starts abruptly as a bright red macular discoloration on the cheeks producing the "slapped-cheek appearance" (Fig. 83-1). The lesions are closely grouped,

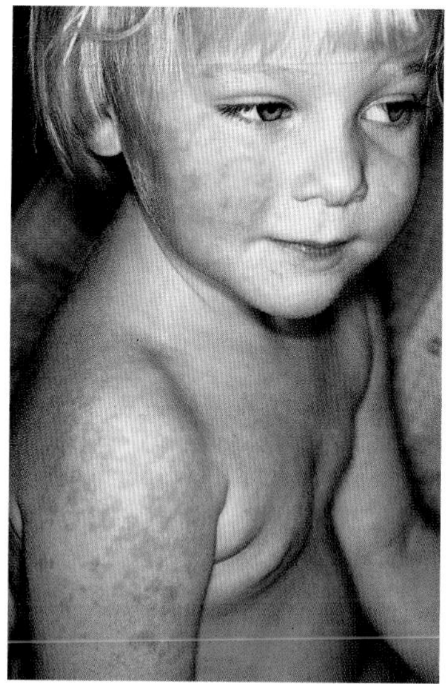

FIGURE 83-1. Erythema infectiosum (fifth disease). Toddler with the classic slapped cheek appearance of fifth disease. Reproduced with permission from Knoop K, Stack L, Storrow A: *Atlas of Emergency Medicine*, 3rd ed. New York: McGraw-Hill Companies, Inc; 2010. Photo contributor: Anne W. Lucky, MD.

tiny papules on an erythematous base with slightly raised edges. The eyelids and chin are characteristically spared. Circumoral pallor is typical. The rash fades after 4 to 5 days. As the illness progresses, and 1 to 2 days after the facial rash appears, a nonpruritic erythematous macular or maculopapular rash appears on the trunk and limbs. This rash may last for 1 week and is not pruritic. As the rash fades, central clearing of the lesions occurs, leaving a lacy reticular appearance. Palms and soles are rarely affected.

The exanthem may recur intermittently in the weeks after the onset of illness. Sun exposure or hot baths may exacerbate the rash. Associated symptoms include fever, malaise, headache, sore throat, cough, coryza, nausea, vomiting, diarrhea, and myalgias. Treatment is supportive.

Eczema Herpeticum

In children with existing eczema, this life-threatening, rare, viral infection can arise. The most frequent etiologic agent is herpes simplex virus. Bacterial superinfection with staphylococci or streptococci is presumed. Clinical manifestations of eczema herpeticum include fever and vesicular eruptions in areas of skin contemporaneously affected by eczematous lesions (Fig. 83-2). Treatment includes **acyclovir** 20 mg/kg/dose PO every

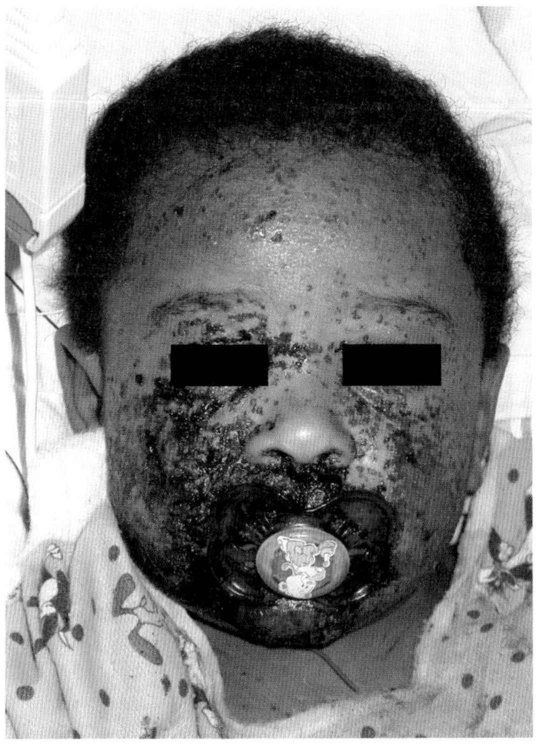

FIGURE 83-2. Typical appearance of eczema herpeticum. Used with permission from University of North Carolina Department of Dermatology.

6 hours and either **trimethoprim-sulfamethoxazole** 5 mg/kg/dose twice daily or **clindamycin** 10 mg/kg/dose three times daily for 10 days. Inpatient admission is often necessary.

Varicella (Chicken Pox)

Due to immunizations, the incidence of varicella has declined dramatically. The etiologic agent is varicella-zoster virus, a herpes virus. It typically occurs in children younger than 10 years but may occur at all ages. Varicella occurs most often in the late winter and early spring. Patients are highly contagious from the prodrome phase of the illness until all lesions are crusted over. The rash starts as faint red macules on the scalp or trunk. Within the first day, lesions begin to vesiculate and develop a red base, producing the characteristic appearance (Fig. 83-3). Over the next few days, groups of lesions develop, producing the classic appearance of crops of lesions in multiple stages of development. Over the next 1 to 2 weeks, lesions become dry and crusted. The rash typically spreads centrifugally (outward from the center). The palms and soles are usually spared. Low-grade fever, malaise, and headache are frequently seen but are typically mild. Treatment is symptomatic and includes

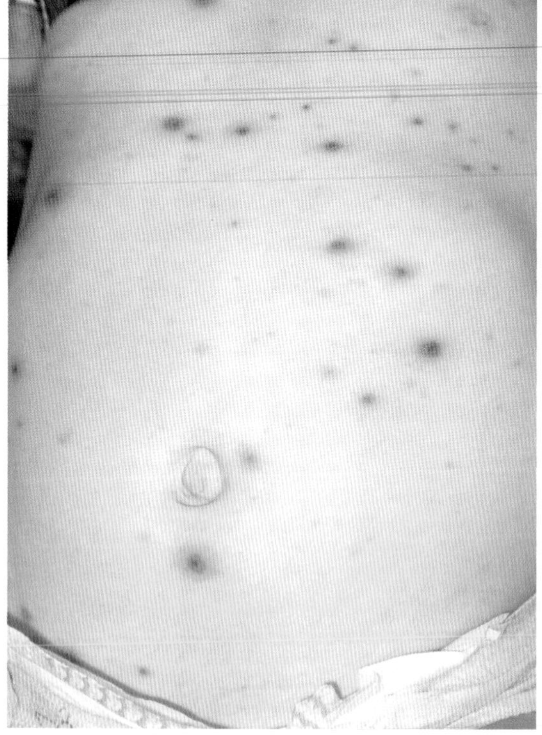

FIGURE 83-3. Typical rash of varicella (chicken pox). Used with permission from University of North Carolina Department of Dermatology.

diphenhydramine 1.25 mg/kg/dose, every 6 hours as needed for itching and **acetaminophen** 15 mg/kg/dose, every 4 hours as needed for fever. Although not needed in healthy children, **varicella-zoster immune globulin** and **acyclovir** 20 mg/kg up to 800 mg PO five times daily may be needed for immunocompromised children.

Roseola Infantum (Exanthem Subitum)

Roseola is a common acute febrile illness in children ages 6 months to 3 years and thought to be caused by human herpesvirus 6. Roseola presents with an abrupt onset, high fever lasting 3 to 5 days. As the fever begins to resolve, blanching macular or maculopapular, rose or pink discrete lesions develop (Fig. 83-4). Areas typically affected include the neck, trunk, and buttocks but the face and proximal extremities may also be involved, though mucous membranes are spared. The rash lasts 1 to 2 days and rapidly fades. Associated symptoms are typically mild and may include irritability when the fever is highest, cough, coryza, anorexia, and abdominal discomfort. The treatment is symptomatic.

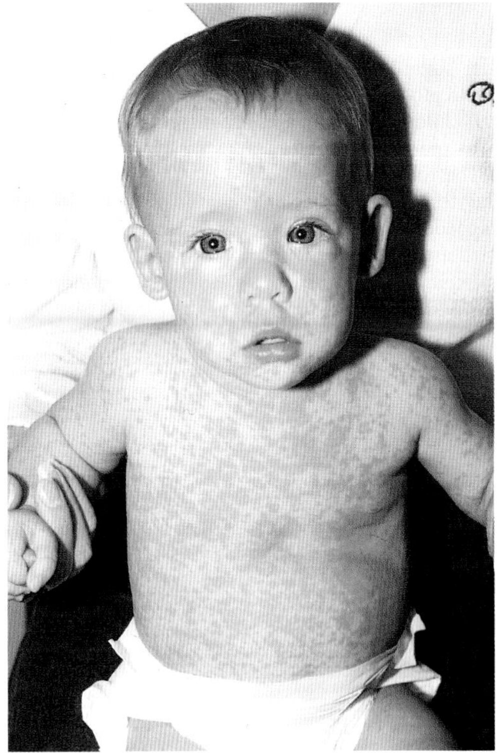

FIGURE 83-4. An infant with roseola infantum. Reproduced with permission from Knoop K, Stack L, Storrow A: *Atlas of Emergency Medicine*, 3rd ed. New York: McGraw-Hill Companies, Inc; 2010. Photo contributor: Raymond C. Baker, MD.

FUNGAL INFECTIONS

Tinea infections are common in infants and children and named for the body parts affected: tinea capitis (scalp), corporis (body), and pedis (foot) are common examples. Tinea infections typically manifest as scaly patches with pruritus of varying intensity. Successful treatment for all but tinea capitis and unguium is usually accomplished with topical creams including those available over-the-counter (**clotrimazole, miconazole, tolnaftate**) or by prescription (**ketoconazole, oxiconazole, ciclopirox, terbinafine**). Treatment is continued for 7 to 10 days after the resolution of lesions. Tinea capitis ranges from mild scalp scaliness with patchy alopecia to a painful, boggy mass known as a kerion. Tinea capitis is treated with oral **griseofulvin** ultramicrosize 15 mg/kg/dose once daily and **selenium sulfide** shampoo. Treatment of tinea capitis is usually for at least 8 weeks and close follow-up is important as treatment response and liver function tests need to be monitored. Tinea unguium is similarly treated with griseofulvin for longer periods of time.

BACTERIAL INFECTIONS

Impetigo

Impetigo is a superficial skin infection, typically caused by group A β-hemolytic streptococci or *Staphylococcus aureus*. The lesions usually occur in small children, often in areas of insect bites or minor trauma. The lesions start as red macules and papules that form vesicles and pustules (Fig. 83-5). The formation of a golden crust results from rupture of the vesicles. The lesions may become confluent. With the exception of regional lymphadenopathy, fever and systemic signs are rare. Most commonly affected areas include the face, neck, and extremities. Diagnosis is

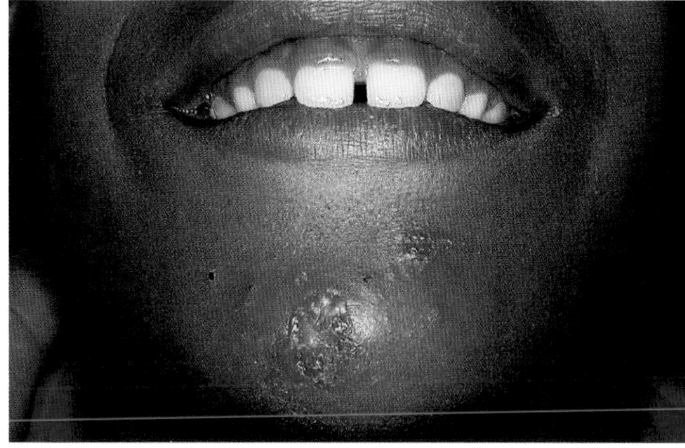

FIGURE 83-5. A young girl with crusting impetiginous lesions on her chin. Reproduced with permission from Knoop K, Stack L, Storrow A: *Atlas of Emergency Medicine*, 3rd ed. New York: McGraw-Hill Companies, Inc; 2010. Photo contributor: Michael J. Nowicki, MD.

based on the appearance of the rash. Localized infections may be treated with mupirocin ointment 2% applied three times daily. Larger infections should be treated with oral **cephalexin** 12.5 to 25 mg/kg/dose four times daily, **trimethoprim-sulfamethoxazole** 5 mg/kg/dose twice daily, or **clindamycin** 10 mg/kg/dose three times daily. Further treatment includes local wound cleaning.

Bullous Impetigo

Bullous impetigo typically occurs in infants and young children. Lesions are superficial, thin-walled bullae that characteristically occur on the extremities, rupture easily, leave a denuded base, dry to a shiny coating, and contain fluid that harbors staphylococci. The diagnosis usually is made by the appearance of the characteristic bullae (see Fig. 83-6). Treatment includes local wound cleaning, topical **mupirocin**, and an oral antistaphylococcal antibiotic such as **clindamycin** 10 mg/kg/dose three times daily or **trimethoprim-sulfamethoxazole** 5 mg/kg/dose twice daily.

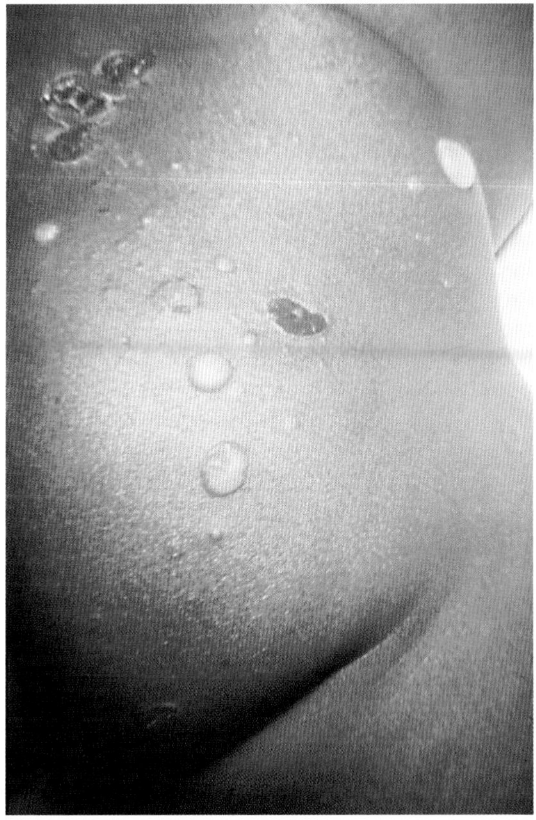

FIGURE 83-6. A child with bullous impetigo. Used with permission from the Centers for Disease Control and Prevention.

Scarlet Fever

A distinctive rash is seen with scarlet fever. The etiologic agent is group A β-hemolytic streptococci (recently group C streptococci also have been implicated). Scarlet fever usually occurs in school-age children and is diagnosed by the presence of exudative pharyngitis, fever, and the characteristic rash (Fig. 83-7). Associated symptoms include sore throat, fever, headache, vomiting, and abdominal pain. The rash starts in the neck, groin, and axillae, with accentuation at flexural creases (Pastia lines). The rash is red and punctate, blanches with pressure, and has a rough sandpaper feel. Early in the course of illness, the tongue has a white coating through which hypertrophic, red papillae project ("white strawberry tongue"). Hemorrhagic spots may be seen on the soft palate. The rash typically develops 1 to 2 days after the illness onset. Facial flushing and circumoral pallor are characteristic. Desquamation occurs with healing approximately 2 weeks after the onset of symptoms.

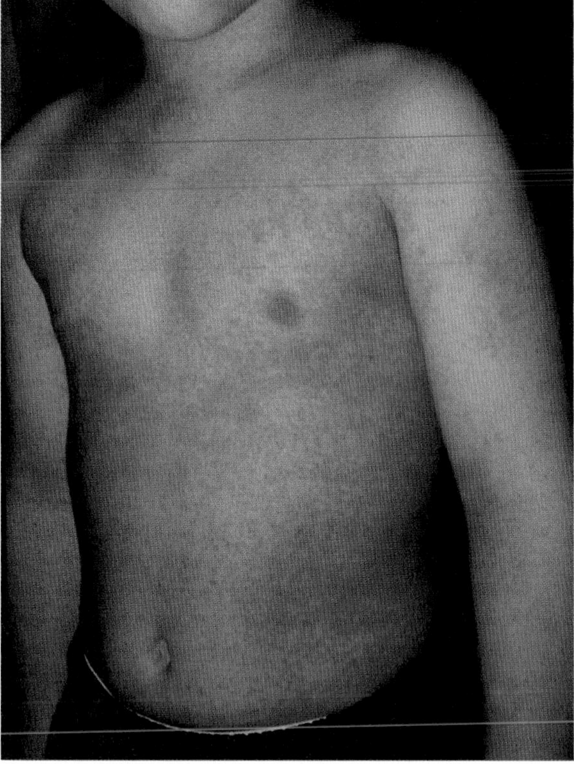

FIGURE 83-7. Scarlatiniform rash of scarlet fever; texture is typically sandpaper-like. Reproduced with permission from Knoop K, Stack L, Storrow A: *Atlas of Emergency Medicine*, 3rd ed. New York: McGraw-Hill Companies, Inc; 2010. Photo contributor: Lawrence B. Stack, MD.

The diagnosis generally is made on clinical grounds. Throat culture typically shows group A β-hemolytic streptococci or group C streptococci. Treatment is with **penicillin V** 16 mg/kg/dose three times daily or **clindamycin** 10 mg/kg/dose three times daily in the penicillin-allergic patient. Antibiotic treatment shortens the course of the illness and reduces the incidence of rheumatic fever.

Cellulitis

Cellulitis manifests a local inflammatory response at the site of infection with erythema, warmth, and tenderness. Fever is uncommon and likely indicates a more serious systemic infection, sepsis, or an unrelated concurrent viral infection. Community-associated methicillin-resistant *Staphylococcus aureus* (CA-MRSA) is becoming an increasingly common cause of cellulitis in children. Traditionally, oral **cephalexin** 12.5 to 25 mg/kg/dose four times daily has been the antibiotic of choice. With the rise of CA-MRSA, **clindamycin** 10 mg/kg/dose three times daily or **trimethoprim-sulfamethoxazole** 5 to 10 mg/kg/dose twice daily are more common choices. Identifying underlying abscesses may require needle aspiration or bedside ultrasonography.

Erysipelas is a cellulitis and lymphangitis of the skin due to group A β-hemolytic streptococci. Fever, chills, malaise, headache, and vomiting are common. The face and extremities are the most common sites, and the lesion typically forms in the area of a skin wound or pimple. The rash starts as a red plaque that rapidly enlarges. Increased warmth, swelling, and a raised, sharply demarcated, indurated border are typical. Diagnosis is by history and the appearance of the rash. Initial treatment may be inpatient with parenteral **penicillin G** 50,000 U/kg/dose, every 6 hours or **clindamycin** 10 mg/kg/dose, every 8 hours in the penicillin-allergic patient. Outpatient treatment includes **cephalexin** 12.5 to 25 mg/kg/dose four times daily, **trimethoprim-sulfamethoxazole** 5 to 10 mg/kg/dose twice daily, or **clindamycin** 10 mg/kg/dose three times daily. Rapid clinical improvement is expected after treatment has begun.

Meningococcemia

Meningococcemia should be suspected in an ill-appearing febrile child with a petechial or purpuric rash. The age distribution is bimodal with increased cases in infants and toddlers 2 years of age and younger and in adolescents 16 to 21 years of age. The etiologic agent is *Neisseria meningitidis* and empiric treatment is **cefotaxime** or **ceftriaxone** 50 mg/kg/dose. Close contacts (those exposed through child care or exposure to oral secretions) should receive chemoprophylaxis such as **rifampin** 5 mg/kg orally every 12 hours for 2 days for neonates; 10 mg/kg up to 600 mg per dose orally every 12 hours for 2 days for children or **ciprofloxacin** 500 mg single dose for adults.

INFESTATIONS

Scabies

Scabies is caused by infestation with the *Sarcoptes scabiei* mite that burrows into the skin resulting in severe pruritus after a 4 to 6 week incubation period. Typical findings in children include a generalized eruption with excoriated linear burrows, papules, pustules, and possibly vesicles. Family members and close contacts may have similar symptoms. Treatment consists of topical **permethrin** cream applied to avoid the mucous membranes and left on for 8 to 12 hours prior to washing it off. **Lindane** is contraindicated in infants and young children and pregnant teens.

Lice

Lice is caused by *Pediculus humanus capitis* and is common among children in school and day care. Lice are more commonly found in long straight hair in which the live mites and egg sacs can be seen. Over-the-counter treatments include **permethrin** 1% lotion, and combination **piperonyl butoxide/pyrethrum** extract shampoo. A fine-toothed comb is usually provided in the product packaging for combing out the egg sacs. Repeat treatment after 1 week is typically indicated.

COMMON NEONATAL RASHES

Erythema Toxicum

This benign, self-limited rash occurs in up to 50% of newborns during the first week of life. The lesions are typically erythematous macules 2 to 3 cm in diameter with central pustules. The rash spontaneously resolves after about a week.

Transient Neonatal Pustular Melanosis

This condition consists of three types of lesions: small pustules on a non-erythematous base that may be present at birth, erythematous macules with a surrounding scale that develop as the pustules rupture, and hyperpigmented brown macules. This may last weeks to months and requires no treatment.

Neonatal Acne

This affects up to 20% of neonates and typically appears around the third week of life. Erythematous papules and pustules are on the face and are typical. No testing or treatment is indicated.

Seborrheic Dermatitis

This rash typically starts between 2 to 6 weeks of life and improves by 6 months of life. Lesions are greasy yellow or red scales and typically involve the scalp (i.e., cradle cap) but may involve the eyebrows, ears, cheeks, and neck. This will typically resolve in weeks to months and can be treated with mineral or olive oil and gentle combing.

Diaper Dermatitis

Diaper rash is a common reason for ED visits in neonates and young infants. There are two main forms of diaper rash: irritant dermatitis and candida dermatitis. Irritant dermatitis is typically caused by prolonged moisture in the sealed diaper. The lesions are typically erythematous and macular or papular with well-demarcated borders. Treatment is frequent diaper changes and the application of a zinc oxide–containing barrier cream. Candida dermatitis is similar to irritant dermatitis in etiology and appearance with the exception of the presence of satellite lesions (small pustules beyond the margins of the main rash). Treatment is frequent diaper changes, the application of a zinc oxide–containing barrier cream, and the application of **nystatin** cream or ointment 100,000 U/g three times per day for 10 to 14 days.

OTHER ETIOLOGIES

Kawasaki's Disease

Kawasaki's disease (mucocutaneous lymph node syndrome) is a generalized vasculitis of unknown cause that typically occurs in children younger than 9 years. Diagnosis depends on the presence of fever for at least 5 days without another source, along with four of the following five criteria: (*a*) conjunctivitis; (*b*) rash; (*c*) lymphadenopathy; (*d*) oropharyngeal changes (injection of the pharynx, cracked lips, and prominent papillae of the tongue); and (*e*) extremity erythema and edema.

Typical rash appearances have been described as erythematous, morbilliform, urticarial, scarlatiniform, and erythema multiforme-like. A perineal rash may be present. Associated findings may include leukocytosis, elevation of acute-phase reactants (e.g., erythrocyte sedimentation rate and C-reactive protein), elevated liver function tests, hypoalbuminemia, anemia, arthritis, arthralgia, and irritability. Later in the illness, findings may include a rise in the platelet count (usually more than 1 million), desquamation of the fingers and toes, and coronary artery aneurysms. One percent to 2% of patients with coronary artery aneurysms develop sudden cardiac death.

Treatment consists of **intravenous immunoglobulin** and **aspirin**. The use of steroids is controversial.

Henoch–Schönlein Purpura

Henoch–Schönlein purpura (HSP) is the most common vasculitis in childhood. There are four main features of HSP: palpable purpura ranging in size from 2 to 10 mm primarily involving the buttocks, thighs, legs, and arms; gastrointestinal symptoms including vomiting, diarrhea, and abdominal pain; polyarthralgias; and hematuria and proteinuria. Children with HSP are generally well appearing and afebrile. HSP is typically self-limited and requires no treatment and no laboratory evaluation other than urinalysis (and renal function tests in the presence of hematuria). Consideration can be given to **prednisone** 1 mg/kg/dose for 2 weeks followed by a 2-week taper for severe joint and gastrointestinal symptoms and **ibuprofen** 10 mg/kg/dose as needed every 6 hours for severe arthralgias and extremity edema.

Erythema Multiforme

Erythema multiforme typically presents with an abrupt onset of rash without pruritis and is characterized by a well-appearing child with target lesions composed of two to three zones consisting of a dark, ruddy-appearing center and a lighter colored area surrounding the center with a red-appearing outer ring. Lesions present as coalescent plaques that frequently involve the palms and soles. Mucous membranes are spared. The etiology can be medication exposure, but is most commonly an infection with a herpes virus (HSV-1 and HSV-2). No treatment is required.

FURTHER READING

For further reading in *Tintinalli's Emergency Medicine: A Comprehensive Study Guide*, 8th ed., see Chapter 141, "Rashes in Infants and Children," by Gary Bonfante and Amy Dunn.

Sickle Cell Anemia in Children

Ilene Claudius

Sickle cell emergencies in children include vasoocclusive crises, hematologic crises, and infections. All children with sickle cell anemia (SCA) presenting with fever, pain, respiratory distress, or a change in neurologic function require a rapid and thorough ED evaluation.

VASOOCCLUSIVE CRISES

Vasoocclusive sickle episodes are due to intravascular sickling, which leads to tissue ischemia and infarction. Bones, soft tissue, viscera, and the central nervous system (CNS) may be affected. Pain may be the only symptom.

PAIN CRISES

Clinical Features

Pain crises are the most common SCA-related presentation to the ED, and typically affect the long bones and back. They can be triggered by stress, extremes of cold, dehydration, hypoxia, or infection, but most often occur without a specific cause. In an individual patient, recurrent pain crises tend to be similar in location and quality to previous episodes. Although, typically, there are no physical findings, pain, local tenderness, swelling, and warmth may occur. Low-grade temperature elevations can occur, but true fever is rare. Infants and toddlers can present initially with dactylitis, a swelling of hands or feet, and low-grade temperature caused by ischemia and infarction of the bone marrow.

Diagnosis and Differential

Differentiating between infection and vasoocclusive crisis can be difficult, particularly since infection can precipitate a pain crisis. Fever, limited range of motion of a joint, and pain that differs in location or quality from previous crises should raise concern for an infection. Pain crises can be associated with leukocytosis; however, a left shift is suspicious for infection. Sedimentation rates are unreliable markers for infections in SCA patients due to anemia. All pain crises represent ischemia, but bony infarcts present with severe, difficult to control pain, significant tenderness, and leukocytosis. Patients with bony infarcts are at risk of fat embolism.

Pain localized to the hip or inguinal area worsening with weight-bearing may be due to avascular necrosis of the femoral head, which may demonstrate flattening and collapse of the femoral head on plain radiograph.

Abdominal pain resulting from vasoocclusive crises is common and is typically abrupt in onset, and poorly localized. Tenderness and guarding may be present on examination. Rebound and rigidity are usually absent. If not typical of a pain crisis, non-SCA-related causes need to be considered (e.g., appendicitis), as well as SCA-related cholelithiasis/cholecystitis (can occur as early as 2 years of age), intrahepatic cholestasis (sudden right upper quadrant pain and tenderness, jaundice, anorexia, hepatomegaly, and sometimes fever), splenic sequestration, or hepatic sequestration (anemia and hepatomegaly). Constipation, urinary tract infection, and peptic ulcer disease are more common in SCA patients. Laboratories, ultrasound, and CT scan may be necessary to differentiate among these etiologies.

Emergency Department Care and Disposition

Pain management must be individualized, using previously effective regimens as a guide. Nonparenteral medications can be used (oral or nasal) to meet the goal of delivering analgesia within an hour of registration.

1. **Mild pain**
   a. Hydration
      i. Oral hydration if possible
      ii. IV hydration at maintenance rate if euvolemic and not tolerating oral fluids
      iii. Correct dehydration
   b. Pain control
      i. Oral NSAIDs, such as **ibuprofen** 10 mg/kg
      ii. Oral narcotics, such as **hydrocodone** 0.15 to 0.2 mg/kg, if needed
2. **Moderate to severe pain**
   a. Hydration
      i. IV hydration, D5½NS at 1 x the age-appropriate maintenance rate
   b. Pain control
      i. Oral or IV NSAIDs, such as **ketorolac** 0.5 mg/kg
      ii. Parenteral narcotics, such as morphine 0.1 to 0.15 mg/kg or **hydromorphone** 0.015 mg/ kg
      iii. Maintain or escalate IV narcotic dose by 25% every 15 to 30 minutes until pain control is achieved for severe pain.
3. Oral antihistamines, if needed.
4. Oxygen for saturation <95%.
5. Heat may be an effective adjunct.
6. Packed red blood cell (PRBC) transfusions are not recommended unless another indication exists.
7. Admission is warranted for poor pain control or inadequate oral fluid intake. Children who have presented repeatedly for the same pain crisis also should be considered for admission.
8. Incentive spirometry should be started in patients receiving narcotic medications.
9. Children discharged from the ED should continue analgesics at home on a scheduled basis with PCP or hematology follow-up the next day.

ACUTE CHEST SYNDROME

Acute chest syndrome (ACS) is believed to represent a combination of pneumonia, pulmonary infarction, and pulmonary emboli from necrotic bone marrow. It is a leading cause of death in all patients with SCA, but especially those older than 10 years.

Clinical Features

Consider ACS in all patients with SCA who present with complaints of chest pain, especially when associated with tachypnea, dyspnea, cough, or other symptoms of respiratory distress. Significant hypoxia and rapid deterioration to respiratory failure can occur.

Diagnosis and Differential

Chest radiographs should be obtained but may be normal during the first hours to days. The diagnosis is made in the setting of a new infiltrate on chest radiograph in the setting of chest pain and respiratory symptoms. Both pneumonia and acute chest syndrome typically cause leukocytosis. Thrombocytopenia may accompany a severe crisis. Sputum and blood cultures are rarely positive. Pneumonia is most commonly due to atypical bacteria (chlamydia, mycoplasma), but can represent community acquired pathogens (*Streptococcus pneumoniae*) as well. Asthma, cardiac volume overload, and, in adulthood, pulmonary hypertension are also commonly associated with SCA.

Emergency Department Care and Disposition

Because deterioration can be rapid, close monitoring is required, typically in the ICU.

1. Initial stabilization: oxygen to maintain saturation >95%, hydration at 50% to 75% maintenance fluids, analgesia (see Pain Crisis).
2. Antibiotics: macrolide, such as **azithromycin** 10 mg/kg PO or IV, and third generation cephalosporin, such as **ceftriaxone** or **cefotaxime** 50 to 100 mg/kg daily IV.
3. Consider simple PRBC transfusion in children with symptomatic ACS who have dropped >1 g/dL from their baseline Hgb. However, raising hemoglobin above 10 g/dL is discouraged, so this recommendation typically applies to patients with a Hgb of <9 g/dL.
4. Consider exchange transfusion for patients with rapid progression of ACS, with saturation <90% despite oxygen, increasing respiratory distress, progressive pulmonary infiltrates, or a declining Hgb despite transfusion.
5. Admit all children with suspected ACS to the hospital.

ACUTE CENTRAL NERVOUS SYSTEM EVENTS

Clinical Features

Consider acute stroke in any patient with SCA who presents with sudden onset headache or neurologic changes, including hemiparesis, seizures, speech defects, visual disturbances, transient ischemic attacks, vertigo, cranial nerve palsies, paresthesias, altered mental status or coma. Children with SCA are at significantly higher risk of acute ischemic stroke than unaffected children.

Diagnosis and Differential

Because of the challenges in diagnosing acute ischemic stroke (e.g., limited availability of MRI, CT negative in acute setting), providers may need to initiate treatment based exclusively on clinical suspicion. As SCA patients age, their risk of a hemorrhagic stroke increases as well, primarily due to aneurysm development. If clinical history is appropriate for a subarachnoid hemorrhage, workup should proceed as for a patient without SCA. Acute chest crisis, sudden severe anemia, and meningitis can cause neurologic symptoms, and appropriate tests should be sent to investigate these possibilities in the appropriate clinical setting.

Emergency Department Care and Disposition

Suspected CNS vasoocclusion necessitates immediate stabilization and careful monitoring. Urgent exchange transfusion is preferred to standard transfusion, and the Hgb should not be raised above 10 g/dL. Transfusion should be initiated with the goal of <30% HbS. As in any ischemic stroke, temperature, glucose, and oxygenation should be monitored and controlled. Limited data exists regarding the use of alteplase, and it currently has no role in the management of SCA-related ischemic stroke in children. Intracranial hemorrhage should be managed in conjunction with a neurosurgeon. All children with suspected stroke should be admitted to the pediatric intensive care unit.

PRIAPISM

Clinical Features and Diagnosis

Priapism, a painful sustained erection >4 hours in the absence of sexual stimulation, occurs when sickled cells accumulate in the corpora cavernosa. It can affect any male with SCA regardless of age, and severe prolonged attacks can cause impotence. Typically, the patient has an edematous and tender penis, with difficulty urinating.

Emergency Department Care and Disposition

Patients with priapism should receive vigorous oral or IV hydration and appropriate analgesia. As in non-SCA priapism, needle aspiration of the corpora cavernosa and administration of a vasoconstrictor, such as 1:1,000,000 epinephrine solution, may be required. Transfusion is not recommended as immediate therapy for priapism. Management and admission decisions should be made promptly in consultation with urology and pediatric hematology.

HEMATOLOGICAL CRISES

Acute Sequestration Crises

Clinical Features and Diagnosis

Intrasplenic trapping of red blood cells primarily affects children under 5 years of age, but can occur in older patients with combined forms of SCA (e.g., SC disease). Often preceded by a viral syndrome, splenic sequestration presents with sudden-onset left upper quadrant pain; pallor and lethargy; tender splenomegaly; and progresses to hypotension, shock, and death. A CBC shows profound anemia, with hemoglobin <6 g/dL, or >2 g/dL lower than the patient's baseline level. Minor episodes can occur with insidious onset of abdominal pain, slowly progressive splenomegaly, and a more gradual fall in hemoglobin level. Generally the hemoglobin level remains >6 g/dL.

Patients may have accompanying mild neutropenia or thrombocytopenia. Less commonly, sequestration can occur in the liver. Clinical features include an enlarged and tender liver with associated hyperbilirubinemia, severe anemia, and elevated reticulocyte count. Cardiovascular collapse is rare in this condition.

Emergency Department Care and Disposition

Hydration, PRBC transfusion, and admission are required for major episodes. Transfusion should be gradual (5 mL/kg), as return of the sequestered RBCs to the intravascular space can occur, causing hyperviscosity. Occasionally, children with minor episodes can be observed, and discharged with close follow-up with a hematologist.

APLASTIC EPISODES

Potentially life-threatening aplastic episodes are precipitated primarily by viral infections, typically parvovirus B19, and present with gradual onset of pallor, dyspnea, and fatigue. The CBC shows an unusually low hemoglobin and reticulocyte count, with normal white blood cell and platelet counts. Recovery is spontaneous within 1 to 2 weeks, and patients can typically be temporized with PRBC transfusion in the ED with close outpatient follow-up in 7 to 10 days for repeat labs or inpatient setting.

HEMOLYTIC CRISES

Bacterial and viral infections in children with SCA can precipitate rapid hemolysis, with sudden-onset of jaundice and pallor. A CBC shows hemoglobin level decreased from baseline, with markedly increased reticulocytosis. Specific therapy is rarely required, though transfusion may be helpful in symptomatic patients. Care should be directed toward treating the underlying infection. Close follow-up to monitor hemoglobin level and reticulocyte count should be arranged if discharged from the ED.

INFECTIONS

Clinical Features

Poor splenic function renders children with SCA particularly susceptible to bacterial infections, particularly in early childhood. Currently, bacteremia rates are 0.3% to 1.1%.

Diagnosis and Differential

Risk factors for sepsis in children with SCA include temperature >40°C, WBC >30,000 or <5000 cells/mm^3, platelet count <100,000/mm^3, Hgb <5 g/dL, ill appearance, and history of pneumococcal sepsis.

Emergency Department Care and Disposition

Children with a temperature above 38.5°C meeting any high-risk feature (see above) should have a CBC, blood culture, reticulocyte count, and, if clinically indicated, a urine culture sent and received a parenteral antibiotic with activity against *Streptococcus pneumoniae* and *Haemophilus influenzae*, such as **ceftriaxone** 50 mg/kg IV or IM, as soon as possible. Vancomycin should be added if the patient is at high risk for penicillin-resistant pneumococcal infection. Septic shock must be managed aggressively with early goal-directed therapy. Patients with any respiratory symptoms should also get a chest radiograph. Well-appearing patients who have reliable next-day follow-up can be discharged following a parenteral dose of ceftriaxone pending culture results. Ill-appearing patients with temperatures >39.5°C should be admitted.

VARIANTS OF SICKLE CELL DISEASE

Sickle cell trait is the carrier state of SCA (heterozygous). These patients are typically asymptomatic and experience sickling only in the presence of extreme hypoxia or high altitude. Baseline microscopic hematuria may exist. *Sickle cell–hemoglobin C disease* is a heterozygous condition characterized by mild to moderate anemia and fewer complications. However, splenomegaly can persist to adulthood, and these patients remain at risk for sequestration crises. *Sickle cell β-thalassemia* disease is a heterozygous condition with variable severity and symptoms.

FURTHER READING

For further reading in *Tintinalli's Emergency Medicine: A Comprehensive Study Guide*, 8th ed., see Chapter 142, "Sickle Cell Disease in Children," by John Marshall.

Hematologic-Oncologic Emergencies in Children

Ilene Claudius

Childhood cancer is a leading cause of death in children, but with improvements in management and outcomes, many patients with new, active, or treated malignancies present to the ED. This chapter covers the most common pediatric malignancies and hematologic issues. More information on malignancy-related complications is provided in Chapter 139 and hemophilia and Von Willebrand's disease are discussed in detail in Chapter 135.

CHILDHOOD LEUKEMIA

Acute lymphoblastic leukemia (ALL) is the most common pediatric malignancy, with a peak incidence between 3 to 5 years of age and a 75% to 80% 5-year survival.

Clinical Features

Patients can present with systemic complaints (fever, weight loss) or any of the following signs or symptoms of bone marrow or extramedullary infiltration: pallor, fatigue, easy bruising or bleeding, fever, or bone pain (particularly nocturnal). Many have hepatomegaly or splenomegaly. Rarely, acute myelogenous leukemia (AML) can present with gingival hyperplasia or subcutaneous masses (chloromas).

Diagnosis and Differential

The complete blood count (CBC) with manual differential is the most useful test, though leukocytosis and blasts may be absent early in the disease process, requiring close follow-up of patients with insidious complaints such as bone pain. White blood cell (WBC) counts below 4000/mL^3, mild anemia, and mild thrombocytopenia should raise suspicion in these cases. Abnormalities of two or more cell lines make leukemia more likely. If the CBC is concerning for acute leukemia, obtain a chest radiograph (for mediastinal mass); electrolytes with creatinine, calcium, uric acid, and phosphate (for evidence of tumor lysis); liver function tests and lactate dehydrogenase, prothrombin time (PT)/partial prothrombin tine (PTT) (looking for disseminated intravascular coagulation); peripheral smear; type and screen if anemic; and blood and urine cultures if febrile.

The differential diagnosis is extensive depending on the patient's presenting symptom. Aplastic anemia and viral infections can cause bone marrow suppression; rheumatologic diseases can overlap with symptoms and findings of leukemia; and idiopathic immune thrombocytopenia can be difficult to differentiate, though classically involves isolated destruction of the platelets without affecting other cell lines.

Emergency Department Care and Disposition

Chemotherapy need not be initiated immediately in most cases. ED care is directed at potential complications and symptoms.

1. Anemia
   a. Irradiated, leukodepleted packed red blood cells (PRBCs) (10 mL/kg) for life-threatening hemorrhage or hemolysis. This will raise hemoglobin (Hb) 2-3 g/dL.
   b. If no hemorrhage or hemolysis, nonemergent transfusions can be given. The clinical picture should determine need for ED transfusions, with a goal hemoglobin (Hb) of >8 to 10 g/dL. This should be done in coordination with an oncologist. A lower Hb should be maintained in hyperleukocytosis if the patient can tolerate this.
2. Thrombocytopenia
   a. Platelets (10 mL/kg) for life-threatening hemorrhage, consumption, or urgent need for invasive procedure (e.g., lumbar puncture). Invasive procedures require platelet count >50,000/mm^3 and surgery 50,000–100,000/mm^3.
   b. If no urgent indication exists, nonemergent transfusions can be given to keep platelets >10,000/mm^3. This does not need to be done in the ED.
3. Infection: Fever (single oral temperature >38.3°C or multiple temperatures >38°C separated by at least an hour) and neutropenia (ANC <500/mm^3 or ANC<1000/mm^3 with anticipated decline) typically become an issue after the initiation of chemotherapy. However, granulocyte function is impaired in newly presenting leukemics, and fever or suspicion of infection in a new leukemic should be treated emergently with broad-spectrum antibiotics regardless of neutrophil count. In children with known neutropenia, consider unusual infections such as perirectal abscess/cellulitis and typhlitis (an appendicitis-like syndrome), as well as bacteremia. Management includes:
   a. Blood cultures
   b. Other studies (e.g., urinalysis) as clinically indicated
   c. Avoid rectal manipulation, including rectal temperatures.
   d. IV **cefepime** (50 mg/kg) or **ceftazidime** (50 mg/kg) or **piperacillin-tazobactam** (80 mg/kg)
   e. If ill-appearing, add IV **gentamycin** (2.5 mg/kg).
   f. If suspicion of gram-positive infection, add IV **vancomycin** (15 mg/kg).
   g. If anaerobic source (e.g., typhlitis), add IV **clindamycin** (10 mg/kg) or **metronidazole** (7.5 mg/kg).
4. Tumor lysis describes the release of intracellular potassium, phosphate, and uric acid, and subsequent decline in serum calcium that occurs from turnover of tumor cells. It typically occurs with chemotherapy, but can occur prior to treatment, particularly in patients with a high tumor burden (ALL or non-Hodgkin's lymphoma). Recognition and treatment of this life- and kidney- threatening condition must begin in the ED, and prevention should be considered in patients with a particularly high WBC count. Check laboratories every 4 hours, treat hyperkalemia in the standard fashion, aggressively hydrate, and consider allopurinol or recombinant urate oxidase (rasburicase) for uric acid management. Hypocalcemia is not treated unless symptomatic. Specifics of management are discussed in Chapter 139.

5. Hyperleukocytosis (WBC >100,000/mm^3) typically requires treatment if symptoms of stasis (e.g., stroke, visual change, dyspnea, priapism) occur, or if the WBC is >200,000/mm^3 for AML and >300,000/mm^3 for ALL in the absence of symptoms. Treatment includes:
   a. Aggressive hydration with normal saline bolus of 20 mL/kg repeated as tolerated.
   b. If patient is symptomatic after hydration, arrange for leukapheresis.
   c. Avoid PRBC transfusions and diuretics if possible.
   d. Anticipate and initiate treatment for tumor lysis syndrome.
   e. If asymptomatic with high levels, consider hydroxyurea which will reduce the WBC count to half in 24 to 48 hours.

LYMPHOMA

Hodgkin's lymphoma is a lymphoid neoplasm preferentially affecting adolescents. Most cases present in the cervical or supraclavicular lymph nodes causing nontender, nonerythematous, rubbery lymphadenopathy chains. Systemic symptoms (e.g., fever, night sweats, weight loss) occur in 39% to 50% of children and teens. A chest radiograph may demonstrate an anterior mediastinal mass. Non-Hodgkin's lymphoma can originate in or outside of the lymphatic system, and occurs across ages, particularly in those with a history of immunosuppression. Because the tumor can occur in any organ, presenting signs and symptoms differ by location. A CBC, electrolytes and creatinine (looking for tumor lysis), and chest radiograph (looking for mediastinal mass) should be performed in the ED. ED care involves management of acute complications, avoidance of steroid therapy except in life-threatening situations, consultation with an oncologist, and recognition of the potential for intrathoracic airway compromise in patients with a mediastinal mass. Compression of the superior vena cava (SVC syndrome) or compression of both SVC and trachea (superior mediastinal syndrome) can occur, with respiratory symptoms, upper body edema, headache, and altered mental status.

CENTRAL NERVOUS SYSTEM TUMORS

Brain tumors are common pediatric malignancies, and typically present with nonspecific symptoms: headaches (especially early morning), irritability, emesis, and behavioral changes related to increased intracranial pressure. In infants, overt signs of increased pressure (e.g., bulging fontanel, sunsetting of eyes) can sometimes be appreciated. Vomiting, ataxia, cranial nerve palsies, or vague neurologic signs and symptoms can occur as well. CT scan or MRI are acceptable imaging studies in the ED. Spinal cord tumors can present with back pain with or without neurological signs and are evaluated by MRI. Seizures should be treated if present, and **dexamethasone** (1 mg/yr of age up to 10 mg) can be given to reduce vasogenic edema in patients not suspected to have leukemia or lymphoma. Further management should be determined by oncology and neurosurgery.

EXTRACRANIAL SOLID TUMORS

Neuroblastoma is a primitive ganglion tumor that can arise along the sympathetic nervous system, most commonly in the adrenal gland, other abdominal location, chest, or neck. Patients can present with a painless mass, hepatomegaly, or symptoms of mass effect from compression of the bowel, bladder, lymphatics, spinal cord, trachea, or superior vena cava. Occasionally, retrobulbar metastasis can cause raccoon eyes and proptosis. Paraneoplastic manifestations can include hypertension, watery diarrhea, and opsoclonus-myoclonus syndrome (rapid, multidirectional eye movements and jerking of the extremities). CBC for evidence of bone marrow infiltration and chest radiograph for mediastinal mass should be obtained in the ED. Urine levels of homovanillic acid and vanillylmandelic acid are helpful diagnostically.

Wilms tumor, or nephroblastoma, primarily affects young children (<10 years of age) and typically presents with an abdominal mass with few symptoms other than those explained by local compression. Many patients present with lung metastasis or hypertension from increased renin production. These masses can rupture with trauma or vigorous palpation.

Germ cell tumors typically present as masses in the ovary or testicle, although extragonadal locations are common in younger children. They are particularly more common in boys with a history of an undescended testicle. Diagnosis is by ultrasound.

Retinoblastoma is a white-grey intraocular malignancy that typically presents in children less than 2 years of age with loss of the normal red reflex (Fig. 85-1). Strabismus, decreased visual acuity, a fixed pupil, glaucoma, or an injected, painful eye are less common presentations.

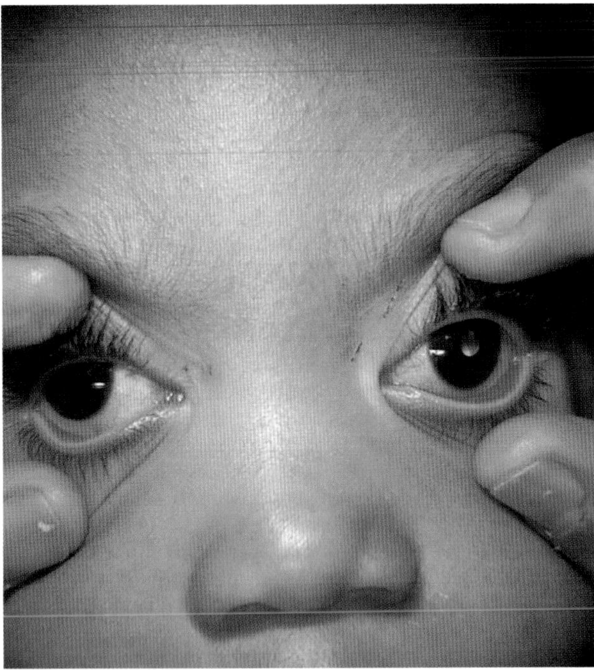

FIGURE 85-1. Typical appearance of leukocoria in a patient with retinoblastoma. Reproduced with permission from Shah BR, Lucchesi M. *Atlas of Pediatric Emergency Medicine.* New York: McGraw-Hill Companies, Inc.; 2006.

One-quarter of cases are bilateral, and diagnosis is made through ophthalmology consultation and CT scan or MRI.

Bone and tissue sarcomas include **rhabdomyosarcoma** (a painless tissue mass), **osteosarcoma** (a bony tumor around the metaphysis of the knee, proximal humerus, pelvis, or mandible), and **Ewing's sarcoma** (a bony tumor of the long bones and axial skeleton). Osteosarcoma and Ewing's sarcoma can present as a dull, aching pain, particularly at night or with activity, a tender mass that seems to appear following a minor trauma, or with systemic symptoms. Diagnosis of rhabdomyosarcoma is by ultrasound or CT scan, while osteosarcoma and Ewing's sarcoma often are seen on plain radiograph, with osteosarcoma demonstrating a mixed sclerotic/lytic "sunburst" appearance of periosteal reaction and Ewing's sarcoma having a destructive, "moth-eaten" appearance.

HEMOPHILIA

Hemophilia is an inherited deficiency of factor 8 (hemophilia A) or factor 9 (hemophilia B) which can be mild (>5% factor activity), moderate (1% to 5% factor activity), or severe (<1% factor activity).

Clinical Features

Appropriate family history or bleeding/bruising out of proportion with injury, recurrent bleeding, or in bleeding into uncommon locations (GI, joints) should raise concern for a bleeding disorder. Common issues in hemophilia are hemarthroses (and resultant destructive arthropathy), muscle bleeds (occasionally causing compartment syndrome), and intracranial hemorrhage.

Diagnosis and Differential

Hemophilia causes an elevated PTT, with normal platelets, bleeding time, and PT. Quantitative factor levels are diagnostic. Other bleeding disorders include thrombocytopenias, vitamin K deficiency bleeding (typically 2 to 14 days after birth in neonates whose parents have refused prophylactic vitamin K administration at birth), and von Willebrand's disease (prolonged bleeding in the face of normal platelet numbers with or without factor 8 deficiency).

Emergency Department Care and Disposition

Treatment is with appropriate factor replacement: up to 100% correction with severe bleeds, and less with more minor bleeds.

ANEMIA

Clinical Features

Anemia may be asymptomatic or accompanied by pallor and fatigue or heart failure.

Diagnosis and Differential

Iron deficiency anemia due primarily to excessive cow's milk intake typically affects children aged 6 months to 3 years of age. Children outside of this age range should be assessed for occult GI bleeding with stool guaiac testing.

Laboratory studies demonstrate anemia with a low reticulocyte count and low mean corpuscular volume (MCV). Hemolytic anemia can be primary or secondary to an underlying infection or intrinsic disorder. Patients have isolated anemia with high MCV, spherocytes and schistocytes on peripheral smear, elevated indirect bilirubin, and a positive direct antibody test.

Emergency Department Care and Disposition

Most asymptomatic or minimally symptomatic patients with iron deficiency anemia can be safely discharged with careful follow-up, reduction of milk intake below 24 oz/d, and initiation of **iron therapy** (2 to 3 mg/kg/dose of elemental iron three times daily). Hemolytic anemia may require more careful observation or transfusion, based on the patient's clinical status and hemoglobin level. Steroids are indicated in the treatment of autoimmune hemolytic anemia. If transfusion is required, patients with very low hemoglobin levels (<5 g/dL) should receive 3 to 5 mL/kg of PRBCs over 2 to 3 hours to start, while patients with a pretransfusion Hb >5 g/dL can receive 10 mL/kg to start.

IDIOPATHIC THROMBOCYTOPENIC PURPURA (ITP)

ITP is an autoimmune disorder of platelet destruction.

Clinical Features

While often an isolated condition in preschool-aged children, ITP can be a feature of rheumatologic disorders (e.g., lupus) or infections (e.g., HIV, hepatitis C), particularly in teens. Patients can present with petechiae or bleeding (nares or gingiva), and, in the younger child without a coexisting condition, ITP often follows a viral infection by days to weeks.

Diagnosis and Differential

Other autoimmune and infectious disorders (lupus, HIV, hepatitis C) should be considered, particularly in the teen. In ITP, other cell lines are not affected and platelets are often below 20,000/mm^3 with a large platelet volume. CBC and blood type should be sent. Disseminated intravascular coagulation and hemolytic-uremic syndrome should be considered in the ill patient with thrombocytopenia.

Emergency Department Care and Disposition

ITP in children carries an excellent prognosis, with 70% resolving spontaneously within 6 months, regardless of treatment. Children with minimal symptoms and platelets >20,000/mm^3 are often followed without intervention. For children with significant bleeding or platelet counts <20,000/mm^3, the following options exist:

1. **Prednisone** 1 to 2 mg/kg/d for 2 to 4 weeks. Steroids should only be started in conjunction with a hematologist once leukemia has been excluded.
2. **Intravenous immunoglobulin (IVIG)** 1 g/kg over 4 to 6 hours. Premedication with acetaminophen and diphenhydramine is recommended.
3. **Anti-Rh (D) immunoglobulin** (WinRho®) 75 μg/kg over 1 hour can be used in patients whose blood type is Rh+. Because these antibodies bind

the RBCs, hemolysis ensues, dropping the Hb 1 to 2 g/dL over the week following treatment. In 2010, a boxed warning was issued by the Food and Drug Administration (FDA) in response to hemolysis-related deaths of primarily older adults following use of WinRho® for ITP, recommending 8 hours of monitoring for signs of hemolysis (back pain, chills, fever, discolored urine) and premedication with acetaminophen and diphenhydramine is recommended.

4. In the case of a life-threatening bleed, single-donor **platelet transfusion** (20 to 30 mL/kg), **IVIG** (1 g/kg over 30 minutes), and high-dose **methylprednisolone** (30 mg/kg) should be considered as a temporizing measure. This platelet dose is much higher than the normal dose of 5 to 10 mL/kg of a single donor pack or 1 U/10 kg of the pooled or "random" donor packs. In a patient without antibodies, this lower dose will increase the platelet level by 30,000 to 50,000/mm^3.

NEUTROPENIA

Neutropenia implies a neutrophil count below 1500/mm^3, but risk of life-threatening infections increases significantly when the count falls in severe neutropenia (<500/mm^3).

Clinical Features

Neutropenia can be asymptomatic or associated with serious bacterial illness.

Diagnosis and Differential

Benign forms of neutropenia include benign transient neutropenia (from viral infections or medications), autoimmune neutropenia, and cyclic neutropenia. More serious forms of neutropenia are chronic and persistent, such as congenital agranulocytosis, or chemotherapy related. Neutropenia can be caused by viral suppression, sepsis-induced bone marrow suppression, medications, isoimmune causes in the neonate, or autoimmune causes (including cyclic neutropenia with recurrent 4- to 6-day episodes on a 21-day cycle) in an older child. It is difficult to differentiate benign from serious causes in the ED.

Emergency Department Care and Disposition

Patients with already diagnosed benign forms of neutropenia and evidence of infection can typically be discharged home, though consultation with the patient's hematologist and a single dose of **ceftriaxone** (50 mg/kg) may be considered depending on the clinical situation. Asymptomatic patients with incidental neutropenia should see a hematologist on an outpatient basis. Febrile children with undifferentiated or nonbenign neutropenia should have blood cultures sent and broad-spectrum antibiotics initiated.

FURTHER READING

For further reading in *Tintinalli's Emergency Medicine: A Comprehensive Study Guide*, 8th ed., see Chapter 143, "Oncologic and Hematologic Emergencies in Children," by Megan E. Mickley, Camilo Gutierrez, and Michele Carney.

Renal Emergencies in Infants and Children

Saranya Srinivasan

Renal emergencies in children represent a large and varied group of disease processes. This chapter focuses on common renal emergencies in children, including acute kidney injury (AKI), nephrotic syndrome, glomerulonephritis, and hemolytic-uremic syndrome.

ACUTE KIDNEY INJURY

Acute kidney injury (AKI), earlier called acute renal failure, is the abrupt loss of renal function resulting in the inability of the body to maintain fluid homeostasis. AKI in children is relatively sporadic and is most often caused by hypoxic injury (e.g., septic shock, dehydration) or nephrotoxins (e.g., antibiotics, contrast dye, NSAIDs).

Clinical Features

The clinical presentation of AKI depends on the underlying cause, such as bloody diarrhea and abdominal pain in hemolytic uremic syndrome or fever, hypotension, and petechiae in sepsis. Ultimately, patients will manifest stigmata of renal failure: nausea and anorexia due to uremia, headache due to hypertension, edema (periorbital, scrotal or labial, dependent, or generalized) resulting in weight gain, and decreased urine output.

Diagnosis and Differential

AKI may be anatomically categorized as prerenal, renal (intrinsic), or postrenal in etiology (Table 86-1). Elevated creatinine and urine output are used to diagnose AKI. Urinalysis (UA) with microscopy can help distinguish between prerenal and renal AKI. In prerenal AKI, the UA may be normal except for a high specific gravity (>1.025). For intrinsic causes

TABLE 86-1 Causes of Acute Kidney Injury in Infants and Children

Prerenal/ Inadequate Renal Perfusion	Renal/Intrinsic Renal Disease or Injury	Postrenal/ Obstruction
Dehydration from GI losses	Glomerular diseases (HSP, glomerulonephritis, nephrotic syndrome, pyelonephritis)	Nephrolithiasis
Blood loss from trauma	Vascular disease (HUS, vasculitides, thrombosis)	Renal vein thrombosis
Capillary leakage due to burns/sepsis, third spacing due to septic shock	Interstitial disease (interstitial nephritis, infections)	Pelvic mass (lymphoma, rhabdomyosarcoma)
Decreased cardiac output in congenital heart disease, myocarditis, cardiogenic shock	Tubular diseases (ischemia, nephrotoxins such as antibiotics, NSAIDs, contrast dye)	Urethral obstruction (posterior urethral valves, ureteropelvic junction obstruction)

such as acute tubular necrosis, hyaline casts may be seen on UA with a low to normal specific gravity. In glomerulonephritis, UA often shows hematuria, casts, and proteinuria while isolated proteinuria is more indicative of nephrotic syndrome. Basic blood tests such as serum electrolytes (including sodium and potassium), BUN and creatinine, and a complete blood count (CBC) should be obtained in all cases of AKI to help identify the cause and guide management. Hyperkalemia and other findings may require emergency interventions. Additional blood tests may be indicated in specific scenarios.

Emergency Department Care and Disposition

Treatment of AKI is based on the etiology. Goals of treatment include identifying the underlying cause and correcting fluid and electrolyte imbalances. Life-threatening complications such as severe hyperkalemia or hypertensive emergency should be addressed immediately. A pediatric nephrologist should be consulted for most cases of AKI as many cases require inpatient admission.

1. For *prerenal AKI*, resuscitate with crystalloid fluids, starting with **10 to 20 mL/kg of normal saline without added potassium**. For prerenal AKI due to hemorrhagic shock, give crystalloid fluids until blood products are available then transfuse packed red blood cells in aliquots of 10 mL/kg.
2. For AKI due to intrinsic renal injury or disease, treatment depends on the clinical state of the patient and the etiology of the AKI. For example, it may be necessary to **fluid restrict** despite oliguria in order to achieve overall fluid balance in hypervolemic patients. It is crucial to monitor the patient's weight and liquid intake and output. Consider discontinuing all nephrotoxic medications and treat hypertension with antihypertensive agents.
3. For postrenal AKI, insert a **Foley catheter** to relieve the obstruction. Antihypertensive agents and/or diuretics may also be necessary to control significant hypertension.

NEPHROTIC SYNDROME

Nephrotic syndrome is a chronic disease that affects glomerular capillary wall permeability causing urinary protein loss. The hallmarks of nephrotic syndrome are significant proteinuria, hypoalbuminemia, hyperlipidemia, and edema.

Clinical Features

Patients most commonly present with edema, which may involve the face, abdomen, scrotum or labia, or lower extremities. Because periorbital edema is nonspecific, patients are often misdiagnosed as having an allergic reaction. Patients may have foamy or bloody urine. Extreme hypoalbuminemia may cause pleural effusions, bowel wall edema, or ascites. Life-threatening complications of nephrotic syndrome include thromboembolic events (arterial and venous) and severe infections due to an immunocompromised state (due to loss of antibodies).

Diagnosis and Differential

Nephrotic syndrome is classified as primary (only affecting the kidney) or secondary (multisystem disease with renal involvement). Primary nephrotic syndromes include minimal change disease, focal segmental sclerosis, membranous nephropathy, membranoproliferative nephritis, and proliferative nephritis (which may be diffuse, focal, or mesangial). Secondary forms of nephrotic syndrome include lupus, Henoch–Schönlein purpura, sickle cell anemia, and drug or toxin exposure (e.g., heavy metals). TORCH infections may cause congenital nephrotic syndrome.

There are four diagnostic criteria for nephrotic syndrome: (1) hypoproteinemia with albumin level <3 g/dL, (2) urine protein to creatinine ratio >2 on first morning void or 24-hour urine protein >50 mg/kg, (3) hypercholesterolemia (>200 mg/dL), and (4) generalized edema. Further testing may be required to distinguish primary from secondary nephrotic syndrome. Renal biopsy is not indicated during initial episodes of acute nephrotic syndrome.

Emergency Department Care and Disposition

In the emergency department (ED), the goal is to treat the acute symptoms. Managing the fluid status of the nephrotic syndrome patient can be challenging since patients may be intravascularly depleted but show signs of fluid overload with significant edema. Treatment principles are as follows:

1. Treat hypovolemic shock with 20 mL/kg **normal saline**.
2. Treat mild to moderate dehydration with small, frequent amounts of a low-salt oral solution.
3. Treat volume overload and edema with **furosemide** 1 to 2 mg/kg/dose. If the serum albumin is extremely low, diuretics may be less effective, so **albumin** 0.5 to 1 g/kg should be administered followed by a dose of furosemide.
4. Definitive treatment of nephrotic syndrome often includes oral corticosteroids; however, steroid therapy should be initiated in conjunction with a pediatric nephrologist.

Many patients with nephrotic syndrome can safely be discharged home on a low-salt diet (< 2 g/d) with close follow-up with their PCP or nephrologist. Indications for admission include severe edema, thrombotic complications, or signs and symptoms of systemic infection.

ACUTE GLOMERULONEPHRITIS

Acute glomerulonephritis (GN) is the result of inflammation leading to glomerular injury and is characterized by hematuria and proteinuria. Glomerulonephritis may be immune-mediated, inherited, or post-infectious, and is classified as primary (isolated renal involvement) or secondary (resulting from a systemic disorder).

Clinical Features

Patients typically present with bloody, foamy (from proteinuria), or tea-colored urine along with oliguria, fatigue, or lethargy. Severe hypertension may result in headaches. In post-*streptococcal* GN, there may be a history of a sore throat, upper respiratory infection (URI), or skin infection preceding the onset of urinary symptoms by 1 to 2 weeks. In IgA nephropathy, children may report a concurrent URI or URI symptoms within the preceding week.

Diagnosis and Differential

Common causes of acute GN include post-infectious etiologies (post-streptococcal GN), Henoch–Schönlein purpura, systemic lupus erythematosus, and IgA nephropathy. Diagnosis of GN is made by examination of the urine. UA with microscopy demonstrates RBC casts, dysmorphic RBCs, and proteinuria. Other laboratory studies should include a CBC, electrolytes, BUN and creatinine, serum albumin, and urine culture. Serum complement levels are low in more than 90% of patients with post-streptococcal GN. Streptococcal serologic tests such as antistreptolysin-O and streptozyme may also be helpful.

Emergency Department Care and Disposition

The treatment of glomerulonephritis is determined by the underlying cause. Treatment of post-streptococcal GN is primarily supportive as symptoms usually resolve within a few weeks. Depending on the severity of disease, immunosuppressive agents may be used to treat inflammation and ACE inhibitors may be required to treat hypertension, particularly in patients with proteinuria. Nephrology consultation is indicated for patients with new-onset GN. Patients with mild disease may be discharged home on a fluid-restricted low-sodium diet with close follow-up.

HEMOLYTIC-UREMIC SYNDROME

Hemolytic-uremic syndrome (HUS) is characterized by acute renal failure, thrombocytopenia, and microangiopathic hemolytic anemia. Approximately 90% of cases are due to Shiga-toxin producing *Escherichia coli* O157:H7, found in unpasteurized milk, undercooked meats, and contaminated produce.

Clinical Features

The majority of patients with HUS present with nausea, vomiting, and bloody diarrhea. Within a week of symptom onset, oliguria, anemia, seizures, and encephalopathy may occur.

Diagnosis and Differential

Diagnosis of HUS is supported by labs. A CBC will demonstrate a hemoglobin level of 5 to 9 g/dL and platelets $<150{,}000/\text{mm}^3$. Peripheral smear shows schistocytes, helmet cells, and burr cells. A stool specimen to test for Shiga toxin and *E. coli* O157:H7 should also be sent.

Emergency Department Care and Disposition

Treatment of HUS in the ED is primarily supportive. Hypovolemia should be treated with 10 to 20 mL/kg boluses of normal saline while monitoring for fluid overload in oliguric patients. Platelet transfusions are not recommended as they increase thrombotic complications. **Antibiotics are contraindicated in pediatric diarrheal illnesses** as they may increase the risk of HUS. **Antiperistaltic agents (e.g., loperamide) are also contraindicated** as they increase the risk for systemic complications of *E. coli* infection. All patients with HUS require hospitalization and up to 70% will require dialysis.

FURTHER READING

For further reading in *Tintinalli's Emergency Medicine: A Comprehensive Study Guide*, 8th ed., see Chapter 134, "Renal Emergencies in Children," by Andrew Dixon and Brandy Stauffer.

SECTION 10

Infectious and Immunologic Diseases

CHAPTER 87

Sexually Transmitted Infections

Jennifer L. Hannum

This chapter covers some of the major sexually transmitted infections that are commonly found in the United States, with the exception of human immunodeficiency virus (HIV), which is discussed in Chapter 92. Vaginitis and pelvic inflammatory disease (PID) are covered separately in Chapters 63 and 64.

GENERAL RECOMMENDATIONS

Sexually transmitted infections are a major public health problem, and emergency medicine providers are commonly called upon to identify, treat, and recommend appropriate follow-up for these conditions. Complications from such infections may contribute to infertility, cancer, or urogenital complications. Due to issues with compliance and the challenge of obtaining consistent follow-up care in some communities, single-dose antibiotic treatment regimens are recommended, when possible. Several of these infections frequently occur together, and providers should consider additional screening for coexisting infections such as HIV, syphilis, and hepatitis. Test for pregnancy, advise treatment of all recent sexual partners, and counsel patients about the appropriate time frame for resuming sexual contact. Treatment regimens listed here are for adult patients who are not pregnant. Updated treatment recommendations are available on the Centers for Disease Control and Prevention (CDC) website (www.cdc.gov) and include specific guidelines for the treatment of children and pregnant patients. The most recent full publication with treatment guidelines for sexually transmitted infections was issued by the CDC in 2010 and is available at https://www.cdc.gov/std/treatment/2010/default.htm.

CHLAMYDIAL INFECTIONS

Clinical Features

Chlamydia trachomatis infections in men present with urethritis, epididymitis, orchitis, proctitis, or Reiter's syndrome (nongonococcal urethritis, conjunctivitis, and rash). Women often have asymptomatic cervicitis, but may also present with vaginal discharge, spotting, or dysuria. Consider chlamydial infection in patients with sterile pyuria. Complications can include PID, ectopic pregnancy, and infertility.

Diagnosis and Differential

Diagnosis of chlamydia is best made with indirect detection methods such as enzyme-linked immunosorbent assay or DNA probes, which have a sensitivity of 75% to 90%. The CDC recommends a nucleic acid amplification test (NAAT) to be used as screening tests for *Chlamydia*. Optimal specimen types for NAAT are vaginal swabs from women and first-catch urine from men.

Emergency Department Care and Disposition

1. **Azithromycin** 1 g PO as a single dose or **doxycycline** 100 mg PO twice daily for 7 days is the treatment of choice for uncomplicated urethritis or cervicitis from chlamydia infection.
2. Alternatives include 7-day treatment with **erythromycin base** 500 mg PO four times daily, **ofloxacin** 300 mg PO twice daily, or **levofloxacin** 500 mg PO daily.
3. Recommend that patients avoid sexual contact for 7 days after completing antibiotic treatment and symptoms have resolved.

GONOCOCCAL INFECTIONS

Clinical Features

Neisseria gonorrhoeae causes urethritis, epididymitis, orchitis, and prostatitis in men and urethritis, cervicitis, PID, and infertility in women. Many gonococcal infections in women are asymptomatic and may coexist with chlamydial infection. Women who are symptomatic may present with nonspecific lower abdominal pain and mucopurulent vaginal discharge with findings of cervicitis or PID. Men often present with dysuria and purulent penile discharge, but can also present with acute epididymitis, orchitis, or prostatitis. Disseminated gonococcemia may present with fever, rash (tender pustules on a red base, usually on the extremities, and may include palms and soles), tenosynovitis, or septic arthritis.

Diagnosis and Differential

The CDC recommends NAAT be performed on cervical, vaginal, urethral, or urine specimens. Culture and nucleic acid hybridization tests require endocervical or urethral swab specimens. Diagnosis of disseminated gonorrhea is challenging because cultures of blood, skin lesions, and joint fluid yield positive results in only 20% to 50% of patients. Culturing the cervix, rectum, and pharynx can be considered for patients suspected of disseminated disease to improve the diagnostic yield.

Emergency Department Care and Disposition

1. For uncomplicated gonorrhea, treat with dual therapy using **ceftriaxone** 250 mg IM AND **azithromycin** 1 g PO single dose or **doxycycline** 100 mg PO twice daily for 7 days.

2. Alternative treatment options include **cefixime** 400 mg PO single dose AND **azithromycin** 1 g PO single dose or **doxycycline** 100 mg PO twice daily for 7 days AND test-of-cure in 1 week.
3. Disseminated gonorrhea is treated initially with parenteral **ceftriaxone** 1 g daily IM/IV AND **azithromycin** 1 g PO single dose. Duration of parenteral therapy varies and should be determined in consultation with an infectious disease specialist.
4. Recommend that patients avoid sexual contact for 7 days after completing antibiotic treatment and symptoms have resolved.

TRICHOMONIASIS

Clinical Features

Patients with *Trichomonas vaginalis* parasite infections can remain asymptomatic or present with a range of symptoms up to severe inflammatory disease. In men this infection is often asymptomatic, but may present as urethritis. Symptoms in women may include vulvar irritation and a malodorous, thin watery discharge with associated burning, pruritus, dysuria, urinary frequency, dyspareunia, or lower abdominal pain.

Diagnosis and Differential

Microscopic visualization of the motile *Trichomonas vaginalis* parasites on a wet preparation of cervical smears or spun urine samples is diagnostic. Motility is only present for 10 to 20 minutes after collection thereby decreasing sensitivity. Culture is the most sensitive and specific test, but may take up to 7 days. DNA probes and monoclonal antibodies are used at some institutions.

Emergency Department Care and Disposition

1. **Metronidazole** 2 g PO, or **tinidazole** 2 g PO in a single dose is the treatment of choice.
2. An alternative treatment regimen is **metronidazole** 500 mg PO twice daily for 7 days.
3. **Metronidazole** (pregnancy category B) 2 g PO in a single dose is the drug of choice for treating symptomatic pregnant patients.
4. Patients should avoid intercourse for 1 week after the last dose of antibiotics.

SYPHILIS

Clinical Features

Treponema pallidum, a spirochete, causes the three stages of syphilis infections: primary, secondary, and tertiary stages. Primary syphilis is characterized by a chancre (Fig. 87-1), a single painless ulcer with indurated borders that develops on the penis, vulva, or other areas of sexual contact. The primary chancre heals and disappears after 3 to 6 weeks, and the secondary stage occurs after several additional weeks. Rash and lymphadenopathy are the most common symptoms of secondary syphilis. The rash consists of nonpruritic dull red or pink papules that begin on the trunk and flexor surfaces of the extremities and subsequently spread to the palms and soles. Constitutional

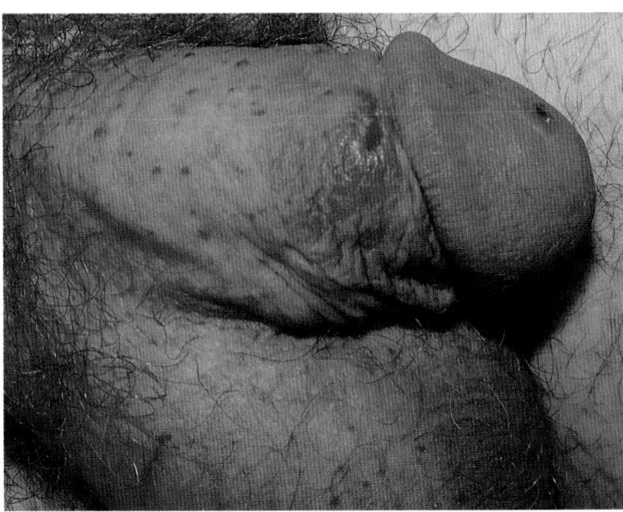

FIGURE 87-1. Syphilis chancre in a male. A painless ulcer caused by syphilis is seen on the distal penile shaft with a smaller erosion on the glans. The ulcer is quite firm on palpation. Reproduced with permission from Wolff K, Johnson RA: Fitzpatrick's Color Atlas and Synopsis of Clinical Dermatology, 7th ed. New York: McGraw-Hill Companies, Inc; 2013.

symptoms such as fever, malaise, headache, and sore throat are common before spontaneous resolution of this second stage. Tertiary or latent syphilis develops in about one-third of patients and can begin 3 to 20 years after the initial infection. Involvement of the nervous system (meningitis, dementia, tabes dorsalis), cardiovascular system (thoracic aneurysm), and widespread granulomatous lesions (gummata) are characteristic of tertiary syphilis.

Diagnosis and Differential

Treponema pallidum cannot be cultured in the laboratory and testing is a challenge because there is no single optimal diagnostic test. The sensitivity and specificity of tests for syphilis depend on the stage of the disease and type of test. Nontreponemal tests such as Venereal Disease Research Laboratory (VDRL) and rapid plasma regain (RPR) detect nonspecific antibodies that are indicative of infection but do not become detectable until 1 to 4 weeks after a chancre appears. Positive results for these screening tests must subsequently be confirmed with an immunoassay specific for *T. pallidum* antibodies. A presumptive diagnosis of syphilis is made if a positive result on a nontreponemal antibody test is supported by a positive confirmatory result on a treponemal antibody test. Direct visualization of organisms using darkfield microscopy is diagnostic for primary, secondary, or early congenital syphilis.

Emergency Department Care and Disposition

1. For primary and secondary syphilis, treat patients with **benzathine penicillin G** 2.4 million units IM as a single dose. Be aware of the

Jarisch–Herxheimer reaction (fever, headache, and myalgias) that may develop within the first 24 hours after treatment.

2. Alternative treatment options for primary, secondary, and early latent syphilis include **doxycycline** 100 mg PO twice daily for 14 days, or **tetracycline** 500 mg PO four times daily for 28 days.
3. Treat tertiary syphilis with **benzathine penicillin G** 2.4 million units IM weekly for 3 weeks.

HERPES SIMPLEX INFECTIONS

Clinical Features

Primary genital herpes simplex virus (HSV) infection often begins with a viral prodrome lasting 2 to 24 hours that is characterized by localized or regional pain, tingling, and burning. Constitutional symptoms such as headache, fever, painful inguinal lymphadenopathy, anorexia, or malaise often follow. Papules and vesicles on an erythematous base appear, with vesicular erosion that occurs over a few hours to several days. In men, painful HSV ulcers often appear on the shaft or glans of the penis (Fig. 87-2), while in

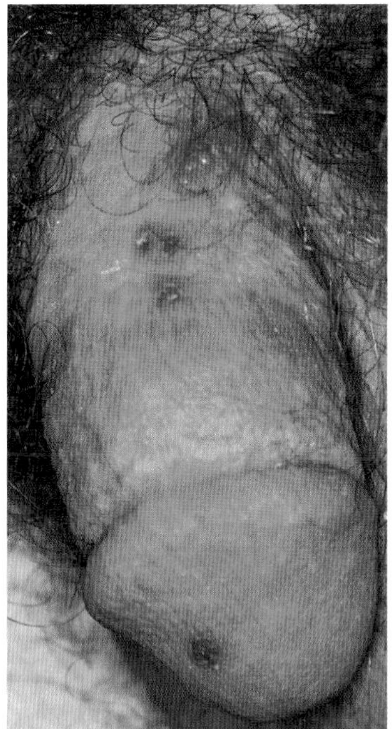

FIGURE 87-2. Genital herpes in a male. Classic vesicles are shown proximally on the penis; several formerly vesicular lesions have crusted over. Reproduced with permission from Goldsmith LA, Katz SI, Gilchrest BA, et al: Fitzpatrick's Dermatology in General Medicine, 8th ed. New York: McGraw-Hill Companies, Inc; 2012.

women, the painful ulcers occur on the introitus, urethral meatus, labia, and perineum. Viral shedding occurs for 10 to 12 days after the onset of the rash, and lesions heal completely within 3 weeks.

Diagnosis and Differential

HSV infection is diagnosed based on a characteristic history and associated physical findings. Viral cultures taken from vesicles or early ulcers are more reliable for confirmation than the classically described Tzanck smear to identify intranuclear inclusions.

Emergency Department Care and Disposition

1. Treat a patient's first episode of HSV with a 7- to 10-day course of **acyclovir** 400 mg PO three times daily, **valacyclovir** 1 g PO twice daily, or **famciclovir** 250 mg PO three times daily. Treatment hastens recovery but does not cure the infection.
2. For proctitis or oral infections, treat with **acyclovir** 400 mg five times daily for 7 to 10 days.
3. Patients with severe disease that require hospitalization should be treated with intravenous **acyclovir** 5 to 10 mg/kg body weight every 8 hours.
4. Recurrent episodes of genital herpes can be treated with a 5-day course of **valacyclovir** 1 g PO daily or **acyclovir** 400 mg PO three times daily. Antiviral therapy may reduce the severity and duration of recurrent episodes of HSV when initiated when symptoms begin.

CHANCROID

Clinical Features

Caused by *Haemophilus ducreyi*, chancroid presents as a painful erythematous papule at the site of infection. This lesion erodes and becomes ulcerated and pustular over the next 2 days (Fig. 87-3). Up to 50% of patients have more than one lesion, with "kissing lesions" occurring from autoinoculation of adjacent areas of skin. Painful lymphadenopathy develops 1 to 2 weeks after primary infection, and if treatment is not initiated these lymph nodes become necrotic and infected buboes.

Diagnosis and Differential

Chancroid is typically diagnosed clinically, with care to consider the diagnoses of syphilis and HSV. Sometimes the organism may be cultured from a swab of an ulcer or bubo, but a special culture medium is required that is not found in many laboratories.

Emergency Department Care and Disposition

1. Treatment regimens include **azithromycin** 1 g PO as a single dose, **ceftriaxone** 250 mg IM as a single dose, **erythromycin base** 500 mg PO three times daily for 7 days, or **ciprofloxacin** 500 mg PO twice daily for 3 days. Symptoms often improve within 3 days, but larger ulcers may require 2 to 3 weeks to heal.
2. Incision and drainage of buboes can be considered for symptomatic relief.

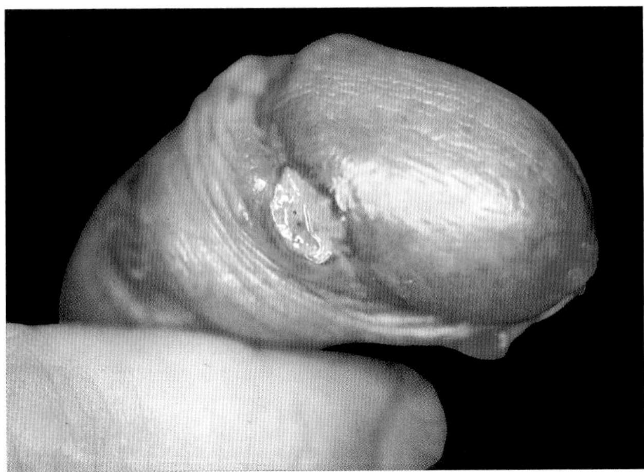

FIGURE 87-3. Chancroid ulcer in a male. The lesion is very painful. The friable base of the ulcer is covered with yellow-gray necrotic exudates. Reproduced with permission from Goldsmith LA, Katz SI, Gilchrest BA, et al: Fitzpatrick's Dermatology in General Medicine, 8th ed. New York: McGraw-Hill Companies, Inc; 2012.

3. Test patients for other sexually transmitted infections such as HSV, syphilis, and HIV.
4. Recommend treatment for all sexual partners in the 10 days prior to diagnosis regardless of whether they have developed symptoms.

FURTHER READING

For further reading in Tintinalli's Emergency Medicine: A Comprehensive Study Guide, 8th ed., see Chapter 149, "Sexually Transmitted Infections," by Flavia Nobay and Susan B. Promes.

CHAPTER 88

Toxic Shock Syndromes

Sorabh Khandelwal

STAPHYLOCOCCAL TOXIC SHOCK SYNDROME

Staphylococcal toxic shock syndrome (TSS) is a severe, life-threatening infection attributed to *Staphylococcus aureus* that can progress rapidly to multisystem dysfunction, severe electrolyte disturbances, renal failure, and shock. Risk factors for TSS include retained foreign bodies (e.g., tampons, female barrier contraceptives), skin and soft tissue infections (e.g., abscess, cellulitis, and mastitis), varicella infection, sinusitis, surgery, trauma, childbirth, and influenza.

Clinical Features

TSS is characterized by high fever, profound hypotension, diffuse macular rash, desquamation (1 to 2 weeks after onset of rash), and multiorgan dysfunction. The details regarding the diagnostic criteria for TSS are listed in Table 88-1. Patients presenting early in the course may exhibit nonspecific symptoms such as fever, chills, malaise, myalgias, headache, sore throat,

TABLE 88-1 Case Definition for Toxic Shock Syndrome

Clinical criteria:

- Fever: temperature ≥ 38.9°C or 102.0°F
- Rash: diffuse macular erythroderma
- Desquamation: 1–2 weeks after onset of rash
- Hypotension: systolic blood pressure ≤ 90 mm Hg (adult) or < 5th percentile by age (children < 16 years of age)
- Multiorgan involvement (≥ 3 organ systems):
  - Gastrointestinal: vomiting and/or diarrhea at onset of illness
  - Muscular: severe myalgia or CPK ≥ 2 times the upper limit of normal
  - Mucous membrane: vaginal, oropharyngeal, or conjunctival hyperemia
  - Renal: BUN or serum Cr ≥ 2 times the upper limit of normal for laboratory or urinary sediment with pyuria (≥ 5 leukocytes per high-power field) in the absence of urinary tract infection
  - Hepatic: total bilirubin, ALT, or AST ≥ 2 times the upper limit of normal
  - Hematologic: platelet count < 100,000/mm^3
  - Central nervous system: disorientation or alterations in consciousness without focal neurologic signs when fever and hypotension are absent

Laboratory criteria: *Negative* results on the following tests, if obtained:

- Blood or cerebrospinal fluid cultures (blood culture may be positive for *Staphylococcus aureus)*
- Serologies for Rocky Mountain spotted fever, leptospirosis, or measles

Case classification:

- Probable: ≥ 4 clinical criteria + laboratory criteria met
- Confirmed: 5 clinical criteria + laboratory criteria met, including desquamation (unless death occurs prior to desquamation)

Abbreviations: ALT, alanine aminotransferase; AST, aspartate aminotransferase; CPK, creatine phosphokinase; Cr, creatinine.

vomiting, diarrhea, or abdominal pain. The rash associated with TSS is described as a "painless sunburn" that typically fades within 3 days and is followed by full-thickness desquamation.

Diagnosis and Differential

TSS is a clinical diagnosis characterized by an acute febrile illness associated with erythroderma, hypotension, and multiorgan involvement. Laboratory evaluation reveals evidence of end-organ damage, and testing often includes CBC, comprehensive metabolic panel, coagulation studies, creatine phosphokinase level, urinalysis, chest radiograph, ECG, blood gas, and cultures of blood and other potential sites of infection. Other infections to consider in the differential diagnosis of TSS include streptococcal toxic shock syndrome (STSS), myonecrosis due to *Clostridium perfringens*, TSS due to *Clostridium sordellii*, staphylococcal scalded skin syndrome, sepsis due to other bacterial organisms, Rocky Mountain spotted fever, leptospirosis, and meningococcemia. Noninfectious illnesses such as Stevens–Johnson syndrome, toxic epidermal necrolysis, and Kawasaki's disease may also be considered in the proper clinical circumstances.

Emergency Department Care and Disposition

TSS is mediated by pyrogenic exotoxins released by certain strains of *S. aureus*, and initial management includes aggressive resuscitation to treat shock and begin treating potential sources of infection. Abscesses should be drained, foreign bodies should be removed, surgical consultation should be considered for debridement of infected tissue, and appropriate broad-spectrum antibiotics are recommended.

1. Resuscitate patients with hypotension and shock using aggressive IV crystalloid intravenous fluids such as normal saline. Use vasopressors to treat persistent hypotension.
2. Treat TSS with suspected methicillin-resistant *Staphylococcus aureus* (MRSA) with **vancomycin** 15 mg/kg IV every 12 hours (maximum dose 2.25 g) or **linezolid** 600 mg IV *plus* **clindamycin** 900 mg IV every 8 hours.
3. Patients with suspected methicillin-sensitive *Staphylococcus aureus* (MSSA) can be treated with **nafcillin** or **oxacillin** 2 g IV every 4 hours, *plus* **clindamycin** 900 mg IV every 8 hours.
4. Consider **IV immunoglobulin** therapy after consultation with infectious disease or critical caire specialists when no clinical improvement is seen after 6 hours of aggressive treatment.

STREPTOCOCCAL TOXIC SHOCK SYNDROME

STSS is a clinical illness characterized by shock and multiorgan failure as a result of invasive infection due to group A *Streptococcus* (*Streptococcus pyogenes*) and other streptococcal pathogens. Risk factors for STSS include the presence of underlying medical conditions such as chronic heart, liver, and kidney disease, diabetes, alcoholism, drug abuse, surgical procedures, traumatic injuries, childbirth, varicella infection, and influenza.

Clinical Features

Similar to TSS, fulminant STSS is often preceded by nonspecific symptoms such as fever, chills, sweats, malaise, arthralgias, cough, sore throat, rhinorrhea, anorexia, nausea, vomiting, abdominal pain, or diarrhea. A rash is seen in a minority of cases. Pain at a localized site, often an extremity or abdomen, that is out of proportion to physical findings is a common presentation of STSS due to the strong association of STSS and necrotizing soft tissue infections. Diagnostic criteria for fulminant STSS are listed in Table 88-2.

Diagnosis and Differential

STSS is a clinical diagnosis characterized by an acute febrile illness associated with hypotension and multiorgan involvement in the setting of a streptococcal infection. Laboratory evaluation is similar to TSS (see above) and findings identify evidence of end-organ damage. The differential diagnosis includes many of the same disease processes as TSS (see above).

Emergency Department Care and Disposition

1. Treat suspected STSS patients with aggressive isotonic fluid resuscitation to restore volume and tissue perfusion. Large volumes of IV crystalloid fluid (10 to 20 L/day) may be required. Use vasopressors or inotropic agents for persistent hypotension.

TABLE 88-2 Case Definition for Streptococcal Toxic Shock Syndrome

Clinical criteria:
- Hypotension: systolic blood pressure ≤90 mm Hg (adult) or < 5th percentile by age (children < 16 years of age)
- Multiorgan involvement (≥ 2 organ systems):
  - Renal: serum Cr ≥ 2 mg/dL (≥ 177 μmol/L) for adults or ≥ 2 times the upper limit of normal for age. In patients with preexisting renal disease, > 2-fold elevation above baseline.
  - Coagulopathy: platelet count ≤ 100,000/mm^3 (≤ 100 × 10^6/L) or disseminated intravascular coagulation, defined by prolonged clotting times, low fibrinogen level, and presence of fibrin degradation products
  - Hepatic: total bilirubin, ALT, or AST ≥ 2 times the upper limit of normal for the patient's age. In patients with preexisting liver disease, > 2-fold elevation above baseline.
  - Acute respiratory distress syndrome: acute onset of diffuse pulmonary infiltrates and hypoxemia in the absence of cardiac failure or by evidence of diffuse capillary leak manifested by acute onset of generalized edema, or pleural or peritoneal effusions with hypoalbuminemia.
  - Skin: generalized erythematous macular rash that may desquamate
  - Soft tissue necrosis, including necrotizing fasciitis or myositis, or gangrene

Laboratory criteria:
- Isolation of group A *Streptococcus*

Case classification:
- Probable: All clinical criteria met + absence of other identified etiology for illness + isolation of group A *Streptococcus* from a nonsterile site
- Confirmed: All clinical criteria met + isolation of group A *Streptococcus* from a sterile site (e.g., blood, cerebrospinal fluid, synovial fluid, pleural fluid, or pericardial fluid)

Abbreviations: ALT, alanine aminotransferase; AST, aspartate aminotransferase; Cr, creatinine.

2. Assess the possible need for airway management, as more than half of patients with STSS will develop ARDS and require intubation and mechanical ventilation.
3. Obtain blood and wound cultures prior to giving antibiotics when possible, as the majority of patients will have positive blood cultures to confirm a streptococcal pathogen.
4. Broad-spectrum antimicrobial therapy is recommended. Treat suspected STSS with **piperacillin-tazobactam** 4.5 g IV *or* **meropenem 1** g IV *plus* IV **clindamycin** 900 mg. Add **vancomycin** 15 mg/kg IV (maximum dose 2.25 g) when MRSA infection is suspected.
5. Administration of IV immunoglobulin remains controversial and consultation should be obtained prior to initiating this therapy.
6. Initiate an emergent surgical consultation for patients with a suspected necrotizing soft tissue infection. Patients with STSS may require debridement, fasciotomy, or amputation as the disease progresses.

FURTHER READING

For further reading in *Tintinalli's Emergency Medicine: A Comprehensive Study Guide*, 8th ed., see Chapter 150, "Toxic Shock Syndromes," by Stephen Y. Liang

CHAPTER 89

Sepsis

John E. Gough

Sepsis is generally defined as a suspected or confirmed infection with evidence of systemic inflammation. Severe sepsis is sepsis with evidence of new organ dysfunction thought to be secondary to tissue hypoperfusion. Septic shock is present when cardiovascular failure occurs, reflected by persistent hypotension or the need for vasopressors despite adequate fluid resuscitation. The majority of sepsis cases are caused by gram-negative and gram-positive bacteria; however, sepsis is a heterogeneous clinical syndrome that can be caused by any class of microorganism including fungi, mycobacteria, viruses, rickettsiae, and protozoa. The most likely microorganisms that cause sepsis varies based on possible patient exposure to drug-resistant microorganisms (e.g., due to recent hospitalization or other health care–associated exposure) and the specific anatomic site of suspected infection. Pneumonia, intraabdominal infection, urinary tract infection, and skin or soft tissue infections are the most common infections that precipitate sepsis.

CLINICAL FEATURES

The presence of sepsis may be apparent on the initial presentation of a critically ill patient. In some cases, however, sepsis can be challenging to identify early in a patient's evaluation. Abnormal vital signs such as hyperthermia or hypothermia, tachycardia, hypotension, and tachypnea may suggest sepsis as a diagnostic possibility in the right clinical circumstances. In particular, up to 40% of patients who present with undifferentiated hypotension are later diagnosed with septic shock when a source of infection is identified through diagnostic testing.

Traditionally sepsis has been categorized as a type of distributive shock associated with peripheral vasodilation, warm extremities, and a compensatory increase in cardiac output. However, this does not accurately reflect the presentation of all patients with sepsis. The combination of intravascular volume depletion and septic cardiomyopathy may also manifest as "cold shock," with impaired peripheral perfusion and cool extremities.

Many different abnormalities are possible with severe sepsis, reflecting different areas of end-organ damage. Severe sepsis is the leading cause of acute lung injury and acute respiratory distress syndrome (ARDS). Widespread inflammation secondary to sepsis commonly affects pulmonary function even in the absence of pneumonia. Refractory hypoxemia, decreased lung compliance, and a chest x-ray demonstrating bilateral pulmonary alveolar infiltrates are commonly found with ARDS. Renal manifestations of severe sepsis include acute renal failure with azotemia, oliguria, and anuria. The most frequent hepatic abnormality is cholestatic jaundice and is associated with elevation in transaminases, alkaline phosphatase, and/or bilirubin. The most frequent hematologic changes associated with sepsis are neutropenia or neutrophilia, thrombocytopenia, and disseminated intravascular coagulation (DIC). Hyperglycemia may develop, and uncontrolled hyperglycemia is a significant risk for adverse outcome. Cutaneous lesions that occur as a result of sepsis can be divided into five categories: direct bacterial involvement of the skin and underlying soft tissues (cellulitis, erysipelas, and fasciitis); lesions from hematogenous seeding of the skin or the underlying tissue (petechiae, pustules, cellulitis, ecthyma gangrenosum); lesions resulting from hypotension and/or DIC (acrocyanosis and necrosis of peripheral tissues); lesions secondary to intravascular infections (microemboli and/or immune complex vasculitis); and lesions caused by toxins (toxic shock syndrome).

DIAGNOSIS AND DIFFERENTIAL

Consider the possibility of sepsis in patients who present with criteria for systemic inflammatory response syndrome (SIRS), as detailed in Table 89-1. Severe sepsis involves these criteria plus evidence of organ dysfunction such as hypotension, elevated serum lactate level, renal dysfunction, hypoxia, hyperbilirubinemia, thrombocytopenia, or coagulopathy. Septic shock involves refractory hypotension, and does not typically reverse with rapid volume replacement of at least 1.5 to 3.0 L of isotonic crystalloid (or 20 to 30 mL/kg in children). History and physical examination findings combined with initial laboratory and radiolographic investigations often identify a presumptive infection source for sepsis, which can guide empiric therapy. Focus particular attention to signs and symptoms of potential infections in the central nervous system, pulmonary system, intraabdominal structures, urinary tract, skin, and soft tissues.

Initial laboratory studies for patients with suspected sepsis often include a CBC with differential and platelet count, lactic acid level, serum electrolytes, liver function panel, renal function panel, arterial blood gas analysis, blood cultures, urinalysis, and urine culture. Consider type and cross-matching blood for patients with acute anemia or refractory hypotension who may need emergent transfusion. A chest x-ray can assess for pneumonia as a potential source of infection. Additional radiographs, CT scans, ultrasound, or lumbar puncture may be utilized in specific patients based on clinical suspicion for potential infectious sources. Other laboratory tests for markers of sepsis may be considered, such as C-reactive protein and procalcitonin.

EMERGENCY DEPARTMENT CARE AND DISPOSITION

Studies have shown that the cornerstones of the initial treatment and stabilization of severe sepsis are early recognition, early reversal of hemodynamic compromise, and early empiric antibiotics for infection control. The goals of resuscitation are to improve preload, tissue perfusion, and oxygen delivery.

1. For patients with hypoxia or respiratory distress, provide supplemental oxygen to keep oxygen saturation greater than 90%, and perform endotracheal intubation if necessary.
2. Initiate IV fluid resuscitation with an initial bolus of crystalloid IV fluid at 20 to 30 mL/kg.
3. Begin vasopressors for patients in septic shock with hypotension that does not respond to aggressive IV fluid bolus therapy. A central venous

TABLE 89-1 Definition of Sepsis in Adults and Children

- **Systemic Inflammatory Response Syndrome (SIRS) criteria:**
  1. Fever (temperature >38.3°C) or hypothermia (temperature <36°C)
  2. Pulse rate (>90 beats/min or >2 SDs above the normal value for age)
  3. Tachypnea (respiratory rate >20 breaths/min)
  4. Leukocytosis (WBC >12,000 cells/μL) *or* leukopenia (WBC <4000 cells/μL), *or* normal WBC with >10% immature forms
- *Sepsis: Infection (documented or suspected), and some of the following:*
- *General Parameters:* Fever (temperature >38.3°C)
- Hypothermia (temperature <36°C)
- Pulse rate (>90 beats/min or >2 SDs above the normal value for age)
- Tachypnea
- Altered mental status
- Significant edema or positive fluid balance (>20 mL/kg during 24 h)
- Hyperglycemia (plasma glucose >140 mg/dL or 7.7 mmol/L) in the absence of diabetes
- **Inflammatory Parameters:**
- Leukocytosis (WBC >12,000 cells/μL)
- Leukopenia (WBC <4000 cells/μL)
- Normal WBC with >10% immature forms
- Plasma C-reactive protein (CRP) >2 SDs above the normal value
- Plasma procalcitonin >2 SDs above the normal value
- **Hemodynamic Parameters:**
- Arterial hypotension (SBP <90 mm Hg, MAP <70 mm Hg, or an SBP decrease >40 mm Hg in adults or <2 SDs below normal for age)
- **Organ Dysfunction Parameters:**
- Arterial hypoxemia (PaO2/FIO2 <300)
- Acute oliguria (urine output <0.5 mL/kg per hour for at least 2 h despite adequate fluid resuscitation)
- Creatinine level increase >0.5 mg/dL
- Coagulation abnormalities (INR >1.5 or aPTT >60 s)
- Ileus (absent bowel sounds)
- Thrombocytopenia (platelet count <100,000 cells/μL)
- Hyperbilirubinemia (plasma total bilirubin >4 mg/dL)
- **Tissue Perfusion Parameters:**
- Hyperlactatemia (above upper limits of laboratory normal levels)
- Decreased capillary refill or mottling
- *Severe Sepsis: Sepsis-induced tissue hypoperfusion or organ dysfunction (any of the following thought to be due to infection)*
- Sepsis-induced hypotension
- Lactate level above upper limits of laboratory normal levels
- Urine output <0.5 mL/kg/h for at least 2 h despite adequate fluid resuscitation
- Acute lung injury with PaO2/FIO2 <250 in the absence of pneumonia as infectious source
- Acute lung injury with PaO2/FIO2 <200 in the absence of pneumonia as infectious source
- Creatinine level >2.0 mg/dL
- Bilirubin level >2 mg/dL
- Platelet count <100,000 cells/μL
- Coagulopathy (INR >1.5)

Abbreviations: aPTT, activated partial thromboplastin time; FIO2, fraction of inspired oxygen; INR, international normalized ratio; MAP, mean arterial pressure; PaO2, arterial partial pressure of oxygen; SBP, systolic blood pressure; SD, standard deviation.

Source: Adapted with permission from Levy M M, Fink MP, Marshall J C, et al: 2001 SCCM/ESICM /ACCP/ATS/SIS International Sepsis Definitions Conference. *Crit Care Med.* April 2003; 31(4): 1250–1256.

line is preferred but large peripheral lines may be used temporarily to begin treatment. Start **norepinephrine** 0.5 to 30 μg/min with a goal mean arterial pressure of 65 mm Hg. Consider **vasopressin** 0.03 or 0.04 U/min as a second-line agent.

4. Consider repeating a serum lactate level after 1 to 2 hours as one way to assess restoration of adequate tissue oxygen perfusion.
5. Initiate appropriate broad-spectrum antibiotics based on the initial suspected source of sepsis (see Table 89-2). Empiric antibiotic therapy is

TABLE 89-2 Empiric Antibiotic Selection in Severe Sepsis and Septic Shock

Host	Likely Pathogens	Initial Antibiotic Selection
Adults (nonneutropenic) without an obvious source of infection	*Staphylococcus aureus*, streptococci, gram-negative bacilli, others	Imipenem, 500 mg every 6 h to 1 g IV every 8 h *or* Meropenem, 1 g IV every 8 h *or* Doripenem, 500 mg IV every 8 h *or* Ertapenem*, 1 g IV every 24 h *plus* Vancomycin†, 15 mg/kg loading dose
Adults (nonneutropenic), suspected biliary source	Aerobic gram-negative bacilli, enterococci	Ampicillin/sulbactam, 3 g IV every 6 h *or* Piperacillin/tazobactam, 4.5 g IV every 6 h *or* Ticarcillin/clavulanate, 3.1 g IV every 4 h
Adults (nonneutropenic), suspected pneumonia	*Streptococcus pneumoniae*, methicillin-resistant *S. aureus*, gram-negative bacilli, *Legionella*	Ceftriaxone, 1–2 g IV every 12 h *plus* Azithromycin, 500 mg IV, then 250 mg IV every 24 h *plus* Levofloxacin, 750 mg IV every 24 h *or* moxifloxacin, 400 mg IV every 24 h *plus* Vancomycin†, 15 mg/kg loading dose
Adults (nonneutropenic), suspected illicit use of IV drugs	*S. aureus*	Vancomycin†, 15 mg/kg loading dose
Adults with petechial rash	*Neisseria meningitidis*, RMSF	Ceftriaxone, 2 g IV every 12 h *or* Cefotaxime, 2 g IV every 4-6 h *Consider* Addition of doxycycline 100 mg IV every 12 h for possible RMSF

(*continued*)

TABLE 89-2 Empiric Antibiotic Selection in Severe Sepsis and Septic Shock (continued)

Host	Likely Pathogens	Initial Antibiotic Selection
Adults (nonneutropenic), suspected intraabdominal source	Mixture of aerobic and anaerobic gram-negative bacilli	Imipenem, 500 mg IV every 6 h to 1 g IV every 8 h *or* Meropenem, 1 g IV every 8 h *or* Doripenem, 500 mg IV every 8 h *or* Ertapenem, 1 g IV every 24 h *or* Ampicillin/sulbactam, 3 g IV every 6 h *or* Piperacillin/tazobactam, 4.5 g IV every 6 h
Adults (nonneutropenic), suspected urinary source (hospitalized with pyelonephritis)	Aerobic gram-negative bacilli, enterococci	Levofloxacin, 750 mg IV every 24 h *or* Moxifloxacin, 400 mg IV every 24 h *or* Piperacillin/tazobactam, 4.5 g IV every 6 h *or* Ceftriaxone, 1–2 g IV every 12–24 h *or* Ampicillin, 1–2 g IV every 4–6 h *plus* gentamicin, 1.0–1.5 mg/kg every 8 h[‡]
Adults (nonneutropenic), suspected urinary source (complicated urinary tract infection/urinary catheter)	Enterobacteriaceae, *Pseudomonas aeruginosa*, entero-cocci, rarely *S. aureus*	Piperacillin/tazobactam, 4.5 g IV every 6 h *or* Imipenem, 500 mg every 6 h to 1 g IV every 8 h *or* Meropenem, 1 g IV every 8 h *or* Doripenem, 500 mg IV every 8 h *or* Ampicillin, 1–2 g IV every 4–6 h *plus* gentamicin, 1.0–1.5 mg/kg every 8 h[‡]
Neutropenic adults	Aerobic gram-negative bacilli, especially *P. aeruginosa, S. aureus*	Ceftazidime, 2 g IV every 8 h *or* Cefepime, 2 g IV every 8 h *or* Imipenem, 500 mg IV every 6 h to 1 g IV every 8 h *or* Meropenem, 1 g IV every 8 h

(*continued*)

TABLE 89-2 Empiric Antibiotic Selection in Severe Sepsis and Septic Shock (continued)

Host	Likely Pathogens	Initial Antibiotic Selection
		or Piperacillin/tazobactam, 4.5 g IV every 6 h *plus* Levofloxacin, 750 mg IV every 24 h *or* moxifloxacin, 400 mg IV every 24 h *plus* Vancomycin†, 15 mg/kg loading dose *and consider* Fluconazole, 400 mg IV every 24 h *or* micafungin, 100 mg every 24 h
Patients with suspected anaerobic source: intraabdominal, biliary, female genital tract infection; necrotizing cellulitis; odontogenic infection; or anaerobic soft tissue infection	Anaerobic bacteria plus gram-negative bacilli	Metronidazole, 15 mg/kg IV load then 7.5 mg/kg every 8 h# *or* Clindamycin, 600–900 mg IV every 8 h
Patients with indwelling vascular devices	Coagulase-negative *Staphylococcus*, methicillin-resistant *S. aureus*	Vancomycin†, 15 mg/kg loading dose
Patients with potential for *Legionella* species infection		Azithromycin, 500 mg IV then 250 mg IV every 24 h *or* Erythromycin, 800 mg IV every 6 h *should be added to the regimen*
Asplenic patients	*S. pneumoniae, N. meningitidis, Haemophilus influenzae, Capnocytophaga*	Ceftriaxone, 1 g IV every 24 h up to 2 g IV every 12 h if meningitis

Abbreviation: RMSF, Rocky Mountain spotted fever.

*Ertapenem has no antipseudomonal coverage and is not recommended in many intensive care units due to concerns of potentiating pseudomonal antimicrobial resistance.

†In most communities in the United States, methicillin-resistant *S. aureus* colonization is extremely high, and consideration should be given to including vancomycin in addition to the antibiotic recommendations given in the table. Although initial vancomycin dosage is typically suggested at 15 mg/kg, this results in delayed time to effective antimicrobial activity, and initial dosages of 25 to 30 mg/kg have been recommended by some authorities. If the patient has an allergy to vancomycin, linezolid 600 mg IV can be substituted.

‡Multiple daily dosing: 2 mg/kg load then 1.7 mg/kg every 8 hours.

#Metronidazole is often prepackaged as 500-mg bags. Dosing at 500 mg IV every 6 or 8 hours to approximate the mg/kg dosing may speed time to antibiotic administration by decreasing pharmacy mixing time.

ideally begun after obtaining cultures, but administration should not be delayed if cultures are difficult to obtain.

6. Remove suspected sources of infection by assessing any indwelling catheters that could be removed and performing incision and drainage of any identified abscesses.

FURTHER READING

For further reading in *Tintinalli's Emergency Medicine: A Comprehensive Study Guide*, 8th ed., see Chapter 151, "Sepsis," by Michael A. Puskarich and Alan E. Jones

Soft Tissue Infections

Jon Femling

Skin and soft tissue infections are common, and their successful evaluation and management involve an understanding of disease severity. Infection and patient characteristics help guide appropriate antibiotic treatment, outpatient or inpatient options, and potential surgical therapy.

METHICILLIN-RESISTANT *STAPHYLOCOCCUS AUREUS*

Community-acquired methicillin-resistant *Staphylococcus aureus* (MRSA) is a common cause of soft tissue infections in adults and children. Understanding treatment guidelines for community-acquired MRSA is important for managing soft tissue infections in the ED.

Clinical Features

Community-acquired MRSA causes skin lesions that are typically warm, red, tender, and commonly associated with soft tissue abscesses that may be spontaneously draining. MRSA lesions are frequently mistaken as spider bites.

Diagnosis and Differential

The diagnosis of MRSA is typically made based on clinical features. Consider the likelihood of community-acquired MRSA for soft tissue infection where *S. aureus* or *Streptococcus* are typically considered common etiologic pathogens. This includes skin and soft tissue infections as well as sepsis and pneumonia. Bedside ultrasound may be helpful to identify abscess collections in cases where physical examination is equivocal.

Emergency Department Care and Disposition

1. For many community-acquired MRSA cutaneous infections where abscesses have developed, local incision and drainage is sufficient treatment to successfully manage these infections. Most patients with normal immune system function will not require additional treatment with antibiotics for small abscesses without accompanying cellulitis or systemic signs of severe illness when the lesions can be successfully incised and drained.
2. For patients with immunocompromise, systemic illness, surrounding cellulitis, or other characteristics prompting antibiotic treatment, consider antibiotics effective against MRSA when appropriate. Options include **clindamycin** 300 mg PO four times daily or **trimethoprim/sulfamethoxazole** double strength two tablets twice a day for 7 to 10 days. Consider adding **cephalexin** 500 mg four times daily to cover *Streptococcus* when using trimethoprim/sulfamethoxazole. For severe infections, **vancomycin** 1 g IV every 12 hours is recommended along with inpatient admission.

3. Patients at the extremes of age, or those who have systemic signs of severe illness, significant comorbidities, or large complicated lesions may benefit from an admission for parenteral antibiotics and surgical consultation when indicated.

NECROTIZING SOFT TISSUE INFECTIONS

Necrotizing soft tissue infections are aggressive and potentially life threatening infections. These infections can present with an insidious onset and early findings may appear deceptively benign. Necrotizing soft tissue infections represent a spectrum of conditions that may be polymicrobial or monomicrobial. Group A *Streptococcus* and *S. aureus* are often the etiologic agents in monomicrobial infections. Clostridial infections are now uncommon secondary to improved hygiene and sanitation.

Clinical Features

Patients present with pain out of proportion to physical findings and a sense of heaviness in the affected part. Physical findings may include a combination of edema, brownish skin discoloration, bullae, malodorous serosanguineous discharge, and crepitus. Patients may have low-grade fever and associated tachycardia out of proportion to the fever. Mental status changes, including delirium and irritability, may accompany necrotizing soft tissue infections and are signs of systemic toxicity.

Diagnosis and Differential

Familiarity with the disease and an appreciation for subtle physical findings early in its development are important factors in making the diagnosis of necrotizing soft tissue infections. Additional findings that may supplement clinical suspicion include gas within soft tissue on plain radiographs, metabolic acidosis, coagulopathy, hyponatremia, leukocytosis, anemia, thrombocytopenia, myoglobinuria, and renal or hepatic dysfunction.

Emergency Department Care and Disposition

1. When necrotizing infections are suspected, IV antibiotics should be administered as soon as possible including **vancomycin** 1 g IV every 12 hours *plus* **meropenem** 500 to 1000 mg IV every 8 hours. Alternatively **piperacillin/tazobactam** 4.5 g IV every 6 hours may be used. **Clindamycin** inhibits toxin synthesis and may also be considered in the treatment regimen.
2. Patients with necrotizing soft tissue infections often need aggressive resuscitation with crystalloid IV fluids. Consider blood transfusion with packed red blood cells if significant anemia from hemolysis occurs.
3. Patients with necrotizing soft tissue infections can rapidly develop septic shock. Patients with hypotension who also have compromised perfusion in an affected extremity can present management challenges when vasoconstrictor use is considered.
4. Tetanus prophylaxis should be administered as indicated (see Chapter 94).
5. Obtain surgical consultation as soon as possible when necrotizing infections are suspected. Patients may require debridement, fasciotomy, or even amputation. Potential roles for hyperbaric oxygen therapy or IV

immunoglobulin remain controversial and may be considered in consultation with surgical colleagues.

CELLULITIS

Cellulitis is a subset of soft tissue infections characterized by a local soft tissue inflammatory response caused by bacterial invasion of the skin. This infection is more common in the elderly, immunocompromised patients, and patients with peripheral vascular disease.

Clinical Features

Cellulitis presents as localized tenderness, erythema, and induration of the skin. Lymphangitis and lymphadenitis can accompany cellulitis and may indicate a more severe infection. Patients may present with associated fever and chills.

Diagnosis and Differential

History and physical examination are often sufficient to make the clinical diagnosis of cellulitis. Obtaining a white cell count or blood cultures rarely changes management of otherwise healthy patients with uncomplicated cellulitis. Cellulitis of the lower extremity may sometimes mimic or be complicated by deep venous thrombosis, and clinical uncertainty may prompt additional studies to evaluate for this possibility. In patients with signs of systemic toxicity, consider additional evaluation for an occult abscess using bedside ultrasound and/or cultures of blood and other suspected areas of infection.

Emergency Department Care and Disposition

1. Consider outpatient treatment of patients with uncomplicated cellulitis in which MRSA is not suspected using **cephalexin** 500 mg PO four times daily, **dicloxacillin** 500 mg PO four times daily, or **clindamycin** 300 PO mg four times daily.
2. When local epidemiology supports a high likelihood of MRSA, treat with antibiotics effective against MRSA (see section "Methicillin-Resistant *Staphylococcus aureus*" above).
3. Recommend follow-up within a few days to evaluate the cellulitis and response to therapy. Skin markers may be helpful to mark the extent of cellulitis for serial evaluations of treatment success.
4. Admit patients with systemic toxicity or evidence of bacteremia to the hospital for IV antibiotics. Consider risks of complications when making treatment decisions for patients with diabetes mellitus, alcoholism, or other immunosuppressive disorders.
5. Initiate IV antibiotics, such as **clindamycin** 600 to 900 mg IV every 8 hours, **cefazolin** 1 to 2 g IV every 8 hours, or **nafcillin** 1 to 2 g IV every 4 hours for patients admitted for inpatient care.

ERYSIPELAS

Erysipelas is a superficial cellulitis with associated lymphatic involvement and is caused primarily by group A *Streptococcus*. Infection is often associated with an initial portal of entry or break in the skin.

Clinical Features

Onset of this infection is often acute and characterized by sudden high fever, chills, malaise, and nausea. Over 1 to 2 days, a small area of erythema with a burning sensation develops. The erythema of erysipelas is sharply demarcated from surrounding skin and is tense and painful. Lymphangitis and lymphadenitis are common.

Diagnosis and Differential

The diagnosis is based primarily on physical findings and history. Although leukocytosis is common, white blood cell counts, cultures, ASO titers, and anti-DNase B titers are of limited use in an acute care setting. Differential diagnosis includes other forms of local cellulitis. Consider surgical consultation for patients with bullae, crepitus, pain out of proportion to examination, or rapidly progressing erythema with signs of systemic toxicity, as these signs and symptoms may suggest necrotizing infection.

Emergency Department Care and Disposition

Guidelines no longer differentiate the treatment of nonpurulent cellulitis from erysipelas. Patients with uncomplicated erysipelas can be treated with antibiotics as detailed above for cellulitis.

CUTANEOUS ABSCESSES

Cutaneous skin abscesses are frequently the result of a breakdown in the cutaneous barrier, with a subsequent focal infection caused by resident bacterial flora. Incision and drainage is often the only necessary treatment for simple skin abscesses.

Clinical Features and Diagnosis

Patients present with an area of swelling, tenderness, and overlying erythema. The area of swelling is often fluctuant. Cutaneous abscesses are usually well-localized infections, although they may cause systemic toxicity in immunosuppressed patients. Evaluate cutaneous abscesses for predisposing injury or foreign bodies. Needle aspiration or bedside ultrasound may be useful when it is unclear whether a patient has an abscess or cellulitis. There are several common abscess types with unique managements discussed below.

Emergency Department Care and Disposition

1. Cutaneous skin abscesses can often be managed with local incision and drainage. In healthy, immunocompetent patients, the routine use of antibiotics following abscess incision and drainage is typically not necessary unless significant surrounding cellulitis or signs of severe disease are present.
2. ***Bartholin gland abscess*** presents as unilateral painful swelling of the labia with a fluctuant 1 to 2 cm mass. Routine antimicrobial treatment is typically not necessary unless there is a suspicion of sexually transmitted disease. Treatment involves incision and drainage along the vaginal

mucosal surface of the abscess, generally followed by the insertion of a Word catheter. The Word catheter can be left in place for up to 4 weeks. Sitz baths are recommended after 2 days. Follow-up with gynecology is recommended within 2 days in patients with severe symptoms and within 1 week in patients with mild symptoms.

3. ***Hidradenitis suppurativa*** is a recurrent chronic infection involving the apocrine sweat glands and commonly occurs in the axilla and groin. Acute abscesses can be treated with incision and drainage. Refer patients with recurrent disease to a surgeon for definitive treatment.
4. ***Infected epidermoid and pilar cysts*** are erythematous, tender, cutaneous nodules that are often fluctuant. Perform a simple incision and drainage and recommend wound rechecks in 2 to 3 days. The cyst contains a capsule that must be removed to prevent recurrence, and this capsule excision is typically done at a later follow-up visit.
5. ***Pilonidal abscess*** presents as a tender, swollen, and fluctuant mass along the superior gluteal fold. Treatment in the acute care setting includes incision and drainage and the patient should be rechecked in 2 to 3 days. Surgical referral is usually necessary for definitive treatment.
6. ***Folliculitis*** is characterized by pruritic erythematous lesions that are usually <5 mm in diameter, with pustules sometimes present at the centers. These inflamed hair follicles are usually caused by bacterial invasion with *S. aureus*. The lesions usually resolve spontaneously with symptomatic care, but can be treated with warm compresses or topical antibiotics such as **bacitracin**. For painful or more extensive cases, oral antibiotics such as **cephalexin**, **dicloxacillin**, or **azithromycin** are recommended.

SPOROTRICHOSIS

Sporotrichosis is caused by traumatic inoculation of the fungus *Sporothrix schenckii*, which is commonly found on plants and in the soil.

Clinical Features

After a 3-week incubation period, three types of infection may occur. The fixed cutaneous type of infection occurs at the site of inoculation and looks like a crusted ulcer or verrucous plaque. The local cutaneous type also remains at the site of inoculation but presents as a subcutaneous nodule or pustule with surrounding erythema. The lymphocutaneous type is the most common of the three and presents as a painless nodule at the site of inoculation with subcutaneous nodules that migrate along lymphatic channels.

Diagnosis and Differential

The diagnosis of sporotrichosis is based on the history and physical examination. Tissue biopsy cultures are often diagnostic but of limited use in the acute care setting. The differential diagnosis includes tuberculosis, tularemia, cat-scratch disease, leishmaniasis, nocardiosis, and staphylococcal lymphangitis.

Emergency Department Care and Disposition

1. **Itraconazole** 100 to 200 mg/d PO for 3 to 6 months is highly effective when treating localized or systemic sporotrichosis.
2. Most cases of cutaneous sporotrichosis can be treated on an outpatient basis. Patients who have systemic symptoms or who are acutely ill with disseminated disease should be admitted for possible treatment with **amphotericin B** 0.5 mg/kg/d.

FURTHER READING

For further reading in *Tintinalli's Emergency Medicine: A Comprehensive Study Guide*, 8th ed., see Chapter 152, "Soft Tissue Infections," by Elizabeth W. Kelly and David Magilner.

Serious Viral Infections

Matthew J. Scholer

Viral illnesses are among the most common reasons that people come to an emergency department. Although many viral illnesses are self-limited, some can be life-threatening, have specific treatments, or have public health implications. This chapter reviews some of the more common specific viral infections.

INFLUENZA

Influenza infections occur worldwide with peak activity found in temperate climates between late December and early March. Influenza virus is transmitted by aerosolized or droplet transmission from the respiratory tract of infected persons or by direct contact. After exposure, the incubation period is about 1 to 4 days, and viral shedding begins 24 hours before the onset of symptoms.

Clinical Features

Symptoms of influenza are often abrupt in onset and include fever with chills or rigors, headache, myalgia, and generalized malaise. Additional symptoms may include cough, rhinorrhea, sore throat, and tender, enlarged cervical lymph nodes. Elderly patients may not have classic symptoms and can present with only fever, malaise, confusion, and/or nasal congestion. Almost 50% of affected children have associated gastrointestinal symptoms, but these are unusual in adults. Fever generally lasts 2 to 4 days, followed by recovery from most of the systemic symptoms within 3 to 7 days. Cough and malaise may persist for several weeks.

Respiratory complications of acute infection include primary influenza pneumonitis, secondary bacterial pneumonia, croup, and exacerbation of chronic obstructive pulmonary disease. Avoid aspirin use in patients with suspected or confirmed influenza due to an association with Reye's syndrome. Other uncommon complications include Guillain–Barré syndrome, myocarditis, and pericarditis.

Diagnosis and Differential

A clinical diagnosis of influenza during a known outbreak can be made using history and physical examination. Rapid antigen assays can give results within 15 minutes but have variable sensitivity (10% to 80%) that can result in higher levels of false-negative results when influenza activity is high. Although specificity is high (90% to 95%), false-positive results can also occur, especially when influenza activity is low. Molecular diagnostic tests are available and are more sensitive and specific than antigen tests.

During influenza season, consider diagnostic testing in the outpatient setting for immunocompetent patients at high risk for influenza complications and within 5 days of symptom onset, and in immunocompromised patients regardless of time since illness onset. Many hospitals implement protocols for influenza testing of patients admitted with respiratory disease. Once influenza has been documented in the local community, influenza testing is not typically indicated for otherwise healthy outpatients with signs and symptoms consistent with influenza, especially during the peak of activity.

Emergency Department Care and Disposition

1. The majority of healthy patients with acute influenza infections will have self-limited, uncomplicated illnesses that can be successfully treated with symptomatic care measures in an outpatient setting.
2. Patients with more severe systemic symptoms or comorbid conditions may require inpatient care with IV fluids, respiratory support, neuraminidase inhibitors, and occasionally vasopressors or other critical care interventions.
3. Treat patients with secondary pneumonia associated with influenza infections with antibiotics that cover methicillin-resistant *S. aureus*.
4. Treatment with neuraminidase inhibitors is generally recommended for any patient with suspected influenza who is hospitalized, has severe, complicated or progressive illness, or is at higher risk for influenza complications. Use of these agents for otherwise healthy adults and children continue to be debated, and clinical benefit is likely limited to patients treated within 48 hours of symptom onset.
5. The most commonly used oral antiviral medication for treating influenza is **oseltamivir** 75 mg by mouth twice daily for 5 days in uncomplicated disease. **Zanamivir** is an inhaled medication that may cause bronchospasm and should be avoided in patients with underlying pulmonary disease. **Peramivir** 600 mg IV is the only intravenous antiviral medication approved for the treatment of influenza.
6. Current Centers for Disease Control and Prevention (CDC) guidelines for the diagnosis and treatment of influenza can be accessed at their website www.cdc.gov/flu.

HERPES SIMPLEX VIRUS

Transmission of herpes simplex virus (HSV) occurs by contact of mucous membranes or open skin with infected bodily fluids from patients with ulcerative lesions or infected individuals who are shedding the virus without overt disease.

Clinical Features

HSV-1 infection most commonly results in orolabial lesions, whereas HSV-2 is most often found in genital herpes. Primary HSV infections typically produce more extensive lesions involving mucosal and extramucosal sites, often accompanied by systemic signs and symptoms. Gingivostomatitis and pharyngitis for 1 to 2 weeks are typical manifestations of primary HSV-1 infection, and these lesions are small thin-walled vesicles on an erythematous base within the mouth. In children younger than 5 years, lesions can be associated with fever and cervical lymphadenopathy. Recurrent HSV-1 infections are typically milder and present as herpes labialis on the lower lip at the outer vermilion border.

Less common manifestations of HSV infection include herpetic whitlow on a finger or herpes gladiatorum elsewhere on the body in wrestlers and other athletes involved in close contact sports. Herpetic keratitis presents as a painful, red eye, and can be identified by characteristic dendritic lesions on fluorescein slit lamp exam. Either HSV-1 or HSV-2 can cause genital lesions, and while genital HSV-2 is more common and has a higher relapse rate, the proportion of genital disease caused by HSV-1 is increasing.

HSV infection within the central nervous system (CNS) is one of the most common viral causes of encephalitis in the United States. This occurs most commonly in patients between 20 and 50 years of age and HSV encephalitis carries a mortality rate >70% if left untreated. HSV encephalitis is associated with fever and neurologic symptoms such as focal motor or cranial nerve deficits, ataxia, seizures, altered mental status, or behavioral abnormalities. Meningitis can occur in up to 25% of females with primary HSV-2 infections, although this typically has a benign course. HSV infections in immunocompromised hosts can lead to widespread dissemination with multi-organ involvement.

Diagnosis and Differential

The diagnosis and initial treatment of suspected HSV infection is often based on clinical findings, as confirmatory testing may take days or weeks before results are available. Because mucocutaneous HSV infection is a lifelong condition, laboratory testing is often recommended for confirmation. Viral culture can be obtained from an unroofed vesicle, or polymerase chain reaction or direct fluorescent antibody testing can be performed on swabbed tissue. A Tzanck test is generally not useful.

Consider the possibility of HSV infection in patients with suspected infection of the CNS, particularly in patients with altered mental status, cognitive deficits, psychiatric symptoms, or seizures (see Chapter 148, "Central Nervous System and Spinal Infections"). Temporal lobe lesions on CT scan or MRI are suggestive of HSV encephalitis and cerebrospinal fluid analysis may demonstrate a lymphocytic pleocytosis and/or erythrocytosis. PCR testing of spinal fluid is the testing modality of choice for HSV when suspected, and the viral DNA can be detected within the first 24 hours, with results remaining positive for a week or longer.

Emergency Department Care and Disposition

1. Treat severe systemic HSV infections, including suspected CNS infection or disseminated disease, with **acyclovir** 10 mg/kg IV every 8 hours. Adjust dosing for immunocompromised patients with severe mucocutaneous involvement to **acyclovir** 5 mg/kg IV every 8 hours based on ideal body weight.
2. Treat mild to moderate HSV infection in immunocompetent patients with oral **acyclovir** 400 mg three times a day, **valacyclovir** 1000 mg every 12 hours, or **famciclovir** 250 mg three times a day. Treatment is most effective when initiated within 48 to 72 hours of symptom onset and is typically continued for 7 to 10 days.
3. Treat recurrent HSV with or **acyclovir** 400 mg three times a day for 5 days, **valacyclovir** 2000 mg every 12 hours for 1 day (labialis) or

500 mg every 12 hours for 3 days (genital), or **famciclovir** 1500 mg for one dose (orolabial) or 1000 mg for one dose (genital). Less severe outbreaks may be treated with topical **5% acyclovir ointment** applied six times per day for 7 days.

VARICELLA AND HERPES ZOSTER

Varicella zoster virus (VZV) is the causative organism for both varicella (chickenpox) and herpes zoster (shingles) infections. Herpes zoster is reactivation of the latent virus within a dorsal root ganglion that can occur with a waning immune response due to advancing age or immunosuppression. The presence of herpes zoster in an otherwise young and healthy person may be a sign of HIV infection or other immunosuppressive disorder.

Clinical Features

Primary varicella infection is a febrile illness with a superficial vesicular rash that appears in crops and is concentrated on the torso and face. Lesions are typically at varying stages of development, including papules, vesicles, and crusted lesions. Headache, malaise, and loss of appetite are often present. Most infections are minor and self-limited with lesions crusting over and sloughing off after 1 to 2 weeks. Varicella is contagious until all of the lesions have crusted over.

Complications are more common in very young and very old patients and those with immunocompromise. Bacterial infections of skin lesions, often with group A streptococci, can cause serious illnesses including necrotizing fasciitis. CNS complications such as cerebellar ataxia, meningitis, and meningoencephalitis have been described. Infection of cerebral arteries resulting in vasculopathy and stroke may also occur. Pneumonitis can be severe and is more common in pregnant women.

Herpes zoster causes lesions similar to those of a primary varicella infection but that occur in a unilateral and dermatomal distribution on the skin. A prodrome of malaise, headache, and photophobia may occur with localized pain, itching, and parasthesias preceding the outbreak of the rash. Although any dermatomal level may be affected, involvement of the trigeminal or thoracic dermatomes are common. Ocular involvement with herpes zoster ophthalmicus may occur when the ophthalmic distribution of the trigeminal nerve is involved (see Chapter 149, "Ocular Emergencies"), and is associated with zoster lesions on the tip or side of the nose (Hutchinson's sign). Consider ophthalmology consultation when these are present or a patient has facial lesions with associated eye symptoms.

Herpes zoster lesions typically last about 2 weeks but may persist for a month. Postherpetic neuralgia is pain that continues 30 days after the initial eruption and occurs more often with advancing age. Rash involving multiple dermatomes or crossing the midline may represent disseminated disease, which can occur in immunocompromised patients when the virus spreads to visceral organs to cause pneumonitis, hepatitis, or encephalitis.

Diagnosis and Differential

Most cases of varicella infection can be diagnosed with history and physical examination findings. Laboratory diagnosis with viral culture, antigen testing, or PCR testing of vesicle fluid may be appropriate in patients with atypical illness or severe disease. Although smallpox has been eradicated, it remains a potential threat as a biologic weapon, and the lesions could be confused with those of varicella. The lesions of smallpox are larger, distributed more on the extremities, and all lesions are at the same stage of development. Obtain a chest radiograph if pneumonitis is suspected. Consider advanced testing when CNS infection is suspected, which may include an MRI of the brain, lumbar puncture, and/or PCR testing.

Emergency Department Care and Disposition

1. Provide supportive care for healthy children with primary varicella infection. Oral **acyclovir** 20 mg/kg (maximum dose of 800 mg) five times a day for 5 days may be considered for high-risk patients such as children >12 years of age, adults, those with chronic skin or pulmonary disorders, those receiving long-term salicylate therapy, and immunocompromised patients.
2. Antiviral agents for the treatment of herpes zoster will hasten lesion resolution, reduce new lesions, reduce viral shedding, and decrease acute pain. Use of antiviral therapy in immunocompromised patients may reduce the risk of disseminated disease. Ideally begin antiviral medication within 72 hours of the onset of rash, although treatment can be considered at >72 hours if new vesicles are developing. Treat with a 7- to 10-day course of oral **acyclovir** 800 mg five times per day, **valacyclovir** 1 g three times daily or **famciclovir** 500 mg three times daily.
3. Provide appropriate analgesia for patients with herpes zoster, as lesions can be very painful.
4. Treat immunocompromised patients with acute varicella infections, severe herpes zoster outbreaks, visceral involvement, or disseminated disease with **acyclovir** 10 mg/kg IV every 8 hours.

EPSTEIN–BARR VIRUS INFECTION

Epstein–Barr virus (EBV) is the causative agent of heterophile-positive infectious mononeucleosis. EBV infection is also associated with cancers such as B-cell lymphoma, Hodgkin's disease, Burkitt's lymphoma, and nasopharyngeal carcinoma.

Clinical Features

Transmission of EBV is via salivary secretions. Close contact is required for transmission, often from an asymptomatic individual. Clinical manifestations depend on age and immune status with peaks of infection in early childhood and young adulthood. Infants and young children are often asymptomatic or have only mild pharyngitis. Teenagers and young adults can develop infectious mononucleosis, which presents with fever, lymphadenopathy, and pharyngitis with tonsillar exudates. Splenomegaly occurs in more than half of patients. Symptoms generally resolve over 2 to 3 weeks, and most patients recover uneventfully.

Epstein–Barr virus can affect nearly all organ systems. Neurologic complications such as encephalitis, meningitis, and Guillain–Barré syndrome have been described. Hepatitis, myocarditis, and hematologic disorders are also known complications. Rarely death results from splenic rupture, CNS complications, and airway obstruction.

Diagnosis and Differential

When infectious mononeucleosis is suspected based on history and physical exam, consider a CBC and a monospot test to provide confirmation, when indicated. Lymphocytosis with >50% lymphocytes and presence of atypical lymphocytes are suggestive of the diagnosis. The monospot test may be negative early in the course of disease, and repeat testing later in the course of illness may be helpful when the diagnosis remains uncertain.

Emergency Department Care and Disposition

1. Rest and analgesia are the mainstays of therapy for EBV infections.
2. Use of corticosteroids is associated with increased complications and is recommended only for patients with severe disease, such as upper airway obstruction, neurologic disease, or hemolytic anemia.
3. Advise patients to avoid all contact sports for a minimum of 3 weeks after illness onset to avoid splenic injury.

MEASLES

Measles is caused by an RNA virus that is highly infectious and is communicable before symptoms begin. Measles outbreaks have occurred recently in communities where children are not appropriately vaccinated.

Clinical Features

Acute measles infection occurs with fever, malaise, cough, runny nose, and conjunctivitis. Small, white Koplik's spots appear on the buccal mucosa early in the illness, followed by a red maculopapular rash that typically begins on the head and spreads throughout the body.

Diagnosis and Differential

The diagnosis of measles is typically made based on clinical findings such as the pathognomonic Koplik's spots and characteristic rash. Confirmatory testing can be done by detection of immunoglobulin M antibodies.

Emergency Department Care and Disposition

1. Treatment for measles is supportive care, with particular attention to ensuring adequate nutrition, especially vitamin A intake.
2. Report suspected measles cases to the local health department. Coordinate with health department officials to identify and offer post-exposure prophylaxis to unvaccinated contacts when appropriate.
3. See http://www.cdc.gov/measles/hcp/ for current CDC guidelines for the diagnosis and treatment of measles.

ARBOVIRAL INFECTIONS

Arboviral infections are spread by mosquito, tick, and fly bites with increased incidence in warmer months due to the breeding patterns of these arthropod vectors. West Nile virus and the viruses that cause La Cross encephalitis, St. Louis encephalitis, eastern equine encephalitis, and western equine encephalitis are found in North America. Other significant arboviral diseases are discussed in Chapter 98, "World Travelers."

Clinical Features

Most arbovirus infections are either asymptomatic or cause a nonspecific mild illness. Only a few infected individuals will develop hemorrhagic fever or encephalitis. Severe human arboviral diseases most commonly manifest as one of four syndromes: fever and myalgia, arthritis and rash, encephalitis, and hemorrhagic fever. Headache is a common symptom of most arboviral infections. Hemorrhagic fever presents with bleeding from the gums, petechiae, and the gastrointestinal tract. The classic presentation of viral encephalitis is fever, headache, and altered level of consciousness. Patients can be lethargic and confused, and occasionally present with seizures.

Diagnosis and Differential

Obtaining a detailed travel and exposure history and knowing local epidemiologic patterns can help when arboviral infections are suspected. Consider neuroimaging as a component of hospitalization for patients diagnosed with encephalitis, recognizing that MRI is more sensitive and may show foci of increased signal intensity. Cerebrospinal fluid typically shows a lymphocytic pleocytosis and a slightly elevated protein level, although these findings are nonspecific. Serologic testing is the primary method for confirming arboviral infections.

Emergency Department Care and Disposition

1. Supportive and symptomatic therapy is the mainstay of management for arboviral infections. Specific antiviral drugs, interferon, and steroids have not been shown to be useful.
2. Early in the course of suspected encephalitis, patients may be treated with empiric antibiotics and acyclovir to cover for possible bacterial infection or HSV encephalitis until confirmatory testing is complete.
3. Admit most patients with acute encephalitis to the hospital for supportive care and additional diagnostic testing.

EBOLA VIRUS AND OTHER HEMORRHAGIC FEVERS

Viral hemorrhagic fevers are rare diseases that can elicit tremendous fear among the public and health care providers, exemplified by the large Ebola virus outbreak in West Africa in 2014. Other examples of hemorrhagic fever include hantavirus pulmonary syndromes and Lassa fever.

Clinical Features

Viral infections leading to hemorrhagic fever illnesses typically begin with nonspecific symptoms such as fever, myalgia, and malaise. Progression of disease leads to gastrointestinal and other organ system involvement, where increased vascular permeability leads to hypotension, pulmonary edema, and renal failure. Abnormalities in the coagulation pathways lead to diffuse hemorrhage with extensive bleeding, organ dysfunction, and shock.

Diagnosis and Differential

Travel to endemic areas of the world and/or contact with a known infected traveler are important clues when suspecting Ebola or other hemorrhagic fever illnesses. Confirm these rare infections using acute serologic testing to identify antibodies or reverse transcriptase polymerase chain reaction of the virus. These tests are typically performed at specialized laboratories such as the CDC.

Emergency Department Care and Disposition

1. Prepare for patients with possible Ebola or other severe viral hemorrhagic fever illnesses by initiating appropriate screening at triage. Patients who have recently traveled to endemic areas who present with fever or symptoms suspicious for these illnesses should be appropriately isolated.
2. Use full contact and droplet precautions including gown, gloves, and facemask with eye protection, as these viruses are spread via contact with infected body fluids such as blood, vomit, and diarrhea.
3. Instruct staff for proper donning and removal of protective equipment to avoid contamination with bodily fluids.
4. Contact appropriate public health organizations when these uncommon infections are clinically suspected. Notify the hospital laboratory to take proper precautions with patient specimens that will need to be sent to specialized labs.
5. Provide supportive care for suspected Ebola and most other viral hemorrhagic fevers using IV fluids, renal replacement, and respiratory support. Experimental serologic treatments and vaccines are under development.

FURTHER READING

For further reading in *Tintinalli's Emergency Medicine: A Comprehensive Study Guide*, 8th ed., see Chapter 153, "Serious Viral Infections," by Sukhjit S. Takhar and Gregory J. Moran.

CHAPTER 92 HIV Infection and AIDS

Sarah Battistich

The human immunodeficiency virus (HIV) and Acquired Immunodeficiency Syndrome (AIDS) remain a major cause of infectious disease deaths worldwide. Despite decades of diagnostic and therapeutic advances, increased life expectancies from highly active antriretrovirals are in general limited to high-income industrialized countries, and morbidity and mortality around the world remains high. The pandemic continues to significantly impact affect Sub-Saharan Africa, where heterosexual transmission is common and as many as 1 in 20 individuals live with HIV and AIDS. In the United States, there are approximately 50,000 new cases annually, with higher incidences in men who have sex with men and young minority populations.

CLINICAL FEATURES

Human immunodeficiency virus is a cytopathic retrovirus that selectively attacks host cells involved in immune function, primarily CD4+ T cells. Infection ultimately results in persistent defects in cellular immunity which permit the development of opportunistic infections and neoplasms. Up to 90% of newly infected individuals have symptoms at the time of an acute HIV infection, most commonly nonspecific influenza-like symptoms that can go unrecognized. Symptoms usually develop 2 to 4 weeks after exposure, and can last for 2 to 10 weeks. The most common symptoms include fever (>90%), fatigue (70% to 90%), sore throat (>70%), rash (40% to 80%), headache (30% to 80%), and lymphadenopathy (40% to 70%).

Seroconversion, which occurs when there is a detectable antibody response to HIV, usually occurs 3 to 8 weeks after infection, although delays of up to 11 months have been reported. This is followed by a long period of asymptomatic infection. The mean incubation time from exposure to the development of AIDS in untreated patients is 8 years in adults and 2 years in children under 5 years of age.

Early symptomatic infection, when CD4 cell counts are 200 to 500 cells/mm^3, is characterized by conditions that are more common and more severe in the presence of HIV infection but are not AIDS-defining conditions. Examples include thrush, persistent vulvovaginal candidiasis, peripheral neuropathy, cervical dysplasia, recurrent herpes zoster, and idiopathic thrombocytopenic purpura. As the CD4 count drops below 200 cells/mm^3, the frequency of opportunistic infections increases. AIDS is defined by the appearance of any indicator condition (Table 92-1) or a CD4 count lower than 200 cells/mm^3. Late symptomatic or advanced HIV infection exists in patients with a CD4 count lower than 50 cells/mm^3 or clinical evidence of end-stage disease, including disseminated *Mycobacterium avium* complex (MAC) or disseminated *Cytomegalovirus* (CMV).

Antiretroviral regimens are effective in suppressing viral loads and maintaining normal CD4 counts, which has favorably changed the long-term prognosis and impact of HIV infection for patients who take these

TABLE 92-1 Stage 3 AIDS-Defining Opportunistic Illnesses in HIV Infection
Bacterial infections, multiple or recurrent[*]
Candidiasis of bronchi, trachea, or lungs
Candidiasis of esophagus
Cervical cancer, invasive[†]
Coccidioidomycosis, disseminated or extrapulmonary
Cryptococcosis, extrapulmonary
Cryptosporidiosis, chronic intestinal (>1 month in duration)
Cytomegalovirus disease (other than liver, spleen, or nodes), onset at age >1 month
Cytomegalovirus retinitis (with loss of vision)
Encephalopathy attributed to HIV
Herpes simplex: chronic ulcers (>1 month in duration) or bronchitis, pneumonitis, or esophagitis (onset at age >1 month)
Histoplasmosis, disseminated or extrapulmonary
Isosporiasis, chronic intestinal (>1 month in duration)
Kaposi's sarcoma
Lymphoma, Burkitt's (or equivalent term)
Lymphoma, immunoblastic (or equivalent term)
Lymphoma, primary, of brain
Mycobacterium avium complex or Mycobacterium kansasii, disseminated or extrapulmonary
Mycobacterium tuberculosis of any site, pulmonary,[†] disseminated, or extrapulmonary
Mycobacterium, other species or unidentified species, disseminated or extrapulmonary
Pneumocystis jirovecii (previously known as *Pneumocystis carinii*) pneumonia
Pneumonia, recurrent[†]
Progressive multifocal leukoencephalopathy
Salmonella septicemia, recurrent
Toxoplasmosis of brain, onset at age >1 month
Wasting syndrome attributed to HIV

[*]Only among children aged <13 years. (CDC. 1994. Revised classification system for human immunodeficiency virus infection in children less than 13 years of age. *MMWR.* 1994;43 [No. RR-12].)

[†]Only among adults and adolescents aged >13 years. (CDC. 1993. Revised classification system for HIV infection and expanded surveillance case definition for AIDS among adolescents and adults. *MMWR.* 1992;41 [No. RR-17].)

medications. Access to medical care, patient compliance, and financial resources to obtain medications are identified barriers to effective treatment in many parts of the world.

DIAGNOSIS AND DIFFERENTIAL

HIV infection can be diagnosed by identifying HIV nucleic acid, detecting viral-specific antigen, detecting antibodies to HIV, or isolating the virus by culture. Mean times from transmission to detection are shortest for viral load (17 days), followed by p24 antigen (22 days), enzyme-linked immunosorbent assay positivity (25 days), and Western blot positivity (31 days). Although viral load assays are not always available in the ED, rapid tests for the detection of the p24 viral antigen enable earlier detection of infection than relying on the development of antibody response alone. The current recommended testing method is detection of antibodies to HIV-1/2 combined with detection of the viral-specific p24 antigen.

Although acute HIV infection is not diagnosed in up to 75% of cases, benefits of early detection include the opportunity to limit transmission to others and for individuals to start antiretroviral medications early.

The spectrum of disease caused by HIV infection varies, from those with asymptomatic infection to those seeking care from involvement of any organ system. In the assessment of patients with known HIV, knowledge of recent CD4 count and HIV viral load can help with management, as CD4 counts below 200 cells/mm^3 and viral load greater than 50,000 copies/mL are associated with an increased risk of AIDS-defining illness. When these levels are unavailable, a total lymphocyte count of <1700 cells/mm^3 is strongly predictive of a CD4 count of <200 cells/mm^3.

Febrile Illness

Systemic symptoms such as fever, weight loss, and malaise are common in HIV-infected patients and account for the majority of HIV-related ED presentations. Laboratory investigation may include electrolytes, complete blood count, blood cultures, urinalysis and culture, liver function tests, and chest radiographs in the appropriate clinical settings. Selected patients may benefit from specific serologic testing for syphilis, cryptococcosis, toxoplasmosis, cytomegalovirus (CMV), and coccidioidomycosis. Consider lumbar puncture after neuroimagingwhen CNS infection is suspected.

In HIV patients without specific signs or symptoms to localize the source of fever, common causes can vary by stage of disease. Patients with CD4 counts higher than 500 cells/mm^3 generally have febrile illnesses from sources similar to those in nonimmunocompromised patients. Those with CD4 counts between 200 and 500 cells/mm^3 are more likely to have bacterial respiratory infections. For patients with CD4 counts lower than 200 cells/mm^3, infections without localizing symptoms or findings can include *Pneumocystis jirovecii* pneumonia (PCP), Mycobacterium avium complex (MAC), *Mycobacterium tuberculosis* (TB), CMV, drug fever, and sinusitis. Other causes may include endocarditis (see Chapter 93), lymphoma, *Histoplasma capsulatum*, and *Cryptococcus neoformans*. Fever caused by the primary HIV infection itself tends to occur in the afternoon or evening and is generally responsive to antipyretics.

Immune reconstitution inflammatory syndrome mimics an autoimmune event, with fever, lymphadenitis, and systemic symptoms that begin weeks to months after starting antiretroviral treatment and often associated with tuberculosis therapy. This rarely requires cessation of medications, but suspected cases should be discussed with an infectious disease specialist.

CMV is a common cause of serious opportunistic viral disease in HIV-infected patients. The most important manifestation is retinitis, which can often be diagnosed via clinical evaluation. Disseminated disease commonly involves the gastrointestinal, pulmonary, and central nervous systems and a specific diagnosis may require a tissue biopsy with histologic evidence of viral inclusions and inflammation. Cultures, antigen-based tests, and nucleic acid testing can be used to confirm CMV infection.

Disseminated MAC occurs predominately in patients with CD4 counts below 100 cells/mm^3 who are not on antiretroviral medications. Persistent fever and night sweats are typical, often with weight loss, diarrhea, malaise, and anorexia. Diagnosis is made with acid-fast stain of stool or other body fluids or culture. Treatment reduces bacteremia and improves symptoms but does not completely eradicate the infection.

Pulmonary Complications

Pulmonary presentations are among the most common reasons for ED visits by HIV-infected patients. Bacterial pneumonia outnumbers opportunistic infections, and *Streptococcus pneumoniae* is the most common cause of pneumonia in HIV-infected patients in the United States and Western Europe. Productive cough, leukocytosis, and the presence of a focal infiltrate suggest bacterial pneumonia. Common HIV-related causes of pulmonary abnormalities include PCP, TB, CMV, *C. neoformans, Histoplasma capsulatum*, and neoplasms. Evaluation may include pulse oximetry, arterial blood gas analysis, sputum culture and Gram stain, acid-fast stain, blood cultures, and chest radiography.

Pneumocystis jirovecii pneumonia is the most frequent opportunistic infection, and the most common identifiable cause of death among AIDS patients in the United States. The symptoms of PCP are often insidious, and include fever, nonproductive cough, and progressive shortness of breath. Chest radiographs typically demonstrate diffuse interstitial infiltrates, although negative radiographs are reported in up to 20% of patients. Elevated lactate dehydrogenase levels, although nonspecific, are often seen. Hypoxia at rest or with exertion and an increased alveolar-arterial oxygen gradient can identify patients at risk, and a presumptive diagnosis of PCP may be made in the setting of unexplained hypoxemia. Definitive diagnosis often requires bronchoscopy.

TB frequently occurs in patients with CD4 T-cell counts of 200 to 500 cells/mm^3. Consider TB in HIV-infected patients with pulmonary symptoms, and initiate appropriate respiratory isolation. As HIV-infection progresses, many patients do not report classic manifestations of TB such as cough with hemoptysis, night sweats, prolonged fevers, weight loss, and anorexia. Classic upper lobe involvement and cavitary lesions are less common, particularly among late-stage AIDS patients. False-negative purified protein derivative TB test results are frequent among AIDS patients due to immunosuppression. Late-stage HIV is also associated with extrapulmonary tuberculosis, typically within lymph nodes, bone marrow, CNS, GI, and urogenital systems.

Consider disseminated fungal infections such as *C. neoformans* and *Aspergillus fumigatus* in severely immunosuppressed patients. Noninfectious causes of pulmonary complaints such as neoplasms and lymphocytic interstitial pneumonitis may also occur.

Neurologic Complications

Neurologic disease may be caused by a variety of opportunistic infections, neoplasms, the HIV virus itself, or even as a side effect of antiretroviral treatment. Headaches, seizures, altered mental status, meningismus, or focal neurologic deficits can be caused by AIDS dementia, *Toxoplasma gondii*, or *C. neoformans*. Consider neuroimaging and lumbar puncture for patients with CD4 <200 and neurologic deficits or headaches. Initial neuroimaging with a noncontrast head computed tomography (CT) scan is appropriate, while a contrast-enhanced CT scan or magnetic resonance imaging (MRI) may also be considered in appropriate clinical circumstances. When obtaining cerebrospinal fluid, measure an opening pressure and order a complete cell count, glucose, protein, Gram stain, India ink stain, bacterial, viral, and fungal cultures, toxoplasmosis and cryptococcus antigen, and coccidioidomycosis titer.

AIDS dementia complex is a progressive process heralded by gradual impairment of recent memory and other cognitive deficits caused by direct HIV infection. Less common CNS infections that may present with neurologic symptoms include bacterial meningitis, histoplasmosis, CMV, progressive multifocal leukoencephalopathy, herpes simplex virus, neurosyphilis, and TB. HIV patients may experience HIV neuropathy characterized by painful sensory symptoms of the feet.

Ophthalmologic Manifestations

CMV retinitis is the most frequent and serious ocular infection and the leading cause of blindness in AIDS patients. Early infection may be asymptomatic, but may progress to changes in visual acuity, visual field abnormalities, photophobia, scotoma, eye redness, or pain. Herpes zoster ophthalmicus is another diagnosis to consider and is recognized by the typical zoster rash in the distribution of the ophthalmic branch of cranial nerve V.

Gastrointestinal Complications

Diarrhea is the most frequent gastrointestinal complaint and is estimated to occur in 50% to 90% of AIDS patients. Common causes include bacteria, parasites, viruses, fungi, and side effects of antiviral therapy. In many cases, a causative organism is never found. Evaluate stool for leukocytes, ova, and parasites, and consider obtaining acid-fast staining and bacterial culture. If bacterial infection is suspected, treat empirically with ciprofloxacin to cover common enteric pathogens. *Cryptosporidium* and *Isospora* are common parasitic causes of diffuse watery diarrhea, and both can be identified by acid-fast staining of a stool specimen. In late-stage AIDS, the most common diarrheal pathogens are MAC and CMV, each requiring biopsy for diagnosis.

Oral candidiasis affects more than 80% of AIDS patients and can be identified by its classic appearance of white plaques easily scraped from an erythematous base. Esophageal involvement may occur with *Candida*, herpes simplex, and CMV. Complaints of odynophagia or dysphagia are usually indicative of esophagitis and may be extremely debilitating and may lead to malnutrition.

Hepatomegaly with elevated alkaline phosphatase occurs in approximately 50% of AIDS patients. Co-infection with hepatitis B and hepatitis C is common, especially among IV drug users.

Anorectal disease is common in AIDS patients. Proctitis is characterized by painful defecation, rectal discharge, and tenesmus. Common causative organisms include *Neisseria gonorrhoeae*, *Chlamydia trachomatis*, syphilis, and herpes simplex.

Cutaneous Manifestations

Generalized conditions such as xerosis, seborrheic eczema, and pruritus are common. Kaposi sarcoma is a rash characterized by painless, raised, non-blanching brown-black or purple papules and nodules and is more common in homosexual men with HIV infection. Common sites are the face, chest, genitals, and oral cavity. Reactivation of varicella-zoster virus is more common in patients with HIV infection and AIDS than in the general population. Herpes simplex virus infections are common. HIV patients may develop bullous impetigo and *Pseudomonas*-associated chronic ulcerations. Bacterial skin infections, scabies, human papillomavirus, and hypersensitivity reactions to medications are also common.

EMERGENCY DEPARTMENT CARE AND DISPOSITION

1. Maintain an awareness of possible undiagnosed HIV infection in all patient populations. ED-based studies have demonstrated that a substantial number of patients have unsuspected HIV infection that cannot be accurately predicted based on demographic factors.
2. Base the decision to admit a patient with AIDS on severity of illness, with attention to new presentation of fever of unknown origin, hypoxia worse than baseline or PaO_2 below 60 mm Hg, suspected PCP, suspected TB, new CNS symptoms, intractable diarrhea, suspected CMV retinitis, herpes zoster ophthalmicus, or a patient unable to perform self-care.
3. Treatment regimens for common HIV-related infections are listed in Table 92-2. Suspected bacterial sepsis and focal bacterial infections should be treated with standard antibiotics (see Chapter 89).

TABLE 92-2 Treatment Recommendations for Common Human Immunodeficiency Virus-Related Infections

Organ System	Infection	Therapy
Systemic	*Mycobacterium avium-intracellulare*	Clarithromycin, 500 mg PO twice a day *and* Ethambutol, 15 mg/kg PO once a day *and* Rifabutin, 300 mg/kg PO once a day
	CMV infection	Ganciclovir, 5 mg/kg IV twice a day for 2 weeks, then 5 mg/kg/d *or* Foscarnet, 90 mg/kg every 12 h for 3 weeks, then 90 mg/kg once a day
Pulmonary	*Pneumocystis jirovecii* (*Pneumocystis carinii*) *pneumonia*	Trimethoprim-sulfamethoxazole dose using 15–20 mg of trimethoprim component per kilogram per day PO or IV in divided doses three times a day for 3 weeks If partial pressure of arterial oxygen is <70 mm Hg or alveolar-arterial gradient is >35 mm Hg, then add Prednisone, 40 mg twice a day for 5 days, then 40 mg once a day for 5 days, then 20 mg once a day for 11 days *or* Pentamidine, 4 mg/kg/d IV or IM for 3 weeks
	Mycobacterium tuberculosis infection*	Isoniazid, 5 mg/kg PO once a day *and* Rifampin, 10 mg/kg PO once a day or rifabutin 5 mg/kg PO once a day *and* Pyrazinamide, 15–30 mg/kg PO once a day *and* Ethambutol, 15–20 mg/kg PO once a day

(*Continued*)

TABLE 92-2 Treatment Recommendations for Common Human Immunodeficiency Virus-Related Infections (Continued)

Organ System	Infection	Therapy
Central nervous	Toxoplasmosis[†]	Pyrimethamine, 200-mg loading dose PO followed by 50–75 mg PO once a day for 6–8 weeks *and* Sulfadiazine, 1–1.5 g PO every 6 h for 6–8 weeks *and* Leucovorin, 10–25 mg once a day
	Cryptococcosis[‡]	Amphotericin B, 0.7 mg/kg IV once a day for 2 weeks *and* Flucytosine, 25 mg/kg IV four times a day for 2 weeks *then* Fluconazole, 400 mg/d PO for 8–10 weeks
Ophthalmologic	CMV infection[§]	Valganciclovir, 900 mg PO twice a day for 14–20 days of induction therapy, then 900 mg PO daily for maintenance therapy *and* Ganciclovir, 2 mg intravitreal injection 1–4 doses over 7–10 days for patients with immediately sight-threatening lesions *or* Foscarnet, 2.4 mg intravitreal injection 1–4 doses over 7–10 days for patients with immediately sight-threatening lesions
GI	Candidiasis (thrush–limited to mouth)	Clotrimazole, 10-mg troches five times a day *or* Nystatin, 500,000 units five times a day, gargle
	Esophagitis (primarily *Candida*)	Fluconazole, 100–400 mg/d PO
	Salmonellosis[†]	Ciprofloxacin, 500 mg PO twice a day for 2–4 weeks
	Cryptosporidiosis	No known effective cure; best results with highly active antiretroviral therapy
Cutaneous	Herpes simplex	Acyclovir, 200 mg PO five times a day for 7 days *or* Famciclovir, 125 mg PO twice a day for 7 days *or* Valacyclovir, 1 g PO twice a day for 7 days or for severe disease Acyclovir, 5–10 mg/kg IV every 8 h for 7 days
	Herpes zoster	Acyclovir, 800 mg PO five times a day for 7–10 days *or* Famciclovir, 500 mg PO three times a day for 7–10 days *or* Valacyclovir, 1 g PO three times a day for 7–10 days *or* for ocular or disseminated disease Acyclovir, 5–10 mg/kg PO every 8 h for 5–7 days

(Continued)

TABLE 92-2 Treatment Recommendations for Common Human Immunodeficiency Virus-Related Infections (Continued)

Organ System	Infection	Therapy
	Candida or *Trichophyton* infection	Topical clotrimazole two or three times a day for 3 weeks *or* Topical miconazole two or three times a day for 3 weeks *or* Topical ketoconazole two or three times a day for 3 weeks

*Specific drug regimen must be adjusted if patient is receiving highly active antiretroviral therapy.
†Maintenance therapy required.
‡Maintenance therapy required; may be discontinued if CD4+ T-cell count is >150 cells/mm^3 for >16 weeks.
§Maintenance therapy required until CD4+ T-cell count is >150 cells/mm^3.
Abbreviation: CMV = cytomegalovirus.

4. Many institutions have guidelines for assessing health care providers with occupational exposures to HIV. Risks for seroconversion include (1) deep injury, (2) visible blood on the injuring device, (3) needle placement in a vein or an artery of the source patient, and (4) a source patient with late-stage HIV infection. Post-exposure prophylaxis should be initiated as quickly as possible, preferably within 2 hours, and should be continued for 28 days. A minimum three-drug regimen is recommended.
5. Although rarely started in the ED, antiretroviral therapy is recommended for CD4+ counts below 350 cells/mm^3 or history of AIDS-defining illness (see Table 92-1) as well as in patients with the following conditions regardless of the CD4 count: pregnancy, HIV-associated neuropathy, and hepatitis B co-infection requiring treatment. Initial treatment includes two nucleoside reverse transcriptase inhibitors plus one or two protease inhibitors or one nonnucleoside reverse transcriptase inhibitor drug. See the Centers for Disease Control and Prevention (CDC) website: http://www.cdc.gov/hiv/.

FURTHER READING

For further reading in *Tintinalli's Emergency Medicine: A Comprehensive Study Guide*, 8th ed., see Chapter 154, "Human Immunodeficiency Virus Infection," by Richard Rothman, Catherine A. Marco, and Samuel Yang.

CHAPTER 93 Infective Endocarditis

Kristin M. Berona

Infective endocarditis is caused by infection and damage to the endocardium of the heart and carries a high morbidity and mortality. This condition is more common in patients with prosthetic heart valves, congenital or acquired structural abnormalities of the heart or valves, or risk factors such as injection drug use, implanted intravascular devices, poor dental hygiene, HIV, or chronic hemodialysis.

Staphylococcus species are the most common cause of infective endocarditis in patients with either native or prosthetic heart valves. *Streptococcus* and *Enterococcus* species are other common infections associated with this condition. Endocarditis with negative blood cultures and no identified causative organism occurs in about 5% of patients. The mitral valve is the most commonly affected valve, followed by aortic, tricuspid, and pulmonic in order of decreasing frequency. Infective endocarditis associated with injection drug use has a predilection for right-sided valvular lesions.

CLINICAL FEATURES

Patients present with symptoms along a continuum, from the fulminant and acute onset of disease associated with fever, a new heart murmur, and acute heart failure, to insidious and indolent symptoms such as malaise and fatigue in a patient with a prosthetic valve. Fever is the most common symptom (80%) followed by chills, weakness, and dyspnea (40%). Other nonspecific symptoms include anorexia, cough, and malaise. The most common findings on physical examination include fever and a heart murmur. Classic skin findings such as tender nodules on pads of fingers and toes (Osler's nodes), painless hemorrhagic plaques on fingers and toes (Janeway lesions), petechiae, and splinter hemorrhages occur in less than 50% of cases.

Patients often present with cardiac, neurologic, and embolic complications. Acute heart failure occurs in approximately 70% of patients due to distortion or perforation of valves or cardiac chambers, or rupture of chordae tendinae. Other less frequent cardiac manifestations include heart blocks and dysrhythmias. Neurologic complications occur in 20% to 40% of patients, including ischemic stroke, brain abscess, cerebral hemorrhage, mycotic aneurysm, or seizure. Other embolic events may occur in the lungs, spleen, intestines, kidneys, and can cause acute limb ischemia.

DIAGNOSIS AND DIFFERENTIAL

Infective endocarditis is difficult to definitively diagnose in the emergency department, given the necessary components for diagnosis are blood culture results, echocardiography, and clinical observation. Consider the diagnosis in patients with unexplained fever and risk factors for the disease, such as injection drug users, patients with prosthetic valves, and those with new or changing murmurs or evidence of arterial emboli. The Duke criteria have long been used to make the diagnosis as detailed in Tables 93-1 and 93-2.

TABLE 93-1 Duke Criteria* for Infective Endocarditis

Major Criteria
Positive blood culture for IE
Typical microorganism consistent with IE from two separate blood cultures* as noted below:
Streptococcus bovis, viridans streptococci, HACEK group
or
Community-acquired *Staphylococcus aureus* or *enterococci* in the absence of a primary focus
or
Microorganisms consistent with IE from persistently positive blood cultures defined as:
At least two positive cultures of blood samples drawn > 12 h apart
or
All of three or a majority of four or more separate blood cultures (with first and last sample drawn at least 1 h apart)
Single positive blood culture for *Coxiella burnetii* or antiphase I immunoglobulin G antibody titer of > 1:800
Evidence of echocardiographic involvement
Positive ECG for IE defined as:
Oscillating intracardiac mass on valve or supporting structures, in the path of regurgitant jets, or on implanted material in the absence of an alternative anatomic explanation
or
Abscess
or
New partial dehiscence of prosthetic valve
New valvular regurgitation (worsening or changing of preexisting murmur not sufficient)
Minor Criteria
Predisposition: predisposing heart condition or injection drug use
Fever: temperature > 38°C (100.4°F)
Vascular phenomena: major arterial emboli, septic pulmonary conjunctival hemorrhages, and Janeway lesions
Immunologic phenomena: glomerulonephritis, Osler nodes, Roth spots, and rheumatoid fever
Microbiologic evidence: positive blood culture but does not meet a major criterion as noted in Table 93-2* or serologic evidence of active infection with organism consistent with IE
Echocardiographic minor findings were eliminated in the modified Duke criteria

*Excludes single positive cultures for coagulase-negative staphylococci and organisms that do not cause IE.

Abbreviations: HACEK, *Haemophilus, Actinobacillus, Cardiobacterium, Eikenella, and Kingella;* IE, infective endocarditis.

When infective endocarditis is suspected as a likely diagnosis, obtain three sets of blood cultures prior to administration of antibiotics from three separate vascular sites, ideally with an hour elapsing between the first and last set of cultures. Obtain an echocardiogram to look for cardiac valve vegetations and to evaluate valvular and overall cardiac function. Transthoracic echocardiography is a common initial modality, although transesophageal echocardiography is more sensitive and specific for valvular pathology and may be necessary if transthoracic images are inconclusive. Additional testing includes electrocardiography, chest X-ray, and laboratory studies. Although nonspecific for infective endocarditis, laboratory abnormalities that may be present are anemia, hematuria, and

TABLE 93-2 Modified Duke Criteria for Infective Endocarditis

Definite Infective Endocarditis
Pathologic criteria
Microorganisms demonstrated by culture or histologic examination of a vegetation or in a vegetation that has embolized, or in an intracardiac abscess
or
Pathologic lesions: vegetation or intracardiac abscess present, confirmed by histology showing active endocarditis
Clinical Criteria, Using Specific Definitions Listed in Table 93-1
Two major criteria
or
One major and three minor criteria
or
Five minor criteria
Possible infective endocarditis
One major criterion and one minor criterion
Three minor criteria
Rejected
Firm alternate diagnosis for manifestations of endocarditis
or
Resolution of manifestations of endocarditis with antibiotic therapy for 4 days or less
or
No pathologic evidence of infective endocarditis at surgery or autopsy after antibiotic therapy for 4 days
Does not meet criteria for possible infective endocarditis

elevations in inflammatory markers. Investigate for potential infections from other sources based on individual presenting complaints.

EMERGENCY DEPARTMENT CARE AND DISPOSITION

1. Focus initial interventions to stabilize any impairments of airway, breathing, and circulation. Patients with acute infective endocarditis may present with respiratory compromise and require emergent airway stabilization.
2. Pulmonary edema may be due to left-sided valvular rupture and may benefit from afterload reduction along with usual care for acute heart failure.
3. Initiate antibiotics to patients with suspected endocarditis as soon as appropriate cultures are obtained. Table 93-3 lists empiric treatment regimens. Definitive therapy is based on culture and sensitivity results and typically requires 4 to 6 weeks of antibiotics.
4. Admit patients with suspected infective endocarditis to the hospital for definitive diagnosis and management. Successful treatment often utilizes a team approach with cardiology, infectious disease, and thoracic surgery. Patients with neurologic or other embolic phenomena may benefit from additional specialist consultation.
5. Guidelines for antibiotic prophylaxis were updated in 2007. Only patients in the highest risk group for infective endocarditis need antibiotic prophylaxis for dental procedures involving manipulation of gingival tissue or procedures on infected skin or soft tissue. These high-risk

TABLE 93-3 Empiric Therapy of Suspected Bacterial Endocarditis*

Patient Characteristics	Recommended Agents, Initial Dose
Uncomplicated history	Ceftriaxone, 1–2 g IV *or* Nafcillin, 2 g IV *or* Oxacillin, 2 g IV *or* Vancomycin, 15 mg/kg *plus* Gentamicin, 1–3 mg/kg IV *or* Tobramycin, 1 mg/kg IV
Injection drug use, congenital heart disease, hospital-acquired, suspected methicillin-resistant *Staphylococcus aureus*, or already on oral antibiotics	Nafcillin, 2 g IV *plus* Gentamicin, 1–3 mg/kg IV *plus* Vancomycin, 15 mg/kg IV
Prosthetic heart valve	Vancomycin, 15 mg/kg IV *plus* Gentamicin, 1–3 mg/kg IV *plus* Rifampin, 300 mg PO

*Based on American Heart Association, endorsed by the Infectious Disease Society of America, http://www.idsociety.org/Organ_System/, accessed April 1, 2014. Because of controversy in the literature regarding the optimal regimen for empiric treatment, antibiotic selection should be based on patient characteristics, local resistance patterns, and current authoritative recommendations.

patients include those with a prior history of infective endocarditis, a prosthetic heart valve, unrepaired or failed repair of a congenital heart defect, or a cardiac transplant recipient with valvular regurgitation due to a structurally abnormal valve. Full antibiotic prophylaxis recommendations may be found at http://circ.ahajournals.org/content/116/15/1736.full.pdf.

FURTHER READING

For further reading in *Tintinalli's Emergency Medicine: A Comprehensive Study Guide*, 8th ed., see Chapter 155, "Infective Endocarditis," by Richard Rothman, Catherine A. Marco, and Samuel Yang.

CHAPTER 94

Tetanus and Rabies

Michael T. Fitch

TETANUS

Tetanus is an acute and frequently fatal disease resulting from an infection with the organism *Clostridium tetani*. The disease is exotoxin mediated and can occur after any of a variety of tissue injuries, including clean and contaminated wounds, elective surgery, burns, puncture wounds, otitis media, dental infections, animal bites, abortion, and pregnancy. Due to successful vaccination campaigns, tetanus is a rare disease in developed countries but remains a significant problem elsewhere in the world.

Clinical Features

C. tetani is prevalent throughout the environment in soil, dust, skin surfaces, and animal and human feces. Spores are resistant to destruction, survive years on environmental surfaces, and are introduced into the body following tissue injury. Anaerobic tissue conditions lead to toxin formation when the spores begin to germinate, and therefore crushed or devitalized tissue, a retained foreign body, or infection can favor growth of the toxin-producing form of *C. tetani*. The incubation period ranges from <24 hours to >1 month, and while most cases occur within 14 days some patients may present several months after injury. Many cases of tetatnus occur in patients where no specific injury is recognized, and injuries are often minor and occur indoors.

Clinically, tetanus is categorized into three forms: local, cephalic, and generalized. Local tetanus is uncommon and presents with persistent muscle contractions in proximity to the injury site. Cephalic tetanus is rare, occurs occasionally with otitis media or head injuries, and has localized involvement of the face and cranial nerves. Generalized tetanus is the most common form (80% of cases) and often presents with a descending pattern of symptoms that begin with pain and stiffness in the jaw. Progression of the symptoms leads to trismus (lockjaw) and development of the classically described facial expression, *risus sardonicus*. Violent spasms and tonic contractions of muscle groups are responsible for the symptoms of the disease including dysphagia, opisthotonos, flexing of the arms, fist clenching, rigidity of abdominal muscles, and extension of the lower extremities. Autonomic symptoms include fever, sweating, hypertension, and tachycardia. Neonatal tetanus is a form of generalized tetanus and can occur due to inadequate maternal immunization and poor umbilical cord care, with symptoms typically presenting by the second week of life and associated with an extremely high mortality rate.

Diagnosis and Differential

Tetanus is diagnosed clinically, and early symptoms may include trismus, neck stiffness or sore throat, and dysphagia. The tetanospasmin toxin interferes with central and peripheral nervous system inhibitory pathways leading to unopposed muscle contraction, seizures, and autonomic nervous system dysfunction. Prior immunization does not eliminate tetanus as a diagnostic possibility. There are no confirmatory laboratory tests. Other potential diagnoses with muscular contraction or other symptoms that may be similar to tetatnus include strychnine poisoning, dystonic reactions to phenothiazine, hypocalcemic tetany, rabies, peritonsillar abscess, peritonitis, and meningitis.

Emergency Department Care and Disposition

1. Patients with tetanus require hospitalization to manage frequent muscle spasms that may last 3 to 4 weeks. Symptoms can be triggered by noise or touch and thus environmental stimuli should be minimized to prevent precipitation of convulsive spasms. The potential for laryngospasm or respiratory muscle spasms are best managed initially in an intensive care unit due to concern for progression to respiratory compromise.
2. Administer **tetanus immune globulin** 3000 to 6000 units IM in a single injection away from the site of tetanus toxoid administration. Give before wound debridement as additional exotoxin may be released during wound manipulation.
3. Administer **tetanus toxoid** 0.5 mL IM at presentation, and 6 weeks and 6 months after presentation.
4. Identify and debride any wound or devitalized tissue where suspected inoculation occurred to minimize further toxin production.
5. Antibiotics are of uncertain value in the treatment of tetanus. **Metronidazole** 500 mg IV every 6 hours is recommended when indicated.
6. Administer benzodiazepines to treat muscle spasms. **Midazolam**, 0.05 to 0.15 mg/kg/h IV may be given in appropriately monitored settings as a continuous drip when needed. **Lorazepam** 2 mg IV to effect may be used in small quantities.
7. Neuromuscular blockade may be required to control ventilation and muscular spasm and to prevent fractures and rhabdomyolysis. In such cases, intubated patients may receive a **vecuronium** bolus of 0.1 mg/kg IV followed by continuous infusion at 1 μg/kg/min. Appropriate sedation during neuromuscular blockade should be provided.
8. **Labetalol** 0.25 to 1 mg/min continuous IV infusion (0.3 to 1 mg/kg/h in children) can be used to treat manifestations of sympathetic hyperactivity. **Magnesium sulfate** 40 mg/kg loading dose followed by 2 g/h IV (1.5 g/h if ≤45 kg) has been suggested as an additional treatment for this condition to maintain blood levels of 2.0–4.0 mmol/L. **Morphine sulfate** 0.5 to 1 mg/kg/h is also useful and may provide sympathetic control without compromising cardiac output. **Clonidine** 0.3 mg every 8 hours PO or NG may be helpful in the management of cardiovascular instability.
9. Patients who recover from clinical tetanus should undergo active immunization as recovery from an active infection does not confer future immunity.

RABIES

Infection with the rabies virus leads to a fatal encephalitis in humans and animals, and is most often transmitted by contact with infected animal saliva via a bite or scratch wound. While most emergency physicians never encounter patients suffering from acute rabies encephalitis, it is very common for patients to present for evaluation and treatment after animal bites or other potential exposures to the rabies virus. In the United States, dog bites, cat bites, and exposure to bats are common reasons that patients present for postexposure prophylaxis. Rabies cases in animals within the United States are most often found in raccoons, bats, skunks, foxes, cats, dogs, and cattle. Ferrets, rabbits, guinea pigs, and squirrels are generally not known to transmit rabies to humans and thus these kinds of exposures are considered very low risk for rabies transmission and providers should contact local public health authorities if there are concerns about how to manage these low-risk exposures.

Clinical Features

Typical incubation periods for rabies virus infections are from 20 to 90 days. However, incubation periods as short as 4 days or as long as 6 years have been reported, emphasizing the importance of postexposure prophylaxis for patients regardless of the amount of time that has elapsed since a suspected exposure. The natural history of clinical rabies in humans is presented in **Table 94-1**.

The viral prodrome associated with human rabies infection includes nonspecific symptoms such as malaise, lethargy, headache, fever, nausea, vomiting, anxiety, and pain at the site of a bite wound. Encephalitic rabies (80% of cases) is characterized by episodic hyperexcitability, disorientation, hallucinations, and bizarre behavior and is associated with autonomic dysfunction, hypersalivation, hyperthermia, tachycardia, and cardiac arrhythmias. Paralytic rabies (20% of cases) generally begins with

TABLE 94-1 Natural History of Clinical Rabies in Humans after Incubation Period

Clinical Stage	Defining Event	Usual Duration	Common Symptoms and Signs*
Prodrome	First symptom	2–10 days	• Pain or paresthesia at site of bite • Malaise, lethargy • Headache • Fever • Nausea, vomiting, anorexia • Anxiety, agitation, depression
Acute neurologic phase	First neurologic sign	2–7 days	• Anxiety, agitation, depression • Hyperventilation, hypoxia • Aphasia, incoordination • Paresis, paralysis • Hydrophobia, pharyngeal spasms • Confusion, delirium, hallucinations • Marked hyperactivity
Coma	Onset of coma	0–14 days	• Coma • Hypotension, hypoventilation, apnea • Pituitary dysfunction • Cardiac arrhythmia, cardiac arrest
Death or recovery (extremely rare)	Death or initiation of recovery	Months (recovery)	• Pneumothorax • Intravascular thrombosis • Secondary infections

*Not every symptom or sign may be present in each case.

progressively worsening extremity paresis and bilateral facial weakness and progresses to coma and organ failure.

Rabies infections lead to coma within 10 days of onset. The clinical course is characterized by complications such as pituitary dysfunction, seizures, respiratory dysfunction, cardiac dysrhythmias, autonomic dysfunction, renal failure, and secondary bacterial infections. Almost all rabies infections are fatal with only a few case reports of patient survival.

Diagnosis and Differential

During the incubation period for rabies infection, there are no definitive diagnostic tests to confirm infection. The diagnosis of rabies infection is therefore clinical, and may be considered for a patient with an unexplained and rapidly progressive encephalitis, especially if autonomic instability, dysphagia, hydrophobia or neurologic symptoms are present. Once symptoms are present, antigen and antibody testing of serum, cerebrospinal fluid (CSF), saliva, and/or tissue biopsies can detect evidence of rabies infection. CSF analysis often demonstrates pleocytosis with a mononuclear predominance. The final diagnosis of rabies is made by postmortem analysis of brain tissue.

Emergency Department Care and Disposition

For the rare patient who presents with an acute rabies infection and symptoms of clinical disease, there are no specific therapies that have demonstrated clinical benefit. Treatment of an active clinical rabies infection is supportive care with admission to a critical care environment where treatment of the associated complications and further diagnostic testing can be completed.

The more typical focus for emergency providers is to assess patients with possible exposure to the rabies virus, manage public health and animal control notification, and appropriately administer postexposure prophylaxis for rabies exposures.

1. Evaluate all patients for potential postexposure prophylaxis who have been bitten, scratched, or exposed to saliva from a wild animal or from a domestic animal that could be rabid.
2. *Exposure to Bats:* Provide postexposure prophylaxis to patients who have had direct contact with a bat unless the person can be certain that a bite, scratch, or mucus membrane exposure did not occur. Consider postexposure prophylaxis for persons who were in the same room as a bat and may have been unaware if a bite or direct contact occurred. When possible, capture and submit animals for testing to the public health department as negative testing means postexposure prophylaxis is not necessary.
3. *Exposures from Healthy-Appearing Domestic Animals that Can Be Observed:* Postexposure prophylaxis may not be immediately necessary if a healthy domestic animal is available for confinement and observation for 10 days after the incident to watch for signs of rabies infection. Consult with local animal control and/or public health officials for guidance in these circumstances.
4. *Exposures from Stray Animals and Wild Animals:* Begin postexposure prophylaxis for exposures from wild animals or stray animals with

uncertain immunization histories that cannot be observed. Report exposures to the appropriate animal control and/or public health authorities.

5. Patients with wounds associated with potential rabies exposures should receive tetanus prophylaxis, wound cleansing with soap and water, irrigation with a dilute solution of povidone-iodine (1 mL povidone-iodine in 9 mL of water or normal saline), antibiotics (if indicated), and rabies prophylaxis.
6. In the United States, postexposure prophylaxis consists of a regimen of one dose of **human rabies immunoglobulin (HRIG)** and four doses of **rabies vaccine** over a 14-day period, except for immunocompromised persons, who should receive a five-dose series of vaccine over a 28-day period. Postexposure prophylaxis recommendations are provided in **Table 94-2**.

TABLE 94-2 Rabies Postexposure Prophylaxis Schedule—United States, 2010

Immunization Status	Treatment	Regimen*
Not previously immunized	Wound cleansing	Cleanse all wounds with soap and water; irrigate wounds with 9:1 diluted solution of povidone-iodine (if available).
	HRIG	Administer **20 IU/kg actual body weight**. If anatomically feasible, infiltrate the *full dose* around the wound(s) and give any remaining volume IM at an anatomic site distant from vaccine administration; do not give HRIG in the same syringe as vaccine. HRIG may partially suppress active production of rabies virus antibody, so **do not give more than the recommended dose**.
	Vaccine	HDCV or PCECV 1.0 mL (deltoid area†), one dose on days 0,‡ 3, 7, and 14.§
Previously immunized‖	Wound cleansing	Cleanse all wounds with soap and water; irrigate wounds with 9:1 povidone-iodine solution.
	HRIG	HRIG should *not* be administered.
	Vaccine	HDCV or PCECV 1.0 mL (deltoid area†), one dose on days 0‡ and 3.

*These regimens are appropriate for all age groups, including children.

†The deltoid area is the only acceptable site of vaccination for adults and older children. For younger children, the outer aspect of the thigh (anterolateral aspect) may be used. Vaccine should never be administered in the gluteal area.

‡Day 0 is the day the first dose of vaccine is administered.

§Day 28 vaccine dose no longer recommended by the Advisory Committee on Immunization Practices, unless the patient is immunocompromised. See http://www.cdc.gov/rabies/resources/acip_recommendations.html.

‖Any persons with a history of preexposure prophylaxis with HDCV or PCECV; prior postexposure prophylaxis with HDCV or PCECV; or previous immunization with any other type of rabies vaccine and a documented history of antibody response to the prior immunization.

Abbreviations: HDCV, human diploid cell vaccine; HRIG, human rabies immunoglobulin; PCECV, purified chick embryo cell culture vaccine.

7. **HRIG** provides passive immunity and is administered once at the beginning of therapy up to the seventh day after the initial exposure. The dose is 20 IU/kg, with as much as possible infiltrated locally at the exposure site and the remainder administered intramuscularly in the deltoid or thigh away from the site where rabies vaccine is given.
8. Provide active immunization with **rabies vaccine** (human diploid cell vaccine or purified chick embryo cell culture vaccine) in the deltoid or lateral thigh given on days 0, 3, 7, and 14 for patients with normal immune systems. Patients with immunocompromise should receive a fifth dose of vaccine on day 28.
9. The Centers for Disease Control and Prevention (CDC) and state or county health departments can provide assistance in the management of postexposure prophylaxis for rabies. The most current information available from the CDC can be accessed at www.cdc.gov/rabies/.

FURTHER READING

For further reading in *Tintinalli's Emergency Medicine: A Comprehensive Study Guide*, 8th ed., see Chapter 156, "Tetanus," by Joel L. Moll and Donna L. Carden; and Chapter 157, "Rabies," by David Weber.

CHAPTER 95 Malaria

Jennifer L. Hannum

Malaria, a protozoan disease transmitted by the bite of the *Anopheles* mosquito, is caused by the genus *Plasmodium*. Five species of the protozoan *Plasmodium* infect humans: *P. falciparum*, *P. vivax*, *P. ovale*, *P. malariae*, and *P. knowlesi*. Consider malaria in patients who have recently traveled to endemic areas and present with an unexplained febrile illness.

Malaria transmission occurs in large areas of Central and South America, the Caribbean, sub-Saharan Africa, the Indian subcontinent, Southeast Asia, the Middle East, and Oceania (e.g., New Guinea, Solomon Islands). More than 50% of malaria cases in the United States, including most cases due to *P. falciparum*, arise from travel to sub-Saharan Africa. Resistance of *P. falciparum* to chloroquine and other drugs continues to spread and strains of *P. vivax* with chloroquine resistance have also been identified.

CLINICAL FEATURES

Plasmodial sporozoites first infect the liver, where asexual reproduction occurs in the exoerythrocytic stage. During this initial incubation stage, which usually lasts 1 to 4 weeks, patients are often asymptomatic. Partial chemoprophylaxis or incomplete immunity can prolong the incubation period to months or even years. The clinical signs of malaria first appear during the erythrocytic stage, which occurs when hepatocyte rupture releases merozoites to invade erythrocytes. In *P. vivax* and *P. ovale* infection, a portion of the intrahepatic forms are not released, but remain dormant as hypnozoites, which can reactivate a malaria infection after months or years.

Early symptoms of malaria are nonspecific, including fever, chills, malaise, myalgias, and headache. Chest pain, cough, abdominal pain, or arthralgias may also be seen. Patients then develop a high fever, followed by diaphoresis and exhaustion when fever abates. Classically, cycles of fever and chills followed by profuse diaphoresis and exhaustion occur at regular intervals, reflecting the ongoing and intermittent hemolysis of infected erythrocytes.

Physical examination findings are nonspecific. During a febrile paroxysm, most patients appear acutely ill, with high fever, tachycardia, and tachypnea. Splenomegaly and abdominal tenderness are common. In *P. falciparum* infections, hepatomegaly, edema, and scleral icterus often occur.

Infections caused by any species of *Plasmodium* can result in hemolysis with anemia, splenic enlargement, and potential splenic rupture. Severe or complicated malaria infections may also occur, and are usually due to *P. falciparum*. Prostration, severe anemia, acidosis, hypoglycemia, acute renal failure, acute respiratory distress syndrome, pulmonary edema, jaundice, shock, and disseminated intravascular coagulation may occur in severe infections. Cerebral malaria is characterized by somnolence, coma, delirium, and seizures. In 2011, 22% of malaria cases imported to the United States were classified as severe. Blackwater fever is a severe complication seen almost exclusively in *P. falciparum* infections, with massive intravascular hemolysis, jaundice, hemoglobinuria, and acute renal failure.

DIAGNOSIS AND DIFFERENTIAL

The diagnosis of malaria relies on a history of potential exposure in an endemic area, along with clinical symptoms, signs, and microscopic examination of thick and thin blood films. A thin blood film is used for counting heavy infections, while a thick blood film detects lower levels of parasitemia. In early infection, especially *with P. falciparum*, parasitemia may be initially undetectable due to hepatic sequestration of organisms. Parasite load in the peripheral circulation fluctuates over time and is highest during an acute rising fever with chills. Initiate appropriate therapy when malaria is suspected, even if the parasite is not detected on initial blood smears. If plasmodia are not initially visualized and malaria is a likely diagnosis, repeat blood smears at least twice daily (preferably during febrile episodes) as long as malaria is suspected or until the patient recovers. Once plasmodia are identified, the smear can further determine the percentage of red blood cells infected (which correlates with prognosis) and species type (in particular *P. falciparum*). Newer techniques for rapid diagnosis and speciation are also available. Sensitivity of such rapid tests is excellent for *P. falciparum* with high parasitemia levels, but poor for the other forms of malaria.

Nonspecific laboratory findings may include normochromic normocytic anemia with findings suggestive of hemolysis, a normal or mildly depressed total leukocyte count, thrombocytopenia, an elevated erythrocyte sedimentation rate, and mild abnormalities of liver and renal functions.

EMERGENCY DEPARTMENT CARE AND DISPOSITION

1. Base treatment decisions on the severity of the illness and the species of the infecting parasite.
2. Admit patients with uncomplicated infection due to *P. falciparum* to the hospital and treat using one of several regimens (see Table 95-1). Artemisinin-containing combination therapies are recommended by the World Health Organization. As of July 2013, the Centers for Disease Control and Prevention (CDC) recommends using chloroquine for *P. falciparum* malaria imported from areas of low chloroquine resistance including Central America (west of the Panama Canal), Haiti, the Dominican Republic, and parts of the Middle East. Dose options are listed at the CDC website (http://www.cdc.gov/malaria/).
3. Uncomplicated malaria infections due to *P. vivax*, *P. malariae*, or *P. ovale* can often be treated as an outpatient. If *P. knowlesi* is suspected, hospital admission is recommended. Recommended treatment for uncomplicated malaria infection due to *P. vivax*, *P. ovale*, *P. malariae*, and *P. knowlesi* is chloroquine. Treat adults with **chloroquine** 600 mg base (= 1 g salt) loading dose, then 300 mg base (= 500 mg salt) in 6 hours, then 300 mg base per day for 2 days (total dose 1550 mg base). Treat children with **chloroquine** 10 mg/kg base to maximum of 600 mg loading dose, then 5 mg/kg base in 6 hours and 5 mg/kg base per day for 2 days.

TABLE 95-1 Drug Options for Therapy of Uncomplicated *Plasmodium falciparum* Malaria

Treatment of Choice Is an Artemisinin-Containing Combination Therapy (ACT)		
Drug	**Adult Dose**	**Pediatric Dose**
Artemether-lumefantrine (CoArtem®; each tablet contains artemether 20 mg and lumefantrine 120 mg)	4 tablets twice daily for 3 days (the first two doses should be about 8 h apart)	• 5–15 kg: 1 tab initially, 1 tablet in 8 h, then 1 tablet every 12 h × 2 days • 15–25 kg: 2 tablets initially, 2 tablets in 8 h, then 2 tablets every 12 h × 2 days • 25–35 kg: 3 tablets initially, 3 tablets in 8 h, then 3 tablets every 12 h × 2 days • >35 kg: follow adult dosing
Artesunate-amodiaquine (where available; not available in the United States; each adult tablet contains artesunate 100 mg and amodiaquine hydrochloride salt 270 mg)	2 tablets once daily for 3 d	• 5 to <9 kg: 1 tablet/day of artesunate (AS) 25 mg/amodiaquine (AQ) 67.5 mg • 9 to <18 kg: 1 tablet/day of AS 50 mg/AQ 135 mg • 18 to <36 kg: 1 tablet/day of AS 100 mg/AQ 270 mg • ≥36 kg: 2 tablets/day of AS 100 mg/AQ 270 mg (adult dose)
Alternatives to ACT		
Drug	**Adult Dose**	**Pediatric Dose**
Atovaquone-proguanil (Malarone®; each adult tablet contains atovaquone 250 mg and proguanil 100 mg; each pediatric tablet contains atovaquone 62.5 mg and proguanil 25 mg)	4 tablets once daily for 3 days. Do not use for treatment if atovaquone-proguanil has been taken as chemoprophylaxis and the patient's current illness is a suspected treatment failure.	• 5–8 kg: 2 pediatric tablets × 3 days • 9–10 kg: 3 pediatric tablets × 3 days • 11–20 kg: 1 adult tablet × 3 days • 21–30 kg: 2 adult tablets × 3 days • 31–40 kg: 3 adult tablets × 3 days • >41 kg: adult dose
Quinine sulfate (plus doxycycline or clindamycin)	650 mg PO every 8 h for 3–7 days	10 mg sulfate salt/kg, up to adult dose PO every 8 h for 3–7 days
Plus		
Doxycycline	100 mg PO every 12 h for 7 days	2.2 mg/kg (up to adult dose of 100 mg) PO every 12 h for 7 days
Or in children under age 8 years		
Clindamycin		7 mg/kg PO every 8 h for 7 days

4. Chloroquine has no effect on the exoerythrocytic forms of *P. vivax* and *P. ovale*, which remain dormant in the liver. Unless treated with primaquine, relapse will occur. This treatment can be given after full recovery from the initial illness. Treat adults with **primaquine phosphate** 30 mg of base per day for 14 days. Treat children with **primaquine phosphate** 0.5 mg/kg base for 14 days. Primaquine should be avoided in patients with glucose-6-phosphate dehydrogenase deficiency because of hemolysis.

TABLE 95-2 Antimalarial Drug Options for Severe (Complicated) Malaria

Drug	Adult Dose	Pediatric Dose
Artesunate* (available from the CDC if quinidine fails to provide improvement; call 770-488-7788)	2.4 mg/kg IV at 0, 8, and 24 h, then daily. Artesunate can be given IM if necessary.	2.4 milligrams/kg IV at 0, 8, and 24 h, then daily. Artesunate can be given IM if necessary.
Quinidine gluconate (plus doxycycline or clindamycin)†	6.25 mg base (= 10 mg salt)/kg IV load over 2 h (maximum, 600 mg), follow with 0.0125 mg base (= 0.02 mg salt)/kg/min continuous infusion.	6.25 mg base (= 10 mg salt)/kg IV load over 2 h (maximum, 600 mg), follow with 0.0125 mg base (= 0.02 mg salt)/kg/min continuous infusion.
Plus		
Doxycycline	2.2 mg/kg IV (up to adult dose of 100 mg) every 12 h for 7 days.	2.2 mg/kg IV (up to adult dose of 100 mg) every 12 h for 7 days
Or in children under age 8 years		
Clindamycin		10 mg base/kg loading dose IV followed by 5 mg base/kg IV every 8 h for 7 days.

*Artesunate is considered the drug of choice by World Health Organization guidelines.

†Quinine dihydrochloride is an alternative to quinidine gluconate (20 mg [salt]/kg infused IV over 2–4 hours, then 10 mg/kg every 8 hours, can be given IM if necessary, as 50 mg/mL solution).

Abbreviation: CDC = Centers for Disease Control and Prevention.

5. For severe or complicated malaria infections, antimalarial drug options are listed in Table 95-2. Continue the treatment by a parenteral route for at least 24 hours. Monitor blood glucose as parenteral quinidine and quinine can cause severe hypoglycemia. These agents are also myocardial depressants, and thus contraindicated in patients with heart disease. Cardiac monitoring is recommended during administration.
6. Provide aggressive supportive care to all hospitalized ill patients, including appropriate IV fluid replacement, correction of metabolic derangements, and advanced support (e.g., dialysis or mechanical ventilation), as necessary.
7. The CDC has a malaria hotline: 770-488-7788 M-F, 9 am to 5 pm EST, and 770-488-7100 after hours, weekends, and holidays. The CDC website can be accessed at http://www.cdc.gov/malaria/ to obtain resistance patterns in various countries and information on malaria prophylaxis and treatment. When resistance patters are uncertain, concern for chloroquine resistance for initial treatment should be considered.

FURTHER READING

For further reading in *Tintinalli's Emergency Medicine: A Comprehensive Study Guide*, 8th ed., see Chapter 158, "Malaria," by Malcolm Molyneaux.

CHAPTER 96

Foodborne and Waterborne Diseases

Benjamin Weston

Foodborne disease may occur after consumption of food contaminated with bacteria, viruses, parasites, chemicals, or biotoxins. Viruses such as norovirus, astrovirus, rotavirus, and enteric adenovirus are the most common sources, with norovirus causing over half of all cases. Bacterial disease is often more severe and includes nontyphoidal *Salmonella*, which is the most common cause for hospitalization and associated death in the United States. Other bacterial causes may include *Clostridium perfringens*, *Campylobacter* spp., *Listeria monocytogenes*, *Shigella* spp., Shiga toxin-producing *Escherichia coli,* and *Staphylococcus aureus*. Parasitic causes include *Giardia lamblia*, *Toxoplasma gondii*, *Entamoeba histolytica,* and *Cryptosporidium.* In addition, patients may experience symptoms of scombroid or ciguatera poisoning after eating some types of fish associated with these toxin-induced syndromes.

Waterborne diseases occur from ingestion or contact with contaminated water. Symptoms are most commonly gastrointestinal or dermatologic in nature. Common organisms include those associated with foodborne illness as well as *Vibrio* species, *Aeromonas* species, *Pseudomonas aeruginosa*, *Yersinia* species, hepatitis A, nontuberculous *Mycobacterium,* and other less common organisms. The most common pathogen responsible for recreational waterborne disease outbreaks is *Cryptosporidium*.

CLINICAL FEATURES

Symptoms of both foodborne and ingested waterborne illness include nausea, vomiting, diarrhea, abdominal cramping, fever, dehydration, and malaise. A history of multiple family members or closely associated individuals with simultaneous symptoms is supportive of a suspected foodborne or ingested waterborne illness. Physical exam may reveal findings of dehydration, and some patients will have stool positive for frank or occult blood. Prolonged illness beyond two weeks suggests protozoan parasites. Shiga-toxin producing *Escherichia coli (E. coli)* infections may present with vomiting, abdominal cramping, bloody diarrhea, and mild fever, and may be complicated by hemolytic uremic syndrome, especially if antibiotic treatment is prescribed.

Patients with scombroid fish or ciguatera poisoning have symptoms similar to other foodborne illnesses and typically present one to six hours after ingestion. In addition to nausea and vomiting, patients with scombroid poisoning frequently have flushing and headache due to a histamine-mediated reaction. Those with ciguatera poisoning may have headaches, muscle aches, paresthesias, reversal of hot and cold sensation, or sensitivity to extreme temperatures, due to sodium channel-mediated nerve depolarizations.

The skin manifestations of waterborne illness may include localized cellulitis, painful indurated plaques of *Mycobacterium marinum*, or necrotizing infections and hemorrhagic bulla associated with *Vibrio vulnificus*. Patients with *Aeromonas hydrophila* skin infections often have a history of trauma associated with freshwater exposure, and may have foul smelling wounds.

DIAGNOSIS AND DIFFERENTIAL

Diagnostic testing is often not indicated as most of these illnesses are self-limited. For those patients who are more acutely ill, or if other significant diagnoses are being entertained, consider stool cultures with Gram stain, the neutrophil marker lactoferrin, electrolytes, and complete blood count. Fecal leukocyte testing is neither sensitive nor specific for invasive disease, and is a poor predictor of response to antibiotic treatment. Shiga toxin-producing *E. coli* and *Vibrio* cultures may require specific laboratory procedures (check local laboratory guidelines). Reserve ova and parasite testing for those patients with symptoms over two weeks, immunocompromise, community waterborne outbreaks, recent travel to endemic areas, or men who have sex with men. *Clostridium difficile* antigen testing may be indicated in those with prolonged symptoms, recent antibiotic use, significant comorbidities, or extremes of age. Likely pathogens to consider in the differential can often be identified based on clinical features of the presenting illness (Table 96-1).

EMERGENCY DEPARTMENT CARE AND DISPOSITION

Most cases are self-limited and improve with supportive treatment.

1. Initiate rehydration with oral fluids, if tolerated. Intravenous rehydration with normal saline will benefit patients who are significantly dehydrated or those with continued vomiting.
2. Antiemetics, such as **metoclopramide** 10 mg PO or IV, or **ondansetron** 4 PO or IV may facilitate oral rehydration. Antihistamines, such as **diphenhydramine** 25 mg PO or IV, may improve the symptoms of scombroid fish poisoning.
3. **Loperamide** 4 mg initially, then 2 mg after every unformed stool up to a maximum of 16 mg per day can be recommended for mild to moderate, nonbloody diarrhea in adults without fever.
4. Antibiotics are recommended for consideration in patients with moderate to severe traveler's diarrhea, symptoms for more than 1 week, patients requiring hospitalization, and immunocompromised hosts. Empiric antibiotics may include **ciprofloxacin** 500 mg PO twice per day for 3 to 5 days or **levofloxacin 500 mg PO once daily for 3 to 5 days**. Antibiotics and antimotility agents are contraindicated in patients with suspected *E. coli 0157:H7* as these can increase the risks of developing hemolytic–uremic syndrome. For specific pathogen treatment protocols, see Tables 159-3 to 159-6 in *Tintinalli's Emergency Medicine: A Comprehensive Study Guide*, 8th edition, Chapter 159.

TABLE 96-1 Clinical Features of Foodborne Infections

Clinical Presentation	Foodborne Pathogens
Gastroenteritis with vomiting as the primary symptom	Viral pathogens: *Norovirus*, *Rotavirus*, and *Astrovirus*; preformed toxins: *Staphylococcus aureus* and *Bacillus cereus*
Noninflammatory diarrhea (watery, nonbloody)	Can be any enteric pathogen, but classically: ETEC *Giardia* *Vibrio cholera* Enteric viruses *Cryptosporidium* *Cyclospora*
Inflammatory diarrhea (grossly bloody, fever)	*Shigella* *Campylobacter* *Salmonella* EIEC Shiga toxin-producing *Escherichia coli* O157:H7 and non-O157:H7 *Vibrio parahaemolyticus* *Yersinia* *Entamoeba*
Persistent diarrhea (>14 days)	Parasites: *Giardia* *Cyclospora* *Entamoeba* *Cryptosporidium*
Neurologic manifestations	Botulism (*Clostridium botulinum* toxin) Scombroid fish poisoning Ciguatera fish poisoning Tetrodotoxin Toxic mushroom ingestion Paralytic shellfish poisoning Guillain–Barré syndrome
Systemic illness	*Listeria monocytogenes* *Brucella* *Salmonella typhi* *Salmonella paratyphi* *Vibrio vulnificus* Hepatitis A and E

Abbreviations: EIEC, enteroinvasive *E. coli*; ETEC, enterotoxigenic *E. coli*.

5. Treat waterborne skin infections with tetanus vaccination and empiric antibiotics (see Table 96-2). Patients with necrotizing infections should have surgical consultation to consider operative debridement.
6. Most patients can be treated as outpatients; admission is indicated in those appearing toxic, those with significant dehydration or uncontrolled vomiting, the immunocompromised, or those at the extremes of age with significant symptoms.

TABLE 96-2 Treatment of Waterborne Skin Infections

Pathogen	Clinical Features of Skin Infection	Treatment
Vibrio vulnificus	Cellulitis with hemorrhagic bullae, septicemia	Doxycycline 100 mg IV twice per day plus fourth-generation cephalosporin; necrotizing infections require emergent surgical debridement
Aeromonas species	Cellulitis, necrotizing wound infections	Mild infections: ciprofloxacin 500 mg PO twice per day; severe infections: ciprofloxacin 400 mg IV twice per day plus an IV antipseudomonal penicillin or fourth-generation cephalosporin; necrotizing infections require emergent surgical debridement
Pseudomonas aeruginosa	Hot-tub folliculitis, cellulitis in immunocompromised/diabetics	Hot-tub folliculitis is usually self-limited. Severe infection: ciprofloxacin 400 mg IV twice per day plus an IV antipseudomonal penicillin or fourth-generation cephalosporin
Mycobacterium marinum	Granulomatous skin infections	Clarithromycin 500 mg PO twice per day or doxycycline 100 mg PO twice per day for 3 months; severe cases: combine with rifampin or ethambutol

FURTHER READING

For further reading in *Tintinalli's Emergency Medicine: A Comprehensive Study Guide*, 8th ed., see Chapter 159, "Food and Waterborne Diseases," by Lane M. Smith and Simon A. Mahler.

CHAPTER 97

Zoonotic Infections

David Gordon

Zoonotic infections are a class of specific diseases and infections that are naturally transmitted between vertebrate animals and humans. Transmission may occur via direct contact with an infected animal or animal product, by ingestion of contaminated water or food products, by inhalation, or through arthropod vectors—most commonly ticks. Diagnosis can be challenging because of the nonspecific nature of symptoms (e.g., fever, headache, and myalgias) which overlap with the presentation of many other infectious and autoimmune diseases. Consider zoonotic infections in patients presenting with viral-like illnesses in conjunction with occupational or geographical risk factors for zoonotic disease exposure and transmission. See Table 97-1 for a list of common systemic zoonotic

TABLE 97-1 Common Systemic Zoonotic Infections

Agent	Animal Reservoir	Physical Findings	Diagnostic Tests	Treatment
Aeromonas species	Fish, reptiles	Nonspecific fever, severe crepitant cellulitis with systemic toxicity, gastroenteritis	—	See Chapter 159, "Food and Waterborne Illnesses," in *Tintinalli's Emergency Medicine: A Comprehensive Study Guide*, 8th ed.
Brucella canis	Dogs	Nonspecific fever	Serologic testing, blood culture	Doxycycline plus gentamicin or rifampin. TMP-SMX plus gentamicin in children
Capnocytophaga	Dogs and cats	Fever, septic shock, and meningitis from infected bite	Culture of bite wound	Amoxicillin-clavulanate or clindamycin. Pip-Tazo or a carbapenem plus clindamycin/vancomycin for shock
Chlamydophila psittaci	Birds	Fever, flu-like illness, pneumonia, endocarditis, sepsis	Serologic testing and sputum culture	Doxycycline. Azithromycin and levofloxacin are alternatives
Coxiella burnetii	Cattle, sheep, goats. Occasionally cats	Fever, pneumonia, hepatitis, meningitis, endocarditis	Serologic testing, PCR	Doxycycline, with the possible alternative of a fluoroquinolone or macrolide
Ehrlichia species	Ticks	Nonspecific fever, sepsis, meningitis, hepatitis	Clinical diagnosis, serologic testing, peripheral blood smear, immunocytologic testing, PCR	Doxycycline recommended for all patients (even children and pregnancy). Rifampin is alternative

(Continued)

TABLE 97-1 Common Systemic Zoonotic Infections (Continued)

Agent	Animal Reservoir	Physical Findings	Diagnostic Tests	Treatment
Leptospira species	Birds, dogs, rodents	Fever, pneumonia, conjunctivitis, lymphadenopathy	Darkfield microscopic examination of body fluids, serologic testing	Penicillin G IV. Ceftriaxone IV alternative. Mild disease: oral doxycycline or amoxicillin or azithromycin
Francisella tularensis	Rabbits, cats, wild animals, biting insects	Fever, sepsis, meningitis, pneumonia, hepatitis, rash	Serologic testing (poses hazards to laboratory staff)	IV aminoglycosides. Alternative: Doxycycline or ciprofloxacin
Rickettsia rickettsii	Ticks	Fever, diarrhea, or typical presentation of Rocky Mountain spotted fever	Clinical diagnosis, rise in antibody titer between acute and convalescent serum, skin biopsy	Doxycycline or chloramphenicol
Salmonella enterica	Dogs, cats (rarely), reptiles (turtles)	Fever, abdominal pain, sepsis, cellulitis, meningitis, endocarditis, septic arthritis	Blood or stool culture	Fluoroquinolones or third-generation cephalosporins
Streptococcus iniae cellulitis	Fish, seafood	Fever, cellulitis	Wound culture, blood culture	β-Lactams except aztreonam. Alternatives: Azithromycin, clindamycin, fluoroquinolones
Yersinia pestis	Dogs, cats, rodents	Bubonic: fever, headache, buboes, or pneumonic: cough, chills, dyspnea, shock	Blood culture, culture of suspected sites	Doxycycline, fluoroquinolone, gentamicin, streptomycin, or chloramphenicol

Abbreviations: PCR, polymerase chain reaction; Pip-Tazo, piperacillin-tazobactam; TMP-SMX, trimethoprim-sulfamethoxazole.

infections and Table 97-2 for specific treatment recommendations for tick-borne diseases.

ROCKY MOUNTAIN SPOTTED FEVER

Rocky Mountain spotted fever (RMSF) is a tick-borne disease caused by *Rickettsia rickettsii*, a pleomorphic obligate intracellular organism. The primary vectors for transmission are the American dog tick (*Dermacentor variabilis*), Rocky Mountain wood tick (*Dermacentor andersoni*) and the brown dog tick (*Rhipicephalus sanguineus*). Most cases occur between April and September with peak occurrences in June and July. While

TABLE 97-2 Tick-borne Zoonotic Infections and Specific Treatment

Tick-borne Zoonotic Infection	Specific Treatment
Rocky Mountain spotted fever	Doxycycline 100 mg PO or IV twice a day for 7 days, or for 2 days after temperature normalizes. Some recommendations exist for an initial loading dose of 200 mg. For children weighing <45 kg, the dose is 2.2 mg/kg twice daily. Although doxycycline is contraindicated for use in pregnancy, it may be warranted in life-threatening situations. Chloramphenicol is an alternative; however, it has multiple toxic effects and contraindications, and may be difficult to obtain. Dosing is 50 mg/kg/d divided into four doses for 7 days.
Lyme disease	Primary stage or mild secondary: 14–21 days of doxycycline (100 mg PO twice a day), amoxicillin (500 mg PO three times a day in adults, 50 mg/kg/d divided three times a day in children), or cefuroxime (500 mg PO twice a day in adults, 30 mg/kg/d divided three times a day in children). Macrolides possible but less effective. Severe illness, CNS positive, or high-degree heart block: ceftriaxone 2 g IV for 14–30 days. A single 200-mg oral dose of doxycycline given within 72 h of a high-risk deer tick bite is effective in preventing Lyme disease.
Tick-borne relapsing fever	Doxycycline (100 mg PO/IV twice a day for 7–10 days). Alternative: erythromycin (500 mg PO/IV four times a day for 7–10 days). Chloramphenicol is an alternate.
Colorado tick fever	Treatment is supportive.
Tularemia	Adults: streptomycin, 1 g IM/IV twice a day, or gentamicin/tobramycin, 5 mg/kg IV divided every 8 h. Treat for 10 days. Children: streptomycin, 15 mg/kg IM twice daily (should not exceed 2 g/d). Mild disease: ciprofloxacin 750 mg PO twice a day or doxycycline 100 mg PO twice a day. Treat for 21 days. Prophylaxis for lab exposures: doxycycline 100 mg PO twice a day or ciprofloxacin 500 mg PO twice a day. Treat for 14 days.
Babesiosis	Atovaquone (750 mg PO every 12 h) plus azithromycin (500 mg PO on day 1, then 250–1000 mg daily). Treat for 10 days. If relapse occurs, treat for the longer duration: 6 weeks or 2 weeks after negative blood smear. Severe disease in adults: clindamycin (1200 mg IV twice a day or 600 mg PO three times a day) + quinine (650 mg PO three times a day). Treat for 7–10 days.
Ehrlichiosis and anaplasmosis	Doxycycline, 100 mg PO twice a day for 7–14 days. For children weighing <45 kg, the dose is 2.2 mg/kg twice a day.

cases have been reported in the majority of the continental United States, more than 60% have originated from five states: North Carolina, Tennessee, Oklahoma, Missouri, and Arkansas.

Clinical Features

Early findings of RMSF include fever, headache, myalgias, and malaise. Patients may also present with lymphadenopathy, nausea, vomiting, and diarrhea. In some patients, particularly children, abdominal pain and edema may be present. Late in the disease course, complications may include meningitis, encephalitis, renal failure, respiratory failure, and myocarditis.

The classic clinical triad for RMSF of fever, rash, and history of tick bite is uncommon as only about 50% of infected patients can recall a tick bite and the rash is absent in about 10% of cases. When the rash does occur, it typically develops 2 to 4 days after the onset of fever as a maculopapular eruption that may subsequently become petechial. Rash often appears on the ankles and wrists and then spreads centripetally to the trunk, usually sparing the face, and characteristically involves the palms and soles.

Diagnosis and Differential

The diagnosis of RMSF is largely clinical, with confirmation coming after treatment is initiated. In the absence of an alternative explanation, consider the possibility of RMSF in a febrile patient with a headache who lives in or recently traveled through an endemic region in the spring or summer seasons with possible exposure to ticks. Laboratory abnormalities are usually nonspecific, but RMSF is suggested by the combination of normal white and red cells, thrombocytopenia, elevated liver function tests, and hyponatremia. RMSF can be confirmed—typically outside of the emergency department setting—with a rise in antibody titer between acute and convalescent sera or via skin biopsy of the rash with immunofluorescence testing.

The differential diagnosis for patients with symptoms of RMSF includes viral illnesses, pneumonia, meningococcemia, ehrlichiosis, Kawasaki's disease, toxic shock syndrome, scarlet fever, and leptospirosis.

Emergency Department Care and Disposition

1. Recommended treatment for adults is **doxycycline** 100 mg PO or IV twice a day. Some recommend an initial loading dose of 200 mg. Treatment should continue for 7 days or until 3 days after resolution of fever.
2. Antibiotic therapy for children weighing <45 kg is **doxycycline** 2.2 mg/kg PO twice a day. Doxycycline has been used for short courses in children without significant staining of the teeth, and is recommended as therapy by both the American Academy of Pediatrics and Centers for Disease Control and Prevention as the treatment of choice for rickettsial diseases in children of all ages.

LYME DISEASE

Lyme disease remains the most common vector-borne zoonotic infection in the United States. The responsible organism is the spirochete *Borrelia burgdorferi* and the vector is the *Ixodes* deer tick (also known as the *black-legged tick*). In highly endemic areas, the transmission rate from a deer tick bite is about 3%, although there is minimal risk if the duration of attachment is <36 hours. Cases have been reported in all 48 continental states, but 95% of cases originate from 13 states in the northeast and northern midwest with peak disease transmission in May through August.

Clinical Features

Lyme disease is typically divided into three distinct stages although some patients may not progress through all stages, and stages may overlap or be separated by periods of remission. The *first stage* involves early localized disease and is characterized by the rash of erythema migrans which may be in conjunction with nonspecific constitutional and rheumatologic symptoms. The characteristic rash occurs within 2 to 30 days in 60% to 80% of cases, often begins at the site of the tick bite, and manifests as an erythematous plaque with central clearing. Other associated symptoms in the first stage of lyme disease include fatigue, headache, fever, neck stiffness, myalgias, arthralgias, and adenopathy.

The *second stage, early disseminated disease*, occurs within a few days to 6 months after initial infection. This stage is characterized by multiple secondary annular target-shaped skin lesions, fever, adenopathy, neuropathies, cardiac abnormalities, and arthritic problems. Approximately 15% of untreated patients develop neurologic complications such as cranial neuritis that may lead to the classically described bilateral facial nerve palsy. Other neurologic manifestations include headache, neck stiffness, difficulty with mentation, cerebellar ataxia, myelitis, encephalitis, motor or sensory radiculoneuritis, and mononeuritis multiplex. Oligoarticular arthritis can occur, usually affecting the large joints such as the knees. In 8% of patients, there are cardiac manifestations such as myopericarditis or varying degrees of atrioventricular (AV) block, which sometimes can require a temporary pacemaker for stabilization.

The *third stage, late disseminated disease*, occurs months to years after initial infection. It can be characterized by chronic arthritis, myocarditis, subacute encephalopathy, axonal polyneuropathy, and leukoencephalopathy. Symptoms can persist for a decade or more.

Diagnosis and Differential

Initial diagnosis of Lyme disease is based primarily on clinical features. Confirmation may be obtained via polymerase chain reaction (PCR) testing, polyvalent fluorescence immunoassay, or western immunoblot testing. Differential diagnosis depends on clinical manifestation of the disease stage, and may include southern tick-associated rash illness (STARI), cellulitis, erythema multiforme, tinea corporis, viral or bacterial meningitis, encephalitis, rheumatic fever, septic arthritis, endocarditis, and other inflammatory or autoimmune conditions.

Emergency Department Care and Disposition

1. Treat primary stage or mild secondary Lyme disease with 14 to 21 days of **doxycycline** 100 mg PO twice a day in adults, 2.2 mg/kg twice daily for children <45 kg, **amoxicillin** 500 mg PO three times a day in adults,

50 mg/kg/d divided three times a day in children, or **cefuroxime** 500 mg PO twice a day in adults, 30 mg/kg/d divided three times a day in children. Macrolides are less effective.

2. Treat severe illness, meningitis, radiculopathy, or high-degree heart block from lyme disease with **ceftriaxone** 2 g IV daily in adults, 50 to 75 mg/kg daily in children for 14 to 30 days.
3. Routine antibiotic prophylaxis for Lyme disease following a tick bite is not recommended. A single dose of **doxycycline** 200 mg in adults and 4 mg/kg in children at least 8 years old may be considered for a deer tick bite in areas highly endemic for Lyme disease when the suspected time of tick attachment is at least 36 hours and prophylaxis can be administered within 72 hours of tick removal.

EHRLICHIOSIS

Ehrlichiosis is a group of zoonotic diseases caused by infection from the *Ehrlichia* genus. These are small, gram-negative pleomorphic coccobacilli that infect circulating leukocytes. The lone star tick (*Amblyomma americanum*) serves as the primary vector while the white-tailed deer is the major animal reservoir in the southeastern United States.

Clinical Features

Symptoms usually develop within 1 to 2 weeks after a tick bite. Clinical manifestations may include fever, headache, malaise, nausea, vomiting, diarrhea, abdominal pain, and arthralgias. Fever is present in a majority of cases (97%). A rash of variable appearance may be present but is not common. A minority of patients progress to serious complications that may include renal failure, respiratory failure, and encephalitis.

Diagnosis and Differential

Diagnosis initially must be made on clinical grounds. Laboratory clues may include leukocytopenia, thrombocytopenia, and elevation of hepatic enzymes. During the first week of illness, a peripheral blood smear may show colonies of bacteria in the white blood cells in 20% of infected patients. PCR offers a specific test for confirmation but is not sensitive enough to be used to exclude illness based only on a negative result. An increase in antibody titer between the acute and convalescent phases of the illness may be used for diagnosis. The gold standard for diagnosis is an immunofluorescence assay.

The differential diagnosis includes RMSF, Lyme disease, babesiosis, anaplasmosis, viral illnesses, cholecystitis/cholangitis, malaria, meningitis, and typhoid.

Emergency Department Care and Disposition

1. **Doxycycline** 100 mg PO twice a day in adults, 2.2 mg/kg twice daily for children <45 kg is first-line treatment for adults and children of all ages. Treatment should continue until 3 to 5 days after fever resolution or 10 to 14 days after resolution of CNS symptoms in severe disease.
2. **Rifampin** 300 mg twice a day for adults can be used for patients with contraindications to doxycycline.

TULAREMIA

Tularemia is caused by *Francisella tularensis*, a small, gram-negative, nonmotile intracellular coccobacillus. The zoonotic vectors are ticks of the *Dermacentor* (wood tick, dog tick) and *Amblyomma* (lone star tick) species. The principal animal reservoirs include rabbits, hares, and deer. Methods of transmission include tick or fly bites, inhalation, and direct inoculation of broken skin or mucosa from the handling of infected animals.

Clinical Features

Clinical features at presentation depend on the route of inoculation. The most common *ulceroglandular* form is characterized by a maculopapular lesion that ulcerates at the site of a tick bite or wound inoculation, followed by painful regional adenopathy and systemic symptoms. *Glandular* tularemia consists of tender regional adenopathy without ulceration. The *typhoidal* form has the highest morbidity and complications such as organ failure, and it presents with fever, chills, headache, and abdominal pain. *Ocular-oropharyngeal* and *pneumonic* forms of the disease result from airborne deposition into the eyes and lungs.

Diagnosis and Differential

Laboratory findings are nonspecific in all forms of tularemia. Diagnosis can be determined by culture, direct fluorescent antibody, or PCR from specimens obtained by skin lesion swabs, lymph node sampling, or sputum. The multiple clinical variations of tularemia lead to a broad differential diagnosis that include pyogenic bacterial infection, syphilis, anthrax, plague, Q fever, psittacosis, typhoid, brucellosis, and rickettsial infection.

Emergency Department Care and Disposition

1. Treat adults with **streptomycin** 1 g IM twice a day or **gentamicin** 5 mg/kg/d IM or IV divided every 8 hours. Treat for 10 days.
2. Treat pediatric patients with **streptomycin** 15 mg/kg IM twice a day (maximum daily dose 2 g), or **gentamycin** 2.5 mg/kg IM/IV two or three times a day. Treat for 10 days.
3. Treat mild disease in adults with **ciprofloxacin** 750 mg PO twice a day or **doxycycline** 100 mg PO twice a day for 21 days.

ANTHRAX

Anthrax is an acute bacterial infection caused by *Bacillus anthracis*, an aerobic gram-positive rod that forms central oval spores. Human infection can result from inhalation of spores, inoculation of broken skin, bites from arthropods (fleas), or ingestion of inadequately cooked meat that is infected with the organism.

Clinical Features

Inhaled or pulmonic anthrax usually results from handling unsterilized, imported animal hides, or imported raw wool. It results in a mediastinitis, rather than a true pneumonia, and is almost always fatal. Initial presentation consists of flu-like symptoms, which progress over 2 to 3 days to include marked mediastinal and hilar edema and respiratory failure. Cutaneous anthrax (*woolsorter's disease*) accounts for 95% of all anthrax infections and begins with a pruritic macule at the inoculation site (most commonly fingers) that then progresses to an ulcerative lesion with multiple infectious serosanguinous vesicles containing the anthrax bacillus. The ulcer eventually progresses to a painless black eschar and falls off within 2 weeks. A small minority of untreated patients develop rapidly fatal bacteremia.

Diagnosis and Differential

Gram stain, direct fluorescent antibody stain, or culture of skin lesions or fluid from vesicles may establish the diagnosis. Blood cultures may also be positive. The differential diagnosis for inhalational anthrax includes influenza, tuberculosis, and other causes of mediastinitis (bacterial, viral, parasitic, sarcoidosis). With symptoms suspicious for cutaneous anthrax, warfarin necrosis, calciphylaxis, ischemic necrosis, tularemia, plague, spider/insect bite, mycobacterial infection, ecthyma gangrenosum, and aspergillosis/mucormycosis may also be considered.

Emergency Department Care and Disposition

1. The initial antibiotic therapy for patients with systemic anthrax with possible or confirmed meningitis consists of **ciprofloxacin** 400 mg IV every 8 hours *plus* **meropenem** 2 g every 8 hours *plus* **linezolid** 600 mg every 12 hours. Also, a one-time infusion of **raxibacumab** 40 mg/kg diluted over 2.25 hours should be considered. Systemic anthrax in patients when meningitis has been excluded can be treated with **ciprofloxacin** 400 mg IV every 8 hours *plus* **clindamycin** 900 mg every 8 hours *or* **linezolid** 600 mg every 12 hours. Consultation with infectious disease specialists is recommended for assistance in managing these patients.
2. Treat cutaneous anthrax without systemic involvement with **ciprofloxacin** 500 mg PO every 12 hours or **doxycycline** 100 mg PO every 12 hours. Duration of treatment is a 7- to 10-day course if naturally acquired from animals with anthrax and not suspected from a bioterrorism-related or aerosolized exposure. Duration of treatment is 60 days for bioterrorism-related cases.
3. A 60-day antibiotic course combined with a three-dose vaccination course may be considered as postexposure prophylaxis for exposed individuals, although the vaccine is not currently FDA approved for this purpose.

PLAGUE

Plague is caused by *Yersinia pestis*, which is a gram-negative aerobic bacillus. In the United States, it is found most often in rock squirrels and ground rodents of the southwest. The rodent flea serves as the primary vector. Transmission to humans occurs through the bite of an infected flea, consuming infected animals, or inhalation of animal secretions.

Clinical Features

An eschar frequently develops at the site of the flea bite and is followed by the development of an enlarged, suppurative, proximal lymph node known as a bubo. Sepsis and pneumonia may develop due to hematologic spread of the bacteria. Bubonic plague often presents with fever, headache, and buboes, while the pneumonic form of the disease is typically associated with cough, chills, dyspnea, and shock. The pneumonic form of the plague is highly contagious and can be transmitted from person to person via aerosolized respiratory secretions and can be rapidly fatal if not treated aggressively.

Diagnosis and Differential

Diagnosis of plague is typically made based on clinical findings in a patient with possible contact with a vector or animal host. Blood culture or culture of suspected sites may reveal organisms, but treatment should be initiated in suspected cases without awaiting culture results. The differential diagnosis includes lymphogranuloma venereum, syphilis, staphylococcal or streptococcal lymphadenitis, other causes of pneumonia, or tularemia.

Emergency Department Care and Disposition

1. Recommended antimicrobials are **gentamicin** 5 mg/kg IM/IV daily or **streptomycin** 15 mg/kg (or 1 g) IM twice a day. Treat for 10 days.
2. Pediatric dosing of **gentamicin** is 2 to 2.5 mg/kg/dose IM/IV every 8 hours.
3. Alternatives include **doxycycline** 100 mg IV twice a day (or 200 mg IV daily), **ciprofloxacin** 400 mg IV twice a day, or **chloramphenicol** 25 mg/kg IV every 6 hours. Treat for 10 days.

FURTHER READING

For further reading in *Tintinalli's Emergency Medicine: A Comprehensive Study Guide*, 8th ed., see Chapter 160, "Zoonotic Infections" by Bryan B. Kitch and John T. Meredith

CHAPTER 98 World Travelers

Bret A. Nicks

Patients returning from travel abroad may present with fever or other symptoms of infection. The evaluation of a potential infectious disease in a returning traveler requires an understanding of the geographical distribution of infections (Table 98-1), risk factors, incubation periods, clinical manifestations, and appropriate laboratory investigations. The Centers for Disease Control and Prevention (CDC) website provides additional health information for travelers based on specific locations around the world: http://wwwnc.cdc.gov/travel/destinations/list/. Some specific disease processes are covered elsewhere in this book: traveler's diarrhea, enteroviral infections, gastroenteritis, giardiasis, salmonellosis, and shigellosis are discussed in Chapters 37 and 96, anthrax and plague are discussed in Chapter 97, and malaria is discussed in Chapter 95. This chapter covers some of the other common infectious diseases that may present in patients returning from travel outside of the United States.

CLINICAL FEATURES

The incubation periods for many diseases are commonly longer than an individual traveler's foreign stay, and therefore travelers who are exposed to infectious diseases often develop symptoms of disease after they return from travel. Ask patients about visits to game parks, farms, caves, health facilities, consumption of exotic foods, activities involving fresh or salt water exposure, insect exposure, sexual activities, reported epidemics in the area visited, contact with ill people, and any pre-trip immunizations and prophylactic antibiotics that have been taken. Determine the chronological history of disease progression, including details about the quality, severity, duration, and episodic nature of fever and chills. When completing a complete history and physical examination, note the presence of any

TABLE 98-1 Regional Tropical Illnesses
Africa: malaria, human immunodeficiency virus, TB, hookworm, tapeworm, roundworm, brucellosis, yellow fever (and other hemorrhagic fevers such as Lassa fever or Ebola), relapsing fever, schistosomiasis, tick typhus, filariasis, strongyloidiasis
Central and South America: malaria, relapsing fever, dengue fever, filariasis, TB, schistosomiasis, Chagas' disease, typhus, Zika virus
Mexico and the Caribbean: dengue fever, hookworm, malaria, cysticercosis, amebiasis, Zika virus
Australia, New Zealand: dengue fever, Q fever, Murray Valley encephalitis, Japanese encephalitis
Middle East: hookworm, malaria, anthrax, brucellosis
Europe: giardiasis, Lyme disease, tickborne encephalitis, babesiosis
China and East Asia: dengue fever, hookworm, malaria, strongyloidiasis, hemorrhagic fever, Japanese encephalitis

Abbreviation: TB, tuberculosis.

TABLE 98-2 Physical Findings in Selected Tropical Infections

Physical Finding	Likely Infection or Disease
Rash	Dengue fever, typhus, syphilis, gonorrhea, Ebola fever, brucellosis, chikungunya, HIV seroconversion, Zika virus
Jaundice	Hepatitis, malaria, yellow fever, leptospirosis, relapsing fever
Lymphadenopathy	Rickettsial infections, brucellosis, HIV, Lassa fever, leishmaniasis, Epstein–Barr virus, cytomegalovirus, toxoplasmosis, trypanosomiasis
Hepatomegaly	Amebiasis, malaria, typhoid, hepatitis, leptospirosis
Splenomegaly	Malaria, relapsing fever, trypanosomiasis, typhoid, brucellosis, kala-azar, typhus, dengue fever, schistosomiasis
Eschar	Typhus, borreliosis, Crimean–Congo hemorrhagic fever, anthrax
Hemorrhage	Lassa, Marburg, or Ebola viruses; Crimean–Congo hemorrhagic fever; meningococcemia, epidemic louse-borne typhus

Abbreviation: HIV, human immunodeficiency virus.

abnormal findings such as fever, skin rash, hepatosplenomegaly, lymphadenopathy, and jaundice (Table 98-2).

DIAGNOSIS AND DIFFERENTIAL

Evaluate the results of laboratory studies to assess for abnormalities suggestive of specific disease processes. On a CBC with differential, look for lymphopenia (dengue, HIV, typhoid), eosinophilia (parasites, fungal disease), or thrombocytopenia (malaria, dengue, acute HIV, typhoid). Consider a blood smear and dipstick antigen test for malaria, if available, for travelers with fever who have recently visited endemic locations. Urinalysis may show proteinuria and hematuria in cases of leptospirosis. Obtain liver function tests if physical examination identifies jaundice. Consider testing for specific diseases suspected by symptoms and risk of exposure. Obtain a chest radiograph when respiratory symptoms are present, and consider a liver ultrasound if amoebic liver abscess is suspected.

EMERGENCY DEPARTMENT CARE AND DISPOSITION

1. **Dengue fever** is commonly known as break-bone fever, and is spread by the day-biting *Aedes aegypti* mosquito and caused by one of four different dengue viruses. Incubation is 4 to 7 days. Symptoms are high fever, headache, nausea, vomiting, myalgias, and rash. Dengue hemorrhagic fever, while classically associated with dengue in Southeast Asia, continues to expand globally and is characterized by high fever, vascular permeability, bleeding, hepatomegaly, and shock. Make the diagnosis using PCR (1 to 8 days after symptom onset) or IgM ELISA (after 4 days of symptoms). Daily blood counts are recommended. Outpatient treatment can be recommended in mild cases, with oral hydration as tolerated and close follow-up for blood work. Avoid aspirin and NSAIDs. Inpatient treatment is recommended for a drop of hemoglobin or platelets, hemorrhagic symptoms, or abnormal vital signs.
2. **Chikungunya** is a common arbovirus infection in returning travelers. Since 2013 when local transmission was first recognized in the

Americas, it has expanded to 45 countries or territories. This disease spreads by day-biting mosquitos (*Aedes aegypti* and *Aedes albopictus*), and presents very much like classic dengue fever with generalized arthralgia that progresses to chronic arthropathy in 5% to 30% of patients. Use PCR to diagnose 1 to 4 days after symptom onset or test for IgM levels after 5 days of symptoms. There is no preventative vaccine and no specific medication to treat chikungunya virus infection. Treatment is supportive and can include rest, fluids, and NSAIDs to relieve pain and fever. People infected with chikungunya should avoid further mosquito exposure during the first week of illness to reduce the risk of local transmission.

3. **Zika virus** is spread through the *Aedes* species mosquito. First discovered in 1947, outbreaks have been reported in Africa, Southeast Asia, and the Pacific Islands—including an outbreak in Brazil and the Americas starting in 2015. Symptoms are commonly fever, rash, joint pain, and conjunctivitis. The illness is usually mild and lasts for less than a week. Development of Guillain-Barré syndrome and congenital microcephaly has been associated with Zika virus infection. Treatment is supportive as no specific antiviral treatment is available for Zika virus disease.
4. **Typhoid fever**, also known as enteric fever, is caused by *Salmonella typhi* and *Salmonella paratyphi*. Transmission is from contaminated food or water, after contact with the infected urine or feces of symptomatic individuals, or asymptomatic carriers. Incubation is 1 to 3 weeks, and typhoid fever commonly lasts more than 10 days in returning travelers. Initial symptoms include fever with headache, and this progresses to high fevers with chills, headache, cough, abdominal distention, myalgias, constipation, and prostration. A classic presentation is a relative bradycardia despite a high fever, but this is often absent. After several days, a pale red macular rash known as "rose spots" appears on the trunk. Complications may include small bowel ulceration, anemia, disseminated intravascular coagulopathy (DIC), pneumonia, meningitis, myocarditis, and renal failure. Diagnosis is made based on clinical findings and can be confirmed by stool culture. Treat with **ceftriaxone** 2 g IV or IM for 14 days, or **ciprofloxacin** 500 to 750 mg PO twice daily for 14 days. For severe typhoid fever complicated by delirium, coma, shock, or DIC, administer an initial dose of **dexamethasone** 3 mg/kg IV. Blood transfusions may be required in severe cases.
5. **Brucellosis** is caused by the bacteria *Brucella*, and is most commonly contracted by contact with cattle, goats, camels, dogs, pigs, or after ingestion of unpasteurized milk or cheese. Symptoms include fever, abdominal pain, back pain, fatigue, headache, joint pain, and loss of appetite. Relapsing fever or a chronic low-grade fever is characteristic. Patients often have lymphadenopathy, hepatomegaly, and splenomegaly, and may develop a septic arthritis. Make the diagnosis based on blood culture results or confirmatory serology testing. Consult infectious disease to align treatment with **doxycycline**, **rifampicin**, **streptomycin** or **gentamicin** for 2 weeks with appropriate follow-up.
6. **Rickettsial spotted fevers** are transmitted by the bite, body fluid, or feces of ixodid arthropod ticks. Mortality without treatment approaches 25%. Scrub typhus (*Rickettsia orientalis*) and African tick

typhus (*R. conorii*) are the most common forms in travelers returning from Southeast Asia and Africa, respectively. Incubation period is 3 to 14 days. Symptoms may include fever, malaise, myalgias, severe headache, rash, nausea, and vomiting followed by lymphadenopathy and splenomegaly. The skin lesion in scrub typhus starts as a papule at the bite site, which later becomes necrotic and forms a crusted black eschar. Make the diagnosis based on clinical findings and use serologic tests to confirm the diagnosis after empiric treatment with **doxycycline** 100 mg twice daily for 7 to 10 days.

7. **Epidemic Louse-Borne Typhus** is common in Mexico, Guatemala, Ethiopia, and the Himalayas, and is caused by *R. prowazekii*. This illness is distinct from the disease caused by *S. typhi*. Incubation period is 8 to 12 days, and patients may or may not be aware of the louse exposure. Symptoms include high fevers, severe headache, and a maculopapular rash between 4 and 7 days. Make the diagnosis based on clinical features and use serologic tests to confirm the diagnosis after empiric treatment with **doxycycline** 100 mg twice daily for 7 to 10 days.
8. **Leptospirosis** occurs after fresh water exposure to *Leptospira interrogans* or after exposure to infected dogs. Incubation period is 2 to 20 days. Symptoms include high fever, severe headache, chills, myalgias, hepatitis, and conjunctival injection. Confirmation of this diagnosis is by serology. Treat mild disease within 3 days of symptoms with **amoxicillin** 500 mg three times daily or **doxycycline** 100 mg twice daily. Treat severe cases with **penicillin G** 5 MU every 6 hours IV, or **ceftriaxone** 1 g IV or IM daily for 7 to 14 days.
9. **Crimean–Congo hemorrhagic fever** is a tick-borne viral disease that is rising in frequency in Africa, Asia, Eastern Europe, and the Middle East. Agricultural workers are at the greatest risk, but this infection can also be acquired from contact with the blood of infected individuals. Symptoms include sudden onset of fever, headache, myalgia, dizziness, and possibly mental confusion. The hemorrhagic period starts the third to fifth day of illness with epistaxis, hemoptysis, GI bleeding, vaginal bleeding, or hematuria. Patients may have laboratory abnormalities such as thrombocytopenia, elevated liver enzymes and creatinine, or prolonged prothrombin time and activated partial thromboplastin time. Make the diagnosis based on clinical findings and confirm with serology. Treatment is supportive and may require transfusions or respiratory support in severe illness. For moderate to severe illness, treat with **ribavirin**.
10. **Yellow fever** is caused by a flavivirus transmitted by a day-biting mosquito, and occurs along a broad equatorial belt in South and Central America and Africa. Symptoms range from a mild flu-like illness to hemorrhagic fever with shock. While only 15% of patients progress to severe disease, these patients have an associated 20% to 50% mortality. After an incubation period of 3 to 6 days, typical early symptoms include fever, headache, myalgias, conjunctival injection, abdominal pain, prostration, facial flushing, and relative bradycardia. Symptoms later progress to jaundice, black emesis, and albuminuria. Severe illness may progress to shock, multiorgan failure, and bleeding. Treatment is supportive including transfusion as needed.

11. **Cysticercosis** is a systemic parasitic infection caused by dissemination of the larval cysts of the pork tapeworm. Humans become infected by ingesting contaminated food or inadvertent contact with contaminated soil. Involvement of almost any tissue can occur. CNS infection is known as neurocysticercosis, and is a common infectious cause of seizures worldwide. Additional symptoms of neurocysticercosis may include headache, visual or mental status changes, stroke, meningoencephalitis, and obstructive hydrocephalus. Noncontrast CT shows calcifications of inactive disease, and may reveal hydrocephalus. Treat with **praziquantel** 17 mg/kg three times daily. Steroids are recommended for those with encephalitis, hydrocephalus, or vasculitis.
12. **African trypanosomiasis (African sleeping sickness)** is caused by the microscopic parasite *Trypanosoma brucei*, and is transmitted by the tsetse fly. After a bite, a localized inflammatory reaction occurs and is followed in 2 to 3 days by a painless chancre that increases in size for 2 to 3 weeks and then gradually regresses. Intermittent fevers then develop with malaise and rash. When CNS infection develops, behavioral and neurologic changes occur with a progression from encephalitis to coma and eventual death. Other complications can include hemolysis, anemia, pancarditis, and meningoencephalitis. Make the diagnosis with rapid evaluation of blood smears for the mobile parasite. The specific drug and treatment course will depend on the type of infection. Consult infectious disease expert for diagnosis and treatment with **pentamidine** or other agents.
13. **Chagas disease (American trypanosomiasis)** is caused by the protozoan *T. cruzi* and is endemic in regions of Latin America and is reported as far north as Texas. This disease is spread by the nocturnal reduviid "kissing bug" or "assassin" bug. Acute phase illness begins with unilateral periorbital edema or painful cutaneous edema at the site of skin penetration (chagoma). The subsequent toxemic phase is characterized by parasitemia with lymphadenopathy and hepatosplenomegaly. The acute phase diagnosis is made by blood culture or examination of peripheral blood smears demonstrating motile parasites. In the chronic phase, serologic tests or tissue biopsy are useful to make the diagnosis. Consult with infectious disease specialists for recommendations to treat with **nifurtimox, benznidazole**, or other agents.
14. **Visceral leishmaniasis** is caused by the intracellular protozoan *Leishmania* that is transmitted by *Lutzomyia* or *Phlebotomus* sandflies. This disease may be found in patients who serve in the military, adventure travelers, field biologists, and emigrants from endemic zones. Visceral leishmaniasis presents with fever, weight loss, hepatosplenomegaly, pancytopenia, and hypergammaglobulinemia. Treat with pentavalent antimonial compounds, such as **sodium stibogluconate** (available through the CDC) or **miltefosine**.
15. **Schistosomiasis** larvae are released into fresh water by snails. Soon after exposure, patients develop a macular-papular pruritic dermatitis over the lower legs. Four to 8 weeks later, fever occurs with headache, cough, urticaria, diarrhea, hepatosplenomegaly, and hypereosinophilia. Worms mature in the venous blood and deposit eggs in the bladder, GI tract, brain, skin, and liver. Diagnosis is suspected from eosinophilia and microscopic identification of eggs in midday urines or stools. Treat

with **praziquantel** 20 mg/kg, two doses in a single day, except with GI involvement, where three doses in a single day are suggested.

16. **Amebiasis** is caused by pathogenic species such as *Entamoeba histolytica* that are endemic to Asia, Africa, and Latin America. Amebiasis is typically spread by asymptomatic carriers whose excrement contains encysted organisms. Incubation is 1 to 3 weeks for colitis, and weeks to months for liver abscess. Symptoms are commonly mild and include loose stool and stomach cramping. Amebic dysentery, a severe form of amebiasis, includes bloody diarrhea, abdominal pain, fever, dehydration, and weight loss. Liver abscess, a rare complication, causes fever, right upper quadrant pain, chronic abdominal pain, and weight loss. Stool for ova and parasites is diagnostic and an ultrasound can identify liver abscess. Treat with **metronidazole** 500 to 750 mg PO three times daily for 10 days.
17. **Ascariasis** is caused by infection with *Ascaris lumbricoides* and can develop after ingestion of street vendor foods or vegetables fertilized by human or animal feces. Symptoms may include a dry cough or pneumonia, as young worms are expectorated and migrate from the lungs to the esophagus and gut. A large worm burden can lead to malnutrition and weakness, and a mass of worms may lead to bowel obstruction. Diagnosis is with stool examination and serology. Treat with **mebendazole** 100 mg PO daily for 3 days or 500 mg PO as a single dose, or **albendazole** 400 mg PO single dose, or **ivermectin** 150 to 200 μg/kg PO single dose.
18. **Enterobiasis (seatworm or pinworm)** infection is typically spread via the fecal-oral route from contaminated objects. Patients experience intense perianal itching, and the diagnosis can be confirmed with a cellophane tape swab of the anus to identify the parasite. Treat with **mebendazole** 100 mg PO single dose and repeat in 2 weeks, or **albendazole** 400 mg PO single dose and repeat in 2 weeks, or **pyrantel pamoate** 11 mg/kg (up to 1 g) PO single dose and repeat in 2 weeks.
19. **Hookworm** infection is caused by *Ancylostoma duodenale* and *Necator americanus* and follows exposure to contaminated soil. Worms may migrate to the lungs, be coughed up, and access the GI tract after being swallowed. Symptoms include abdominal pain, severe anemia, and cutaneous larva migrans with red burrows visible underneath the skin. Treat with **albendazole** 400 mg PO single dose, **mebendazole** 100 mg PO twice daily for 3 days or 500 mg PO single dose, or **pyrantel pamoate**, 11 mg/kg (up to 1 g) PO daily for 3 days.
20. **Tapeworm Infections** occur after ingestion of undercooked pork (*Taenia solium*), beef (*Taenia saginata*), or fish (*Diphyllobothrium latum*). Symptoms include diarrhea, abdominal pain, bowel obstruction, and taenia cysts in eye, heart, and brain. Diagnosis is by stool examination or serology. Treat with **praziquantel** 5 to 10 mg/kg PO single dose.

FURTHER READING

For further reading in *Tintinalli's Emergency Medicine: A Comprehensive Study Guide*, 8th ed., see Chapter 161, "Global Travelers," by Raghu Venugopal and Shawn D'Andrea.

CHAPTER 99 The Transplant Patient

Sarah E. Unterman

Management of patients with transplanted organs in the emergency department (ED) involves three general areas: (1) disorders specific to certain transplanted organs, (2) disorders common to many different kinds of transplant patients due to an immunosuppressed state or antirejection medications, and (3) disorders not specifically related to a transplanted organ but where special care may be warranted due to associated medications or altered physiology. Disorders specific to the transplanted organ are manifestations of acute rejection, surgical complications specific to the procedure performed, and altered physiology (most important in cardiac transplantation). The most common conditions that prompt transplant patients to present to the ED are infections (39%), noninfectious gastrointestinal (GI) or genitourinary pathology (15%), dehydration (15%), electrolyte disturbances (10%), cardiopulmonary pathology (10%) or injury (8%), and rejection (6%).

POSTTRANSPLANT INFECTIOUS COMPLICATIONS

Posttransplant infections are the most common presenting diagnosis to the ED for this patient population, in part due to the ongoing immunosuppression required for transplant recipients. Additional infection risk factors include diabetes mellitus, advanced age, obesity, and other host factors. Table 99-1 lists the broad array of potential infections and the time after transplant they are most likely to occur.

TABLE 99-1 Infections Stratified by Posttransplant Period

Period after Transplant/ Conditions	Infection	Comments
<1 mo: resistant organisms	• MRSA • Vancomycin-resistant *Enterococcus faecalis* • *Candida* species (including non-albicans)	Opportunistic infections are generally absent during this period as full effect of immunosuppression not complete. MRSA important in HSCT patients.
<1 mo: complications of surgery and hospitalization	• Aspiration • Catheter infection • Wound infection • Anastomotic leaks and ischemia • *C. difficile* colitis	*Clostridium difficile* common during this period. Early graft injuries may abscess. Unexplained early signs of infection such as hepatitis, encephalitis, pneumonitis, or rash may be donor derived.
<1 mo: colonization of transplanted organ or HSCT neutropenia	• *Aspergillus* • *Pseudomonas* • *Klebsiella* • *Legionella*	Microbiologic analysis of aspirates or biopsy from surgery essential for therapeutic decisions.

(Continued)

TABLE 99-1 Infections Stratified by Posttransplant Period (Continued)

Period after Transplant/ Conditions	Infection	Comments
<1 mo: HSCT-specific infections	• Additional bacterial pathogens: *Streptococcus viridans* and enterococci • Viral infections include respiratory syncytial virus and HSV	Neutropenia and mucocutaneous injury increase risk for HSCT patients. Lungs, bloodstream, and GI tract most commonly affected sites.
1–6 mo: in patients with *Pneumocystis jirovecii* pneumonia and antiviral (CMV, HBV) prophylaxis	• Polyomavirus BK infection, nephropathy • *C. difficile* colitis • HCV infection • Adenovirus infection, influenza • *Cryptococcus neoformans* infection • *Mycobacterium tuberculosis* infection • Anastomotic complications	Activation of latent infections, relapse, residual, and opportunistic infections occur during this period. Viral pathogens and allograft rejection cause the majority of febrile episodes during this period. Polyomavirus BK, adenovirus infections, and recurrent HCV are becoming more common.
1–6 mo: in patients without prophylaxis	• *Pneumocystis* • Infection with herpesviruses (HSV, varicella-zoster virus, CMV, Epstein–Barr virus) • HBV infection • Infection with *Listeria, Nocardia, Toxoplasma, Strongyloides, Leishmania, Trypanosoma cruzi*	Discontinuation of prophylaxis at the end of this period may prompt active infection, especially CMV. Graft-versus-host disease and mucocutaneous injury increase risk for HSCT patients.
>6 mo: general	• Community-acquired pneumonia and urinary tract infections • Infection with *Aspergillus*, atypical molds, *Mucor* species • Infection with *Nocardia, Rhodococcus* species	Community-acquired organisms dominate during this period. Transplant recipients have a persistently increased risk of infection due to community-acquired pathogens.
>6 mo: late viral infections	• CMV infection (colitis and retinitis) • Hepatitis (HBV, HCV) • HSV encephalitis • Community-acquired viral infections (severe acute respiratory syndrome, West Nile) • JC polyomavirus infection (progressive multifocal leukoencephalopathy) • Skin cancer, lymphoma (PTLD)	In some patients, chronic viral infections may cause allograft injury (e.g., cirrhosis from HCV infection in liver transplant recipients, bronchiolitis obliterans in lung transplant recipients, accelerated vasculopathy in heart transplant recipients with CMV infection) or a malignant condition such as PTLD or skin or anogenital cancers.

Abbreviations: CMV, cytomegalovirus; HBV, hepatitis B virus; HCV, hepatitis C virus; HSCT,hematopoietic stem cell transplant; HSV, herpes simplex virus; MRSA, methicillin-resistant *Staphylococcus aureus*; PTLD, posttransplantation lymphoproliferative disorder.

Clinical Features

The most common reason for transplant recipients to present to the ED is fever, although as many as half of transplant patients with serious infections can present without fever. When fever is present, the underlying cause in addition to a possible infection can be drug side effects, hypersensitivity reactions, rejection, or malignancy.

Diagnosis and Differential

Pneumonia and urinary tract infections are the most common infections found in this population. Blood counts, inflammatory markers, and tests of renal and liver function may be helpful to obtain in this group of complex patients. Maintain a low threshold for obtaining chest radiographs. Obtain appropriate cultures of urine, blood, and other bodily fluids based on patient symptoms, presentation, physical examination findings, and disease severity. Consider the possibility of central nervous system infections such as meningitis or encephalitis and perform lumbar puncture when appropriate. Liver transplant patients are especially susceptible to intraabdominal infections during the first postoperative month. Lung transplant patients are prone to pneumonia. Cardiac transplant patients may develop mediastinitis during the first postoperative month.

Emergency Department Care and Disposition

1. When an infection is diagnosed in a patient with an organ transplant, consider consultation with the transplant team to help determine recommended treatment medications and duration.
2. For infections of skin and superficial wounds, a broad-spectrum antibiotic plus an agent specific to MRSA is recommended. Common treatment options include **imipenem** 500 mg IV every 6 hours, *or* **meropenem** 1 g IV every 8 hours, *or* **piperacillin/tazobactam** 3.375 IV every 6 hours *plus* **vancomycin** 1 g IV every 12 hours *or* **linezolid** 600 mg IV every 12 hours.
3. Pneumonia may be caused by a wide variety of organisms from common to atypical to opportunistic. Treatment options include **imipenem** 500 mg IV every 6 hours, **meropenem** 1 g IV every 8 hours, **cefotaxime** 1 to 2 g IV every 6 to 8 hours *plus* **gentamicin** 1 to 2 mg/kg IV every 8 hours, *or* **piperacillin/tazobactam** 3.375 g IV every 6 hours. Add MRSA-specific therapy, listed above, and fungal therapy, listed below, if suspected.
4. Intraabdominal infections may be due to enteric gram-negative aerobic, obligate anaerobic bacilli and facultative bacilli, or enteric gram-positive streptococci. Recommended coverage is to combine **metronidazole** 500 mg IV every 12 hours *plus* one of the following agents: **imipenem** 500 mg IV every 6 hours, **meropenem** 1 g IV every 8 hours, **doripenem** 500 mg IV every 8 hours, *or* **piperacillin/tazobactam** 3.375 g IV every 6 hours.
5. The initial treatment of suspected fungal disease is **fluconazole** 400 mg daily IV; **amphotericin B** 0.7 mg/kg/d IV has been a mainstay of treatment but has more toxicity than fluconazole. For oral or esophageal *Candida*, treat with **fluconazole** 200 mg PO on day 1 followed by 100 mg PO daily.

6. Suspected CMV disease is treated with **ganciclovir** 5 mg/kg IV twice daily. For bone marrow transplant patients, add immunoglobulin.
7. Disseminated or ocular varicella and herpes simplex virus are typically treated with **acyclovir** 800 mg IV five times a day. Adjust dosing in the presence of renal insufficiency. Alternatives include **valacyclovir** 1000 mg every 8 hours *or* **famciclovir** 500 mg every 8 hours.
8. Treatment for *Pneumocystis jirovecii* pneumonia starts with prednisone 80 mg/d followed immediately by antimicrobial therapy. First choice is **trimethoprim/sulfamethoxazole** (TMP-SMX) 15 mg/kg/d IV divided every 8 hours while critically ill. Oral therapy is TMP-SMX double strength (DS) two tablets PO every 8 hours for 3 weeks of total therapy. **Pentamidine** 4 mg/kg/d IV *or* IM for 3 weeks, *or* **clindamycin** 600 mg IV *plus* **primaquine** 30 mg orally daily are reserved as alternative therapies if TMP-SMX is not tolerated.
9. Toxoplasmosis can be treated initially with **pyrimethamine** 200 mg PO initially *then* 50 to 75 mg PO daily *plus* **sulfadiazine** 1 to 4 g PO daily *plus* **folinic acid** 10 mg PO daily.
10. Urinary tract infections (see Chapter 53), invasive gastroenteritis (due to *Salmonella, Campylobacter*, and *Listeria*, see Chapter 37 and Chapter 96), and diverticulitis (see Chapter 44) can be treated with commonly recommended antimicrobial agents.

COMPLICATIONS OF IMMUNOSUPPRESSIVE AGENTS

Therapeutic immunosuppression is associated with a number of adverse effects and complications. These adverse effects are typically gradual in onset and may include pancreatitis, bleeding, hypoglycemia or hyperglycemia, bradycardia or tachycardia, hyperkalemia, hypertension or hypotension, cardiotoxicity, pulmonary edema, seizures, thromboembolic events, and thrombocytopenia. Medication side effects such as fever or rigors may be similar to symptoms that would otherwise suggest an infection. A headache syndrome often indistinguishable from migraine is common in transplant recipients and usually develops within the first two months of immunosuppression, and may require an initial workup to exclude life-threatening conditions such as a mass lesion or infection. As the number of immunosuppressive drugs has increased dramatically, a complete listing of adverse effects is beyond the scope of this manual. Please refer to the parent textbook, referenced at the end of this chapter, or to web resources for a more complete listing of side effects of these medications.

An illness that prevents a transplant patient from successfully taking his or her immunosuppressive therapy may warrant hospital admission for IV therapy. Consider discussing new medications with a member of the patient's transplant team, as starting even simple medications can precipitate complications.

CARDIAC TRANSPLANTATION

Heart transplantation results in a denervated heart that does not respond with centrally mediated tachycardia in response to stress or exercise, but does respond appropriately to circulating catecholamines. Patients therefore may experience fatigue or shortness of breath at the onset of exercise before an appropriate increase in heart rate occurs over time to meet the metabolic demand. A donor heart is implanted with its sinus node intact to preserve normal atrioventricular conduction, and therefore a normal heart rate is typically 90 to 100 beats/min. However, electrocardiograms frequently will have two distinct P waves as the technique of cardiac transplantation also preserves the recipient's native sinus node at the superior cavoatrial junction. The sinus node of the donor heart is easily identified by its constant 1:1 relation to the QRS complex, whereas the native P wave appears independently through the donor heart rhythm.

Clinical Features

Because the heart is denervated, patients experiencing myocardial ischemia do not present with angina. Instead, heart transplant recipients may present with heart failure secondary to silent myocardial infarctions. Evaluate transplant recipients who have new-onset shortness of breath, chest fullness, or symptoms of congestive heart failure with an electrocardiogram and serial troponin levels to evaluate for the possible presence of myocardial ischemia or infarction.

Although most episodes of acute cardiac transplant rejection are asymptomatic, the most common symptoms that do occur are dysrhythmias and generalized fatigue. Consider the possibility of transplant rejection for patients who present with atrial or ventricular dysrhythmia or symptoms of acute heart failure. In children, rejection may present with low-grade fever, fussiness, and poor feeding.

Emergency Department Care and Disposition

1. Treat acute rejection with **methylprednisolone** 1 g IV after consultation with a representative from the transplant center. Treatment for rejection is typically begun after biopsy confirmation unless the patient is hemodynamically unstable.
2. **Atropine** has no effect on a denervated heart and is not recommended for bradydysrhythmias in heart transplant patients. Instead, administer **isoproterenol** 2 to 10 μg/min IV infusion.
3. Treat hypotension with inotropic agents such as **dopamine** 2 to 20 μg/kg/min IV or **dobutamine** 2 to 20 μg/kg/min IV.
4. Symptoms concerning for acute rejection or another illness requiring hospitalization should prompt transfer to a transplantation center, when possible.

LUNG TRANSPLANTATION

Clinical Features

A lung transplant patient suffering rejection may develop cough, chest tightness, fever, and hypoxemia. Infection, such as interstitial pneumonia, may present with a clinical picture similar to acute rejection. Acute rejection can manifest very quickly, with a severe and rapid decline in patient status and in some circumstances an isolated fever may be the only initial finding. Spirometry may show a >10% drop in forced expiratory volume in 1 second, and physical examination may reveal rales and adventitious sounds. Chest radiograph may demonstrate bilateral interstitial infiltrates or effusions but may be normal in some patients, particularly when rejection occurs longer than 6 weeks after transplant. The further removed a patient is from transplant, the less classic a chest radiograph may appear for acute rejection. Bronchoscopy with a transbronchial biopsy is usually needed to confirm rejection and exclude infection.

Diagnosis and Differential

To assess a lung transplant patient for findings of infection or acute rejection, clinicians may obtain a chest radiograph, pulse oximetry, arterial blood gas analysis, spirometry, complete blood cell count, serum electrolytes, creatinine and magnesium levels, and appropriate drug levels.

Emergency Department Care and Disposition

1. Initiate empiric antibiotics for suspected infection (see above recommendations).
2. Treat acute rejection with **methylprednisolone** 1 g IV after consultation with a representative from the transplant center.
3. Symptoms concerning for acute rejection or another illness requiring hospitalization should prompt transfer to a transplantation center, when possible.

RENAL TRANSPLANT

Clinical Features

Renal transplant recipients with symptoms of acute rejection complain of vague tenderness over the allograft, which is typically located in the left or right iliac fossa. Patients also may describe decreased urine output, rapid weight gain from fluid retention, low-grade fever, and generalized malaise. Physical examination may reveal worsening hypertension, allograft tenderness, and peripheral edema. The absence of these symptoms and signs, however, may not entirely exclude the possibility of acute rejection, as an asymptomatic decline in renal function may be the only initial finding to suggest acute rejection.

Diagnosis and Differential

Even small changes in creatinine values may be important in assessing a renal transplant patient's risk of acute rejection. When rejection is suspected, obtain a urinalysis, renal ultrasonography, levels of immunosuppressive drugs, and a thorough history and examination. Interpret changes in renal function in the context of prior data such as trends of recent serum creatinine levels, recent history of rejection, or other causes of allograft dysfunction. In addition to considering acute rejection, evaluate for other potential causes of decreased renal function such as dehydration or cyclosporine-induced nephrotoxicity.

Imaging may be helpful to evaluate the graft. Renal ultrasound can detect urinary obstruction. MRI can be used to detect hematomas and fluid collections, vascular abnormalities, and infarctions caused by medication-induced vasculitis. Discuss imaging options with the transplant team, particularly before using gadolinium-based contrast agents in a renal transplant patient.

Emergency Department Care and Disposition

1. Treat acute rejection with **methylprednisolone** 1 g IV after consultation with a representative from the transplant center.
2. Symptoms concerning for acute rejection or another illness requiring hospitalization should prompt transfer to a transplantation center, when possible.

LIVER TRANSPLANT

Clinical Features

Although frequently subtle in presentation, a syndrome of acute liver transplant rejection includes fever, liver tenderness, lymphocytosis, eosinophilia, liver enzyme elevation, and a change in bile color or production. In the perioperative period, the differential diagnosis also includes infection, acute biliary obstruction, or vascular insufficiency. Diagnosis can be made with certainty only by hepatic ultrasound and biopsy, which usually requires referral back to the transplant center for diagnosis and management of this complication.

Possible postsurgical complications in liver transplant patients include biliary obstruction, biliary leakage, and hepatic artery thrombosis. Biliary obstruction follows three typical presentations: (1) intermittent episodes of fever and fluctuating liver function tests, (2) a gradual worsening of liver function tests without symptoms, and (3) acute bacterial cholangitis with fever, chills, abdominal pain, jaundice, and bacteremia. These complications can be difficult to distinguish clinically from rejection, hepatic artery thrombosis, CMV infection, or a recurrence of a preexisting disease such as hepatitis.

If a postsurgical biliary complication is suspected, obtain a chest radiograph, complete blood count, serum chemistry levels, liver function tests, basic coagulation studies, and lipase levels. Consider cultures of blood, urine, bile, or ascites, as appropriate. An abdominal ultrasound can evaluate for fluid collections, thrombosis of the hepatic artery or portal vein, and dilatation of the biliary tree. Alternatively, abdominal computed tomography can be used. Some patients may benefit from cholangiography or ERCP if biliary obstruction is suspected.

Biliary leakage is associated with 50% mortality and occurs most frequently in the third or fourth postoperative week. This high rate of mortality may be related to concomitant hepatic artery thrombosis, infection of leaked bile, or difficult repair when the tissue is inflamed. Patients most often have peritoneal signs and fever, but these signs may be masked by use of steroids and immunosuppressive agents. Laboratory studies may reveal elevated prothrombin time and transaminase levels with little or no bile production. This complication also may present as acute graft failure, liver abscess, unexplained sepsis, or biliary tract leakage, obstruction, abscess, or breakdown of the anastomosis.

Emergency Department Care and Disposition

1. Treat acute rejection with **methylprednisolone** 1 g IV after consultation with a representative from the transplant center.
2. Symptoms concerning for acute rejection or another illness requiring hospitalization should prompt transfer to a transplantation center, when possible.

3. Surgical complications are best managed at the original transplant center, when possible. Biliary obstruction is managed with balloon dilatation, and all patients should receive broad-spectrum antibiotics against gram-negative and gram-positive enteric organisms, such as **metronidazole** 500 mg IV every 12 hours *plus* one of the following agents: **imipenem** 500 mg IV every 6 hours *or* **piperacillin/tazobactam** 3.375 g IV every 6 hours. Biliary leakage is treated surgically, and hepatic artery thrombosis may require retransplantation.

HEMATOPOIETIC STEM CELL TRANSPLANT

Hematopoietic stem cell transplant (HSCT) is performed for a variety of conditions, including hematopoietic malignancies, severe anemia, and other conditions. The most common complication of HSCT is graft-versus-host disease, affecting approximately 50% of HSCT patients.

Clinical Features

A HSCT recipient presenting to the ED with nonspecific maculopapular rash (see Fig. 99-1) should be evaluated for possible graft-versus-host disease. The rash may be pruritic or painful, and frequently demonstrates a

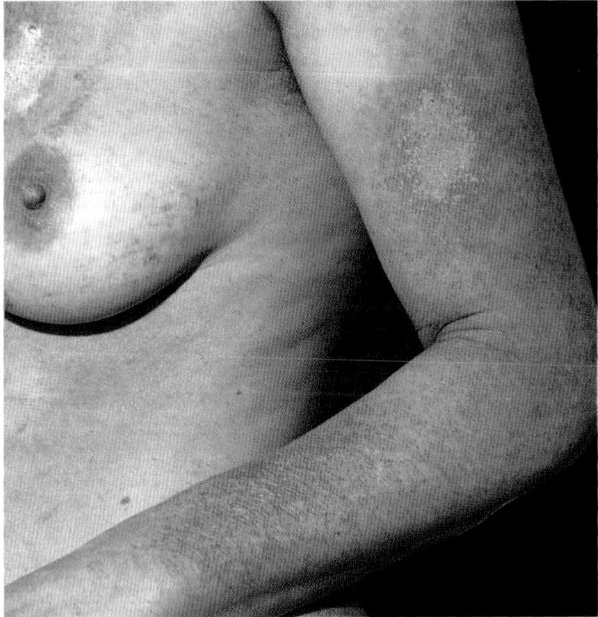

FIGURE 99-1. Rash of acute cutaneous graft-versus-host disease. The maculopapular lesions have acquired a brownish hue and there is slight scaling. Reproduced with permission from Wolff KL, Johnson R, Suurmond R. *Fitzpatrick's Color Atlas & Synopsis of Clinical Dermatology.* 6th ed. New York: McGraw-Hill; 2009.

brownish hue with slight scaling. The distribution varies greatly but often involves palms and soles initially, and later progresses to cheek, ears, neck, trunk, chest, and upper back. In the more severe forms, skin involvement is erythrodermic or may show bullae formation. Mucositis has been reported to occur in 35% to 70% of patients.

The second most common presentation of graft-versus-host disease is diarrhea. Upper GI symptoms such as anorexia, nausea, and emesis are common. The patient may develop painful cramping, ileus, and, sometimes, life-threatening hemorrhage from the colon.

Diagnosis and Differential

The initial diagnosis of graft-versus-host disease is made on clinical grounds. A patient with a significant GI hemorrhage in the early posttransplant period may have coagulation deficits, especially thrombocytopenia. The differential diagnosis of GI bleeding in this setting includes all the usual causes in addition to infection. Hepatic involvement presents with hyperbilirubinemia and elevated liver function tests.

Emergency Department Care and Disposition

1. Most patients with graft-versus-host disease will need supportive care in consultation with the patient's transplant team for management including possible admission or transfer to the transplant center.
2. Initiate **prednisone** 60 mg PO daily, or **methylprednisolone** at 1 to 2 mg/kg IV daily.
3. If other immunosuppressants have recently been tapered or discontinued, these are generally increased or reinstituted in the setting of a new diagnosis of graft-versus-host disease.

FURTHER READING

For further reading in *Tintinalli's Emergency Medicine: A Comprehensive Study Guide*, 8th ed., see Chapter 297, "The Transplant Patient," by J. Hayes Calvert.

SECTION 11

Toxicology and Pharmacology

CHAPTER 100 General Management of the Poisoned Patient

L. Keith French

Death from unintentional poisoning is a growing problem worldwide and prevention requires a multi-disciplinary approach. Knowledge of appropriate decontamination techniques and timely administration of antidotes coupled with excellent supportive care may positively alter the outcome of poisoned patients.

CLINICAL FEATURES

A detailed history is essential in the evaluation of a potentially poisoned patient. In the conscious, cooperative person, the specific agent(s), time, route, amount, and intent of exposure need to be determined. In the uncooperative or altered patient, adjunctive information from friends, family, prehospital providers, police, or bystanders may provide more accurate details. Environmental clues such as drug paraphernalia, empty pill bottles, odors, or suicide notes may aid in the diagnosis. If available, review hospital records for recent prescriptions or any history of psychiatric illness. Loose pills with imprint codes may be identified by the pharmacy or Poison Center.

A thorough exam begins with a completely disrobed patient. Review all vital signs and perform a comprehensive physical examination. Focus on the general appearance, level of consciousness, pupil size, mucous membranes, respiratory rate, breath sounds, presence of bowel sounds, skin temperature, and muscle tone as the combination of findings may suggest a specific toxidrome (Table 100-1). Important clinical features in the poisoned patient include hypoglycemia, cardiac dysrhythmias, seizures, agitation, and temperature alterations.

DIAGNOSIS AND DIFFERENTIAL

A diagnosis of poisoning is established primarily through the history, though the physical examination may provide clues when a history is not possible. Specific toxicology screens may be available, but are, in general, of limited utility and seldom impact care or outcome (Table 100-2). False-negative or false-positive results for drugs of abuse may be confusing and

TABLE 100-1 Common Toxidromes

Toxidrome	Examples of Agents	Examination Findings (most common in bold)
Anticholinergic	Atropine, *Datura* spp., antihistamines, antipsychotics	**Altered mental status, mydriasis, dry flushed skin, urinary retention, decreased bowel sounds, hyperthermia, dry mucous membranes** Seizures, arrhythmias, rhabdomyolysis
Cholinergic	Organophosphate and carbamate insecticides Chemical warfare agents (Sarin, VX)	**Salivation, lacrimation, diaphoresis, vomiting, urination, defecation, bronchorrhea, muscle fasciculations, weakness** Miosis/mydriasis, bradycardia, seizures
Ethanolic	Ethanol	**Central nervous system depression, ataxia, dysarthria, odor of ethanol**
Extrapyramidal	Risperidone, haloperidol, phenothiazines	**Dystonia, torticollis, muscle rigidity** Choreoathetosis, hyperreflexia, seizures
Hallucinogenic	Phencyclidine Psilocybin, mescaline Lysergic acid diethylamide	**Hallucinations, dysphoria, anxiety** Nausea, sympathomimetic signs
Hypoglycemic	Sulfonylureas Insulin	**Altered mental status, diaphoresis, tachycardia, hypertension** Dysarthria, behavioral change, seizures
Neuromuscular malignant	Antipsychotics	**Severe muscle rigidity, hyperpyrexia, altered mental status** Autonomic instability, diaphoresis, mutism, incontinence
Opioid	Codeine Heroin Morphine	**Miosis, respiratory depression, central nervous system depression** Hypothermia, bradycardia
Salicylate	Aspirin Oil of Wintergreen (methyl salicylate)	**Altered mental status, respiratory alkalosis, metabolic acidosis, tinnitus, tachypnea, tachycardia, diaphoresis, nausea, vomiting** Hyperpyrexia (low grade)
Sedative/hypnotic	Benzodiazepines Barbiturates	**Central nervous system depression, ataxia, dysarthria** Bradycardia, respiratory depression
Serotonin	SSRIs MAOIs Tricyclic antidepressants Amphetamines Fentanyl St. John's wort	**Altered mental status, hyperreflexia and hypertonia (>lower limbs), clonus, tachycardia, diaphoresis** Hypertension, flushing, tremor
Sympathomimetic	Amphetamines Cocaine Cathinones	**Agitation, tachycardia, hypertension, hyperpyrexia, diaphoresis** Seizures, acute coronary syndrome

Abbreviations: MAOI = monoamine oxidase inhibitor; SSRI = selective serotonin reuptake inhibitor.

TABLE 100-2 Drug Concentrations That May Assist Patient Assessment or Management

Acetaminophen	Methanol
Carbamazepine	Methotrexate
Carbon monoxide	Paraquat
Digoxin	Phenobarbital
Ethanol	Phenytoin
Ethylene glycol	Salicylate
Iron	Theophylline
Lithium	Valproic acid
Methemoglobin	

potentially distracting. Consider empiric testing for acetaminophen and aspirin in all potentially poisoned patients. Complementary testing includes blood glucose concentration, serum lactate/electrolytes, renal/liver function, urine HCG, and electrocardiography.

EMERGENCY DEPARTMENT CARE AND DISPOSITION

1. Gross decontamination should occur **prior** to patient entry into the ED. Observe universal precautions and don personal protective gear. Ensure that the victim's clothing and jewelry are removed/bagged.
2. The primary goal in management is **resuscitation**. Focus on assessment and stabilization of the airway, breathing, and circulation. Supportive care is often the only required intervention in the poisoned patient. Early **endotracheal intubation** may be necessary given the anticipated clinical course of some toxidromes. Treat hypotension with IV crystalloid infusions (10 to 20 mL/kg in children) before initiating pressors. Treat ventricular dysrhythmias according to standard ACLS/PALS protocols. Potentially useful medications in the management of toxin-induced cardiac arrest are listed in Table 100-3.
3. The **proper** and timely use of antidotes (Table 100-4) is paramount in the management for select poisoned patients. Rarely, however, does antidotal therapy trump standard resuscitation steps. Focus first on resuscitation measures as listed above.
4. Altered mental status and coma are common presentations of many intoxicants. Reasonable empiric treatments include supplemental oxygen, naloxone (0.2 to 2 mg IV/IO/IM), glucose (1 to 1.5 g/kg IV/IO), and thiamine (10 to 100 mg IV/IO) in the adult patient.
5. Seizures from toxins generally respond to benzodiazepines (first-line) or barbiturates (second-line). Isoniazid (INH) poisoning may precipitate seizures which are refractory to benzodiazepines or barbiturates. Treatment for INH poisoning requires pyridoxine. Hypoglycemia and hyponatremia should be excluded as the etiology for seizures. Phenytoin is not effective in toxin-induced seizures and is not recommended.

TABLE 100-3 Potential Interventions in Toxin-Induced Cardiac Arrest

Toxin or Toxin/Drug Class	Intervention
Toxins with a specific antidote (examples) Digoxin Organophosphates Envenomation	Antidote Digoxin Fab Atropine Antivenom
Sodium channel blocker or wide-complex tachycardia	Sodium bicarbonate
Calcium channel blocker or β-blocker	High-dose insulin
Local anesthetic agents Lipophilic cardiotoxins	IV lipid emulsion
Other Therapies to Consider	
Cardiac pacing Intra-aortic balloon pump Extracorporeal membrane oxygenation	

TABLE 100-4 Common Antidotes: Initial Dosages and Indications

Antidote	Pediatric Dose	Adult Dose	Indication
Calcium chloride 10% 27.2 mg/mL elemental Ca	0.2–0.25 mL/kg IV	10 mL IV	Calcium channel antagonists
Calcium gluconate 10% 9 mg/mL elemental Ca	0.6–0.8 mL/kg IV	10–30 mL IV	Hypermagnesemia Hypocalcemia
Cyanide antidote kit Amyl nitrite	Not typically used	1 ampule O_2 chamber of ventilation bag 30 s on/30 s off	Cyanide Hydrogen sulfide (use only sodium nitrite)
Sodium nitrite (3% solution)	0.33 mL/kg IV	10 mL IV	Cyanide
Sodium thiosulfate (25% solution)	1.65 mL/kg IV	50 mL IV	Cyanide
Dextrose (glucose)	0.5 g/kg IV	1 g/kg IV	Insulin Oral hypoglycemics
Digoxin Fab Acute toxicity	1–2 vials IV	5–10 vials	Digoxin and other cardioactive steroids
Flumazenil	0.01 mg/kg IV	0.2 mg IV	Benzodiazepines
Glucagon	50–150 μg/kg IV	3–10 mg IV	Calcium channel blockers β-Blockers
Hydroxocobalamin	70 mg/kg IV (maximum 5 g). Can be repeated up to 3 times. Administer with sodium thiosulfate.		Cyanide Nitroprusside

(continued)

TABLE 100-4 Common Antidotes: Initial Dosages and Indications (continued)

Antidote	Pediatric Dose	Adult Dose	Indication
IV lipid emulsion 20%	1.5 mL/kg IV bolus over 1 min (may be repeated two times at 5-min intervals), followed by 0.25 mL/kg per minute	100-mL IV bolus over 1 min, followed by 400 mL IV over 20 min	Local anesthetic toxicity Rescue therapy for lipophilic cardiotoxins
Methylene blue	1–2 mg/kg IV Neonates: 0.3–1.0 mg/kg IV	1–2 mg/kg IV	Oxidizing toxins (e.g., nitrites, benzocaine, sulfonamides)
Naloxone	As much as required Start: 0.01 mg IV	As much as required Start: 0.1–0.4 mg IV	Opioids Clonidine
Pyridoxine	Gram for gram if amount isoniazid ingested is known		Isoniazid *Gyromitra esculenta* Hydrazine
	70 mg/kg IV (maximum 5 g)	5 g IV	
Sodium bicarbonate	1–2 mEq/kg IV bolus followed by 2 mEq/kg per h IV infusion		Sodium channel blockers Urinary alkalinization
Thiamine	5–10 mg IV	100 mg IV	Wernicke's syndrome Wet beriberi

6. Once stabilized, **surface decontamination** is the next priority in care. If not previously done, completely disrobe the patient. Dermal toxins must be removed from the skin by irrigation. Ocular exposure often requires pain control with topical agents. Copiously irrigate the eye with isotonic crystalloid. This may require several liters before restoration of physiologic pH. Ophthalmology consultation is recommended for all ocular alkali injuries.
7. Gastrointestinal decontamination is achieved via removal of the toxin from the stomach, binding toxin within the GI tract, or enhancing transit time through the gut. The particular method(s) utilized, if any, depends on the route, timing, amount, and nature of the toxin. Consider GI decontamination if (1) the exposure is expected to cause significant toxicity, (2) GI decontamination is expected to positively affect clinical outcome, and (3) the risk/benefit ratio favors GI decontamination. GI decontamination should only be instituted when an airway is patent/protected. Table 100-5 lists the indications, contraindications, and complications of several GI decontamination modalities.
   a. Inducing emesis with syrup of ipecac is no longer recommended for routine use in the ED. **Orogastric lavage (OG)** is now rarely used in the management of poisoned patients due to potentially serious consequences and unproven benefit. Only consider OG lavage when the poison was ingested within an hour of presentation and the nature/dose of the poison is likely to cause clinical deterioration despite supportive care or antidotal therapy. This procedure requires advance-

TABLE 100-5 Indications, Contraindications, and Complications of Gastrointestinal Decontamination Procedures

Orogastric Lavage	
Indications	Rarely indicated Consider for recent (<1 h) ingestion of life-threatening amount of a toxin for which there is no effective treatment once absorbed
Contraindications	Corrosive/hydrocarbon ingestion Supportive care/antidote likely to lead to recovery Unprotected airway Unstable, requiring further resuscitation (hypotension, seizures)
Complications	Aspiration pneumonia/hypoxia Water intoxication Hypothermia Laryngospasm Mechanical injury to gastrointestinal tract Time consuming, resulting in delay instituting other definitive care
Activated Charcoal	Adults 50 g orally, children 1 g/kg orally
Indications	Ingestion within the previous hour of a toxic substance known to be adsorbed by activated charcoal, where the benefits of administration are judged to outweigh the risks
Contraindications	Nontoxic ingestion Toxin not adsorbed by activated charcoal Recovery will occur without administration of activate charcoal Unprotected airway Corrosive ingestion Possibility of upper gastrointestinal perforation
Complications	Vomiting Aspiration of the activated charcoal Impaired absorption of orally administered antidotes
Whole-Bowel Irrigation	Polyethylene glycol 2 L/h in adults, children 25 mL/kg per hour (maximum 2 L/h)
Indications (potential)	Iron ingestion >60 mg/kg with opacities on abdominal radiograph Life-threatening ingestion of diltiazem or verapamil Body packers or stuffers Slow-release potassium ingestion Lead ingestion (including paint flakes containing lead) Symptomatic arsenic trioxide ingestion Life-threatening ingestions of lithium
Contraindications	Unprotected airway Gastrointestinal perforation, obstruction or ileus, hemorrhage Intractable vomiting Cardiovascular instability
Complications	Nausea, vomiting Pulmonary aspiration Time consuming; possible delay instituting other definitive care

ment of a 36F to 40F orogastric tube into the stomach while the patient lies in a left lateral position. The head of the bed should be tilted down 20°. Aliquots of roughly 200 mL (10 mL/kg in children) of warm tap water are instilled into the stomach, then removed via gravity or suction. The procedure continues until the effluent is clear.

b. Activated charcoal (AC) binds a large number of xenobiotics and prevents their absorption across the GI tract. AC does not effectively absorb metals, corrosives, or alcohols. AC is not recommended for routine use, and an individual risk assessment needs to be made before administration. Consider using if the xenobiotic is still available for adsorption or >60 minutes after ingestion for xenobiotics that slow GI motility (e.g., anticholinergics) or form bezoars (e.g., salicylates). The recommended dose is 1 g/kg.

c. **Whole-bowel irrigation** (WBI) is accomplished through drinking or NG tube instillation of **polyethylene glycol.** The infusion is continued until the rectal effluent is clear or passage of foreign body (e.g., drug packet) occurs. Do not use WBI if bowel sounds are absent or if ileus/obstruction is suspected (Table 100-5).

8. Considerations for enhanced elimination depend on the specific toxin and response to standard treatment. Multi-dose activated charcoal, urinary **alkalinization,** and **extracorporeal removal** (hemodialysis) are the three of the most commonly utilized modalities. Indications and contraindications to use are listed in Tables 100-6 and 100-7.

TABLE 100-6 Indications, Contraindications, and Complications or Enhanced Elimination Procedures

Multidose Activated Charcoal	Initial dose: 50 g (1 g/kg children), repeat dose 25 g (0.5 g/kg children) every 2 h
Indications	Carbamazepine coma (reduces duration of coma) Phenobarbital coma (reduces duration of coma) Dapsone toxicity with significant methemoglobinemia Quinine overdose Theophylline overdose if hemodialysis/hemoperfusion unavailable
Contraindications	Unprotected airway Bowel obstruction Caution in ingestions resulting in reduced gastrointestinal motility
Complications	Vomiting Pulmonary aspiration Constipation Charcoal bezoar, bowel obstruction/perforation
Urinary Alkalinization	
Indications	Moderate to severe salicylate toxicity not meeting criteria for hemodialysis Phenobarbital (multidose activated charcoal superior) Chlorophenoxy herbicides (2-4-dichlorophenoxyacetic acid and mecoprop): requires high urine flow rate 600 mL/h to be effective Chlorpropamide: supportive care/IV dextrose normally sufficient

(continued)

TABLE 100-6 Indications, Contraindications, and Complications or Enhanced Elimination Procedures (continued)

Multidose Activated Charcoal	Initial dose: 50 g (1 g/kg children), repeat dose 25 g (0.5 g/kg children) every 2 h
Contraindications	Preexisting fluid overload Renal impairment Uncorrected hypokalemia
Complications	Hypokalemia Volume overload Alkalemia Hypocalcemia (usually mild)

TABLE 100-7 Indications, Contraindications, and Complications of Extracorporeal Removal Techniques

Hemodialysis	Movement of solute down a concentration gradient across a semipermeable membrane	
Toxin requirements	Low volume of distribution, low protein binding, low endogenous clearance, low molecular weight	
Indications	**Life-threatening poisoning by:** Lithium Metformin lactic acidosis Phenobarbital Salicylates Valproic acid	Methanol/ethylene glycol Metformin-induced lactic acidosis Potassium salts Theophylline
Contraindications	Hemodynamic instability Infants (generally)	Poor vascular access Significant coagulopathy
Hemoperfusion	Movement of toxin from blood, plasma, or plasma proteins onto a bed of activated charcoal (or other adsorbent)	
Toxin requirements	Low volume of distribution, low endogenous clearance, bound by activated charcoal	
Indications	**Life-threatening poisoning caused by:** Theophylline (high-flux hemodialysis is an alternative) Carbamazepine (multidose activated charcoal or high-efficiency hemodialysis also effective) Paraquat (theoretical benefit only if instituted early after exposure)	
Contraindications	Hemodynamic instability Infants (generally) Poor vascular access	Significant coagulopathy Toxin not bound to activated charcoal
Continuous Renal Replacement Therapies	Movement of toxin and solute across a semipermeable membrane in response to hydrostatic gradient. Can be combined with dialysis	
Indications (potential)	Life-threatening ingestions of toxins when hemodialysis or hemoperfusion is indicated, but is unavailable, or hemodynamic instability precludes their utilization	
Contraindications	Hemodialysis or hemoperfusion is available Poor vascular access Significant coagulopathy	

(continued)

TABLE 100-7 Indications, Contraindications, and Complications of Extracorporeal Removal Techniques (continued)

Complications of Extracorporeal Removal Techniques	
Fluid/metabolic disruption	Limited by hypotension (not continuous renal replacement therapy)
Removal of antidotes	Infection/bleeding at catheter site
Limited availability	Intracranial hemorrhage secondary to anticoagulation

9. Intravenous Lipid Emulsion Therapy (ILET) is a potentially beneficial option for the management of life-threatening cardiotoxicity precipitated by lipid soluble xenobiotics (e.g., local anesthetics, tricyclic antidepressants, lipophilic beta-blockers) when conventional therapies have failed to improve the patient's condition.
10. Disposition depends on the nature of the intoxicant. Medical management is the priority and special attention must be made for exposures that may result in delayed toxicity.
11. Consider early consultation with a toxicologist and Poison Center for all poisonings. Consult with a mental health specialist for all intentional overdoses. Consider neglect or abuse in pediatric exposures.

FURTHER READING

For further reading in *Tintinalli's Emergency Medicine: A Comprehensive Study Guide*, 8th ed., see Chapter 176, "General Management of Poisoned Patients," by Shaun Greene

CHAPTER 101

Anticholinergic Toxicity

O. John Ma

CLINICAL FEATURES

Clinical findings include hypotension or hypertension, tachycardia, hypoactive or absent bowel sounds, urinary retention, flushed skin, hyperthermia, dry skin and mucus membranes, mydriasis, confusion, agitation, disorientation, and auditory and visual hallucinations. Table 101-1 compares muscarinic and antimuscarinic effects.

DIAGNOSIS AND DIFFERENTIAL

The diagnosis is primarily clinical. In isolated anticholinergic toxicity, routine laboratory studies should be normal, and routine toxicology screening is often of little value. Nonetheless, check electrolytes, glucose, and creatine phosphokinase levels. The differential diagnosis includes viral

TABLE 101-1 Muscarinic and Antimuscarinic Effects

Organ	Stimulation or Muscarinic Effect	Antagonism or Antimuscarinic Effect
Brain	Complex interactions Possible improvement in memory	Complex interactions Impairs memory Produces agitation, delirium, and hallucinations Fever
Eye	↓ pupil size (miosis) ↓ intraocular pressure ↑ tear production	↑ pupil size (mydriasis) ↑ intraocular pressure Loss of accommodation (blurred vision)
Mouth	↑ saliva production	↓ saliva production Dry mucous membranes
Lungs	Bronchospasm ↑ bronchial secretions	Bronchodilation
Heart	↓ heart rate Slows atrioventricular conduction	↑ heart rate Enhances atrioventricular conduction
Peripheral vasculature	Vasodilation (modest)	Vasoconstriction (very modest)
GI	↑ motility ↑ gastric acid production Produces emesis	↓ motility ↓ gastric acid production
Urinary	Stimulates bladder contraction and expulsion of urine	↓ bladder activity Promotes urinary retention
Skin	↑ sweat production	↓ sweat production (dry skin) Cutaneous vasodilation (flushed appearance)

encephalitis, Reye syndrome, head trauma, other intoxications, neuroleptic malignant syndrome, delirium tremens, acute psychiatric disorders, and sympathomimetic toxicity.

EMERGENCY DEPARTMENT CARE AND DISPOSITION

Treatment is primarily supportive. The goal is to prevent life-threatening complications, which include status epilepticus, hyperthermia, cardiovascular collapse, and rhabdomyolysis.

1. Place the patient on a cardiac monitor and secure intravenous or intraosseous access.
2. **Activated charcoal** may decrease drug absorption, even beyond 1 hour of ingestion.
3. Monitor temperature. Treat hyperthermia using conventional methods.
4. Hypertension usually does not require intervention, but should be treated conventionally as necessary.
5. Standard antidysrhythmics are usually effective, but avoid class IA medications (e.g., procainamide). Treat dysrhythmias, widened QRS complexes, and hypotension from sodium blocking agents (e.g., cyclic antidepressants) with IV **sodium bicarbonate** 1 mEq/kg.
6. Treat agitation with benzodiazepines, such as **lorazepam** 2 to 4 mg IV or 0.1 mg/kg). Avoid use of phenothiazines.
7. Treat seizures with benzodiazepines, such as lorazepam 2 mg IV or 0.1 mg/kg.
8. **Physostigmine** treatment is controversial. It is indicated if conventional therapy fails to control seizures, severe agitation, unstable dysrhythmias, coma with respiratory depression, malignant hypertension, or hypotension. The initial dose is 0.5 to 2 mg IV (0.02 mg/kg in children, maximum dose 2 mg), slowly administered over 5 minutes. When effective, a significant decrease in agitation may be apparent within 15 to 20 minutes. Physostigmine may worsen cyclic antidepressant toxicity and lead to bradycardia and asystole. It is contraindicated in patients with cardiovascular or peripheral vascular disease, bronchospasm, intestinal or bladder obstruction, cardiac conduction disturbances, and suspected concomitant sodium channel antagonist poisoning. Observe the patient for cholinergic excess.
9. If diagnosis of anticholinergic poisoning is unclear, then do not administer a diagnostic challenge of physostigmine in order to avoid the small but increased risk of adverse effects in patients without anticholinergic toxicity.
10. Patients with mild anticholinergic toxicity can be discharged after 6 hours of observation if their symptoms have resolved. Admit more symptomatic patients for 24 hours of observation. Patients who receive physostigmine usually require a 24-hour admission.

FURTHER READING

For further reading in *Tintinalli's Emergency Medicine: A Comprehensive Study Guide*, 8th ed., see Chapter 202, "Anticholinergics," by Dan Quan and Frank Lovecchio.

CHAPTER 102 Psychopharmacologic Agents

Shan Yin

CYCLIC ANTIDEPRESSANTS

Cyclic antidepressants inhibit reuptake of norepinephrine and serotonin, block sodium channels, and antagonize postsynaptic serotonin receptors. They can produce severe toxicity in overdose. Their use has declined as newer, safer agents have been developed.

Clinical Features

Toxicity may present with altered mental status, seizures, cardiac conduction or rhythm disturbances, hypotension, respiratory depression, and, in severe cases, coma. If serious toxicity is going to develop, it generally develops within 6 hours of the ingestion.

Diagnosis

The diagnosis is clinical. Characteristic ECG changes include sinus tachycardia; right axis deviation of the terminal 40 ms; PR, QRS, and QT interval prolongation. Right bundle-branch block, A-V blocks, and the Brugada pattern are less common. Amoxapine can notably cause toxicity without characteristic ECG changes.

Emergency Department Care and Disposition

Care is primarily supportive.

1. Obtain IV access, and initiate cardiac rhythm and ECG monitoring.
2. Consider using 1 g/kg of **activated charcoal** PO if no contraindications exist.
3. Hypotension is treated with isotonic crystalloids. **Norepinephrine or epinephrine** is indicated if hypotension persists.
4. Treat conduction disturbances and ventricular dysrhythmias with **sodium bicarbonate** as an IV bolus of 1 to 2 mEq/kg, repeated until the patient improves or until blood pH is 7.50 to 7.55. A continuous IV infusion (150 mEq added to 1 L of 5% dextrose in water) may be used at a rate of 2 to 3 mL/kg/h.
5. Treat torsades de pointes with 2 g of IV **magnesium sulfate**.
6. Control agitation with **benzodiazepines**. Avoid physostigmine.
7. Treat seizures with **benzodiazepines**. **Phenobarbital**, starting at 10 to 15 mg/kg IV, may be required for refractory seizures.
8. Patients who remain asymptomatic after 6 hours do not need admission for toxicologic reasons. Admit symptomatic patients to a monitored bed or intensive care unit (ICU).

ATYPICAL ANTIDEPRESSANTS, SEROTONIN REUPTAKE INHIBITORS, AND SEROTONIN SYNDROME

Newer antidepressants include trazodone, bupropion, mirtazapine, selective serotonin reuptake inhibitors, and serotonin/norepinephrine reuptake inhibitors. They are safer than older agents but can still cause toxicity, including the serotonin syndrome.

TRAZODONE

Clinical Features

Symptoms of toxicity include central nervous system depression, ataxia, dizziness, seizures, orthostatic hypotension, vomiting, and abdominal pain. ECG abnormalities include QT interval prolongation, sinus bradycardia and tachycardia, and torsades de pointes. Priapism can be seen at therapeutic doses.

Emergency Department Care and Disposition

Supportive care is generally sufficient in isolated overdoses.

1. Initiate cardiac rhythm monitoring and obtain a 12-lead ECG.
2. Consider single-dose **activated charcoal if no contraindications exist**.
3. Treat hypotension with isotonic IV fluids, followed by **norepinephrine**.
4. Treat torsades de pointes with IV **magnesium sulfate** or **overdrive pacing**.
5. Discharge patients who remain asymptomatic for at least 6 hours, with psychiatric evaluation as indicated. Admit those with neurologic and/or cardiac symptoms to a monitored bed.

BUPROPION

Clinical Features

Toxicity manifests as agitation, dizziness, tremor, vomiting, drowsiness, and tachycardia. Seizures are more common than with other atypical antidepressants and can be the initial presenting sign. ECG changes include sinus tachycardia, QRS interval widening, and QT interval prolongation.

Emergency Department Care and Disposition

Seizures should be anticipated.

1. Start a peripheral IV line and initiate cardiac rhythm monitoring.
2. Consider activated charcoal if no contraindications exist.
3. Treat seizures with **benzodiazepines**, followed by **phenobarbital**.
4. Administer IV sodium bicarbonate for QRS prolongation.
5. Consider IV lipid emulsion for refractory cardiovascular instability.
6. Observe asymptomatic patients for 8 hours. Monitor patients ingesting >450 mg of sustained-release bupropion for up to 24 hours. Admit those with seizures, persistent tachycardia, or lethargy.

MIRTAZAPINE

Clinical Features

Toxicity causes sedation, confusion, sinus tachycardia, and hypertension. Coma and respiratory depression are seen in severe cases or with co-ingestion of other sedatives.

Emergency Department Care and Disposition

1. Isolated overdoses can generally be managed with supportive care.
2. Consider single-dose **activated charcoal if no contraindications exist**.
3. Admit symptomatic patients to a monitored bed. Discharge asymptomatic patients after 6 hours.

SELECTIVE-SEROTONIN REUPTAKE INHIBITORS

Clinical Features

Selective-serotonin reuptake inhibitors (SSRIs) include fluoxetine, fluvoxamine, paroxetine, sertraline, citalopram, and escitalopram. Signs and symptoms may include vomiting, sedation, tremor, sinus tachycardia, mydriasis, seizures, diarrhea, and hallucinations. Sinus bradycardia is more common with fluvoxamine than with other SSRIs. QRS and QT interval prolongation has been reported in citalopram and escitalopram ingestions.

Emergency Department Care and Disposition

Supportive care is generally sufficient.

1. Establish IV access and initiate cardiac monitoring.
2. Single-dose **activated charcoal** is appropriate for most ingestions if there are no contraindications.
3. **Benzodiazepines** are recommended for management of seizures.
4. Administer IV **sodium bicarbonate** for QRS prolongation.
5. Observe patients for at least 6 hours. Admit patients who are tachycardic, have altered mental status, have conduction abnormalities, or have signs of serotonin syndrome.

SEROTONIN-NOREPINEPHRINE REUPTAKE INHIBITORS

Clinical Features

Serotonin-norepinephrine reuptake inhibitors (SNRIs) include venlafaxine, duloxetine, levomilnacipran, and desvenlafaxine. Overdose may cause hypotension, diaphoresis, tremor, mydriasis, sedation, coma, and seizures. ECG changes include sinus tachycardia and QRS or QT interval widening. Rhabdomyolysis has been reported with venlafaxine overdoses with and without seizures.

Emergency Department Care and Disposition

There are no established guidelines for treating SNRI overdoses.

1. Initiate peripheral IV access and cardiac monitoring.
2. Consider single-dose **activated charcoal if no contraindications exist**. Consider whole-bowel irrigation for venlafaxine overdoses >4000 mg.

3. **Benzodiazepines** are the anticonvulsants of choice.
4. Treat hypotension with fluids and a direct-acting vasopressor.
5. Administer IV **sodium bicarbonate** for QRS prolongation.
6. Administer IV fluid for rhabdomyolysis.
7. All patients require at least 6 hours of observation, or 24 hours for those ingesting extended-release preparations. Admit symptomatic patients to a monitored bed.

SEROTONIN SYNDROME

Serotonin syndrome is a potentially life-threatening adverse reaction to serotoninergic medications. It can be produced by any drug or combination of drugs that increase central serotonin neurotransmission, most commonly antidepressants.

Clinical Features

Signs and symptoms are altered mental status, hyperthermia, seizures, and increased muscle tone, particularly myoclonus. Hyperthermia is the most common cause of death.

Diagnosis

Symptoms are nonspecific, and there are no confirmatory laboratory tests. Diagnostic criteria emphasize exposure to a serotoninergic drug and presence of myoclonus.

Emergency Department Care and Disposition

Treatment is supportive. Watch patients for rhabdomyolysis and metabolic acidosis.

1. Endotracheal intubation and ventilatory support may be required in severe cases.
2. Use **benzodiazepines** to decrease discomfort and promote muscle relaxation.
3. The antiserotonergic agent **cyproheptadine** may be given at an initial dose of 4 to 12 mg PO, repeated with 2 mg doses at 2-hour intervals if no response.
4. Admit all patients until symptoms resolve. Severely ill patients require admission to an ICU. Discontinue serotonergic drugs.

MONOAMINE OXIDASE INHIBITORS

Monoamine oxidase inhibitors (MAOIs) are used to treat refractory depression. They cause accumulation of neurotransmitters such as norepinephrine in presynaptic nerve terminals and increased systemic availability of dietary amines, such as tyramine. MAOIs can lead to fatal food and drug interactions and cause severe toxicity in overdose.

Clinical Features

Symptoms include headache, agitation, palpitations, chest pain, and tremor. Signs include sinus tachycardia, hyperreflexia, diaphoresis, fasciculations, mydriasis, hyperventilation, nystagmus, flushing, muscle rigidity, and hypertension. Signs and symptoms often are delayed after ingestion and the delay can be up to 24 hours. Coma, seizures, bradycardia, hypotension, hypoxia, and hyperthermia may develop. Death usually results from multi-organ failure.

Diagnosis and Differential

Diagnosis is made on clinical grounds. Laboratory tests can identify complications, including rhabdomyolysis, renal failure, hyperkalemia, metabolic acidosis, and disseminated intravascular coagulation. The differential diagnosis includes drugs and conditions that produce a hyperadrenergic state, altered mental status, and/or muscle rigidity.

Emergency Department Care and Disposition

Treatment consists of supportive care and management of complications.

1. Obtain IV access and initiate cardiac rhythm monitoring.
2. Consider **activated charcoal if no contraindications exist**.
3. Hypertension may be treated with **phentolamine**, 2.5 to 5 mg IV every 10 to 15 minutes, followed by an infusion. An alternative agent is **nitroprusside**. Avoid beta-blockers.
4. **Nitroglycerin** is indicated for anginal chest pain and signs of myocardial ischemia.
5. Treat hypotension with isotonic IV fluid boluses, followed by **norepinephrine**.
6. Treat ventricular dysrhythmias with **lidocaine** or **procainamide**.
7. Treat bradycardia with **atropine**, **isoproterenol**, **dobutamine**, and **pacing**.
8. Treat seizures with **benzodiazepines**. General anesthesia and muscle paralysis using vecuronium, with ongoing EEG monitoring, may be necessary.
9. Treat hyperthermia with benzodiazepines to reduce muscle rigidity plus cooling measures. Chemical paralysis with a nondepolarizing agent may be needed for severe rigidity. **Dantrolene** 0.5 to 2.5 mg/kg IV every 6 hours could be considered if other measures have failed.
10. Patients who have ingested >1 mg/kg require ICU admission. Those who have ingested less can be admitted to a monitored bed. Observe asymptomatic patients for 24 hours.

ANTIPSYCHOTICS

Antipsychotics are used to treat psychosis, agitation, nausea, headaches, hiccups, and involuntary motor disorders. Their therapeutic action involves blockade of dopamine receptors.

Clinical Features

Central nervous system effects include lethargy, ataxia, dysarthria, confusion, and coma. Seizures are more common with loxapine and clozapine. Antimuscarinic toxicity may be seen. Cardiovascular manifestations include orthostatic hypotension; sinus tachycardia; PR, QRS, and QT interval prolongation; and ST and T wave abnormalities. Extrapyramidal symptoms such as dystonia, akathisia, and tardive dyskinesia can be seen during therapeutic use.

Neuroleptic malignant syndrome is a rare but potentially fatal idiosyncratic reaction to antipsychotic agents. It typically develops over 1 to 3 days. It is characterized by fever, muscular rigidity, autonomic dysfunction, and altered mental status (Table 102-1). Death results from complications of muscle rigidity, such as rhabdomyolysis, renal failure, or cardiac or respiratory failure.

Diagnosis

Diagnostic studies should include a complete blood count, basic chemistries, a pregnancy test for women of childbearing age, and an ECG. Also obtain a creatine kinase level and liver function tests in patients with neuroleptic malignant syndrome.

Emergency Department Care and Disposition

Treatment is largely supportive.

1. Establish IV access and initiate cardiac rhythm monitoring.
2. Ventilatory support may be necessary for patients with respiratory depression.

TABLE 102-1 Diagnostic Criteria for Neuroleptic Malignant Syndrome

	Caroff and Mann*	Levenson†	American Psychiatric Association‡
Major criteria	Fever >38°C (100.4°F) Muscle rigidity	Fever Muscle rigidity Elevated CK level	Fever Muscle rigidity
Minor criteria	Change in mental status Tachycardia Hypertension or hypotension Tachypnea or hypoxia Diaphoresis or sialorrhea Tremor Incontinence Increased CK level or myoglobinuria Leukocytosis Metabolic acidosis	Tachycardia Abnormal blood pressure Tachypnea Leukocytosis Diaphoresis Altered mental status	Diaphoresis Dysphagia Tremor Incontinence Altered mental status Mutism Tachycardia Labile blood pressure Leukocytosis Elevated CK level
Diagnostic requirement	Both major and at least five minor criteria must be present, and treatment with an antipsychotic must have been within 7 days of symptom onset (or 2–4 weeks with a depot agent).	All three major criteria or two major and four minor criteria must be present.	Both major and at least two minor criteria must be present.

*Caroff SN, Mann SC. Neuroleptic malignant syndrome. *Med Clin North Am.* 1993;77:185.

†Levenson J. Neuroleptic malignant syndrome. *Am J Psychiatry.* 1985;142:1137.

‡ American Psychiatric Association. *Diagnostic and Statistical Manual of Mental Disorders.* 4th ed., text revision. Washington, DC: American Psychiatric Association; 2000:795–798.

Abbreviation: CK, creatine kinase.

3. Treat seizures with a **benzodiazepine**.
4. Treat hypotension with fluid resuscitation and **norepinephrine or phenylephrine**.
5. Treat intraventricular conduction delay and ventricular dysrhythmias with IV **sodium bicarbonate**. Lidocaine is an alternative for ventricular dysrhythmias.
6. Consider IV lipid emulsion for severe quetiapine overdoses with cardiovascular instability refractory to conventional therapy.
7. Treatment of neuroleptic malignant syndrome includes cooling measures and benzodiazepines to reduce muscle rigidity. Intubation and paralysis with a nondepolarizing agent may facilitate cooling. Consider **dantrolene** (1 to 2.5 mg/kg IV load) when muscle rigidity is pronounced. **Bromocriptine** may possibly shorten the duration.
8. Observe patients for 6 hours post-ingestion. Admit symptomatic patients to a monitored bed. Patients with neuroleptic malignant syndrome warrant ICU admission.

LITHIUM

Lithium is used to treat bipolar disorder and mania. Toxicity results from overdose or altered renal clearance. Death is usually from respiratory or cardiac failure.

Clinical Features

Patients may present with tremor, muscle fasciculations or weakness, clonus, ataxia, agitation, peripheral neuropathy, lethargy, or coma. Acute renal failure may be noted, especially in the elderly and those with preexisting renal impairment, diabetes, hypertension, or dehydration. Gastrointestinal symptoms are common in acute and chronic toxicity. Cardiac abnormalities are more common in acute toxicity and include conduction disturbances and ventricular dysrhythmias. Nephrogenic diabetes insipidus and hypothyroidism can be noted as adverse effects from chronic therapeutic use.

Diagnosis

Acute overdoses present with more GI than neurologic toxicity. Serum lithium levels may not correlate well with symptoms. Patients with chronic toxicity display more neurologic effects at lower levels. In this setting, serum lithium levels correlate better with toxicity. Acute-on-chronic ingestions have aspects of both. ECG abnormalities include QT interval prolongation and T wave inversions.

Emergency Department Care and Disposition

Stabilization includes securing the airway and ventilatory and hemodynamic support.

1. Obtain IV access, and initiate cardiac rhythm and ECG monitoring.
2. Initial laboratory studies should include renal function tests, electrolyte levels, complete blood count, thyroid-stimulating hormone and thyroid hormone levels if altered level of consciousness, and serum levels of lithium and other possible ingestants.

3. Treat seizures with IV **benzodiazepines**, followed by **phenobarbital**.
4. Activated charcoal does not adsorb lithium but may be helpful for other ingestions.
5. **Whole-bowel irrigation** may be helpful, especially for sustained-release lithium products.
6. IV administration of **normal saline** is important. In most adults, a 2-L IV bolus is given over 30 to 60 minutes followed by a continuous infusion at 1.5 to 2 times the maintenance rate.
7. **Sodium polystyrene sulfonate** (Kayexalate®) can bind lithium and increase the elimination but can only be given orally. Hypokalemia and constipation may develop as well.
8. **Hemodialysis** is indicated when serum lithium levels are >4 mEq/L in acute overdose, or if there is severe toxicity as evidenced by coma, seizures, or life-threatening dysrhythmias. Patients with renal failure and rising lithium levels, and those who have ingested sustained-release preparations may also benefit.
9. Monitor patients with acute ingestions for 4 to 6 hours. Admit those with lithium levels >1.5 mEq/L and patients who have ingested a sustained-release preparation. Treat patients with mild chronic toxicity with IV normal saline for 6 to 12 hours, and discharge or refer for psychiatric evaluation once their lithium level decreases to <1.5 mEq. Admit patients with more severe chronic toxicity.

FURTHER READING

For further reading in *Tintinalli's Emergency Medicine: A Comprehensive Study Guide*, 8th ed., see Chapter 177, "Cyclic Antidepressants," by Frank LoVecchio; Chapter 178, "Atypical and Serotonergic Antidepressants" by Frank LoVecchio and Erik Mattison; Chapter 179, "Monoamine Oxidase Inhibitors," by Frank LoVecchio; Chapter 180, "Antipsychotics" by Michael Levine and Frank LoVecchio; and Chapter 181, "Lithium," by Sandra M. Schneider, Daniel J. Cobaugh, and Benjamin D. Kessler

CHAPTER 103 Sedatives and Hypnotics

Shan Yin

Sedative and hypnotic medications are commonly used pharmaceuticals. The three classes include barbiturates, benzodiazepines, and nonbenzodiazepines (buspirone, carisoprodol, meprobamate, chloral hydrate, γ-hydroxybutyrate, melatonin, ramelteon, zaleplon, zolpidem, and zopiclone).

BARBITURATES

Clinical Features

Among the sedative-hypnotic class of medications, barbiturates are associated with the greatest morbidity and mortality. Owing to safer alternatives for seizure management, the clinical use of barbiturates has declined.

Barbiturates cause a dose-dependent spectrum of central nervous system depression. With mild to moderate ingestions, toxicity resembles that of ethanol or other sedative-hypnotic medications: confusion, ataxia, slurred speech, drowsiness, and disinhibition. Gastrointestinal motility may be slowed. The toxic dose will vary depending on route, speed of administration, and patient tolerance. Severe intoxication follows a tenfold overdose, and loss of deep tendon and corneal reflexes may occur. Hypothermia, hypotension, and respiratory depression are common. Complicating features of the toxicity include hypoglycemia, aspiration pneumonia, pulmonary edema, and acute lung injury.

Barbiturate withdrawal syndrome may occur in the habituated patient who suddenly stops taking their medication. The syndrome occurs within 24 hours of cessation and begins with mild symptoms, which may become severe over the next 2 to 8 days. Short-acting barbiturates generally cause a more robust withdrawal syndrome than the long-acting products. Minor symptoms include anxiety, restlessness, depression, insomnia, anorexia, nausea, and vomiting. Major symptoms include psychosis, hallucinations, delirium, generalized seizures, hyperthermia, and cardiovascular collapse. Barbiturate withdrawal has a high mortality and gradual inpatient withdrawal of the addicting agent is recommended.

Diagnosis and Differential

Serum barbiturate levels may help establish an etiology for altered mental status in a comatose patient; however, decisions regarding management are based primarily on clinical grounds. Mixed sedative-hypnotic ingestions may be inappropriately ascribed to the barbiturate alone. Due to variability among patients with barbiturate overdoses, heart rate, pupil size and reactivity, and nystagmus are not clinically distinguishing signs. Skin bullae ("barbiturate blisters") are rarely evident and are not specific to barbiturates. Myocardial depression is more common with barbiturates than benzodiazepines.

Bedside glucose measurement is imperative in the patient with altered mental status and may help narrow the differential diagnosis. Other useful diagnostic testing includes arterial or venous blood gas analysis, electrocardiogram, liver function tests, salicylate and acetaminophen concentrations, blood urea nitrogen and creatinine levels, complete blood count, and creatinine phosphate kinase.

Emergency Department Care and Disposition

Treatment begins with airway management and supportive care. Once pulmonary and cardiovascular function have been adequately assessed and stabilized, enhancing elimination can be considered.

1. Stabilize the airway. **Endotracheal intubation** in the severely poisoned patients is commonly required and should be initiated early in the ED course.
2. Due to the potential for myocardial depression, place two large-bore IVs and initiate fluid resuscitation with isotonic saline for hypotension.
3. Consider empiric treatment with naloxone and thiamine early in the management.
4. **Dopamine** or **norepinephrine** may be needed if fluid boluses fail to reverse hypotension. Hypothermia between 30°C (86°F) and 36°C (96.8°F) requires standard rewarming techniques.
5. **Activated charcoal** helps reduce absorption. In the awake, cooperative patient, 50 to 100 g orally (1 g/kg in children) should be administered. For sedated or unconscious patients, airway protection should precede the administration of activated charcoal. Multidose charcoal may reduce serum levels, but has not been shown to change clinical outcome.
6. Forced diuresis is not indicated due to risks of sodium and fluid overload and a lack of proven efficacy.
7. Urinary alkalinization is not considered first-line therapy. While it may enhance the clearance of phenobarbital and primidone, it is less effective than multidose charcoal alone, and has no role in the management of short-acting barbiturates.
8. **Hemodialysis**, hemoperfusion, and hemodiafiltration are reserved for patients who deteriorate despite aggressive medical support, but are only effective with phenobarbital toxicity.
9. Disposition depends on the degree of intoxication: evidence of toxicity greater than 6 hours from time of arrival requires hospital admission. Obtain psychiatric consult for intentional overdose. Toxicology or poison center consultation is recommended to assist with management.

BENZODIAZEPINES

Clinical Features

Benzodiazepine overdoses are common but carry a low mortality rate in isolation. There is, however, variation in the clinical outcome among agents due to differences in potency. Parenteral administration in the ED may produce significant complications. Benzodiazepines, when mixed with other sedative-hypnotics, may produce profound toxicity including respiratory depression, hypotension, and death.

The primary effect of benzodiazepines is central nervous system depression and is characterized by somnolence, dizziness, slurred speech, confusion, ataxia, incoordination, and general impairment in intellectual function. Neurologic effects in the elderly, very young, or malnourished may be prolonged or enhanced. Disinhibition, extrapyramidal reactions, and paradoxical excitation are uncommon but reported. Short-term, anterograde amnesia is a common, sometimes desirable, effect with the administration of certain benzodiazepines.

Chronic use of benzodiazepines is associated with physiologic addiction. Withdrawal from benzodiazepines may occur following abrupt cessation. Symptoms are more intense following withdrawal from short-acting agents. Clinical findings may mimic alcohol withdrawal and include anxiety, irritability, insomnia, nausea, vomiting, tremor, and sweating. Serious manifestations include hallucinations, psychosis, disorientation, and seizures. Treatment begins with reintroduction of a benzodiazepine with subsequent, gradual tapering.

Diagnosis and Differential

There is limited value in toxicological testing as serum levels do not correlate well with clinical findings. Qualitative urine screening is unreliable and a positive test does not prove causation of clinical signs as clinical features are nonspecific and may be seen with overdose of any sedative-hypnotic.

Emergency Department Care and Disposition

1. Priorities include assessment and stabilization of the airway, breathing, and circulation (see the preceding section on barbiturates for guidance regarding initial management, resuscitation, and laboratory monitoring).
2. Do not induce emesis. **Activated charcoal** (1 g/kg in children or 50 to 100 g in adults) will adsorb benzodiazepines. Exercise caution in the sedated patient, and secure the airway before administration. Multidose charcoal is not indicated. Gastric lavage, forced dieresis, enhanced elimination, hemodialysis, and hemoperfusion are ineffective and unnecessary.
3. **Flumazenil** is a unique, selective antagonist of the central effects of benzodiazepines. Unlike naloxone, flumazenil should not be used empirically for the undifferentiated sedative-hypnotic toxidrome as it may precipitate seizures (Table 103-1). The ED applications of flumazenil are generally limited to the setting of respiratory depression following procedural sedation with benzodiazepines. The dose is 0.2 mg IV and titrated every minute to a maximum total dose of 3 mg (0.01 to 0.02 mg/kg in children). The half-life of flumazenil is approximately 1 hour and rebound sedation can occur in the setting of overdose with long-acting benzodiazepines.
4. In general, care is supportive. Admit patients with significant alterations of mental status, respiratory depression, or hypotension. Consultation with mental health specialists may be appropriate.

TABLE 103-1 Contraindications to Flumazenil

Overdose of unknown agents
Suspected or known physical dependence on benzodiazepines
Suspected cyclic antidepressant overdose
Coingestion of seizure-inducing agents
Known seizure disorder
Suspected increased intracranial pressure

NONBENZODIAZEPINE SEDATIVES

Clinical Features

The hallmark of all sedative-hypnotic medications, regardless of subclass, is sedation. Exposure to nonbenzodiazepine agents is common and coingestion with other sedatives may be synergistic and produce profound sedation. Three agents, ethchlorvynol, glutethimide, and methaqualone, have been removed from the markets in the United States and Canada.

Buspirone

Buspirone has a complex mechanism of action and rapid absorption. Side effects include sedation, GI distress, vomiting, and dizziness. The symptoms with overdose are exaggerations of the side effects noted with therapeutic dosing. The drug is generally well tolerated in overdose, and treatment is primarily supportive. Due to effects on the serotoninergic system, serotonin syndrome has been reported. Seizures, hypotension, priapism, and dystonia are rare complications.

Carisoprodol and Meprobamate

Carisoprodol and its active metabolite, meprobamate, are marketed as central-acting muscle relaxants and anxiolytics, respectively. In overdoses, both may cause sedation, coma, and cardiopulmonary depression. Carisoprodol, but not meprobamate, can cause myoclonus, which may be a clue in an unknown overdose. Meprobamate has been associated with pharmacobezoars, and may be a cause of prolonged toxicity.

Chloral Hydrate

Chloral hydrate is the oldest sedative-hypnotic available today. At therapeutic doses, chloral hydrate produces mental status depression without loss of airway and respiratory reflexes. Vomiting and paradoxical excitation can occur in a small percentage of children. In overdose, coma and respiratory depression can occur. Chloral hydrate is a myocardial sensitizer and cardiac dysrhythmias, decreased cardiac contractility, and asystole have been reported. When combined with alcohol, a potent, "knock-down" cocktail known as a "Mickey Finn" is created. A withdrawal syndrome similar to ethanol has been described.

Chloral hydrate may produce a characteristic pear-like odor. Abdominal radiographs may aid in the diagnosis of pharmacobezoars, as chloral hydrate is radiopaque. Respiratory depression and coma are treated supportively. **Treat ventricular dysrhythmias with IV β-blockers**.

γ -Hydroxybutyrate

γ-Hydroxybutyrate (GHB) has been marketed as a muscle builder, fat burner, antidepressant, anxiolytic, hypnotic, and cholesterol-lowering medication. The only approved use in the United States is for the treatment of narcolepsy and is prescribed as its sodium salt (sodium oxybate). GHB is often used illicitly and has street names including "liquid ecstasy," "Georgia home boy," "G," and "grievous bodily harm." GHB has a narrow therapeutic window and may produce a range of toxicity from mild sedation to coma. Seizures, bradycardia, hypothermia, and cardiac depression may occur. Rapid sedation with abrupt recovery 6 to 12 hours later is a common feature with GHB. Due to its amnestic effects and rapid sedation, GHB has been illicitly used for drug-facilitated sexual assault. Two compounds, 1,4 butanediol and γ-butyrolactone are GHB precursors and have been abused to produce similar effects. Treatment is primarily supportive with focus on airway management. Physostigmine and neostigmine should be avoided. Rapid awaking and self-extubation may be a clue to GHB intoxication. Toxicologic detection of GHB is difficulty owing to its very short half-life and rapid elimination. Withdrawal from GHB mimics alcohol withdrawal and may be severe, lasting from 3 days to 2 weeks.

Melatonin

The endogenous hormone melatonin is secreted by the pineal gland and is believed to help regulate the sleep–wake cycle. Melatonin can be purchased without prescription. Side effects following therapeutic dosing include headache, dizziness, fatigue, and irritability. Overdose data are limited, and signs and symptoms exaggerate the side effects from therapeutic doses.

Ramelteon

Ramelteon is a relatively new medication used to treat insomnia. It binds to melatonin receptors in the brain. Absorption following oral dosing is rapid. In overdose, sedation is common and treatment is supportive. Abuse and withdrawal have not been reported.

Tasimelteon

Tasimelteon is used to treat non-24-hour sleep–wake disorder. It peaks quickly following ingestion. There is no data on overdoses currently. Abuse and withdrawal have not been reported.

Zolpidem, Zaleplon, and Zopiclone

Zolpidem, zaleplon, and zopiclone have gained increased popularity for the treatment of insomnia. Though initially thought to produce little or no psychomotor impairment, addiction or withdrawal, experience has proved otherwise. Zaleplon appears to be less likely to cause withdrawal than zolpidem or zopiclone. Side effects in therapeutic doses include nausea and somnolence. Sedation would be the expected primary effect after overdose. Vivid dreams, sleep-walking, and driving have been reported with zolpidem. Fatalities following zolpidem overdoses have been reported, but are usually associated with mixed ingestions. Methemoglobinemia and hemolytic anemia have been reported after large zoplicone overdoses.

Emergency Department Care and Disposition

1. In general, management for the nonbenzodiazepines is supportive (see the preceding section on benzodiazepines for treatment priorities).
2. For ventricular dysrhythmias in the setting of chloral hydrate intoxication, **IV β-blockers** (e.g., **propranolol** 1 mg IV or 0.01 to 0.1 mg/kg IV in children) are first-line agents.
3. Disposition is largely guided by the degree of symptoms. Have a low threshold for admission of any patient with altered mental status, abnormal vital signs, or dysrhythmias. Consult psychiatric services when appropriate.

FURTHER READING

For further reading in *Tintinalli's Emergency Medicine: A Comprehensive Study Guide*, 8th ed., see Chapter 182, "Barbiturates," by Chip Gresham and Frank LoVecchio; Chapter 183, "Benzodiazepines," by Dan Quan; and Chapter 184, "Nonbenzodiazepine Sedatives," by Michael Levine and Dan Quan.

CHAPTER 104

Alcohols

Michael Levine

All alcohols are potentially toxic and cause clinical inebriation. Ethanol and isopropanol are the most commonly ingested alcohols and cause direct toxicity, while methanol and ethylene glycol cause toxicity as a result of conversion to toxic metabolites.

ETHANOL

Ethanol is the most commonly abused drug in the world. While acute toxicity may result in death due to respiratory depression, the majority of morbidity and mortality is due to trauma owing to impaired cognitive function. Blood ethanol levels correlate poorly with the degree of intoxication due to the development of tolerance. On an average, nondrinkers metabolize ethanol at a rate of 20 mg/dL/h, whereas chronic alcoholics metabolize ethanol at a rate of 30 mg/dL/h.

Clinical Features

Signs and symptoms of ethanol intoxication include disinhibited behavior, slurred speech, impaired coordination, followed later by respiratory and central nervous system (CNS) depression.

Diagnosis and Differential

Head injury and hypoglycemia can present similarly to ethanol intoxication, and these diagnoses may coexist. Glucose should be measured in all patients with altered mental status. In those patients without a clear explanation for their altered mental status, serum ethanol levels may help confirm intoxication, although the value may be difficult to interpret. For patients with comorbid disease or injury, additional labs that may be helpful include the following: electrolytes may demonstrate an anion gap acidosis; liver enzymes may reveal hepatic damage. Obtain imaging as indicated by external signs of trauma in the inebriated patient.

Emergency Department Care and Disposition

1. The mainstay of treatment is observation. A careful physical examination should be performed to evaluate for complicating injury or illness.
2. Treat hypoglycemia with IV **dextrose**. **Thiamine** 100 mg IV or IM may be given concurrently if Wernicke encephalopathy is suspected.
3. Consider secondary causes of deterioration or lack of improvement during observation and manage accordingly.
4. Discharge the patient once sober enough to pose no threat to self or others.

ISOPROPANOL

Isopropanol is commonly found in rubbing alcohol, solvents, skin and hair products, paint thinners, and antifreeze. Acetone is the principal toxic metabolite.

Clinical Features

Clinically, isopropanol intoxication is similar to that of ethanol but produces a greater degree of intoxication than ethanol. Severe poisoning presents as coma, respiratory depression, and hypotension. Hemorrhagic gastritis is common and causes nausea, vomiting, abdominal pain, and upper gastrointestinal (GI) bleeding.

Diagnosis and Differential

A glucose level should be measured in all patients with altered mental status. Laboratory studies may reveal an elevated osmolal gap, ketonemia, and ketonuria, without acidosis. In the setting of upper GI bleeding, coagulation studies, a complete blood count, and a type and screen should be obtained. When available, serum isopropanol and acetone levels confirm the diagnosis, but are not required for management.

Emergency Department Care and Disposition

1. Treat hypotension with aggressive infusion of IV crystalloids, although persistent hypotension may require vasopressors. Treat significant bleeding from hemorrhagic gastritis with transfusion of packed red blood cells and plasma as indicated.
2. Do not administer metabolic blockade with fomepizole or ethanol since acetone, the metabolite of isopropanol, is no more toxic than the parent compound.
3. Hemodialysis removes both isopropanol and acetone, and may be indicated for refractory hypotension due to isopropanol.
4. Patients with prolonged CNS depression require admission. Those who are asymptomatic after 6 to 8 hours of observation can be discharged or referred for psychiatric evaluation if indicated.
5. Charcoal does not bind alcohols, and is useful only if there is coingestion of an absorbable substance.

METHANOL AND ETHYLENE GLYCOL

Methanol is commonly found in windshield washing fluid, solid fuel for stoves, and solvents. Ethylene glycol is commonly found in antifreeze. Toxicity from these alcohols results from the formation of toxic metabolites, which produce a significant anion gap metabolic acidosis. Methanol leads to the formation of toxic formic acid, while ethylene glycol is metabolized into the toxic compounds glycolic acid, glyoxylic acid, and oxylic acid with subsequent formation of calcium oxylate crystals.

Clinical Features

The clinical features of methanol toxicity include metabolic acidosis, CNS depression, and visual changes (classically, a complaint of looking at a snowstorm). The onset of symptoms may be delayed with concurrent ethanol consumption. Funduscopic examination may reveal retinal edema or hyperemia of the optic disk.

Ethylene glycol poisoning often exhibits three distinct clinical phases after ingestion. First, within 12 hours, CNS effects predominate: the patient appears intoxicated without the odor of ethanol on the breath. Second,

12 to 24 hours after ingestion, cardiopulmonary effects predominate: elevated heart rate, respiratory rate, and blood pressure are common. Congestive heart failure, respiratory distress syndrome, and circulatory collapse may develop. Third, 24 to 72 hours after ingestion, renal effects predominate which are characterized by flank pain, costovertebral angle tenderness, and acute tubular necrosis with acute renal failure. Hypocalcemia may result from precipitation of calcium oxalate into tissues leading to tetany and typical ECG changes.

Diagnosis and Differential

The diagnosis is based on clinical presentation and laboratory findings of an elevated osmol gap, and/or an anion gap metabolic acidosis (which may take hours to develop). Elevated levels of methanol or ethylene glycol can confirm toxicity. An elevated osmolal gap is present early, and may be useful when methanol or ethylene glycol testing is not immediately available. Basic laboratory investigations include a bedside glucose, electrolytes, renal function arterial blood gas, urinalysis, and methanol or ethylene glycol level. Ethylene glycol poisoning differs from methanol poisoning in that visual disturbances and fundoscopic abnormalities are absent and calcium oxalate crystals may be present in the urine.

The differential diagnosis includes other causes of an anion gap metabolic acidosis such as salicylate or isoniazid toxicity, diabetic ketoacidosis, alcoholic ketoacidosis, uremia, and lactic acidosis.

Emergency Department Care and Disposition

Treatment is based on metabolic blockade and removing toxic metabolites from the body. Both fomepizole and ethanol have a greater affinity for alcohol dehydrogenase than methanol and ethylene glycol. Indications for metabolic blockade are listed in Table 104-1.

1. Administer **fomepizole** 15 mg/kg IV load followed by 10 mg/kg every 12 hours for four additional doses. Subsequent doses should be at 15 mg/kg. Fomepizole is a potent inhibitor of alcohol dehydrogenase with greater affinity and fewer side effects than ethanol. If fomepizole is not available, use ethanol 800 mg/kg IV load, followed by a continuous

TABLE 104-1 Indications for Metabolic Blockade with Fomepizole or Ethanol

1. Elevated plasma levels: methanol >20 mg/dL (>6 mmol/L) or ethylene glycol > 20 mg/dL (>3 mmol/L)
2. If methanol or ethylene glycol level not available: A. Documented or suspected significant methanol or ethylene glycol ingestion with ethanol level lower than approximately 100 mg/dL (22 mmol/L) B. Coma or altered mental status in patient with unclear history and: Unexplained serum osmolar gap of >10 mOsm/L *or* Unexplained metabolic acidosis *and* ethanol level of <100 mg/dL (<22 mmol/L)*

*If serum ethanol level is >100 mg/dL (>22 mmol/L), patient will be protected from the formation of toxic metabolites by coingestion of ethanol, and specific metabolic blockade treatment can be delayed until toxic alcohol level is available. If the ethanol level is likely to fall to <100 mg/dL before the toxic alcohol results are back, then initiate metabolic blockade.

infusion of 100 mg/kg/h in the average drinker and 150 mg/kg/h in the heavy drinker. Adjust the infusion accordingly to maintain a blood ethanol level at 100 to 150 mg/dL. If resources are limited, oral therapy with commercial 80 proof liquor can be initiated. A load of 3 to 4 oz with maintenance of 1 to 2 oz/h is a typical dose for a 70-kg patient.

2. Monitor serum glucose during treatment with ethanol as hypoglycemia may be induced, especially in children. Treat hypoglycemia with 1 mL/kg **50% dextrose in water** in adults and 5 mL/kg **10% dextrose in water** in children.
3. Dialysis eliminates both methanol and ethylene glycol and their toxic metabolites. Indications include metabolic acidosis or evidence of end organ impairment (e.g., blindness, renal failure). Fomepizole or ethanol treatments do not alter the indications for dialysis; however, both fomepizole and ethanol are dialyzed and, therefore, increase the dosing interval of fomepizole to every 4 hours. Double the infusion rate of ethanol during dialysis and adjust accordingly to maintain the level at 100 to150 mg/dL.
4. Continue dialysis, fomepizole, or ethanol treatment until the methanol or ethylene glycol level is <20 mg/dL and the metabolic acidosis has resolved.
5. In methanol poisoning, administer **folinic acid** (**leucovorin**) 50 mg IV. In ethylene glycol poisoning, administer **pyridoxine** 100 mg IV and **thiamine** 100 mg IV.
6. Administer **sodium bicarbonate** 1 to 2 mEq/kg and titrated to maintain a normal pH in methanol toxicity to increase renal excretion of formic acid. Sodium bicarbonate may also be given to an ethylene glycol toxic patient with metabolic acidosis.
7. Treat documented and symptomatic hypocalcemia in ethylene glycol toxicity with calcium gluconate or calcium chloride.
8. Consult a medical toxicologist or regional poison control center (800 222-1222) to aid in the management of symptomatic methanol or ethylene glycol ingestion.
9. Patients with suspected ethylene glycol or methanol ingestion who are asymptomatic after 6 hours with no ethanol detected and no osmolar gap or metabolic acidosis may be safely discharged. In the setting of co-ingestion with ethanol, it is important to ensure no metabolic acidosis develops 6 hours after ethanol has been metabolized. Patients with significant signs and symptoms should be admitted to an intensive care unit.

FURTHER READING

For further reading in *Tintinalli's Emergency Medicine: A Comprehensive Study Guide*, 8th ed., see Chapter 185, "Alcohols," by Jennifer P. Cohen and Dan Quan.

CHAPTER 105

Drugs of Abuse

D. Adam Algren

OPIOIDS

The term *opioid* refers to any drug that is active at the opioid receptor, while *opiates* refers to naturally occurring derivatives of the opium plant, such as morphine. *Narcotic* is a legal term and generically refers to any drug that causes sedation. Emergency physicians commonly utilize opioids as analgesics and must be familiar with the clinical presentation and treatment of opioid toxicity.

Clinical Features

Opioid overdose produces a clinical toxidrome: miosis, and central nervous system (CNS) and respiratory depression. However, normal or large pupils may be seen with diphenoxylate, meperidine, pentazocine, and propoxyphene toxicities. Severe hypoxia or co-ingestants could also produce mydriasis. Severe opioid overdose, especially with heroin, may be associated with acute lung injury. Seizures have been reported with tramadol, propoxyphene, and meperidine overdoses. Meperidine, tramadol, and dextromethorphan have been associated with serotonin syndrome when combined with other serotonergic agents. Methadone may prolong the QT interval and result in torsade de pointes. Opioid withdrawal is manifest by abdominal pain, nausea, vomiting, diarrhea, dysphoria, piloerection, and lacrimation.

Diagnosis and Differential

The diagnosis is clinical. Qualitative immunoassay urine drug screens are commonly available but must be interpreted with caution as there are numerous agents that produce false-positive and false-negative results for opioids. Toxicity from clonidine, guanfacine, and imidazolines mimics opioid intoxication and produces varying degrees of miosis and CNS/respiratory depression. Because response to naloxone with these agents is less reliable, consider clonidine intoxication in patients who appear opioid poisoned but do not respond to naloxone. Other possible causes of CNS depression and miosis include pontine hemorrhage and toxicity from organophosphates/carbamates, antipsychotics, and sedative-hypnotics (i.e., GHB).

Emergency Department Care and Disposition

1. **Naloxone** is the primary treatment for opioid toxicity. Administer a small dose of 0.1 to 0.4 mg IV, SC, or IM initially for CNS and respiratory depression to avoid precipitating withdrawal. Larger doses of 2 mg could be used in apneic patients. Repeat doses may be administered every 3 minutes. The pediatric dose is 0.1 mg/kg. Given the relatively short duration of action of naloxone, monitor closely for recurrent toxicity.

2. In large overdoses, consider an infusion of naloxone: two-thirds of the dose required to initially "wake up" the patient per hour.
3. Consider endotracheal intubation in patients who respond poorly to naloxone and those with acute lung injury from overdose.
4. Patients with heroin overdose who are awake and asymptomatic 2 hours after the last naloxone dose can be discharged. Patients with immediate-acting opioid exposures require observation for at least 6 hours, or 6 hours following naloxone administration if given. Patients with exposure to long-acting opioids (sustained release morphine/oxycodone, methadone, and buprenorphine) require admission for prolonged observation.
5. Treatment of opioid withdrawal is supportive (i.e., fluids, antiemetics). **Clonidine** 0.1 to 0.3 mg PO may be used to treat withdrawal.

COCAINE AND AMPHETAMINES

Cocaine and amphetamines are widely used drugs of abuse and produce similar clinical manifestations.

Clinical Features

Cocaine and amphetamines induce euphoria and produce complications secondary to the enhanced release and blockade of catecholamines at the synaptic receptors. Onset of effect via intranasal, inhalational (crack use), and intravenous use is rapid. Repeated drug administration leads to prolonged effects and increased toxicity. Symptoms of sympathomimetic overdose include mydriasis, hypertension, tachycardia, diaphoresis, agitation, rhabdomyolysis, acute kidney injury, and hyperthermia.

Cardiovascular complications include dysrhythmias, myocardial ischemia, cardiomyopathy, and aortic/coronary artery dissection. Chest pain is common and often atypical. Patients are at risk of developing an acute coronary syndrome (STEMI and NSTEMI) related to vasospasm and increased thrombogenesis. Cocaine dysrhythmias result from sodium and potassium blockade. Following cocaine use patients may develop supraventricular tachycardia (SVT), atrial fibrillation/flutter along with wide complex tachycardia/dysrhythmias similar to tricyclic antidepressants. The Brugada pattern and prolonged QT may also be seen with cocaine. Although amphetamines may result in SVT, other dysrhythmias are less commonly seen.

Neurologic complications of cocaine and amphetamines include seizures, spinal cord infarctions, cerebral vasculitis, and ischemic/hemorrhagic cerebrovascular accidents. Choreoathetoid movements and dystonic reactions may occur. A "washout" syndrome following heavy use may result in CNS depression that generally resolves within 24 hours. Amphetamine users may develop severe psychosis.

Cocaine users can develop pulmonary complications including pneumomediastinum, pneumothorax, bronchospasm, and pulmonary edema and hemorrhage. Cocaine abuse during pregnancy increases risk for spontaneous abortion, abruptio placentae, fetal prematurity, and intrauterine growth retardation. "Body stuffers" (hasty ingestion of drugs to avoid police) and "body packers" (ingestion of large amounts of tightly packed pure drug for importation) may be asymptomatic or demonstrate signs of severe cocaine toxicity if a bag ruptures.

Diagnosis and Differential

Diagnosis of cocaine, amphetamine, or stimulant intoxication is usually clinical. Urine drug screening for cocaine is reliable and can detect exposure within 72 hours. Urine screens for amphetamines are less specific and have high false-negative and false-positive results.

Additional laboratory evaluation for intoxicated patients includes a complete metabolic panel to assess acid/base status, kidney function, and a creatine kinase (CK) to assess for rhabdomyolysis. The evaluation of altered mental status or seizure may include a head CT to exclude intracranial hemorrhage. Consider ECG, chest radiograph, and cardiac enzymes in cocaine- or amphetamine-intoxicated patients presenting with chest pain.

The differential diagnosis includes drug intoxications (anticholinergic, PCP, serotonin syndrome), sedative-hypnotic withdrawal, stroke, CNS infections, hypoglycemia, hyponatremia, and thyrotoxicosis. Concomitant use of substances such as alcohol or opioids may significantly alter the presentation.

Emergency Department Care and Disposition

1. Benzodiazepines are the mainstay of treatment for cardiovascular and CNS effects. Administer **lorazepam** 2 mg IV, or 0.1 mg/kg in children; or **diazepam** 5 mg for agitation, hypertension, and tachycardia, and titrate to effect. Judicious use of antipsychotic medications can be considered for those with refractory agitation and violent behavior.
2. Treat seizures with benzodiazepines as noted above. In addition, **phenobarbital** 15 to 20 mg/kg, **propofol,** and neuromuscular blockade with continuous EEG monitoring may be necessary for status epilepticus.
3. Treat cardiac ischemia or acute coronary syndrome with aspirin, nitrates, morphine, and benzodiazepines. **Diltiazem** 20 mg IV can be used in those with ischemic ST changes. β-blockers are contraindicated due to unopposed β-receptor stimulation. Although coronary angiography is preferred for persistent, concerning ST changes, fibrinolytic therapy may be used in those without contraindications.
4. Treat cocaine-induced wide complex tachydysrhythmia and QRS interval prolongation with sodium bicarbonate 1 to 2 mEq/kg titrated to a serum pH of 7.45 to 7.55. **Diltiazem** 20 mg IV can be used to treat SVT. Torsades de pointes can be treated with magnesium and/or overdrive pacing. Consider **lipid emulsion therapy** 1.5 mL/kg IV over 2 minutes then 0.25 mL/kg/min until improvement; maximum dose 10 mL/kg for those with severe, refractory cardiac toxicity.
5. Treat hypertension unresponsive to benzodiazepines with **nitroprusside** 0.3 μg/kg/min IV or **phentolamine** 2.5 to 5 mg IV.
6. Treat "body stuffers" with activated charcoal and supportive care as above. Treat asymptomatic "body packers" with activated charcoal and whole-bowel irrigation using **polyethylene glycol**. Symptomatic "body packers" with presumed rupture of ingested packets are treated for acute toxicity as above and require immediate surgical consultation

for possible laparotomy. Endoscopy should be avoided due to risk of rupture.

7. Patient disposition depends on initial presentation, response to treatment, stimulant involved, and expected duration of effect. Amphetamines have a longer duration of effect than cocaine and may require longer periods of observation or hospital admission. Patients with mild toxicity that resolves completely during observation may be discharged. Admit "body packers" and those patients with more severe toxicity or who remain symptomatic.

HALLUCINOGENS

Clinical Features

Table 105-1 summarizes the classification, features, complications, and specific treatments of commonly abused hallucinogens.

Diagnosis and Differential

Diagnosis is primarily clinical. Routine drug screens will not detect LSD, psilocybin, or mescaline. Urine tests for phencyclidine (PCP) are unreliable. Some amphetamine screens will detect methylenedioxymethamphetamine (MDMA). Urine tests for marijuana are unreliable indicators of acute use because patients may be positive for days to weeks after their last use. Check glucose, electrolytes, renal function, CK, and urinalysis to evaluate for hyponatremia, rhabdomyolysis, and acute kidney injury.

Exclude other causes of altered mental status, including traumatic injuries, hypoglycemia, and infection in patients with hyperthermia. The differential diagnosis of hallucinogen intoxication includes alcohol and benzodiazepine withdrawal, hypoglycemia, anticholinergic poisoning, thyrotoxicosis, CNS infections, structural CNS lesions, and acute psychosis.

Emergency Department Care and Disposition

Most hallucinogen intoxications are managed by monitoring, providing a calm environment, and the use of benzodiazepines for agitation and sympathomimetic symptoms. Antipsychotic medications should be used with caution as these may lower seizure threshold. β-Blockers should not be used as noted above.

1. Treat agitation, hyperthermia, seizures, tachycardia, and hypertension with **lorazepam** 1 to 2 mg IV or PO, or 0.1 mg/kg in children; or **diazepam** 5 to10 mg IV or PO. Repeat dosing as needed. Consider propofol, intubation, and paralysis for severe, refractory toxicity.
2. Consider **nitroprusside** or **phentolamine** for severe hypertension refractory to benzodiazepines.
3. Treat rhabdomyolysis with aggressive isotonic IV fluid administration.
4. Most patients with hallucinogen intoxication can be safely discharged from the ED after a period of observation. Admit patients with persistent altered mental status or serious medical complications, such as severe hyperthermia, hypertension, seizures, and rhabdomyolysis.

TABLE 105-1 Common Hallucinogens

Drug	Typical Hallucinogenic Dose	Duration of Action	Clinical Features	Complications	Specific Treatment
Lysergic acid diethylamide	20–80 μg	8–12 h	• Mydriasis • Tachycardia • Anxiety • Muscle tension	• Coma • Hyperthermia • Coagulopathy • Persistent psychosis • Hallucinogen persisting perception disorder	• Reassurance • Benzodiazepines
Psilocybin	5–100 mushrooms 4–6 mg of psilocybin	4–6 h	• Mydriasis • Tachycardia • Muscle tension • Nausea and vomiting	• Seizures (rare) • Hyperthermia (rare)	• Reassurance • Hydration • Benzodiazepines
Mescaline	3–12 "buttons" 200–500 mg of mescaline	6–12 h	• Mydriasis • Abdominal pain • Nausea/vomiting • Dizziness • Nystagmus • Ataxia	• Rare	• Supportive • Benzodiazepines
Methylenedioxymethamphetamine ("Ecstasy")	50–200 mg	4–6 h	• Mydriasis • Bruxism • Jaw tension • Ataxia • Dry mouth • Nausea	• Hyponatremia • Hypertension • Seizures • Hyperthermia • Dysrhythmias • Rhabdomyolysis	• Benzodiazepines • Hydration • Active cooling • Dantrolene • Specific serotonin antagonists

(Continued)

TABLE 105-1 Common Hallucinogens (Continued)

Drug	Typical Hallucinogenic Dose	Duration of Action	Clinical Features	Complications	Specific Treatment
Synthetic cathinone derivatives ("bath salts")	50–300 mg of mephedrone	2–4 h	• Agitation • Tachycardia • Hypertension • Diaphoresis • Mydriasis	• Paranoia • Panic reactions • Hyperthermia • Seizures • Hyponatremia • Rhabdomyolysis	• Benzodiazepines • Hydration • Active cooling
Phencyclidine ("angel dust")	1–9 mg	4–6 h	• Small or midsized pupils • Nystagmus • Muscle rigidity • Hypersalivation • Agitation • Catatonia	• Coma • Seizures • Hyperthermia • Rhabdomyolysis • Hypertension • Hypoglycemia	• Benzodiazepines • Hydration • Active cooling
Marijuana (cannabis)	5–15 mg of tetrahydrocannabinol	2–4 h	• Tachycardia • Conjunctival injection	• Acute psychosis (rare) • Panic reactions (rare)	• Supportive • Benzodiazepines
Synthetic cannabinoids ("K2," "Spice")	2–5 mg of JWH-018	3–4 h	• Tachycardia • Conjunctival injection	• Acute psychosis • Panic reactions • Seizures (rare) • Dysrhythmias (rare)	• Supportive • Benzodiazepines
Bromo-benzodifuranyl-isopropylamine (Bromo-DragonFLY)	200–800 μg	10–14 h	• Agitation • Hallucinations	• Seizures • Vasoconstrictor with necrosis and gangrene	• Supportive • Benzodiazepines

FURTHER READING

For further reading in *Tintinalli's Emergency Medicine: A Comprehensive Study Guide*, 8th ed., see Chapter 186, "Opioids" by Guillermo Burillo-Putze and MiroOscar; Chapter 187, "Cocaine and Amphetamines" by Jane M. Prosser and Jeanmarie Perrone; and Chapter 188, "Hallucinogens" by Katherine M. Prybys and Karen N. Hansen.

CHAPTER 106

Analgesics

Joshua N. Nogar

Over-the-counter analgesics, such as salicylates (ASA) and acetaminophen (APAP), can result in fatal overdose, but early identification of toxicity and initiation of appropriate treatment can significantly reduce mortality from these exposures. Nonsteroidal anti-inflammatory drug (NSAID) overdoses are rarely fatal and typically require only supportive care. The widespread availability of these medications in over-the-counter preparations, and in other products (e.g., ASA in oil of wintergreen, APAP in cough and cold preparations), can lead to both intentional and accidental toxicity.

ASPIRIN AND SALICYLATES

Clinical Features

The features of aspirin (ASA) toxicity are summarized in Table 106-1. Chronic or "therapeutic" (repeated dose) poisonings are generally more serious and associated with higher mortality than acute overdoses, and are typically encountered in elderly patients with multiple medical problems. Chronic toxicity develops at lower drug levels compared to acute overdoses. The duration of symptoms is often prolonged and there may be a delay in diagnosis because the clinical picture can mimic infection. Chronic salicylism should be considered in any patient with unexplained nonfocal neurologic and behavioral abnormalities, especially with coexisting acid–base disturbance, tachypnea, dyspnea, fever, or noncardiogenic pulmonary edema.

In children, acute ASA overdoses generally present within hours of ingestion. Children younger than 4 years of age tend to develop early metabolic acidosis (pH <7.38), whereas children older than 4 years usually manifest a mixed acid–base disturbance as seen in adults.

Diagnosis and Differential

ASA toxicity is a clinical diagnosis made in conjunction with the patient's acid–base status. Respiratory alkalosis with an anion-gap metabolic acidosis, and hypokalemia are the classic features of this poisoning. ASA blood concentrations correlate poorly with toxicity, and relying on ASA levels as a sole measure of toxicity is the most common pitfall in the management of ASA poisonings.

TABLE 106-1 Severity Grading of Salicylate Toxicity in Adults

	Mild	Moderate	Severe
Acute ingestion (dose)	<150 mg/ kg	150–300 mg/kg	>300 mg/kg
End-organ toxicity	Tinnitus Hearing loss Dizziness Nausea/vomiting	Tachypnea Hyperpyrexia Diaphoresis Ataxia Anxiety	Abnormal mental status Seizures Acute lung injury Renal failure Cardiac dysrhythmias Shock

Check bedside glucose levels in all patients with altered mental status. Additional laboratory studies include electrolytes, blood urea nitrogen (BUN), creatinine, complete blood count (CBC), prothrombin time (PT), ASA level, APAP level (to exclude coingestion), and blood gas. Hypoglycemia or hyperglycemia may be seen with severe or chronic toxicity.

The differential diagnosis of ASA toxicity includes diabetic ketoacidosis, sepsis, meningitis, acute iron poisoning, caffeine overdose, theophylline toxicity, and Reye's syndrome.

Emergency Department Care and Disposition

1. Institute cardiac monitoring and support the ABCs. Establish intravenous access early. Careful airway management is critical in ASA-poisoned patients as a sudden drop in serum pH due to respiratory failure will immediately exacerbate ASA toxicity, and aggressive ventilation guided by acid–base status is essential in the intubated patient. Respiratory acidosis often occurs shortly after a mechanical ventilator is set to "normal" rate/volume parameters, and is typically a premorbid event.
2. Administer **activated charcoal** 1 g/kg PO, NG, or OG. Whole-bowel irrigation may effectively decontaminate the GI tract in the setting of large overdose, enteric-coated, or sustained-release preparations.
3. Administer IV normal saline (NS) to patients with evidence of volume depletion. During initial resuscitation, monitor urine pH, ASA level, electrolytes (especially potassium), glucose, and acid–base status hourly. Add dextrose to parenteral fluids after initial NS resuscitation. Consider 10% dextrose in the setting of hypoglycemia or neurologic symptoms. Add **potassium** 40 mEq/L after establishing adequate urine output (1 to 2 mL/kg/h), if not contraindicated by initial electrolytes and renal function.
4. Alkalinize the serum and urine to enhance ASA protein binding and urinary elimination. Administer a bolus of **sodium bicarbonate** 1 to 2 mEq/kg, then administer a bicarbonate infusion (three ampules of either 44 or 50 mEq/ampule of sodium bicarbonate added to 1L of 5% dextrose in water) at two to three times the patient's maintenance rate; adjust the infusion to maintain urine pH >7.5, if possible. Bicarbonate may worsen hypokalemia and precipitate dysrhythmias; potassium should be aggressively repleted.
5. Consider hemodialysis for all patients with ASA levels in excess of 100 mg/dL. In the setting of chronic toxicity, hemodialysis is needed at lower ASA levels: 60 to 80 mg/dL. Also consider hemodialysis for clinical deterioration despite supportive care and alkalinization, renal insufficiency or failure, severe acid–base disturbance, altered mental status, or adult respiratory distress syndrome. Check serial ASA levels every 2 hours until they begin to fall, then every 4 to 6 hours until the level is nontoxic.
6. Enteric-coated and sustained-release preparations result in delayed peak serum levels from 0 to 60 hours postingestion and their ingestion requires admission for at least 24 hours to ensure declining serial ASA levels and improving clinical status.
7. Discharge a patient from the ED if there is progressive clinical improvement, no significant acid–base abnormality, and a decline in serial ASA levels toward the therapeutic range. In deliberate overdoses, obtain a psychiatric consultation before discharge.

ACETAMINOPHEN (APAP)

Clinical Features

Acute APAP toxicity can present in four classic stages outlined in Table 106-2. Massive APAP ingestions (4-hour APAP level >800 micrograms/mL) may cause early coma or agitation and lactic acidosis, as opposed to delayed symptom onset seen in the majority of APAP overdoses.

Diagnosis and Differential

Toxic exposure to APAP is likely when a patient >6 years old ingests either: (a) >10 g or 200 mg/kg in a single ingestion or over a 24-hour period, or (b) >6 g or 150 mg/kg/d for two consecutive days. For children <6 years old, either: (a) >200 mg/kg in a single ingestion or over an 8-hour period, or (b) 150 mg/kg/day for two consecutive days would be considered toxic. Confirm toxicity with a serum APAP concentration and an exact time of ingestion. Plot the serum APAP level on the Rumack–Matthew nomogram (Fig. 106-1); this nomogram applies only to the setting of a single acute exposure during the window between 4 hours and 24 hours postingestion. Obtain additional laboratory studies including electrolytes, glucose, BUN, creatinine, transaminases, CBC, PT, ASA, urine toxicology screen, and ECG as clinically indicated (e.g., potential coingestion in the suicidal patient).

Emergency Department Care and Disposition

1. Early administration of **activated charcoal** 1 g/kg PO, NG, or OG if possible.
2. **N-acetylcysteine** (NAC) is the antidote for APAP poisoning. The treatment algorithm is depicted in Fig. 106-2 and dosing of NAC is outlined in Table 106-3.

TABLE 106-2 Clinical Stages of Acute Acetaminophen Toxicity

	Stage 1	Stage 2	Stage 3	Stage 4
Timing	First 24 h	Days 2 to 3	Days 3 to 4	After day 5
Clinical manifestations	Anorexia Nausea Vomiting Malaise	Improvement in anorexia, nausea, and vomiting Abdominal pain Hepatic tenderness	Recurrence of anorexia, nausea, and vomiting Encephalopathy Anuria Jaundice	Clinical improvement and recovery (7–8 days) *or* Deterioration to multi-organ failure and death
Laboratory abnormalities	Hypokalemia	Elevated serum transaminases Elevated bilirubin and prolonged prothrombin time if severe	Hepatic failure Metabolic acidosis Coagulopathy Renal failure Pancreatitis	Improvement and resolution *or* Continued deterioration

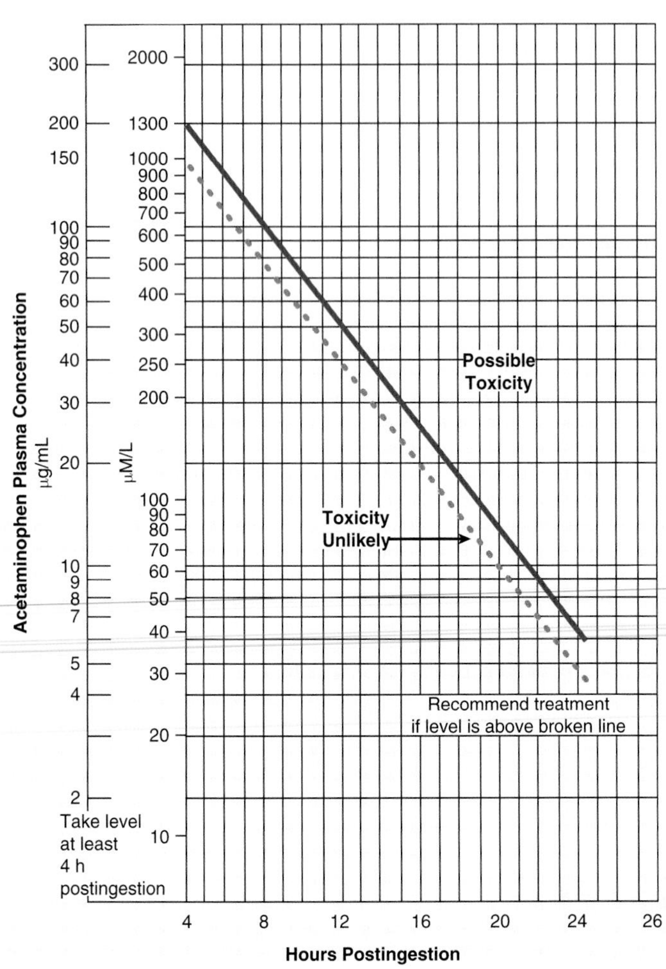

FIGURE 106-1. Rumack–Matthew nomogram.

3. If APAP is still detectable after the dosing regimens described in Table 106-3 are complete, continue NAC until APAP is undetectable in serum.
4. Treat abnormalities related to fulminant hepatic failure by correcting coagulopathy and acidosis, managing cerebral edema, and supporting multi-organ failure. Consider early transfer to a transplant center.
5. Patients with nontoxic APAP levels based on the Rumack–Matthew nomogram may be medically cleared from the ED if there is no evidence of other drug ingestion. Admit all patients receiving NAC therapy.

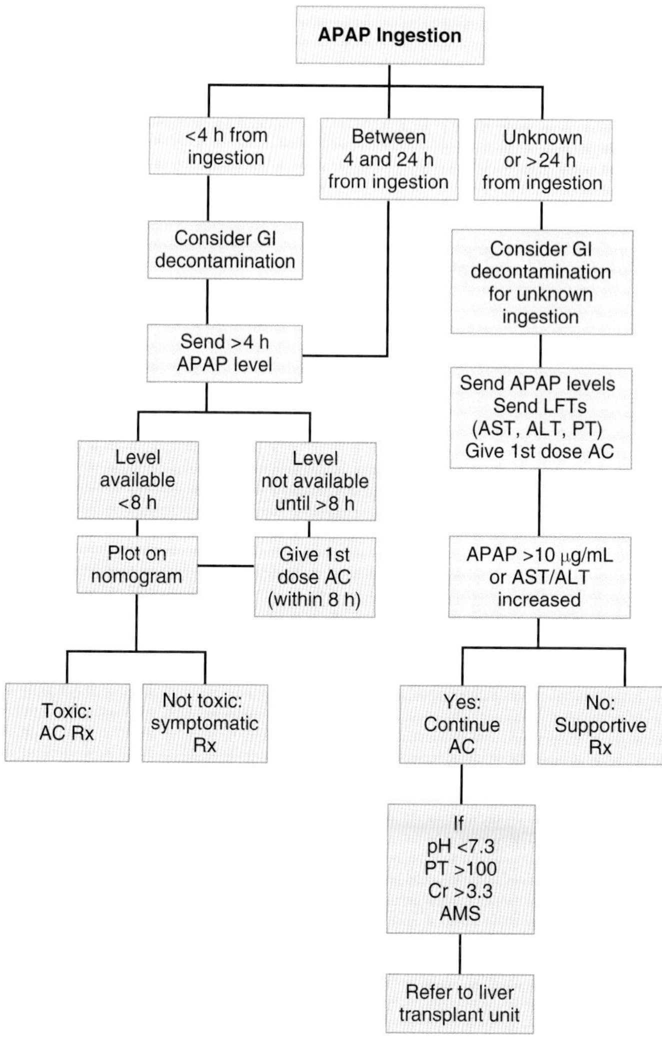

FIGURE 106-2. Treatment guidelines for acetaminophen (APAP) ingestion. All times noted are postingestion. AC, acetylcysteine; ALT, alanine aminotransferase; AMS, altered mental status; AST, aspartate aminotransferase; Cr, creatinine; LFTs, liver function tests; PT, prothrombin time; Rx, treatment.

NONSTEROIDAL ANTI-INFLAMMATORY DRUGS (NSAIDS)

Clinical Features

NSAID toxicity is more commonly associated with chronic therapeutic use as opposed to acute overdoses. The clinical features of acute NSAID toxicity are outlined in Table 106-4.

TABLE 106-3 Acetylcysteine Dosing Regimens

	Oral	IV Adult	IV Pediatric (<40 kg)
Preparation	Available as 10% and 20% solutions Dilute to 5% solution for oral administration	Available as 20% solution	Available as 20% solution Dilute to 2% solution by mixing 50 mL in 450 mL 5% dextrose in water
Loading dose	140 mg/kg	150 mg/kg in 200 mL 5% dextrose in water infused over 15–60 min	150 mg/kg (7.5 mL/kg) infused over 15 to 60 min
Maintenance dose	70 mg/kg every 4 h for 17 doses	50 mg/kg in 500 mL 5% dextrose in water infused over 4 h *followed by* 100 mg/kg in 1000 mL 5% dextrose in water infused over 16 h	50 mg/kg (2.5 mL/kg) infused over 4 h *followed by* 100 mg/kg (5 mL/kg) infused over 16 h
Duration of therapy	72 h	20 h	20 h
Comments	Dilute with powdered drink mix, juice, or soda Serve chilled Drink through a straw to reduce disagreeable smell	Monitor for drug-related adverse effects and anaphylactoid reactions	Monitor for drug-related adverse effects and anaphylactoid reactions 500 mL of the 2% solution prepared as described above is enough to treat a 33-kg child for the full 20-h course

Diagnosis and Differential

The manifestations of NSAID toxicity are generally nonspecific. NSAID levels are not readily available or clinically useful in assessing toxicity. Laboratory evaluation should include electrolytes, glucose, renal and hepatic function tests, and an APAP level. Consideration of evaluation for co-ingestions should be made. Bedside glucose determination is indicated for altered mental status or seizures.

TABLE 106-4 NSAID Toxicity After an Acute Overdose

Initial symptoms within 4 h of ingestion	Abdominal pain, nausea, vomiting
Central nervous system	Headache, nystagmus, diplopia, altered mental status, coma, muscle twitching, and seizures (mefenamic acid)
Cardiovascular	Hypotension, shock, bradydysrhythmia
Electrolyte	Hyperkalemia, hypocalcemia, hypomagnesemia
GI and hepatic	Continued abdominal pain, nausea, vomiting, hepatic injury, pancreatitis (rare)
Renal	Acute kidney injury

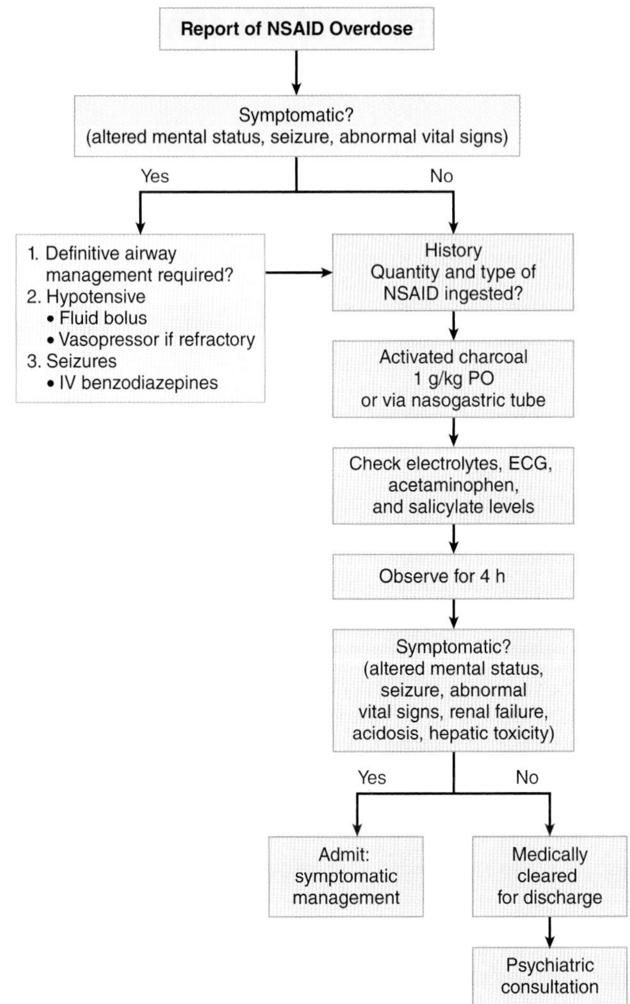

FIGURE 106-3. Approach to treatment of acute NSAID overdose.

Emergency Department Care and Disposition

A general algorithm for acute NSAID overdoses is outlined in Fig. 106-3.

FURTHER READING

For further reading in *Tintinalli's Emergency Medicine: A Comprehensive Study Guide*, 8th ed., see Chapter 189, "Salicylates," by Rachel Levitan and Frank Lovecchio; Chapter 190, "Acetaminophen," by Oliver L. Hung and Lewis S. Nelson; and Chapter 191, "Nonsteroidal Anti-Inflammatory Drugs," by Joseph G. Rella and Wallace A. Carter.

CHAPTER 107

Xanthines and Nicotine

Robert J. Hoffman

XANTHINES

Theophylline, theobromine, and caffeine are methylxanthines.

Theophylline was once widely used for the management of asthma and chronic obstructive pulmonary disease, and continues to be used for apnea of prematurity. Caffeine is the most widely used psychoactive drug in the world, and is consumed primarily from beverages such as coffee, tea, and energy drinks, but is also contained in medications and dietary supplements. Caffeine is used medically in the management of apnea of prematurity, and as an analgesic adjunct.

Clinical Features

Methylxanthine toxicity can cause life-threatening cardiac, neurologic, and metabolic abnormalities. Even therapeutic concentrations of theophylline can cause significant side effects in some individuals. Elderly patients with concomitant medical problems are more susceptible to life-threatening toxicity during chronic therapeutic use than are younger patients with acute overdose.

Cardiac side effects usually include sinus tachycardia, and may include atrial and/or ventricular dysrhythmias. Ventricular dysrhythmias are more common with severe toxicity, chronic toxicity, in the elderly, and those with underlying cardiac dysfunction. Hypotension may also occur as a result of peripheral Beta 2 induced vasodilation.

Neurologic toxicity includes agitation, headache, irritability, sleeplessness, tremors, hallucinations, and seizures. Methylxanthine-induced seizures can be severe and refractory to standard treatment.

Metabolic side effects include hypokalemia, hyperglycemia, and metabolic acidosis. Rhabdomyolysis has been reported with theophylline and caffeine overdose. Compartment syndrome resulting from an unclear etiology is also a rare, but well-described occurrence in theophylline toxicity. Gastrointestinal (GI) effects commonly include nausea and vomiting. Nausea and vomiting are often severe, and poorly responsive to less potent antiemetics.

Diagnosis and Differential

Therapeutic serum theophylline levels of 20 μg/mL can produce toxic effects. In acute poisoning, severity of symptoms typically correlates with serum concentration, but with chronic or acute on chronic toxicity symptom severity correlates more poorly with concentration.

In cases of chronic or acute on chronic toxicity, life-threatening side effects can occur with little warning and before lesser symptoms manifest. Smoking cessation, cirrhosis, and numerous medications, such as cimetidine and erythromycin, increase the half-life of theophylline and increase risk of chronic toxicity. Investigations recommended for theophylline or caffeine toxicity includes serial measurement of the serum theophylline or caffeine concentration, serum electrolytes, and a 12-lead ECG. The differential diagnosis includes other sympathomimetic overdose (e.g., amphetamines, cocaine) as well as anticholinergic toxicity.

Emergency Department Care and Disposition

Treatment of methylxanthine poisoning consists of stabilization, gastric decontamination and elimination, treatment of life-threatening toxic effects, and, in severe cases, hemoperfusion or dialysis.

1. Table 107-1 lists appropriate methods of GI decontamination and elimination in methylxanthine toxicity.
2. Place all patients on cardiac monitors and establish intravenous (IV) or intraosseous (IO) access.
3. Treat nausea and vomiting with **ondansetron** 4 to 8 mg IV or PO (0.1 to 0.15 mg/kg). Consider ranitidine for gastric hypersecretion but **avoid cimetidine, which can prolong the half-life of theophylline.**
4. Treat seizures with benzodiazepines, barbiturates, or even propofol. Rapid escalation of anticonvulsant treatment is warranted when a benzodiazepine treatment fails. **Lorazepam** 0.1 mg/kg IV, or 1 to 2 mg empirically for adults may be used as initial treatment, repeated within 5 to 10 minutes if seizures do not cease. **Phenobarbital** 20 mg/kg or **pentobarbital** 5 mg/kg may be used in cases of benzodiazepine failure. Anticipate respiratory depression and the need for ventilator assistance when using phenobarbital after a benzodiazepine. **Phenytoin is contraindicated in theophylline toxicity**. Due to the common occurrence of severe seizures and status epileptics, use phenobarbital to prophylax against seizures in cases of acute toxicity with theophylline concentration of 80 μg/dL or chronic toxicity with serum concentrations of >40 μg/dL.
5. Administer IV isotonic crystalloid for hypotension. Consider cardioselective beta blockers such as esmolol or metoprolol in patients with hypotension unresponsive to IV fluids or conventional vasopressors.
6. Treat cardiac dysrhythmias with cardioselective blockers such as metoprolol and esmolol. Consider a calcium channel blocker such as diltiazem for atrial fibrillation. Hypokalemia may be severe but is typically

TABLE 107-1 GI Decontamination for Methylxanthine Toxicity

GI Decontamination Technique	Indication*	Dosing
Activated charcoal (single dose)	Acute ingestion	<12 y old: 0.5–1 g/kg PO >12 y old: 25–100 g PO
Multidose activated charcoal (requires close observation)	Acute ingestion	Normal activated charcoal loading dose, followed by: 0.25–0.5 g/kg PO every 2–4 h for 12 h (frequency and duration may vary)
Whole-bowel irrigation using iso-osmolar polyethylene glycol electrolyte solution	Acute ingestion of sustained-release preparations	9 mo–6 y: 25 mL/kg/h 6–12 y old: 1000 mL/h >12 y old: 1500–2000 mL/h Duration: 4–6 h or until clear rectal effluent

*Consider contraindications; for details see http://www.clintox.org/positionstatements.cfm.

unresponsive or poorly responsive to potassium supplementation because the force driving potassium intracellularly continues despite potassium supplementation. In cases of potassium supplementation, hyperkalemia may occur as massive quantities of potassium move extracellularly as the effect of theophylline or caffeine abates. Therefore, potassium supplementation is not recommended unless the patient experiences a dysrhythmia likely to be the result of hypokalemia or empirically if the serum potassium is <2.5 mmol/L

7. Consider hemodialysis or hemoperfusion in a symptomatic patient with a serum theophylline level >90 μg/mL after acute ingestion, or >40 μg/mL in the setting of chronic toxicity and in patients with life-threatening seizures or dysrhythmias.
8. Admit patients with seizures or ventricular dysrhythmias to an intensive care unit. Patients with mild symptoms and theophylline levels below 25 μg/mL usually do not require admission or specific treatment other than symptomatic care. Decrease the dose or discontinue theophylline or caffeine. Symptomatic patients using theophylline with serum concentrations >30 μg/mL may be given 1 to 2 doses of **oral activated charcoal**, regardless of when the last ingestion of theophylline medication occurred, as activated charcoal works by "gut dialysis" to draw theophylline from the blood across the GI surface and into the charcoal sink, effectively lowering serum concentration.

NICOTINE

Nicotine is present in tobacco products and smoking cessation medications, and is also used as an outdoor pesticide. Pediatric exposures to nicotine gum or discarded cigarette butts placed in a beverage such as a soda can are relatively common. Nicotine is rapidly absorbed through the lungs, mucous membranes, intestinal tract, and skin. Once absorbed, it binds to nicotinic receptors throughout the body including the central nervous system, autonomic system, and neuromuscular junction.

Clinical Features

Nicotine toxicity affects the GI, neurologic, cardiovascular, and respiratory systems. Nausea, vomiting, bradycardia, dysrhythmias, hypoventilation, coma, and seizures can occur. In severe poisoning, nicotine can result in paralysis and respiratory arrest. Table 107-2 lists the clinical effects of nicotinic receptor stimulation.

Diagnosis and Differential

Diagnosis of acute nicotine toxicity is largely based on history and physical examination. The differential diagnosis for nicotine toxicity is primarily cholinergic poisoning by other substances, such as organophosphate and carbamate pesticides, as well as cholinergic medication overdose.

Emergency Department Care and Disposition

1. Place patients on a cardiac monitor and establish vascular access.
2. In cases of dermal exposure to nicotine from a pesticide product, perform decontamination as for other HAZMAT substances. This is

TABLE 107-2 Clinical Effects of Nicotine Toxicity

Organ System	Signs and Symptoms of Nicotine Toxicity*	
	Immediate (<1 h)	Delayed (>1 h)
GI	Hypersalivation Nausea Vomiting	Diarrhea
Cardiovascular	Tachycardia Hypertension	Dysrhythmias Bradycardia Hypotension
Neurologic	Tremor Headache Ataxia	Hypotonia Seizure Coma
Respiratory	Bronchorrhea	Hypoventilation Apnea

*Onset of toxicity is varied and can be delayed for hours following dermal exposure.

typically done in a dedicated location, often external to the ED. GI decontamination for nicotine exposure is not recommended, and **urine acidification is contraindicated**.

3. Treat nausea and vomiting with **ondansetron** 4 to 8 mg IV or PO (0.15 mg/kg).
4. Treat seizures or agitation with **lorazepam** 2 mg IV (0.1 mg/kg).
5. Administer isotonic crystalloid for hypotension.
6. Anticipate neuromuscular weakness or respiratory depression in severe toxicity and be prepared for endotracheal intubation and mechanical ventilation.
7. Patients who remain asymptomatic at least 3 hours after ingestion of nicotine-containing products can be discharged. However, patients who ingest intact transdermal patches should be monitored for at least 6 hours.

FURTHER READING

For further reading in *Tintinalli's Emergency Medicine: A Comprehensive Study Guide*, 8th ed., see Chapter 192, "Methylxanthines and Nicotine," by Chip Gresham and Daniel E. Brooks.

CHAPTER 108 Cardiac Medications

Michael Levine

DIGITALIS GLYCOSIDES

Digoxin is used to treat atrial fibrillation, especially with concurrent congestive heart failure. Other cardiac glycosides are found in plants such as foxglove, oleander, and lily of the valley.

Clinical Features

Toxicity can occur following acute ingestion or develop during chronic therapy (Table 108-1). *Acute toxicity* typically presents with abrupt onset of nausea and vomiting. Characteristic cardiac effects include bradydysrhythmias and/or supraventricular tachycardia with atrioventricular block. Severe toxicity can result in ventricular dysrhythmias. *Chronic toxicity* is more common in the elderly and often occurs as a result of renal failure or diuretic therapy. Neuropsychiatric symptoms are more common with chronic toxicity, though cardiac effects are similar to those seen with acute toxicity.

Diagnosis and Differential

Hyperkalemia is often seen in acute poisoning, but may be absent in chronic toxicity. Serum digoxin levels are neither sensitive nor specific for toxicity. However, those patients with higher levels (>2 ng/mL) are more likely to experience toxicity. Almost any dysrhythmia, except for rapidly conducted atrial dysrhythmias, may be seen with toxicity; however, the

TABLE 108-1 Clinical Presentation of Digitalis Glycoside Toxicity

Acute toxicity	
Clinical history	Intentional or accidental ingestion
GI effects	Nausea and vomiting
Central nervous system effects	Headache, dizziness, confusion, coma
Cardiac effects	Bradydysrhythmias or supraventricular tachydysrhythmias with atrioventricular block
Electrolyte abnormalities	Hyperkalemia
Digoxin level	Marked elevation (if obtained within 6 h)
Chronic toxicity	
Clinical history	Typically in elderly cardiac patients taking diuretics; may have renal insufficiency
GI effects	Nausea, vomiting, diarrhea, abdominal pain
Central nervous system effects	Fatigue, weakness, confusion, delirium, coma
Cardiac effects	Almost any dysrhythmia, other than a rapidly conducted atrial fibrillation, can occur; ventricular dysrhythmias are common
Electrolyte abnormalities	Normal, low, or high serum potassium, hypomagnesemia
Digoxin level	Minimally elevated or within "therapeutic" range

most common finding is premature ventricular beats. The differential diagnosis includes sinus node disease or toxicity from calcium channel blockers, β-blockers, class IA antidysrhythmics, clonidine, other cardiotoxic plants, or intrinsic conduction disease.

Emergency Department Care and Disposition

All patients require continuous cardiac monitoring, intravenous (IV) access, and frequent reevaluation (Table 108-2).

1. Administer **activated charcoal** 1 g/kg in cases of acute toxicity in which the patient is awake and cooperative.
2. Use **atropine** 0.5 to 1 mg (0.02 mg/kg, minimum dose 0.1 mg) IV to treat bradydysrhythmias.
3. Administer **digoxin-specific Fab** for ventricular dysrhythmias, hemodynamically significant bradydysrhythmias, and hyperkalemia greater than 5.5 mEq/L. Dosing of digoxin-specific Fab is calculated according to Table 108-3.
4. Hyperkalemia that is thought to be due to cardiac glycoside toxicity is best treated with Fab fragments. Hyperkalemia that is felt to be due to intrinsic renal disease may be treated with dextrose followed by insulin;

TABLE 108-2 Treatment of Digitalis Glycoside Poisoning

Asymptomatic patients
Obtain accurate history
Continuous cardiac monitoring
IV access
GI decontamination (for awake, cooperative patients within 1 h of ingestion): activated charcoal, 1 g/kg orally
Frequent reevaluation
Calculate digoxin-specific Fab antibody fragment dose in anticipation of potential need: may bring to drug bedside, depending on ready availability
Symptomatic patients
Obtain accurate history
IV access
Continuous cardiac monitoring
GI decontamination (for awake, cooperative patients within 1 h of ingestion): activated charcoal, 1 g/kg orally
Life-threatening dysrhythmias
Digoxin-specific Fab antibody fragments: IV infusion
Atropine (for symptomatic bradycardia): 0.5 to 1 mg IV (0.02 mg/kg, minimum dose 0.1 mg)
Pacer: external or transvenous

Abbreviation: Fab, antigen-binding fragment.

TABLE 108-3 Calculation of Digoxin-Specific Fab Antibody Fragment Dose*

Acute life-threatening ingestion with unknown digoxin level and unknown amount ingested: 10 vials intravenous digoxin-specific Fab
A simple and accurate variation using serum digoxin level Number of vials = [serum digoxin level (ng/mL) × patient's weight (kg)]/100

*The digoxin-specific Fab antibody fragments commercially available in the United States contain 38 or 40 mg per vial, depending on the manufacturer, but both bind approximately 0.5 mg of digoxin.

Abbreviation: Fab, antigen-binding fragment.

other options are sodium bicarbonate, potassium-binding resin, or hemodialysis. Historically, IV calcium use has been discouraged because of reports of ventricular dysrhythmias. However, recent evidence suggests that IV calcium use is likely safe.

5. Admit patients with signs of mild toxicity to a monitored setting and manage those with significant toxicity in an intensive care unit. Repeated digoxin levels following digoxin Fab are not accurate and should not be obtained.

β-BLOCKERS

β-Blockers are used in the management of hypertension, acute coronary syndromes, dysrhythmias, congestive heart failure, thyrotoxicosis, social phobias, migraines, and glaucoma. In overdose, their negative inotropic and chronotropic effects result in progressive bradycardia and hypotension.

Clinical Features

Toxicity usually develops within 6 hours of ingestion of an immediate-release product. With sustained-release preparations toxicity is generally seen within 8 hours of ingestion. The cardiovascular system is the primary organ system affected; however, other noncardiac manifestations may occur (Table 108-4). Sotalol, unlike other β-blockers, is also a class III antidysrhythmic, and thus may cause QT-interval prolongation and torsades de pointes. The onset of toxicity from sotalol may be delayed up to 12 hours postingestion.

Diagnosis and Differential

The diagnosis is made based on clinical findings. An ECG should be obtained in all cases. Laboratory studies are directed at identifying underlying medical conditions or complications. Specific drug levels are not commonly available and correlate poorly with clinical effects. Table 108-5 lists other agents that result in bradycardia and hypotension.

TABLE 108-4 Common Findings with β-Blocker Toxicity
Cardiac
Hypotension
Bradycardia
Conduction delays and blocks
Ventricular dysrhythmias (seen with sotalol)
Asystole
Decreased contractility
Central nervous system
Depressed mental status
Coma
Psychosis
Seizures
Pulmonary
Bronchospasm
Endocrine
Hypoglycemia

TABLE 108-5 Toxicologic Causes of Bradycardia and Hypotension

Causes	Differentiating Features
β-Blockers	Relative or absolute hypoglycemia
Calcium channel blockers	Marked hyperglycemia
Naturally occurring cardiac glycosides (oleander, foxglove, lily of the valley, rhododendron, and toad-derived bufotoxin)	Ventricular ectopy Hyperkalemia May cross-react with digoxin immunoassay
Class IC antidysrhythmic drugs (propafenone)	Wide-complex bradycardia
Clonidine	Opioid-like manifestations: coma, miosis, decreased respirations
Digoxin (acute)	Hyperkalemia Elevated level on digoxin immunoassay
Organophosphates	Muscarinic toxidrome

Emergency Department Care and Disposition

The goal of therapy is to restore cardiac output by increasing heart rate and improving myocardial contractility (Fig. 108-1). Establish continuous cardiac monitoring and IV access. IV fluids may be administered for hypotension.

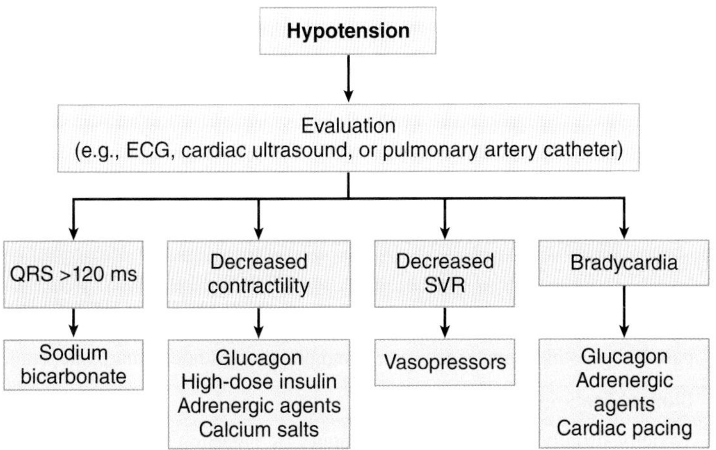

FIGURE 108-1. Management strategies in β-blocker toxicity. Cardiac function is evaluated using ECG and cardiac ultrasound and/or a pulmonary artery catheter. For patients with a wide QRS interval, consider sodium bicarbonate therapy. For patients with impaired myocardial contractility, consider glucagon, norepinephrine, insulin and glucose, and/or calcium therapy. For patients with preserved cardiac contractility, administer IV fluids. For patients with decreased systemic vascular resistance, consider norepinephrine. For patients with bradycardia, consider atropine, glucagon, and/or cardiac pacing. (See the text for details.) IVF, IV fluids; SVR, systemic vascular resistance.

1. Administer **activated charcoal** 1 g/kg within 1 to 2 hours of ingestion if no contraindications exist.
2. **Glucagon** has inotropic and chronotropic effects and is the agent of choice for the treatment of toxicity. Administer as an IV bolus of 3 to 10 mg (0.05 mg/kg). Follow with a continuous infusion of 1 to 5 mg/h. Nausea and vomiting are common side effects. Pretreatment with antiemetics is recommended.
3. Use vasopressors, such as **norepinephrine** 2 to 30 μg/kg/min or **epinephrine** 1 to 20 μg/kg/min, for refractory bradycardia and hypotension. Significantly higher doses may be necessary.
4. Calcium may be of limited benefit in cases of refractory hypotension as either **calcium gluconate** or **calcium chloride**: 10 mL of 10% (0.15 mL/kg) repeated three to six times as necessary. Although calcium chloride contains more elemental calcium than calcium gluconate, it is irritating to soft tissues and should be administered via central line.
5. **Hyperinsulinemia-euglycemia (HIE)** therapy may improve myocardial contractility. Bolus **regular insulin** IV 1 U/kg followed by a continuous infusion of 1 U/kg/h. Serum glucose should be supplemented as needed and monitored frequently to avoid hypoglycemia. Monitor serum potassium for severe hypokalemia.
6. Cardiac pacing may be attempted but it is often unsuccessful. Aggressive measures include extracorporeal circulation or intra-aortic balloon pump placement. Hemodialysis may be of benefit in cases involving acebutolol, atenolol, nadolol, or sotalol.
7. **Isoproterenol,** a pure β-agonist, may provide benefit.
8. Use **magnesium sulfate**, **lidocaine**, and **overdrive pacing** to treat **sotalol-induced** ventricular dysrhythmias.
9. Symptomatic patients should be admitted to an ICU. Asymptomatic patients who ingest can be medically cleared 6 hours after an ingestion of an immediate-release drug or 8 hours after an ingestion of a sustained release drug. Patients who ingest sotalol should be observed for 12 hours.

CALCIUM CHANNEL BLOCKERS

Calcium channel blockers are used in the treatment of hypertension, vasospasm, and rate control of supraventricular tachydysrhythmias. Three widely used classes of calcium channel blockers are the phenylalkylamines (verapamil), benzothiazepines (diltiazem), and dihydropyridines (nifedipine, etc.).

Clinical Features

Toxicity usually develops within 6 hours of ingestion of an immediate-release product. With sustained-release preparations toxicity can be delayed 12 to 24 hours. Toxicity primarily affects the cardiovascular system causing sinus bradycardia, atrioventricular block, and hypotension. Verapamil and diltiazem have a proportionally greater effect on the myocardium than the dihydropyridines. Dihydropyridine overdose can result in reflex tachycardia. With severe toxicity, all classes of calcium channel blockers can cause bradycardia, depressed myocardial contractility, and vasodilatation. Hyperglycemia, lactic acidosis, and noncardiogenic pulmonary edema may occur. Central nervous system effects are due to hypoperfusion and other etiologies should be sought if the blood pressure is normal.

Diagnosis and Differential

The diagnosis is based on clinical findings. Laboratory studies help identify complications. Hyperglycemia is common and helps distinguish calcium channel blocker from β-blocker toxicity, which is associated with hypoglycemia. The differential diagnosis for bradycardia and hypotension is listed in Table 108-5.

Emergency Department Care and Disposition

Treatment is supportive, with an emphasis on increasing cardiac output and systemic vascular resistance (Fig. 108-2). Establish continuous cardiac monitoring and IV access. Administer IV fluids for hypotension.

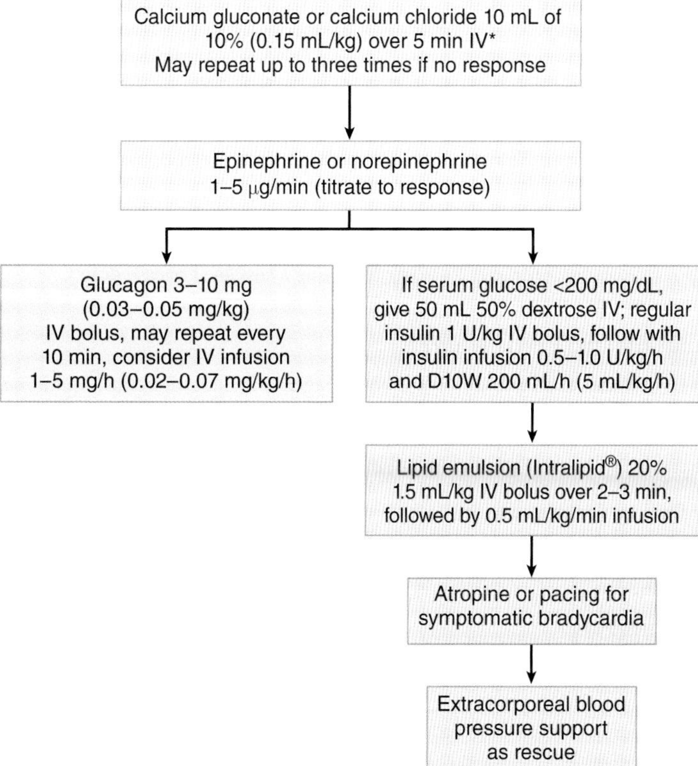

FIGURE 108-2. Treatment algorithm for severe calcium channel blocker toxicity showing recommended progression in therapy at each step if no response occurs. All listed modalities have been shown to be potentially beneficial and in severe cases can be started simultaneously. D10W, 10% dextrose in water. The use of lipid emulsion therapy should be reserved for those patients with verapamil ingestion who have progression of symptoms, refractory to optimal medical management. *Calcium chloride provides three times as much elemental calcium as calcium gluconate; it should be used with caution in cases of digoxin toxicity.

1. Administer **activated charcoal** 1 g/kg within 1 to 2 hours of ingestion if no contraindications exist.
2. Give **atropine** 0.5 to 1 mg IV (0.02 mg/kg, minimum dose 0.1 mg).
3. **Calcium gluconate** or **calcium chloride** can be administered, but typically do not result in significant improvements in hemodynamics. Calcium chloride should be administered via a central line.
4. Use **norepinephrine** 2 to 30 μg/kg/min or **epinephrine** 1 to 20 μg/kg/min for refractory bradycardia and hypotension. Much higher doses may be required.
5. **Hyperinsulinemia-euglycemia (HIE)** therapy can improve myocardial contractility and blood pressure (Table 108-6). Bolus regular insulin 1 U/kg IV followed by continuous infusion (1 U/kg/h). Monitor serum glucose and potassium frequently.
6. **Glucagon** is variably successful in the treatment of calcium channel blocker toxicity. Administer as an IV bolus of 3 to 10 mg (0.05 mg/kg) followed by continuous infusion of 1 to 5 mg/h. Pretreatment with antiemetics is recommended.
7. **IV fat emulsion** (20% solution) may be beneficial in the case of verapamil overdose. Its use should be reserved for those failing standard therapy. Administer as a bolus of 1.5 mL/kg IV followed by a continuous infusion of 0.25 mL/kg/min for 30 to 60 minutes.
8. Symptomatic patients should be admitted to an ICU. Asymptomatic patients may be medically cleared following 6 hours of observation for immediate release drugs, or after 24 hours following a sustained release drug.

ANTIHYPERTENSIVES

Commonly available antihypertensive agents include diuretics, clonidine, angiotensin-converting enzyme inhibitors, and angiotensin II receptor antagonists (Table 108-7). Acute overdose of diuretics are not expected to result in life-threatening clinical toxicity.

Clinical Features

Thiazides and loop diuretics (hydrochlorothiazide, furosemide) can cause mild hypotension, tachycardia, and hypokalemia.

TABLE 108-6 Protocol for Hyperinsulinemia-Euglycemia Therapy in Severe Calcium Channel Blocker Overdose
Administer 50 mL of 50% dextrose (0.5 g/mL) in water IV.
Administer regular insulin 1 U/kg IV bolus.
Begin regular insulin infusion at 1 U/kg/h.
Supplemental dextrose [10% solution (0.1 g/mL) in water at 200 mL/h (adult) or 5 mL/kg/h (pediatric)] may be required.
Monitor serum glucose every 20 minutes. Titrate dextrose infusion rate to maintain serum glucose level between 150 and 300 mg/dL.
Once infusion rates have been stable for 60 minutes, glucose monitoring may be decreased to hourly.
Monitor serum potassium level and start IV potassium infusion if serum potassium level is <2.8 mEq/L.

TABLE 108-7 Summary of Antihypertensive Drugs

Class	Drug	Mechanism of Action	Clinical Presentation of Toxicity	Comments
Diuretics	Acetazolamide	Inhibition of proximal tubule sodium–hydrogen exchange	Hypovolemia Nonanion gap metabolic acidosis	
	Chlorothiazide Chlorthalidone Hydrochlorothiazide Indapamide Metolazone	Inhibition of distal tubule sodium chloride absorption	Hypovolemia Hypercalcemia	
	Bumetanide Furosemide	Inhibition of sodium-potassium chloride symporter in renal loop of Henle	Hypovolemia Hypocalcemia Hypokalemia Hypomagnesemia	
	Amiloride Triamterene	Inhibition of sodium absorption and potassium elimination in renal distal collecting duct	Hypovolemia Hyperkalemia	
	Eplerenone Spironolactone	Mineralocorticoid antagonist	Hypovolemia Hyperkalemia	
Sympatholytics	Doxazosin Prazosin Tamsulosin Terazosin	α_1-Adrenergic receptor antagonist	Orthostatic hypotension	Phenylephrine may be used for refractory hypotension.
	Clonidine Guanabenz	α_2-Adrenergic receptor agonist Imidazoline receptor agonist	Hypotension Bradycardia	Hypotension may respond to high-dose naloxone.
	Guanfacine Oxymetazoline Tetrahydrozoline	μ-Receptor opioid agonist	Neurologic depression	Phenylephrine may be used for refractory hypotension.

(Continued)

TABLE 108-7 Summary of Antihypertensive Drugs (Continued)

Class	Drug	Mechanism of Action	Clinical Presentation of Toxicity	Comments
ACE inhibitors	Benazepril Captopril	Inhibition of angiotensin-converting enzyme Inhibition of bradykininase	Hypotension (rare)—most are asymptomatic Hyperkalemia	
	Enalapril Fosinopril Moexipril Perindopril Quinapril Trandolapril		Angioedema (idiosyncratic) Cough (idiosyncratic)	
Angiotensin receptor blockers	Candesartan Eprosartan Irbesartan Losartan Telmisartan Valsartan	Angiotensin II receptor antagonist	Hypotension Hyperkalemia Angioedema (less common than with ACE inhibitors)	
Vasodilators	Hydralazine	Arteriolar vasodilation	Hypotension	
	Minoxidil		Tachycardia Increased myocardial oxygen demand Lupus-like syndrome (idiosyncratic reaction to hydralazine)	
	Sodium nitroprusside	Arteriolar and venous vasodilation (via nitric oxide release)	Hypotension Tachycardia Thiocyanate toxicity (after prolonged infusion) Cyanide toxicity (very rare)	Thiosulfate should be administered if cyanide toxicity is considered.

Abbreviation: ACE, angiotensin-converting enzyme.

Potassium-sparing diuretics (spironolactone, triamterene, and amiloride) can cause hyperkalemia and hypovolemia.

Emergency Department Care and Disposition

Management is supportive, including correction of electrolyte abnormalities. Establish continuous cardiac monitoring and IV access in all patients.

1. Administer **activated charcoal** 1 g/kg within 1 to 2 hours of ingestion if no contraindications exist, and the patient is awake, cooperative, and able to drink charcoal.
2. Administer IV normal saline to correct hypovolemia.
3. Start **norepinephrine** for hypotension refractory to volume resuscitation.
4. Correct potassium abnormalities using standard measures. Patients with severe hyperkalemia from potassium-sparing diuretics may require dialysis.
5. Most patients can be medically cleared after a 4- to 6-hour observation period. Patients with hypotension or electrolyte abnormalities require admission.

CLONIDINE

Clonidine is a centrally acting α-agonist used for the management of hypertension and opiate withdrawal.

Clinical Features

Clonidine toxicity causes miosis, hypotension, and bradycardia, as well as CNS and respiratory depression.

Emergency Department Care and Disposition

Management is supportive though respiratory depression and apnea, most commonly seen in children, may infrequently require endotracheal intubation. Establish continuous cardiac monitoring and IV access in all patients.

1. Administer IV normal saline for hypotension.
2. Use **norepinephrine** 2 to 30 μg/kg/min for hypotension refractory to fluid resuscitation.
3. Give **atropine** 0.5 to 1 mg (0.02 mg/kg, minimum dose 0.1 mg) for symptomatic bradycardia.
4. **Naloxone** anecdotally may be effective for cases of refractory hypotension or altered mental status, but convincing data supporting naloxone in this setting are lacking.
5. Patients who remain asymptomatic after a 6-hour observation period can be medically cleared. Admit symptomatic patients to a monitored setting.

ANGIOTENSIN-CONVERTING ENZYME INHIBITORS

Agents include captopril, enalapril, and lisinopril. Most patients with ACE-inhibitor overdose remain asymptomatic. The primary toxicity in overdose is hypotension, which may be treated with IV normal saline and vasopressors. Patients should be observed for the onset of hypotension.

ANGIOTENSIN II RECEPTOR ANTAGONISTS

Agents include iosartan, valsartan, and candesartan. As with ACE inhibitors, most patients remain asymptomatic. However, hypotension or hyperkalemia may occur. Therapy is supportive and includes IV fluid administration, correction of electrolyte disturbances, and cardiac monitoring for at least 6 hours.

FURTHER READING

For further reading in *Tintinalli's Emergency Medicine: A Comprehensive Study Guide*, 8th ed., see Chapter 193, "Digitalis Glycosides," by Michael Levine and Aaron B. Skolnik; Chapter 194, "β-Blockers," by Jennifer L. Englund and William P. Kerns II; Chapter 195, "Calcium Channel Blockers," by Alicia B. Minns and Christian Tomaszewski; and Chapter 196, "Antihypertensives" by Frank Lovecchio and Dan Quan.

CHAPTER 109

Anticonvulsants

Robert J. Hoffman

PHENYTOIN

Intentional phenytoin overdose rarely leads to death, provided adequate supportive care is administered. Most phenytoin-related deaths have been caused by rapid IV administration and hypersensitivity reactions. Phenytoin toxicity may occur after single acute exposure, and also may occur in patients chronically using phenytoin. In patients using phenytoin, toxicity occurs after lesser ingestions because a large quantity of phenytoin is already present in the body.

Clinical Features

The toxic effects of phenytoin depend on the duration of exposure, dosage taken, and route of administration. Life-threatening effects such as hypotension, bradycardia, and asystole are seen with IV administration and are likely secondary to the diluent, propylene glycol. Morbidity can be avoided by slowing the rate of administration during infusion. Extravasation of phenytoin, but not fosphenytoin, may result in catastrophic injury with significant loss of soft tissue or even loss of digits or the hand.

Clinical manifestations in overdose are typically dose related and are listed in Table 109-1. The primary clinical features of overdose are related to acute CNS effects while cardiovascular toxicity almost exclusively results from IV administration. Supratherapeutic phenytoin levels commonly result

TABLE 109-1 Clinical Features of Phenytoin Toxicity

Central nervous system	Dizziness, tremor (intention), visual disturbance, horizontal and vertical nystagmus, diplopia, miosis or mydriasis, ophthalmoplegia, abnormal gait (bradykinesia, truncal ataxia), choreoathetoid movements, irritability, agitation, confusion, hallucinations, fatigue, coma, encephalopathy, dysarthria, meningeal irritation with pleocytosis, seizures (rare)
Peripheral nervous system	Peripheral neuropathy, urinary incontinence
Hypersensitivity (anticonvulsant hypersensitivity syndrome)	Eosinophilia, rash, pseudolymphoma (diffuse lymphadenopathy), systemic lupus erythematosus, pancytopenia, hepatitis, pneumonitis
Gastrointestinal	Nausea, vomiting, hepatotoxicity
Dermatologic	Hirsutism, acne, rashes (including Stevens–Johnson syndrome)
Other organs	Fetal hydantoin syndrome, gingival hyperplasia, coarsening of facial features, hemorrhagic disease of the newborn, hyperglycemia, hypocalcemia
Parenteral toxicity	May cause hypotension, bradycardia, conduction disturbances, myocardial depression, ventricular fibrillation, asystole, and tissue necrosis from infiltration

TABLE 109-2 Correlation of Plasma Phenytoin Level and Side Effects

Total Plasma Level (μg/mL)	Toxic Effects
<10	Usually none
10–20	Occasional mild nystagmus
20–30	Nystagmus
30–40	Ataxia, slurred speech, nausea and vomiting
40–50	Lethargy, confusion
>50	Coma, seizures

in cerebellar symptoms of dizziness, ataxia, and nystagmus. Skin and soft tissue injury may be seen with IM injection or after extravasation from IV infusion. Therapeutic use has been associated with hypersensitivity reactions and gingival hyperplasia. Phenytoin is teratogenic.

Diagnosis and Differential

Diagnosis is made by history, clinical exam, and serum drug levels. The therapeutic range is 10 to 20 μg/mL and toxicity generally correlates with increasing plasma levels (Table 109-2). Absorption is erratic, and serial levels should be obtained in cases of suspected ingestion. Electrocardiographic changes in toxicity include increased PR interval, widened QRS interval, and altered ST-wave and T-wave segments.

Emergency Department Care and Disposition

1. Place patients on monitor and obtain IV access.
2. Treat acute oral overdose or severe supratherapeutic toxicity with multidose of oral **activated charcoal** (1 g/kg) every 4 to 6 hours for the first 24 hours.
3. Correct acidosis to decrease free serum phenytoin.
4. Treat hypotension from IV administration of phenytoin with IV isotonic crystalloid and discontinuation of the infusion.
5. Treat bradydysrhythmias with atropine or cardiac pacing.
6. Treat seizures with a benzodiazepine or phenobarbital.
7. Admit patients with serious complications (e.g., seizures, coma, altered mental status, and ataxia). Consider a patient's ability to safely ambulate when determining admission or discharge status. Generally, ability to safely ambulate is required for safe discharge. Observe patients with mild symptoms until serum levels are declining; cardiac monitoring after isolated oral ingestion is unnecessary.
8. Discontinue phenytoin in cases of toxicity. The number of days to withhold phenytoin depends on the serum level. Generally, at least 1 or 2 days without phenytoin are needed, and after 2 to 3 days the patient can return to a medical provider to have his or her serum phenytoin level rechecked.

CARBAMAZEPINE

Clinical Features

Carbamazepine's anticholinergic properties delay GI motility and can cause delayed clinical deterioration. Manifestations of acute toxicity include ataxia, nystagmus, miosis or mydriasis, ileus, bowel obstruction, hypertonicity, increased deep tendon reflexes, dystonic reactions, and an anticholinergic toxidrome. Severe toxicity may result in coma and respiratory failure, and seizures can occur at high serum concentrations. Though rare, carbamazepine can widen the QRS interval and cause cardiac dysrhythmias. Patients taking carbamazepine therapeutically will develop toxicity with lesser acute ingestions because a large quantity of carbamazepine is already present in the body.

Diagnosis and Differential

Serum carbamazepine concentrations do not correlate with severity of poisoning, though concentrations >40 μg/mL may be associated with an increased risk of complications, and those more than 60 to 80 μg/mL may be fatal. A false-positive tricyclic antidepressant result on urine drug screen can occur.

Emergency Department Care and Disposition

1. Consider activated charcoal in the awake patient within 1 hour of ingestion or in patients chronically taking carbamazepine therapeutically.
2. Consider hemodialysis or hemodiafiltration for life-threatening overdose.
3. Obtain an ECG to evaluate for QRS interval widening. Treat QRS interval widening with sodium bicarbonate.
4. Patients can be discharged if asymptomatic, with declining serum levels (below 15 μg/mL), and a normal ECG.

VALPROATE

Clinical Features

In acute overdose, valproate causes central nervous system depression. Other findings include respiratory depression, hypotension, hypoglycemia, hypernatremia, hypophosphatemia, and anion gap metabolic acidosis that may persist for days. Liver toxicity, cerebral edema, hyperammonemia, pancreatitis, and thrombocytopenia have been reported after acute overdose. Hepatic failure (microvesicular steatosis) occurs in about 1 in 20,000 patients on long-term therapy, with children <3 years of age on multiple antiepileptics at greatest risk.

Diagnosis and Differential

Obtain a serum valproate level. The therapeutic range is 50 to 100 μg/mL; adverse effects increase at concentrations >150 μg/mL and frank coma may occur with levels above 800 μg/mL. Check serum ammonia and bedside glucose in patients with altered level of consciousness. Consider liver function tests, electrolytes, and a CBC.

Emergency Department Care and Disposition

1. Consider multidose activated charcoal after ingestion of enteric-coated, delayed-release preparations and measure serial concentrations to account for delayed peak serum concentration. Consider whole-bowel irrigation in any enteric-coated or extended-release preparations.

2. **L-carnitine**, 50 mg/kg/day, may hasten recovery in patients with acute intoxication and increase survival from hepatotoxicity.
3. Hemodialysis may be useful in toxicity associated with very high serum concentrations >800 μg/mL. Hemoperfusion and hemodiafiltration can be used to treat severe overdose.
4. All symptomatic patients, other than those with mild symptoms, require admission. Asymptomatic patients with declining serum levels can be discharged.

SECOND-GENERATION ANTICONVULSANTS

As a group, the second-generation anticonvulsants possess little toxicity in acute overdose.

- Felbamate may cause aplastic anemia and hepatic failure and can crystallize in the kidney, leading to acute renal failure in large overdose.
- Gabapentin may cause drowsiness, ataxia, nausea, and vomiting that generally resolve in about 10 hours. Gabapentin is increasingly abused for its benzodiazepine-like effects.
- Lacosamide may cause dizziness, headache, nausea, and diplopia during therapeutic use.
- Lamotrigine has been associated with autoimmune reactions during therapeutic use and drowsiness, vomiting, ataxia, and dizziness in overdose. Seizures, coma, cardiac toxicity (QRS and QT-interval prolongation), and acute pancreatitis have been reported. Treatment includes sodium bicarbonate.
- Levetiracetam may cause lethargy, coma, and respiratory depression.
- Oxcarbazepine may cause hyponatremia and a drug rash during therapeutic use.
- Pregabalin has been reported to cause somnolence and dizziness during long-term therapeutic use. Overdose may cause depressed level of consciousness. Pregabalin is increasingly abused for its benzodiazepine-like effects.
- Rufinamide may cause headache, dizziness, fatigue and somnolence during long-term therapy.
- Tiagabine may cause the rapid neurologic toxicity, including lethargy, coma, seizures, myoclonus, muscular rigidity, and delirium.
- Topiramate may cause nephrolithiasis and glaucoma during therapeutic use. In overdose, somnolence, vertigo, agitation, mydriasis, and seizures have been reported. Topiramate can produce a metabolic acidosis, which can last up to 7 days due to the long half-life of the drug.
- Zonisamide may promote renal stone formation and cause a drug rash during therapeutic use.

FURTHER READING

For further reading in *Tintinalli's Emergency Medicine: A Comprehensive Study Guide*, 8th ed., see Chapter 197, "Anticonvulsants" by Frank LoVecchio.

CHAPTER 110 Iron

O. John Ma

CLINICAL FEATURES

Iron toxicity from an intentional or accidental ingestion is a common poisoning. Based on clinical findings, iron poisoning can be divided into five stages.

The first stage develops within the first few hours of ingestion. Direct irritative effects of iron on the gastrointestinal (GI) tract produce abdominal pain, vomiting, and diarrhea. Vomiting is the clinical sign most consistently associated with acute iron toxicity. The absence of these symptoms within 6 hours of ingestion essentially excludes a diagnosis of significant iron toxicity.

During the second stage, which may continue for up to 24 hours following ingestion, the patient's GI symptoms may resolve, providing a false sense of security despite toxic amounts of iron absorption. While patients may be asymptomatic, they often appear ill and may have abnormal vital signs reflecting hypovolemia and metabolic acidosis.

The third stage may appear early or develop hours after the second stage as shock and a metabolic acidosis evolve. Iron-induced coagulopathy may cause bleeding and worsen hypovolemia. Hepatic dysfunction, cardiomyopathy, and renal failure may also develop.

The fourth stage develops 2 to 5 days after ingestion and is characterized by elevation of aminotransferase levels and possible progression to hepatic failure.

The fifth stage, which occurs 4 to 6 weeks after ingestion, reflects the corrosive effects of iron on the pyloric mucosa and may cause gastric outlet obstruction.

DIAGNOSIS AND DIFFERENTIAL

The diagnosis of iron poisoning is based on the clinical picture and the history provided by the patient, significant others, caretakers, or EMS providers. When determining a patient's potential for toxicity, the total amount of elemental iron must be used in calculations. Table 110-1 reviews the predicted clinical effects based on the amount of iron ingested.

Laboratory evaluation includes serum electrolytes, renal studies, serum glucose, coagulation studies, complete blood count, hepatic enzymes, and a serum iron level. A single serum iron level does not reflect what iron levels have been previously, what direction they are going, or the degree of iron toxicity in tissues; a single low serum level does not exclude the diagnosis of iron poisoning since there are variable times to peak level following ingestion of different iron preparations. Serum iron levels have limited use in directing management since toxicity is primarily intracellular rather than in the blood. The total iron binding capacity (TIBC) becomes falsely elevated in the presence of elevated serum iron levels or deferoxamine, and is of no clinical value.

TABLE 110-1 Predicted Toxicity of Iron Ingestion

Predicted Clinical Effects	Elemental Iron Dose*	Serum Iron Concentration†
Nontoxic or mild GI symptoms	<20 mg/kg	<300 μg/dL (<54 μM/L)
Expected significant GI symptoms and potential for systemic toxicity	20–60 mg/kg	300–500 μg/dL (54–90 μM/L)
Moderate to severe systemic toxicity	>60 mg/kg	>500 μg/dL (>90 μM/L)
Severe systemic toxicity and increased morbidity		>1000 μg/dL (>180 μM/L)

*Elemental iron dose by history.

†Serum iron concentration obtained within 4 to 6 hours of ingestion.

Plain radiographs may reveal iron in the GI tract; however, many iron preparations are not radiopaque, so normal radiographs do not exclude iron ingestion.

EMERGENCY DEPARTMENT CARE AND DISPOSITION

Patients who have remained asymptomatic for 6 hours after ingestion of iron, have not ingested a potentially toxic amount, and who have a normal physical examination do not require medical treatment for iron toxicity. Patients whose symptoms resolve after a short period of time, and who have normal vital signs, usually have mild toxicity and require only supportive care. This subset of patients still requires an observation period. Figure 110-1 is an algorithm for the clinical management of patients after an acute iron ingestion.

Patients who are symptomatic or demonstrate signs of hemodynamic instability after iron ingestion require aggressive management in the ED.

1. Place the patient on supplemental oxygen and a cardiac monitor, and establish two large-bore IV lines.
2. Administer vigorous **intravenous (IV) crystalloid infusion** to help correct hypovolemia and hypoperfusion.
3. Perform **gastric lavage** in patients who present within 60 minutes of ingestion. Activated charcoal is not recommended.
4. Whole-bowel irrigation with a **polyethylene glycol** solution is efficacious. Administration of 250 to 500 mL/h in children or 2 L/h in adults via nasogastric tube may clear the GI tract of iron pills before absorption occurs.
5. Administer antiemetics such as **ondansetron** 4 mg IV in adults (0.1 mg/kg to a maximum dose of 4 mg in pediatric patients) or **promethazine** 25 mg IV in adults.
6. Correct coagulopathy with **vitamin K_1** 5 to 10 mg SC and **fresh frozen plasma** 10 to 25 mL/kg in adults (10 mL/kg in pediatric patients). Order blood for type and screen or crossmatch as necessary.
7. **Deferoxamine** is a chelating agent that can remove iron from tissues and free iron from plasma. Deferoxamine is safe to administer to children and pregnant women. Deferoxamine therapy is indicated in patients

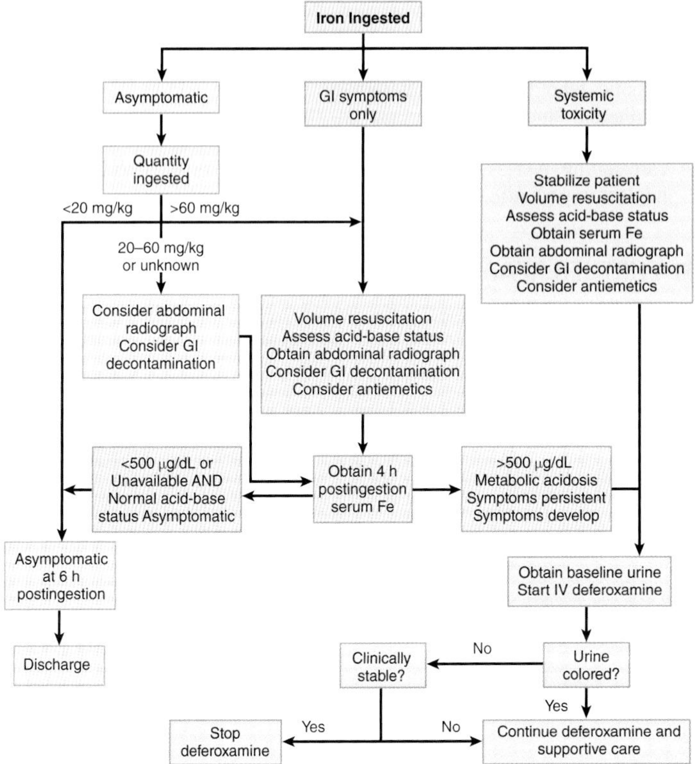

FIGURE 110-1. Algorithm for clinical management of patients following iron ingestion.

with systemic toxicity, metabolic acidosis, worsening symptoms, or a serum iron level predictive of moderate to severe toxicity.

Intravenous infusion is the preferred route of **deferoxamine** administration because IM absorption is unpredictable in the hypovolemic patient. The recommended initial dose is 50 mg/kg in children to an adult dose of 1000 mg IV. Since hypotension is the rate-limiting factor for IV infusion, it is recommended to begin with a slow IV infusion at 5 mg/kg/h. The deferoxamine infusion rate can be increased to 15 mg/kg/h, as tolerated, within the first hour of treatment. The recommended total amount of deferoxamine is 360 mg/kg or 6 g during the first 24 hours. Initiate deferoxamine therapy without waiting for the serum iron level in any clinically ill patient with a known iron ingestion.

Evaluate the efficacy of deferoxamine treatment through serial urine samples. As ferrioxamine is excreted, urine changes to a classic *vin rose* appearance. Clinical recovery is the most important factor guiding the termination of deferoxamine therapy.

8. Patients who remain asymptomatic after 6 hours of observation, have a normal physical examination, and have a reliable history of an insignificant ingestion may be considered for discharge. Patients initially symptomatic who become asymptomatic should be admitted for further evaluation since this may represent the second stage of iron toxicity. Admit all patients who receive deferoxamine therapy to an intensive care setting. Assess all patients for suicide risk. Consider child abuse or neglect in pediatric cases.

FURTHER READING

For further reading in *Tintinalli's Emergency Medicine: A Comprehensive Study Guide*, 8th ed., see Chapter 198, "Iron," by Stephanie H. Hernandez and Lewis S. Nelson.

Hydrocarbons and Volatile Substances

Allyson A. Kreshak

Products containing hydrocarbons are found in many household and workplace settings and include fuels, lighter fluids, paint removers, pesticides, polishers, degreasers, and lubricants. Some volatile substances may be recreationally abused. Exposure may cause mild to severe toxicity and, rarely, sudden death.

CLINICAL FEATURES

Toxicity depends on route of exposure, physical characteristics, chemical characteristics, and the presence of toxic additives (e.g., lead or pesticides). See Table 111-1 for clinical features.

Chemical pneumonitis is the most common pulmonary complication and is most likely to occur following aspiration of a hydrocarbon with low viscosity (ability to resist flow), high volatility (tendency for a liquid to become a gas), and low surface tension (cohesive force between molecules). Symptoms occur quickly and include cough, gagging, choking, and dyspnea. Physical examination may reveal tachypnea, wheezing, grunting, and an elevated temperature. Radiographic abnormalities do not always occur. If radiographic findings occur, they may lag behind the clinical picture by 4 to 24 hours, but most are apparent within 6 hours.

Cardiac toxicity manifests as potentially lethal dysrhythmias resulting from myocardial sensitization to circulating catecholamines ("sudden sniffing death syndrome"). Halogenated hydrocarbon solvents are most frequently implicated, but all classes of hydrocarbons have been associated with dysrhythmias.

TABLE 111-1 Clinical Manifestations of Hydrocarbon Exposure

System	Clinical Manifestations
Pulmonary	Tachypnea, grunting respirations, wheezing, retractions
Cardiac	Ventricular dysrhythmias (may occur after exposure to halogenated hydrocarbons and aromatic hydrocarbons)
Central nervous	Slurred speech, ataxia, lethargy, coma
Peripheral nervous	Numbness and paresthesias in the extremities
GI and hepatic	Nausea, vomiting, abdominal pain, loss of appetite (mostly with halogenated hydrocarbons)
Renal and metabolic	Muscle weakness or paralysis secondary to hypokalemia in patients who abuse toluene
Hematologic	Lethargy (anemia), shortness of breath (anemia), neurologic depression/syncope (carbon monoxide from methylene chloride), cyanosis (methemoglobinemia from amine-containing hydrocarbons)
Dermal	Local erythema, papules, vesicles, generalized scarlatiniform eruption, exfoliative dermatitis, "huffer's rash," cellulitis

Central nervous system toxicity may present as intoxication, ranging from initial giddiness, agitation, and hallucinations to seizures, slurred speech, ataxia, and coma. Chronic exposure may cause recurrent headaches, cerebellar ataxia, and mood lability.

Gastrointestinal toxicity can include vomiting (which can lead to aspiration), abdominal pain, anorexia, and hepatic damage (particularly from halogenated hydrocarbons such as carbon tetrachloride, methylene chloride, trichloroethylene, and tetrachloroethylene).

Dermal toxicity includes contact dermatitis and blistering with progression to full-thickness burns. Injection of hydrocarbons can cause tissue necrosis. Burns can result after cutaneous contact with hot tar and asphalt.

Less common acute toxicities include hematologic disorders such as hemolysis, methemoglobinemia, carboxyhemoglobinemia (from methylene chloride), and renal dysfunction.

DIAGNOSIS AND DIFFERENTIAL

Diagnosis is made by history and physical examination findings, bedside monitoring, laboratory tests, and chest radiograph. An abdominal radiograph may reveal ingestion of radiopaque substances (e.g., chlorinated hydrocarbons).

EMERGENCY DEPARTMENT CARE AND DISPOSITION

1. Secure the airway and maintain ventilation support in patients with respiratory insufficiency or neurologic depression. Administer oxygen to symptomatic patients and place them on a cardiac monitor (see Table 111-2). An EKG should be obtained.
2. Treat hypotension with intravenous crystalloid infusion. Avoid catecholamines except in cases of cardiac arrest. Treat tachydysrhythmias with propranolol, esmolol, or lidocaine. Avoid class IA and III agents.
3. Follow standard hazardous material measures for decontamination of the patient. Initial decontamination should ideally be done at the scene and should include removal of the patient from the exposure (including clothing or dermal contact). Skin may be irrigated with soap and water. Activated charcoal is not indicated following isolated hydrocarbon ingestions. The use of gastric emptying is not beneficial, and this decontamination technique is not regularly employed following ingestion.
4. Meticulous wound care with potential surgical debridement is indicated for dermal exposures. Treat tar and asphalt injuries with immediate cooling and cold water, and application of ointment combined with surface-active agents (e.g., Polysorbate 80).
5. Prophylactic antibiotics are not generally indicated. Corticosteroid use is not indicated.
6. Admit symptomatic patients, those exposed to hydrocarbons capable of producing delayed toxicity (e.g., halogenated hydrocarbons), and those exposed to hydrocarbons with toxic additives (e.g., pesticides or organic metal compounds). Patients with severe respiratory distress may need

TABLE 111-2 Management of Hydrocarbon Exposures

Airway and breathing	Secure airway. Antidotes: Administer oxygen for carboxyhemoglobinemia and methylene blue for methemoglobinemia. Provide supplemental oxygen if wheezing. Administer inhaled β_2-agonists if wheezing. Ventilatory support: Provide positive end-expiratory pressure or continuous positive airway pressure as needed to achieve adequate oxygenation.
Cardiac	Circulation: Administer IV crystalloid fluid for initial volume resuscitation of hypotensive patients. Do not use catecholamines in cases of halogenated hydrocarbon exposure. Consider propranolol, esmolol, or lidocaine for ventricular dysrhythmias induced by halogenated hydrocarbon exposure. Consult the poison control center, toxicologist, and other appropriate specialists as needed.
Decontamination	Dermal: Remove hydrocarbon-soaked clothes, decontaminate skin with soap and water, and decontaminate eyes with saline irrigation. GI: Not indicated.
Other	Laboratory tests: Order CBC, basic metabolic panel, liver function tests (serum transaminase, bilirubin, albumin levels), prothrombin time, partial thromboplastin time, carboxyhemoglobin level, methemoglobin level, and/or radiologic studies as indicated (see the text). Correct electrolyte abnormalities. Do not give steroids. Administer blood products as needed.

intubation and mechanical ventilation with high levels of PEEP. Patients exposed to nonhalogenated aliphatic hydrocarbons that are asymptomatic and with a normal chest radiograph may be discharged with return precautions after 6 to 8 hours of observation.

FURTHER READING

For further reading in *Tintinalli's Emergency Medicine: A Comprehensive Study Guide*, 8th ed., see Chapter 199, "Hydrocarbons and Volatile Substances," by C. William Heise and Frank LoVecchio.

CHAPTER 112

Caustics

Jennifer Cullen

Caustics are substances that can cause histological and functional damage on contact and include both alkalis (pH >7) and acids (pH <7). The most common alkali exposure is household bleach (sodium hypochlorite with hydroxide), which is usually benign except in intentional ingestions. The most common acid exposures are drain cleaners (sulfuric acid), automobile batteries, and masonry cleaners (hydrochloric acid).

CLINICAL FEATURES

Common features of caustic ingestions include dysphagia, odynophagia, epigastric pain, and vomiting with gastrointestinal (GI) tract injuries. Dysphonia, stridor, and respiratory distress can be seen with laryngotracheal injury. Esophageal injuries are graded by direct endoscopic visualization: (1) edema and hyperemia; (2) ulcerations, blisters, and exudates (2a—noncircumferential; 2b—circumferential); (3) deep ulceration and necrosis. Intentional ingestions are associated with higher-grade injury that can lead to the development of strictures. Most ingestions with serious injury are symptomatic with stridor, drooling, or vomiting, although distal GI injury without oral or facial burns is possible. Disc battery ingestions are often asymptomatic, though batteries >15 mm in diameter can become lodged in the esophagus and cause pressure necrosis.

Caustic exposures to the cornea are particularly serious if they involve alkalis. Dermal exposures to caustics usually produce only local pain and irritation. However, alkali and sodium hydrofluoric acid burns can penetrate deeply. Alkali exposures lead to liquefactive necrosis, which is more severe than the coagulation necrosis caused by most acids. Hydrofluoric acid can cause systemic hypocalcemia, hypomagnesemia, and hyperkalemia with subsequent ventricular dysrhythmias.

DIAGNOSIS AND DIFFERENTIAL

The diagnosis is clinical. Routine laboratory tests are recommended for severely affected patients and include electrolytes, assessment of acid–base status, and monitoring for potential gastrointestinal bleeding. Monitor serum calcium and magnesium levels and perform an ECG in patients with hydrofluoric acid exposures, especially ingestions. Consider chest and/or abdominal radiographs in symptomatic caustic ingestions to assess for free air or to investigate for foreign body in cases of suspected disc battery ingestion. Noncontrast CT of the chest and abdomen may be useful if perforated viscus is suspected, especially after ingestion of strong acids. Early endoscopic evaluation (ideally <12 hours after ingestion) is indicated for intentional caustic ingestions, and unintentional cases presenting with stridor, oral burns, vomiting, drooling, or inability to tolerate oral intake.

EMERGENCY DEPARTMENT CARE AND DISPOSITION

Focus treatment on decontamination, early anticipatory airway management, stabilization of hemodynamic status, and delineation of extent of injury.

Decontamination

1. Remove contaminated clothing and irrigate exposed skin with copious amounts of water. Alkali burns may require local debridement and removal of devitalized tissue followed by additional irrigation.
2. Perform aggressive ocular decontamination with normal saline for a minimum of 15 minutes with frequent monitoring of ocular pH until a pH of 7.5 to 8.0 is achieved.
3. **Gastric decontamination in the form of activated charcoal, ipecac, or gastric lavage is contraindicated.**

Supportive Care

1. Perform early oral intubation with direct visualization in symptomatic patients with stridor, significant drooling, or dysphonia. Blind nasotracheal intubation is contraindicated.
2. Obtain IV access and administer isotonic IV fluids for hypotension.
3. Obtain surgical consultation for suspected or confirmed peritonitis or free air.

Special Considerations

1. Treat hydrofluoric acid dermal exposures with topical **calcium gluconate** gel (3.5 g mixed with 150 mL water-soluble lubricant). Consider intradermal 5% calcium gluconate for large burns and calcium gluconate infusion into the radial artery over 4 hours or given as a Bier block (10 mL of 10% calcium gluconate in 40 mL saline or 5% dextrose) for refractory distal extremity burns.
2. Oral ingestions of hydrofluoric acid within an hour can be suctioned via nasogastric tube followed by instillation of up to 300 mL of 10% calcium gluconate. High doses of IV calcium and magnesium may be needed to treat systemic deficiencies and dysrhythmias.
3. Disc batteries lodged in the esophagus require emergent endoscopic removal.
4. Laundry detergent pod ingestions in young children may produce serious toxicity including caustic injury, respiratory distress, and neurologic depression. Treat supportively with airway protection as needed.

FURTHER READING

For further reading in *Tintinalli's Emergency Medicine: A Comprehensive Study Guide*, 8th ed., see Chapter 200, "Caustic Ingestions," by Nicole C. Bouchard and Wallace A. Carter.

CHAPTER 113 Pesticides

Charles W. O'Connell

Pesticides include insecticides, herbicides, and rodenticides. In addition to active toxic ingredients, many pesticides also contain "inert" products such as petroleum distillates, which may be toxic as well. Although the mainstay of treatment is supportive care, some antidotes are essential.

INSECTICIDES

Clinical Features

Organophosphate insecticides include agents such as diazinon, acephate, malathion, parathion, and chlorpyrifos. Absorption occurs through ingestion, inhalation (e.g., nerve gas agents), and dermal routes. Toxicity is produced through binding and inhibition of acetylcholinesterase, causing excess accumulation of acetylcholine and stimulation of cholinergic receptors, of both the muscarinic and nicotinic receptor types. The muscarinic receptor agonism results in a cholinergic crisis known as "SLUDGE" and "DUMBELS" effects (Table 113-1).

Onset of symptoms, ranging from minutes to hours, varies based on amount and route of exposure. Most patients become symptomatic within 8 hours of acute exposure, though some fat-soluble agents (e.g., fenthion) can cause delayed symptoms with dermal exposure. Nicotinic receptor stimulation leads to fasciculations and muscle weakness, which is most pronounced in the respiratory muscles, which leads to worsening of pulmonary dysfunction caused by bronchorrhea from muscarinic effects. Nicotinic effects can also cause tachycardia and mydriasis, paradoxical to the

TABLE 113-1 SLUDGE, DUMBELS, and "Killer Bees" Mnemonics for the Cholinergic Effects of Cholinesterase Inhibition

S	Salivation
L	Lacrimation
U	Urinary incontinence
D	Defecation
G	GI pain
E	Emesis
D	Defecation
U	Urination
M	Muscle weakness, miosis
B	Bradycardia, bronchorrhea, bronchospasm
E	Emesis
L	Lacrimation
S	Salivation
Killer Bees	Bradycardia, bronchorrhea, bronchospasm

expected muscarinic cholinergic effects. Central nervous system (CNS) effects, which often predominate in children, include tremor, restlessness, confusion, seizures, and coma.

A variety of subacute and chronic effects are associated with organophosphate insecticide poisoning. An intermediate syndrome, 1 to 5 days after acute poisoning, may present with paralysis or weakness of neck, facial, and respiratory muscles, which can result in respiratory arrest if not treated. Organophosphate-induced delayed neuropathy can occur 1 to 3 weeks after acute poisoning, resulting in a distal motor-sensory polyneuropathy with leg weakness and paralysis.

Diagnosis and Differential

Organophosphate poisoning is typically a clinical diagnosis based on the toxidrome and history of exposure (Table 113-1); laboratory cholinesterase assay can aid in confirmation. An ECG may be useful to monitor for prolonged QT, which is associated with increased morbidity and mortality in organophosphate poisoning.

Emergency Department Care and Disposition

Treatment of organophosphate poisoning is listed in Table 113-2, and should not be delayed pending confirmatory tests.

1. In symptomatic patients, administer 100% oxygen and focus on airway management, with gentle suctioning of secretions. Nondepolarizing agents should be used for rapid sequence intubation. The use of succinylcholine for intubation, which is metabolized by plasma cholinesterase, may result in prolonged paralysis.
2. The key in treatment is large amounts of **atropine** titrated to attenuation of tracheobronchial secretions. Tachycardia and dilated pupils are not contraindications to additional atropine. Of note, atropine will only reverse the muscarinic effects, but not the nicotinic effects of excess

TABLE 113-2 Treatment for Organophosphate Poisoning

Decontamination	Protective clothing must be worn to prevent secondary poisoning of health care workers Handle and dispose of all clothes as hazardous waste. Wash patient with soap and water Handle and dispose of water runoff as hazardous waste
Monitoring	Cardiac monitor, pulse oximeter, 100% oxygen
Gastric lavage	No proven benefit
Activated charcoal	No proven benefit
Urinary alkalinization	No proven benefit
Atropine	1 mg or more IV in an adult or 0.01 to 0.04 mg/kg (but never <0.1 mg) IV in children. Repeat every 5 min until tracheobronchial secretions attenuate
Pralidoxime	1 to 2 g for adults or 20 to 40 mg/kg (up to 1 g) in children, mixed with normal saline and infused IV over 5 to 10 min Continuous infusion may be employed
Seizures	Benzodiazepines

TABLE 113-3 Nonorganophosphate Insecticide Poisoning

Agent	Example	Clinical Feature	Diagnosis	Treatment
Carbamates	Carbaryl, pirimicarb, propoxur, trimethacarb	Similar to organophosphates	Depressed cholinesterase levels	Atropine
Organochlorines	Chlordane, heptachlor, dieldrin, aldrin	Neurological: excitability, seizures	History, special lab	Benzodiazepine, cooling
Pyrethroids	Pyrethrins	parasthesia, vomiting, oropharyngeal irritation, allergic hypersensitivty	History	Bronchodilators and antihistamines, supportive
Neonicotinoids	Imidacloprid	Nausea, headache, sedation	History	Supportive
N,N-Dietyl-3-methylbenzamide	DEET	Seizures	History	Benzodiazepines

acetylcholine. **Glycopyrrolate** or high-dose **diphenhydramine** can be substituted for atropine if it is not available.

3. Minimal exposures require only 6 to 8 hours of observation. Recrudescence can occur due to reexposure to contaminated clothing, particularly leather. Significant poisonings require intensive care monitoring.
4. Other commonly encountered pesticides and their treatment are listed in Table 113-3.

HERBICIDES

Herbicides are agents used to kill weeds. In addition to intrinsic toxicity, they may also be packaged with surfactants or solvents with their own toxic effects. The most dangerous are bipyridyl herbicides, namely paraquat and diquat. Nonbipyridyl herbicides and their treatments are depicted in Table 113-4.

TABLE 113-4 Nonbipyridyl Herbicides

Agent	Example	Clinical Feature	Treatment
Chlorophenoxy	2,4-dichlorophenoxyacetic acid	Mucous membrane irritation, pulmonary edema, muscle toxicity, hyperthermia	Urine alkalization Hemodialysis
Glyphosate		Mucous membrane irritation, erosions, multiorgan failure, respiratory distress	Observe asymptomatic patients for 6 h
Urea-substituted	Chlorimuron, diuron, fluomenturon, isoproturon	Methemoglobinemia	Methylene blue
Organophosphates	Butiphos	SLUDGE	Same as pesticides
N,N-Dietyl-3-methylbenzamide	DEET	Seizures	Benzodiazepines

Paraquat is especially toxic with lethality seen with oral doses of 10 to 20 mL in an adult and 4 to 5 mL in children of 20% solution. Both agents are toxic via inhalation, dermal exposure, or ingestion. Due to their caustic properties, ulceration of skin and mucous membranes and gastrointestinal corrosion can occur. Paraquat ingestions result in renal, cardiac, and hepatic failure along with progressive pulmonary fibrosis from oxidative damage. Due to the latter, treatment often includes restriction of supplemental oxygen except for severe hypoxia. Decontamination of skin is important to prevent continued absorption. Early after ingestion, GI decontamination with **activated charcoal, fuller's earth,** or **bentonite** may be helpful. Charcoal hemoperfusion may remove paraquat. Because of poor prognosis, especially with paraquat ingestions, admit patients with ingestion for further observation and treatment.

RODENTICIDES

The most commonly used rodenticides are superwarfarins, including brodifacoum, difenacoum, and bromadiolone. Coagulopathy typically develops within 48 hours and lasts for weeks to months due to the long half-lives of these agents. Single small ingestions in children usually do not result in toxic effects. Acute intentional or repeated ingestions may present with delayed hemorrhage, including hematuria, gastrointestinal hemorrhage, or epistaxis. Screening for toxic effect can be performed with an INR obtained 24 to 48 hours after ingestion. If the INR is elevated (>2), then start oral **vitamin K_1**, typically at doses of 20 mg/d in adults (1 to 5 mg for children), which can be continued for up to 10 months until the anticoagulant effect is cleared. Acute hemorrhage requires more aggressive therapy with volume replacement, fresh frozen plasma or four-factor prothrombin complex, IV vitamin K_1, and supportive care. Nonanticoagulant rodenticides are described in Table 113-5.

TABLE 113-5 Nonanticoagulant Rodenticides

Agent	Toxicity	Clinical Effects	Treatment
Arsenic	Severe	Vomiting and diarrhea, cardiovascular collapse	Supportive care, BAL for acute poisoning, Succimer
Barium carbonate	Severe	Vomiting and diarrhea, dysrhythmia, respiratory failure, hyopkalemia, paralysis	Gastric lavage with sodium or magnesium sulfate; potassium replacement
White phosphorus	Severe	Burns, cardiovascular collapse	Lavage with potassium permangante
N-3-Pyridylmethyl-*N*′-p-nitrophenyl urea (Vacor)	Severe	GI symptoms, insulin deficient hyperglycemia and DKA	Nicotinamide IV
Sodium fluroacetate	Severe	Vomiting, respiratory depression, impaired conciousness, twitching, seizure	Supportive care
Strychnine	Severe	Awake seizure like activity	Benzodiazepines

(Continued)

TABLE 113-5 Nonanticoagulant Rodenticides (Continued)

Agent	Toxicity	Clinical Effects	Treatment
Thallium	Severe	Early GI irritation, respiratory failure and dysrhythmias	Oral Prussian blue
Metal phosphides	Severe	Vomiting, shock, hypocalcemia	Intragastric alkalization
α-Napthyl-thiourea	Moderate	Pulmonary edema	Supportive care
Cholecalciferol	Moderate	Hypercalcemia	Saline, furosemide, steroids
Bromethalin	Low	Tremors, focal seizures	Benzodiazepines
Norbormide	Low	Vasoconstrictive tissue hypoxia	Supportive care
Red squill	Low	Vomiting, diarrhea, hyperkalemia, heart block with ventricular dysrhythmias	Supportive care

FURTHER READING

For further reading in *Tintinalli's Emergency Medicine: A Comprehensive Study Guide*, 8th ed., see Chapter 201, "Pesticides," by Burillo-Putze Guillermo and Xarau Santiago Nogue.

CHAPTER 114 Metals and Metalloids

D. Adam Algren

Metal and metalloid poisoning, although uncommon, can result in morbidity and mortality if unrecognized. Toxicity results from occupational, recreational, or environmental exposures and results in multi-system organ involvement.

LEAD POISONING

Clinical Features

Lead poisoning manifests with signs and symptoms affecting a variety of organ systems (Table 114-1).

Diagnosis and Differential

Suspect lead poisoning in any individual demonstrating a combination of abdominal pain, nausea, vomiting, and neurologic symptoms (particularly children with encephalopathy), especially in the setting of anemia. A complete blood count (CBC) may demonstrate normocytic or microcytic anemia with hemolysis and basophilic stippling; however, hematologic findings are neither sensitive nor specific for lead poisoning. Lead toxicity is confirmed by an elevated blood lead level, though results are often not immediately available. Radiographs may identify metaphyseal long-bone lead lines, radiopaque material in the GI tract, or retained bullet fragments. The differential diagnosis of toxicity is broad and includes meningitis, encephalitis, metabolic abnormalities, hypoxia, drug intoxications, arsenic, mercury, and carbon monoxide poisoning.

TABLE 114-1 Clinical Features of Lead Poisoning

System	Clinical Manifestations
Central nervous	Acute toxicity: encephalopathy, seizures, altered mental status, papilledema, optic neuritis, ataxia Chronic toxicity: headache, irritability, depression, fatigue, mood and behavioral changes, memory deficit, sleep disturbance
Peripheral nervous	Paresthesias, motor weakness (classic is wrist drop), depressed or absent deep tendon reflexes, sensory function intact
GI	Abdominal pain (mostly with acute poisoning), constipation, diarrhea, toxic hepatitis
Renal	Acute toxicity: Fanconi's syndrome (renal tubular acidosis with aminoaciduria, glucosuria, and phosphaturia) Chronic toxicity: interstitial nephritis, renal insufficiency, hypertension, gout
Hematologic	Hypoproliferative and/or hemolytic anemia; basophilic stippling (rare and nonspecific)
Reproductive	Decreased libido, impotence, sterility, abortions, premature births, decreased or abnormal sperm production

TABLE 114-2 Guidelines for Chelation Therapy in Lead-Poisoned Patients*

Severity (Blood Lead Level [μg/dL])	Dose
Encephalopathy	Dimercaprol, 75 mg/m² (or 4 mg/kg) IM every 4 h for 5 days *and* Edetate calcium disodium, 1500 mg/m² per day via continuous infusion or in 2–4 divided doses IV for 5 days; start 4 h after dimercaprol
Symptomatic and/or Adults: blood lead >100 Children: blood lead >69	Dimercaprol *and* Edetate calcium disodium (as described above) *or* Edetate calcium disodium (alone) *or* Succimer (as described below)
Asymptomatic Adults: blood lead 70–100 Children: blood lead 45–69	Succimer, 350 mg/m² (or 10 mg/kg) PO every 8 h for 5 days, then every 12 h for 14 days
Asymptomatic Adults: blood lead <70 Children: blood lead <45	Routine chelation not indicated; remove patient from source of exposure

*General guidelines. Consult with medical toxicologist or regional poison center for specifics and dosing.

Emergency Department Care and Disposition

1. Address life-threatening problems with advanced airway management and fluid resuscitation.
2. Decontaminate the GI tract with **whole-bowel irrigation** using polyethylene glycol solution in those with retained lead flecks in the GI tract. Larger foreign bodies may require endoscopic or surgical removal.
3. Treat seizures aggressively with benzodiazepines, followed by barbiturates and/or propofol, and/or general anesthesia. Avoid lumbar puncture in the setting of lead-induced encephalopathy as this can precipitate herniation.
4. Chelation therapy is the mainstay of treatment and often must be started empirically (Table 114-2). Dimercaprol (BAL) can only be administered intramuscularly and is contraindicated in those with peanut allergies.
5. Admit patients requiring parenteral chelation therapy or those who cannot avoid further environmental lead exposure. Arrange follow up for patients started on succimer (DMSA).

ARSENIC POISONING

Clinical Features

Arsenic is used in a variety of insecticides and herbicides as well as mining and smelting processes. Acute ingestion results in profound vomiting and diarrhea within hours of exposure. Hypotension and tachycardia may develop secondary to hypovolemia and direct myocardial dysfunction. Encephalopathy, acute lung injury, and acute kidney injury may develop. Arsenic toxicity can prolong the QT interval and cases of torsades de

TABLE 114-3 Guidelines for Chelation Therapy in Arsenic-Poisoned Patients

Chelator	Dose
Dimercaprol	3–5 mg/kg IM every 4 h for 2 days, followed by 3–5 mg/kg IM every 6–12 h until able to switch to succimer
Succimer	10 mg/kg PO every 8 h for 5 days, followed by 10 mg/kg PO every 12 h

pointes have been reported. Chronic poisoning causes peripheral neuropathy, malaise, and confusion. Skin findings include alopecia, hyperpigmentation, keratoses, and transverse white nail lines (Mees' lines).

Diagnosis and Differential

An exposure history is most useful in identifying arsenic poisoning. However, consider the diagnosis in patients with hypotension preceded by profound vomiting and diarrhea. The CBC may demonstrate leukocytosis with acute poisoning. An ECG may show QT-interval prolongation. The diagnosis is confirmed by documenting an elevated 24-hour urine arsenic level. Other diagnoses to consider include gastroenteritis, septic shock, encephalopathy, peripheral neuropathy, Addison's disease, and lead, thallium, or mercury poisoning.

Emergency Department Care and Disposition

1. Support the ABCs: endotracheal intubation may be required to protect the airway; treat hypotension with volume resuscitation and vasopressors, but avoid overresuscitation that may result in pulmonary or cerebral edema. Manage dysrhythmias according to ACLS/PALS protocols, but avoid agents that prolong the QT interval (class IA, IC, and III antidysrhythmics). Magnesium sulfate, isoproterenol, and/or overdrive pacing should be considered for treatment of torsades de pointes.
2. Decontaminate the gastrointestinal tract with **whole-bowel irrigation** using polyethylene glycol solution in those with radiopaque GI fragments.
3. Treat symptomatic patients empirically with chelation therapy (Table 114-3) using **dimercaprol IM**. **Succimer** PO is preferred for clinically stable patients who can tolerate oral intake.
4. Hospitalize acutely poisoned patients, patients requiring dimercaprol, or those with suspected suicidal or homicidal intent. Discharge stable patients with subacute or chronic poisoning if follow-up is ensured.

MERCURY POISONING

Mercury poisoning can result from exposure to elemental, inorganic, or organic mercury compounds.

Clinical Features

Elemental mercury exposure is most likely to occur after contact with a broken thermometer, light bulb or other mercury spills. Mercury is primarily absorbed via inhalation (especially with heating or vacuuming). Ingestions of elemental mercury are nontoxic in those with normal GI tracts. Vapor exposure results in cough, fever, dyspnea, vomiting, and headache.

TABLE 114-4 Guidelines for Chelation Therapy in Mercury-Poisoned Patients

	Elemental and Inorganic Mercury	Organic Mercury
Severe acute poisoning	Dimercaprol, 5 mg/kg IM every 4 h for 2 days, followed by 2.5 mg/kg IM every 6 h for 2 days, followed by 2.5 mg/kg IM every 12–24 h until clinical improvement occurs or until able to switch to succimer therapy	Succimer, 10 mg/kg PO every 8 h for 5 days, then every 12 h for 14 days
Mild acute poisoning and chronic poisoning	Succimer, 10 mg/kg PO every 8 h for 5 days, then every 12 h for 14 days	No proven benefit for chelation therapy

Acute lung injury can progress to respiratory failure. Classic findings include tremor, rash, and hypertension. *Inorganic mercury* is used as a disinfectant and in manufacturing. Ingestion of inorganic mercury results in corrosive injury to the GI tract, with vomiting, diarrhea, abdominal pain, and GI bleeding early, followed by acute kidney injury. *Organic mercury* is found in some fungicides and pesticides and can be absorbed when ingested. Poisoning tends to occur with chronic exposures and results in profound central nervous system dysfunction.

Diagnosis and Differential

A history of exposure to mercury is key to diagnosis and is confirmed by an elevated 24-hour urine mercury level when toxicity is due to elemental or inorganic mercury; an elevated whole blood mercury level is necessary in cases of organic mercury exposure. The differential diagnosis is extensive and includes causes of metal fume fever (elemental), encephalopathy or tremor (elemental/inorganic/organic), thyroid disease, metabolic encephalopathy, stroke, and tumor. Consider alternative causes of corrosive gastroenteritis (ingestion of iron, arsenic, phosphorus, acids, and alkalis) if mercury salt ingestion is suspected.

Emergency Department Care and Disposition

1. Support the ABCs with airway management and crystalloid infusion.
2. Consider gastric lavage in cases of *inorganic* mercury ingestion or activated charcoal in cases of *organic* mercury ingestion.
3. Begin chelation therapy prior to confirming the diagnosis (Table 114-4). **Dimercaprol** is preferred for *elemental* and *inorganic* mercury poisonings. **Succimer** is the agent of choice in *organic* mercury poisonings and in cases of mild or chronic elemental/inorganic mercury toxicity.
4. Admit patients with respiratory symptoms following elemental mercury vapor exposure, those with inorganic mercury ingestions, or patients requiring dimercaprol chelation. Ensure prompt environmental assessment in cases of elemental mercury vapor exposures to prevent further toxicity.

POISONING WITH OTHER METALS

Less common toxic heavy metals include bismuth, cadmium, chromium, cobalt, copper, silver, thallium, and zinc. Unique manifestations and treatments of these exposures are outlined in Table 114-5.

TABLE 114-5 Miscellaneous Metal Poisoning: Unique Manifestations and Treatments of Patients Poisoned by Less Common Metals

Metal	Poisoning Source	Acute Clinical Manifestations	Chronic Clinical Manifestations	Specific Treatment
Bismuth	Antidiarrheals (bismuth subsalicylate), impregnated surgical packing paste	Abdominal pain, acute kidney injury	Myoclonic encephalopathy	Dimercaprol (limited evidence)
Cadmium	Contaminated soil in cadmium-rich areas; alloys used in welding, soldering, jewelry, and batteries	Ingestion: hemorrhagic gastroenteritis Inhalation: pneumonitis, acute lung injury	Proteinuria, osteomalacia (itai-itai or ouch-ouch disease), lung cancer (questionable)	Ingestion: succimer (limited evidence; not generally indicated) Pneumonitis: chelation not indicated
Chromium	Corrosion inhibitors (e.g., heating systems), pigment production, leather tanning, metal finishing, dietary supplements, prosthetic joints	Skin irritation and ulceration, contact dermatitis; GI irritation, renal and pulmonary failure	Mucous membrane irritation, perforation of nasal septum, chronic cough, contact dermatitis, skin ulcers ("chrome holes"), lung cancer	Acetylcysteine (animal studies suggest efficacy as chelator)
Cobalt	"Hard metal dust" (tungsten–cobalt mixture), flexible magnets, drying agents, prosthetic joints	Contact dermatitis, asthma	Hard metal lung disease (spectrum ranging from alveolitis to fibrosis), cardiomyopathy, thyroid hyperplasia	Acetylcysteine (animal studies suggest efficacy as chelator)
Copper	Leaching from copper pipes and containers; fungicide (copper sulfate); welding (copper oxide)	Ingestion: resembles iron poisoning; blue vomitus (copper salts), hepatotoxicity, hemolysis, methemoglobinemia Inhalation: metal fume fever (self-limited fever, chills, cough, dyspnea)	Hepatotoxicity (childhood cirrhosis or idiopathic copper toxicosis)	Dimercaprol for hepatic or hematologic toxicity Succimer in mild poisoning

(Continued)

TABLE 114-5 Miscellaneous Metal Poisoning: Unique Manifestations and Treatments of Patients Poisoned by Less Common Metals (Continued)

Metal	Poisoning Source	Acute Clinical Manifestations	Chronic Clinical Manifestations	Specific Treatment
Silver	Colloidal (metallic) silver used for medicinal purposes as oral solutions, aerosols, and douches; cauterizing and antiseptic agent (silver nitrate); jewelry, wire	Mucosal irritation (silver oxide and nitrate)	Argyria (permanent skin discoloration due to silver deposition and melanocyte stimulation)	Selenium (possible role)
Thallium	Rodenticides (use prohibited in the United States); contaminated herbal products; medical radioisotope (miniscule dose); most poisonings related to homicide	Early: nausea, vomiting, abdominal pain, tachycardia Intermediate (>24 h): painful ascending neuropathy, cardiac dysrhythmias, altered mental status Delayed (2 weeks): alopecia	Sensorimotor neuropathy, psychosis, dermatitis, hepatotoxicity	Multidose activated charcoal Prussian blue, 125 mg/kg PO every 12 h (usually dissolved in 50 mL of 15% mannitol)
Zinc	Smelting, electroplating, military smoke bombs, zinc lozenges, welding/galvanizing (zinc oxide)	Ingestion: nausea, vomiting, abdominal pain (resembles iron poisoning) Inhalation: mucosal irritation, metal fume fever (zinc oxide)	Copper deficiency, sideroblastic anemia, neutropenia	Edetate calcium disodium Supportive care for metal fume fever

FURTHER READING

For further reading in *Tintinalli's Emergency Medicine: A Comprehensive Study Guide*, 8th ed., see Chapter 203, "Metals and Metalloids," by Heather Long and Lewis S. Nelson.

CHAPTER 115 Industrial Toxins

Landen Rentmeester

There are over 50,000 hazardous chemicals used in various industrial processes throughout the United States. Exposures are inevitable and the emergency physician must be prepared to appropriately care for these patients. Material Safety Data Sheets, regional poison control centers and medical toxicologists are valuable resources for information on specific hazards, optimal management, and patient disposition. Children and pregnant women are patient populations who require special attention, the former due to differences in respiratory, dermatologic, and gastrointestinal physiology and the latter requiring a focus on maternal care in order to optimize fetal well-being.

RESPIRATORY TOXINS

Clinical Features

Phosgene, chlorine, nitrogen dioxide, and ammonia are significant respiratory toxins seen in industrial exposures, and are further described in Table 115-1. Hydrocarbons, cyanide, and carbon monoxide are also inhalational toxins that can have systemic effects.

TABLE 115-1 Toxic Industrial Exposures That Cause Respiratory Symptoms

Agent	Irritant	Signs/Symptoms/Findings	Treatment
Phosgene	Mild/none	I—Eye and upper airway irritation; possibly none	Supplemental oxygen if hypoxemic (Sa_{O2} <92%)
		D—Dyspnea, noncardiogenic pulmonary edema	Respiratory supportive care Nebulized β-agonists Mandatory rest Ocular supportive care
Chlorine	Yes	I—Eye and upper airway irritation, nausea and vomiting (low-level exposure)	Humidified oxygen Respiratory supportive care
		D—Pulmonary edema (high-level exposure)	Nebulized β-agonists Nebulized sodium bicarbonate Ocular care
Nitrogen dioxide	Yes	I—Dyspnea with transient improvement	Humidified oxygen
		D—Worsening dyspnea due to pulmonary edema 24–72 hours after exposure; methemoglobinemia	Respiratory supportive care Early corticosteroid treatment
Ammonia	Yes	I—Coughing, hoarseness, bronchospasm, eye and upper airway irritation	Humidified oxygen Nebulized β-agonists Nebulized anticholinergics Respiratory supportive care Ocular supportive care

Abbreviations: D = delayed; I = immediate; Sa_{O2} = arterial oxygen saturation.

Diagnosis and Differential

Examine the upper airway for evidence of singed nasal hair, soot in the oropharynx, facial or oropharyngeal burns, stridor, hoarseness, dysphagia, cough, carbonaceous sputum, tachypnea, retractions, accessory muscle use, wheezing, or cyanosis. Diagnostic workup includes arterial blood gas analysis with carboxyhemoglobin, methemoglobin, serum lactate concentration, chest radiography, electrocardiogram, and cardiac monitoring.

Emergency Department Care and Disposition

1. Give supplemental oxygen for hypoxemia and inhaled bronchodilators for bronchospasm. A low threshold for endotracheal intubation is appropriate in cases of upper airway injury.
2. Irrigation of the eyes and skin if necessary.
3. Prophylactic antibiotics and steroids are NOT routinely indicated following toxic gas inhalation, except in cases of nitrogen dioxide exposure, but can be considered in patients with toxin-induced bronchospasm or underlying reactive airway disease.

PHOSGENE

Clinical Features

Phosgene, once used in chemical warfare, is a precursor in the production of plastics, pharmaceuticals, dyes, polyurethane, and pesticides. It is also produced when chlorinated fluorocarbons are heated, a potential danger for those who work in the refrigeration or air-conditioning industries. Initial symptoms include upper airway and mucous membrane irritation, with an accompanying odor of freshly mown hay. Upon reaching the lower airways, phosgene converts to carbon dioxide and hydrochloric acid, in which the latter causes caustic injury, capillary leakage, and noncardiogenic pulmonary edema. Clinically, this process is manifested as chest tightness and dyspnea. Pulmonary edema may be delayed up to 24 hours, while onset within 4 hours suggests a poor prognosis. Diagnosis is typically made on history of exposure and clinical symptoms.

Emergency Department Care and Disposition

1. Respiratory failure requires intubation and ventilation with low tidal volumes, low plateau pressures, and high positive end expiratory pressure. Otherwise, refrain from supplemental oxygen unless hypoxia is present.
2. Nebulized Beta agonists may be beneficial if administered early.
3. Instruct the patient to minimize physical exertion.
4. Observe all patients with phosgene exposures for a minimum of 24 hours.

CHLORINE

Clinical Features

Chlorine is used in a variety of industrial and water treatment processes. It has a very characteristic acrid, pungent odor and may disperse as a dense green yellow gas. Upon exposure to water, chlorine acid derivatives are produced, leading to irritation of the mucous membranes of the eyes and upper airway. With increasing exposure, the more distal airways are affected, leading to pulmonary edema and acute respiratory distress syndrome, which may be delayed up to 6 hours.

Emergency Department Care and Disposition

1. Treat respiratory symptoms with humidified oxygen and bronchodilators.
2. Nebulized sodium bicarbonate may be of benefit within 4 hours of exposure.
3. Consider steroids, either intravenous or inhaled. However, there is insufficient evidence of improved outcomes with steroid therapy.
4. Evaluate for dermal and corneal burns in patients with significant exposure.
5. Monitor patients with moderate symptoms for 24 hours.

NITROGEN DIOXIDE

Clinical Features

Nitrogen dioxide and nitrogen oxides are typically encountered in silo gas and military ordinance, and are formed in any instance of air-based combustion. A triphasic clinical course is often observed, manifested initially as dyspnea and flu-like symptoms, followed by transient improvement, then increasing dyspnea 12 hours post-exposure due to pulmonary edema. Methemoglobinemia has also been reported. Diagnosis is typically made by clinical history.

Emergency Department Care and Disposition

1. Initial treatment is supportive, ensuring airway integrity and adequate oxygenation/ventilation.
2. Give supplemental humidified oxygen and bronchodilators if bronchospasm is present.
3. Because the respiratory effects of NO_2 exposure are delayed, patients may present with minimal symptoms despite significant exposure, and early intubation should be considered.
4. Early corticosteroids may reduce the risk of delayed pulmonary edema.
5. Most patients require hospitalization for 24 to 48 hours.

AMMONIA

Clinical Features

Ammonia is found in many household chemicals, fertilizers, and plastic production. It has a characteristic pungent odor and rapidly irritates the mucous membranes of the upper airway. Lower airway injury may occur with massive exposure. Diagnosis is typically made by clinical history.

Emergency Department Care and Disposition

1. Treat exposed patients supportively with humidified oxygen, bronchodilators, and anticholinergics.
2. Provide copious irrigation and corneal burn evaluation for patients with eye discomfort.

CYANIDE

Clinical Features

Cyanide is an extremely toxic chemical generated during the combustion of synthetic materials, wool, and silk. It is used in vermin extermination, precious metal reclamation, and chemical laboratories. It is also found naturally in seeds of the *Prunus* species. Toxicity is caused by inhibition of cytochrome oxidase, which subsequently disrupts oxidative phosphorylation and ATP production. Patients with significant exposure present with altered consciousness, hyperventilation, hypotension, and bradycardia. They will typically have normal oxygen saturation on co-oximetry. A smell of bitter almonds may be detected. Cherry-red skin is an uncommon finding.

Diagnosis and Differential

A severe, unexplained anion gap metabolic acidosis is characteristic of cyanide exposure and is due to lactic acid production from anaerobic metabolism. The PaO_2 of venous blood will approach that of arterial blood as a result of impaired tissue oxygen consumption. An elevation of carboxyhemoglobin may also be seen in fire victims. Whole blood cyanide levels confirm exposure, but are not rapidly available. The diagnosis is made clinically and treatment initiated as soon as possible.

Emergency Department Care and Disposition

1. Treat cyanide poisoning with aggressive supportive care and antidotal therapy, outlined in Tables 115-2 and 115-3. Nitrites induce the formation of methemoglobin, which binds and removes cyanide to allow reactivation of oxidative phosphorylation. Sodium thiosulfate provides a sulfate group that is transferred to cyanide to create less toxic thiocyanate. Hydroxocobalamin directly binds cyanide, removing it from cytochrome oxidase, and forming cyanocobalamin. Nitrite therapy is not contraindicated in patients with hypotension from severe cyanide

TABLE 115-2 Treatment of Cyanide Poisoning in Adults

100% supplemental oxygen	
IV crystalloids and vasopressors for hypotension	
Sodium bicarbonate for acidemia	
AND	
Cyanide antidote kit	Amyl nitrite inhaler; crack vial and inhale over 30 s.* Sodium nitrite 3% solution: 10 mL (300 mg) IV given over no less than 5 min.† Sodium thiosulfate 25% solution: 50 mL (12.5 g) IV. Repeat sodium thiosulfate once at half dose (25 mL) if symptoms persist.
OR	
Hydroxocobalamin	5 g IV over 15 min. If needed, may repeat 5 g for a total of 10 g.

*Not necessary if IV is in place.

†Avoid nitrites in the presence of severe hypotension if diagnosis is unclear; consider sodium thiosulfate or hydroxocobalamin.

TABLE 115-3 Treatment of Cyanide Poisoning in Children

100% oxygen	
IV crystalloids and vasopressors for hypotension	
Sodium bicarbonate for acidemia	
AND	
Cyanide antidote kit	Amyl nitrite inhaler; crack vial and hold in front of nose for 15–30 s.[*],[†]
	Sodium nitrite 3% solution: adjusted according to hemoglobin level, given IV over no less than 5 min[‡] (monitor methemoglobin level <30%)
Hemoglobin (g/100 mL)	**Sodium Nitrite 3% Solution (mL/kg)**
7	0.19
8	0.22
9	0.25
10	0.27
11	0.30
12	0.33
13	0.36
14	0.39
Sodium thiosulfate 25% solution: 1.65 mL/kg IV.	
Repeat sodium thiosulfate once at half dose (0.825 mL/kg) if symptoms persist.	

[*]Not necessary if IV is in place.

[†]Consider withholding nitrites if suspected concomitant carbon monoxide poisoning.

[‡]Avoid nitrites in the presence of severe hypotension if diagnosis is unclear.

toxicity. However, nitrites are relatively contraindicated in hypotensive patients with an uncertain exposure history and in victims of smoke inhalation who may have concomitant carbon monoxide poisoning. The latter contraindication is due to reduced oxygen delivery from induced methemoglobinemia. In these instances, hydroxocobalamin is the ideal antidote; however, sodium thiosulfate may also be used while omitting the use of nitrites from the cyanide antidote kit.

2. Consider activated charcoal in patients with a history of cyanide ingestion who present within 1 hour, are alert, and have a patent airway.
3. Admit patients receiving antidotal therapy or who may have ingested a substance with the potential for delayed toxicity.

HYDROGEN SULFIDE

Clinical Features

Hydrogen sulfide is a colorless, flammable gas found in petroleum processing, as a byproduct of organic matter decomposition, and can be made from household products. The mechanism of toxicity is the same as cyanide, except that the inhibition of oxidative phosphorylation quickly ceases when removed from exposure. A characteristic rotten egg's odor is frequently described. Mucous membrane irritation is common, and with significant exposure, rapid loss of consciousness, seizures, delayed pulmonary edema, corneal injury, and death may occur.

Emergency Department Care and Disposition

1. Removal from the source of hydrogen sulfide is the most important aspect of care, followed by aggressive supportive care with humidified oxygen and decontamination.
2. Treat patients with persistent mental status changes or cardiovascular instability with sodium nitrite.

FURTHER READING

For further reading in *Tintinalli's Emergency Medicine: A Comprehensive Study Guide*, 8th ed., see Chapter 204, "Industrial Toxins," by Chip Gresham and Frank LoVecchio

CHAPTER 116

Vitamins and Herbals

Janna H. Villano

Over-the-counter vitamin and herbal preparations are widely used and considered innocuous by most of the public. Many of these products, however, can produce significant toxicity, especially if used in excess. In addition, many patients neglect to mention or are reluctant to divulge that they are taking these products.

CLINICAL FEATURES

Hypervitaminosis most commonly occurs with supratherapeutic dosing, in part due to lack of public awareness of the harms of excessive use. Ingestion of large doses of fat-soluble vitamins A, D, and E can produce subacute or chronic toxicity. Water-soluble vitamins associated with toxicity include niacin, pyridoxine, and vitamin C. Common symptoms of vitamin toxicities are listed in Table 116-1.

TABLE 116-1 Symptoms of Hypervitaminosis

Vitamin	Symptoms
Vitamin A	Subacute toxicity: red peeling rash, headache, vomiting Chronic toxicity: blurred vision, appetite loss, abnormal skin pigmentation, hair loss, dry skin, pruritus, long-bone pain, bone fractures, rare cases of pseudotumor cerebri, hypercalcemia, and hepatic failure
Vitamin D	Subacute toxicity: hypercalcemia, anorexia, nausea, abdominal pain, lethargy, weight loss, polyuria, constipation, confusion, and coma
Vitamin E	Chronic toxicity: coagulopathy in patients on warfarin, nausea, fatigue, headache, weakness, and blurred vision
Vitamin K	Acute toxicity: anaphylactoid reactions if given in parenteral form (rare)
Vitamin B_1 (thiamine)	No toxicity observed with ingestion of large doses
Vitamin B_2 (riboflavin)	No toxicity observed with ingestion of large doses
Vitamin B_3 (niacin)	Acute toxicity: niacin flush, dose >100 mg, redness, burning, and itching of the face, neck, and chest; rarely hypotension Chronic toxicity: doses >2000 mg/day, abnormalities of liver function, impaired glucose tolerance, hyperuricemia, skin dryness, and discoloration
Vitamin B_6 (pyridoxine)	Subacute and chronic toxicity: doses >1–3 g/day orally or more over several weeks, peripheral neuropathy with unstable gait, numbness of the feet, similar symptoms in the hands and arms, marked loss of position and vibration senses
Vitamin B_{12}	No toxicity observed with ingestion of large doses. With large IV doses: erythema of skin, mucous membranes, serum, and urine. Rare anaphylactoid reactions. Possible interference with serum colorimetric lab studies.

(Continued)

TABLE 116-1 Symptoms of Hypervitaminosis (Continued)

Vitamin	Symptoms
Folate	No toxicity observed with ingestion of large doses. Masking of macrocytic anemia from vitamin B_{12} deficiency with large doses of folate.
Vitamin C (ascorbate)	Chronic toxicity: nephrolithiasis (controversial), intrarenal deposition of oxalate crystals with renal failure; large doses can produce diarrhea and abdominal cramps.

Many popular herbal preparations have potential for serious toxicity and medication interactions, despite being considered by many to be natural and safe alternatives to Western pharmaceuticals. Lack of regulation of these products raises the potential for toxic contaminants that may independently cause acute poisoning. While generally safe, chamomile, glucosamine, and Echinacea rarely cause anaphylaxis. Other commonly used agents, their uses, and associated adverse events are listed in Table 116-2.

TABLE 116-2 Commonly Used Herbal Agents and Potential Adverse Effects

Agent	General Use	Adverse Effect
Black cohosh†	Menopause	Nausea, vomiting, dizziness, weakness
Chondroitin*	Arthritis	May cause GI upset
Ephedra†	Weight loss	Hypertension; contraindicated for patients with hypertension, diabetes, or glaucoma Drug interactions: monoamine oxidase inhibitors, sympathomimetics
Garlic*	Hypertension, colic, hyperlipidemia	Hypotension, rash, nausea, vomiting, diarrhea; death has been reported in massive doses in children
Gingko*	Dementia, vertigo, peripheral arterial disease	May inhibit platelet aggregation and increase bleeding risk May cause GI upset Drug interactions: aspirin, warfarin
Ginseng*	Impotence, fatigue, ulcers, stress	May interact with warfarin Lowers blood glucose May cause insomnia, nervousness
Juniper†	Diuretic	Hallucinogenic; may also cause renal toxicity, nausea, and vomiting
Nutmeg†	Dyspepsia, muscle aches, arthritis	Hallucinations, GI upset, agitation, coma, miosis, and hypertension
Pennyroyal†	Rubefacient, delaying menses, abortifacient	Hepatotoxicity
St. John's wort*	Depression	Phototoxicity May interact with serotonin reuptake inhibitors; avoid tyramine-containing foods Many drug interactions including cyclosporine (transplant rejection), digoxin, indinavir

(Continued)

TABLE 116-2 Commonly Used Herbal Agents and Potential Adverse Effects (Continued)

Agent	General Use	Adverse Effect
Wormwood (Absinthe)†	Dyspepsia	Absinthism: restlessness, vertigo, tremor paresthesias, delirium
Yohimbine†	Aphrodisiac	Hallucinations, weakness, hypertension, paralysis Drug interactions: clonidine, cyclic antidepressants

*Considered generally safe; rare adverse effects.

†Increased potential for toxicity, adverse effects more common.

DIAGNOSIS AND DIFFERENTIAL

Diagnosis is usually made clinically. A history of massive acute ingestion or chronic supratherapeutic use should be sought. Laboratory studies that may be helpful include a complete blood count, basic metabolic panel, hepatic enzymes, coagulation studies, bleeding time, creatine phosphokinase, toxicology screen, and urine pregnancy test. An ECG may be indicated if signs of sympathomimetic stimulation are present.

EMERGENCY DEPARTMENT CARE AND DISPOSITION

Basic supportive care and discontinuation of the vitamin or herbal preparation are usually all that are needed to treat mild toxicity.

1. Consider **activated charcoal** 1 g/kg PO for large vitamin A or vitamin D ingestions.
2. Treat hypercalcemia from vitamin A or D overdose with normal saline, loop diuretics, and corticosteroids (to reduce GI absorption). Refractory cases may require adjunctive treatments, such as bisphosphonates and calcitonin.
3. Consider diagnostic and therapeutic lumbar puncture to treat idiopathic intracranial hypertension (pseudotumor cerebri) from hypervitaminosis A.
4. Administer **diphenhydramine** 25 to 50 mg IV (1 mg/kg in children) or PO to patients with "niacin flush" symptoms.
5. Consider ***N*-acetylcysteine** 140 mg/kg PO or IV for treating severe hepatotoxicity from herbal preparations such as pennyroyal oil.

FURTHER READING

For further reading in *Tintinalli's Emergency Medicine: A Comprehensive Study Guide*, 8th ed., see Chapter 205, "Vitamins and Herbals," by Rick Tovar.

CHAPTER 117 Dyshemoglobinemias

Chulathida Chomchai

Dyshemoglobinemias result from the alteration of the hemoglobin molecule, which prevents it from carrying oxygen. Carboxyhemoglobin is created following exposure to carbon monoxide, which is usually considered an environmental emergency and is discussed in Chapter 127. Table 117-1 lists common pharmaceuticals capable of causing the formation of methemoglobin.

CLINICAL FEATURES

Methemoglobinemia presents with grayish-brown discoloration of the skin that is recognized as cyanosis. Children up to the age of 4 months lack the enzyme activity that normally reduces methemoglobin, thus making them susceptible to oxidant stress-induced methemoglobinemia. Three scenarios occur with some frequency: children with acute gastroenteritis and increased nitrate production from bacteria in the GI tract; children exposed to nitrates in water of agricultural areas where fertilizer runoff contaminates water sources; and overconsumption of nitrogenous vegetables such as spinach.

In drug-induced methemoglobinemia, the slate-gray to blue discoloration of the skin is apparent with levels of 10% to 15%. Symptoms occur in proportion to declining oxygen delivery. Headache, nausea, and fatigue

TABLE 117-1 Drugs Commonly Implicated in Patients with Methemoglobinemia

Oxidant	Comments
Analgesics	Commonly reported
Phenazopyridine	Rarely used
Phenacetin	
Antimicrobials	Common
Antimalarials	Hydroxylamine metabolite formation is inhibited by cimetidine
Dapsone	
Local anesthetics	Most commonly reported of the local anesthetics
Benzocaine	Rare
Lidocaine	Common in topical anesthetics
Prilocaine	Rare
Dibucaine	
Nitrates/nitrites	Cyanide antidote kit used to enhance sexual encounters
Amyl nitrite	Used to enhance sexual encounters
Isobutyl nitrite	Cyanide antidote kit
Sodium nitrite	Cold packs
Ammonium nitrae	Excessive topical use
Silver nitrate	Problem in infants, due to nitrate fertilizer runoff
Well water	Rare
Nitroglycerin	
Sulfonamides	Uncommon
Sulfamethoxazole	

occur at lower levels (20% to 30%). Levels above 50% can cause loss of consciousness, myocardial ischemia, dysrhythmias, seizures, and metabolic acidosis. Levels above 70% may be lethal. In patients with cardiopulmonary disease in which there is impaired oxygen delivery, the symptoms will be manifested at lower methemoglobin levels.

DIAGNOSIS AND DIFFERENTIAL

The diagnosis of methemoglobinemia should be considered in patients presenting with cyanosis that does not improve with administration of oxygen. During venipuncture, blood may appear chocolate brown, a visible effect that is easily identified when the blood is placed on filter paper with a normal patient's blood for comparison. Levels are measured by co-oximetry on an arterial blood gas analyzer, with either an arterial or venous sample. Standard pulse oximetry will give an erroneously high oxygen saturation level at approximately 85% and does not change despite administration of 100% oxygen. Pulse co-oximeters are available that can noninvasively measure both methemoglobin and carboxyhemoglobin.

EMERGENCY DEPARTMENT CARE AND DISPOSITION

Methemoglobinemia should be treated initially with close monitoring and high concentrations of inspired oxygen (Table 117-2). Methemoglobinemia at levels above 25% and symptomatic patients with lower levels should be treated with **methylene blue**. The initial dose of methylene blue is 1 to 2 mg/kg as a 10% solution IV, given over 15 minutes. Clinical improvement should occur within 20 minutes, after which the dose may be repeated if improvement has not occurred. Failure to respond to a second dose is usually due to one of five causes (in order or likelihood of occurrence):

1. Glucose-6-phosphate dehydrogenase deficiency (G6PD): Consider transfusion of packed red blood cells for severely elevated methemoglobin levels in patients with suspected G6PD deficiency.
2. Dapsone: Compounds with long half-life, such as dapsone, can produce prolonged oxidative stress. Activated charcoal should be given. Treat dapsone-induced methemoglobinemia with a repeated dose of methylene blue; consider the addition of IV **cimetidine** to impede the metabolism of dapsone to its oxidant metabolite, hydroxylamine.

TABLE 117-2 Management of Methemoglobinemia

Management of Methemoglobinemia
Assess airway, breathing, and circulation
Place an IV line
Administer oxygen
Attach the patient to a cardiac and pulse oximetry monitor
Obtain an ECG
Decontaminate the patient as needed
Administer methylene blue—if symptomatic or methemoglobin >25%
Consider: cimetidine for patients taking dapsone

3. NADPH-methemoglobin reductase deficiency: Patients with congenital absence of this enzyme are not chronically cyanotic, nor do they have resting methemoglobin levels above normal. However, they lack the ability to convert methylene blue to its active metabolite. As with G6PD deficiency, consider packed red cell or exchange transfusions for severe cases, especially those with hemolysis.
4. Methylene blue-induced hemolysis: Paradoxically, methylene blue can be a source of oxidant stress. Methylene blue doses, therefore, should not exceed 7 mg/kg/d.
5. Sulfhemoglobinemia: This rare drug-induced dyshemoglobinemia can occur with sulfur-containing pharmaceuticals and phenacetin. Patients appear cyanotic at sulfhemoglobin levels of 5%, and pulse oximetry may read in the 70% to 80% range, but are rarely symptomatic. Treat sulfhemoglobinemia with supplement oxygen.

FURTHER READING

For further reading in *Tintinalli's Emergency Medicine: A Comprehensive Study Guide*, 8th ed., see Chapter 207, "Dyshemoglobinemias," by Brenna M. Farmer and Lewis S. Nelson.

SECTION 12

Environmental Injuries

CHAPTER 118

Cold Injuries

Gerald (Wook) Beltran

NONFREEZING COLD INJURIES

Trench foot is a direct soft tissue injury that results from prolonged exposure to nonfreezing cold and moisture. The foot is initially pale, mottled, pulseless, and anesthetic and does not improve quickly with rewarming. Several hours after rewarming, the foot becomes hyperemic and painful as perfusion returns after 2 to 3 days. Bullae and edema are late findings. Anesthesia may persist for weeks or even permanently. Hyperhidrosis and sensitivity to cold are late features and may last for months to years. Chilblains (pernio) are painful inflammatory lesions typically affecting the ears, hands, and feet caused by chronic exposure to intermittent damp, nonfreezing conditions. Localized edema, erythema, and cyanosis appear up to 12 hours after the exposure and are accompanied by pruritis and burning paresthesias. Tender blue nodules may form after rewarming and can persist for several days. Treatment of trench foot and chilblains includes drying, elevation, warming, and bandaging of the affected body part. With chilblains, add **nifedipine** 20 mg PO three times daily, **pentoxifyline** 400 mg PO three times daily, or **limaprost** 20 μg PO three times daily, as well as topical corticosteroids, such as **0.025% fluocinolone cream**.

FROSTBITE

Clinical Features

Freezing of tissue causes frostbite. Patients initially complain of stinging, burning, and numbness. Frostbite injuries are classified by the depth of injury and amount of tissue damage based on appearance after rewarming. First-degree frostbite (frostnip) is characterized by partial thickness skin freezing, erythema, edema, lack of blistering, and no tissue loss. Second-degree frostbite is characterized by deeper, full-thickness skin freezing and results in the formation of clear bullae. The patient complains of numbness, followed by aching and throbbing. Deep cold injury or third-degree frostbite involves freezing of the skin and subdermal plexus leading to hemorrhagic bullae and skin necrosis. Fourth-degree frostbite extends into muscle, tendon, and bone with mottled skin, nonblanching cyanosis, and eventual dry, black, mummified eschar formation. Early injuries are better classified as superficial or deep because it is difficult to initially evaluate the depth of injury. Laboratory testing and imaging are not needed to diagnose frostbite.

Treatment

1. Provide rapid **rewarming** in circulating water at 37°C to 39°C (98.6°F to 102.2°F) for 20 to 30 minutes until tissue is pliable and erythematous.
2. Debridement of clear blisters and aspiration of hemorrhagic blisters are controversial. Consult with a surgeon for local preference.
3. Apply topical **aloe vera** every 6 hours.
4. Provide pain management, local wound care, and dressing. Splint and elevate the affected extremities. Patients may require parenteral opioids initially, followed by oral NSAIDs.
5. Provide tetanus immunoprophylaxis, if needed.
6. Patients with superficial, local frostbite may be discharged home with close follow-up arranged.
7. Patients with deeper injuries require admission for ongoing care.
8. The use of prophylactic bacitracin ointment, antibiotics, and silver sulfadiazine is controversial.

HYPOTHERMIA

Hypothermia, a core body temperature of <35°C (<95°F), results from heat loss through conduction, convection, radiation, or evaporation.

Clinical Features

The features of hypothermia represent a continuum. Mild hypothermia (32°C to 35°C [90°F to 95°F]) can present with tachycardia, tachypnea, hypertension, shivering, and a normal level of consciousness. As core temperatures fall below 32°C (90°F), shivering ceases and heart rate and blood pressure decrease. As temperature decreases further, patients become confused, lethargic, and then comatose. Pupillary reflexes are lost. Respiratory rate decreases, gag and cough reflexes are diminished, and bronchorrhea occurs. Aspiration is common. Impaired renal concentration results in a cold diuresis and hemoconcentration. The cardiac effects of worsening hypothermia progress from sinus bradycardia, to atrial fibrillation with slow ventricular response, to ventricular fibrillation, to asystole. At temperatures <32°C (<90°F), the risk for dysrhythmias increases. As core body temperature falls below 28°C (below 82°F), the risk for cardiac arrest increases as the potential for malignant cardiac dysrhythmias become more pronounced.

Diagnosis and Differential

The diagnosis of hypothermia is based on core temperature and may not be initially obvious, especially in cases where a history of prolonged environmental exposure is missing. Low-reading thermometers are required to measure and monitor temperature. Along with the history and physical exam, laboratory investigation is directed at determining the underlying cause and complications. Helpful laboratory studies may include glucose, complete blood count (CBC), electrolytes, thyroid-stimulating hormone, random cortisol level, clotting profile, lactic acid, lipase, creatinine, blood gas, and electrocardiogram (ECG). Acid-base disorders are common, but do not follow a predictable pattern. Intravascular thrombosis, embolism, and disseminated intravascular coagulation (DIC) may occur. Electrocardiographic changes include PR, QRS, and QT prolongations, T-wave inversion, and a slow positive deflection at the end of the QRS (Osborn J wave). In addition to environmental exposure, causes of hypothermia include hypoglycemia, hypothyroidism, hypoadrenalism, hypopituitarism, central nervous system (CNS) dysfunction, drug intoxication, sepsis, and dermal disease.

Emergency Department Care and Disposition

1. Place patient in a warm environment. Initiate continuous monitoring of vital signs, pulse oximetry, and core temperature (rectal, bladder, or esophageal thermometer). Indications for intubation are similar to those for normothermic patients. Initiate warmed intravenous fluids titrated to a rate based on the patient's volume status. Remove wet clothing, dry, and cover patients.
2. Handle patients gently to avoid precipitation of a lethal dysrhythmia.
3. Attempt to palpate a pulse and detect respirations for 30 to 45 seconds. If none is detected, initiate cardiopulmonary resuscitation (CPR). Alternatively, use bedside ultrasonography to help determine cardiovascular status and need for CPR.
4. Sinus bradycardia, atrial fibrillation, and atrial flutter usually require no therapy and will resolve with rewarming. Ventricular fibrillation is typically refractory to therapy until the patient is rewarmed, although the American Heart Association guidelines do recommend a single defibrillation attempt.
5. Rewarming techniques include passive rewarming, active external rewarming, and active core rewarming (Table 118-1). Choice of technique depends primarily on cardiovascular status. Temperature is a secondary

TABLE 118-1 Staging and Treatment of Accidental Hypothermia

Stage	Clinical Symptoms	Typical Core Temperature	Treatment
Mild (HT I)	Conscious, shivering	35–32°C	Warm environment and clothing, warm sweet drinks, and active movement (if possible) HT I patients with significant trauma or comorbidities or those suspected of secondary hypothermia should receive HT II treatment
Moderate (HT II)	Impaired consciousness* (may or may not be shivering)	<32–28°C	Active external and minimally invasive rewarming techniques (warm environment; chemical, electrical, or forced air heating packs or blankets; warm parenteral fluids) Cardiac and core temperature monitoring Minimal and cautious movements to avoid arrhythmias Full-body insulation, horizontal position, and immobilization

(Continued)

TABLE 118-1 Staging and Treatment of Accidental Hypothermia (Continued)

Stage	Clinical Symptoms	Typical Core Temperature	Treatment
Severe (HT III)	Unconscious,* vital signs present	<28°C	HT II management plus: Airway management as required Preference to treat in an ECMO/CPB center, if available, due to the high risk of cardiac arrest Consider ECMO/CPB in cases with cardiac instability that is refractory to medical management Consider ECMO/CPB for comorbid patients who are unlikely to tolerate the low cardiac output associated with HT III
HT IV	Vital signs absent	Cardiac arrest is possible below 32°C; the risk increases substantially below 28°C and continues to increase with ongoing cooling	CPR and up to three doses of epinephrine and defibrillation (further dosing guided by clinical response) Airway management Transport to ECMO/CPB† Prevent further heat loss (insulation, warm environment, do not apply heat to head) Active external and minimally invasive rewarming (see HT II) during transport is recommended but controversial; do not apply heat to head

Abbreviations: CPB, cardiopulmonary bypass; CPR, cardiopulmonary resuscitation; ECMO, extracorporeal membrane oxygenation; HT, hypothermia.

*Consciousness may be impaired by comorbid illness (e.g., trauma, CNS pathology, toxic ingestion) independent of core temperature.

†Transfering an HT IV patient to an ECMO/CPB center may reduce mortality by 40% to 90% (number needed to treat, approximately 2); if ECMO/CPB is not available within a few hours of transport, consider on-site rewarming with hot packs or forced air blankets, warm IV fluid, ± warm thoracic lavage, ± warm bladder lavage, and ± warm peritoneal lavage; do not apply heat to the head.

consideration. Patients with a stable cardiovascular status (including sinus bradycardia and atrial fibrillation) and temperature above 30°C (above 90°F) may be passively rewarmed. All patients with cardiovascular instability require rapid core rewarming; extracorporeal circuit rewarming (e.g., extracorporeal membrane oxygenation or cardiopulmonary bypass) is the technique of choice for these patients. Invasive rapid core rewarming in patients without cardiac instability is controversial.

6. Continue resuscitative efforts until the core temperature reaches 32°C (90°F).
7. Address and treat underlying causes (e.g., **dextrose** 50 mL IV for hypoglycemia; treat suspected hypothyroidism and hypoadrenalism with hormone replacement).
8. Admit all patients with symptomatic hypothermia or with hypothermia secondary to an underlying condition. Healthy patients with mild environmental hypothermia that resolves quickly may be discharged home if social circumstances allow (Fig. 118-1).

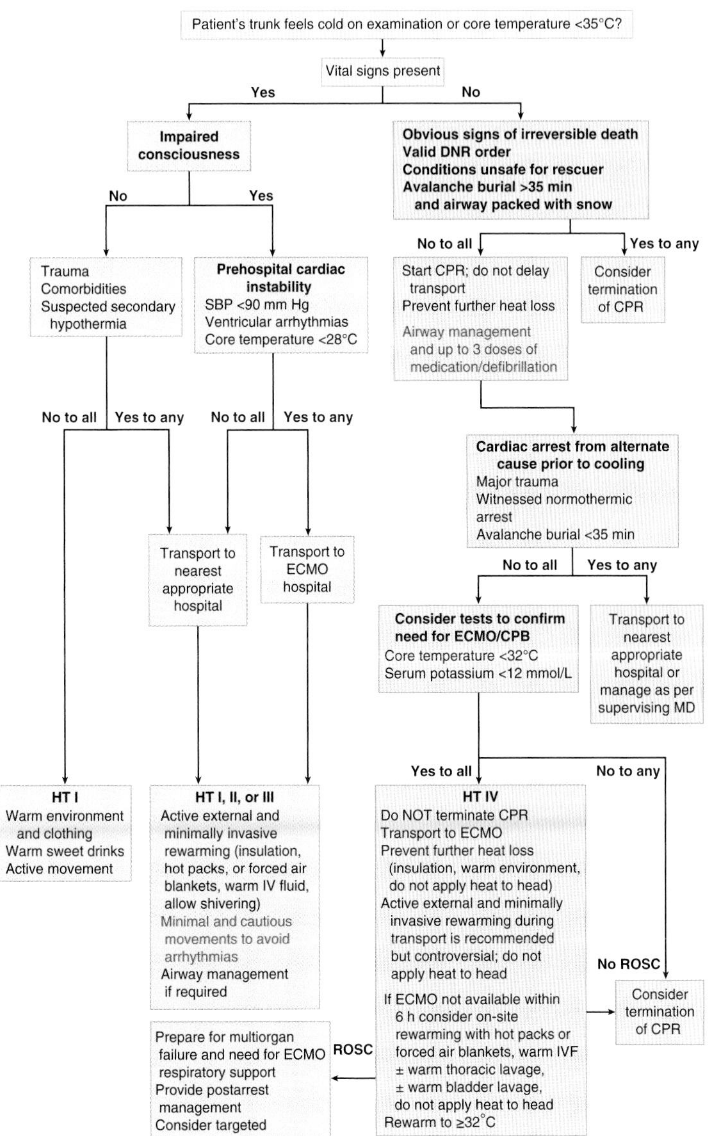

FIGURE 118-1. Transport and management of accidental hypothermia. CPB, cardiopulmonary bypass; DNR, do not resuscitate; ECMO, extracorporeal membrane oxygenation; HT, hypothermia; ROSC, return of spontaneous circulation; SBP, systolic blood pressure. Used with permission from Doug Brown, MD, FRCPC.

FURTHER READING

For further reading in *Tintinalli's Emergency Medicine: A Comprehensive Study Guide*, 8th ed., see Chapter 208, "Cold Injuries," by Michael T. Paddock; Chapter 209, "Hypothermia," by Doug Brown.

CHAPTER 119 Heat Emergencies

Eric Kraska

Heat-related illness is a spectrum of disease ranging from minor heat disorders, such as prickly heat and heat cramps, to severe heat imbalance that results in life-threatening heat stroke.

CLINICAL FEATURES

Malignant Heat Illnesses

Heat stroke develops in the setting of unmitigated heat imbalance. The cardinal features are hyperthermia (core temperature >40°C [104°F]) and end-organ injury. Height of the temperature and duration of heat exposure dictate degree of injury. Neural tissue, hepatocytes, nephrons, and vascular endothelium are most sensitive to heat stress. Prominent neurologic abnormalities include confusion, agitation, bizarre behavior, ataxia, seizures, and coma. Other bedside findings include hyperventilation, vomiting, diarrhea, and oliguria. Anhidrosis or profuse sweating may be seen. When coagulopathy/DIC develops, patients may have purpura, hemoptysis, or GI bleeding.

Heat stroke is further classified as exertional and nonexertional. Physical activity during high heat/humidity produces exertional heat stroke. Evaporation is the principal mechanism of heat loss, but is ineffective when humidity exceeds 75%. Nonexertional heat stoke is seen in the debilitated, chronically ill, and persons who are otherwise unable to escape from hot environments (e.g., closed vehicles, heavily bundled in crib, or isolated in a hot residence).

Minor Heat Illnesses

Heat syncope results from volume depletion, peripheral vasodilation, and decreased vasomotor tone. It occurs most commonly in the elderly and poorly acclimatized individuals. Postural vital signs may or may not be demonstrable on presentation to the emergency department. Exclude other causes of syncope.

Heat cramps are characterized by painful muscle spasms, especially in the calves, thighs, and shoulders during athletic events. They usually occur when individuals replace evaporative losses with free water but not with salt. Core body temperature may be normal or elevated.

Heat edema and *heat rash* are usually self-limited symptoms during the first few days of heat exposure and are characterized by swelling of dependent extremities (e.g., hands and feet) or rash found commonly over clothed areas of the body.

DIAGNOSIS AND DIFFERENTIAL

The differential diagnosis includes infection (e.g., sepsis, meningitis, encephalitis, malaria, typhoid, tetanus), endocrine disorders (e.g., diabetic ketoacidosis, thyroid storm), neurologic disorders (e.g., cerebrovascular accident, status epilepticus), and toxicologic causes (e.g., amphetamines for ADHD, dietary supplements, anticholinergics, sympathomimetics, salicylates, serotonin syndrome, malignant hyperthermia, neuroleptic malignant syndrome, alcohol or benzodiazepine withdrawal).

EMERGENCY DEPARTMENT CARE AND DISPOSITION

Malignant Heat Illnesses

Acute care requires accurate identification of hyperthermia with end-organ injury and rapid mitigation of the heat imbalance. Initial diagnostic studies are directed at detecting end-organ damage and excluding other disease processes. Early laboratory abnormalities associated with heat stroke include hypoglycemia, hypophosphatemia, hypokalemia, elevated liver enzymes, hypercalcemia, elevated hematocrit along with elevated creatine phosphokinase and myoglobin from rhabdomyolysis. Laboratory abnormalities of DIC and renal failure may develop with time. Obtain an EKG and CXR. Neuroimaging studies and other evaluations (e.g., septic workup, toxicology screens) can be individualized as clinically indicated.

1. Supportive care is required for airway, breathing, and circulation. Intubate patients with significantly altered mental status, diminished gag reflex, or hypoxia. Continuously monitor vital signs and core temperature (rectal, bladder, or esophageal thermometer). Provide high flow oxygen and begin IV crystalloids to maintain mean arterial pressure above 80 to 90 mm Hg. Avoid volume overload. Vasopressors may be required.
2. Initiate rapid cooling until core temperature reaches 38°C (100.4°F). External cooling is most effective. Place patient on cooling blanket, wet skin and dry with fan to optimize evaporative cooling, and place ice packs to the groin/axilla/neck. Cold water immersion is effective, but not practical. Internal cooling measures include infusing room temperature IVF, central catheter heat exchange methods, and in extreme cases, cardiopulmonary bypass. Gastric, rectal, and bladder lavage are unlikely to be more effective than external cooling measures (Table 119-1).
3. Seizures and excessive shivering can be treated with benzodiazepines, such as lorazepam 1 to 2 mg IV or diazepam 5 mg IV.
4. Treat rhabdomyolysis with IV hydration. To date, no prospective control studies have shown improved outcomes from alkalinization of the urine or forced diuresis with mannitol or loop diuretics.
5. Monitor serum electrolytes every hour initially. Treat hyperkalemia and DIC with standard regimens.
6. Antipyretics (e.g., acetaminophen, ibuprofen, and dantrolene) are ineffective and should not be used.
7. Most heat stroke patients require admission to the ICU.

Minor Heat Illnesses

Symptoms usually resolve independent of treatment and patients are typically discharged home. Heat edema treatment consists of elevation of the extremities or compressive stockings. Diuretics may exacerbate volume depletion and should be avoided. Heat rash may improve with antihistamines,

TABLE 119-1 Summary of Cooling Techniques

Cooling Method	Advantages	Disadvantages	Recommendations
Evaporative cooling	Provides effective cooling Readily available Practical Well tolerated	Can cause shivering Less effective in humid environments Makes it difficult to maintain electrode positions	Strongly recommended
Immersion cooling	Provides effective cooling	Can cause shivering Poorly tolerated Not compatible with resuscitation settings	Recommended
Ice packs on neck, axillae, and groin	Practical Can be added to other cooling methods	Cooling times longer than other modalities Poorly tolerated	Can be used as adjunct cooling method
Cardiopulmonary bypass	Provides fast and effective cooling	Invasive Not readily available Setup is labor intensive	Recommended in severe or resistant cases when available
Cooling blankets	Easy to apply	Have limited cooling efficacy Impede use of other cooling methods	Not recommended when other methods available
Cold water gastric, urinary bladder, rectal, or peritoneal lavage	–	Invasive Labor intensive May lead to water intoxication Human experience is limited	Effectiveness and safety not established

low-potency topical corticosteroids, or calamine lotion. Advise patients to wear light, loose fitting clothing. Treatment of heat syncope and heat cramps consists of rest and oral or IV rehydration.

FURTHER READING

For further reading in *Tintinalli's Emergency Medicine: A Comprehensive Study Guide*, 8th ed., see Chapter 210, "Heat Emergencies," by Frank LoVecchio.

CHAPTER 120

Bites and Stings

Michael Levine

WASPS, BEES, AND STINGING ANTS (HYMENOPTERA)

Wasps, bees, and stinging ants are members of the order Hymenoptera. Local and generalized reactions may occur in response to an encounter. Systemic toxicity may result from an allergic reaction or from massive envenomation as occurs classically with the so-called Africanized bees, which often attack in large numbers. Fire ant venom may cross-react in individuals sensitized to other Hymenoptera stings.

Clinical Features

Local reactions consist of pain, erythema, edema, and pruritus at the sting site. Severe local reactions may increase the likelihood of serious systemic reactions if the patient is reexposed. The local reaction to a fire ant sting consists of a sterile pustule that evolves over 6 to 24 hours, sometimes resulting in necrosis and scarring. *Systemic reactions* may include urticaria, angioedema, hypotension, and bronchospasm. In addition, those with massive envenomation may develop severe vomiting, diarrhea, rhabdomyolysis, myocardial injury, hepatic failure, and renal failure. *Delayed reactions*, which manifest 5 to 14 days post-envenomation, infrequently occur, but resemble serum sickness. Such illness is characterized by fever, malaise, headache, urticaria, lymphadenopathy, and polyarthritis.

Emergency Department Care and Disposition

1. In addition to fluid resuscitation, patients with anaphylactic or anaphylactoid reactions should receive the following:
   a. **Epinephrine** 1:1000 concentration (0.3 to 0.5 cc IM in adults or 0.01 mg/kg up to a maximal dose of 0.5 cc in pediatrics). Patients whose symptoms persist despite IM epinephrine or those with evidence of shock should receive IV epinephrine as a continuous infusion.
   b. Endotracheal intubation should be performed if needed for airway edema.
   c. Steroids, such as **methylprednisolone** 2 mg/kg, with a maximal single dose of 125 mg, or **prednisone** 1 mg/kg orally, with a maximal single dose of 60 mg.
   d. H_1 antagonists, such as **diphenhydramine** 1 mg/kg IV with a maximal single dose of 50 mg.
   e. H_2 receptor antagonists, such as famotidine 0.5 mg/kg IV with a maximal dose of 40 mg.
   f. Bronchospasm should be treated with *beta* agonists, such as **albuterol** 2.5 to 5 mg via nebulization.
2. Patients with urticaria, but no other systemic manifestations, should be treated with H_1 and H_2 blockers and steroids, but without epinephrine or albuterol.
3. The stinger should be removed after the patient has been stabilized.

4. Patients with a single sting who have only minor symptoms can be discharged home after a period of observation.
5. For patients with multiple stings, disposition is as follows:
   a. Admit if more than 100 stings, substantial comorbidities, extremes of age, or severe systemic manifestations
   b. Patients with <100 stings, and who remain asymptomatic without laboratory evidence of complications (e.g., no rhabdomyolysis and normal renal function) following an observation period of 6 hours can be discharged from the Emergency Department.
6. Refer all patients with Hymenoptera reactions to an allergist for further evaluation, prescribe a premeasured epinephrine injector (EpiPen®), and advise them to carry allergy alert identification. Instruct patients to use epinephrine at the first sign of a systemic reaction.

BROWN RECLUSE SPIDER (*LOXOSCELES RECLUSA*)

Clinical Features

The initial *L. reclusa* bite is painless. It evolves into a firm erythematous lesion that heals over several days to weeks. Occasionally, a severe reaction with immediate pain, hemorrhagic blister formation, and local blanching may occur. These lesions often become necrotic over the next 3 to 4 days and form significant eschars. *Loxoscelism* is a common systemic reaction following the bite of some South American *Loxosceles* species, but occurs infrequently following the bite of *L. reclusa*. Systemic symptoms, which are more common in children, typically occur 1 to 3 days post-envenomation, and are characterized by fever, chills, vomiting, arthralgias, myalgias, petechiae, and hemolysis. Severe cases progress to seizures, renal failure, disseminated intravascular coagulation, and death.

Diagnosis and Differential

Loxosceles species are distinguished by three sets of paired eyes; most other spiders have eight eyes in two rows. A pigmented, violin-shaped pattern on the cephalothorax of the brown recluse is characteristic but unreliable. The diagnosis of *L. reclusa* envenomation is commonly clinical since the bite is rarely witnessed. Assays to confirm *L. reclusa* poisoning are not clinically available. Patients with significant envenomation may exhibit hemolysis, coagulopathy, or abnormal renal function. Local abscesses are frequently misdiagnosed as *Loxosceles* envenomation

Emergency Department Care and Disposition

1. Treatment of a brown recluse spider bite includes supportive measures, such as pain medication, tetanus prophylaxis, and antibiotics if infection is present. In the United States, antivenom is not commercially available and is usually not needed.
2. Most wounds heal without intervention. Dapsone, which was once advocated for treatment of these envenomations, has not been clearly proven to be beneficial. Due to the risk of significant adverse events and the lack of proven efficacy, its use in this setting is not recommended. Arrange serial wound evaluations for outpatients.

3. Patients with systemic reactions and hemolysis should be hospitalized.
4. Surgery is reserved for lesions larger than 2 cm and is deferred for 2 to 3 weeks after the bite.

HOBO SPIDER (*TEGENARIA AGRESTIS*)

The hobo spider, also known as the Northwestern brown spider, causes clinical signs and symptoms that are similar to those of the brown recluse spider bite. The skin site is initially painless before developing induration, erythema, blistering, and necrosis. Patients may experience headache, vomiting, and fatigue. There is no specific diagnostic test or therapeutic intervention for hobo spider bites. Surgical repair for severe ulcerative lesions is delayed until the necrotizing process is complete.

BLACK WIDOW SPIDER (*LATRODECTUS MACTANS*)

Clinical Features

Black widow spider bites induce an immediate pinprick sensation that may quickly spread to the entire extremity. Erythema at the site appears within 1 hour and often forms a "target" lesion. Systemic manifestations may include diffuse myalgias, especially involving the larger muscle groups, including the back, abdomen, and trunk. Severe pain may wax and wane for several days. Other signs and symptoms include hypertension, tachycardia, muscle fasciculations, headache, nausea, vomiting, and diaphoresis. The fasciculations and diaphoresis may be localized or diffuse. Serious, albeit rare, acute complications include myocarditis, priapism, and dyspnea.

Emergency Department Care and Disposition

1. Initial therapy includes local wound treatment and supportive care. Liberal dosing of analgesics and benzodiazepines will relieve pain and cramping.
2. ***Lacrodectus* antivenom**, derived from horse serum, is rapidly effective for severe envenomation even when the presentation is delayed. Fatal cases of anaphylaxis have been described with this therapy, and its use should be reserved for severe cases refractory to opioid analgesics and benzodiazepines. The package insert provides dosing instructions.
3. Patients receiving antivenom may be discharged after a short observation period if symptoms of envenomation resolve.

TARANTULAS

When threatened, tarantulas may flick barbed hairs into their victim. Although North American tarantula hairs rarely penetrate human skin, they can embed deeply into the conjunctiva and cornea and cause an inflammatory response. Any patient complaining of ocular symptoms after exposure to a tarantula should undergo a thorough slit lamp examination to search for embedded hairs. Treatment includes topical steroids and consultation with an ophthalmologist for surgical removal of the hairs.

Tarantula bites may also occur. They are painful, and cause local erythema and edema. Provide local wound care and analgesia.

SCORPION (SCORPIONIDA)

Clinical Features

Although highly toxic species are found in the Caribbean, Asia, and Africa, the only North American scorpion that produces systemic toxicity is the bark scorpion (*Centruroides sculpturatus*). Venom from *C. sculpturatus* causes immediate pain and paresthesia. A positive "tap test" (exquisite local tenderness when the area is lightly tapped) may be seen. Systemic effects are relatively infrequent and occur mainly in children. Systemic manifestations include diffuse motor involvement and/or cranial nerve dysfunction, the latter of which may result in roving eye movements, diplopia, and difficulty swallowing. Systemic symptoms may last 24 to 48 hours without antivenom therapy.

Emergency Department Care and Disposition

1. Most patients require only oral analgesics and/or benzodiazepines.
2. Patients with systemic manifestations may require IV benzodiazepines and opiates.
3. While uncommon, patients with significant hypersalivation and stridor may warrant endotracheal intubation. Atropine has been used to help with secretions, although data supporting its use for this purpose are lacking.
4. A **F(ab) equine antivenom** is available and highly effective for those patients with high-grade, systemic toxicity.
5. Patients without systemic symptoms may be observed briefly and discharged with analgesics.

SCABIES (*SARCOPTES SCABIEI*)

Clinical Features

Scabies bites are often concentrated in the web spaces between fingers and toes. Other common areas include the axilla and genital area, children's faces and scalps, and the female nipple. Transmission is typically by direct contact. The distinctive feature of scabies infestation is intense pruritus with "burrows." The female mite is easily scraped out with a blade edge. Associated vesicles, papules, crusts, and eczematization may obscure the diagnosis.

Emergency Department Care and Disposition

Advise patients to apply permethrin cream from the neck down; infants may require additional application to the scalp, temple, and forehead. The patient should bathe before application, apply the medication, and then bathe again in 12 hours. Reapplication is necessary only if mites are found 2 weeks after treatment, although the pruritus may last for several weeks after successful therapy. **Ivermectin**, 200 μg/kg PO, followed by a second dose in 10 days, is an alternative treatment.

TICKS

The spectrum of tick borne illness includes Lyme disease, Rocky Mountain spotted fever, ehrlichiosis, babesiosis, Colorado tick fever, tularemia, and tickborne encephalitis. Certain species of ticks have a neurotoxin capable of inducing tick paralysis, a symmetric ascending flaccid paralysis nearly identical to Guillain–Barré syndrome. Indeed, a diagnosis of Guillain–Barré syndrome should not be considered until a thorough search rules out the presence of an engorged tick. The recommended method of tick removal involves grasping the tick with forceps near the point of attachment and pulling with steady, gentle traction. Since disease transmission is time dependent, prompt tick removal is essential.

CHIGGERS (TROMBICULIDAE)

Clinical Features

Chiggers are tiny mite larvae that cause intense pruritus when they feed on host epidermal cells. They tend to attach to skin in areas of tight-fitting clothing such as near waistbands. Children who have been sitting on lawns are prone to chigger lesions in the genital area. Itchiness begins within a few hours, followed by a papule that enlarges to a nodule ("chigger bite") over the next 1 to 2 days. Single bites may cause soft tissue edema, whereas infestation has been associated with fever and erythema multiforme. The diagnosis of chigger bites is based on typical skin lesions and intense pruritus in the context of known outdoor exposure.

Emergency Department Care and Disposition

Treatment is symptomatic with oral or topical antihistamines, although oral steroids may be required in more severe cases. Annihilation of the mites requires topical application of permethrin or other topical scabicides. The package insert provides techniques for proper use.

FLEAS (SIPHONAPTERA)

Flea bites are frequently found in zigzag lines, especially on the legs and waist. They are intensely pruritic lesions with hemorrhagic puncta, surrounding erythema, and urticaria. Discomfort is relieved with calamine lotion, cool soaks, and oral or topical antihistamines. Severe irritation may require topical steroid creams. Patients who develop impetigo and other local infections should be treated with topical or oral antibiotics.

LICE (ANOPLURA)

Body lice concentrate on the waist, shoulders, axillae, and neck. Their bites produce red spots that progress to papules and wheals. They are so intensely pruritic that linear scratch marks are suggestive of infestation. The white ova of *head lice* are adherent to the hair shaft and therefore can be distinguished from dandruff. *Pubic lice* are spread by sexual contact. They cause intense pruritus, and their small white eggs (nits) are visible on hair shafts. As with scabies, permethrin is the primary treatment for body lice infestation. Treatment of any hair-borne infestation requires application of pyrethrin with piperonyl butoxide after hair washing, with reapplication in 10 days. Wet combing hair with a fine-tooth comb will remove dead lice and nits. Clothing, bedding, and personal articles should be washed in hot (>52°C [125.6°F]) water to prevent reinfestation.

KISSING BUGS AND BED BUGS (HEMIPTERA)

Kissing bugs, also known as reduviid or conenose beetles, and bed bugs feed on blood of a sleeping victim. The initial bite is painless. Bedbug bites are often linear. Bites are often multiple and result in wheals or hemorrhagic papules and bullae. Dark lines of bedbug excrement on bed linens may be seen. Treatment consists of local wound care, topical steroids, and oral antihistamines. Allergic reactions may occur in sensitized individuals.

SNAKE BITES

Venomous snake bites in North America are typically caused by pit vipers (Crotaline-rattlesnakes, copperhead, water moccasin, and massasauga) or coral snakes (Elapidae).

PIT VIPER (CROTALINAE) BITES

Crotaline snakes, commonly known as pit vipers, are identified by their two retractable fangs and by heat-sensitive depressions ("pits") located bilaterally between each eye and nostril. Only 25% of bites result in envenomation.

Clinical Features

The effects of crotaline envenomation depend on the size and species of snake, the age and size of the victim, the time elapsed since the bite, and the characteristics of the bite itself. The hallmark of pit viper envenomation is the presence of one or more fang marks combined with pain, and progressive edema extending from the site. Tender lymphadenopathy in the envenomated extremity is common. Nausea, vomiting, and a metallic taste are often described in those patients with envenomations. Severe systemic manifestations may rarely occur, and include hypotension, tachycardia, and shock. Thrombocytopenia, coagulopathy, and hypofibrinogenemia may be observed.

Diagnosis and Differential

The diagnosis of crotaline envenomation is based on the presence of the aforementioned local injuries, systemic symptoms or hematologic abnormalities. The absence of any of these findings after 8 to 12 hours indicates a dry bite.

Minimal envenomation is defined as local swelling, no systemic signs, and no laboratory abnormalities. *Severe* envenomation causes extensive swelling, potentially life-threatening systemic signs, and markedly abnormal coagulation parameters. Initially mild envenomation syndromes may progress to severe syndromes over several hours. Pertinent laboratory tests include a complete blood count, coagulation tests, urinalysis, and blood typing.

Emergency Department Care and Disposition

1. Consultation with a medical toxicologist or poison control center is recommended for all pit-viper bites.
2. Cardiac monitoring and IV access in the non-envenomated extremity should be established.

3. Provide local wound care and tetanus immunization. Measure limb circumference at several sites above and below the wound and check every 30 to 60 minutes.
4. Treat patients with progressive local swelling, systemic effects, or coagulopathy immediately with antivenom therapy, **Polyvalent Crotalidae Immune Fab (FabAV)**, a sheep-derived antivenin. Administer an "initial control" dose of **FabAV** 4 to 6 vials IV; there is no need for prior skin testing. "Initial control" is defined as cessation of progression of all components of envenomation: local effects, systemic effects, and laboratory parameters (coagulopathy and/or thrombocytopenia). The initial dose of FabAV, as well as any subsequent dose, is diluted in 250 mL normal saline and infused IV over 1 hour. The goal of therapy is to neutralize existing venom; the dose of FabAV is the same for children and adults although the amount of diluent may need to be decreased in small children. If an allergic reaction occurs, stop the infusion and treat with epinephrine and antihistamines, as indicated.
5. If the "initial control" is not achieved with the first infusion, give a repeat dose of 4 to 6 vials.
6. Monitor blood count and coagulation studies every 4 hours or after each course of antivenom, whichever is more frequent. Monitor renal function.
7. The endpoint of antivenom therapy is the arrest of progressive symptoms and coagulopathy. Maintenance therapy includes administration of an additional 2-vial dose at 6, 12, and 18 hours after "initial control" is achieved. The antivenom package insert will guide in administration. The administration of antivenom must continue until complete control of the envenomation is achieved.
8. *Compartment syndrome* rarely occurs secondary to envenomation. Treatment includes limb elevation and additional 4 to 6 vials of IV antivenom. Fasciotomy should only be performed if compartment syndrome is suspected and elevated compartment pressures persist despite elevation and additional antivenom. Discussion with a toxicologist or poison control center is recommended.
9. Active bleeding due to severe coagulopathy may require blood component therapy, although FabAV remains the mainstay of treatment for coagulopathy or thrombocytopenia not associated with overt hemorrhage.
10. Observe all patients with a pit viper bite for at least 6 to 8 hours. Admit patients with severe bites and those receiving antivenin to the intensive care unit. Patients with no evidence of envenomation after 8 hours may be discharged, although some advocate admitting all children with lower extremity bites for 24 hours due to possibility of delayed recognition of lower extremity edema. All patients who receive FabAV should be counseled regarding the 5% risk of serum sickness. The standard treatment for serum sickness is oral **prednisone**, 1 mg/kg/d tapering over 1 to 2 weeks.

CORAL SNAKE BITE

Clinical Features

Venomous coral snakes in the United States are brightly colored with adjacent red and yellow bands. In the United States, only bites from the eastern coral snake (*Micrurus fulvius fulvius*) require significant treatment as its venom is a potent neurotoxin that causes tremor, salivation, respiratory paralysis, seizures, and bulbar palsies (e.g., dysarthria, diplopia, and dysphagia). Bites of the Sonoran (Arizona) coral snake are mild and only need local care.

Emergency Department Care and Disposition

1. Consultation with a medical toxicologist or poison control center is recommended.
2. The toxic effects of toxic coral snake venom may be preventable, but they are not easily reversed. All patients who have been bitten should receive 3 to 5 vials of **antivenom (*M. fulvius*)** *at the first sign of toxicity.* Additional antivenom doses are required if symptoms appear. Access to coral snake antivenom is extremely limited, as it is no longer manufactured in the United States.
3. Follow pulmonary function parameters and neurological exams (e.g., inspiratory pressure and vital capacity) and admit to the hospital for 24 to 48 hours of observation.

GILA MONSTER BITE

Gila monster bites result in pain and swelling. Systemic toxicity is rare but may consist of diaphoresis, paresthesia, weakness, hypertension, and angioedema. The biting animal may be tenacious, and the reptile should be removed as soon as possible. If the reptile is still attached, it may loosen its bite when placed on a solid surface where it is not suspended in midair. Once removed, perform standard wound care including a search for implanted teeth. No further treatment is required. Patients should be observed for airway edema for at least 6 hours after the Gila monster is removed. Those without systemic manifestations, including angioedema, can be discharged home.

FURTHER READING

For further reading in *Tintinalli's Emergency Medicine: A Comprehensive Study Guide*, 8th ed., see Chapter 211, "Bites and Stings," by SchneirAaron and ClarkRichard F.; and Chapter 212, "Reptile Bites," by Richard C. Dart and Julian White.

Trauma and Envenomation from Marine Fauna

Christian A. Tomaszewski

The population growth along coastal areas has made exposure to hazardous marine fauna increasingly common. The popularity of home aquariums generates additional exposures inland. Marine fauna can inflict injury through direct traumatic bite or envenomation, usually via a stinging apparatus.

CLINICAL FEATURES

Major marine trauma includes bites from sharks, great barracudas, moray eels, seals, crocodiles, needlefish, wahoos, piranhas, and triggerfish. Shark bites may also cause substantial tissue loss, particularly the legs, with hemorrhagic shock. Minor trauma is usually due to cuts and scrapes from coral which can cause local stinging pain, erythema, urticaria, and pruritus.

Marine wounds can be infected with routine skin flora, such as *Staphylococcus* and *Streptococcus* species, along with bacteria unique to the marine environment. The most serious halophilic organism is the gram-negative bacillus *Vibrio*, which can cause rapid infections marked by pain, swelling, hemorrhagic bullae, vasculitis, and even necrotizing fasciitis and sepsis. Immunosuppressed patients, particularly those with liver disease, are susceptible to sepsis and death (up to 60%) from *Vibrio vulnificus*. Another bacterium, *Erysipelothrix rhusiopathiae,* implicated in fish-handler's disease, can cause painful, marginating plaques after cutaneous puncture wounds. The unique marine bacterium *Mycobacterium marinum*, an acid-fast bacillus, can cause a chronic cutaneous granuloma 3 to 4 weeks after exposure.

Numerous invertebrate and vertebrate marine species are venomous. The invertebrates belong to five phyla: Cnidaria, Porifera, Echinodermata, Annelida, and Mollusca.

The four classes of Cnidaria all share stinging cells, known as nematocysts, which deliver venom subcutaneously when stimulated. The most common effect is local pain, swelling, pruritus, urticaria, and even blistering and necrosis in severe cases. Some can cause systemic reactions due to toxic effects. The Hydrozoans include hydroids, *Millepora* (fire corals), and *Physalia* (Portuguese man-of-war). The latter causes a linear erythematous eruption and rarely can cause respiratory arrest, possibly from anaphylaxis. In addition to local tissue injury, the Scyphozoans (true jellyfish) include Atlantic Ocean larval forms that can cause a persistent dermatitis under bathing suits lasting days after exposure (Seabather's eruption). The Cubozoans (box jellyfish), in particular *Chironex fleckeri* in Australia and *Chiropsalmus* in the Gulf of Mexico, can cause a cardiotoxic death after severe stings. A Hawaiian box jellyfish, *Carybdea*, has been implicated in painful stings but no deaths. Another Australian box jellyfish, *Carukia barnesi*, can cause Irukandji's syndrome, characterized by diffuse pain, hypertension, tachycardia, diaphoresis, and even pulmonary edema. The most innocuous Cnidaria are the anthozoans (anemones) that occasionally cause a mild local reaction.

Porifera (the sponges) can produce a stinging, pruritic dermatitis. Spicules of silica or calcium carbonate can become embedded in the skin along with toxic secretions from the sponge. Echinodermata include sea urchins and sea stars. Sea urchin spines produce immediate pain with trauma; some contain venom that leads to erythema and swelling. Retained spines can lead to infection and granuloma formation. The crown-of-thorns sea star, *Acanthaster planci*, has sharp rigid spines that cause burning pain and local inflammation. Another class of echinoderms are sea cucumbers, which can cause mild contact dermatitis. Annelida include bristle and fire worms, which embed bristles in the skin, causing pain and erythema. Mollusca include gastropods and octopuses. Both the Indo-Pacific cone shell, *Conus*, and the blue-ringed octopus, *Hapalochlaena*, can deliver paralytic venom that can quickly lead to respiratory paralysis.

Vertebrate envenomations are primarily due to stingrays (order Rajiformes) and spined venomous fish (scorpion fish, lionfish, catfish, and weeverfish). The stingray whip tail has venomous spines, which puncture or lacerate causing an intense painful local reaction. The spines of venomous fish have glands that force venom into the wound after puncture and cause local pain, erythema, and edema. Retention of a spine tip can lead to infection. In tropical Indo-Pacific waters, bites by venomous sea snakes, although rare, can cause neurotoxicity and myotoxicity, and even death from ascending paralysis.

EMERGENCY DEPARTMENT CARE AND DISPOSITION

1. Copiously irrigate lacerations, punctures, and bite wounds; explore for foreign matter and debride devitalized tissue. Soft tissue radiographs or ultrasound may help locate foreign bodies, which usually require removal especially if intraarticular. Leave lacerations open for delayed primary closure. Update tetanus, if needed.
2. Prophylactic antibiotic therapy is not indicated for routine minor wounds in healthy patients but may be considered in selected patients (Table 121-1). Antibiotic therapy for infected wounds is first directed toward likely pathogens and later by culture and sensitivity results. Treat *Staphylococcus* and *Streptococcus* species with a first-generation cephalosporin, such as **cephalexin** 500 mg (10 to 25 mg/kg in children) four times daily PO or **cefazolin** 1 to 2 g (25 mg/kg in children) every 8 hours IV; alternatively **doxycycline** 100 mg PO/IV twice daily for MRSA coverage may be used in adults. Addition of a third-generation cephalosporin, such as **ceftriaxone** 1 g (50 mg/kg in children) IV daily or **cefotaxime** 2 g (50 mg/kg in children) IV every 8 hours, or a fluoroquinolone, such as **levofloxacin** or **ciprofloxacin** 500 mg PO/IV daily will cover ocean-related infections from *Vibrio* (avoid use in children). A **fluoroquinolone** or **third-generation cephalosporin**, or **trimethoprim-sulfamethoxazole double strength, 1 tablet (4 mg/kg trimethoprim component in children) PO twice each day**, or **imipenem, 500 mg (10 to 25 mg/kg**

TABLE 121-1 Recommendations for Antibiotic Treatment of Marine-Associated Wounds

No Antibiotics Indicated	Prophylactic/Outpatient Antibiotics	Hospital Admission for IV Antibiotics
Healthy patient	Late wound care	Predisposing medical conditions
Prompt wound care	Large lacerations or injuries	Long delays before definitive wound care
No foreign body	Early or local inflammation	Deep wounds, significant trauma
No bone or joint involvement		Wounds with retained foreign bodies
Small or superficial injuries		Progressive inflammatory change Penetration of periosteum, joint space, or body cavity Major injuries associated with envenomation Systemic illness

in children) IV every 6 hours, will cover fresh water infections from *Aeromonas*. Granulomas from *Mycobacterium marinum* require several months of treatment with **clarithromycin** or **rifampin plus ethambutol**.

3. Treatment of jellyfish stings is controversial and may be species dependent. Regardless, initial irrigation with seawater to remove nematocyst-laden tentacles may be beneficial. **Hot water (111°F (43.3°C) to 114°F (45.6°C)**) and **topical lidocaine** may lessen local venom effects. See Table 121-2 summarizing early treatment of all marine envenomations.

TABLE 121-2 Early Treatment of Marine Envenomations

Marine Organism	Detoxification	Further Treatment
Penetrating Envenomations		
Catfish, lionfish, scorpionfish, stingray	Hot water immersion*; lidocaine infiltration.	Usual wound care.† Assess for stingray spines (x-ray or exploration). Observe for development of systemic symptoms.
Stonefish	Hot water immersion*; lidocaine infiltration	Usual wound care.† Administer stonefish antivenin if severe systemic reaction.
Sea snake	—	Pressure immobilization. Administer antivenom if severe systemic reaction. Observe 8 h for myotoxicity or neurotoxicity.
Australian blue-ringed octopus	—	Use pressure immobilization. Provide supportive care.

(Continued)

TABLE 121-2 Early Treatment of Marine Envenomations (Continued)

Marine Organism	Detoxification	Further Treatment
Cone snail	—	Use pressure immobilization. Provide supportive care.
Sea urchin	Hot water immersion*; topical lidocaine	Explore wound and remove any spines.
Fireworms	Topical 5% acetic acid (vinegar).	Consider topical corticosteroids. Remove bristles.
Nonpenetrating Envenomations		
Fire coral, hydroids, anemones	Irrigate with seawater or saline.	Topical corticosteroid for itching.
Portuguese man-of-war, blue bottles, and non-box jellyfish	Hot water immersion,* sea water irrigation, topical lidocaine. Remove tentacles and nematocysts.	Topical corticosteroid for itching. Observe for development of systemic symptoms. Supportive care.
Box jellyfish	Hot water immersion.* Irrigate with saline or seawater. Topical 5% acetic acid (vinegar). Remove tentacles and nematocysts. Topical lidocaine.	Topical corticosteroid for itching. Observe for development of systemic symptoms. Supportive care. Administer *Chironex* antivenin.
Irukandji's syndrome	Irrigate with saline or seawater. Hot water immersion.* Remove tentacles and nematocysts.	Parenteral opioids for pain. Magnesium for cardiac arrest.

*Hot water immersion = 111°F (43.3°C) to 114°F (45.6°C) water until pain relieved.

†Usual wound care = irrigate, explore, debride, consider antibiotics and analgesi.

FURTHER READING

For further reading in *Tintinalli's Emergency Medicine: A Comprehensive Study Guide*, 8th ed., see Chapter 213, "Marine Trauma and Envenomation," by John J. Devlin and Kevin Knoop.

CHAPTER 122

High-Altitude Disorders

Shaun D. Carstairs

High-altitude disorders are due primarily to hypoxia; the rapidity and height of ascent influence the risk of occurrence.

ACUTE MOUNTAIN SICKNESS

Clinical Features

Acute mountain sickness (AMS) is usually seen in nonacclimated people making a rapid ascent to higher than 2000 m (6560 ft) above sea level. Symptoms resembling a hangover may develop within 6 hours after arrival at altitude but may be delayed as long as one day. Typical symptoms include bifrontal headache along with a combination of GI disturbance, dizziness, fatigue, or sleep disturbance. Worsening headache, vomiting, oliguria, dyspnea, and weakness indicate progression of AMS. Physical examination findings in early AMS are limited. Postural hypotension and peripheral and facial edema may occur. Localized rales are noted in up to 20% of cases. Funduscopy shows tortuous and dilated veins; retinal hemorrhages are common at altitudes higher than 5000 m (16,500 ft). Resting S_aO_2 is typically normal for altitude and correlates poorly with the diagnosis of AMS.

Diagnosis and Differential

The differential diagnosis includes hypothermia, carbon monoxide poisoning, pulmonary or central nervous system infections, migraine, dehydration, and exhaustion. The diagnosis is based largely on history of rapid ascent and symptoms.

Emergency Department Care and Disposition

The goals of treatment are to prevent progression, abort the illness, and improve acclimatization.

1. Terminate further ascent until symptoms resolve. For mild AMS, symptomatic therapy includes an analgesic, such as **acetaminophen** or an NSAID, and an antiemetic, such as **ondansetron** disintegrating tablets, 4 to 8 mg every 4 to 6 hours PO. Mild AMS usually improves or resolves in 12 to 36 hours if ascent is stopped.
2. A decrease in altitude of 300 to 1000 m should provide prompt relief of symptoms. Immediate descent and treatment are indicated for patients with moderate AMS or if there is a change in the level of consciousness, ataxia, or pulmonary edema.
3. Low-flow **oxygen** also relieves symptoms.
4. Consider hyperbaric therapy for moderate AMS if descent is not possible.
5. Pharmacologic therapy for moderate AMS includes **acetazolamide** 125 to 250 mg in adults and 2.5 mg/kg in children, PO twice daily, until

symptoms resolve and **dexamethasone** 4 mg PO, IM, or IV every 6 hours with a taper over several days.

a. Indications for acetazolamide are (a) history of altitude illness, (b) abrupt ascent higher than 3000 m (9840 ft), (c) AMS, and (d) symptomatic periodic breathing during sleep at high altitude.
b. Acetazolamide pharmacologically produces an acclimatization response by inducing a bicarbonate diuresis and metabolic acidosis. Acetazolamide is effective for both prophylaxis and treatment.
c. Acetazolamide should be avoided in sulfa-allergic patients.

6. Patients who respond well to treatment may be discharged. Provide counseling on preventing future episodes: graded ascent, prophylaxis using acetazolamide, and avoidance of overexertion, alcohol, and respiratory depressants. Begin prophylaxis with acetazolamide a day before ascent and continue for at least two days after reaching high altitude.

HIGH-ALTITUDE PULMONARY EDEMA

Risk factors for high-altitude pulmonary edema (HAPE) include rapid ascent, heavy exertion, cold, pulmonary hypertension, and use of a sleep medication. Children with acute respiratory infections may be more susceptible to HAPE. HAPE may be fatal if not recognized and treated early.

Clinical Features

HAPE usually begins on the second to fourth night at a new altitude and may progress quickly from dry cough and impaired exercise capacity to resting dyspnea, productive cough, severe weakness, and cyanosis. Physical examination findings include tachycardia, tachypnea, localized or generalized rales, and signs of pulmonary hypertension, such as a prominent P_2 and right ventricular heave. Resting SaO_2 is low for altitude and drops significantly with exertion. CXR abnormalities progress from interstitial to localized to generalized alveolar infiltrates. Right axis deviation and a right ventricular strain pattern are seen on EKG with progressive disease.

Diagnosis and Differential

The differential diagnosis includes pneumonia, acute asthma, congestive heart failure, myocardial ischemia, and pulmonary embolism. Decreased exercise performance and dry cough are enough to suspect early HAPE. A key to diagnosis is response to treatment.

Emergency Department Care and Disposition

Early recognition of HAPE is essential to prevent progression. General measures include rest and keeping patients warm.

1. Initiate supplemental **oxygen** and titrate to $SaO_2 \geq 90\%$.
2. **Immediate descent** is the treatment of choice. Exertion by the patient must be minimized during descent. Hyperbaric treatment may be used if descent is not an option. Patients with very mild cases of HAPE may be managed with bed rest and oxygen alone.

3. Pharmacologic treatment is usually unnecessary if descent and oxygen are available. In such cases (field conditions), options include **nifedipine** 20 to 30 mg extended release PO every 12 hours, or **tadalafil** 10 mg PO twice daily. Tadalafil blunts hypoxic pulmonary vasoconstriction. Nifedipine or tadalafil may also be used for HAPE prophylaxis in persons with prior episodes. Inhaled **albuterol** 2 to 4 puffs every 4 to 6 hours may be used for both prophylaxis and treatment but is not well studied.
4. Patients may be discharged if clinical and radiographic improvements are noted and room air SaO_2 remains >90%.

HIGH-ALTITUDE CEREBRAL EDEMA

Clinical Features

High-altitude cerebral edema (HACE) is defined as progressive neurologic deterioration with AMS or HAPE. Patients present with altered mental status, ataxia, stupor, and progress to coma if untreated. Focal neurologic signs such as third and sixth cranial nerve palsies may be present.

Diagnosis and Differential

The differential diagnosis includes stroke or transient ischemic attack, tumor, meningitis, encephalitis, or metabolic disturbance. Increased T2 signaling in the splenium of the corpus callosum is seen on MRI. Laboratory testing to rule out other diagnoses may be considered but should not delay treatment.

Emergency Department Care and Disposition

1. Initiate supplemental oxygen and titrate to $SaO_2 \geq 90\%$. Comatose patients require intubation and ventilation.
2. **Immediate descent** is needed. Initiate hyperbaric therapy if descent is not possible.
3. Administer **dexamethasone** 8 mg PO, IM or IV, followed by 4 mg PO, IM or IV every 6 hours.
4. In intubated patients, monitor arterial blood gases, taking care to avoid lowering $PaCO_2$ below 30 mmHg. Monitor intracranial pressures and cerebral blood velocities by transcranial Doppler US, if possible.
5. Patients remaining ataxic or confused after descent require admission.

FURTHER READING

For further reading in *Tintinalli's Emergency Medicine: A Comprehensive Study Guide*, 8th ed., see Chapter 221, "High-Altitude Disorders," by Peter H. Hackett and Christopher B. Davis.

CHAPTER 123

Dysbarism and Complications of Diving

Christian A. Tomaszewski

Dysbarism is commonly encountered in scuba divers and refers to complications associated with changes in environmental ambient pressure and with breathing compressed gases. These effects are governed by three gas laws: Boyle's law states that pressure and volume are inversely related; Henry's law states that, at equilibrium, the quantity of gas in solution is proportional to the partial pressure of that gas; Dalton's law states that total pressure exerted by a mixture of gases is the sum of the partial pressures of each gas.

CLINICAL FEATURES

Barotrauma is the most common diving-related affliction and is caused by the direct mechanical effects of pressure, as gas-filled cavities in the body contract or expand with pressure changes. The most common form of barotrauma occurs during descent and is middle ear squeeze, or barotitis media. It is caused by inability to equalize pressure causing tympanic membrane bleeding or rupture and may result in conductive hearing loss. A forceful Valsalva during equalization can cause inner ear barotrauma with rupture of the round or oval window. Symptoms include tinnitus, sensorineural hearing loss, and vertigo. If the sinus ostia are occluded on descent, an impending squeeze can cause bleeding from the maxillary or frontal sinuses, resulting in pain and epistaxis.

Barotrauma during ascent is due to expansion of gas in body cavities. In the middle ear, the pressure differential from asymmetrical expansion can cause alternobaric vertigo. Although rare, "reverse squeeze" may affect the ear or sinuses during ascent with rupture. Pulmonary overinflation and even burst lung can occur during rapid, panicked ascents if divers fail to exhale or if intrinsic pulmonary air trapping exists (e.g., COPD) resulting in pneumomediastinum, subcutaneous emphysema, or pneumothorax. The most serious consequence is cerebral arterial gas embolism (CAGE). Neurologic symptoms occur on ascent or immediately upon surfacing and include loss of consciousness, seizure, blindness, disorientation, hemiplegia, or other signs of stroke.

Divers using compressed air, caisson (tunnel) workers, and high-altitude pilots can all present with decompression sickness (DCS). In divers, this usually results from exceeding the dive table limits for depth and time. DCS can occur within minutes to hours of surfacing, rarely days later. Excessive bubble formation in tissue or circulation from saturated gas can cause both acute occlusive and delayed inflammatory effects. Type I DCS, "pain-only," includes mottled skin and deep pain of the joints, usually the shoulder or knee, and is unaffected by movement. Type II, "serious," DCS involves the central nervous system, typically the spine. Patients may initially complain of truncal constriction with ascending paralysis. Prolonged exposure at depth can lead to cardiopulmonary "chokes" with cough and hemoptysis or vestibular "staggers" with vertigo and hearing loss. Because DCS and

CAGE can be difficult to distinguish, or present simultaneously, the term "decompression illness" is now typically used for both.

DIAGNOSIS AND DIFFERENTIAL

Dive profile (depth, duration, and repetitiveness) and time of symptom onset are the most useful historical factors in distinguishing dysbarism from other disorders. During descent, the most common maladies are the squeezes. A fistula test, insufflation of the tympanic membrane on the affected side causing the eyes to deviate to the contralateral side, may help diagnose inner ear barotrauma. During ascent, barotrauma or alternobaric vertigo is most likely to occur. A chest x-ray may reveal pneumomediastinum, pneumothorax or subcutaneous air after pulmonary overinflation. If accompanied by early neurological symptoms, CAGE should be considered. Laboratory testing may reveal elevated hematocrit from hemoconcentration or elevated creatine phosphokinase from circulatory distribution of bubbles.

The differential diagnosis for DCS is broad. Musculoskeletal complaints could be due to joint strain or symptomatic herniated cervical disk. Chest pain may represent cardiac ischemia from overexertion. Immersion pulmonary edema from noncardiogenic causes can occur during strenuous dives, particularly in cold water. Seizures at depth can result from breathing enriched mixtures of oxygen exceeding 1.4 atmospheres absolute. Regardless, DCS should be suspected in patients with vague pain or neurological symptoms especially if safe diving limits, depth and time, were exceeded. If DCS is suspected, an early trial of pressure with hyperbaric oxygen usually results in some improvement.

EMERGENCY DEPARTMENT CARE AND DISPOSITION

1. **Decompression Illness (DCS/CAGE):**
   a. Administer **100% oxygen** and **IV fluids**.
   b. If CAGE is suspected, place the patient in the supine position; place in the left lateral decubitus position if vomiting occurs.
   c. Rapidly arrange for **recompression therapy with hyperbaric oxygen**. Divers Alert Network (1-919-684-9111) may help provide chamber locations.
   d. **Lidocaine** 1 mg/kg IV bolus followed by a continuous infusion at 1 mg/min may provide neuroprotection in CAGE.
2. Treat middle ear barotitis with **decongestants** and **analgesics**. Consider antibiotics if infection is suspected. Advise patients against diving until healing is completed. Inner ear barotrauma requires bed rest with the head upright until otolaryngologic evaluation for possible surgical exploration.
3. Pulmonary overinflation with ascent may require **needle decompression** or **tube thoracostomy** acutely if a pneumothorax develops.

FURTHER READING

For further reading in *Tintinalli's Emergency Medicine: A Comprehensive Study Guide*, 8th ed., see Chapter 214, "Diving Disorders," by Brain Snyder and Tom Neuman.

CHAPTER 124

Near Drowning

Richard A. Walker

Drowning is submersion in a liquid resulting in respiratory distress or failure. Prognosis after submersion injuries depends on the degree of pulmonary and central nervous system injury and, therefore, is highly dependent on early rescue and resuscitation. Prevention is the most important means to reduce associated morbidity and mortality.

CLINICAL FEATURES

Up to 20% of patients who suffer submersion injuries do not aspirate water, but sustain injury due to asphyxia. Patients who aspirate water into their lungs have washout of surfactant, resulting in diminished alveolar gas transfer, atelectasis, ventilation perfusion mismatch, and hypoxia. Noncardiogenic pulmonary edema results from moderate to severe aspiration. Physical examination findings at presentation vary. Lungs may be clear or have rales, rhonchi, or wheezes. Mental status ranges from normal to comatose. Patients are at risk for hypothermia even in "warm water" submersions.

DIAGNOSIS AND DIFFERENTIAL

Evaluate patients for associated injuries (e.g., traumatic injuries to the brain or spinal cord) and underlying precipitating disorders including syncope, seizures, hypoglycemia, and acute myocardial infarction or dysrhythmias. Respiratory acidosis may be present early followed by metabolic acidosis later. Early electrolyte disturbances are unusual. A chest radiograph (CXR) is usually obtained but is frequently normal in patients who are otherwise asymptomatic. Without a history of diving or associated trauma, routine cervical immobilization and computerized tomography (CT) of the brain are not necessary.

EMERGENCY DEPARTMENT CARE AND DISPOSITION

1. Treatment for submersion events is summarized in Figure 124-1.
2. Measure core temperature. Treat hypothermia if present. (See Chapter 118, "Frostbite and Hypothermia.") Hypothermic victims of cold-water submersion with cardiac arrest should undergo prolonged and aggressive resuscitation maneuvers until they are normothermic or considered not viable.
3. Data do not support routine antibiotic prophylaxis for pulmonary aspiration.
4. Efforts at "brain resuscitation," including the use of mannitol, loop diuretics, hypertonic saline, fluid restriction, mechanical hyperventilation, controlled hypothermia, barbiturate coma, and intracranial pressure monitoring, have not shown benefit.

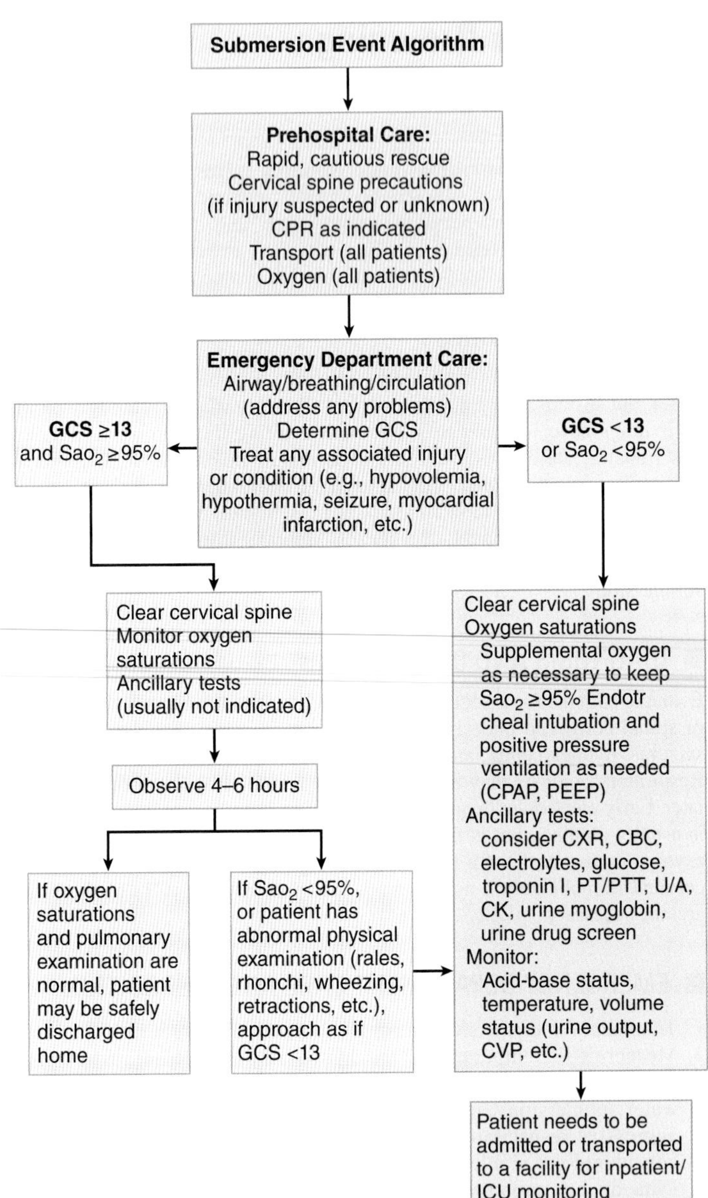

FIGURE 124-1. Drowning event algorithm. CBC = complete blood count; CK = creatine kinase; CPAP = continuous positive airway pressure; CVP = central venous pressure; CXR = chest radiograph; GCS = Glasgow Coma Scale; ICU = intensive care unit; PEEP = positive end-expiratory pressure; PT = prothrombin time; PTT = partial thromboplastin time; Sao_2 = oxygen saturation (via pulse oximetry); U/A = urinalysis.

5. Patients who arrive in the emergency department in asystole or cardiac arrest after warm water submersion and are normothermic have a poor prognosis for recovery without significant neurologic handicaps.

FURTHER READING

For further reading in *Tintinalli's Emergency Medicine: A Comprehensive Study Guide*, 8th ed., see Chapter 215, "Drowning," by Stephen John Cico and Linda Quan.

CHAPTER 125

Thermal and Chemical Burns

Sandra L. Werner

THERMAL BURNS

The majority of burn patients are treated and released from the ED. Of those hospitalized, more than 60% are admitted to one of the country's 127 burn centers. The risk of death from a major burn is associated with larger burn size, advanced age, concomitant inhalation injury, and female sex.

Clinical Features

Burns are categorized by their size and depth. Burn size is calculated as the percentage of body surface area (BSA) involved. The most common method to estimate this is the Rule of Nines (Fig. 125-1). A more accurate tool, especially in infants and children, is the Lund and Browder burn diagram (Fig. 125-2). For smaller burns, the patient's hand can be used to estimate the size of the burn. The area of the back of the patient's hand represents approximately 1% of BSA, and the number of "hands" represents the BSA burned.

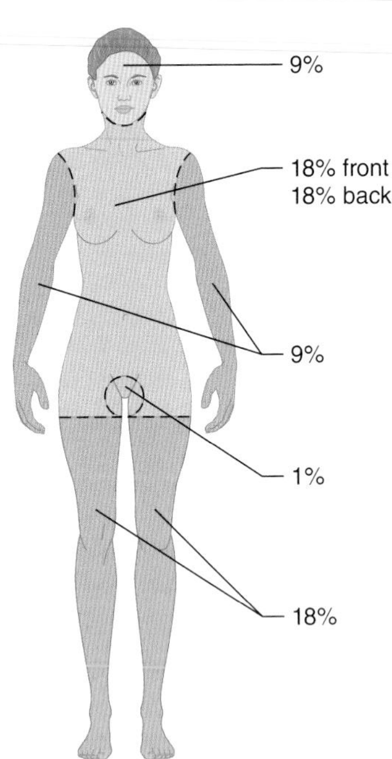

FIGURE 125-1. Rule of Nines to estimate the percentage of burn.

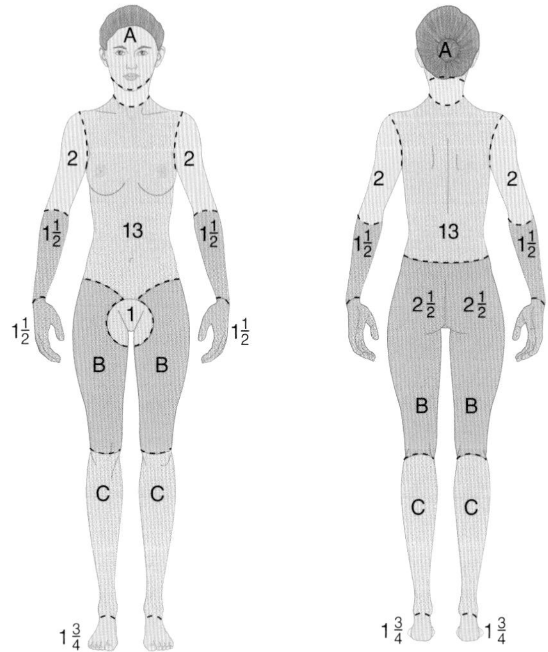

Relative percentages of areas affected by growth (age in years)

	0	**1**	**5**	**10**	**15**	**Adult**
A: half of head	$9\frac{1}{2}$	$8\frac{1}{2}$	$6\frac{1}{2}$	$5\frac{1}{2}$	$4\frac{1}{2}$	$3\frac{1}{2}$
B: half of thigh	$2\frac{3}{4}$	$3\frac{1}{4}$	4	$4\frac{1}{4}$	$4\frac{1}{2}$	$4\frac{3}{4}$
C: half of leg	$2\frac{1}{2}$	$2\frac{1}{2}$	$2\frac{3}{4}$	3	$3\frac{1}{4}$	$3\frac{1}{2}$

Second-degree ____________________ and

Third-degree ____________________ =

Total percent burned ________

FIGURE 125-2. Lund and Browder diagram to estimate the percentage of a burn.

Burn depth historically has been described in degrees: first, second, third, and fourth. A more clinically relevant classification scheme categorizes burns as superficial partial thickness, deep partial thickness, and full thickness. Table 125-1 summarizes the characteristics of each type of burn.

Inhalation injury occurs most frequently in closed-space fires and in patients with decreased cognition (intoxication, overdose, head injury). Both the upper and lower airway can be injured by heat, particulate matter, and toxic gases. Thermal injury is usually limited to the upper airway, and can result in acute airway compromise. Particulate matter can reach

TABLE 125-1 Burn Depth Features Classified by Degree of Burn

Burn Depth	Histology/Anatomy	Example	Healing
Superficial (first degree)	Epidermis No blisters, painful	Sunburn	7 days
Superficial partial-thickness (superficial second degree)	Epidermis and superficial dermis Blisters, very painful	Hot water scald	14–21 days, no scar
Deep partial-thickness (deep second degree)	Epidermis and deep dermis, sweat glands, and hair follicles Blisters, very painful	Hot liquid, steam, grease, flame	3–8 weeks, permanent scar
Full-thickness (third degree)	Entire epidermis and dermis charred, pale, leathery; no pain	Flame	Months, severe scarring, skin grafts necessary
Fourth degree	Entire epidermis and dermis, as well as bone, fat, and/or muscle	Flame	Months, multiple surgeries usually required

the terminal bronchioles and lead to bronchospasm and edema. Clinical indicators of inhalation injury include facial burns, singed nasal hair, soot in the upper airway, hoarseness, carbonaceous sputum, and wheezing. Carbon monoxide poisoning should be suspected in all patients with inhalation injuries. Hydrogen cyanide poisoning should be considered in fires involving nitrogen-containing polymer products such as wool, silk, polyurethane, and vinyl.

Diagnosis and Differential

The American Burn Association (ABA) classifies burns into major, moderate, and minor. Table 125-2 summarizes the ABA burn classifications.

TABLE 125-2 Burn Depth Features: American Burn Association Burn Classification

Burn Classification	Burn Characteristics	Disposition
Major burn	Partial-thickness >25% BSA, age 10–50 years Partial-thickness >20% BSA, age <10 years or >50 years Full-thickness >10% BSA in anyone Burns involving hands, face, feet, or perineum Burns crossing major joints Circumferential burns of an extremity Burns complicated by inhalation injury Electrical burns Burns complicated by fracture or other trauma Burns in high-risk patients	Burn center treatment

(continued)

TABLE 125-2 Burn Depth Features: American Burn Association Burn Classification (continued)

Burn Classification	Burn Characteristics	Disposition
Moderate burn	Partial-thickness 15–25% BSA, age 10–50 years Partial-thickness 10–20% BSA, age <10 years or >50 years Full-thickness burns ≤10% BSA in anyone No major burn characteristics present	Hospitalization
Minor burn	Partial-thickness <15% BSA, age 10–50 years Partial-thickness <10% BSA, age <10 years or >50 years Full-thickness <2% in anyone No major burn characteristics present	Outpatient treatment

Abbreviation: BSA, body surface area.

Emergency Department Care and Disposition

Management of patients with *moderate to major* burns is divided into three phases: prehospital care, ED resuscitation and stabilization, and transfer to a burn center. Prehospital burn care consists of stopping the burning process, establishing an airway, initiating fluid resuscitation, relieving pain and protecting the burn wound.

1. In the ED, reevaluate the airway, administer **100% O_2**, and intubate and ventilate the patient if there are signs of airway compromise, an airway burn, or respiratory distress. Obtain an ABG, carboxyhemoglobin level, and CXR. Monitor vital signs and oxygen saturation.
2. Establish 2 IV lines in unburned areas. Use a burn formula, such as the Parkland/Baxter formula, to guide initial **fluid resuscitation** (Table 125-3). Ongoing fluid resuscitation is further guided by vital signs, cerebral and peripheral perfusion, and adequate urine output.
3. Evaluate and treat traumatic injuries using standard trauma resuscitation guidelines (Chapter 156, "Trauma in Adults"; Chapter 157, "Trauma in Children"; Chapter 158, "Trauma in the Elderly").

TABLE 125-3 Parkland Formula for Fluid Resuscitation

Adults
LR 4 mL × weight (kg) × % BSA burned* over initial 24 h Half over the first 8 h from the time of burn Other half over the subsequent 16 h Example: 70-kg adult with 40% second- and third-degree burns: 4 mL × 70 kg × 40 = 11,200 mL over 24 h
Children
LR 3 mL × weight (kg) × % BSA burned* over initial 24 h plus maintenance Half over the first 8 h from the time of burn Other half over the subsequent 16 h

*Partial- and full-thickness burns only.

Abbreviations: BSA, body surface area; LR, lactated Ringer's solution.

4. After initiating resuscitative measures, address burn wound care. Apply cool compresses to small burns. Cover large burns with sterile dry sheets as saline soaked dressings may induce hypothermia. Administration of empiric antibiotics and application of topical antimicrobials during resuscitation are not recommended.
5. Administer intravenous opioid analgesia early and titrate to pain.
6. Treat inhalation injuries with humidified oxygen, endotracheal intubation and mechanical ventilation, bronchodilators, and pulmonary toilet. **Hyperbaric oxygen therapy** is used for severe carbon monoxide poisoning.
7. Circumferential burns of the neck, chest, or limbs may compromise breathing and circulation. **Escharotomy** may be required.
8. Update tetanus prophylaxis, if needed.
9. Hospitalize patients with moderate and major burns. The ABA's criteria for referral to a burn unit are listed in Table 125-4.
10. Table 125-5 summarizes the care of minor burns. Patients with minor burns may be discharged after ED treatment, provided close follow-up is available.

CHEMICAL BURNS

More than 25,000 products are capable of producing chemical burns. Chemical burn injuries represent a smaller percentage of burn injuries but account for 30% of burn deaths.

TABLE 125-4 American Burn Association Burn Unit Referral Criteria
Full-thickness/third-degree burns in any age group
Electrical burns, including lightning injury
Chemical burns
Inhalation injury
Burn injury in patients with preexisting medical disorders that could complicate management, prolong recovery, or affect mortality
Burn injury in any patients with concomitant trauma (such as fractures) in whom the burn injury poses the greatest risk of morbidity or mortality
Burn injury in children in hospitals without qualified personnel or equipment to care for children
Burn injury in patients who will require special social, emotional, or long-term rehabilitative intervention
Burn injury in children <10 years and adults >50 years of age

TABLE 125-5 ED Care of Minor Burns
Provide appropriate analgesics before burn care and for outpatient use
Cleanse burn with mild soap and water or dilute antiseptic solution
Debride wound as needed
Apply topical antimicrobial:
1% silver sulfadiazine cream (not on the face or in patients with a sulfa allergy)
Bacitracin ointment
Triple-antibiotic ointment (neomycin, polymyxin B, bacitracin zinc)
Consider use of synthetic occlusive dressings
Provide detailed burn care instructions with follow-up in 24–48 h

Clinical Features

Clinical features depend on the type of agent, concentration, volume, duration of exposure, and extent of penetration. Alkalis usually produce more damage than acids. Acids typically cause coagulation necrosis, which produces an eschar that limits further damage. Alkalis produce liquefaction necrosis, allowing deeper damage to occur. Hydrofluoric (HF) acid is a special case as it rapidly penetrates intact skin and can cause progressive pain and deep tissue destruction without obvious superficial tissue damage. Systemic toxicity, including hypotension, acidosis, and shock, may occur if certain chemicals are absorbed.

Chemical burns of the eye are true ocular emergencies. Acid ocular burns quickly precipitate proteins in the superficial eye structures resulting in a "ground glass" appearance of the cornea. Alkali ocular burns are more severe due to deeper ongoing penetration. Lacrimators (tear gas and pepper mace) cause ocular, mucous membrane, and pulmonary irritation.

Diagnosis and Differential

The diagnosis of chemical burn usually is made by history of exposure to a chemical agent. Chemical topical exposures should be considered in all cases of skin irritation and/or pain. For ocular exposures, pH paper can distinguish alkali from acid exposure.

Emergency Department Care and Disposition

1. The first priority in the treatment of chemical burns is to terminate the burning process. Remove garments. Brush off dry chemical particles. **Immediately irrigate the skin copiously with water**. Cover elemental metals (sodium, lithium, calcium, and magnesium) with **mineral oil** because exposure to water may cause a severe exothermic reaction.
2. For ocular burns, begin irrigation of each involved eye with 1 to 2 L of normal saline. In patients with acid or alkali burns, continue irrigation until the pH is normal. Patients with alkali burns may require prolonged irrigation. *Visual acuity check and pH testing should follow, not precede, initial ocular irrigation.* Consult with an ophthalmologist.
3. Treatment for specific chemical burns is provided in Table 125-6. Options for treating cutaneous HF acid burns are provided in Table 125-7.

TABLE 125-6 Treatment of Select Chemical Burns

Chemical	Treatment	Comments
Acids		
All acid burns require prompt decontamination and copious irrigation with water		
Acetic acid	Copious irrigation	Consider systemic antibiotics for extensive scalp burns
Phenol (carbolic acid)	Copious irrigation Sponge with undiluted polyethylene glycol 200–400	Isopropyl alcohol may also be used
Chromic acid	Copious irrigation	Observe for systemic toxicity

(continued)

TABLE 125-6 Treatment of Select Chemical Burns (continued)		
Chemical	Treatment	Comments
Formic acid	Copious irrigation	Dialysis may be needed for severe toxicity
Hydrofluoric acid	Copious irrigation	Consider intradermal injection of 10% calcium gluconate or intraarterial calcium gluconate for severe cases
	10% calcium gluconate intradermal	Monitor serum calcium and magnesium in severe exposure
	Topical calcium gluconate gel	25 mL of 10% calcium gluconate in 75 mL of sterile water-soluble lubricant (K-Y jelly or US jelly)
Nitric acid	Copious irrigation	Consult with burn specialist
Oxalic acid	Copious irrigation IV calcium may be required	Evaluate serum electrolytes and renal function Cardiac monitoring for serious dermal exposure
Alkalis		
All alkali burns require prompt decontamination and copious, prolonged irrigation with water		
Portland cement	Prolonged copious irrigation	May need to remove cement particles with a brush, such as a preoperative scrubbing brush
Elemental Metals		
Water is generally contraindicated in extinguishing burning metal fragments embedded in the skin		
Elemental metals (sodium, lithium, potassium, magnesium, aluminum, and calcium)	Cover metal fragments with sand, foam from a class D fire extinguisher, or mineral oil Excise metal fragments that cannot be wiped away	
Hydrocarbons		
Gasoline	Decontamination	
Tar	Cool before removal Remove using antibiotic ointment containing polyoxylene sorbitan (polysorbate)	Baby oil can be used
Vesicants		
Mustards	Decontaminate Copious irrigation	If limited water supply, adsorbent powders (flour, talcum powder, fuller's earth) can be applied to the mustard and then wiped away with a moist towel
Reducing Agents		
Alkyl mercury compounds	Copious irrigation Debride, drain, and copiously irrigate blisters	Blister fluid is high in metallic mercury content

(*continued*)

TABLE 125-6 Treatment of Select Chemical Burns (continued)

Chemical	Treatment	Comments
Lacrimators		
Tear gas	Copious irrigation	May cause respiratory symptoms if inhaled
Pepper spray	Copious irrigation	May cause respiratory symptoms if inhaled
Miscellaneous		
White phosphorus	Remove clothing Copious irrigation, keep exposed skin areas wet or submerged until all particles have been removed due to risk of ignition when exposed to air Debride visible particles	Systemic toxicity is a significant concern
Airbag	Prolonged copious irrigation	

TABLE 125-7 Options for Treatment of Hydrofluoric Acid Skin Burns

1. Copious irrigation for 15–30 min immediately.
2. Application of calcium gluconate gel, 25 mL of 10% calcium gluconate in 75 mL of water-soluble lubricant.
3. Further treatment options as dictated by patient response:
   a. Dermal injection of 10% calcium gluconate at the rate of 0.5 mL/cm^2 of skin surface using a small-gauge needle.
   b. Arterial infusion over 4 h (40 mL of 5% dextrose in water with 10 mL of 10% calcium gluconate).
   c. Consider supplemental magnesium and calcium IV.

Consult with a plastic surgeon for patients with HF acid burns of the hands, feet, digits, or nails.

4. After initial decontamination measures, initiate IV fluid resuscitation, analgesia, tetanus prophylaxis, and address systemic toxicity, as needed.

FURTHER READING

For further reading in *Tintinalli's Emergency Medicine: A Comprehensive Study Guide*, 8th ed., see Chapter 216, "Thermal Burns," by E. Paul DeKoning; Chapter 217, "Chemical Burns," by Anthony F. Pizon and Michael J. Lynch.

CHAPTER 126

Electrical and Lightning Injuries

Norberto Navarrete

ELECTRICAL INJURIES

Electrical injuries occur with a wide spectrum of damage, from superficial skin burns to multisystem injury. Electrical injuries are arbitrarily classified as those of low voltage ($\leq$1000 V) and high voltage ($>$1000 V).

Clinical Features

Electricity-induced injuries can occur via several mechanisms: (1) direct tissue damage from the electrical energy, (2) tissue damage from thermal energy, and (3) mechanical injury from trauma induced by a fall or muscle contraction. Patients may sustain immediate cardiac dysrthymias including ventricular fibrillation, respiratory arrest, or seizures. Cardiac complications are more commonly seen in high-voltage injuries. Temporary loss of consciousness is common. Severe burns may result from contact with high-voltage lines. The size of the skin injury does not correlate well with internal injuries. Traumatic injuries frequently accompany electrical injuries. The details of specific immediate and delayed systemic injuries and complications are summarized in Table 126-1.

TABLE 126-1	Immediate and Delayed Complications of Electrical Injuries
Cardiovascular	Sudden death (ventricular fibrillation, asystole), chest pain, dysrhythmias, ST-T segment abnormalities, bundle branch block, myocardial damage, myocardial infarction (rare), hypotension (volume depletion), hypertension (catecholamine release)
Neurologic	Altered mental status, agitation, coma, seizures, cerebral edema, hypoxic encephalopathy, headache, aphasia, weakness, paraplegia, quadriplegia, spinal cord dysfunction (may be delayed), peripheral neuropathy, cognitive impairment, insomnia, emotional lability
Cutaneous	Electrothermal contact injuries, noncontact arc and "flash" burns, secondary thermal burns (clothing ignition, heating of metal)
Vascular	Thrombosis, coagulation necrosis, disseminated intravascular coagulation, delayed vessel rupture, aneurysm, compartment syndrome
Pulmonary	Respiratory arrest (central or peripheral, e.g., muscular tetany), aspiration pneumonia, pulmonary edema, pulmonary contusion, inhalation injury
Renal/metabolic	Acute renal failure (due to heme pigment deposition and hypovolemia), myoglobinuria, metabolic (lactic) acidosis, hypokalemia, hypocalcemia, hyperglycemia
Gastrointestinal	Perforation, stress ulcer (Curling ulcer), GI bleeding, GI tract dysfunction, various reports of lethal injuries at autopsy
Muscular	Myonecrosis, compartment syndrome

(Continued)

TABLE 126-1	Immediate and Delayed Complications of Electrical Injuries (Continued)
Skeletal	Vertebral compression fractures, long bone fractures, shoulder dislocations (anterior and posterior), scapular fractures
Ophthalmologic	Corneal burns, delayed cataracts, intraocular hemorrhage or thrombosis, uveitis, retinal detachment, orbital fracture
Auditory	Hearing loss, tinnitus, tympanic membrane perforation (rare), delayed mastoiditis or meningitis
Oral burns	Delayed labial artery hemorrhage, scarring and facial deformity, delayed speech development, impaired mandibular/dentition development
Obstetric	Spontaneous abortion, fetal death

Abbreviation: GI, gastrointestinal.

Diagnosis and Differential

The diagnosis of electrical injury is usually based on the history of contact with an electrical source and the typical skin or oral lesions in children. However, patients with amnesia or any other type of altered mental status, with no skin injuries, must undergo an interview and a more detailed physical examination, especially for possible thunderstorm incidents. Laboratory and radiographic evaluation of high-voltage injures should follow standard trauma guidelines. Atrial or ventricular arrhythmias, bradyarrthymias, prolonged QT intervals or ST-T wave abnormalities may be noted on the ECG. An elevated serum CK, myoglobin or urine myoglobin suggests extensive muscle injury and rhabdomyolysis. Assessment and treatment of complications associated with electrical injuries are summarized in Table 126-2.

TABLE 126-2	Assessment and Treatment of Complications of Electrical Injuries
Circulatory	Order cardiac monitoring and ECG. Assess indications for admission for cardiac monitoring.
Renal	Initiate fluid resuscitation and monitor urine output with a Foley catheter.
Nervous system	Order head CT as needed for altered mental status; assess for spinal cord and peripheral nerve injury.
Skin	Assess and treat cutaneous burns.*
Musculoskeletal	Perform a careful assessment of spine, pelvis, long bones, and joints. Assess for compartment syndrome and need for fasciotomy.†
Vascular	Spasm may occur leading to delayed thrombosis, aneurysm formation, or muscle damage.
Coagulation	Treat coagulation disorders by eliminating the precipitating factor through early surgical debridement. If hemorrhage is present, replace coagulation factors.
Lungs	Assess for inhalation injury, carbon monoxide, alveolar injury from blast.
Eyes	Document complete eye examination. Delayed cataracts may develop.

(Continued)

TABLE 126-2	Assessment and Treatment of Complications of Electrical Injuries (Continued)
Ears	Assess for blast injury. Document hearing. Middle and inner ear disorders and hearing loss may occur.
GI	Intra-abdominal injury may occur from current or blast.
Lips and oral cavity	Watch for delayed bleeding.

*Refer to Chapter 125, "Thermal and Chemical Burns."

†Refer to Chapter 51, "Rhabdomyolysis."

The differential diagnosis includes other causes of arrhythmias, such as myocardial ischemia and neurologic dysfunction, such as stroke, closed head injury, and spinal cord injury.

Emergency Department Care and Disposition

1. Victims should be treated as blunt multiple trauma patients with attention to advanced life-support protocols and cervical and spine immobilization.
2. Assess and stabilize the airway. In facial burns due to electric flash, burn injury of the airway is not common, and the need to control the airway even less so. Provide high-flow oxygen and monitor with pulse oximetry.
3. Treat ventricular fibrillation, asystole, or ventricular tachycardia using standard ACLS protocols. Other dysrhythmias are usually transient and do not need immediate therapy.
4. Seizures occur immediately after the electric shock. A new seizure requires standard therapy and it is necessary to consider focal cerebral injury.
5. In compartment syndrome, consultation with a general surgeon, trauma surgeon, or burn surgeon must be requested in a priority manner.
6. Monitor for hyperkalemia, rhabdomyolysis, and the potential to develop acute kidney injury. Monitor urine output with a Foley catheter. Initiate crystalloid resuscitation in patients with large burns or extensively damaged muscle. The usual fluid replacement formulas used for burn patients often underestimate fluid requirements. In severe rhabdomyolysis or myoglobinuria, use aggressive fluid rehydration aiming for a urine output of 2 mL/kg/h and continuing until the serum creatine kinase level is less than five times normal or urine myoglobin measurements return to normal.
7. Burns need to be covered with dry sterile dressings. Prophylactic systemic antibiotics are usually not necessary unless there are large open contaminated wounds.
8. Administer tetanus prophylaxis, if not up to date.
9. Provide pain control with opioids.
10. Reduce and immobilize fractures and dislocations.
11. For pregnant patients, consult an obstetrician for fetal monitoring and admission.
12. Patients with more than a minor low-voltage injury should be admitted for further monitoring (Table 126-3).

TABLE 126-3 Indications for Admission for Patients with Electrical Injuries
High voltage >600 V
Symptoms suggestive of systemic injury
Cardiovascular: chest pain, palpitations
Neurologic: loss of consciousness, confusion, weakness, headache, paresthesias
Respiratory: dyspnea
Gastrointestinal: abdominal pain, vomiting
Evidence of neurologic or vascular injury to a digit or extremity
Burns with evidence of subcutaneous tissue damage
Dysrhythmia or abnormal electrocardiogram
Suspected foul play, abuse, suicidal intent, or unreliable social situation
Pregnancy
Associated injuries requiring admission
Comorbid diseases (cardiac, renal, neurologic)

13. Children with isolated oral injuries or isolated hand wounds can usually be discharged home after consultation with an ENT specialist or plastic surgeon. Provide parents with instructions for controlling delayed labial artery bleeding. Arrange close follow-up with the consulting surgeon to assess scarring and stricture.
14. Asymptomatic patients who sustained a low-voltage injury (≤240 V) and have a normal ECG on presentation and normal physical exam may be discharged home.

INJURIES DUE TO ELECTRONIC CONTROL DEVICES

Electronic control devices, such as the cattle prod, stun gun, and the TASER®, deliver high-voltage, low-amperage electrical pulses that induce involuntary muscle contraction, neuromuscular incapacitation, and/or pain. The likelihood of electrical injury is minimal. Injuries are usually limited to superficial punctures, and minor lacerations and cutaneous burns. The majority of deaths that have followed the use of these devices have occurred in persons who were extremely ill and agitated due to psychosis, stimulant drugs, or other conditions. Ill-appearing and agitated patients should be evaluated and treated in the same way as all patients who may have sustained blunt trauma or who have ingested unknown substances. Cardiac monitoring and other testing are not needed just because a TASER® has been used.

LIGHTNING INJURIES

Lightning is a unidirectional extremely high-voltage current that causes substantially different injuries from those caused by high-voltage AC electricity. Lightning often travels over the skin, rather than through the body (*flashover*), which may explain why most people survive. However, a significant number may have permanent sequelae.

Clinical Features

Clinical events occur at multiple levels due to the electric effect, the high temperature generated, and mechanical effects due to the shock wave. The

TABLE 126-4 Complications Associated with Lightning Injuries

System	Injury
Cardiovascular	Dysrhythmias (asystole, ventricular fibrillation/tachycardia, premature ventricular contractions), electrocardiographic changes, myocardial infarction (unusual)
Neurologic	Immediate or delayed, permanent or transient; loss of consciousness, confusion, amnesia, intracranial hemorrhage, hemiplegia, amnesia, respiratory center paralysis, cerebral edema, neuritis, seizures, parkinsonian syndromes, cerebral infarction, myelopathy, progressive muscular atrophy, progressive cerebellar syndrome, transient paralysis, paresthesias, myelopathy, autonomic dysfunction
Cutaneous	Burns (first to third degree), scars, contractures
Ophthalmologic	Cataracts (often delayed), corneal lesions, uveitis, iridocyclitis, vitreous hemorrhage, macular degeneration, optic atrophy, diplopia, chorioretinitis, retinal detachment, hyphema
Otologic	Tympanic membrane rupture, temporary or permanent deafness, tinnitus, ataxia, vertigo, nystagmus
Renal	Myoglobinuria, hemoglobinuria, renal failure (rare)
Obstetric	Fetal death, placental abruption
Miscellaneous	Secondary blunt trauma, compartment syndrome, disseminated intravascular coagulation

most common immediate cause of death after lightning strike is primary or secondary hypoxic cardiac arrest due to respiratory arrest. In the patient with spontaneous circulation, hypertension and tachycardia are caused by sympathetic activation. Patients may experience temporary loss of consciousness, confusion, and amnesia. Feathering or fern-shaped burns on the skin are pathognomonic of lightning but are transient and rarely seen. Tympanic membrane rupture may occur by blast effect. Deep tissue injuries, myoglobinuria, and renal failure are uncommon. The details of specific immediate and delayed systemic injuries and complications are summarized in Table 126-4.

Diagnosis and Differential

The diagnosis of lightning injury is based on history and should be considered in any critically ill patient found outside during or after a thunderstorm. While increasingly rare, indoor exposures to lightning may occur via indoor pools, use of hard-wired telephones, or in poorly constructed structures. Carefully assess patients for neurologic and cardiovascular complications, otologic and ophthalmologic injuries, and blunt trauma. Burns are uncommon. Laboratory and radiographic evaluation of lightning injures should follow standard trauma guidelines. Differential diagnosis includes stroke or intracranial hemorrhage, seizure disorder, and cerebral, spinal cord, or other neurologic trauma.

Emergency Department Care and Disposition

1. Victims should be treated as blunt multiple trauma patients with attention to advanced life-support protocols and cervical and spine immobilization.

2. In the event of mass casualties, in contrast to standard triage, provide aggressive resuscitation in patients with respiratory and cardiac arrest due to lightning strike. Respiratory arrest may outlast initial cardiac arrest and adequate ventilation can prevent hypoxic injury until return of spontaneous circulation.
3. Treat arrhythmias using standard ACLS protocols.
4. Provide continuous monitoring of vital signs, heart rate and rhythm, and pulse oximetry. Provide high-flow oxygen and begin IV crystalloids.
5. Hypertension is frequent but transient and is not an indication for therapy. Hypotension is unexpected and should prompt investigation for hemorrhage.
6. Early seizures are probably due to early anoxia. Persistent seizures require standard therapy and it is necessary to consider focal cerebral injury.
7. Keraunoparalysis, transient weakness in limbs following a lightning strike, should be a diagnosis of exclusion. Always investigate for other possible causes of paresis secondary to blunt trauma. In pulseless extremities, fasciotomies are only indicated with high intracompartmental pressure.
8. In patients with burns and wounds, administer tetanus prophylaxis, if not up to date. Prophylactic antibiotics are not indicated unless there is contamination with organic material.
9. Admit patients with persistent musculoskeletal symptoms, neurologic, cardiac rhythm, or vascular abnormalities, or significant burns to a critical care unit. Consult with a general surgeon, trauma surgeon, or burn surgeon. All pregnant patients require obstetric consultation and referral for fetal monitoring.
10. Patients with minor injuries and a negative workup may be discharged with outpatient follow-up to assess delayed effects of lightning injury.

FURTHER READING

For further reading in *Tintinalli's Emergency Medicine: A Comprehensive Study Guide*, 8th ed., see Chapter 218, "Electrical and Lightning Injuries" by Caitlin Bailey

CHAPTER 127 Carbon Monoxide

Jon B. Cole

Carbon monoxide is a colorless, odorless, nonirritating gas that displaces oxygen from hemoglobin, resulting in early tissue hypoxia and delayed neurologic damage. Sources of exposure to carbon monoxide include the incomplete combustion of any carbonaceous fuel (e.g., gasoline, kerosene, natural gas, and charcoal) or the metabolism of inhaled methylene chloride (paint stripper).

CLINICAL FEATURES

A history of exposure to gas- or propane-powered motors or heaters, smoke inhalation, or multiple victims with altered mental status, acidosis, or coma should alert one to the possibility of carbon monoxide poisoning. The clinical features of carbon monoxide poisoning are highly variable and primarily relate to hypoxic effects on the cardiovascular and neurologic systems (Table 127-1). Symptoms range from "flu-like," such as headache, dizziness, nausea, and vomiting, to coma. The "classic finding" of cherry red lips is rarely seen in living patients. Patients with significant poisoning may experience long-term neurological and cognitive problems.

DIAGNOSIS AND DIFFERENTIAL

Blood cooximetry is the most reliable test to diagnose carbon monoxide poisoning. Although elevated carboxyhemoglobin (COHb) levels confirm exposure, they do not necessarily correlate with symptoms or prognosis. Baseline COHb may be as high as 5% in nonsmokers and 10% in smokers. Higher levels are suggestive of CO exposure. The use of bedside pulse cooximetry in the ED to screen for CO exposure is still under investigation.

TABLE 127-1 Signs and Symptoms of Acute Carbon Monoxide Poisoning
Headache
Visual disturbances
Vomiting
Confusion
Ataxia
Dyspnea/tachypnea
Seizure
Ischemic ECG changes and/or dysrhythmias
Syncope
Retinal hemorrhage
Chest pain
Bullous skin lesions
Focal neurologic deficit

Standard pulse oximetry is unreliable in the presence of increasing COHb as oxygen saturation readings will be artificially high or normal. Additional laboratory and imaging abnormalities seen in symptomatic patients may include elevated anion gap metabolic acidosis, elevated lactate, elevated creatine phosphokinase, elevated troponin, ECG changes consistent with ischemia, and bilateral globus pallidus lesions on brain imaging.

The differential diagnosis is wide due to the nonspecific nature of the symptoms and includes flu-like illness, gastroenteritis, exposure to other toxins, and infectious causes of mental status changes. Cardiovascular compromise after poisoning may represent a concomitant myocardial infarction.

EMERGENCY DEPARTMENT CARE AND DISPOSITION

Remove patients from the source of exposure and address airway, breathing, and circulation.

1. Begin treatment in all patients suspected of CO poisoning with the **highest concentration of supplemental oxygen** available (e.g., 100% oxygen via facemask with reservoir) and continue until the patient is asymptomatic. Provide continuous monitoring of vital signs, heart rate, and rhythm. Establish IV access.
2. Guidelines for **hyperbaric oxygen therapy** (HBO) in patients with severe poisoning are listed in Table 127-2. Indications for pediatric and adult HBO are similar. The threshold COHb for initiating HBO in pregnant patients is lower because of concerns for the fetus. Consult with a hyperbaric specialist. Patients must have a secure airway and stable hemodynamics before transport and treatment with HBO as access may be limited en route and in the hyperbaric chamber.
3. Guidelines for disposition are listed in Table 127-3. Ensure that the home or work environment is no longer a source of carbon monoxide exposure.

TABLE 127-2 Commonly Utilized Indications for Referral for Hyperbaric Oxygen Treatment

Syncope
Confusion/altered mental status
Seizure
Coma
Focal neurologic deficit
Pregnancy with carboxyhemoglobin >15%
Carboxyhemoglobin >25% in any patient
Evidence of acute myocardial ischemia

TABLE 127-3 Disposition Considerations

Symptom Severity	Disposition	Comments
Minimal or no symptoms	Home	Assess safety issues
Headache	Home after symptom resolution	Administer 100% oxygen in ED
Vomiting		Observe 4 h
Elevated carbon monoxide level		Assess safety issues
Ataxia, seizure, syncope, chest pain, focal neurologic deficit, dyspnea, ECG changes	Hospitalize	Administer 100% oxygen in ED
	Consult with hyperbaric specialist	Carbon monoxide level, comorbid conditions, including pregnancy, age, and stability of the patient must be considered if considering transfer for hyperbaric oxygen

FURTHER READING

For further reading in *Tintinalli's Emergency Medicine: A Comprehensive Study Guide*, 8th ed., see Chapter 222, "Carbon Monoxide," by Gerald Maloney.

CHAPTER 128 Mushroom and Plant Poisoning

Chulathida Chomchai

MUSHROOMS

Mushroom poisoning occurs in four population groups: foragers who purposefully harvest mushrooms or plants for food; teenagers and young adults who use mushrooms to get "high"; preschool-age children who accidentally ingest mushrooms while playing outdoors; and, rarely, victims of attempted homicide or suicide.

Clinical Features

Mushroom toxicity is divided into those with early onset, defined as within 2 hours after ingestion, and delayed onset, defined as 6 hours to 20 days after ingestion. It is important to determine if patients ingested only one type or multiple types of mushrooms and the time elapsed from ingestion to symptoms. Foragers may be able to provide a description of the mushroom. Clinical features of common mushroom poisonings are listed in Table 128-1.

Diagnosis and Differential

Most patients who develop GI symptoms within 2 hours of ingestion have a reassuring clinical course and do not develop major organ failure (Table 128-1). An exception to this is *Amanita smithiana* ingestion, which results in early GI symptoms and delayed renal failure. Mushrooms with potential liver, kidney, and CNS effects are often associated with onset of vomiting that is delayed for 6 or more hours after ingestion. Toxic species include species of genera *Amanita*, *Galerina*, *Gyromitra*, and *Lepiota*. Ingestions may be misdiagnosed as viral gastrointestinal illness or food poisoning if a history of mushroom ingestion is not pursued.

Emergency Department Care and Disposition

Consultation with a poison center is advised as regional differences in mushrooms types and toxicity exist.

1. Treatment regimens for mushroom poisonings are listed in Table 128-1.
2. Admit all patients with delayed onset of vomiting or diarrhea for ongoing monitoring of renal and liver function and fluid status for 48 hours.
3. Rapid progression to hepatic encephalopathy, hepatorenal syndrome, or coagulopathy are indications for liver transplantation. Consider transfer to a liver transplant center early in the course of mushroom ingestion.
4. Patients who ingest hallucinogenic mushrooms or mushrooms with muscarinic effects only may be discharged when symptoms subside.

TABLE 128-1 Mushrooms: Symptoms, Toxicity, and Treatment

Symptoms	Mushrooms	Toxicity	Treatment
Gastrointestinal symptoms			
Onset <2 h	*Chlorophyllum molybdites* *Omphalotus illudens* *Cantharellus cibarius*	Nausea, vomiting, diarrhea (occasional bloody)	IV hydration Antiemetics
Onset 6–24 h	*Amanita smithiana* (delayed renal failure) *Amanita phalloides,* *Amanita verna,* *Amanita virosa* *Lepiota* sp. (delayed liver failure) *Gyromitra esculenta (delayed onset seizures)*	Initial: nausea, vomiting, diarrhea Day 2: rise in AST, ALT Day 3: hepatic failure coagulopathy renal failure hemolysis As above + headache, tremor, ataxia, seizures	IV hydration; closely monitor electrolytes, glucose, renal, hepatic, and coagulation functions For *Amanita* and *Lepiota*: Acetylcysteine, load with 140 mg/kg PO/NG Penicillin G 300,000 to 1,000,000 U/kg IV per day Silymarin 5 mg/kg IV over 1 h, then 20 mg/kg IV per day (available PO in the United States) For *Gyromitra,* treat seizures with both benzodiazepines AND pyridoxine 5 g IV
Muscarinic (SLUDGE) syndrome Onset <30 min	*Inocybe* sp. *Clitocybe* sp.	Salivation, lacrimation, diarrhea, gastrointestinal distress, emesis	Supportive, atropine 0.01 mg/kg IV repeated as needed for severe secretions
CNS excitement Onset <30 min	*Amanita muscaria* *Amanita pantherina* *Amanita gemmata*	Intoxication, dizziness, ataxia, visual disturbances, seizures, tachycardia, hypertension, warm dry skin, dry mouth, mydriasis (anticholinergic effects)	Supportive, sedation with diazepam 2–5 mg IV as needed for adults
Hallucinations Onset <30 min	*Paneolus* *Psilocybe* sp. *Gymnopillus spectabilis*	Visual hallucinations, ataxia	Supportive, sedation with or diazepam 2–5 mg IV for adults
Disulfiram	*Coprinus atramentarius*	Headache, flushing, tachycardia, hyperventilation, palpitations	Supportive IV hydration
Onset 2–72 h after mushroom, and <30 min after alcohol	*Clitocybe clavipes*		

Abbreviations: ALT, alanine aminotransferase; AST, aspartate aminotransferase; BUN, blood urea nitrogen; CNS, central nervous system; IV, intravenous; PT, prothrombin time; PTT, partial thromboplastin time; SLUDGE syndrome, salivation, lacrimation, urination, defecation, gastrointestinal hypermotility, and emesis.

PLANTS

Most patients with plant-related exposures and ingestions require no treatment and may be discharged after a short period of observation. Tables 128-2 and 128-3 describe the clinical symptoms and treatment regimens of common and severe poisonous plant ingestions.

TABLE 128-2 Symptoms and Treatment of Severely Poisonous Plant Ingestions

Plant	Symptoms	Treatment
Castor bean (*Ricinus communis*)	Delayed gastroenteritis, delirium, seizures, coma, death	Whole-bowel irrigation Supportive care
Coyotillo (*Karwinskia humboldtiana*)	Ascending paralysis	Supportive care
Foxglove (*Digitalis purpurea*)	Nausea, vomiting, diarrhea, abdominal pain, confusion, cardiac dysrhythmias	GI decontamination with activated charcoal Monitoring of potassium level Antidysrhythmics Digoxin-specific Fab antibody for dysrhythmias
Jequirity bean (*Abrus precatorius*)	Delayed gastroenteritis, delirium, seizures, coma, death	Whole-bowel irrigation Supportive care
Oleander (*Nerium oleander*)	Nausea, vomiting, diarrhea, abdominal pain, confusion, cardiac dysrhythmias	GI decontamination with activated charcoal Monitoring of potassium level Antidysrhythmics Digoxin-specific Fab antibody for dysrhythmias
Poison hemlock (*Conium maculatum*)	Tachycardia, tremors, diaphoresis, mydriasis, muscle weakness, seizures, neuromuscular blockade	GI decontamination with activated charcoal Supportive care
Water hemlock (*Cicuta maculata*)	Nausea, vomiting, abdominal pain, delirium, seizures, death	GI decontamination Supportive care
Yew (*Taxus* species)	Common: nausea, vomiting, abdominal pain Rare: seizures, cardiac dysrhythmias, coma	GI decontamination with activated charcoal Consider whole-bowel irrigation Supportive care

TABLE 128-3 Symptoms and Treatment of Common Poisonous Plant Ingestions or Exposures

Plant	Symptoms	Treatment
Ackee (*Blighia sapida*)	Hypoglycemia	Glucose
Aloe (*Aloe barbadensis*)	Abdominal pain, diarrhea, red urine, nephritis	Supportive care
Azalea (*Rhododendron* species)	Usually minor symptoms Severe intoxication: salivation, lacrimation, bradycardia, hypotension, progressive paralysis	GI decontamination with activated charcoal Atropine for symptomatic bradycardia Fluids or vasopressors for hypotension

(Continued)

TABLE 128-3 Symptoms and Treatment of Common Poisonous Plant Ingestions or Exposures (Continued)

Plant	Symptoms	Treatment
Cactus	Pain and irritation from embedded spines	Removal of spines Rubber cement peel
Caladium species	Usually minor symptoms Severe intoxication: burning and irritation of oral mucosa, swelling, drooling, dysphagia, respiratory compromise	Ingest cold milk or ice cream for oral burning bradycardia Fluids or vasopressors for hypotension
Colchicum (autumn crocus, meadow saffron, glory lily)	Delayed and severe gastroenteritis → severe multi-system organ failure	GI decontamination with activated charcoal Aggressive fluid resuscitation
Dumbcane (*Dieffenbachia amoena*)	Usually minor symptoms Severe intoxication: burning and irritation of oral mucosa, swelling, drooling, dysphagia, respiratory compromise	Ingest cold milk or ice cream for oral burning Analgesics Consider steroids if severe symptoms
Fava beans (*Vicia faba*)	In persons with glucose-6-phosphate dehydrogenase deficiency: GI upset, fever, headache, hemolytic anemia, hemoglobinuria, jaundice	Treatment varies depending on degree of hemolysis seen
Henbane (*Hyoscyamus niger*)	Anticholinergic symptoms: hallucinations, mydriasis, tachycardia, agitation, seizures, coma	Consider physostigmine in severe cases
Jimsonweed (*Datura* species)	Anticholinergic symptoms: hallucinations, mydriasis, tachycardia, agitation, seizures, coma	GI decontamination with activated charcoal Consider whole-bowel irrigation Supportive care
Lily of the valley (*Convallaria majalis*)	Nausea, vomiting, diarrhea, abdominal pain, confusion, cardiac arrhythmias	GI decontamination with activated charcoal Monitoring of potassium level Antiarrhythmics Digoxin-specific Fab antibody for arrhythmias
Monkshood (*Aconitum* species)	Bradycardia, heart block, torsades de pointes, ventricular fibrillation	GI decontamination with activated charcoal Supportive care
Nettle (stinging nettle, bull nettle) (*Urtica* species)	Localized burning	Symptomatic care
Nightshade, common or woody (*Solanum* species)	Nausea, vomiting, diarrhea, abdominal pain; with larger doses: delirium, hallucinations, coma	Supportive care
Nightshade, deadly (*Atropa belladonna*)	Anticholinergic symptoms: hallucinations, mydriasis, tachycardia, agitation, seizures, coma	GI decontamination with activated charcoal Supportive care

(Continued)

TABLE 128-3 Symptoms and Treatment of Common Poisonous Plant Ingestions or Exposures (Continued)

Plant	Symptoms	Treatment
Peach, apricot, pear, crab apple, yam bean, and hydrangea (pits or seeds)	Acute cyanide toxicity if large amounts are ingested: diaphoresis, nausea, vomiting, abdominal pain, lethargy	GI decontamination with activated charcoal Whole-bowel irrigation Cyanide antidote therapy
Pepper (*Capsicum* species)	Irritation and pain on contact	Copious irrigation with water Milk or ice cream for oral irritation Analgesics
Philodendron species	Usually minor symptoms Severe intoxication: burning and irritation of oral mucosa, swelling, drooling, dysphagia, respiratory compromise	Cold milk or ice cream for oral irritation Analgesics Consider steroids
Pokeweed (*Phytolacca americana*)	Mucosal irritation, abdominal pain, nausea, vomiting, profuse diarrhea Severe intoxication: coma, death	GI decontamination with activated charcoal Supportive care
Potato, eggplant (raw) (*Solanum* species)	Nausea, vomiting, diarrhea, abdominal pain With larger doses: delirium, hallucinations, coma	Supportive care
Pothos (devil's ivy, *Epipremnum* species)	Usually minor symptoms Severe intoxication: burning and irritation of oral mucosa, swelling, drooling, dysphagia, respiratory compromise	Cold milk or ice cream for oral irritation Analgesics Consider steroids
Yellow sage (*Lantana camara*)	Dilated pupils, vomiting, diarrhea, weakness, coma	GI decontamination with activated charcoal Fluids
Toxicodendron species (poison ivy, oak, and sumac)	Dermatitis	Skin protection Antipruritic and topical therapies Systemic steroids for facial, genital, or widespread involvement
Holly (*Ilex* species)	Gastroenteritis Can be fatal if significant ingestion	GI decontamination with activated charcoal Supportive care
Poinsettia (*Euphorbia pulcherrima*)	Occasional local irritation	—
American mistletoe (*Phoradendron flavescens*)	Gastroenteritis	GI decontamination with activated charcoal Supportive care
Easter lily (*Lilium longiflorum*)	Toxicity has not been reported in humans	No treatment necessary

FURTHER READING

For further reading in *Tintinalli's Emergency Medicine: A Comprehensive Study Guide*, 8th ed., see Chapter 219, "Mushroom Poisoning," by Anne F. Brayer and Lynette Froula; and Chapter 220, "Poisonous Plants," by Betty C. Chen and Lewis S. Nelson.

SECTION 13

Endocrine Emergencies

Diabetic Emergencies

Michael P. Kefer

HYPOGLYCEMIA

Hypoglycemia in diabetics is usually a complication of treatment with insulin or sulfonylureas (chlorpropamide, glyburide, glipizide). Hypoglycemia is unlikely due to the glitizones (rosiglitazone, pioglitazone), glinides (repaglinide, nateglinide), alpha-glucosidase inhibitors (acarbose, miglitol), and rare, if ever, due to the biguanide metformin, the incretin analogues (exenatide, liraglutide), or the amylin analogue pramlintide.

Clinical Features

Typical signs and symptoms of hypoglycemia include sweating, shakiness, anxiety, nausea, dizziness, palpitations, slurred speech, blurred vision, headache, seizure, focal neurologic deficits, and altered mental status ranging from confusion to coma.

Diagnosis and Differential

The diagnosis is based on detecting low blood glucose during the occurrence of typical signs and symptoms which resolve with treatment. Hypoglycemia can easily be misdiagnosed as a neurologic or psychiatric condition. The differential diagnosis includes stroke, seizure disorder, head injury, multiple sclerosis, psychosis, depression, and alcohol or drug intoxication.

Emergency Department Care and Disposition

1. Administer glucose. Provide a carbohydrate meal when the patient can tolerate PO. Treat patients with altered mental status with **50% dextrose** 50 mL IV. A continuous infusion of **10% dextrose** solution may be required to maintain the blood glucose above 100 mg/dL.
2. Administer **glucagon** 1 mg IM or SC if there is no IV access.
3. Treat refractory hypoglycemia secondary to the sulfonylureas with **octreotide** 50 to 100 μg SC. A continuous infusion of 125 μg/h may be required.
4. Repeat blood glucose every 30 minutes initially to monitor for rebound hypoglycemia.

5. Disposition depends on the patient's response to treatment, cause of hypoglycemia, comorbid conditions, and social situation. Most insulin reactions respond rapidly. Patients can be discharged with instructions to continue carbohydrate intake and monitor their glucose. Patients with hypoglycemia due to the sulfonylureas or long acting insulins should be admitted due to the risk of rebound from these agents. See Table 129-1 for admission guidelines.

TABLE 129-1 Disposition/Guidelines for Hospital Admission
Inpatient care for type 2 diabetes mellitus is generally appropriate for the following clinical situations:
Life-threatening metabolic decompensation such as diabetic ketoacidosis or hyperglycemic hyperosmolar nonketotic state
Severe chronic complications of diabetes, acute comorbidities, or inadequate social situation
Hyperglycemia (>400 mg/dL [>22 mmol/L]) associated with severe volume depletion or refractory to appropriate interventions
Hypoglycemia with neuroglycopenia (altered level of consciousness, altered behavior, coma, seizure) that does not rapidly resolve with correction of hypoglycemia
Hypoglycemia resulting from long-acting oral hypoglycemic agents
Fever without an obvious source in patients with poorly controlled diabetes

DIABETIC KETOACIDOSIS

Diabetic ketoacidosis (DKA) results from a relative insulin deficiency and counter-regulatory hormone excess causing hyperglycemia and ketonemia. Table 129-2 lists important causes.

TABLE 129-2 Important Causes of Diabetic Ketoacidosis
Omission or reduced daily insulin injections
Dislodgement/occlusion of insulin pump catheter
Infection
Pregnancy
Hyperthyroidism, pheochromocytoma, Cushing's syndrome
Substance abuse (cocaine)
Medications: steroids, thiazides, antipsychotics, sympathomimetics
Heat-related illness
Cerebrovascular accident
GI hemorrhage
Myocardial infarction
Pulmonary embolism
Pancreatitis
Major trauma
Surgery

Clinical Features

Hyperglycemia causes an osmotic diuresis resulting in dehydration, hypotension, and tachycardia. Ketonemia causes an acidosis with myocardial depression, vasodilation, and compensatory Kussmaul respiration. Nausea, vomiting, and abdominal pain are common. The absence of fever does not exclude infection. Acetone, formed from oxidation of ketone bodies, causes the characteristic fruity odor of the patient's breath.

Diagnosis and Differential

Diagnosis of DKA is based on laboratory values of glucose >250 mg/dL, anion gap >10 mEq/L, bicarbonate <15 mEq/L, pH <7.3, and a moderate ketonemia/ketonuria. Beware of "euglycemic ketoacidosis" where blood glucose is only mildly elevated but the other criteria are present. This may occur if the patient has just taken insulin, has impaired gluconeogenesis (alcoholics), or takes a sodium-glucose cotransporter 2 inhibitor, such as canaglifozin.

An anion gap metabolic acidosis results from formation of ketone bodies. In DKA, the conversion of acetoacetate to β-hydroxybutyrate is favored which can result in low acetoacetate levels and high β-hydroxybutyrate levels. If the nitroprusside test is used to detect serum or urine ketones, it may be falsely low or negative as it only detects acetoacetate, not β-hydroxybutyrate.

Osmotic diuresis results in loss of sodium, chloride, calcium, phosphorus, and magnesium. Serum and urine glucose and ketones are elevated. Pseudohyponatremia is common: for each 100 mg/dL increase in blood glucose, the sodium decreases by 1.6 mEq/L, though some recommend this correction factor be 2.4, especially if glucose >400 mg/dL. Serum potassium may be low from osmotic diuresis and vomiting, normal, or high from acidosis. In acidosis, potassium is driven extracellularly. Note the acidotic patient with normal or low potassium has marked depletion of total body potassium.

Laboratory investigation includes serum pH, glucose, electrolytes, blood urea nitrogen, creatinine, phosphorus, magnesium, complete blood count, urinalysis (and pregnancy if indicated), electrocardiogram, and chest radiograph to assess the severity of DKA and search for the underlying cause. Determine pH using venous blood. The difference between venous and arterial pH (0.03) is not clinically significant, so the risk and pain of arterial puncture is unnecessary.

The differential diagnosis includes hypoglycemia, hyperosmolar hyperglycemic state, alcoholic or starvation ketoacidosis, renal failure, lactic acidosis, and ingestions such as salicylate, methanol, ethylene glycol, iron, or isoniazid.

Emergency Department Care and Disposition

1. The goal of treatment is to correct the volume deficit, acid–base imbalance, and electrolyte abnormalities, administer insulin, and treat the underlying cause (Fig. 129-1). See Table 129-1 for admission guidelines.

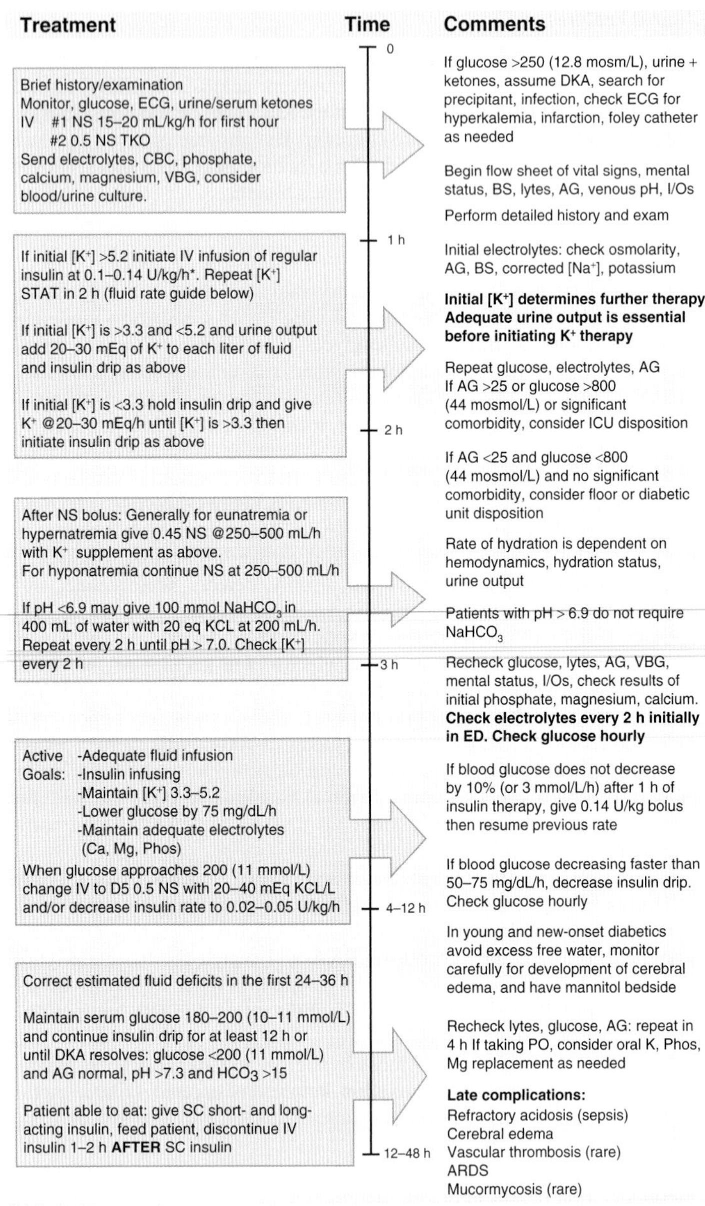

FIGURE 129-1. Timeline for the typical adult patient with suspected diabetic ketoacidosis. *IV insulin infusion <1.0 U/kg/h may require a bolus dose of regular insulin (0.1 U/kg). AG, anion gap; ARDS, acute respiratory distress syndrome; BS, blood sugar; ECG, electrocardiogram; ICU, intensive care unit; I/Os, inputs/outputs; NS, normal saline; TKO, to keep vein open; VBG, venous blood gas.

2. Administer bicarbonate when the pH ≤6.9. Then, the benefits of correcting the effects of acidosis (vasodilation, hyperkalemia, depression of cardiac, respiratory, and CNS systems) outweigh the risk of bicarbonate treatment (paradoxical CSF acidosis, hypokalemia, impaired oxyhemoglobin dissociation, rebound alkalosis, sodium overload).
3. Monitor glucose, anion gap, potassium, and bicarbonate hourly until recovery is established: glucose <200 mg/dL, bicarbonate ≥18, and pH >7.3.
4. Cerebral edema is a complication of treatment. Young age and new-onset diabetes are risk factors. If there is any change in neurologic status early in therapy, begin treatment with **mannitol** 1 g/kg before obtaining the diagnostic CT scan. Avoiding rapid correction of sodium, glucose, and hypovolemia may reduce risk.

HYPEROSMOLAR HYPERGLYCEMIC STATE

Hyperosmolar hyperglycemic state (HHS) occurs in type 2 diabetics. Causes are similar to DKA (Table 129-2). Insulin deficiency or resistance combined with physiologic stress results in an inflammatory state with elevated counterregulatory hormones causing hyperglycemia. The resulting osmotic diuresis causes hypovolemia and electrolyte losses.

Clinical Features

The typical patient is elderly with type 2 diabetes and presents with nonspecific complaints of weakness, dyspnea, chest or abdominal pain, or mental status changes, and has preexisting lung, heart, renal, or neurologic disease.

Physical examination reveals signs of dehydration with orthostasis, dry skin and mucous membranes, and altered mental status. Focal deficits and seizures may occur.

Diagnosis and Differential

Hyperosmolar hyperglycemic state is defined by laboratory values of glucose >600 mg/dL, calculated serum osmolality (formula: Osm = 2 [Na+] + glucose/18) >315 mOsm/kg, bicarbonate >15 mEq/L, pH >7.3, and negative to mildly positive ketones. Marked elevation in glucose and serum osmolality and the absence of a significant ketosis help distinguish HHS from DKA. Further laboratory investigation is similar to that for DKA discussed above.

Emergency Department Care and Disposition

Treatment consists of correcting the volume deficit, electrolyte imbalance, and hyperosmolality, and treating the underlying cause (Fig. 129-2). See Table 129-1 for admission guidelines.

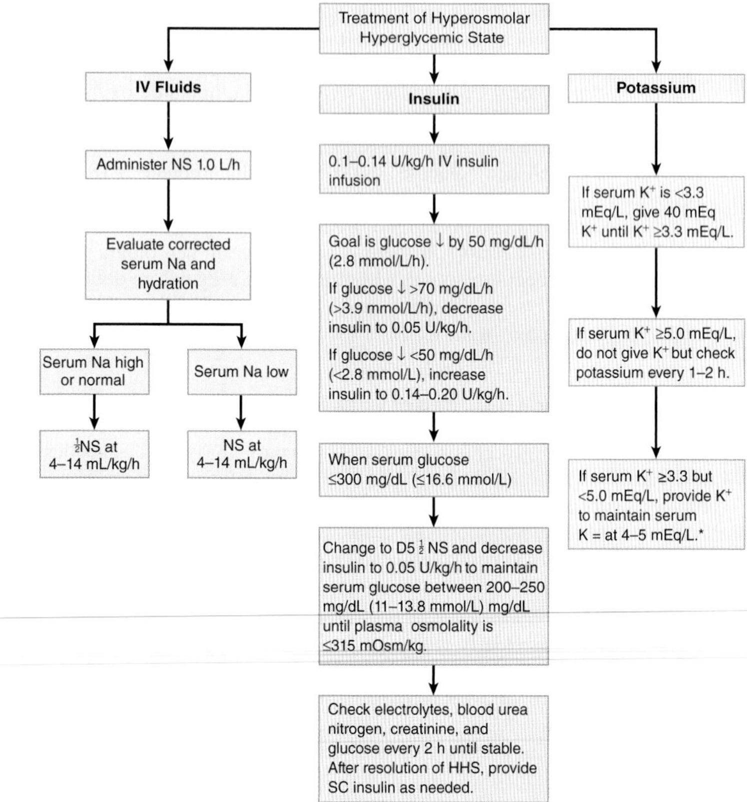

FIGURE 129-2. Protocol for the management of severely ill adult patients with hyperosmolar hyperglycemic state (HHS). *Concentrations of $K^+ \geq 20$ mEq/L should be administered via central line. D5 1/2 NS, 5% dextrose in half normal saline; HHS, hyperosmolar hyperglycemic state; NS, normal saline.

DIABETIC FOOT ULCERS

These are classified and managed as nonlimb-threatening, limb-threatening, or life-threatening (Table 129-3). Recommended antibiotic therapy is listed in Table 129-4.

TABLE 129-3 Clinical Practice Pathways for Diabetic Foot Ulcer and Infection

Extent of Infection	Characteristics	Diagnostic Procedures	Treatment
Non-limb-threatening infection	<2 cm cellulitis	Cultures from base of ulcer (with tissue specimen if possible)	Outpatient management with follow-up in 24–72 h
	Superficial ulcer	Diagnostic imaging (radiography, MRI, nuclear scans as indicated)	Debridement of all necrotic tissue and callus
	Mild infection	Serologic testing	Wound care/dressing
	No systemic toxicity	CBC with differential	Empiric antibiotic coverage, modified by culture findings
	No ischemic changes	ESR	Appropriate off-loading of weight-bearing
	No bone or joint involvement	Comprehensive metabolic panel	Wound care continued with packs, dressings, and debridement as needed
	Does not probe to bone		Hospital admission if infection progresses or systemic signs or symptoms develop
			Refer to podiatrist for follow-up care, special shoes, and prostheses as needed
Life- or limb-threatening infection	>2 cm cellulitis	Deep culture from base of ulcer/wound with tissue specimen if possible	Hospital admission
	Deep ulcer	Diagnostic imaging (radiography, MRI, nuclear scan, bone scan, leukocyte scan, arteriography)	Surgical debridement with resection of all necrotic bone and soft tissue
	Odor or purulent drainage from wound	Serologic testing	Exploration and drainage of deep abscess
	Fever	CBC with differential	Empiric antibiotic coverage, modified by culture findings
	Ischemic changes	ESR	Surgical resection of osteomyelitis
	Lymphangitis, edema	Comprehensive metabolic panel	Wound care continued with packs, dressings, debridement as needed
	Sepsis or septic shock	Blood cultures	Foot-sparing reconstructive procedures
			Refer to podiatrist for follow-up care, special shoes, and prostheses as needed

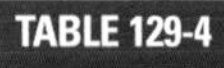

TABLE 129-4 Antimicrobial Therapy in Infected Diabetes-Related Lower Extremity Ulcers

Non-limb-threatening*
Cephalexin, 500 mg PO every 6 h, 10-day course
Or
Clindamycin, 300–450 mg PO every 6–8 h, 10-day course
Or
Dicloxacillin, 500 mg PO every 6 h, 10-day course
Or
Amoxicillin-clavulanate, 875/125 mg PO every 12 h, 10-day course
Or
Clarithromycin 500 mg PO every 12 h (in severe penicillin allergy)
Limb-threatening*
Oral regimen†:
(Ciprofloxacin or levofloxacin or moxifloxacin) plus clindamycin
Or
Trimethoprim-sulfamethoxazole plus amoxicillin-clavulanate
IV regimens:
Ampicillin-sulbactam, 3 g every 6 h
Or
Piperacillin-tazobactam 4.5 g every 6–8 h
Or
Clindamycin, 900 mg every 6 h plus (ciprofloxacin, 400 mg every 8–12 h or ceftriaxone, 1 g every 12 h)
Life-threatening*
IV regimens:
Imipenem-cilastatin, 500 mg every 6 h
Or
Meropenem 1 g every 8 h
Or
Vancomycin, 15–20 mg/kg every 12 h, plus metronidazole, 500 mg every 8 h, plus aztreonam, 2 g every 6–8 h or ciprofloxacin 400 mg every 8–12 h)
(if MRSA coverage is warranted)

*See the section "Foot and Lower Extremity Complications" for definitions in *Tintinalli's Emergency Medicine: A Comprehensive Study Guide*, 8th ed., Chapter 224.

†This approach is acceptable under special circumstances with close follow-up.

Abbreviation: MRSA, methicillin-resistant *Staphylococcus aureus.*

Note: Adjust all dosages for renal/hepatic function and monitor blood levels where appropriate.

FURTHER READING

For further reading in *Tintinalli's Emergency Medicine: A Comprehensive Study Guide*, 8th ed., see Chapter 223, "Type 1 Diabetes Mellitus," by Nikhil Goyal and Adam B. Schlichting; Chapter 224, "Type 2 Diabetes Mellitus," by Mohammad Jalili and Mahtab Niroomand; Chapter 225, "Diabetic Ketoacidosis," by Andrew L. Nyce, Cary L. Lubkin, and Michael E. Chansky; Chapter 227, "Hyperosmolar Hyperglycemic State," by Charles S. Graffeo.

CHAPTER 130

Alcoholic Ketoacidosis

Michael P. Kefer

Alcoholic ketoacidosis (AKA) results from heavy alcohol intake, either acute or chronic. Glycogen stores are depleted, activating lipolysis to supply energy. Lipolysis and alcohol metabolism generate ketoacids, causing an anion gap metabolic acidosis.

CLINICAL FEATURES

The patient typically presents with nausea, vomiting, and abdominal pain after heavy alcohol intake. The patient appears acutely ill, dehydrated, and has abdominal tenderness that is nonspecific or is the result of other causes related to alcohol, such as gastritis, hepatitis, or pancreatitis.

DIAGNOSIS AND DIFFERENTIAL

Laboratory investigation reveals an anion gap metabolic acidosis. However, the serum pH may vary as these patients often have mixed acid–base disorders such as a metabolic acidosis from AKA and a metabolic alkalosis from vomiting and dehydration. Blood glucose is low to mildly elevated. The alcohol level is usually low or undetected as symptoms limit intake. Serum ketones, acetoacetate, and its reduced form, beta-hydroxybutyrate, are elevated. If the nitroprusside test is used to measure serum and urine ketones, acetoacetate is detected, but beta-hydroxybutyrate is not. The redox state may be such that most, or all, acetoacetate is reduced to beta-hydroxybutyrate resulting in a falsely low- or false-negative result, respectively.

Diagnostic criteria for AKA are listed in Table 130-1. The differential diagnosis of an anion gap metabolic acidosis is listed in Table 130-2.

TABLE 130-1 Diagnostic Criteria for Alcoholic Ketoacidosis*

Low, normal, or slightly elevated serum glucose
Binge drinking ending in nausea, vomiting, and decreased intake
Wide anion gap metabolic acidosis
Positive serum ketones*
Wide anion gap metabolic acidosis without alternate explanation

*The absence of ketones in the serum based on the nitroprusside test does not exclude the diagnosis.

TABLE 130-2 The Differential Diagnosis of an Anion Gap Metabolic Acidosis Is Recalled by the Acronym MUDPILES

- Methanol
- Uremia
- Diabetic ketoacidosis
- Paraldehyde
- Iron, isoniazid, inhalants
- Lactic acidosis
- Ethanol, ethylene glycol
- Salicylates

EMERGENCY DEPARTMENT CARE AND DISPOSITION

1. Administer **D5NS IV** until rehydrated, then **D5 0.45NS** IV for maintenance. The isotonic crystalloid solution restores intravascular volume. The glucose stimulates the patient's endogenous insulin release, which inhibits ketosis (insulin is not administered, unlike treatment for DKA).
2. **Thiamine** 100 mg IV before glucose administration may prevent precipitation of Wernicke's disease.
3. Supplement electrolytes and other vitamins as indicated.
4. Continue treatment until the acidosis clears and oral intake is tolerated.
5. Consider other causes of an anion gap acidosis if the gap does not close with treatment.
6. Consider **sodium bicarbonate** if, despite treatment, the pH remains <7.0.

FURTHER READING

For further reading in *Tintinalli's Emergency Medicine: A Comprehensive Study Guide*, 8th ed., see Chapter 226 "Alcoholic Ketoacidosis," by William A. Woods and Debra G. Perina.

CHAPTER 131 Thyroid Disease Emergencies

Aziz Darawsha

HYPOTHYROIDISM AND MYXEDEMA COMA

Hypothyroidism may be caused by multiple factors. Myxedema coma (also called myxedema crisis) is a rare, life-threatening expression of hypothyroidism. It may be precipitated by infection, cold exposure, trauma, medications, or myocardial infarction. It classically occurs during the winter months in elderly women with undiagnosed or undertreated hypothyroidism.

Clinical Features

The presentation of hypothyroidism is summarized in Fig. 131-1. Patients with myxedema coma have hypothyroidism and present with metabolic and multi-organ decompensation, including hypothermia, bradycardia, hypotension, and altered mental status. Respiratory insufficiency and altered mental status can result from CO_2 narcosis, and a difficult airway may be encountered due to macroglossia, glottic, and oropharyngeal edema. Laboratory abnormalities include hypoglycemia and hyponatremia.

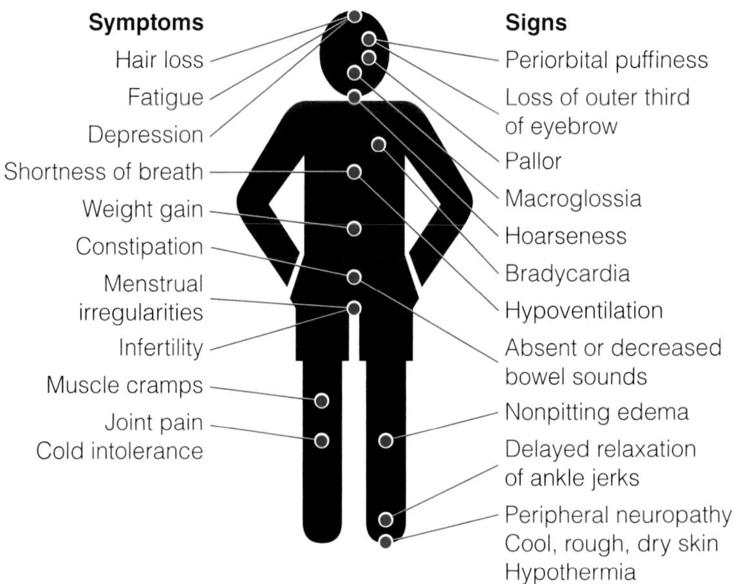

FIGURE 131-1. Symptoms and signs of hypothyroidism.

Diagnosis and Differential

The diagnosis of myxedema coma is clinical. Send confirmatory thyroid studies, but do not delay treatment for test results. Low free thyroxine (FT4) and triiodothyronine (FT3), and elevated thyroid stimulating hormone (TSH) are diagnostic. The differential diagnosis includes sepsis, depression, adrenal crisis, congestive heart failure, hypoglycemia, stroke, hypothermia, meningitis, and drug overdose.

Emergency Department Care and Disposition

Management of myxedema coma includes:

1. Supportive care with airway stabilization, mechanical ventilation, and cardiac monitoring. Treat hypotension with fluid resuscitation. Vasopressors may be ineffective until thyroid hormone replacement is initiated. Passively rewarm hypothermic patients.
2. Seek out and treat precipitating causes. Administer **hydrocortisone**100 mg IV for suspected adrenal insufficiency. Correct hypoglycemia.
3. Thyroid replacement therapy: **Levothyroxine (T4)** 4 μg/kg, followed in 24 hours by 100 μg IV, then 50 μg IV until oral medication is tolerated or **liothyronine** (T3) 20 μg IV followed by 10 μg IV every 8 hours until the patient is conscious for severe myxedema coma. Start with no more than 10 μg IV in the elderly and patients with cardiovascular disease. Switch to levothyroxine 50 to 200 μg/day PO when the patient is ambulatory.
4. Admit patients to a monitored or ICU setting.
5. Identify and treat precipitating factors
   - Infections
   - Sedatives
   - Anesthetic agents (e.g., etomidate)
   - Cold exposure
   - Trauma
   - Myocardial infarction or congestive heart failure
   - Cerebrovascular accident
   - GI hemorrhage
   - Contributing metabolic conditions include hypoxia, hypercapnia, hyponatremia, and hypoglycemia

THYROTOXICOSIS AND THYROID STORM

Hyperthyroidism refers to excess circulating hormone due to thyroid gland hyperfunction, whereas thyrotoxicosis refers to excess circulating thyroid hormone from any cause. Thyroid storm is an acute, life-threatening state of thyrotoxicosis that is most common in patients with antecedent Graves' disease.

Clinical Features

The clinical features of thyrotoxicosis are manifestations of enhanced adrenergic activity. Signs and symptoms are shown in Table 131-1. As for thyroid storm, the leading signs and symptoms are constitutional (fever), central nervous system related (agitation, confusion, delirium, stupor, coma, and seizure), and cardiovascular (tachycardia, arrhythmia, and heart failure).

TABLE 131-1 Symptoms and Signs of Thyrotoxicosis

Affected System	Symptoms	Signs
Constitutional	Lethargy Weakness Heat intolerance	Diaphoresis Fever Weight loss
Neuropsychiatric	Emotional lability Anxiety Confusion Coma Psychosis	Fine tremor Muscle wasting Hyperreflexia Periodic paralysis
Ophthalmologic	Diplopia Eye irritation	Lid lag Dry eyes Exophthalmos Ophthalmoplegia Conjunctival infection
Endocrine: thyroid gland	Neck fullness Tenderness	Thyroid enlargement Bruit
Cardiorespiratory	Dyspnea Palpitations Chest pain	Widened pulse pressure Systolic hypertension Sinus tachycardia Atrial fibrillation or flutter Congestive heart failure
GI	Diarrhea	Hyperactive bowel sound
Reproductive	Oligomenorrhea Decreased libido	Gynecomastia Telangiectasia
Gynecologic	Menorrhagia Irregularity	Sparse pubic hair
Hematologic	Pale skin	Anemia Leukocytosis
Dermatologic	Hair loss	Pretibial myxedema* Warm, moist skin Palmar erythema Onycholysis

*Pretibial myxedema may be present in 5% of patients with Graves' disease.

Diagnosis and Differential

An elevated FT4 or FT3 level and a suppressed TSH level are diagnostic of thyrotoxicosis. Thyroid storm is a clinical diagnosis. Fever and tachycardia are cardinal features; laboratory tests cannot distinguish it from thyrotoxicosis. The differential diagnosis for thyroid storm includes sepsis, heat stroke, delirium tremens, neuroleptic malignant syndrome, serotonin syndrome, pheochromocytoma, and sympathomimetic drug overdose.

Emergency Department Care and Disposition

Treatment includes:

1. Supportive care, including airway stabilization, supplemental oxygen, and cardiac monitoring. Cooling is indicated for hyperthermia. Administer **acetaminophen** 325 to 650 mg PO/PR every 4 to 6 hours. Correct

dehydration with IV fluids. Provide nutritional support: glucose, multivitamins, thiamine, folate.

2. Inhibit thyroid hormone release with thioamides: **PTU** loading dose of 600 to 1000 mg PO and follow with 200 to 250 mg every 4 hours or **methimazole** 40 mg PO as loading dose and follow with 25 mg every 4 hours. PTU is preferred as it also blocks peripheral conversation of T4 to T3.
3. Inhibit new thyroid hormone production (at least 1 hour after step 3) with **Lugol solution** 8-10 drops PO every 6-8 h or **potassium iodide** 5 drops PO every 6 h or **IV iopanoic** acid 1 gram every 8 h for the first 24 h, then 500 mg twice a day or **ipodate** 0.5 - 3 g/day for 3 days or **lithium carbonate** 300mg PO every 6 h.
4. Provide peripheral β-adrenergic receptor blockade using **propranolol** IV in slow 1 to 2 mg boluses and repeat every 10 to 15 minutes or **esmolol** 500 mcg/kg IV bolus followed by 50 to 200 mcg until desired effect is achieved. **Propranolol** 20 -120 mg PO may be used in patients with less toxicity. Avoid propranolol and esmolol in patients with bronchospastic disease or severe congestive heart failure.
5. Prevent peripheral conversion of T4 to T3 using **hydrocortisone** 100 mg initially, followed by three times daily until stable or **dexamethasone** 2 mg every 6 h.
6. Evaluate and treat precipitating causes. Search for an infectious source in febrile patients and administer appropriate antibiotics for identified infections.
7. Admit patients to a monitored or ICU setting.

FURTHER READING

For further reading in *Tintinalli's Emergency Medicine: A Comprehensive Study Guide*, 8th ed., see Chapter 228, "Hyperthyroidism" by Alzamani Mohammad Idrose; Chapter 229, "Hyperthyroidism," by Alzamani Mohammad Idrose.

CHAPTER 132

Adrenal Insufficiency

Michael P. Kefer

Adrenal insufficiency results when the physiologic demand for glucocorticoids and mineralocorticoids exceeds the supply from the adrenal cortex. The pituitary secretes adrenocorticotropin hormone (ACTH) and associated melanocyte stimulating hormone (MSH). ACTH stimulates the adrenal cortex to secrete cortisol. Cortisol has negative feedback on the pituitary to inhibit secretion of ACTH and MSH.

CLINICAL FEATURES

Primary adrenal insufficiency is due to adrenal gland failure, resulting in low cortisol and aldosterone production. Clinical features include weakness, dehydration, hypotension, anorexia, nausea, vomiting, weight loss, and abdominal pain. Hyperpigmentation of skin and mucous membranes occurs as a result of uninhibited MSH secretion in conjunction with ACTH.

Secondary adrenal insufficiency results from inadequate secretion of ACTH with resultant cortisol deficiency. Aldosterone levels are not affected because of regulation by the renin-angiotensin axis and serum potassium levels. Therefore, hyperpigmentation and hyperkalemia do not occur.

Adrenal crisis is the acute, life-threatening form of adrenal insufficiency. Clinical features described above are severe and accompanied by shock and altered mental status.

DIAGNOSIS AND DIFFERENTIAL

All patients with adrenal insufficiency have low plasma cortisol levels. The ACTH level is high in primary and low in secondary adrenal insufficiency. Cortisol and ACTH levels are usually not available in the emergency department, so the diagnosis of primary adrenal insufficiency is based on the presence of the clinical features and lab findings of hyponatremia, hyperkalemia, hypoglycemia, anemia, metabolic acidosis, and prerenal azotemia. Secondary adrenal insufficiency is similarly diagnosed, but hyperkalemia is not seen as aldosterone secretion is normal.

The most common cause of acute adrenal insufficiency is adrenal suppression from prolonged steroid use with either abrupt steroid withdrawal or exposure to increased physiologic stress such as injury, illness, or surgery. It may take up to 1 year for the hypothalamic-pituitary-adrenal axis to recover following prolonged suppression with steroid treatment. Tables 132-1 and 132-2 list causes of primary and secondary adrenal insufficiency, respectively. Consider the diagnosis of adrenal crisis in any patient with unexplained hypotension refractory to pressors, especially if one of the causes listed is known to exist.

TABLE 132-1 Causes of Primary Adrenal Insufficiency

Primary Adrenal Insufficiency	Examples
Autoimmune	Isolated adrenal insufficiency or associated with polyglandular insufficiencies (polyglandular autoimmune syndrome type I or II)
Adrenal hemorrhage or thrombosis	Necrosis caused by meningococcal sepsis Coagulation disorders Overwhelming sepsis (Waterhouse–Friderichsen syndrome)
Drugs	*Adrenal enzyme inhibitors (affect those with limited pituitary or adrenal reserve)* Etomidate Aminoglutethimide (can be used by body builders) Mitotane (orphan drug used to treat adrenocortical carcinoma) Ketoconazole
Infections	Tuberculosis Fungal, bacterial sepsis Acquired immunodeficiency syndrome involving adrenal glands
Infiltrative disorders	Sarcoidosis Hemochromatosis Amyloidosis Lymphoma Metastatic cancer
Surgery	Bilateral adrenalectomy Bariatric surgery
Hereditary	Adrenal hypoplasia Congenital adrenal hyperplasia Adrenoleukodystrophy Familial glucocorticoid deficiency

TABLE 132-2 Causes of Secondary Adrenal Insufficiency

Secondary Adrenal Insufficiency (hypothalamic-pituitary dysfunction)	Examples
Sudden cessation of prolonged glucocorticoid therapy	Chronic use of steroid inhibits CRH and ACTH production
Pituitary necrosis or bleeding	Postpartum pituitary necrosis (Sheehan's syndrome)
Exogenous glucocorticoid administration	Causes decreased production of CRH at hypothalamus and ACTH at pituitary
Brain tumors	Pituitary tumor Hypothalamic tumor Local invasion (craniopharyngioma)
Pituitary irradiation Pituitary surgery Head trauma involving the pituitary gland	Disrupts CRH and ACTH production capacity in hypothalamic-pituitary axis

(Continued)

TABLE 132-2 Causes of Secondary Adrenal Insufficiency (Continued)

Secondary Adrenal Insufficiency (hypothalamic-pituitary dysfunction)	Examples
Infiltrative disorders of the pituitary or hypothalamus	Sarcoidosis Hemosiderosis Hemochromatosis Histiocytosis X Metastatic cancer Lymphoma
CNS infections involving hypothalamus or pituitary	Tuberculosis Meningitis Fungus Human immunodeficiency virus

Abbreviations: ACTH, adrenocorticotropic hormone; CRH, corticotropin-releasing hormone.

EMERGENCY DEPARTMENT CARE AND DISPOSITION

1. **Five percent dextrose in normal saline** is the fluid of choice to correct hypoglycemia, hyponatremia, and hypotension.
2. **Hydrocortisone** 100 mg IV provides glucocorticoid and mineralcorticoid activity. If an ACTH stimulation test is planned, use **dexamethasone** 4 mg IV instead, which will not affect the test result.
3. **Vasopressors** are added when shock is refractory to the above.
4. Patients on chronic steroid therapy for adrenal insufficiency with minor illness or injury should have their glucocorticoid dose tripled daily with prompt follow-up.

FURTHER READING

For further reading in *Tintinalli's Emergency Medicine: A Comprehensive Study Guide*, 8th ed., see Chapter 230, "Adrenal Insufficiency," by Alzamani Mohammad Idrose.

SECTION 14

Hematologic and Oncologic Emergencies

Evaluation of Anemia and the Bleeding Patient

Rita K. Cydulka

Anemia may be chronic and unrelated to the chief complaint, or it may result from acute blood loss as seen in trauma, gastrointestinal bleeding, or other acute hemorrhage. Suspect underlying bleeding disorders in patients presenting with spontaneous bleeding from multiple sites, bleeding from nontraumatized sites, delayed bleeding several hours after injury, or bleeding into deep tissues or joints.

CLINICAL FEATURES

The rate of the development of the anemia, the extent of the anemia, the age of the patient, and the ability of the cardiovascular system to compensate for the decreased oxygen-carrying capacity determine the severity of the patient's symptoms and clinical presentation. Patients may complain of weakness, fatigue, palpitations, orthostatic symptoms, and dyspnea with minimal exertion. Patients may have pale conjunctiva, skin, and nail beds. Tachycardia, hyperdynamic precordium, and systolic murmurs may be present. Tachypnea at rest and hypotension are late signs. Use of ethanol, prescription drugs, and recreational drugs may alter the patient's ability to compensate for the anemia.

Patients with bleeding may or may not have an obvious site of hemorrhage. A history of excessive or abnormal bleeding in the patient and other family members may indicate an underlying bleeding disorder. Historical data about liver disease and drug use, such as use of ethanol, aspirin, nonsteroidal anti-inflammatory drugs, warfarin, and antibiotics should be gathered. Mucocutaneous bleeding (including petechiae, ecchymoses, purpura, and epistaxis), gastrointestinal, genitourinary, or heavy menstrual bleeding are features associated with qualitative or quantitative platelet disorders. Patients with deficiencies of coagulation factors often present with delayed bleeding, hemarthroses, or bleeding into potential spaces between fascial planes and into the retroperitoneum. Patients with combination abnormalities of platelets and coagulation factors, such as disseminated intravascular coagulation, present with both mucocutaneous and potential space bleeding.

Acquired hemolytic anemia may be autoimmune or drug-induced. Microangiopathic syndromes include thrombotic thrombocytopenic purpura (TTP) and hemolytic-uremic syndrome (HUS). The classic pentad of TTP is CNS abnormalities, renal disease, fever, microangiopathic hemolytic anemia, and thrombocytopenia. HUS consists of acute nephropathy or renal failure, microangiopathic hemolytic anemia, and thrombocytopenia. Macrovascular hemolysis can be caused by prosthetic heart valves.

DIAGNOSIS AND DIFFERENTIAL

A decreased red blood count, hemoglobin, and hematocrit are diagnostic for anemia. The initial evaluation of newly diagnosed anemia includes a complete blood count, review of RBC indices, reticulocyte count, stool hemoccult examination, urine pregnancy test in females, and examination of the peripheral blood smear. The mean corpuscular volume (MCV) and reticulocyte count can assist in classifying the anemia and can aid in differential diagnosis (Fig. 133-1).

Laboratory studies used to diagnose bleeding disorders can be divided into the following three categories: (a) those that test the initial formation of a platelet plug (primary hemostasis); (b) those that assess the formation of cross-linked fibrin (secondary hemostasis); and (c) those that test the fibrinolytic system, which is responsible for limiting the size of the fibrin clots formed (see Tables 133-1 and 133-2). Initial studies to evaluate the patient with suspected bleeding disorders include complete blood count with platelet count, prothrombin time, and partial thromboplastin time and international normalized ratio (INR). If there is a suspicion for a hemolytic anemia, further studies may be warranted (Table 133-3).

EMERGENCY DEPARTMENT CARE AND DISPOSITION

1. Type and crossmatch blood in patients with anemia and ongoing blood loss so that it is available for transfusion, if necessary.
2. Consider immediate transfusion of **packed RBCs** in symptomatic patients who are hemodynamically unstable or have evidence of tissue hypoxia.
3. Admit patients with anemia and ongoing blood loss for further evaluation and treatment. Admit patients with chronic anemia or newly diagnosed anemia with unclear etiology if they are hemodynamically unstable, hypoxic, acidotic, or demonstrate cardiac ischemia.
4. Consider **hematology consultation** to assist in evaluation of those patients with anemia of unclear etiology, anemic patients with concomitant abnormalities of platelets and white blood cell counts, and patients with suspected bleeding disorders.

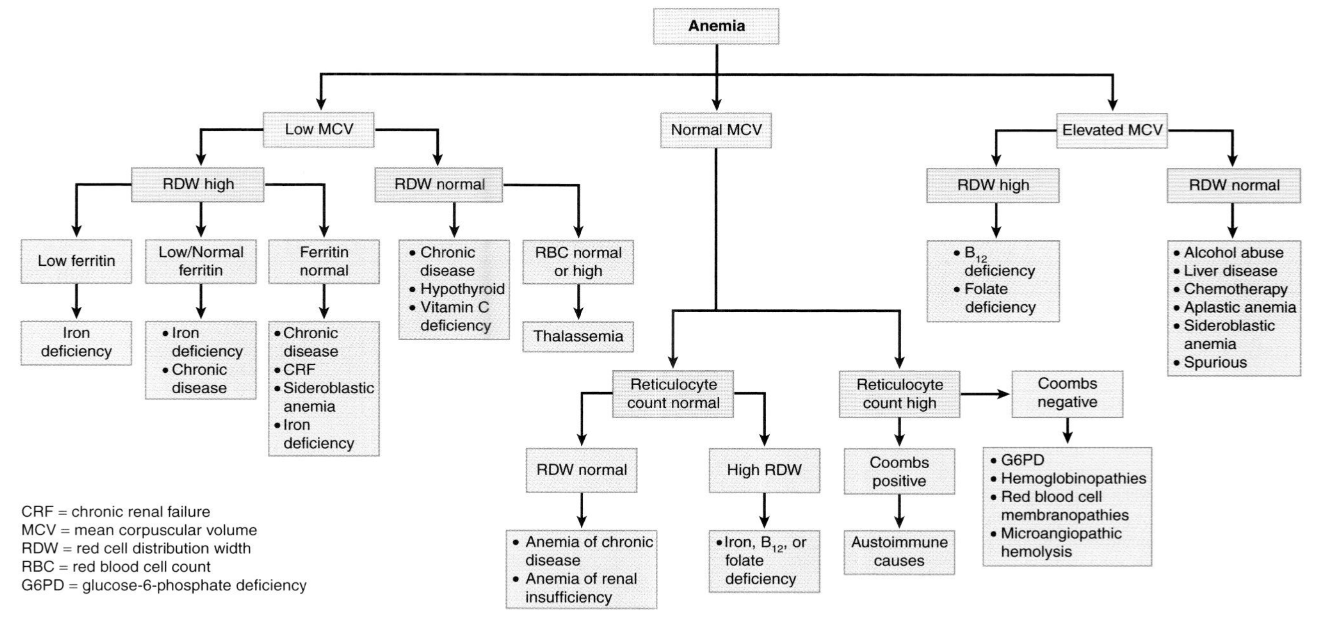

FIGURE 133-1. Flowchart for the evaluation of anemia.

TABLE 133-1 Initial Tests of Hemostasis

Screening Tests	Reference Value	Component Measured	Clinical Correlations
Primary Hemostasis			
Platelet count	150–400/mm^3 (150–400 × 10^9/L)	Number of platelets per mm^3	*Decreased platelet count (thrombocytopenia)*: bleeding usually not a problem until platelet count is <50,000/mm^3 (50 × 10^9/L); high risk of spontaneous bleeding, including CNS bleeding, seen with count of <10,000/mm^3 (10 × 10^9/L); usually due to decreased production or increased destruction of platelets *Elevated platelet count (thrombocytosis)*: commonly a reaction to inflammation or malignancy, and occurs in polycythemia vera; can be associated with hemorrhage or thrombosis
Bleeding time (BT)	Variable Typically 2.5–10.0 min using a BT template	Interaction between platelets and the subendothelium	*Prolonged BT* caused by: Thrombocytopenia (platelet count <50,000/mm^3 or 50 × 109/L) Abnormal platelet function (von Willebrand's disease, antiplatelet drugs, uremia, liver disease)
Secondary Hemostasis			
Prothrombin time (PT) and international normalized ratio (INR)	PT: 11–13 s; depends on reagent INR: 1.0	Extrinsic system and common pathway—factors VII, X, V, prothrombin, and fibrinogen INR = 1.7 corresponds to approximately 30% activity of coagulation factors as a whole	*Prolonged PT* most commonly caused by: Warfarin (inhibits production of vitamin K–dependent factors II, VII, IX, and X) Liver disease with decreased factor synthesis Antibiotics that inhibit vitamin K–dependent factors (moxalactam, cefamandole, cefotaxime, cefoperazone)

Activated partial thromboplastin time (aPTT)	22–34 s Depends on type of thromboplastin reagent used "Activated" with kaolin	Intrinsic system and common pathway—factors XII, XI, IX, VIII, X, V, prothrombin, and fibrinogen	*Prolonged aPTT* most commonly caused by: Heparin therapy Factor deficiencies (factor levels have to be <30% of normal to cause prolongation)
Fibrinogen level	Slightly variable according to specific test	Protein made in liver; converted to fibrin as part of normal coagulation cascade	Low levels seen in disseminated intravascular coagulation
Thrombin clotting time (TCT)	10–12 s	Conversion of fibrinogen to fibrin monomer	*Prolonged TCT* caused by: Low fibrinogen level Abnormal fibrinogen molecule (liver disease) Presence of heparin, fibrin degradation products, or a paraprotein (multiple myeloma); these interfere with the conversion Occasionally seen in hyperfibrinogenemia
"Mix" testing	Variable	Performed when results on one or more of the above screening tests is prolonged; the patient's plasma ("abnormal") is mixed with "normal" plasma and the screening test is repeated	*If the mixing corrects* the screening test result: one or more factor deficiencies are present *If the mixing does not correct* the screening test result: a circulating inhibitor is present

TABLE 133-2 Additional Hemostatic Tests

Test	Reference Value	Component Measured	Clinical Correlations/ Comments
Fibrin degradation product (FDP) and d-dimer levels	FDP: variable depending on specific test, typically <2.5–10 μg/mL (2.5–10 mg/L) D-Dimer: variable depending on specific test, typically <250–500 ng/mL (250–500 μg/L)	FDP test: measures breakdown products from fibrinogen and fibrin monomer D-Dimer test: measures breakdown products of cross-linked fibrin	Levels are elevated in diffuse intravascular coagulation, venous thrombosis, pulmonary embolus, and liver disease, and during pregnancy
Factor level assays	60–130% of reference value (0.60–1.30 units/mL)	Measures the percent activity of a specified factor compared to normal	To identify specific deficiencies and direct therapeutic management
Protein C level	Variable Typically 60–150% of reference value	Level of protein C in the blood	Vitamin K dependent Increases with age Values higher in males than females Deficiency associated with thromboembolism in people <50 years of age
Protein S level	Variable Typically 60–150% of reference value	Level of protein S in the blood	Vitamin K dependent Increases with age Values higher in males than females Deficiency associated with thromboembolism in people <50 years of age
Factor V Leiden (FVL)	Variable	Screening test looks for activated protein C resistance, and confirmatory test analyzes DNA sequence of factor V gene Screening assay uses activated partial thromboplastin time with and without added activated protein C	FVL not inactivated by activated protein C Heterozygotes have 7× and homozygotes have a 20× increased lifetime risk of venous thrombosis Mutation associated with thromboembolism in people <50 years of age

TABLE 133-3 Basic Tests and Findings in the Evaluation of Hemolytic Anemia

Purpose	Test	Finding
Confirm anemia/blood loss	Hemoglobin Hematocrit	Decreased Decreased
Confirm compensatory RBC production	Reticulocyte count	Increased
Confirm hemolysis	Peripheral smear	Schistocytes—intravascular hemolysis, RBCs fragmented by shear mechanism Spherocytes—extravascular hemolysis, RBC phagocytosis by macrophages
Confirm hemolysis	Lactate dehydrogenase Potassium	Increased, released by RBCs Increased, released by RBCs
Confirm hemolysis	Haptoglobin Free haemoglobin Hemoglobinuria	Decreased, indicative of intravascular hemolysis Increased, indicative of intravascular hemolysis Present
Confirm hemoglobin breakdown	Total bilirubin Indirect (unconjugated) bilirubin Urinary urobilinogen	Increased Increased (hepatic conjugation of bilirubin overwhelmed) Increased

Abbreviation: RBC, red blood cell.

FURTHER READING

For further reading in *Tintinalli's Emergency Medicine: A Comprehensive Study Guide*, 8th ed., see Chapter 231, "Anemia," by John C. Ray and Robin R. Hemphill; Chapter 232, "Tests of Hemostasis," by Stephen John Cico and Robin R. Hemphill; Chapter 237, "Acquired Hemolytic Anemia," by Laurie Ann Dixon and Robin R. Hemphill.

CHAPTER 134 Acquired Bleeding Disorders

Alisheba Hurwitz

Platelet abnormalities, drugs, systemic illnesses, and endogenous anticoagulants can cause acquired bleeding disorders.

ACQUIRED PLATELET DEFECTS

Clinical Features

Patients with platelet disorders commonly present with petechiae or mucosal bleeding. Splenomegaly may be noted in patients experiencing platelet sequestration.

Diagnosis and Differential

Acquired platelet abnormalities include quantitative and qualitative defects. *Quantitative platelet disorders* may be caused by decreased platelet production (marrow infiltration, aplastic anemia, drugs, viral infections, and chronic alcohol use), or increased platelet destruction (idiopathic thrombocytopenic purpura (ITP), thrombotic thrombocytopenic purpura (TTP), hemolytic uremic syndrome, disseminated intravascular coagulation (DIC), viral infections, drugs, and HELLP syndrome). Other causes include acute hemorrhage, hemodialysis, and splenic sequestration. *Qualitative platelet disorders* are commonly associated with renal disease, liver disease, DIC, drugs (aspirin, NSAIDs, clopidogrel), and myeloproliferative disorders.

Emergency Department Care and Disposition

1. Circulatory stabilization of the acutely bleeding patient is paramount, including volume resuscitation, packed red cell transfusion, and pressors as necessary.
2. Perform a focused history and physical; order appropriate laboratory studies. Most evaluations of bleeding patients will include a CBC with peripheral smear. Other studies to consider include PT/INR, PTT, basic metabolic panel, type and screen, and fibrinogen.
3. Consider platelet transfusion in patients with a platelet count $<10{,}000/\text{mm}^3$ or active bleeding with platelets $<50{,}000/\text{mm}^3$.
4. Consult with a hematologist, as subtleties in diagnosis and treatment exist. For example, some conditions may be worsened by platelet transfusion (DIC and TTP).

BLEEDING IN IMMUNE THROMBOCYTOPENIA

Emergency Department Care and Disposition

In general, patients with a platelet count $>50{,}000/\text{mm}^3$ require no treatment. Patients with a platelet count $<30{,}000/\text{mm}^3$ and patients with a platelet count of $<50{,}000/\text{mm}^3$ with bleeding typically require treatment.

1. Treatment options include corticosteroids, such as **prednisone 60 to 100 mg PO** daily (onset of action 4 to 14 days).

2. **Immunoglobulin 1 g/kg daily IV** (onset of action 1 to 3 days) is usually reserved for patients with very low platelet counts and bleeding.
3. **If transfusing platelets, generally two to three times the usual dose** is required due to circulating antibodies.

ACQUIRED COAGULATION DEFECTS

Coagulation disorders often present with significant hemorrhage and frequently involve platelet defects as well.

Bleeding in Liver Disease

Patients with liver disease have an increased risk of bleeding for multiple reasons including decreased synthesis of vitamin K-dependent coagulation factors (II, VII, IX, and X), thrombocytopenia, and increased fibrinolysis.

Emergency Department Care and Disposition

1. Transfuse **red cells** as needed.
2. Transfuse **platelets** for thrombocytopenia <60,000/mm^3.
3. Consider transfusion of **fresh frozen plasma 15 mL/kg IV with caution**. It may increase the risk of thrombotic complications, and it may increase portal hypertension thus worsening variceal bleeding.

Bleeding in Renal Disease

A variety of hemostatic defects are associated with renal disease including platelet dysfunction due to anemia, deficiency of coagulation factors, and thrombocytopenia.

Emergency Department Care and Disposition

1. Transfuse **red cells** as needed.
2. **Desmopressin 0.3 μg/kg SC or IV** improves platelet function rapidly.
3. **Hemodialysis** improves platelet function transiently for 1 to 2 days.
4. Transfuse **platelets** and **cryoprecipitate** for life-threatening bleeding only.

Disseminated Intravascular Coagulation

The clinical features of DIC are a result of simultaneous hemorrhage and thrombosis and vary according to the underlying illness. Bleeding typically predominates and can range from petechiae to diffuse hemorrhaging from GI/GU tracts, surgical wounds, and venipuncture sites.

Emergency Department Care and Disposition

1. Treat the underlying illness and provide hemodynamic support including pressors and packed red cells as necessary.
2. Transfuse **platelets** if counts <20,000/mm^3, or <50,000/mm^3 with active bleeding.
3. Transfuse **fresh frozen plasma (15 mL/kg)** for bleeding patient with PT or PTT that are >1.5 times the upper limit of normal, or with fibrinogen level <150 mg/dL.

4. Transfuse **fibrinogen concentrate** to patients with hypofibrinogenemia and active bleeding, with the goal of raising fibrinogen levels to 100 to 150 mg/dL.
5. Administer **vitamin K IV** to bleeding patients with elevated PT.
6. Consider heparin use for patients with a clinical picture dominated by thrombosis.
7. **Tranexamic acid** should be given only in the setting of DIC due to trauma.

Bleeding Due to Circulating Anticoagulants

Patients with acquired factor VIII inhibitors (acquired hemophilia A) present with spontaneous bruising and hematomas. Consult with a hematologist for management guidance. Treatment options for acute bleeding episodes include **recombinant factor VIIa** and **activated prothrombin complex concentrate**.

FURTHER READING

For further reading in *Tintinalli's Emergency Medicine: A Comprehensive Study Guide*, 8th ed., see Chapter 233, "Acquired Bleeding Disorders," by Robert W. Shaffer and Sally A. Santen

CHAPTER 135

Hemophilias and von Willebrand Disease

Colin G. Kaide

HEMOPHILIAS

The most common hemophilias are caused by genetic deficiencies of factor VIII (hemophilia A) or factor IX (hemophilia B).

Clinical Features

Bleeding complications depend on the severity of the disease. Patients with severe disease (factor VIII or factor IX activity level <1%) experience spontaneous bleeds and difficult to control bleeding after trauma. Patients with moderate disease (1% to 5% factor activity level) may bleed spontaneously but more commonly bleed after trauma. Patients with mild disease (5% to 40% factor activity level) usually only bleed after trauma. Easy bruising, recurrent hemarthrosis, and muscle hematomas are the most common clinical manifestations. Central nervous system (CNS) bleeding accounts for the most common cause of death. Retroperitoneal, gastrointestinal (GI), and soft tissue bleeding can occur. Mucocutaneous bleeding (dental bleeding, epistaxis, GI tract bleeding, lungs bleeding) can occur, although this is rare. Neck hematomas may obstruct the airway. Unless there is another underlying disease, most patients with hemophilia do not have problems with minor cuts or abrasions. Almost all cases of hemophilia occur in men with women being genetic carriers of the disease. The unlikely exception occurs when a hemophiliac man reproduces with a woman who is a carrier of the hemophilia gene; hemophiliac females can result. Owing to spontaneous mutations and lyonization of the X chromosome women may develop varying degrees of decreased factor levels.

A rare form of hemophilia occurs when a person develops a spontaneous antibody to their intrinsic factor VIII. It is often (40%) associated with other conditions such as autoimmune diseases, cancers, certain drugs, the postpartum period. It usually happens in the sixth or seventh decade and affects men and women equally. Widespread purpura and internal bleeding are common with hemarthrosis less common.

Diagnosis and Differential

Clinically, it is impossible to differentiate between hemophilias A and B. Laboratory testing in patients with hemophilia most often shows a normal prothrombin time (PT), prolonged partial thromboplastin time (PTT), and a normal bleeding time. However, if greater than 30% to 40% of factor activity is present, the PTT may be normal. Specific factor assays may be used to differentiate between the types of hemophilia. Ten percent to 25% of patients with hemophilia A and 1% to 2% of patients with hemophilia B will develop an inhibitor, which is an antibody against the deficient factor. The presence of an inhibitor makes treatment more difficult, requiring alternative, pre-activated factors such as recombinant factor VIIa or factor eight inhibitor bypassing activity (FEIBA).

Emergency Department Care and Disposition

The mainstay of therapy is early factor replacement. Replacement factor products are listed in Table 135-1.

1. Determine the type of hemophilia and the presence or absence of inhibitor. See Table 135-2 for factor replacement guidelines. Factor replacement may need to be instituted before definitive imaging after head trauma and other life-threatening injuries. If an inhibitor is present, use therapy as outlined in Table 135-3.
2. Determine the desired factor activity level. Factor activity level determines how much factor replacement is required. Calculate the amount of factor needed using the patient's weight and the desired increase in factor:
   Factor VIII required = (Target factor − Base line factor) × Weight (kg) × 0.5
   Factor IX required = (Target factor − Base line factor)× Weight (kg)
   For severe hemophilia, assume 0% intrinsic activity. The half-life of factor VIII is approximately 8 to 12 hours. For hemophilia B, the half-life of factor IX is approximately 16 to 24 hours.
3. Treat patients with undiagnosed bleeding disorders with fresh frozen plasma (FFP). FFP contains 1 unit of factor VIII/mL. Specific factor assays should guide further therapy.

TABLE 135-1 Replacement Factor Products for Hemophilia Treatment

Hemophilia Type	Available Products* (Manufacturer/Distributor)
Hemophilia A	*Recombinant Factor VIII Concentrates*
	Advate® (Baxter)
	Helixate FS® (Bayer/CSL Behring)
	Kogenate FS® (Bayer)
	Recombinate® (Baxter)
	Xyntha® (Pfizer)
	Human Plasma-Derived Factor VIII Concentrates
	Hemofil M® (Baxter)
	Monoclate-P® (CSL Behring)
	Human Plasma-Derived Factor VIII Concentrates That Contain von Willebrand Factor
	Alphanate® (Grifols)
	Humate-P® (CSL Behring GmbH)
	Koate-DVI® (Grifols/Kedrion Biopharma)
Hemophilia B	*Recombinant Factor IX Concentrate*
	BeneFIX® (Pfizer)
	Human Plasma-Derived Factor IX Concentrates
	AlphaNine SD® (Grifols)
	Mononine® (CSL Behring)

*Commercial trade names provided for ease of specific identification.

TABLE 135-2 Initial Factor Replacement Guidelines in Severe Hemophilia

Severity and Site	Desired Factor Level to Control Bleeding	Hemophilia A Initial Dose (IU/ kg)	Hemophilia B Initial Dose (IU/ kg)	Comments
Minor: skin (deep laceration)	–	–	–	Abrasions and superficial lacerations usually do not require factor replacement. Treat with pressure and topical thrombin.
Minor: early hemarthrosis, mild muscle bleeding, mild oral bleeding	0.2–0.4 IU/mL (20%–40%)	10–20	20–30	Repeat dose every 12–24 h for 1–3 days until bleeding episode is resolved. Typical duration of replacement is 1–3 days.
Moderate: definite hemarthrosis, moderate muscle bleeding, moderate oral bleeding	0.3–0.6 IU/mL (30%–60%)	15–30	25–50	Orthopedic consult may be required for splinting, physical therapy, and follow-up. Typical duration of replacement is 3–5 days.
Major: retropharyngeal, GI, intra-abdominal, intrathoracic, retroperitoneal	0.6–1.0 IU/mL (60%–100%)	30–50	30–50	Repeat dose every 8–24 h until resolution of bleeding episode. May require replacement for up to 10 days.
CNS	1.0 IU/mL (100%)	50	50–100	Treat before CT. Early neurosurgical consultation.

TABLE 135-3 Replacement Therapy for Hemophilia A and B in Patients with Inhibitors

Type of Product*	Initial Dose	Dosing Interval	Comments
Human plasma-derived activated prothrombin complex concentrate FEIBA NF® (Baxter)	50–100 units/kg	6–12 h	Total daily doses should not normally exceed 200 units/kg.
Recombinant activated factor VII NovoSeven RT® (Novo Nordisk)	90 μg/kg	2 h	Repeat until hemostasis achieved or therapy judged ineffective.

*Commercial trade names provided for ease of specific identification.

4. Treat minor bleeding in patients with mild hemophilia A with **desmopressin (DDAVP)** 0.3 μg/kg IV over 15 to 30 minutes or **DDAVP** 150 μg single spray in each nostril (for children >5 years, **DDAVP** 150 μg single spray in one nostril). Very mild mucosal bleeding can also be treated with antifibrinolytic agents, such as **e-aminocaproic acid (EACA)** 75 to 100 mg/kg (up to 6 g) IV/PO every 6 hours or tranexamic acid 10 to 25 mg/kg IV every 6 hours.
5. Indications for admission include bleeding involving the head, neck, pharynx, retropharynx, or retroperitoneum, potential compartment syndrome, and inability to control pain, and treatment requiring multiple factor replacement.

VON WILLEBRAND DISEASE

Clinical Features

von Willebrand disease (vWD) is a group of disorders caused by a defect or deficiency of von Willebrand factor (vWF). vWF is a cofactor for platelet adhesion and a carrier protein for factor VIII in the plasma. Type 1 vWD is most common; patients have 20% to 50% of normal vWF levels and usually manifest with skin and mucosal bleeding symptoms. Patients with type 2 vWF have abnormal and dysfunctional vWF. Patients with type 3 vWF have complete vWF deficiency and have clinical presentations similar to hemophilia. Patients with mild vWF are frequently unaware of the disease until bleeding occurs after a traumatic episode or surgical procedure.

Diagnosis and Differential

The PT and PTT are usually normal. The bleeding time is prolonged and vWF activity is low. Bleeding time, however, is rarely used anymone and has been suplanted by more specific platelet activation and aggregation studies. Variability in vWF levels can make it difficult to distinguish vWD from hemophilia A.

Emergency Department Care and Disposition

The treatment of vWD depends on the type of disease and the severity of bleeding. Indications for admission are similar to patients with hemophilia.

1. The mainstay of treatment for bleeding in type 1 vWD is **desmopressin (DDAVP)** 0.3 μg/kg (up to 20 μg) SC/IV every 12 to 24 hours for up to four doses or **DDAVP** 150 μg single spray in each nostril (for children >5 years, **DDAVP** 150 μg single spray in 1 nostril). If there is no response to DDAVP, administer factor VIII concentrate or cryoprecipitate as described for type 2 and 3 vWD.
2. Factor VIII concentrate containing vWF is used to treat bleeding in patients with type 2 or 3 disease (Table 135-1).
3. **Cryoprecipitate** 10 bags IV every 12 to 24 hours can be used for type 1 refractory to DDAVP or type 2 or 3 vWD. There is, however, a risk of viral transmission.
4. Platelet transfusions may benefit patients with type 3 vWD who do not respond to vWF-containing plasma products.

5. Oral contraceptives may help increase vWF levels and limit menstrual bleeding in women with vWD and menorrhagia.
6. Patients who have sustained dental injuries or who require dental procedures may need **e-aminocaproic acid (EACA)** 75 to 100 mg/kg (up to 6 grams) PO every 6 hours or **tranexamic acid mouthwash** for 5 to 10 days.

FURTHER READING

For further reading in *Tintinalli's Emergency Medicine: A Comprehensive Study Guide*, **8th** ed., see Chapter 235, "Hemophilias and von Willebrand's Disease," by Robin R. Hemphill.

CHAPTER 136

Sickle Cell Disease and Other Hereditary Hemolytic Anemias

Colleen Fant

Inherited anemias stem from abnormal hemoglobin structure or production or from abnormal RBC structure or metabolism. Anemia occurs when destruction of red blood cells exceeds production. Most patients with dyshemoglobinemia are aware of their status.

SICKLE CELL DISEASE

Clinical Features

Most patients with sickle cell disease (SCD) (homozygous (HbSS)) or sickle trait (heterozygous (HbAS)) present with symptoms related to vasoocclusive crisis, or with pain, weakness, or infections. Physical examination findings commonly include pallor, venous stasis changes, jaundice, hepatosplenomegaly, cardiac flow murmurs, cardiomegaly, and high-output congestive heart failure (CHF).

Painful vasooclusive crisis in the musculoskeletal system or, in some cases, organ-specific symptoms are the most common presentations to the ED. Crisis occurs when sickled RBCs mechanically obstruct blood flow, causing ischemia, organ damage, and infarction. Crisis-causing stresses include fever or infection (especially encapsulated organisms *Haemophilus influenzae* or *Pneumococcus*), cold exposure or high altitude, dehydration or overexertion, medication noncompliance, or drug use.

Acute symptomatic anemia results from splenic sequestration, bone marrow failure (aplastic crisis), or hemolysis due to infection and presents with fatigue, weakness, dyspnea, chronic heart failure, or shock.

Life or limb-threatening events seen in SCD patients include acute chest syndrome (vasoocclusive pulmonary insult), stroke, renal infarct, mesenteric infarcts, sepsis, avascular necrosis, osteomyelitis, pneumonia, or priapism.

Diagnosis and Differential

The degree of illness guides the evaluation of an acute crisis. Although workups should be individualized, the more common, vague complaints (pain, weakness, fever) must include a search for an underlying, treatable event. See Table 136-1.

Anemia due to splenic sequestration may present as splenomegaly with or without left-upper quadrant pain and elevated reticulocyte count. Anemia due to bone marrow failure may be suggested by a depressed reticulocyte count. Leukocytosis or left shift with increased bands suggests infection. Assessment of electrolytes will allow evaluation of dehydration and renal function. Liver function tests and lipase may help evaluate abdominal pain. Perform a pregnancy test on women. Febrile SCD patients without localizing symptoms should have blood cultures, urinalysis, and chest radiographs performed.

TABLE 136-1 Guidelines for the Assessment and Management of Acute Vasoocclusive Crisis

History	Duration and location of pain History of fever History of focal swelling or redness Precipitating factors for acute episode Medications taken for pain relief
Physical examination	Assess degree of pain Inspect sites of pain, looking for swelling, warmth, redness General: respiratory distress, pallor, hydration, jaundice, rash Vital signs: especially temperature, pulse oximetry Respiratory: lung sounds Heart: cardiomegaly and systolic murmur common with chronic anemia Abdomen: tenderness, organomegaly
Ancillary tests	If moderate to severe pain, focal pathology is present, or pain is atypical for acute episode Obtain CBC, leukocyte differential, reticulocyte count, urinalysis Chest radiograph, if signs of lower respiratory tract pathology Blood cultures and additional blood tests: as indicated by clinical condition
General management	Bed rest, provide warmth and a calm, relaxing atmosphere Distractions where appropriate: television, music, etc. Oral fluids: typically about 3 L/d IV fluids to correct dehydration or if reluctant to drink or vomiting is present Oxygen: not routinely required unless hypoxemia is present Encourage deep breathing, incentive spirometry Consider adjuvant therapy: anxiolytic, tinzaparin, antiemetic

Pain management	Use analgesics appropriate to degree of pain
	Acetaminophen for mild pain
	NSAID for mild to moderate pain (avoid if renal insufficiency is present)
	Opioids for moderate to severe pain, typical initial doses include:
	  Morphine, 0.3 mg/kg PO or 0.1–0.15 mg/kg IV
	  Hydromorphone, 0.06–0.08 mg/kg PO or 0.015–0.020 mg/kg IV
	Reassess response in 15–30 minutes, may repeat with one-fourth to one-half initial dose, consider patient's known effective dose

Disposition and follow-up	Consider admission to the hospital if:
	  Acute chest syndrome is suspected
	  Sepsis, osteomyelitis, or other serious infection is suspected
	  Hemoglobin is <5 g/dL
	  White blood cell count is >30,000/mm3
	  Platelet count is <100,000/mm3
	Consider discharge if:
	  Pain is under control and patient can take oral fluids and medications
	  Appropriate oral analgesics are available
	  Patient is able to comply with home care instructions
	  Patient has resources for follow-up

Abbreviations: CBC, complete blood count; NSAID, nonsteroidal anti-inflammatory drug.

Patients presenting with symptoms of acute chest syndrome (chest pain, cough, fever, dyspnea) need immediate evaluation (Table 136-2). Chest radiographs are important to identify the presence of a new infiltrate. Assess oxygenation; type and cross for possible exchange transfusion.

Radiographs of the skeleton are indicated for atypical focal bone pain. Advanced imaging for abdominal pain or for neurologic manifestations will help to assess these symptoms.

TABLE 136-2 Assessment and Treatment of Acute Chest Syndrome

History	Major presenting symptom: dyspnea, fever, cough Accompanying chest, rib, bone, or joint pain Assess degree or severity of pain Recent or previous sepsis, infection, pneumonia, or hospitalization Prior history of acute chest syndrome, especially if required intubation and ventilatory support Potentially infectious contacts Current medications Immunization history: especially pneumococcal and *Haemophilus influenzae* type b Baseline hemoglobin level and arterial oxygenation saturation
Physical examination	General: respiratory distress, pallor, hydration, jaundice, rash Vital signs: especially temperature, pulse oximetry Respiratory: chest wall, lung sounds Heart: cardiomegaly and systolic murmur common with chronic anemia Abdomen: tenderness, organomegaly
Ancillary tests	Complete blood count, leukocyte differential, reticulocyte count, urinalysis Cross-match sample: if red blood cell transfusion is contemplated Arterial blood gas: if moderate to severe respiratory distress and/or hypoxemia on pulse oximetry Chest radiography Blood cultures Additional blood tests: as indicated by clinical condition
Treatment	Oxygen: adjust according to pulse oximetry Oral hydration: preferable IV hydration: use hypotonic fluids, use a rate and dose at approximately 1.5 times of maintenance (overaggressive IV fluids can worsen acute chest syndrome) Analgesics: if needed, generally potent parenteral opioids are used; monitor for signs of respiratory suppression Antibiotics: empiric antibiotics recommended to treat community acquired pneumonia Bronchodilators: nebulized β_2-adrenergic agonists Chest physiotherapy Transfusion: use if severe acute anemia is present
Exchange transfusion	Consider when Severe acute chest syndrome on admission and past history of requiring ventilatory support: useful to prevent intubation Deterioration despite above management: useful to prevent intensive care unit admission Patient already intubated and on ventilatory support: useful to shorten duration of ventilatory need Suspected or confirmed fat or bone marrow embolism

The differential diagnosis for musculoskeletal pain includes osteomyelitis, bony infarcts, cellulitis, and acute arthritides. For abdominal pain, the differential includes pancreatitis, hepatitis, cholecystitis, pelvic inflammatory disease, and pyelonephritis. Chest pain may be due to acute chest, pneumonia, or pulmonary embolus. Neurologic symptoms may be due to meningitis, cerebral infarct, ischemia, or hemorrhage.

Emergency Department Care and Disposition

Initial management for acute crisis in SCD patients is primarily supportive and includes pain management and an assessment for the underlying cause of the crisis (see Tables 136-1 and 136-2).

1. Encourage oral **rehydration** if dehydration is suspected. IV crystalloid may be used as an alternative, up to 1.5 times maintenance. Hypotonic fluids may reduce the tendency for sickling.
2. Administer **opioid pain medications** for severe pain. Individualized **treatment plans** are warranted for patients with frequent relapses.
3. Administer supplemental **oxygen** for hypoxia.
4. **ECG** and **cardiac monitoring** are appropriate for patients with cardiopulmonary symptoms.
5. For symptoms of acute infection, **cultures** should be obtained and **broad-spectrum antibiotics** administered. For patients with suspected acute chest, antibiotics should be targeted toward community-acquired pneumonia.
6. Consider **exchange transfusion** for acute crisis or complications in specific circumstances—aplastic crisis, cardiopulmonary decompensation, pregnancy, stroke, respiratory failure, general surgery, and priapism (requires urologic consultation). Exchange transfusion is typically reserved for patients with severe crises, that is, PaO_2 <60 mm Hg.
7. Patients with priapism lasting >4 hours should additionally receive corporal aspiration and injection of dilute α-adrenergic agonist.
8. Admission criteria include pulmonary, neurologic, aplastic, or infectious crises; splenic sequestration; intractable pain; persistent nausea and vomiting; or an uncertain diagnosis.
9. Patients able to be discharged should receive oral analgesics, close follow-up, and instructions to return immediately for temperature above 38°C or worsening symptoms.

VARIANTS OF SICKLE CELL DISEASE

Other genetic variants of hemoglobinopathies exist and vary in presentation, from asymptomatic to SCD-like and depend upon the specific abnormality and whether homozygous, heterozygous, or combined with sickle cell trait.

Thalassemias

Thalassemias are hereditary disorders caused by defective synthesis of globin chains, resulting in microcytic, hypochromic, hemolytic anemia. The degree of illness depends upon the type and number of genetic abnormalities.

Patients with β-thalassemia minor have mild microcytic anemia and are generally asymptomatic. Patients with β-thalassemia major (Cooley's anemia) develop hepatosplenomegaly, jaundice, and bony changes. They are at increased risk for infection and may develop severe anemia requiring blood transfusions. Iron overload from transfusions can cause significant morbidity and mortality.

Glucose-6-Phosphate Dehydrogenase Deficiency

Glucose-6-phosphate dehydrogenase (G6PD) deficiency is the most common enzymopathy of RBCs. This causes hemoglobin precipitation, RBC removal by the spleen, and hemolysis. The amount of hemolysis depends on degree of enzyme abnormality. Most patients are asymptomatic until an exposure to an oxidative stress (e.g., medication, infection, fava beans) causes hemolysis. A serious complication of G6PD deficiency is severe neonatal jaundice that presents in the first week of life. Evaluation includes a complete blood count and reticulocyte count, bilirubin levels, serum aminotransferases, and lactate dehydrogenase. Treatment is determined by the patient's overall clinical condition and includes early treatment of infection and may include blood transfusion for severe anemia.

Hereditary Spherocytosis

Hereditary spherocytosis results from an erythrocyte membrane defect creating small inflexible RBCs that are unable to pass through the spleen resulting in an increased rate of destruction and a compensatory increase in RBC production. Complications include aplastic or megaloblastic crises, cholecystitis or cholelithiasis, splenomegaly, hemolytic crisis, and neonatal hemolysis with jaundice. Treatments include blood transfusions and splenectomy in severe cases.

FURTHER READING

For further reading in *Tintinalli's Emergency Medicine: A Comprehensive Study Guide*, 8th ed., see Chapter 236, "Sickle Cell Disease and Hereditary Hemolytic Anemias," by Jean Williams-Johnson and Eric Williams.

CHAPTER 137 Transfusion Therapy

Özlem Köksal

Patients are typically transfused in the emergency department to treat acute blood loss and/or circulatory shock. The goal of transfusion is to improve oxygen delivery to tissues, provide intravascular volume expansion, and replace missing or depleted clotting factors. Great care must be taken to ensure that the correct blood product is delivered to the correct patient.

WHOLE BLOOD

There are few indications for the use of whole-blood transfusion. Although whole-blood transfusion would seem ideal to replace acute blood loss, storage of whole blood inactivates platelets and other factors. Therefore, whole blood is fractionated to its components for transfusion.

PACKED RED BLOOD CELLS

Packed red blood cells (PRBCs) are prepared from whole blood by removing most platelets and/or white cells. A single unit of PRBC has 250 mL and raises an adult's hemoglobin by 1 g/dL (hematocrit by 3%). In children, 10 to 15 mL/kg of PRBCs raises the hemoglobin level by approximately 2 to 3 g/dL (hematocrit by 6% to 9%). PRBCs increase oxygen-carrying capacity in anemic patients.

The decision to transfuse PRBC is based on individual clinical judgment, taking into account patient's hemodynamic status, underlying medical condition, tolerance for anemia, and risk of end-organ ischemic injury. Adequate oxygen delivery in healthy normovolemic patients can be maintained with hemoglobin levels as low as 7 g/dL, although patients with comorbid conditions may require transfusion at higher levels of hemoglobin. The usual indications for PRBC transfusion include (a) acute blood loss about 30% of blood volume (1500 mL in adult), (b) acute hemorrhage, (c) unstable trauma patients based on inadequate response to an initial 2-L bolus of IV crystalloid or 40 mL/kg in children; and (d) symptomatic anemia with hemoglobin <7 g/dL or being at-risk for ischemic events, such as patients with hemoglobin <8 to 9 g/dL who have sepsis or ischemic heart or brain injury.

Type and cross-match assesses ABO/Rh blood type, the presence of antibodies, and patient and donor blood compatibility. Blood type can be determined in approximately 15 minutes, whereas it takes about 45 to 60 minutes to perform a serologic cross-match.

In critical situations, where there is no time to perform a complete ABO/Rh-typing, group O/Rh-negative blood ("universal donor") can be given to patients without waiting for a complete type and cross-match. Type O/Rh-positive blood may be used if Rh-negative blood is unavailable, but should be avoided in girls and women of childbearing potential. Before transfusion, blood for baseline laboratory tests, type, and crossmatching should be obtained.

Packed red blood cells may be further treated to minimize complications in special patient populations, such as neonates, transplant and patients on transplant list, patients who have received prior transfusions, pregnant patients, immunocompromised patients, and patients with hypersensitivity to plasma. Options include leukocyte-reduced, irradiated, frozen deglycerolized, washed, and *Cytomegalovirus*-negative PRBCs.

One unit of PRBC is generally transfused over 1 to 2 hours. PRBCs should be transfused more rapidly in patients with hemodynamic instability. Single-unit PRBC transfusions should not exceed 4 hours to prevent contamination. Micropore filters are used to filter out microaggregates of platelets, fibrin, and leukocytes. Normal saline solution is the only crystalloid compatible with PRBCs. Blood warmers or concurrently administered warmed saline solution (39°C to 43°C or 102.2°F to 109.4°F) can be used to prevent hypothermia.

MASSIVE TRANSFUSION

Massive transfusion is the replacement of one blood volume or approximately 10 units of PRBCs in an adult within a 24-hour period. The best ratio of PRBCs to platelets to fresh frozen plasma (FFP) during a massive transfusion is controversial. Some experts advocate a 1:1:1 ratio, although lower ratios of platelets to FFP have been used without clear evidence of inferiority. Complications of massive transfusion include coagulopathy, citrate toxicity, hypocalcemia, hypomagnes, emia, and hypothermia. See Table 137-1 for recognition, management, and evaluation of selected acute transfusion reactions.

PLATELETS

Platelet transfusions may be used in thrombocytopenic patients to prevent bleeding or to help stop active bleeding. Platelet transfusion is usually not helpful in cases of bleeding from platelet dysfunction (e.g., uremia) or from thrombocytopenia due to increased consumption/sequestration until the underlying disorder (e.g., DIC) is corrected. General indications for platelet transfusion include platelet count $< 5{,}000/mm^3$ in asymptomatic patients, platelet count $< 20{,}000/mm^3$ with a coagulation disorder, low-risk procedure, during outpatient treatment, platelet count $< 50{,}000/mm^3$ with active bleeding or invasive procedure within 4 hours, platelet count $< 100{,}000/mm^3$ with neurologic or cardiac surgery, or as part of a massive transfusion protocol.

One apheresis single-donor platelet unit will increase the platelet count by up to $50{,}000/mm^3$. Typical dose is 1 unit or 5 mL/kg. Typical dose of pooled donor platelet is 6 units or 5 mL/kg.

ABO-type specific platelets are preferable. Platelets may also be washed or irradiated. The platelet count should be checked at 1 and 24 hours after transfusion. Transfused platelets survive 3 to 5 days unless there is a platelet- consumptive process.

TABLE 137-1 Transfusion Reactions

Reaction Type	Signs and Symptoms	Management	Evaluation
Acute intravascular hemolytic reaction	Fever, chills, low back pain, flushing, dyspnea, tachycardia, shock, hemoglobinuria	Immediately stop transfusion. IV hydration to maintain diuresis; diuretics may be necessary. Cardiorespiratory support as indicated.	Retype and repeat cross-match. Direct and indirect Coombs test. CBC, creatinine, prothrombin time, activated partial thromboplastin time. Haptoglobin, indirect bilirubin, lactate dehydrogenase, plasma free hemoglobin. Urine for hemoglobin.
Delayed extravascular hemolytic reaction	Often have low-grade fever but may be entirely asymptomatic	Usually presents days to weeks after transfusion. Rarely causes clinical instability.	Hemolytic workup as above to investigate the possibility of intravascular hemolysis.
Febrile nonhemolytic transfusion reaction	Fever, chills	Stop transfusion. Initially manage as in intravascular hemolytic reaction (above) because one cannot initially distinguish between the two. Can treat fever and chills with acetaminophen. Usually mild but can be life-threatening in patients with tenuous cardiopulmonary status. Consider infectious workup. Premedication with acetaminophen can mask this reaction.	Hemolytic workup as above because may not be able to initially distinguish febrile from hemolytic transfusion reactions.
Allergic reaction	Mild: urticaria, pruritus Severe: dyspnea, bronchospasm, hypotension, tachycardia, shock	Stop transfusion. If mild, reaction can be treated with diphenhydramine; if symptoms resolve, can restart transfusion. If severe, may require cardiopulmonary support; do not restart transfusion.	For mild symptoms that resolve with diphenhydramine, no further workup is necessary, although blood bank should be notified. For severe reaction, do hemolytic workup as above because initially may be indistinguishable from a hemolytic reaction.

FRESH FROZEN PLASMA

Fresh frozen plasma contains all coagulation factors and fibrinogen. FFP is used for replacement of multiple coagulation deficiencies (liver failure, warfarin-induced over-anticoagulation and massive transfusion) and to correct coagulation defects for which no factor is available. FFP is also administered prior to high-risk invasive procedures if PT/INR > 1.5X normal, aPTT > 1.5X top of normal range, or coagulation factor assay < 25% normal activity. FFP is not indicated to treat a prolonged INR in the absence of active bleeding.

Fresh frozen plasma needs to be thawed for 20 to 40 minutes before it can be used. Each 200 to 250 mL pack of FFP contains 1 unit/mL of each coagulation factor and 2 mL fibrinogen. In general, 1 unit of FFP will increase most coagulation factors by 3% to 5% in a 70-kg adult. FFP should be ABO-type compatible. Type AB is the universal donor for FFP, and in emergencies, universal donor FFP can be given minutes after thawing. Starting dose is 15 mL/kg (or 4 units in a 70-kg adult). If rapid reversal of a vitamin K antagonist coagulopathy is needed, prothrombin complex concentrate or recombinant activated factor VII is faster and more reliable.

CRYOPRECIPITATE

Cryoprecipitate is derived from FFP. One bag of cryoprecipitate contains 80 units factor VIII, 200 to 300 mL von Willebrand factor, 40 to 60 units fibrinogen, factor XIII, and variable amounts of fibronectin.

Cryoprecipitate is indicated for (a) active bleeding in patients with afibrinogenemia or hypofibrinogenemia (fibrinogen levels < 100 mL/dL) as a result of a pathological process (DIC, severe liver disease, abruptio placentae, amniotic fluid embolus, massive transfusion); (b) active bleeding in patients with von Willebrand disease when desmopressin (DDAVP) is not effective or in patients with von Willebrand disease type 2B, or if factor VIII concentrate containing von Willebrand factor is not available; and (c) hemophilia type A when virally inactivated factor VIII concentrates are not available. Cryoprecipitate can also be used as fibrin surgical adhesives in surgical patients.

Cryoprecipitate should be ABO-compatible. The volume of each unit is 20 to 50 mL. The usual dose is 1 unit/5 kg of body weight (10 to 14 units for an adult) and will raise fibrinogen concentration to 75 mL/dL.

FIBRINOGEN CONCENTRATE

Fibrinogen concentrate is derived from pooled human plasma. It used to treat bleeding episodes in patients with congenital fibrinogen deficiency.

Fibrinogen is dosed according to the patient's fibrinogen baseline level, the target level (usually >150 mL/dL), volume of distribution, and body weight. If the baseline level is unknown, the initial dose is **fibrinogen concentrate** 70 mL/kg.

Prothrombin complex concentrate (PCC) is a blood-derived concentration of vitamin K-dependent clotting factors (factors II, VII, IX, and X). Some PCC formulations may also contain the anticoagulant proteins C, S, and antitrombin, as well as heparin. PCC administration does not necessitate ABO-compatibility testing.

COAGULATION FACTOR VIIA (RECOMBINANT)

Coagulation factor VIIa is primarily used for treatment of hemophilia A and B in patients who have developed inhibitor antibodies to factors VII or IX, respectively.

SPECIFIC FACTOR REPLACEMENT THERAPY

Table 137-2 outlines therapy for congenital coagulation factor deficiencies.

COMPLICATIONS OF TRANSFUSIONS

Acute complications include febrile nonhemolytic transfusion reaction (most common), acute hemolytic reaction, ABO incompatibility, allergic reaction and anaphylaxis, and transfusion related acute lung injury (TRALI).

TABLE 137-2 Replacement Therapy for Congenital Factor Deficiencies

Coagulation Factor	Approximate Incidence*	Replacement Therapy
Factor I (fibrinogen)	1 per million	Cryoprecipitate Fibrinogen concentrate
Factor II (prothrombin)	1 per 2 million	3- or 4-factor PCC for major bleeding
Factor V	1 per million	FFP
Factor VII	1 per 500,000	4-factor PCC for major bleeding Coagulation factor VIIa (recombinant)
Factor VIII†	1 per 5000–10,000 males	Recombinant factor VIII Desmopressin for mild hemophilia
Von Willebrand's disease‡	Up to 1 per 100 persons	Desmopressin or factor VIII concentrates (or cryoprecipitate if either unavailable)
Factor IX†	1 per 30,000 males	Recombinant factor IX 3- or 4-factor PCC
Factor X	1 per million	FFP for minor bleeding episodes 3- or 4-factor PCC for major bleeding
Factor XI‡	3 per 10,000 Ashkenazi Jews 1 per million in general population	FFP
Factor XII	25 per 1000	No bleeding manifestations, replacement not required
Factor XIII	1 per million	FFP or cryoprecipitate

Abbreviations: FFP, fresh frozen plasma; PCC, prothrombin complex concentrate.

**Source:* van Herrewegen F, Meijers JC, Peters M, van Ommen CH: Clinical practice: the bleeding child. Part II: disorders of secondary hemostasis and fibrinolysis. *Eur J Pediatr.* 2012;171:207.

†See Chapter 235, "Hemophilias and von Willebrand's Disease," in *Tintinalli's Emergency Medicine: A Comprehensive Study Guide*, 8th ed.

‡Factor XI levels correlate poorly with bleeding complications; many patients have low levels but no bleeding complications.

Two important first steps in any confirmed or suspected transfusion reaction are to (1) immediately stop the transfusion, and (2) contact the blood bank that issued the transfusion product. (3) Table 137-1 summarizes the clinical presentation, evaluation, and management of acute transfusion reactions.

Delayed transfusion complications present days or weeks after the index transfusion and include delayed hemolytic transfusion reaction, transfusion associated graft versus host disease, posttransfusion purpura, and infectious disease transmission.

FURTHER READING

For further reading in *Tintinalli's Emergency Medicine: A Comprehensive Study Guide*, 8th ed., see Chapter 238, "Transfusion Therapy," by Clinton J. Coil and Sally A. Santen.

CHAPTER 138

Anticoagulants, Antiplatelet Agents, and Fibrinolytics

Jessica L. Smith

Antithrombotic therapy is used to treat acute coronary syndrome, deep venous thrombosis (DVT), pulmonary embolism (PE), transient ischemic attack, and ischemic stroke. These agents are also used to prevent occlusive vascular events in patients at risk. Detailed management strategies and dosing regimens are provided in Chapter 18, "Acute Coronary Syndromes: Management of Myocardial Infarction and Unstable Angina," Chapter 25, "Thromboembolism," and Chapter 141, "Stroke and Transient Ischemic Attack." This chapter provides an overview of antithrombotic agents.

ORAL ANTICOAGULANTS

The goals of anticoagulant therapy include (1) stop further acute thrombosis, (2) reduce the risk of embolism from a thrombus, and (3) prevent the formation of de novo thrombus in patients at risk.

Warfarin is the most commonly used oral anticoagulant in the United States. It preferentially inhibits vitamin K-dependent cofactors in the extrinsic coagulation cascade. Dosing is guided by measuring the international normalized ratio (INR), and most patients are therapeutic in a range of 2 to 3. Patients with mechanical heart valves or antiphospholipid antibody syndrome require an INR of 2.5 to 3.5. It takes about 3 to 4 days to reach full anticoagulation upon initiating treatment. A parenteral anticoagulant should be used until the INR is maintained in the desired range for 2 days, as warfarin therapy causes a transient state of thrombogenesis for 24 to 36 hours at the start of therapy. Parenteral bridging is crucial in patients with prosthetic heart valves or those who are at high risk for catastrophic complications of intravascular thrombosis when initiating warfarin. Warfarin use is contraindicated during pregnancy due to teratogenicity. Complications of warfarin use include skin necrosis (associated with protein C deficiency) and increased bleeding risk in patients with hypertension, anemia, prior cerebrovascular disease, gastrointestinal (GI) lesions, or renal disease. A number of medications, foods, or disease states interfere with warfarin absorption or metabolism and cause clinically significant consequences. There are three approaches for warfarin reversal depending on the intensity of therapy and the patient's risk for recurrent thromboembolism: stop the warfarin, administer vitamin K, and replace deficient coagulation factors. Figure 138-1 describes the management of warfarin-induced coagulopathy.

Direct thrombin inhibitors like dabigatran, and factor Xa inhibitors like rivaroxaban, apixaban, and edoxaban, are used in nonvalvular atrial fibrillation to reduce systemic embolism and stroke risk. A normal thrombin clotting time excludes significant coagulopathy due to dabigatran. **Idarucizumab, 5 g IV**, can be used for dabigatran reversal. It may be repeated once, if needed No other reversal agent is currently available.

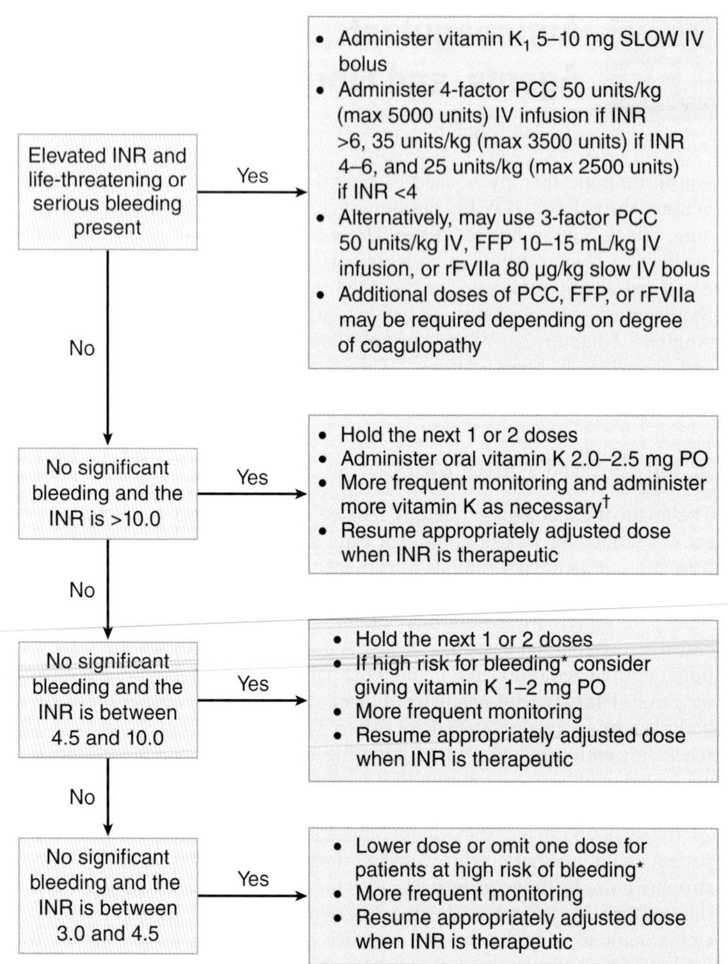

FIGURE 138-1. Management of prolonged INR (warfarin-induced coagulopathy). *High risk of bleeding: age >75 years, concurrent antiplatelet drug use, polypharmacy, liver or renal disease, alcoholism, recent surgery, or trauma. †There are no validated tools to predict risk of short-term major bleeding in patients with severe over-anticoagulation. The decision to admit for observation relies on physician judgment. FFP = fresh frozen plasma; IU = international unit; PCC = prothrombin complex concentrate; rFVIIa = recombinant activated factor VII.

Hemodialysis can remove 60% or more of dabigatran, but hemodialysis is not effective in removing rivaroxaban. If emergency reversal is needed for dabigatran or rivaroxaban, activated prothrombin complex concentrate or recombinant activated factor VII can be used. Fresh frozen plasma can also be used to reverse rivaroxaban, but has not been shown to have a major benefit in dabigatran reversal.

HEPARINS, POLYSACCHARIDES, AND HIRUDINS

Parenteral agents include unfractionated heparin (UFH), low-molecular-weight heparin (LMWH) (e.g., enoxaparin, dalteparin), Xa inhibitors (fondaparinux), and direct thrombin inhibitors (e.g., hirudin, lepirudin, bivalirudin, argatroban). UFH and LMWH are used to treat and prevent DVT, as well as PE, unstable angina, and acute myocardial infarction. Dosing regimens for UFH and LMWH are weight based. UFH requires monitoring of the activated partial thromboplastin time. Therapeutic range is 1.5 to 2.5 "normal" value. Heparin and LMWH may be used during pregnancy. Enoxaparin 1 mg/kg SC every 12 hours may be used in outpatient management of DVT. The two major complications of heparin are bleeding and heparin-induced thrombocytopenia (HIT). Hirudin, lepirudin, and argatroban can be used for anticoagulation in patients with HIT.

Although protamine can reverse the anticoagulation effects of heparin, the adverse effects of protamine are significant. LMWH carries a lower bleeding risk than UFH, but a higher bleeding risk in patients with renal disease. LMWH may also cause pruritis, local skin reaction, or rarely, skin necrosis.

ANTIPLATELET AGENTS

Oral agents include aspirin, clopidogrel, prasugrel, ticagrelor, dipyridamole, and cilostazol. Aspirin is an irreversible cyclooxygenase inhibitor; its effects last for the life of the platelet. Nonenteric-coated aspirin (162 to 325 mg) should be administered in the setting of ACS, although it is contraindicated during active GI hemorrhage, it is generally considered safe to give to closely monitored patients with guaiac positive stool. Nonsteroidal anti-inflammatories have the potential to reduce the efficacy of aspirin. Clopidogrel, prasugrel, and ticagrelor inhibit platelet activation by rendering the fibrinogen receptor ineffective. An oral loading dose of clopidogrel 600 mg results in full antiplatelet effect by 2 hours, and sustained effects last up to 48 hours. Side effects of aspirin are mainly GI and dose related. Complications of clopidogrel include dyspepsia, rash, or diarrhea. Omeprazole reduces clopidogrel's efficacy.

GPIIb/IIIa parenteral medications alter the common final pathway receptor in platelet aggregation. These agents should be used in consultation with the interventional cardiologist. Patients receiving GPIIb/IIIa agents are at increased risk of bleeding complications during cardiac catheterization or coronary artery bypass surgery, but are not at increased risk of intracranial hemorrhage.

FIBRINOLYTICS

Fibrinolytic agents include streptokinase, anistreplase, alteplase/tPA, reteplase, and tenecteplase. Although mechanisms of action vary, each agent eventually converts plasminogen to plasmin, which breaks down the

TABLE 138-1 General Contraindications to Fibrinolytic Therapy

Absolute
- Active or recent (<14 days) internal bleeding
- Ischemic stroke within the past 2–6 months
- Any prior hemorrhagic stroke
- Intracranial or intraspinal surgery or trauma within the past 2 months
- Intracranial or intraspinal neoplasm, aneurysm, or arteriovenous malformation
- Known severe bleeding diathesis
- Current anticoagulant treatment (e.g., warfarin with INR >1.7 or heparin with increased aPTT)
- Current use of a direct thrombin inhibitor or direct factor Xa inhibitor with evidence of anticoagulant effect by laboratory tests
- Platelet count <100,000/mm^3 (<100 × 10^9/L)
- Uncontrolled hypertension (i.e., blood pressure >185/110 mm Hg)
- Suspected aortic dissection or pericarditis
- Pregnancy

Relative*
- Active peptic ulcer disease
- Cardiopulmonary resuscitation for longer than 10 min
- Hemorrhagic ophthalmic conditions
- Puncture of noncompressible vessel within the past 10 days
- Significant trauma or major surgery within the past 2 weeks to 2 months
- Advanced renal or hepatic disease

*Concurrent menses is not a contraindication.

Abbreviation: aPTT = activated partial thromboplastin time.

fibrin in a thrombus. Alteplase/tPA theoretically causes less systemic fibrinolysis, without the antigenic side effects of streptokinase and anistreplase that prevent retreatment within 6 months and preclude treatment within 12 months of a streptococcal infection. Strict adherence to established guidelines and informed consent is essential. Hemorrhagic complications, including intracranial hemorrhage, may occur. Streptokinase and anistreplase may cause hypotension or anaphylaxis. Contraindications to fibrinolytic therapy are listed in Table 138-1.

COMPLICATIONS OF ANTITHROMBOTIC USE

Emergency treatment of bleeding complications of antithrombotic therapy is listed in Table 138-2.

TABLE 138-2 Emergency Treatment of Bleeding Complications of Antithrombotic Therapy

Agent	Management
Heparins	
Minor bleeding	Immediate cessation of heparin administration. Supratherapeutic aPTT not always present. Anticoagulation effect lasts up to 3 h from last IV dose. Observation with serial aPTT may be sufficient.

(Continued)

TABLE 138-2 Emergency Treatment of Bleeding Complications of Antithrombotic Therapy (Continued)

Agent	Management
Major bleeding	Protamine 1 mg IV per 100 units of total amount of IV UFH administered within the past 3 h. Protamine is given slowly IV over 1–3 min with a maximum of 50 mg over any 10-min period. Protamine has an anaphylaxis risk. Protamine does not completely reverse low-molecular-weight heparin. Enoxaparin: Protamine 1 mg IV (maximum dose, 50 mg) for every 1 mg of enoxaparin given in the previous 8 h. If 8–12 h since last enoxaparin dose, give protamine 0.5 mg IV for every 1 mg of enoxaparin given. Dalteparin and tinzaparin: Protamine 1 mg IV per every 100 units of dalteparin or tinzaparin given. If aPTT (measured 2–4 h after the protamine infusion) remains prolonged, give a second dose of protamine 0.5 mg IV per 100 units of dalteparin or tinzaparin.
Pentasaccharides	
Fondaparinux	Antithrombotic effect of fondaparinux is 24–30 h. For life-threatening bleeding, anecdotal evidence suggests rFVIIa 90 μg/kg IV is effective.
Oral Direct Thrombin Inhibitors	
Dabigatran	Oral activated charcoal if recent or excessive ingestion. Maintain urine output. Consider hemodialysis or charcoal hemoperfusion. For life-threatening bleeding, consider in descending order: aPCC, rFVIIa, or PCC. For severe bleeding or urgent reversal, administer Idarucizumab 5 g IV. Dose may be repeated x 1.
Oral Factor Xa Inhibitors	
Rivaroxaban	For major bleeding, experimental evidence suggests PCC can reverse the antithrombotic effect of rivaroxaban.
Apixaban	For major bleeding, administer andexanet alfa (when available), dose not established.
Oral Antiplatelet Agents	
Aspirin	Desmopressin 0.3–0.4 μg/kg IV over 30 min. Platelet transfusion to increase count by 50,000/mm^3 (typically requires one single donor apheresis-collected platelet concentrate or six units of random donor platelets). Aspirin-induced platelet inhibition may last for 7 days, so repeat platelet transfusions are sometimes required.
Other antiplatelet agents: clopidogrel, prasugrel, ticagrelor	Platelet transfusion to increase count by 50,000/mm^3 (typically requires one single donor apheresis-collected platelet concentrate or six units of random donor platelets). Desmopressin 0.3–0.4 μg/kg IV over 30 min. NSAID-induced platelet inhibition typically lasts <1 day. Clopidogrel-, prasugrel-, or ticagrelor-induced platelet inhibition may last up to 5–7 days.

(Continued)

TABLE 138-2 Emergency Treatment of Bleeding Complications of Antithrombotic Therapy (Continued)

Agent	Management
Fibrinolytics	
Minor external bleeding	Manual pressure.
Significant internal bleeding	Immediate cessation of fibrinolytic agent, antiplatelet agent, and/or heparin. Reversal of heparin with protamine as above. Typed and cross-matched blood ordered with verification of aPTT, CBC, thrombin clotting time, and fibrinogen level. Volume replacement with crystalloid and packed red blood cells as needed.
Major bleeding or hemodynamic compromise	All measures listed for significant internal bleeding. Fibrinogen concentrate 70 mg/kg IV, and recheck fibrinogen level; if fibrinogen level <100 mg/dL, repeat fibrinogen concentrate dose. If bleeding persists after fibrinogen concentrate or despite fibrinogen level >100 mg/dL, administer FFP two units IV. If bleeding continues after FFP, administer an antifibrinolytic such as aminocaproic acid 5 g IV over 60 min followed by 1 g/h continuous IV infusion for 8 h or until bleeding stops, or tranexamic acid 10 mg/kg IV every 6–8 h. Consider platelet transfusion.
Intracranial hemorrhage	All measures listed for significant internal and major bleeding with hemodynamic compromise. Immediate neurosurgery consultation.

Abbreviations: aPCC = activated prothrombin complex concentrate (not available in the United States); aPTT = activated partial thromboplastin time; FFP = fresh frozen plasma; NSAID = nonsteroidal anti-inflammatory drug; PCC = prothrombin complex concentrate; rFVIIa = recombinant activated factor VII; UFH = unfractionated heparin.

FURTHER READING

For further reading in *Tintinalli's Emergency Medicine: A Comprehensive Study Guide*, 8th ed., see Chapter 239, "Thrombotics and Antithrombotics," by David E. Slattery and Charles V. Pollack Jr.

CHAPTER 139

Emergency Complications of Malignancy

Ross J. Fleischman

Oncologic emergencies arise from the underlying malignancy or as complications of therapy.

AIRWAY OBSTRUCTION

Patients with tumors of the upper and lower respiratory tract may experience acute airway compromise due to edema, bleeding, infection, or loss of protective mechanisms. Presenting symptoms and signs include dyspnea, tachypnea, wheezing, and stridor. Imaging involves plain radiographs, CT scan, and/or endoscopic visualization. Emergency measures include humidified oxygen, optimal patient positioning, and possibly administration of a helium–oxygen mixture. If intubation is required, an "awake look" with a fiber optic bronchoscope with a 5-0 or 6-0 endotracheal tube is preferred. A surgical airway such as cricothyroidotomy, transtracheal jet ventilation, or tracheotomy may be needed.

BONE METASTASES AND PATHOLOGIC FRACTURES

Patient with solid tumors, most commonly in breast, lung, and prostate, may present with bony metastases and pathologic fractures, usually in the axial skeleton and proximal limbs. Plain radiographs may only identify half of metastases, so negative films should be followed by CT with contrast or MRI. Control pain with opioid analgesia. Most pathologic fractures require surgical intervention. Painful bone metastases are treated with radiotherapy.

SPINAL CORD COMPRESSION

Spinal cord compression from metastases to the vertebral bodies may cause weakness, radicular pain, and bowel or bladder dysfunction. MRI is the imaging study of choice. The presentation, evaluation, and management of malignant spinal cord compromise are described in Table 139-1.

Consider giving corticosteroids if imaging will be delayed. **Malignant spinal cord compression is a radiotherapy emergency.**

MALIGNANT PERICARDIAL EFFUSION

Malignant pericardial effusions are usually asymptomatic but can progress to life-threatening cardiac tamponade. Symptoms depend on the rate of accumulation (see Chapter 24, "The Cardiomyopathies, Myocarditis, and Pericardial Disease"). Patients with symptomatic effusions may present with chest heaviness, dyspnea, cough, and syncope. Physical examination findings include tachycardia, narrowed pulse pressure, hypotension, distended neck veins, muffled heart tones, and pulsus paradoxus.

TABLE 139-1 Malignant Spinal Cord Compression

Suspect	Most common cancers: lung, breast, prostate. Thoracic location: 70%. Progressive pain and worse when supine. Motor weakness: proximal legs. Sensory changes and bladder or bowel dysfunction: late findings.
Imaging	MRI: modality of choice, image entire vertebral column. Plain radiographs: may detect vertebral body metastases but less sensitive and specific for malignant spinal cord compression. CT myelography: used when MRI is not available.
Corticosteroids	Dexamethasone, 10 mg IV followed by 4 mg PO or IV every 6 h. Consider starting in ED if imaging is delayed.
Radiotherapy	Beneficial in approximately 70% of cases. Prognosis highly dependent on pretreatment neurologic function.
Surgery	Consider in highly selected cases, such as: Patient in good general condition and able to undergo extensive surgery Appropriate prognostic life expectancy Rapidly progressive symptoms Clinical worsening during radiotherapy Unstable vertebral column

Echocardiography is the test of choice as it can demonstrate the presence of tamponade. Chest radiograph may demonstrate an enlarged cardiac silhouette or pleural effusion. ECG may show sinus tachycardia, low QRS amplitude, or electrical alternans. The differential diagnosis includes cardiomyopathy related to chemotherapy, such as doxorubin and radiation therapy. Asymptomatic effusions do not require specific treatment. Symptomatic effusions are treated with ultrasound-guided pericardiocentesis.

SUPERIOR VENA CAVA SYNDROME

Superior vena cava (SVC) syndrome most commonly occurs due to external compression of the superior vena cava by an external malignant mass such as lung cancer or lymphoma. It is less commonly caused by intravascular thrombosis. The most common symptoms are face or arm swelling, distended neck veins, dyspnea, cough, and chest pain. CT of the chest with IV contrast is the diagnostic procedure of choice. CXR will usually show a mediastinal mass.

Patients with neurologic symptoms require urgent treatment including supplemental oxygen and elevation of the head and upper body. **Dexamethasone** 20 mg IV or **methylprednisolone** 125 to 250 mg IV may be beneficial in patients with increased intracranial pressure or lymphoma. In patients without neurologic symptoms, SVC syndrome usually does not cause rapid deterioration and can await consultation regarding chemotherapy, radiation, or intravascular stenting. Patients with intravascular thrombosis may require anticoagulation, fibrinolysis, or catheter removal.

HYPERCALCEMIA OF MALIGNANCY

Hypercalcemia is most commonly seen with breast cancer, lung cancer, and multiple myeloma. The symptoms are nonspecific and include polydipsia, polyuria, generalized weakness, lethargy, anorexia, nausea, constipation, abdominal pain, volume depletion, and altered mentation.

Signs and symptoms are related to the rate of rise and may occur above 12 mg/dL (ionized >5.5 mg/dL). ECG may show shortened QT interval, ST depression, and atrioventricular blocks.

Normal saline infusion to restore normovolemia followed by an infusion of 250 mL/h if the patient can tolerate is the mainstay of treatment. Furosemide is not recommended unless needed to prevent volume overload in patients with cardiac or renal failure. Further treatment should be discussed with the patient's oncologist. Bisphosphonates such as **zoledronic acid** 4 mg IV over 15 minutes or **pamidronate** 60 to 90 mg IV over 4 to 24 hours can prevent bone resorption. **Calcitonin** 4 IU/kg SC or IM causes a more rapid decrease in calcium levels. **Glucocorticoids** may be helpful in lymphoma and multiple myeloma. Consider hemodialysis for patients with profound mental status changes and renal failure, or those who cannot tolerate a normal saline infusion (see Chapter 4, "Fluids, Electrolytes, and Acid Base Disorders").

HYPONATREMIA DUE TO SYNDROME OF INAPPROPRIATE ANTI-DIURETIC HORMONE (SIADH)

Inappropriate anti-diuretic hormone secretion is most commonly associated with bronchogenic lung cancer, but can also occur from chemotherapy or medications. Symptoms include anorexia, nausea, headache, altered mentation, and seizures. Mild hyponatremia (>125 mEq/L) is usually asymptomatic.

SIADH should be suspected in patients with cancer who present with normovolemic hyponatremia. Laboratory abnormalities include serum osmolality <280 mOsm/L, urine osmolality >100 mOsm/L, and urine sodium >20 mEq/L. The differential diagnosis includes hypothyroidism, renal failure, cirrhosis, adrenal crisis, and hypovolemia/hypervolemia.

Mild hyponatremia >125 mEq/L is treated with a water restriction of 500 mL/d and close follow-up. More severe hyponatremia is treated with **furosemide** 0.5 to 1 mg/kg PO with normal saline infusion to maintain normovolemia. **Three percent hypertonic saline** is reserved for severe hyponatremia <120 mEq/L with seizures or coma. An infusion of 25 to 100 mL/h should be titrated to a correction of 0.5 to 1 mEq/h with a maximum of 12 mEq/L/d (see Chapter 4, "Fluids, Electrolytes, and Acid Base Disorders").

ADRENAL CRISIS

Adrenal crisis is most commonly caused by acute physiologic stress in the face of exogenous steroid-induced adrenal suppression or malignant infiltration of adrenal tissue. Symptoms include weakness or nausea, and hypotension unresponsive to fluids. Laboratory abnormalities may include hypoglycemia, hyponatremia, and hyperkalemia. A serum cortisol level is ideally drawn before giving steroids. Treat acute adrenal insufficiency empirically with stress-dose **hydrocortisone** 100 to 150 mg IV, **methyl-prednisolone** 20 to 30 mg IV, or **dexamethasone** 4 mg IV, IV crystalloids, and supportive care (see Chapter 132, "Adrenal Insufficiency and Adrenal Crisis").

TUMOR LYSIS SYNDROME

Tumor lysis syndrome occurs when massive quantities of potassium, phosphate, and uric acid are released. It usually occurs 1 to 3 days after chemotherapy for acute leukemia or lymphoma. The resulting hyperuricemia, hyperkalemia, hyperphosphatemia, and hypocalcemia may cause uric acid precipitates and calcium phosphate deposits in the kidney with renal failure, life-threatening arrhythmias, tetany, and seizures. Laboratory evaluation should include 12-lead ECG, basic electrolyte levels, complete blood count, uric acid, and phosphorus.

Preventative measures reduce the incidence of tumor lysis syndrome. Hyperkalemia is the most immediate life threat. Treatment of hyperkalemia is with **insulin, glucose, bicarbonate** (if acidotic), and **albuterol** (see Chapter 4, "Fluids, Electrolytes, and Acid Base Disorders"). Avoid calcium unless ventricular arrhythmias or widened QRS complexes are seen, as it may worsen calcium phosphate precipitation in the kidney. Aggressive infusion of **isotonic fluids** reverses volume depletion and helps to prevent renal deposition of uric acid and calcium phosphate crystals. Manage hyperphosphatemia with IV **insulin** and **glucose**. Phosphate binders have a limited effect. Consider hemodialysis for potassium levels above 6.0 mEq/L, uric acid levels above 10.0 mg/dL, phosphate levels above 10 mg/dL, creatinine levels above 10 mg/dL, symptomatic hypocalcemia, or volume overload. Patients with tumor lysis syndrome should be admitted to an intensive care unit.

FEBRILE NEUTROPENIA

Febrile neutropenia is defined by temperatures above 38°C for an hour or a single temperature above 38.3°C with an absolute neutrophil count below 1000 cells/mm^3. Neutrophil counts typically reach a nadir 10 to 15 days after chemotherapy and rebound 5 days later.

Febrile neutropenic patients often lack localizing signs and symptoms because of an attenuated immune response. Meticulous attention must be paid to all skin surfaces, mucosal areas, and vascular access sites in which the patient may have an occult infection. Digital rectal examination is often withheld until after initial antibiotic administration because of the fear of inducing bacteremia.

Laboratory evaluation includes complete blood count with differential, blood cultures obtained through all lumens of indwelling catheters as well as a peripheral site, urinalysis, urine culture, and CXR, electrolytes, renal, and liver function tests. Additional studies based on symptoms may include stool culture (diarrhea), sputum culture (cough), lumbar puncture (headache, stiff neck, altered mental status), wound culture (drainage), and CT or ultrasound (abdominal pain).

The decision for empiric antibiotics and admission should be made with the patient's oncologist. Empiric antibiotics (Table 139-2) are generally

TABLE 139-2 Initial Empiric Antibiotic Therapy in Febrile Neutropenia

Circumstance	Drug and Adult Dosage	Comments
Outpatient	Ciprofloxacin, 500 mg PO every 8 h *and* Amoxicillin/clavulanate, 500 mg PO every 8 h	Useful for low-risk patients with daily assessments by a medical provider for the initial 3 days.
Monotherapy	Cefepime, 2 g IV every 8 h *or* Ceftazidime, 2 g IV every 8 h *or* Imipenem/cilastatin, 1 g IV every 8 h *or* Meropenem, 1 g IV every 8 h *or* Piperacillin/tazobactam, 4.5 g IV every 6 h	Monotherapy with these broad-spectrum agents appears to be as good as dual-drug therapy in most circumstances.
Dual therapy	One of the monotherapy agents *plus* Gentamicin, 1.7 mg/kg IV every 8 h *or* Tobramycin, 1.7 mg/kg IV every 8 h *or* Amikacin, 5 mg/kg IV every 8 h	Potential advances include synergistic effects against some gram-negative bacteria and reduced emergence of drug resistance. There is an increased risk for adverse effects, including nephrotoxicity, ototoxicity, and hypokalemia.
Risk factors for severe gram-positive infection (see text)	Vancomycin, 1 g IV every 12 h *plus* Cefepime, 2 g IV every 8 h *or* Ceftazidime, 2 g IV every 8 h *or* Imipenem/cilastatin, 1 g IV every 8 h *or* Meropenem, 1 g IV every 8 h	Vancomycin is not usually necessary for initial empiric antibiotic therapy. Vancomycin may be incorporated into initial therapeutic regimens of high-risk patients in institutions with increased gram-positive infection rates.

indicated for an ANC <500/mm^3. For neutrophil counts between 500 and 1000, the decision is based on the patient's presentation. Add **vancomycin** for severe mucositis, catheter site infection, recent use of fluoroquinolone prophylaxis, hypotension, residence in an institution with hospital-associated methicillin-resistant *Staphylococcus aureus*, or known colonization with resistant gram-positive organisms.

HYPERVISCOSITY SYNDROME

Hyperviscosity syndrome refers to impaired blood flow due to abnormal elevations of paraproteins or blood cells. It is most common in patients with dysproteinemia (e.g., Waldenstrom's macroglobulimenia and multiple myeloma), acute leukemia, or polycythemia. Hematocrits above 60% and WBC counts above 100,000/mm^3 may cause hyperviscosity syndromes.

Initial symptoms include fatigue, abdominal pain, headache, blurry vision, dyspnea, fever, or altered mental status. Thrombosis or bleeding may occur. Physical exam findings may include retinal hemorrhages, exudates, and "sausage-linked" vessels. Elevated serum viscosity (>4) or rouleaux formation (red cells stacked like coins) support the diagnosis. Serum viscosity measurement will not identify hyperviscosity caused by polycythemia or leukemia.

Initial therapy consists of intravenous **isotonic fluids** and **plasmapheresis** or **leukopheresis** in consultation with a hematologist. A temporizing measure in patients with coma is 1000 mL **phlebotomy** with simultaneous infusion of 2 to 3 L normal saline.

THROMBOEMBOLISM

Thromboembolism is the second leading cause of death in cancer patients. See Chapter 25 for discussion of the diagnosis and management of deep vein thrombosis and pulmonary embolism. Low-molecular-weight heparin (LMWH) is the recommended initial treatment for cancer patients with venous thromboembolism and is usually continued for the duration of treatment for the clot. There is insufficient experience with the new oral anticoagulants to recommend them.

NAUSEA AND VOMITING

Chemotherapy commonly causes nausea and vomiting. Other causes of nausea and vomiting include radiation enteritis, bowel obstruction, infection or tumor infiltration, and increased intracranial pressure. Treatment consists of rehydration, administration of antiemetics, and correction of electrolyte derangements (Table 139-3).

TABLE 139-3 Antiemetic Agents for Chemotherapy-Induced Vomiting

Class and Agent	Adult Dose	Comments
Dopamine receptor antagonists		
Metoclopramide	10 mg IV or IM	Dose-related extrapyramidal side effects
Promethazine	25 mg IV or IM	IV use common but not approved by the FDA
Serotonin antagonists		
Dolasetron	0.35 mg/kg IV, max 12.5 mg over 5 min	Constipation, headaches (all)
Granisetron	10 μg/kg IV over 5 min	
Ondansetron	0.15 mg/kg IV, max 16mg over 15 min	
Corticosteroids		
Dexamethasone	20 mg IV	Mechanism unknown, no immunosuppression
Benzodiazepines		
Lorazepam	1 to 2 mg IV	Sedation, anxiolysis
Histamine receptor antagonists		
Diphenhydramine	50 mg IV or IM	Minor therapeutic effect

Abbreviation: FDA, Food and Drug Administration.

EXTRAVASATION OF CHEMOTHERAPEUTIC AGENTS

Clinical manifestations of extravasation include pain, erythema, and swelling, usually within hours of the infusion. Consult with the patient's oncologist to discuss the use of antidotes for extravasation of anthracyclines, vinca alkaloids, mitomycin, cisplatin, mechlorethamine, and paclitaxel.

FURTHER READING

For further reading in *Tintinalli's Emergency Medicine: A Comprehensive Study Guide*, 8th ed., see Chapter 240, "Emergency Complications of Malignancy," by J. Stephan Stapczynski.

SECTION 15

Neurology

CHAPTER 140 Headache

Steven Go

CLINICAL FEATURES

Headache is a common complaint for patients presenting to an emergency department (ED). The majority of headaches have benign causes (96%), although evaluating patients for potential high-risk features may be useful when screening for headaches associated with significant morbidity or mortality (see Table 140-1).

TABLE 140-1 High-Risk Features for Headache: Clinical "Red Flags"

Onset	Sudden Trauma Exertion
Symptoms	Altered mental status Seizure Fever Neurologic symptoms Visual changes
Medications	Anticoagulants/antiplatelets Recent antibiotic use Immunosuppressants
Past history	No prior headache Change in headache quality, or progressive headache worsening over weeks/months
Associated conditions	Pregnancy or postpregnancy status Systemic lupus erythematosus Behçet's disease Vasculitis Sarcoidosis Cancer
Physical examination	Altered mental status Fever Neck stiffness Papilledema Focal neurologic signs

DIAGNOSIS AND DIFFERENTIAL

Identify patients with high-risk features, such as patients older than 50 years with a new or worsening headache. Sudden onset of a maximum intensity headache, often described as a "thunderclap headache," is associated 10% to 14% of the time with a high-risk etiology (see Table 140-2).

Assess headache quality, pattern, frequency, intensity, location, and any associated symptoms such as fever or visual changes. Additional information such as medication history, potential toxic exposures, prior headache history, substance abuse, comorbid conditions, or family history of headaches may be useful.

Tailor the physical examination based on patient history to identify potential causes of headache. Specific physical examination findings may help to focus potential diagnoses, such as the presence of fever, hypertension, sinus or temporal artery tenderness, papilledema or elevated intraocular pressure, neck stiffness, or neurologic abnormalities.

While laboratory testing is often of limited value in the workup of an acute headache, erythrocyte sedimentation rate (ESR) and/or C-reactive protein (CRP) are useful when temporal arteritis is suspected. When indicated, a noncontrast head CT scan can be useful to evaluate for intracranial hemorrhage, subdural hematoma, space-occupying lesion, signs of potentially elevated intracranial pressure, or subarachnoid hemorrhage. Additional diagnostic studies may be indicated when the head CT is negative, for example, if clinical suspicion remains for a subarachnoid hemorrhage. Depending on clinical suspicion, other imaging modalities may be useful, such as MRI to assess for cerebral venous thrombosis, and MR or CT angiography to evaluate for arterial dissection or small subarachnoid hemorrhage. Lumbar puncture can be utilized when meningitis or encephalitis is suspected (see Chapter 148, "Central Nervous System and Spinal Infections") or to look for evidence of subarachnoid hemorrhage after a negative CT scan (see Chapter 141, "Stroke Syndromes and Spontaneous Subarachnoid Hemorrhage").

Consider **subdural hematoma** or **intracerebral hemorrhage** as potential sources of headache in elderly patients, alcoholics, substance abusers, and in patients taking antiplatelet or anticoagulation medications. Consider

TABLE 140-2 Causes of Thunderclap Headache

Hemorrhage	Intracranial hemorrhage "Sentinel" aneurysmal hemorrhage Spontaneous intracerebral hemorrhage
Vascular	Carotid or vertebrobasilar dissection Reversible cerebral vasoconstriction syndrome (RCVS) Cerebral venous thrombosis Posterior reversible encephalopathy syndrome (PRES)
Other causes	Coital headache Valsalva-associated headache Spontaneous intracranial hypotension Acute hydrocephalus (e.g., colloid cyst obstructing third ventricle) Pituitary apoplexy

cerebellar hemorrhage when headache is associated with vestibular symptoms as this may need surgical consultation.

Headaches associated with **brain tumors** may be bilateral, unilateral, constant, or intermittent. These are classically described as worse upon awakening, worsened by Valsalva maneuver, positional, and associated with nausea and vomiting. Consider the possibility of primary or metastatic brain lesions in patients with known cancer diagnoses, seizures, or mental status changes.

Risk factors for **cerebral venous thrombosis** include patients with hypercoagulable states due to oral contraceptive use, postpartum or perioperative status, clotting factor deficiencies, or polycythemia. Papilledema may be present, and neurological findings can wax and wane. Lumbar puncture may demonstrate an increased opening pressure, and MR venography is most useful for diagnosis.

Temporal arteritis (see Table 140-3) presents most commonly in patients over the age of 50 and its incidence increases with age. Associated symptoms may include fatigue, fever, jaw claudication, and vision changes. The involved temporal artery may be tender, nonpulsatile, or have a diminished pulse, but can also be normal. ESR and CRP can be helpful in establishing the diagnosis, and a temporal artery biopsy allows a definitive diagnosis.

Migraine headaches are the most common benign cause of headache in ED patients. These generally have a gradual onset, last 4 to 72 hours, and are typically unilateral, pulsating, and worsened by physical activity. Nausea and vomiting, photophobia, and phonophobia are frequently present, and the headache may be associated with or without an aura.

Idiopathic intracranial hypertension, also known as pseudotumor cerebri, is most common in obese women ages 20 to 44. This may present with headaches, transient vision disturbances, back pain, and pulsatile tinnitus, and when left untreated can lead to permanent vision loss. The diagnosis is most often made by the presence of papilledema, a normal neurological examination, and elevated lumbar puncture opening pressure.

Intracranial hypotension can occur after a procedure that violates the dura such as lumbar puncture or epidural anesthesia. This headache is typically worsened with upright posture and improved with lying down. Alterations in hearing or vision, nausea, and vomiting may occur.

TABLE 140-3 American College of Rheumatology Criteria for Diagnosis of Temporal Arteritis

Clinical Features	Comments
Age at disease onset ≥50 years	
New headache	Onset or type
Temporal artery abnormality	Tenderness to palpation of temporal arteries Decreased pulsation of temporal arteries
Erythrocyte sedimentation rate ≥50 mm/h	Westergren method
Abnormal artery biopsy (can be done after initiating steroids)	Vasculitis Predominance of mononuclear cell infiltration or granulomatous inflammation Multinucleated giant cells

Cluster headaches are uncommon and present with severe pain that is unilateral and located in the orbital, supraorbital, or temporal area. These are frequently associated with lacrimation, nasal congestion, rhinorrhea, conjunctival injection, and pacing in the exam room. These symptoms tend to occur daily for weeks, with periods of remission that may last for for weeks to years.

EMERGENCY DEPARTMENT CARE AND DISPOSITION

1. Assess patients with an initial history and physical examination. When indicated, utilize appropriate diagnostic testing and/or neuroimaging based on risk factors, patient history, and physical findings. Disease-specific treatment and specialty consultation are indicated in the appropriate clinical circumstances.
2. When temporal arteritis is suspected in patients without vision loss, begin empiric treatment with oral **prednisone** 60 mg daily. Consult with an ophthalmologist or other appropriate specialist to arrange a temporal artery biopsy to confirm the diagnosis and for appropriate follow-up and continued treatment.
3. Treat patients with migraine headache with medications for symptom relief that may include **dihydroergotamine (DHE)**, **sumatriptan**, and dopamine-antagonist antiemetics such as **metoclopramide**, **chlorpromazine**, or **prochlorperazine** (see Table 140-4). Consider **dexamethasone** 6 to 10 mg IV as an adjunctive therapy that may reduce migraine recurrence.
4. Treat patients with idiopathic intracranial hypertension with a starting dose of oral **acetazolamide** 250 to 500 mg twice a day and recommend weight loss for obese patients. During a diagnostic lumbar puncture, excess cerebrospinal fluid can be removed to reduce intracranial pressure to 15 to 20 cm H_2O. Consult with a neurologist and/or ophthalmologist for ongoing evaluation and treatment.
5. Patients with intracranial hypotension due to lumbar puncture or epidural anesthesia often respond well to symptomatic treatment. Evidence of efficacy for intravenous fluids and caffeine is limited. The most effective treatment is an epidural blood patch, typically performed by an anesthesiologist.
6. Treat cluster headaches with high-flow oxygen delivered at 12 L/min for 15 minutes via a nonrebreathing facemask. Consider **sumitriptan** 6 mg subcutaneous injection for pain that is unresolved with oxygen therapy.
7. Consult with appropriate specialists based on the suspected underlying cause of headache, if symptom control is not adequately achieved in the ED, or if admission for further diagnostic testing or treatment may be needed.
8. When patients are discharged home, discuss indications for return and reassessment such as worsening of symptoms, failure to improve, or the development of new symptoms such as fever, neck stiffness, vision changes, or neurological abnormalities. Advise patients about expected side effects of medications prescribed or given in the ED. Recommend appropriate follow-up and outpatient management instructions based on the suspected diagnosis.

TABLE 140-4 Treatment Options for Migraine Headache

Drug	Dosing	Contraindications	Precautions and Pregnancy Category	Notes
Ketorolac	30 mg IV or IM	History of peptic ulcer disease (especially in elderly)	Pregnancy Category B Avoid in third trimester	
Prochlorperazine	5–10 mg IV or PR		Pregnancy Category C Drowsiness Dystonic reactions	**Antiemetic** Concurrent: diphenhydramine
Metoclopramide	10 mg IV		Pregnancy Category B Drowsiness Dystonic reactions	**Antiemetic** Concurrent: diphenhydramine
Droperidol	2.5 mg IV slow, or 2.5 mg IM		Pregnancy Category C QT interval prolongation and/or torsade de pointes	Concurrent: diphenhydramine
Chlorpromazine	7.5 mg IV		Pregnancy not classified Hypotension Drowsiness Dystonic reactions	**Antiemetic** Pretreat with: normal saline bolus to minimize hypotension Concurrent: diphenhydramine
Magnesium sulfate	2 g IV over 30 min		Pregnancy Category D but effective in pre-eclampsia and eclampsia	Nonvalidated
Methylprednisolone	125 mg IV or IM		Rescue therapy	Nonvalidated
Dexamethasone	6–10 mg IV		Rescue therapy	Adjunctive therapy to reduce recurrence
Sumatriptan	6 mg SC	Ischemic Heart Disease Uncontrolled hypertension Basilar or hemiplegic migraine	Pregnancy Category C	
Dihydroergotamine (DHE)	1 mg IV over 3 min	Pregnancy Uncontrolled hypertension Ischemic Heart Disease Recent sumatriptan use (within 24 h) Basilar or hemiplegic migraine	Pregnancy Category X Nausea Vomiting Diarrhea Abdominal pain	Pretreat with antiemetic
Valproate	500 mg IV	Pregnancy	Pregnancy Category X	Nonvalidated

FURTHER READING

For further reading in *Tintinalli's Emergency Medicine: A Comprehensive Study Guide*, 8th ed., see Chapter 165, "Headache" by Michael Harrigan and Ana C.G. Felix.

Stroke Syndromes and Spontaneous Subarachnoid Hemorrhage

Steven Go

Stroke encompasses any disease process that interrupts normal blood flow to the brain. Ischemic strokes (87%) are more common than intracerebral hemorrhage (10%) or nontraumatic subarachnoid hemorrhage (SAH) (3%) (Table 141-1). A transient ischemic attack (TIA) is a transient episode of neurological dysfunction caused by ischemia but without an acute infarction of brain tissue. TIA episodes typically lasts less than 1 to 2 hours, but duration of symptoms alone can be unreliable in discriminating between TIA and stroke as they are similar disease processes on a continuum of severity.

CLINICAL FEATURES

Specific findings in patients with ischemic or hemorrhagic stroke depend on the regions of the brain that are compromised and the severity of the insult (Table 141-2).

Typical symptoms of anterior cerebral artery involvement include contralateral leg weakness and sensory changes. A middle cerebral artery stroke presents with contralateral hemiparesis (arm > leg), facial plegia, and sensory loss. Aphasia is often present if the dominant hemisphere (usually left) is affected. Inattention, neglect, and dysarthria without aphasia are all signs of nondominant hemisphere involvement.

A posterior circulation stroke can present with subtle clinical findings. Unilateral limb weakness, dizziness, vertigo, blurry vision, headache, dysarthria, visual field loss, gait ataxia, cranial nerve VII dysfunction, lethargy, and sensory deficits can occur alone or in various combinations. Basilar artery occlusion can produce these symptoms, as well as oculomotor signs, Horner's syndrome, and rarely, a "locked-in" state. Cerebellar strokes present similarly to other posterior stroke syndromes, but these patients can deteriorate rapidly if a hematoma or edema is present.

Cervical artery dissection can involve either the anterior or posterior arterial systems and symptoms reflect the area of compromised brain tissue. A patient with an internal carotid dissection may present with unilateral head pain (68%), neck pain (39%), or face pain (10%). Vertebral artery dissections may present with neck pain (66%) and headache (65%), which can be unilateral or bilateral.

Intracranial hemorrhages may be clinically indistinguishable from cerebral infarction on physical examination and patients may present with similar neurological deficits. SAH is classically described as a sudden onset of headache at its maximal intensity ("thunderclap" headache), although patients with severe headaches and significant changes in intensity or quality from previous experiences may prompt consideration for this or other intracranial abnormalities in appropriate clinical circumstances. Approximately 20% of patients who presented with SAH had onset of symptoms

TABLE 141-1 Stroke Classification

Stroke Type	Mechanism	Major Causes	Clinical Notes
Ischemic			
Thrombotic	Narrowing of a damaged vascular lumen by an in situ process—usually clot formation	Atherosclerosis Vasculitis Arterial dissection Polycythemia Hypercoagulable state Infection (human immunodeficiency virus infection, syphilis, trichinosis, tuberculosis, aspergillosis)	Symptoms often have gradual onset and may wax and wane. Common cause of transient ischemic attack.
Embolic	Obstruction of a normal vascular lumen by intravascular material from a remote source	Valvular vegetations Mural thrombi Paradoxical emboli Cardiac tumors (myxomas) Arterial-arterial emboli from proximal source Fat emboli Particulate emboli (IV drug use) Septic emboli	Typically sudden in onset. Account for 20% of ischemic strokes.
Hypoperfusion	Low–blood flow state leading to hypoperfusion of the brain	Cardiac failure resulting in systemic hypotension	Diffuse injury pattern in watershed regions. Symptoms may wax and wane with hemodynamic factors.
Hemorrhagic			
Intracerebral	Intraparenchymal hemorrhage from previously weakened arterioles	Hypertension Amyloidosis Latrogenic anticoagulation Vascular malformations Cocaine use	Intracranial pressure rise causes local neuronal damage. Secondary vasoconstriction mediated by blood breakdown products or neuronal mechanisms (diaschisis) can cause remote perfusion changes. Risks include advanced age, history of stroke, and tobacco or alcohol use. More common in those of Asian or African descent.
Nontraumatic subarachnoid	Hemorrhage into subarachnoid space	Berry aneurysm rupture Vascular malformation rupture	May be preceded by a sentinel headache ("warning leak").

associated with activities known to elevate blood pressure, such as sexual intercourse, weight lifting, defecation, or coughing. Loss of consciousness, seizure, diplopia, vomiting, photophobia, nuchal irritation, low-grade fever, and altered mental status all may occur. The presence or absence of focal neurological findings depends on the location of the aneurysm.

TABLE 141-2 Anterior and Posterior Circulation of the Brain

Circulation	Major Arteries	Major Regions of Brain Supplied
Anterior (internal carotid system)	Ophthalmic	Optic nerve and retina
	Anterior cerebral	Frontal pole Anteromedial cerebral cortex Anterior corpus callosum
	Middle cerebral	Frontoparietal lobe Anterotemporal lobe
Posterior (vertebral system)	Vertebral Posteroinferior cerebellar Basilar Posterior cerebral Medial temporal lobe	Brainstem Cerebellum Thalamus Auditory/vestibular structures Visual occipital cortex

DIAGNOSIS AND DIFFERENTIAL

Patients with stroke may present variably and sometimes subtly. Assess for stroke risk factors based on age and comorbidities such as atrial fibrillation, hypertension, diabetes, smoking, coronary atherosclerosis, valvular replacement, and recent myocardial infarction. Risk factors for SAH include excessive alcohol consumption, polycystic kidney disease, family history of SAH, Marfan's syndrome, and Ehlers–Danlos syndrome. Inquire about a history of drug use, chiropractic manipulation, or recent activities associated with blood-pressure elevation. Consider alternative diagnoses that may mimic stroke (Table 141-3). If ischemic stroke is the primary working diagnosis and thrombolytic therapy is being considered, it is essential to obtain an accurate determination of the time the patient was last known to be at their neurological baseline and whether the patient may be a candidate for thrombolytic therapy (Tables 141-4 and 141-5).

Focus patient assessment on the neurological examination, with particular emphasis on detecting motor weakness, sensory deficits, and cerebellar dysfunction. Depending on clinical circumstances, investigate other findings such as meningismus, carotid bruits, signs of embolic disease, papilledema, or preretinal hemorrhage. Calculate a National Institutes of Health Stroke Scale (NIHSS) score if thrombolytic therapy may be considered. Appropriately expedite the history, physical examination, laboratory, and radiographic imaging.

An emergent noncontrasted CT scan of the brain (best interpreted by a neuroradiologist) is essential to determine whether hemorrhage or a stroke mimic is present. Most acute ischemic strokes will not be visualized on a CT scan in the early hours of a stroke.

The differential diagnosis for SAH is broad and includes intracranial hemorrhage, drug toxicity, ischemic stroke, meningitis, encephalitis, intracranial tumor, venous sinus thrombosis, and primary headache syndromes. Modern CT scanners are reported to be 98% sensitive to detect SAH within 6 to 12 hours of symptom onset, 91% to 93% at 24 hours, and 50% at 1 week. If SAH is suspected and the CT is negative, many clinicians recommend a lumbar puncture to assess for the presence of red blood cells or xanthochromia as evidence of subarachnoid blood that was not visualized on CT scan. However, some recent studies have challenged this position and suggest that

TABLE 141-3 Stroke Mimics

Disorder	Distinguishing Clinical Features
Seizures/postictal paralysis (Todd's paralysis)	Transient paralysis following a seizure, which typically disappears quickly; can be confused with transient ischemic attack. Seizures can be secondary to a cerebrovascular accident.
Syncope	No persistent or associated neurologic symptoms.
Meningitis/encephalitis	Fever, immunocompromised state may be present, meningismus, detectable on lumbar puncture.
Complicated migraine	History of similar episodes, preceding aura, headache.
Brain neoplasm or abscess	Focal neurologic findings, signs of infection, detectable by imaging.
Epidural/subdural hematoma	History of trauma, alcoholism, anticoagulant use, bleeding disorder; detectable by imaging.
Subarachnoid hemorrhage	Sudden onset of severe headache.*
Hypoglycemia	Can be detected by bedside glucose measurement, history of diabetes mellitus.
Hyponatremia	History of diuretic use, neoplasm, excessive free water intake.
Hypertensive encephalopathy	Gradual onset; global cerebral dysfunction, headache, delirium, hypertension, cerebral edema.
Hyperosmotic coma	Extremely high glucose levels, history of diabetes mellitus.
Wernicke's encephalopathy	History of alcoholism or malnutrition; triad of ataxia, ophthalmoplegia, and confusion.
Labyrinthitis	Predominantly vestibular symptoms; patient should have no other focal findings; can be confused with cerebellar stroke.
Drug toxicity (lithium, phenytoin, carbamazepine)	Can be detected by particular toxidromes and elevated blood levels. Phenytoin and carbamazepine toxicity may present with ataxia, vertigo, nausea, and abnormal reflexes.
Bell's palsy	Neurologic deficit confined to isolated *peripheral* seventh nerve palsy; often associated with younger age.
Ménière's disease	History of recurrent episodes dominated by vertigo symptoms, tinnitus, deafness.
Demyelinating disease (multiple sclerosis)	Gradual onset. Patient may have a history of multiple episodes of neurologic findings in multifocal anatomic distributions.
Conversion disorder	No cranial nerve findings, nonanatomic distribution of findings (e.g., midline sensory loss), inconsistent history or examination findings.

*Although subarachnoid hemorrhage is a type of stroke, it has special considerations in terms of diagnosis and management. See Chapter 166, "Spontaneous Subarachnoid and Intracerebral Hemorrhage," in *Tintinalli's Emergency Medicine: A Comprehensive Study Guide*, 8th ed.

TABLE 141-4 American Heart Association (AHA)/American Stroke Association (ASA) 2013 Inclusion/Exclusion Criteria for IV Recombinant Tissue Plasminogen Activator (rtPA) in Acute Ischemic Stroke

Inclusion Criteria	
Measurable diagnosis of acute ischemic stroke	Use of NIHSS score recommended. Major strokes (NIHSS score >22) are more likely to have poor outcomes.
Onset of symptoms <3 h prior to rtPA administration	Must be *well established* and is defined as the time of the witnessed onset of symptoms or the time the patient was last known at baseline.
Age ≥18 years	No clear upper age limit.
Exclusion Criteria	
Significant head trauma or prior stroke in previous 3 months Symptoms suggest subarachnoid hemorrhage Arterial puncture at noncompressible site ≤7 days ago History of previous intracranial hemorrhage Intracranial neoplasm, arteriovenous malformation, or aneurysm* Recent intracranial or intraspinal surgery* Pretreatment systolic blood pressure >185 mm Hg *or* diastolic blood pressure >110 mm Hg despite therapy Active internal bleeding*	
Platelet count <100,000/mm^3	If patient has no history of thrombocytopenia, rtPA may be given before this lab result is available; however, rtPA should be stopped if the platelet count is <100,000/mm^3
Use of heparin within preceding 48 h *and* a prolonged activated partial thromboplastin time (aPTT) greater than upper limit of normal	
International normalized ratio (INR) >1.7 or partial thromboplastin time (PTT) >15 s	Oral anticoagulant use in and of itself is not a contraindication to rtPA. If patient is not taking oral anticoagulant or heparin, rtPA may be given before this lab result is available; however, rtPA should be stopped if these lab tests come back elevated above normal limits.
Current use of direct thrombin inhibitors or direct factor Xa inhibitors with elevated sensitive laboratory tests (such as aPTT, INR, platelet count, and ecarin clotting time [ECT]; thrombin time [TT]; or appropriate factor Xa activity assays)*	
Blood glucose level <50 mg/dL (2.7 mmol/L)	
Non–contrast-enhanced CT (NECT) demonstrates multilobar infarction (hypodensity >1/3 cerebral hemisphere)	Do not give rtPA if CT shows acute intracranial hemorrhage or neoplasm.

(Continued)

TABLE 141-4 American Heart Association (AHA)/American Stroke Association (ASA) 2013 Inclusion/Exclusion Criteria for IV Recombinant Tissue Plasminogen Activator (rtPA) in Acute Ischemic Stroke (Continued)

Relative Exclusion Criteria	
Only minor or rapidly improving stroke symptoms (clearing spontaneously)	Some patients may have a lower NIHSS score but have a potentially disabling condition (e.g., aphasia, hemianopia). Some studies have shown poor outcomes for untreated minor strokes.
Pregnancy	No randomized controlled trials have been published regarding safety or efficacy of rtPA for ischemic stroke in pregnancy. Case series have reported mixed results.
Seizure at onset with postictal residual neurologic impairments	rtPA can be given if the residual impairments are thought to be secondary to the stroke as opposed to the seizure.
Major surgery or serious trauma within preceding 14 days†	
Previous GI or urinary tract hemorrhage within preceding 21 days†	
Previous myocardial infarction within preceding 3 months†	Rationale for this criterion was a statement indicating that myocardial rupture can result if rtPA is given within a few days of acute myocardial infarction.
Former Exclusion Criteria from 2007 AHA/ASA Guidelines	
Evidence of acute trauma (fracture)	
Failure of the patient or responsible party to understand the risks and benefits of, and alternatives to, the proposed treatment after a full discussion	

*New exclusion criteria for 2013 AHA/ASA guidelines.

†Changed from absolute contraindication from 2007 AHA/ASA guidelines.

Abbreviation: NIHSS, National Institutes of Health Stroke Scale.

a lumbar puncture may be unnecessary if a third-generation CT scan done within 6 hours of symptom onset is interpreted as negative by a neuroradiologist. A growing body of literature is exploring the combination of a negative noncontrast CT with CT angiography to exclude SAH or an associated aneurysm, with a 99.4% reported negative predictive value of this combination. However, potential downsides to this diagnostic strategy are the additional ionizing radiation exposure and possible detection of incidental cerebral aneurysms.

Other diagnostic tests may be useful in certain patients to exclude stroke mimics or concurrent conditions. Tests such as bedside glucose, complete blood count, ECG, pulse oximetry, electrolyte and coagulation studies, cardiac enzyme levels, toxicology screen, blood alcohol level, echocardiogram, carotid duplex scanning. MRI, MR angiogram, and CT angiogram may be of value when the suspicion for alternative disease entities is high.

TABLE 141-5 American Heart Association (AHA)/American Stroke Association (ASA) 2013 Additional Inclusion/Exclusion Criteria for IV Recombinant Tissue Plasminogen Activator (rtPA) in Acute Ischemic Stroke for Patients Presenting within 3 to 4.5 Hours after Onset

Additional Inclusion Criteria
Measurable diagnosis of acute ischemic stroke Onset of stroke symptoms 3–4.5 h before initiation of rtPA administration
Additional Exclusion Criteria
Age >80 years Severe stroke as assessed clinically (e.g., NIHSS score >25) or by appropriate imaging techniques (i.e., involving >1/3 of middle cerebral artery territory) Taking an oral anticoagulant regardless of international normalized ratio History of previous ischemic stroke and diabetes mellitus
Exclusion Criterion from ECASS III Not Included in Current AHA/ASA Guidelines
Blood glucose >400 mg/dL

Abbreviations: ECASS III, European Cooperative Acute Stroke Study III; NIHSS, National Institutes of Health Stroke Scale.

EMERGENCY DEPARTMENT CARE AND DISPOSITION

1. For patients presenting with acute neurological deficits, rapidly assess and stabilize any airway, breathing, and circulation abnormalities, establish IV access, obtain rapid bedside glucose testing, and place on cardiac monitoring and pulse oximetry. Supplemental oxygen is recommended only when patients are hypoxic to keep pulse oxygenation >94%.
2. Use patient history, prehospital provider information, and family member or bystander information to determine the last time patient was known to be at baseline neurological status.
3. Once the patient's clinical condition is stabilized, immediately obtain a noncontrasted head CT and appropriate laboratory testing, including coagulation studies.
4. American Heart Association (AHA) and American Stroke Association (ASA) recommendations for the care of patient with suspected acute ischemic stroke include time goals from the time of emergency department (ED) arrival for physician evaluation (10 minutes), activation of stroke team (15 minutes), beginning head CT (25 minutes), completing head CT interpretation (45 minutes), beginning thrombolytic therapy (if given, 1 hour), and admission to stroke unit (3 hours).
5. For a patient with acute ischemic stroke who is not a candidate for thrombolysis, current guidelines recommend permissive hypertension with no active blood pressure management unless systolic blood pressure is >220 mm Hg or diastolic blood pressure is >120 mm Hg. If blood pressure control is needed, target a systolic blood pressure reduction of 15% during the first 24 hours.
6. If a patient is a candidate being considered for intravenous thrombolysis, guidelines recommend that the patient's blood pressure should be managed to achieve a target blood pressure of SBP ≤185 mm Hg and DBP ≤110 mm Hg using **labetalol** 10 to 20 mg IV over 1 to 2 minutes (may repeat one time) or **nicardipine** infusion 5 mg/h titrated to a maximum of

15 mg/h and when desired blood pressure is attained, reduced to 3 mg/h. If blood pressure cannot be adequately controlled with these measures, the patient not a good candidate to consider for thrombolytic therapy.

7. The U.S. Food and Drug Administration (FDA) has approved the use of IV recombinant tissue plasminogen activator (rtPA) for patients with acute ischemic stroke ≤3 hours duration since symptom onset. In 2009, the AHA and the ASA recommended expansion of the treatment window to 4.5 hours for selected patients; however, this use is considered "off-label" because the FDA has denied approval for this indication. If thrombolysis is being considered, carefully review rtPA inclusion and exclusion criteria prior to administration of rtPA (Table 141-4). If the therapeutic window is to be extended to 3 to 4.5 hours, then use the additional European Cooperative Acute Stroke Study III (ECASS III) exclusion criteria (Table 141-5) as well.
8. Obtain informed consent from the patient or their designee prior to thrombolytic therapy. Although thrombolytic treatment of ischemic stroke may be associated with improved outcomes, the risk of symptomatic intracerebral hemorrhage is reported to be 6.4% (45% mortality) when rtPA is given within ≤3 hours of symptom onset, and 7.9% (NINDS definition) between 3 and 4.5 hours.
9. **The total dose of rtPA is 0.9 mg/kg IV, with a maximum dose of 90 mg; 10% of the dose is administered as a bolus, with the remaining amount infused over 60 minutes**. No aspirin or heparin should be administered in the initial 24 hours after treatment. Closely monitor blood pressures for patients who receive rtPA and treat as necessary. Intracerebral bleeding may be the cause of any neurologic worsening, and an emergent repeat noncontrasted head CT is indicated in these circumstances.
10. For patients diagnosed with TIA, treatment with **aspirin** 75 to 325 mg PO daily, **clopidogrel** 75 mg PO daily, or the combination of **aspirin** plus **extended-release dipyridamole** 25 mg PO and 200 mg PO twice daily, respectively.
11. For patients with acute ischemic stroke, **aspirin** 325 mg PO is recommended within 24 to 48 hours, although patients should not receive any antiplatelet medications in the first 24 hours after rtPA. Current guidelines do not recommend starting heparin or warfarin in the acute treatment of TIA or ischemic stroke in the ED, even in the presence of atrial fibrillation.
12. All patients with stroke should receive appropriate supportive care in the ED, including aspiration prevention, normalization of glucose level, fall precautions, and treatment for comorbidities. Admit all patients with acute stroke to monitored care units familiar with the care of stroke patients, preferably specialized units at designated centers.
13. For patients with SAH, the risk of rebleeding is greatest in the first 24 hours and can be reduced by adequate blood pressure control at a patient's prehemorrhage blood pressure or a MAP <140 mm Hg if the baseline blood pressure is unknown. If blood pressure management is necessary, administer an IV titratable antihypertensive such as **labetalol** 10 to 20 mg IV bolus over 1 to 2 minutes or continuous infusion starting at 2 mg/min, titrated to effect; or **nicardipine** continuous infusion beginning at 5 mg and titrated by 2.5 mg/h to a maximum dose of 15 mg/h.

14. Admit patients with SAH to an intensive care unit in consultation with a neurosurgeon. Administer **nimodipine** 60 mg PO every 4 hours, which may produce modest improvements by decreasing vasospasm. Seizure prophylaxis is controversial and should be discussed with the admitting specialist. Reverse any coagulopathy with vitamin K, fresh frozen plasma, and/or prothrombin concentrates.
15. Patients with intracerebral hemorrhage should be admitted to a monitored critical care area for treatment with antiepileptic medications if seizures occur, management of hyperglycemia, blood pressure management, and reversal of coagulopathy with vitamin K, fresh frozen plasma, and/or prothrombin concentrates. Patients with evidence of increased intracranial pressure (ICP) should be treated with head elevation to 30°, analgesia, and sedation. If more aggressive ICP reduction is indicated, such as with osmotic diuretics or intubation with neuromuscular blockade with mild hyperventilation, invasive monitoring of ICP by neurosurgery may be necessary
16. Appropriate use of neurology, neurosurgery, and neurocritical care specialists early in the evaluation of patients with stroke can be helpful. Emergent neurology consultation may be helpful in stroke cases as the indications for intravenous thrombolysis and endovascular therapy are evolving rapidly. Early neurosurgical consultation is appropriate for patients with SAH and intracerebral hemorrhage when evidence of increased ICP, location of bleeding, or other conditions suggest that surgical intervention may be indicated. Consider transfer to a designated stroke center, as admission to specialized stroke units is associated with improved outcomes.
17. The ABCD^2 scoring system has been recommended for use to predict stroke risk in TIA patients (Table 141-6). Using this system, the 2-day risks of subsequent stroke are as follows: 1% (ABCD^2 score 0 to 3); 4.1% (4 to 5); and 8.1% (6 to 7). While definitive evidence-based thresholds for admission have not yet been determined, some experts

TABLE 141-6 ABCD^2 Score to Predict Very Early Stroke Risk after Transient Ischemic Attack

Criteria	Points
Age ≥60 years	0 = Absent 1 = Present
Blood pressure ≥140/90 mm Hg	0 = Absent 1 = Present
Clinical features	0 = Absent 1 = Speech impairment without unilateral weakness 2 = Unilateral weakness (with or without speech impairment)
Duration	0 = Absent 1 = 10–59 min 2 = ≥60 min
Diabetes	0 = Absent 1 = Present
	Total Score: 0–7

recommend admission for most TIA patients for further evaluation and observation. Others recommend beginning the workup in the ED, starting antiplatelet therapy in appropriate patients, providing education about risk modification, and giving explicit return precautions. An individualized approach to select low-risk, asymptomatic patients may depend on medical factors, available healthcare resources, and a favorable social situation.

FURTHER READING

For further reading in *Tintinalli's Emergency Medicine: A Comprehensive Study Guide*, 8th ed., see Chapter 166, "Spontaneous Subarachnoid and Intracerebral Hemorrhage," by Jeffrey L. Hackman, Anna M.Nelson, and O. John Ma; and Chapter 167, "Stroke Syndromes," by Steven Go and Daniel J. Worman.

CHAPTER 142

Altered Mental Status and Coma

C. Crawford Mechem

Mental status is the clinical state of emotional and intellectual functioning of an individual. Patients presenting with altered mental status in the ED can include the diagnoses of delirium, dementia, and coma.

DELIRIUM

Clinical Features

Delirium is a transient disorder characterized by impaired attention, perception, thinking, memory, and cognition. Typically, delirium develops over a time course of days. Sleep–wake cycles may be disrupted, with patients exhibiting increased somnolence during the day and agitation characteristic of sundowning at night. Levels of alertness may be reduced, and activity levels may fluctuate rapidly. Different caregivers witnessing completely different patient behaviors within a brief time span may complicate making the diagnosis. Tremor, asterixis, tachycardia, sweating, hypertension, emotional outbursts, and hallucinations may be present. Features of delirium, dementia, and psychiatric disorders are listed in Table 142-1.

Diagnosis and Differential

The acute onset of attention deficits and cognitive abnormalities fluctuating throughout the day and worsening at night is characteristic of delirium. A detailed medication history should be obtained, as well as a mental status evaluation. ED evaluation is directed at identifying an underlying process contributing to the development of delirium such as infection (Table 142-2). Ancillary tests may include basic metabolic panel, hepatic studies, ammonia level, urinalysis, complete blood count, and chest radiograph. Cranial CT should be performed if a mass lesion is suspected, and clinicians may consider doing a lumbar puncture if meningitis or subarachnoid hemorrhage is suspected and an alternative diagnosis is not established.

TABLE 142-1 Features of Delirium, Dementia, and Psychiatric Disorder

Characteristic	Delirium	Dementia	Psychiatric Disorder
Onset	Over days	Insidious	Sudden
Course over 24 h	Fluctuating	Stable	Stable
Consciousness	Reduced or hyperalert	Alert	Alert
Attention	Disordered	Normal	May be disordered
Cognition	Disordered	Impaired	May be impaired
Orientation	Impaired	Often impaired	May be impaired
Hallucinations	Visual and/or auditory	Often absent	Usually auditory
Delusions	Transient, poorly organized	Usually absent	Sustained
Movements	Asterixis, tremor may be present	Often absent	Absent

TABLE 142-2 Important Medical Causes of Delirium

Infectious	Pneumonia Urinary tract infection Meningitis or encephalitis Sepsis
Metabolic/toxic	Hypoglycemia Alcohol ingestion Electrolyte abnormalities Hepatic encephalopathy Thyroid disorders Alcohol or drug withdrawal
Neurologic	Stroke or transient ischemic attack Seizure or postictal state Subarachnoid hemorrhage Intracranial hemorrhage CNS mass lesion Subdural hematoma
Cardiopulmonary	Congestive heart failure Myocardial infarction Pulmonary embolism Hypoxia or carbon dioxide narcosis
Drug related	Anticholinergic drugs Alcohol or drug withdrawal Sedatives-hypnotics Narcotic analgesics Selective serotonin or serotonin-norepinephrine reuptake inhibitors Polypharmacy

Emergency Department Care and Disposition

1. Direct treatment at the underlying medical illness that is causing delirium. Environmental manipulation such as adequate lighting and emotional support may help patient condition.
2. Treat acute episodes of agitation with **haloperidol**, 5 to 10 mg PO or IM, with reduced dosing in the elderly. **Lorazepam**, 0.5 to 2 mg PO, IM, or IV, may also be considered.
3. Consider inpatient admission for patients diagnosed with delirium unless a readily reversible cause for the acute mental status change is discovered, treatment is initiated, and improvement is seen.

DEMENTIA

Clinical Features

Dementia implies a loss of mental capacity over time. Psychosocial level and cognitive abilities deteriorate and behavioral problems develop. The largest categories of dementia are Alzheimer's disease and vascular dementia, and onset is typically insidious with gradual and progressive impairment of memory, especially recent memory. Hallucinations, delusions, and repetitive behaviors may be present. Other features of dementia include naming problems, forgetting items, loss of reading and direction, disorientation, inability to perform self-care tasks, and personality changes. Anxiety, depression, and speech difficulties may be observed. Patients with vascular dementia may be noted to have exaggerated or asymmetric deep tendon reflexes, gait abnormalities, or extremity weakness.

Diagnosis and Differential

While dementia typically develops slowly over time, physical examination may identify a precipitant or underlying cause of an acute or subacute change in a patient's level of functioning. Focal neurologic signs suggest the possibility of vascular dementia or a mass lesion. Increased motor tone and other extrapyramidal signs may suggest Parkinson's disease. Consider normal pressure hydrocephalus if urinary incontinence and gait disturbance are noted. This is further suggested by excessively large ventricles on head CT. Diagnostic studies may include a complete blood count, basic metabolic profile, urinalysis, thyroid profile, serum vitamin B_{12} level, testing for syphilis, erythrocyte sedimentation rate, serum folate level, human immunodeficiency virus testing, and chest radiography. Consider head CT or MRI as well as lumbar puncture if the diagnosis is not readily apparent and intracranial processes or central nervous system infections are suspected causes. The differential diagnosis includes delirium, depression, and other treatable causes.

Emergency Department Care and Disposition

1. Initiate an appropriate workup to assess for medical causes of worsening mental function.
2. Use antipsychotic drugs to manage persistent psychosis or severely disruptive or dangerous behavior, keeping in mind potential adverse reactions.
3. Aim treatment of vascular dementia at addressing risk factors, such as hypertension.
4. Many patients with newly diagnosed dementia will need inpatient admission for further evaluation and treatment. Discharge is appropriate for those patients who have longstanding and stable symptoms, consistent caregivers, and reliable follow-up for outpatient evaluation.

COMA

Clinical Features

Coma is a state of reduced alertness and responsiveness from which the patient cannot be aroused. Severity can be quantified using the Glasgow Coma Scale (Table 142-3) and the FOUR (Full Outline of UnResponsiveness) score. Pupillary findings, cranial nerve testing, findings of hemiparesis, and response to stimulation can help the clinician to determine a probable general category: diffuse CNS dysfunction such as a toxic-metabolic coma or focal CNS dysfunction characteristic of structural coma. Toxic-metabolic coma is characterized by lack of focal physical examination findings. The pupils are typically small and reactive, but may be large in severe sedative poisoning as from barbiturates.

Coma from supratentorial lesions or masses may present with progressive hemiparesis or asymmetric muscle tone and reflexes. Coma without

TABLE 142-3 Glasgow Coma Scale

Component	Score	Adult	Child <5 years	Child >5 years
Motor	6	Follows commands	Normal spontaneous movements	Follows commands
	5	Localizes pain	Localizes to supraocular pain (>9 months)	
	4	Withdraws to pain	Withdraws from nail bed pressure	
	3	Flexion	Flexion to supraocular pain	
	2	Extension	Extension to supraocular pain	
	1	None	None	
Verbal	5	Oriented	Age-appropriate speech/vocalizations	Oriented
	4	Confused speech	Less than usual ability; irritable cry	Confused
	3	Inappropriate words	Cries to pain	Inappropriate words
	2	Incomprehensible	Moans to pain	Incomprehensible
	1	None	No response to pain	
Eye opening	4	Spontaneous	Spontaneous	
	3	To command	To voice	
	2	To pain	To pain	
	1	None	None	

lateralizing signs may result from decreased cerebral perfusion from increased intracranial pressure (ICP). In addition, reflex changes in blood pressure and heart rate may be observed, such as the Cushing reflex (hypertension and bradycardia). Coma from posterior fossa or infratentorial lesions may be abrupt in onset, with abnormal extensor posturing and loss of pupillary reflexes and extraocular movements. Brainstem compression with loss of brainstem reflexes may develop rapidly. Pontine hemorrhage, another infratentorial cause of coma, may present with pinpoint pupils.

Pseudocoma or psychogenic coma is a diagnostic challenge. History taking and observation of responses to stimulation reveal findings that differ from typical syndromes. Pupillary responses, extraocular movements, muscle tone, and reflexes are intact. Valuable tests include responses to manual eye opening (there should be little or no resistance in an unresponsive patient) and extraocular movements. If avoidance of gaze is consistently seen with the patient always looking away from the examiner, or if nystagmus is demonstrated with caloric vestibular testing, this is strong evidence for nonphysiologic or feigned unresponsiveness.

Diagnosis and Differential

History, examination, laboratory studies, and neuroimaging will often identify potential causes for a comatose state. Abrupt onset of coma suggests a catastrophic stroke or status epilepticus. Gradual onset suggests a metabolic process or progressive lesion such as a tumor or a slowly developing intracranial bleed. Examination may reveal signs of trauma or suggest other possibilities, such as toxidromes. Fine neurologic testing is not feasible with a comatose patient, but asymmetric findings on pupillary examination, assessment of corneal reflexes, and testing of oculovestibular reflexes may suggest focal CNS lesions. Extensor or flexor posturing suggests profound CNS dysfunction. A head CT should be obtained followed by lumbar puncture if the scan is nondiagnostic and a subarachnoid hemorrhage or infection is suspected. Basilar artery thrombosis may be a concern in a comatose patient with a nondiagnostic head CT and an absence of alternative diagnoses; MRI or cerebral angiography may be considered to evaluate for this potential diagnosis. Patients who have had seizures and remain unresponsive may be having electrical seizures without motor activity (nonconvulsive status epilepticus), and an EEG should be performed if this is suspected. Consider toxic ingestions, infections, and nonaccidental trauma in comatose children. The differential diagnosis of coma includes primary CNS disorders (Table 142-4) and generalized disease processes that also affect the brain.

TABLE 142-4 Differential Diagnosis of Coma
Coma from causes affecting the brain diffusely
Encephalopathies
• Hypoxic encephalopathy
• Metabolic encephalopathy
• Hypertensive encephalopathy
Hypoglycemia
Hyperosmolar state (e.g., hyperglycemia)
Electrolyte abnormalities (e.g., hypernatremia or hyponatremia, hypercalcemia)
Organ system failure
• Hepatic encephalopathy
• Uremia/renal failure
Endocrine (e.g., Addison's disease, hypothyroidism, etc.)
Hypoxia
Carbon dioxide narcosis
Toxins
Drug reactions (e.g., neuroleptic malignant syndrome)
Environmental causes—hypothermia, hyperthermia
Deficiency state—Wernicke's encephalopathy
Sepsis
Coma from primary CNS disease or trauma
Direct CNS trauma
• Diffuse axonal injury
• Subdural hematoma
• Epidural hematoma
Vascular disease
• Intraparenchymal hemorrhage (hemispheric, basal ganglia, brainstem, cerebellar)
Subarachnoid hemorrhage
Infarction
• Hemispheric, brainstem
CNS infections
Neoplasms
Seizures
• Nonconvulsive status epilepticus
• Postictal state

Emergency Department Care and Disposition

Treatment of coma involves supportive care and identification of the underlying cause.

1. Stabilize the airway, breathing, and circulation.
2. Identify and treat reversible causes, such as hypoglycemia and opioid toxicity. Consider empiric naloxone. Administer thiamine before glucose in hypoglycemic patients with a history of alcohol abuse or malnutrition.
3. Consider nonconvulsive status epilepticus in patients who have had a seizure and have not returned to baseline neurological function.
4. If increased ICP is suspected, elevate the head of the bed to 30°. Consider giving **mannitol,** 0.5 to 1.0 g/kg. **Dexamethasone**, 10 mg IV reduces vasogenic brain edema associated with a tumor. Hyperventilation may transiently lower ICP. Avoid lowering $PaCO_2$ below 35 mm Hg.
5. Discharge patients with readily reversible causes of coma if home care and follow-up care are adequate and a clear cause of the episode is found and reversed. Admit all other patients for further evaluation and management.

FURTHER READING

For further reading in *Tintinalli's Emergency Medicine: A Comprehensive Study Guide*, 8th ed., see Chapter 168, "Altered Mental Status and Coma," by J. Stephen Huff.

CHAPTER 143

Ataxia and Gait Disturbances

Ross J. Fleischman

Ataxia is uncoordinated movement while a gait disorder is an abnormal pattern or style of walking. Both of these are findings that can be associated with many different disease processes, and thus clinicians evaluating patients with these abnormalities should view them in the context of individual clinical circumstances.

CLINICAL FEATURES

When initially evaluating a patient with ataxia or a gait distubance, consider whether the observed abonormalities are secondary manifestations of systemic disease rather than primary neurologic processes. Key symptoms that may suggest systemic disease include headache, nausea, fever, and decreased level of alertness. The physical examination may also show abnormalities outside of the nervous system, such as orthostatic vital sign changes that can point to hypovolemia or other systemic illness. Some forms of nystagmus may be suggestive of a central nervous system (CNS) disease process.

When evaluating ataxia that is suspected as a primary problem, differentiate between motor and sensory causes. One finding that suggests a cerebellar motor lesion is dysmetria, which can be elicited by finger to nose testing where patients may undershoot or overshoot their movements. Dysdiadochokinesia may be elicited by having the patient alternately flip their palms and backs of their hands on their thighs where clumsy rapid alternating movements can be observed. Heel to shin testing by having the patient slide one heel down the opposite shin can be useful for distinguishing between primary cerebellar disease and other sensory processing abnormalities. Overshoot of the knee or ankle signifies cerebellar disease, while a wavering course down the shin suggests a deficit of proprioception.

The Romberg test is primarily a test of sensation and can help to distinguish sensory ataxia from motor disease. Unsteadiness with the eyes open suggests a cerebellar motor ataxia, whereas worsening symptoms with eyes closed suggests a sensory ataxia that is unmasked with the removal of visual input. Test the posterior columns of the spinal cord by evaluating vibration and position sense in the lower extremities. Abnormalities attributed to posterior column degeneration can occur in tabes dorsalis (neurosyphilis) and vitamin B_{12} deficiency.

Observe patient ambulation in the emergency department to fully evaluate potential ataxia or gait disturbances. Subtle proximal or distal weakness can be identified by observing the patient rise from a chair and walk on heels and toes. Tandem heel-to-toe walking may elicit subtle ataxia. Broad-based, unsteady steps are characteristic of a motor ataxic gait, while a sensory ataxia with loss of proprioception may be notable for abrupt movements and slapping of the feet with each impact. A senile gait that is slow, broad based, and with a shortened stride may be seen with aging, but also with neurodegenerative disease such as Parkinson's disease and normal pressure hydrocephalus. Patients with Parkinson's disease often develop a narrow-based festinating gait with small shuffling steps that become more rapid. Weakness of the peroneal muscle weakness can manifest as foot drop, and is known as an equine gait.

DIAGNOSIS AND DIFFERENTIAL

Table 143-1 shows common causes of acute ataxia and gait disturbances.

Tailor the extent of ED evaluation based on the acuity and severity of symptoms. Patients with an acute onset of new symptoms or recent progression of symptoms will often undergo a more extensive diagnostic workup. Obtain radiographic imaging with CT scan or MRI when clinically indicated. Obtain a lumbar puncture to analyse cerebrospinal fluid when a CNS infection is suspected.

Wernicke's encephalopathy is characterized by ataxia, altered mental status, and ophthalmoplegia. While it is classically associated with alcoholics, this disease can be seen in any malnourished individual. Nystagmus is the most common ocular finding. Vestibular damage may cause unsteadiness

TABLE 143-1 Common Etiologies of Acute Ataxia and Gait Disturbances
Systemic conditions
Intoxications with diminished alertness
Ethanol
Sedative-hypnotics
Intoxications with relatively preserved alertness (diminished alertness at higher levels)
Phenytoin
Carbamazepine
Valproic acid
Heavy metals—lead, organic mercurials
Other metabolic disorders
Hyponatremia
Inborn errors of metabolism
Wernicke's disease
Disorders predominantly of the nervous system
Conditions affecting predominantly one region of the CNS
Cerebellum
Hemorrhage
Infarction
Degenerative changes
Abscess
Cortex
Frontal tumor, hemorrhage, or trauma
Hydrocephalus
Subcortical
Thalamic infarction or hemorrhage
Parkinson's disease
Normal pressure hydrocephalus
Spinal cord
Cervical spondylosis and other causes of spinal cord compression
Posterior column disorders
Conditions affecting predominantly the peripheral nervous system
Peripheral neuropathy
Vestibulopathy

while standing still, cerebellar damage may cause motor ataxia, and sensory neuropathy may also be present. Confabulation characterizes the memory loss of Korsakoff's syndrome. Consider vitamin B_{12} deficiency in patients with loss of position sense in the second toe and a positive Romberg test. A serum cyanocobalamin level and complete blood count are the initial steps in evaluation, although neurologic manifestations often precede macrocytic anemia. Neurosyphilis will cause similar symptoms of posterior column disease and can be screened for with VDRL or RPR tests. Gait impairments can also present in elderly patients as manifestations of Parkinson's disease or normal pressure hydrocephalus.

Ingestions are a common cause of acute ataxia in children. Ataxia in a 2- to 4-year-old may follow recent immunizations, viral illnesses, or varicella. Cranial nerve abnormalities or motor dysfunction along with cerebellar abnormalities may be present with posterior fossa mass lesions. Chaotic eye movements (opsoclonus) and myoclonic jerks of the head and chest are most commonly associated with neuroblastomas of the chest or abdomen. In the absence of post-varicella ataxia or another identifiable cause, clinicians can consider neuroimaging, lumbar puncture, and consultation as clinically indicated.

EMERGENCY DEPARTMENT CARE AND DISPOSITION

1. Administer **thiamine** 100 mg IV to alcoholics and other malnourished adults who might have Wernicke–Korsakoff syndrome.
2. Admit patients with an acute unexplained inability to walk for further evaluation and diagnostic testing.

FURTHER READING

For further reading in *Tintinalli's Emergency Medicine: A Comprehensive Study Guide*, 8th ed., see Chapter 169, "Ataxia and Gait Disturbances," by J. Stephen Huff.

CHAPTER 144

Acute Vertigo

Steven Go

CLINICAL FEATURES

Vertigo is a perception of movement when none exists that results from a mismatch between the visual, vestibular, and proprioceptive sensory systems. Symptoms of vertigo are classically described by patients as a sensation that "the room is spinning," but can also include atypical sensations of other types of movement. Vertigo is classified as peripheral or central (Table 144-1). **Peripheral vertigo** (involving the vestibular apparatus and eighth cranial nerve) usually has a sudden onset with intense symptoms that include nausea, vomiting, intolerance of head movement, and diaphoresis. **Central vertigo** (involving central structures such as the brainstem or cerebellum) can present either abruptly or gradually, but usually is characterized by less severe symptoms that are not well characterized by patients. Clinicians can work to discriminate between these two types of vertigo during a care encounter in the Emergency Department (ED) while recognizing that some overlap may exist between these two types of vertigo.

DIAGNOSIS AND DIFFERENTIAL

The differential diagnosis for an episode of vertigo (Table 144-2) may be extensive, and providers should evaluate for the presence or absence of some

TABLE 144-1 Differentiating Peripheral from Central Causes of Acute Undifferentiated Vertigo

	Peripheral	Central
Onset	Sudden or insidious	Sudden
Severity of vertigo	Intense spinning	Ill defined, less intense
Prodromal dizziness	Occurs in up to 25%; often single episode	Occurs in up to 25%; recurrent episodes suggest transient ischemic attacks
Intolerant of head movements/ Dix–Hallpike maneuver	Yes	Sometimes
Associated nausea/diaphoresis	Frequent	Variable
Auditory symptoms	Points to peripheral causes	May be present
Proportionality of symptoms	Usually proportional	Often disproportionate
Headache or neck pain	Unusual	More likely
Nystagmus	Rotatory-vertical, horizontal	Vertical
CNS symptoms/signs	Absent	Usually present
Head impulse test	Abnormal	Usually normal
HINTS examination (combined horizontal head impulse test, nystagmus, and test of skew)	Peripheral signs on all three bedside tests	Central signs on at least one of three bedside tests

TABLE 144-2 Causes of Acute Undifferentiated Vertigo

Vestibular/otologic	Benign paroxysmal positional vertigo Traumatic: following head injury Infection: labyrinthitis, vestibular neuronitis, Ramsay Hunt syndrome
Systemic conditions with vestibular/otologic effects	Ménière's syndrome Neoplastic Vascular Otosclerosis Paget's disease Toxic or drug-induced: aminoglycosides
Neurologic	Vertebrobasilar insufficiency or vertebral artery dissection Lateral Wallenberg's syndrome Anterior inferior cerebellar artery syndrome Neoplastic: cerebellopontine angle tumors Cerebellar disorders: hemorrhage, degeneration Basal ganglion diseases Multiple sclerosis Infections: neurosyphilis, tuberculosis Epilepsy Migraine headaches Cerebrovascular disease
General	Hematologic: anemia, polycythemia, hyperviscosity syndrome Toxic: alcohol Chronic renal failure Metabolic: thyroid disease, hypoglycemia

key features during the history and physical examination. Inquire about the speed of symptom onset, severity, duration, temporal pattern, head or neck trauma, chiropractic manipulation, and any associated symptoms such as headache, neck pain, or loss of consciousness. Assess risk factors for stroke such as age, hypertension, cardiovascular disease, and coagulopathy. Physical examination should include eye (e.g., nystagmus), ear, vestibular, and neurological examinations, with particular attention to potential abnormalities of the cranial nerves or cerebellar function. Since focal deficits are not universal in central vertigo, further specialized neurological tests may be of value in some patients. HINTS testing consists of the Head Impulse test (evaluation of the vestibulo-ocular reflex), examination for Nystagmus direction that changes with gaze direction, and Test of Skew (vertical ocular misalignment during the cover-uncover eye test). The presence of one or more findings on the HINTS exam that are consistent with central vertigo has been reported to be sensitive and specific for stroke when completed by experts, although it is unclear whether this specific testing is useful for physicians without special training. If benign paroxysmal positional vertigo (BPPV) is suspected, a Dix–Hallpike maneuver may be useful to help make the diagnosis (sensitivity 75% to 82%). Physical examination maneuvers that involve head or neck twisting should not be used if cervical artery dissection, vertebrobasilar insufficiency, or spinal pathology are suspected.

Laboratory investigations are not typically indicated in the routine workup for patients with symptoms consistent with peripheral vertigo, unless there is strong suspicion of a specific cause where laboratory analysis would be helpful. Neuroimaging studies such as an emergent CT scan,

CT angiogram, MRI, or MR angiogram are not routinely indicated when peripheral vertigo is suspected, but may be useful when specific causes of central vertigo are significant concerns. Consider neuroimaging in elderly patients with signs or symptoms concerning for central vertigo (such as cranial nerve or cerebellar findings), significant stroke risks, coagulopathy (e.g., taking anticoagulant medications), headache, head or neck trauma, or intractable or persistent (>72 hours) symptoms. Figure 144-1 illustrates an approach to patients with vertigo.

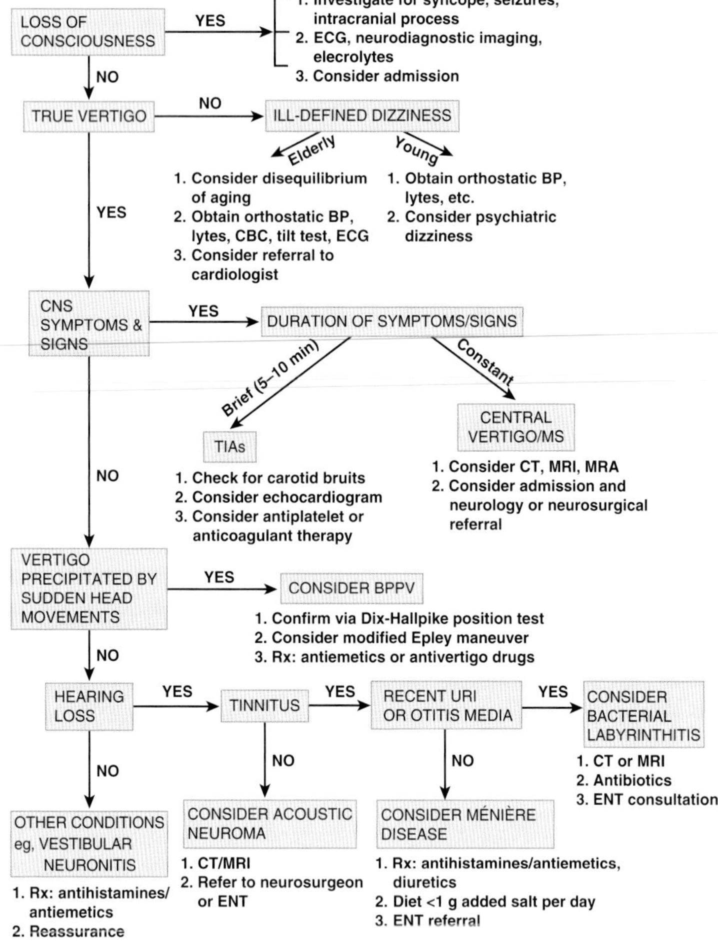

FIGURE 144-1. Approach to a patient with vertigo. BP, blood pressure; BPPV, benign paroxysmal positional vertigo; CBC, complete blood count; CNS, central nervous system; ENT, ear, nose, and throat; MRA, magnetic resonance angiography; MS, multiple sclerosis; Rx, treatment; TIAs, transient ischemic attacks; URI, upper respiratory infection.

CAUSES OF PERIPHERAL VERTIGO

Benign paroxysmal positional vertigo (BPPV) is believed to be caused by loose otoconia that most commonly enter the posterior semicircular canal and cause the inappropriate sensation of motion. Findings suggestive of BPPV are listed in Table 144-3. The Dix–Hallpike maneuver can support the diagnosis. To perform this physical examination maneuver, begin with the patient seated with the head turned 45° to the right. Rapidly lower the patient to a supine position, with the head hanging over the edge of the bed and the neck in 20° of extension. A positive test is when patients experience a short-lived rotatory nystagmus, with rapid eye beating toward the affected (dependent) ear that is associated with an acute episode of vertigo. After any nystagmus or symptoms resolve, slowly return the patient to the sitting position. Repeat the maneuver with the head turned 45° to the left. The side with the positive test serves as the starting point for the potentially curative Epley maneuver (see below).

Ménière's syndrome is characterized by recurrent bouts of vertigo associated with unilateral tinnitus and a sense of fullness and diminished hearing in the affected ear. Because the diagnosis requires multiple episodes of attacks with progressive hearing loss, Ménière's syndrome is not typically diagnosed on the first presentation of vertigo.

A **perilymph fistula** presents with sudden onset of vertigo during activities that can cause barotrauma such as flying, scuba diving, heavy lifting, and coughing. Infection can also cause a perilymph fistula, and the diagnosis can be confirmed by nystagmus elicited by pneumatic otoscopy.

Vestibular neuronitis is characterized by the sudden onset of severe vertigo sometimes associated with unilateral tinnitus and hearing loss. It is the second most common cause of peripheral vertigo, and is thought to be viral in nature. Symptoms last several days to weeks before they resolve spontaneously without recurrence.

Vestibular ganglionitis causes vertigo when a neurotrophic virus such as varicella zoster reactivates. The most famous variant is Ramsay Hunt syndrome (deafness, vertigo, and facial nerve palsy), which is associated with vesicles inside the external auditory canal.

Labyrinthitis, although commonly viral, can also be caused by bacterial infection from otitis media, meningitis, and mastoiditis. Patients with labyrinthitis present with a sudden onset of vertigo with hearing loss and middle ear findings.

Ototoxicity may induce hearing loss and vertigo. Common offenders causing peripheral ototoxicity include NSAIDs, salicylates, aminoglycosides,

TABLE 144-3 Supportive Findings in Benign Paroxysmal Positional Vertigo

Latency period of <30 sec between the provocative head position and onset of nystagmus.
The intensity of nystagmus increases to a peak before slowly resolving.
Duration of vertigo and nystagmus ranges from 5 to 40 sec.
If nystagmus is produced in one direction by placing the head down, then the nystagmus reverses direction when the head is returned to the sitting position.
Repeated head positioning causes both the vertigo and accompanying nystagmus to fatigue and subside.
Abnormal horizontal head impulse test indicating abnormal vestibulo-ocular reflex function.
HINTS testing not indicative of stroke.

Abbreviation: HINTS, horizontal head impulse test, nystagmus, and test of skew.

loop diuretics, and cytotoxic agents. Anticonvulsants, tricyclic antidepressants, neuroleptics, hydrocarbons, alcohol, and phencyclidine may cause centrally mediated vertigo.

Tumors of the eighth cranial nerve and cerebellopontine angle, such as meningiomas, acoustic neuromas, and acoustic schwannomas, may present with hearing loss and subsequent gradual onset of mild vertigo. Ataxia, ipsilateral facial weakness, loss of the corneal reflex, and cerebellar signs can also occur.

Vertigo may occur after closed head injury (e.g., basilar skull fracture) and tends to resolve over several weeks. In the acute setting, injuries with an associated intracranial hemorrhage should be excluded with neuroimaging. Postconcussive syndrome can also develop subacutely and may include an unsteady gait with dizziness.

CAUSES OF CENTRAL VERTIGO

Cerebellar hemorrhage or infarction typically causes moderate vertigo symptoms and can be associated with headache, nausea, and vomiting. Cerebellar findings such as truncal ataxia, abnormal Romberg testing, and tandem gait abnormalities are often present.

Lateral medullary infarction of the brainstem (Wallenberg syndrome) causes vertigo and ipsilateral facial numbness, loss of the corneal reflex, Horner syndrome, dysphagia, and dysphonia. Contralateral loss of pain and temperature sensation in the extremities also occur.

Vertebrobasilar insufficiency may result in sudden vertigo due to brainstem transient ischemic attack that typically lasts from minutes to 24 hours. Diplopia, dysphagia, dysarthria, vision changes, and syncope may also be present. Unlike other causes of central vertigo, vertebrobasilar insufficiency may be induced by movement of the head that is caused by positional decreases in vertebral artery blood flow.

Vertebral artery dissection can be caused by mechanisms that induce a sudden rotation of the head such as a motor vehicle crash, chiropractic adjustments, or violent sneezing. Patients present with central vertigo, headache, neck pain, and a unilateral Horner's syndrome.

Other potential causes of central vertigo include multiple sclerosis, neoplasms of the fourth ventricle, and vestibular migraine.

EMERGENCY DEPARTMENT CARE AND DISPOSITION

1. For most causes of peripheral vertigo, pharmacologic therapies in the ED may include anticholinergics and antihistamines (Table 144-4). **Diphenhydramine** 25 to 50 mg IM, IV, or PO and **meclizine** 25 mg PO are often effective in providing symptomatic relief. Transdermal **scopolamine** 0.5 mg is often recommended, but may be less useful for acute treatment due to its prolonged onset of action (4 to 8 hours). It may be most useful when prescribed as a discharge medication.
2. Second-line pharmacologic agents to consider when other medications are inadequate include calcium channel blockers, neuroleptics (avoid in orthostatic patients), and antiemetics such as **ondansetron** 4 mg IV. **Benzodiazepines** prevent the process of vestibular rehabilitation and can be used sparingly for symptomatic relief.

TABLE 144-4 Pharmacotherapy of Vertigo and Dizziness

Category	Drug	Dosage	Indications	Advantages	Disadvantages
Anticholinergics	Scopolamine	0.5 mg transdermal patch (behind ear) three to four times a day	Vertigo, nausea	Useful if patient is vomiting	Sometimes difficult to obtain
Antihistamines	Dimenhydrinate	50–100 mg IM, IV, or PO every 4 h	Vertigo, nausea	Inexpensive	Drowsiness/anticholinergic effect
	Diphenhydramine	25–50 mg IM, IV, or PO every 4 h	Vertigo, nausea	Inexpensive	Drowsiness/anticholinergic effect
	Meclizine	25 mg PO two to four times a day	Vertigo, nausea		Drowsiness/anticholinergic effect
Antiemetics	Hydroxyzine	25–50 mg PO four times a day	Vertigo, nausea	Inexpensive	Drowsiness/anticholinergic effect
	Metoclopramide	10–20 mg IV, PO three times a day	Vertigo, nausea	Effective, versatile	Occasional extrapyramidal effect
	Ondansetron	4 mg IV two to three times a day; 8 mg PO twice a day			
	Promethazine	25 mg IM, PO, or PR three to four times a day	Vertigo, nausea	Useful if vomiting	Occasional extrapyramidal effect
Benzodiazepines	Diazepam	2–5 mg PO two to four times a day	Central vertigo, anxiety related to peripheral vertigo	Inexpensive	Dependency, may impair vestibular compensation
	Clonazepam	0.5 mg PO two times a day	Central vertigo, anxiety related to peripheral vertigo	Inexpensive	Dependency, may impair vestibular compensation
Calcium antagonists	Cinnarizine	25 mg PO two to three times a day	Peripheral vertigo, vestibular migraine	Nonsedating	Lesser clinical experience
	Nimodipine	30 mg PO two times a day	Peripheral vertigo, vestibular migraine	Nonsedating	Lesser clinical experience
	Flunarizine	20 mg PO two times a day	Ménière's syndrome	Well tolerated	Not available in the United States

(Continued)

TABLE 144-4 Pharmacotherapy of Vertigo and Dizziness (Continued)

Category	Drug	Dosage	Indications	Advantages	Disadvantages
Vasodilators	Betahistine	48 mg PO three times a day for up to 6–12 months	Ménière's syndrome	Well tolerated	Little evidence of efficacy for other causes of peripheral vertigo
Corticosteroids	Methylprednisolone	100 mg/d tapered by 20 mg/d every fourth day	Vestibular neuronitis	Well tolerated	Efficacy largely unproven; adverse effects associated with corticosteroids
Antivirals	Valacyclovir	1000 mg three times a day for 7 days	Vestibular neuronitis	Well tolerated	Efficacy largely unproven
Anticonvulsants	Carbamazepine	200–600 mg/d	Vestibular paroxysmia	Inexpensive	Monitor CBC and liver function tests
	Topiramate	50–100 mg/d	Vestibular migraine prophylaxis	Well tolerated	Not well evaluated; does not abort acute vertigo
	Valproic acid	300–900 mg/d	Vestibular migraine prophylaxis	Well tolerated	Not well evaluated; does not abort acute vertigo
	Gabapentin	300 mg four times per day	MS-associated dizziness	Reduces acquired pendular nystagmus of multiple sclerosis	Known adverse effect profile
β-Blockers	Metoprolol	100 mg/d	Vestibular migraine prophylaxis	Long experience	Known adverse effect profile

3. Treat patients with suspected posterior canal BPPV with the **Epley maneuver** to move the otoconia out of the semicircular canal. With the patient seated, turn the head 45° toward the affected ear. (The affected ear is determined by the direction in which the Dix–Hallpike position test is positive.) Quickly bring the patient to the recumbent position with the head hanging 20° below the examining table. After nystagmus and symptoms resolve (or 30 to 60 seconds) gently rotate the head 90° to the unaffected side. After nystagmus and symptoms resolve (or 30 to 60 seconds), roll the patient onto the shoulder of the unaffected side as the head turns a further 90° so it is nearly facedown. After nystagmus and symptoms resolve (or 30 to 60 seconds), return the patient to a sitting position with legs dangling off the side of the table and the head to the midline. The patient may experience vertigo during any step of this procedure. The Epley maneuver may be repeated if necessary. If the Epley maneuver is not successful in relieving symptoms, consider instructing the patient in vestibular rehabilitation exercises.
4. Treat vestibular neuronitis symptomatically. Methylprednisolone and antivirals are of no proven benefit in this condition.
5. Treat vestibular ganglionitis with antiviral agents and bacterial labyrinthitis with appropriate antibiotics.
6. Most patients with peripheral vertigo may be discharged home with follow-up. Referral to an ENT specialist is indicated for patients with suspected perilymph fistula or labyrinthitis of suspected bacterial etiology.
7. Patients with suspected central vertigo should have imaging studies performed and emergent specialty referral. Consult neurosurgery for patients with posterior fossa hemorrhage or brain tumors. Other emergent causes of central vertigo such as ischemic stroke or vertebral artery dissection should receive appropriate neurology consultation.

FURTHER READING

For further reading in *Tintinalli's Emergency Medicine: A Comprehensive Study Guide*, 8th ed., see Chapter 170, "Vertigo," by Brian Goldman.

CHAPTER 145 Seizures and Status Epilepticus in Adults

C. Crawford Mechem

A seizure is an episode of abnormal neurologic function caused by the inappropriate electrical discharge of brain neurons. Primary seizures are those without an identified specific cause. Secondary seizures result from another identifiable neurologic condition, such as a mass, head injury, or stroke (Table 145-1).

CLINICAL FEATURES

Seizures are classified as *generalized* or *partial*. Generalized seizures are characterized by widespread involvement of the entire cerebral cortex and are typically associated with an abrupt loss of consciousness. Generalized tonic-clonic seizures (*grand mal*) often begin with a sudden onset of muscle rigidity where the trunk and extremities are extended and the patient falls to the ground. This rigid (tonic) phase is followed by a symmetric and rhythmic (clonic) jerking of the trunk and extremities. Generalized seizures are commonly associated with incontinence and an immediate postictal period where the patient remains flaccid and unconscious. A typical episode may last from 60 to 90 seconds with a gradual return of consciousness afterwards, although postictal confusion may persist for hours. Absence (*petit mal*) seizures are a subclass of generalized seizures typically seen in

TABLE 145-1 Common Causes of Provoked (Secondary) Seizures

- Trauma (recent or remote)
- Intracranial hemorrhage (subdural, epidural, subarachnoid, intraparenchymal)
- Structural CNS abnormalities
- Vascular lesion (aneurysm, arteriovenous malformation)
- Mass lesions (primary or metastatic neoplasms)
- Degenerative neurologic diseases
- Congenital brain abnormalities
- Infection (meningitis, encephalitis, abscess)
- Metabolic disturbances
- Hypo- or hyperglycemia
- Hypo- or hypernatremia
- Hyperosmolar states
- Uremia
- Hepatic failure
- Hypocalcemia, hypomagnesemia (rare)
- Toxins and drugs (many)
- Cocaine, lidocaine, antidepressants, theophylline, isoniazid
- Mushroom toxicity (*Gyromitra* spp.)
- Hydrazine (rocket fuels)
- Alcohol or drug withdrawal
- Eclampsia of pregnancy (may occur up to 8 weeks postpartum)
- Hypertensive encephalopathy
- Anoxic-ischemic injury (cardiac arrest, severe hypoxemia)

school-aged children and often last only a few seconds. Patients suddenly lose consciousness without losing postural tone and appear confused, detached, or withdrawn. An absence seizure typically ends abruptly with a return to normal functioning.

Partial seizures are due to electrical discharges that begin in a localized region of the cerebral cortex. These seizures may remain localized to one area of the brain or may later spread to other regions. Partial seizures are described as *simple*, in which consciousness is not affected, or *complex*, in which consciousness is altered. Complex partial seizures are often due to discharges in the temporal lobe (also termed *temporal lobe seizures*) and may include automatisms, visceral complaints, hallucinations, memory disturbances, distorted perception, and affective disorders.

Status epilepticus is defined as a single seizure lasting for longer than 5 minutes, or as two or more seizures that occur sequentially without an intervening recovery of consciousness. *Nonconvulsive status epilepticus* is characterized by altered mental status without perceptible muscular convulsive activity and is confirmed by electroencephalogram (EEG).

Eclampsia is a disorder found in pregnant women from 20 weeks gestation up to 8 weeks postpartum and is characterized by generalized seizures, hypertension, edema, and proteinuria.

DIAGNOSIS AND DIFFERENTIAL

When a patient presents with seizure-like activity, obtain a detailed history and inquire about the presence of preceding aura, abrupt or gradual onset, progression of motor activity, incontinence, whether the activity was local or generalized, symmetry of symptoms, duration of the episode, and presence of postictal confusion or lethargy. When a patient has a previously diagnosed seizure disorder, inquire about their baseline seizure pattern, common precipitants, and any recent changes in antiepileptic regimen. For those patients without a history of seizures, ask about recent or remote head injury. Consider the possibility of intracranial pathology if persistent, severe, or sudden-onset headaches are present. Consider eclampsia in patients with a current or recent pregnancy. Other factors that may predispose to seizures include metabolic or electrolyte abnormalities, hypoxia, systemic illness, cancer, sequelae of coagulopathy or anticoagulation, exposure to industrial or environmental toxins, drug ingestion or withdrawal, and alcohol use. Seizures are a common manifestation of central nervous system (CNS) disease in patients with the human immunodeficiency virus.

Evaluate each patient for findings of physical injuries that may have occurred during the seizure, perform a neurologic exam, and closely follow the level of consciousness. A transient focal deficit following a simple or complex focal seizure is referred to as *Todd's paralysis* and typically resolves within 48 hours. Initiate appropriate further testing for neurologic findings that are new or cannot be readily attributed to a benign cause.

Laboratory testing should be individualized and may not be indicated in all circumstances. In a patient with a known seizure disorder who has had a typical seizure, a glucose level and pertinent anticonvulsant levels may be appropriate. In an adult with a first seizure, additional studies are often used to assess for medical causes of seizure and may include serum glucose, basic metabolic panel, calcium, magnesium, a pregnancy test, and toxicology studies, as indicated. A noncontrast head CT is appropriate for a patient with a first seizure or a change in seizure pattern to identify a structural lesion or an acute intracranial process. Additional neuroradiographic imaging may be indicated based on CT scan results or clinical circumstances. MRI is typically not necessary on an emergent basis, but is often recommended as an aspect of non-emergent outpatient follow-up for patients with a first-time seizure. Lumbar puncture is indicated if CNS infection or subarachnoid hemorrhage is suspected.

The differential diagnosis of seizures includes syncope, pseudoseizures, hyperventilation syndrome, movement disorders, and migraines.

EMERGENCY DEPARTMENT CARE AND DISPOSITION

1. During an active seizure, take measures to protect the patient from injury or aspiration. IV anticonvulsants are often not needed during an uncomplicated seizure that resolves spontaneously.
2. In patients with a known seizure disorder whose anticonvulsant levels are low or who have missed doses of prescribed medications, supplemental doses may be appropriate.
3. Oral loading of **phenytoin** 20 mg/kg divided into three doses given every 2 to 4 hours is time-consuming and results in a delay in reaching therapeutic levels. Alternatively, **phenytoin** 20mg/kg IV may be administered at a rate of 25 mg/min. The loading dose of **fosphenytoin** is 20 phenytoin equivalents (PE)/kg at a maximum IV rate of 150 PE/min.
4. Administer IV **magnesium sulfate** to patients with suspected eclampsia. Consult an obstetrician early in the patient's care.
5. Patients in status epilepticus should have IV access, cardiac monitoring, and pulse oximetry. Endotracheal intubation may be required. If a paralytic agent is used, a short-acting drug is preferred so that any ongoing seizure activity can be monitored. Otherwise, EEG monitoring should be initiated. See Fig. 145-1 for anticonvulsant medication options. **Lorazepam** is considered the initial anticonvulsant of choice, followed by **phenytoin**, **fosphenytoin, or levetiracetam**. In refractory cases, consider IV **midazolam, propofol, phenobarbital, pentobarbital, or ketamine**. Early neurology consultation should be requested.
6. Patients with a first seizure who have a normal neurologic examination, no acute or chronic medical comorbidities, normal diagnostic testing including neuroimaging, and a normal mental status can be discharged from the ED with appropriate recommendations for outpatient follow-up. Initiation of antiepileptic medication, brain MRI, and other additional testing may be deferred to the outpatient setting.
7. Instruct discharged patients to take precautions that minimize the risks for injury from further seizures. Swimming, working with hazardous tools or machines, and working at heights should be prohibited. Patients should not drive vehicles until cleared by a neurologist or primary care physician, and driving privileges should conform to state laws.

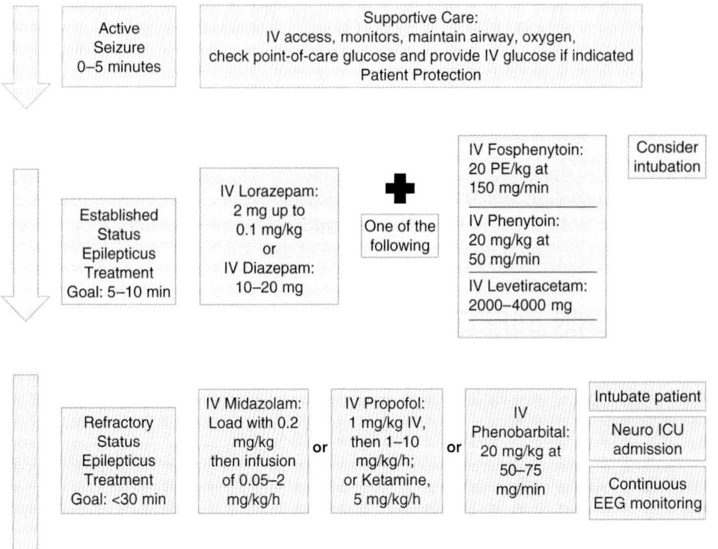

FIGURE 145-1. Guidelines for management of active seizures and status epilepticus. ICU = intensive care unit; PE = phenytoin equivalent.

FURTHER READING

For further reading in *Tintinalli's Emergency Medicine: A Comprehensive Study Guide*, 8th ed., see Chapter 171, "Seizures," by Joshua G. Kornegay.

CHAPTER 146 Acute Peripheral Neurologic Lesions

Nicholas E. Kman

A systematic approach to evaluating neurologic symptoms includes localizing the problem anatomically and distinguishing peripheral disorders from those with a central etiology. Peripheral nerve disorders may affect sensory, motor, and autonomic functions (Table 146-1).

GUILLAIN-BARRÉ SYNDROME

Clinical Features

Guillain-Barré syndrome (GBS) is an acute polyneuropathy characterized by immune-mediated peripheral nerve myelin sheath or axon destruction. It can be associated with a viral or febrile illness, *Campylobacter jejuni* infection, or vaccination.

Diagnosis and Differential

Although numerous variants exist, the typical presentation from GBS includes ascending symmetric weakness or paralysis and loss of deep tendon reflexes. Respiratory failure and significant autonomic fluctuations may occur. Cerebrospinal fluid (CSF) analysis typically shows high protein and a normal cell count (Table 146-2).

TABLE 146-1 Differentiating Central Nervous System from Peripheral Nervous System Disorders

	Central	Peripheral
History	Cognitive changes Sudden weakness Nausea, vomiting Headache	Weakness confined to one limb Weakness with associated pain Posture- or movement-dependent pain Weakness after prolonged period in one position
Physical Examination		
Reflexes	Brisk reflexes (hyperreflexia) Babinski's sign Hoffman's sign	Hypoactive reflexes Areflexia
Motor	Asymmetric weakness of ipsilateral upper and lower extremity Facial droop Slurred speech	Symmetric proximal weakness
Sensory	Asymmetric sensory loss in ipsilateral upper and lower extremity	Reproduction of symptoms with movement (compressive neuropathy) All sensory modalities involved
Coordination	Discoordination without weakness	Loss of proprioception

TABLE 146-2 Diagnostic Criteria for Classic Guillain-Barré Syndrome

Required	
	Progressive weakness of more than one limb
	Areflexia
Suggestive	
	Progression over days to weeks
	Recovery beginning 2–4 weeks after cessation of progression
	Relative symmetry of symptoms
	Mild sensory signs and symptoms
	Cranial nerve involvement (Bell's palsy, dysphagia, dysarthria, ophthalmoplegia)
	Autonomic dysfunction (tachycardia, bradycardia, dysrhythmias, wide variations in blood pressure, postural hypotension, urinary retention, constipation, facial flushing, anhydrosis, hypersalivation)
	Absence of fever at onset
	Cytoalbuminologic dissociation of cerebrospinal fluid (high protein and low white cell count)
	Typical findings on electromyogram and nerve conduction studies

Emergency Department Care and Disposition

1. Initial treatment includes supportive care which may include respiratory support as the disease progresses.
2. Consultation with a neurologist for admission to a monitored setting is recommended.
3. Administration of IV **immunoglobulin** and **plasmapheresis** may shorten the time to recovery.

BELL'S PALSY

Clinical Features

Bell's palsy causes seventh cranial nerve dysfunction. Patients may complain of facial weakness, articulation problems, difficulty keeping an eye closed, or inability to keep food in the mouth on one side.

Diagnosis and Differential

Physical examination findings demonstrate weakness on one side of the face, including the forehead, without other focal neurologic findings. The differential diagnosis includes stroke, Lyme disease, GBS, parotid tumors, middle ear lesions, cerebellopontine angle tumors, eighth cranial nerve lesions, HIV, and vascular disease. Inspect the ear for ulcerations caused by cranial herpes zoster activation, which is diagnostic for Ramsey–Hunt syndrome. Bell's Palsy is not likely if muscle strength is retained in the forehead on examination, and such a finding suggests a possible central neurologic lesion warranting radiographic imaging of the brain.

Emergency Department Care and Disposition

1. Systemic corticosteroids increase the frequency of complete recovery. Prescribe **prednisone** 1 mg/ kg per day PO for 7 days.
2. There is no proven benefit from administering antiviral medications unless evidence of Ramsey–Hunt syndrome is noted.

3. Treat patients with Ramsey–Hunt syndrome with antiviral medications, such as **famciclovir** 500 mg PO three times a day for 7 days or **valacyclovir** 1 g PO three times a day for 7 days.
4. Advise patients to use an **ophthalmic moisturizing ointment** at night to prevent corneal drying from incomplete eye closure.
5. Arrange follow-up with a primary care physician or ENT specialist to ensure appropriate resolution.

FOCAL MONONEUROPATHIES

Clinical Features

Focal mononeuropathies are most often due to focal nerve compression, although some systemic processes may also lead to mononeuropathy. Examples include carpal tunnel syndrome, resulting from compression of the median nerve at the wrist, and cubital tunnel syndrome, resulting from compression of the ulnar nerve at the elbow.

Diagnosis and Differential

Carpal tunnel syndrome causes pain, paresthesias, and numbness in the distribution of the medial nerve. The presence of Tinel's sign (light percussion over median nerve at wrist results in electric shock sensation shooting into hand) and use of Phalen's maneuver (holding wrists in flexion for 60 seconds worsens symptoms) may help confirm the diagnosis. Cubital tunnel syndrome causes tingling in the fifth and lateral fourth fingers that may progress to paralysis and wasting of the intrinsic hand muscles. Other common focal neuropathies include deep peroneal entrapment (causing foot drop and numbness between the first and second toes), meralgia paresthetica (entrapment of the lateral femoral cutaneous nerve causing numbness and pain of the anterolateral thigh), and mononeuritis multiplex (dysfunction of multiple peripheral nerves separated temporally and anatomically).

Emergency Department Care and Disposition

1. Conservative treatment is recommended, including anti-inflammatory medications.
2. Consider applying an appropriate splint for comfort. For carpal tunnel syndrome, splint the wrist in neutral position.
3. Direct additional treatment at the underlying cause of the neuropathy.

PLEXOPATHIES

Plexopathies can be caused by trauma, surgery, neoplasm, or radiation therapy. Brachial plexopathy causes weakness in the arm or shoulder girdle followed by pain and paresthesias. Patients have weakness in various distributions of the brachial plexus. ED evaluation is directed at identifying acutely reversible causes, such as joint dislocation or traumatic injury, and referral for other causes, such as neoplasm. Lumbosacral plexopathy is less likely due to injury and can be caused by radiation, diabetic amyotrophy, aortic aneurysm, retroperitoneal hemorrhage, or arteriovenous malformations. Symptoms are weakness, decreased sensation, and possibly decreased reflexes in the areas innervated by the affected portions of the plexus. Plain radiographs, MRI, and abdominal CT may be useful in determining the etiology. Direct specific treatment at the underlying cause.

NEUROMUSCULAR JUNCTION DISORDERS

Botulism is a toxin-mediated disorder of the neuromuscular junction that is caused by *Clostridium botulinum* toxin. Foodborne botulism typically comes from improperly preserved canned foods. In infantile botulism, organisms arise from ingested spores, often in honey, and produce a systemically absorbed toxin. Clinical features appear 6 to 48 hours after ingestion and may be preceded by nausea, vomiting, and diarrhea. Consider wound botulism in patients with a wound or a history of intravenous drug use. Early complaints involve the eye or bulbar musculature and progress to symmetric descending weakness and potential respiratory insufficiency. Treatment includes respiratory support, **trivalent botulinum antitoxin** 10 mL IV, and admission. For infants, **human botulism immunoglobulin** decreases mechanical ventilation requirements and length of intensive care unit stays.

FURTHER READING

For further reading in *Tintinalli's Emergency Medicine: A Comprehensive Study Guide*, 8th ed., see Chapter 172, "Acute Peripheral Neurologic Disorders," by Phillip Andrus and J. Michael Guthrie.

CHAPTER 147

Chronic Neurologic Disorders

Michael T. Fitch

Patients with chronic neurologic disorders may present to the emergency department with complications of their underlying medical conditions. Emergency management of these disorders often centers on evaluation of potential respiratory complications and an assessment for appropriate inpatient or outpatient management of acute illness or exacerbation of chronic disease.

AMYOTROPHIC LATERAL SCLEROSIS

Clinical Features

Patients with amyotrophic lateral sclerosis (ALS) experience progressive muscle atrophy and weakness. Limb spasticity, hyperreflexia, and emotional lability are common symptoms of upper motor neuron demyelination, while lower motor neuron dysfunction can cause muscle weakness, atrophy, fasciculations, dysarthria, dysphagia, and difficulty with mastication. In the early phase of disease, symptoms may be asymmetric. Respiratory muscle weakness causes progressive respiratory difficulty that presents as dyspnea with exertion or at rest. Sensory and cognitive function is often spared, although up to 15% of patients may also develop dementia and Parkinsonism.

Diagnosis and Differential

The diagnosis early in the course of illness can be challenging, which contributes to a median time to diagnosis of 14 months. Clinicians may suspect ALS when signs are found of upper and lower motor neuron dysfunction without other central nervous system dysfunction. Other diagnoses to consider that may have ALS-like symptoms are systemic illnesses such as diabetes, thyroid and parathyroid dysfunction, vitamin B_{12} deficiency, heavy metal toxicity, vasculitis, and CNS tumors.

Emergency Department Care and Disposition

1. A new diagnosis of ALS is uncommon to make in the emergency department. Stable patients with suspicious symptoms should be referred for appropriate testing by a neurologist if an initial workup does not reveal an emergent cause of neurologic symptoms.
2. Patients with a known diagnosis of ALS may present for emergency care with complications such as respiratory failure, aspiration pneumonia, choking episodes, or traumatic injuries.
3. Optimize pulmonary function based on an individual patient's respiratory status and comorbidities using interventions such as nebulizer treatments, steroids, antibiotics, and intubation, as indicated. While a blood gas may not reliably predict impending respiratory failure, a forced vital capacity <25 mL/kg or 50% decreased from predicted

normal increases the likelihood of pneumonia and respiratory failure in these patients.

4. Patients with pneumonia, inability to handle secretions, respiratory distress, or need for ventilator support should be admitted to an appropriate level of inpatient care.

MYASTHENIA GRAVIS

Clinical Features

Myasthenia gravis is an autoimmune disorder of the neuromuscular junction that is characterized by muscle weakness and fatigue. Most patients have weakness of proximal extremity muscles, neck extensors, and facial or bulbar muscles. Ptosis and diplopia are common presenting symptoms, and symptoms typically worsen as the day progresses and improve with rest. Severe respiratory muscle weakness causing respiratory failure is characteristic of a myasthenic crisis.

Diagnosis and Differential

The symptoms of myasthenia gravis can mimic those seen in many other disorders, including Lambert-Eaton syndrome, botulism, thyroid disorders, and stroke. The diagnosis can be established through administration of **edrophonium** (an acetylecholinesterase inhibitor), electromyography, and serum testing for acetylcholine receptor antibodies. **Edrophonium** or **neostigmine** is expected to improve muscle strength in objectively weak limb and ocular or pharyngeal muscles and can help make an initial diagnosis.

Emergency Department Care and Disposition

1. Myasthenia gravis can be treated with the acetylcholinesterase inhibitors **pyridostigmine** or **neostigmine**, thymectomy, immune suppression with steroids or **azathioprine**, and immune modulation with plasma exchange or IV immunoglobulin.
2. Many drugs used in the emergency department have the potential to impact neuromuscular function. Check carefully for drug interactions when treating patients with myasthenia gravis (Table 147-1).
3. Respiratory failure can occur in patients with infection, recent surgery, or recent changes in immunosuppressant medications. When possible, avoid depolarizing or nondepolarizing paralytic agents if intubation is required.
4. Myasthenic crisis requiring emergent intervention may occur in undiagnosed patients with myasthenia gravis, or in patients with known disease who have acute exacerbations or inadequate treatment.
5. Administration of **edrophonium** 1 mg slow IV can help to distinguish a myasthenic crisis (inadequately treated myasthenia gravis) from a cholinergic crisis (often from overmedication). Resolution of muscle weakness within a few minutes suggests a myasthenia exacerbation that can be further treated with **neostigmine** 0.5 to 2 mg IM, IV, SC or in increments of 15 mg PO.

TABLE 147-1 Drugs to Avoid in Myasthenia Gravis

Steroids	Adrenocorticotropic hormone,* methylprednisolone,* prednisone*
Anticonvulsants	Phenytoin, ethosuximide, trimethadione, paraldehyde, magnesium sulfate, barbiturates, lithium
Antimalarials	Chloroquine,* quinine*
IV fluids	Sodium lactate solution
Antibiotics	Aminoglycosides, fluoroquinolones,* neomycin,* streptomycin,* kanamycin,* gentamicin, tobramycin, dihydrostreptomycin,* amikacin, polymyxin A, polymyxin B, sulfonamides, viomycin, colistimethate,* lincomycin, clindamycin, tetracycline, oxytetracycline, rolitetracycline, macrolides, metronidazole
Psychotropics	Chlorpromazine,* lithium carbonate,* amitriptyline, droperidol, haloperidol, imipramine
Antirheumatics	D-Penicillamine, colchicine, chloroquine
Cardiovascular	Quinidine,* procainamide,* β-blockers (propranolol, oxprenlol, practolol, pindolol, sotalol), lidocaine, trimethaphan; magnesium; calcium channel blockers (verapamil)
Local anesthetics	Lidocaine,* procaine*
Analgesics	Narcotics (morphine, hydrmorphone, codeine, Pantopon, meperidine)
Endocrine	Thyroid replacement*
Eye drops	Timolol,* echothiophate
Others	Amantadine, diphenhydramine, emetine, diuretics, muscle relaxants, central nervous system depressants, respiratory depresants, sedatives, procaine,* phenothiazines
Neuromuscular blocking agents	Tubocurarine, pancuronium, rocuronium, gallamine, dimthyl tubocurarine, succinylcholine, decamethonium

Note: See also discussion on eMedicine from WebMD by William D. Goldenberg, MD, available at: http://emedicine.medscape.com/article/793136-overview#a1.

*Case reports implicate drugs in exacerbations of myasthenia gravis.

MULTIPLE SCLEROSIS

Clinical Features

Multiple sclerosis (MS) is caused by multifocal areas of CNS demyelination and manifests with motor, sensory, visual, and/or cerebellar dysfunction. Types of MS include relapsing and remitting (90%), relapsing and progressive, and chronically progressive. Lhermitte sign is commonly experienced and is described as an electric shock sensation, vibration, or pain radiating down the back and often into the arms or legs from neck flexion. Physical examination may show decreased strength, increased tone, hyperreflexia, clonus, decrease in vibratory sense and joint proprioception, a positive Babinski reflex, and reduced pain and temperature sense. Optic neuritis with loss of central vision is a presenting symptom in 30% of cases and may cause an afferent papillary defect (Marcus–Gunn pupil). Bilateral internuclear ophthalmoplegia causes abnormal eye adduction and horizontal nystagmus, and its presence is strongly suggestive of MS. Cognitive and emotional problems are common as the disease progresses.

Diagnosis and Differential

A diagnosis of MS is suspected when a patient experiences two or more prolonged episodes of neurologic dysfunction that suggest white matter pathology in more than one location in the brain and/or spinal cord. MRI shows multiple discrete lesions in the supratentorial white matter, homogeneous borders around the ventricles, or infratentorial or spinal cord lesions. CSF protein and γ-globulin levels are often elevated. Other conditions that mimic symptoms of MS include systemic lupus erythematosus, Lyme disease, neurosyphilis, HIV disease, and Guillain-Barré syndrome.

Emergency Department Care and Disposition

1. Consult with a neurologist for assistance in managing a patient with MS and suspected exacerbation. Refer patients with new symptoms suspicious for MS to a neurologist for further evaluation.
2. High-dose **methylprednisolone** therapy, 500 to 1000 mg per day, shortens the duration of exacerbations.
3. Consider testing for urinary tract infections in the appropriate clinical setting, especially for patients with known bladder dysfunction and post-void residuals >100 mL.
4. Evaluate for potential sources of infection when fever is present. Fever reduction measures can help to minimize the muscle weakness that is associated with temperature elevations.
5. Consider inpatient admission for patients with significant exacerbations who may require IV steroids or antibiotics.

LAMBERT-EATON MYASTHENIC SYNDROME

Lambert-Eaton myasthenic syndrome is an autoimmune disorder with fluctuating proximal limb muscle weakness and fatigue. It is classically described in older men with lung cancer. Strength improves with sustained or repeated exercise (Lambert sign). Patients complain of myalgias, stiffness, paresthesias, metallic tastes, and autonomic symptoms. Eye movements are unaffected. Electromyography is abnormal, and serum tests are specific for antibodies to voltage-gated calcium channels. Treatment is mostly supportive, but neuromuscular transmission can also be enhanced with **3,4-diaminopyridine**. Immunosuppressive drugs may reduce symptom severity.

PARKINSON'S DISEASE

Clinical Features

Parkinson's disease is a progressive extrapyramidal movement disorder with four classic signs: resting tremor, cogwheel rigidity, bradykinesia or akinesia, and impaired posture and equilibrium. Initially, many patients develop a unilateral resting upper extremity tremor, referred to as a "pill rolling" tremor, which improves with intentional movement.

Diagnosis and Differential

The diagnosis of Parkinson's disease is clinical and based on the presence of the four classic signs. Parkinsonism can secondarily develop from exposure to illicit drugs, toxins, neuroleptic medications, hydrocephalus, head trauma, and other rare neurologic conditions. Drug-induced Parkinson's disease most commonly presents with akinesia. No radiographic imaging or laboratory study is pathognomonic for making the diagnosis.

Emergency Department Care and Disposition

Most patients with known Parkinson's disease are treated with medications that increase central dopamine, have anticholinergic properties, or act as central dopamine receptor agonists. Medication side effects may include psychiatric or sleep disturbances, anorexia, nausea, vomiting, cardiac dysrhythmias, orthostatic hypotension, dyskinesias, and dystonia. Patients being treated with medication for Parkinson's disease who present with new motor or psychiatric disturbances or decreased drug efficacy, a "drug holiday" for 1 week can be considered in consultation with a neurologist.

POLIOMYELITIS AND POSTPOLIO SYNDROME

Clinical Features

Poliomyelitis is caused by an enterovirus infection that can lead to paralysis by motor neuron destruction and muscle denervation in some patients. Most acutely infected patients are asymptomatic or have a mild viral syndrome without paralysis. Major illness occurs in only 1% to 2% of infections and most commonly involves the spinal cord, resulting in asymmetric proximal limb weakness and flaccidity, absent tendon reflexes, and fasciculations. Maximal paralysis occurs within 5 days and is followed by muscle atrophy. Paralysis will resolve within 1 year in most patients. Other sequelae include autonomic dysfunction, speech and swallowing dysfunction, and encephalitis. Polio was eradicated from the United States in 1979 but is still endemic in Nigeria, Pakistan, Afghanistan, and India.

Postpolio syndrome is the recurrence of motor symptoms after a latent period of several decades in a patient who has a history of acute paralytic poliomyelitis. Symptoms may include muscle fatigue, joint pain, or weakness of new and previously affected muscle groups. Patients may have new bulbar, respiratory, or sleep difficulties.

Diagnosis and Differential

Consider an acute polio virus infection when an at-risk patient from an endemic area presents with an acute febrile illness, aseptic meningitis, and asymmetric flaccid paralysis with loss of deep tendon reflexes and preserved sensation. The diagnosis can be made by evaluating cerebrospinal fluid (CSF), which will demonstrate a pleocytosis and positive viral cultures for poliovirus, or from throat or rectal swab testing.

Other diseases with similar neurologic symptoms include Guillain-Barré syndrome, peripheral neuropathies associated with other disorders (e.g., mononucleosis, Lyme disease, or porphyria), abnormal electrolyte levels, toxins, inflammatory myopathies, and other viral infections (e.g., Coxsackie, mumps, echovirus, and various enteroviruses).

Emergency Department Care and Disposition

Acute care for patients suffering from a postpolio syndrome is supportive, with analgesics and anti-inflammatory medications. Muscle training and daily exercise regimens are helpful. **Lamotrigine** may improve quality of life for patients with postpolio syndrome. Consultation with a neurologist is recommended for disposition and continued follow-up treatment.

FURTHER READING

For further reading in *Tintinalli's Emergency Medicine: A Comprehensive Study Guide*, 8th ed., see Chapter 173, "Chronic Neurologic Disorders" by Daniel A. Handel and Sarah Andrus Gaines.

CHAPTER 148

Central Nervous System and Spinal Infections

Michael T. Fitch

Identifying infections in the central nervous system (CNS) can be challenging for clinicians in the Emergency Department (ED), as invasive testing is often required for definitive diagnoses. Bacterial meningitis, viral encephalitis, brain abscess, and spinal epidural abscess are life-threatening emergencies that can initially present with a spectrum of nonspecific symptoms that may make early diagnosis difficult. Differentiating these conditions from viral meningitis or other conditions that can be treated with supportive care is important when a CNS infection is suspected.

MENINGITIS AND ENCEPHALITIS

Clinical Features

Meningitis is inflammation of the membranes surrounding the brain and spinal cord. Bacterial meningitis is inflammation caused by infection, often with encapsulated organisms, and is a life-threatening emergency. Even with appropriate and timely treatment this emergent CNS infection can have significant morbidity and mortality. Aseptic meningitis is diagnosed when such inflammation is due to causes other than bacterial infection, such as drug reactions, rheumatologic conditions, or nonbacterial infections such as fungi or viruses. Enteroviruses and echoviruses are the most common causes of aseptic meningitis.

The classically described clinical triad of meningitis is fever, neck stiffness, and altered mental status, although less than half of patients will initially present with all three of these features. Headache is a common symptom and fever is often present. Many initial symptoms such as headache, fever, neck pain, nausea, and vomiting are nonspecific and overlap with other more common conditions, which can make early diagnosis a challenge especially in very young and very old patients.

Physical findings often include fever, and when CNS infection is suspected clinicians should evaluate for the presence of meningeal signs such as nuchal rigidity (severe neck stiffness), Kernig's sign (pain in the back and legs with flexing the hip and extending the knee), and Brudzinski's sign (flexion of the hips with passive flexion of the neck), although these classically described findings have been demonstrated to have poor sensitivity for meningitis. Evaluate mental status and look for potential neurological deficits that may accompany CNS infections such as cranial nerve palsies or other focal findings. Examine the skin for petechiae, splinter hemorrhages, or other findings concerning for systemic infection.

Encephalitis is an infection of the brain parenchyma that causes inflammation within the CNS and is often caused by viral infection. This can be caused by a number of different viral pathogens including herpes simplex virus (HSV), which is the most treatable cause of encephalitis. Patients with acute viral encephalitis will present with many of the same signs and symptoms as bacterial meningitis, such as fever, stiff neck, or headache. Additionally, patients diagnosed with encephalitis typically present with altered mental status, cognitive deficits, psychiatric symptoms, or seizures.

Diagnosis and Differential

A promptly performed lumbar puncture (LP) to obtain cerebrospinal fluid (CSF) is the appropriate diagnostic procedure for patients with suspected meningitis or encephalitis. Consider a CT scan of the brain before the procedure when altered mental status, new onset seizures, immunocompromise, focal neurologic signs, or papilledema are present. The goal for imaging in this circumstance is to identify possible contraindications to LP such as an occult mass or signs of brain shift or herniation (see Fig. 148-1).

Send CSF for cell count and differential, protein and glucose levels, and a Gram's stain and bacterial culture. Consider additional CSF studies for immunocompromised patients or if a specific CNS infection is suspected based on the initial CSF testing results. HSV or enterovirus PCR, bacterial antigen testing, or specialized fungal testing can be considered as additional testing in appropriate clinical situations. Consider other laboratory studies such as a complete blood count (CBC), serum glucose and electrolytes, blood urea nitrogen (BUN), and creatinine to assess for other potential diagnoses. A blood culture may be helpful to identify bacterial pathogens, particularly when empiric antibiotics are given prior to lumbar puncture. See Table 148-1 for classically described findings in bacterial, viral, fungal, and neoplastic meningitis, although several studies have demonstrated that no single laboratory finding can accurately categorize the cause of CSF pleocytosis in all patients. Although not typically part of an ED workup, characteristic findings on MRI in the medial temporal and inferior frontal lobes are suggestive of HSV infection.

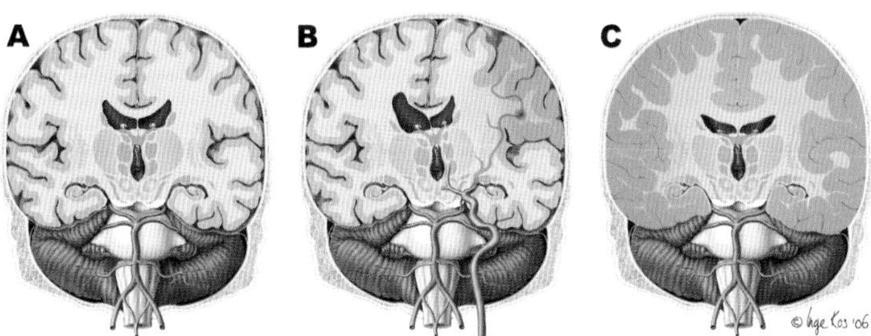

FIGURE 148-1. Cranial imaging to evaluate potential contraindications for lumbar puncture should be focused on identifying signs of a focal space-occupying lesion, evidence of brain shift, and/or signs of severe diffuse brain swelling: **(A)** normal brain, **(B)** meningitis-associated cerebral infarct causing pronounced brain shift, and **(C)** diffuse brain swelling associated with severe infection. Initial lumbar puncture should not be done when CT findings of significant brain shift are found, and empiric therapy for meningitis should be continued in such patients. Reproduced with permission from Fitch MT, van de Beek D. Emergency diagnosis and treatment of adult meningitis. *Lancet Infect Dis*. 2007 Mar;7(3):191–200.

TABLE 148-1 Cerebrospinal Fluid (CSF) Diagnostic Evaluation

	Opening Pressure (<170 mm H_2O)*	Color (Clear)	Gram Stain (Negative)	Cell Count (<5 WBC, 0 PMN)	Glucose (>40 mg/dL)	Protein (<50 mg/dL)	Cytology (Negative)
Bacterial	Elevated	Cloudy, turbid	Positive (60%–80% before antibiotic, 7%–41% after antibiotic)	>1000–2000/mm^3 WBC, neutrophilic predominance, >80% PMN	<40 mg/dL, CSF/ blood glucose ratio <0.3–0.4	>200 mg/dL	Negative
Viral	Normal	Clear or bloody	Negative	<300/mm^3 WBC, lymphocytic predominance, <20% PMN	Normal	<200 mg/dL	Negative
Fungal	Normal to elevated	Clear or cloudy	Negative	<500/mm^3	Normal to slightly low	>200 mg/dL	Negative
Neoplastic	Normal	Clear or cloudy	Negative	<300/mm^3	Normal to slightly low	>200 mg/dL	Positive

*Normal values and findings are in parentheses.

Abbreviation: PMN, polymorphonuclear lymphocyte.

The differential diagnosis for patients with findings concerning for meningitis or encephalitis may include subarachnoid hemorrhage, meningeal neoplasm, brain abscess, cerebral toxoplasmosis, and other systemic viral or bacterial infections.

Emergency Department Care and Disposition

1. When bacterial meningitis is a likely diagnosis, begin empiric antibiotic therapy based on patient risk factors and most likely causative pathogens. Start antibiotics as soon as possible after a promptly performed LP, or immediately after blood cultures are drawn if neuroimaging or other diagnostic testing will be performed.
2. When administering empiric antibiotics for suspected bacterial meningitis, adults less than 50 years old should receive a third-generation cephalosporin such as **ceftriaxone** 2 g IV plus **vancomycin** 15 mg/kg IV. Patients at risk for *Listeria monocytogenes* infection (e.g., age 50 years or older, pregnant women, alcoholics, immunocompromised patients) should additionally receive **ampicillin** 2 g IV.
3. For patients with bacterial meningitis, adjunctive corticosteroids treatment started before or at the same time as the first dose of antibiotics may decrease mortality and neurologic sequelae for some subsets of patients. Consider **dexamethasone** 10 mg IV every 6 hours for 4 days in adults or 0.15 mg/kg IV every 6 hours for 4 days in children 3 months and older when it is initiated before or at the same time antibiotics are given.
4. Patients with suspected encephalitis should be started on **acyclovir** 10 mg/kg IV to cover for possible HSV or herpes zoster virus infections. Cytomegalovirus encephalitis can be treated with **ganciclovir** 5 mg/kg IV. Most other causes of viral encephalitis have no specific antimicrobial treatment that will impact patient outcomes, and recommended treatment in these circumstances is supportive care.
5. Patients with suspected bacterial meningitis or encephalitis should be admitted to the hospital for intravenous antimicrobial agents and further care.

BRAIN ABSCESS

Clinical Features

A brain abscess is caused by a bacterial infection of the brain parenchyma and is composed of a central purulent cavity ringed by a layer of granulation tissue and an outer fibrous capsule. Presenting signs and symptoms are often nonspecific and may include headache, neck stiffness, fever, vomiting, confusion, or changes in mental status. Patient symptoms may reflect the origin of the infection (e.g., ear or sinus pain), and symptoms may be present for 1 to 8 weeks before the diagnosis is made.

Diagnosis and Differential

Neuroimaging is needed to make the diagnosis of a brain abscess. A CT scan of the head without contrast may identify abnormalities or evidence of surrounding edema, but a CT scan with contrast is more likely to accurately identify an abscess with thin rings of enhancement surrounding a low-density center. MRI is another sensitive test for making the diagnosis. Avoid lumbar puncture if a brain abscess or other mass lesion is suspected or identified. Routine laboratory studies are usually nonspecific. When possible, obtain blood cultures or cultures of other sites of infection to guide future management.

The differential diagnosis includes cerebrovascular disease, meningitis, brain neoplasm, subacute cerebral hemorrhage, and other focal brain infections, such as toxoplasmosis.

Emergency Department Care and Disposition

1. Early empiric antibiotic therapy is recommended based on the likely source of infection (see Table 148-2).
2. Consult with a neurosurgeon for admission to the hospital as many patients will require surgery for diagnosis, pathogen identification, and definitive treatment.

EPIDURAL ABSCESS

Clinical Features

Spinal epidural abscess is a rare infection consisting of pyogenic material that accumulates in the epidural space. Up to half of these infections originate from hematogenous spread of bacteria from soft tissue, urine, or

TABLE 148-2 Guidelines for Empiric Treatment of Brain Abscess Based on Presumed Source

Presumed Source	Primary Empiric Therapy	Alternative Therapy
Otogenic	Cefotaxime 2 g IV every 4–6 h or ceftriaxone 2 g IV every 12 h PLUS metronidazole 500 mg IV every 8 h	Piperacillin/tazobactam 4.5 g IV every 6 h
Odontogenic	Penicillin G 4 million units IV every 4 h	Ceftriaxone 2 g IV every 12 h PLUS metronidazole 500 mg IV every 6 h
Sinogenic	Cefotaxime 2 g IV every 6 h or ceftriaxone 2 g IV every 12 h PLUS metronidazole 500 mg IV every 8 h	No recommendation
Penetrating trauma	Cefotaxime 2 g IV every 6 h or ceftriaxone 2 g IV every 12 h PLUS metronidazole 500 mg IV every 8 h ± rifampin 10 mg/kg every 24 h	No recommendation
After neurosurgical procedure	Vancomycin loading dose 25–30 mg/kg IV loading dose or linezolid 600 mg IV every 12 h PLUS ceftazidime 2 g IV every 8 h ± rifampin 10 mg/kg every 24 h	Can substitute linezolid 600 mg IV every 12 h instead of vancomycin. Can substitute meropenem 2 g IV every 8 h OR piperacillin/tazobactam 4.5 g IV every 6 h OR cefepime 2 g IV every 8 h for ceftazidime.
Unknown source	Cefotaxime 2 g IV every 6 h PLUS metronidazole 500 mg IV every 6 h	No recommendation

Note: See also http://www.hopkins-abxguide.org; accessed June 18, 2014.

respiratory sources. Most of these infections occur in the thoracic and lumbar spine.

The classic triad of back pain, fever, and neurological symptoms is present in a minority of patients, although back pain itself is very common and found in 70% to 90% of cases. Fever is also a common symptom. The typical course of an untreated epidural abscess occurs in four stages: (1) back pain, fever, and localized spinal tenderness; (2) spinal irritation with radicular pain, hyperreflexia, and nuchal rigidity; (3) fecal or urinary incontinence plus focal neurological deficits; and (4) motor paralysis of the lower extremities.

Diagnosis and Differential

Assess patient's epidural abscess risk factors such as immunocompromised states, intravenous drug abuse, spinal surgery, or recent procedures such as lumbar puncture or epidural anesthesia. Physical examination findings may include midline spine tenderness to palpation or percussion. Assess for neurologic findings and findings concerning for cauda equina syndrome. For example, decreased rectal tone has a reported sensitivity of 60% to 80%, while decreased perineal sensation has a sensitivity of 75%.

This challenging diagnosis is often delayed due to nonspecific presenting symptoms and the rarity of this condition. Laboratory studies such as CBC, erythrocyte sedimentation rate, and C-reactive protein may be helpful. Blood cultures are positive in 40% of cases and can be helpful to guide treatment after admission to the hospital. Neuroimaging with a gadolinium MRI is the preferred imaging modality for diagnosis, although a CT scan with myelography may be helpful if an MRI is not possible.

Emergency Department Care and Disposition

1. Emergent consultation with a spine surgeon is important when an epidural abscess is identified. While conclusive data regarding operative versus IV antibiotic therapy alone are not available, many patients do receive surgical debridement.
2. Begin empiric antibiotic therapy if a patient with an epidural abscess exhibits neurological dysfunction, signs of sepsis or systemic illness, or if immediate surgery is not available. Initial antibiotic dosing in the ED includes **vancomycin** 25 to 30 mg/kg IV along with **ceftazidime** 2 g IV or **cefepime** 2 g IV. Consider additional coverage with **gentamycin** 5 mg/kg IV in a patient with a recent neurosurgical procedure.
3. Patients with epidural abscess should be admitted to the hospital for IV antibiotics, close monitoring, neurological checks, and possible surgical debridement.

FURTHER READING

For further reading in *Tintinalli's Emergency Medicine: A Comprehensive Study Guide*, 8th ed., see Chapter 174, "Central Nervous System and Spinal Infections," by Mary E. Tanski and O. John Ma.

SECTION 16

Eye, Ear, Nose, Throat, and Oral Emergencies

CHAPTER 149 Eye Emergencies

Steven Go

INFECTIONS AND INFLAMMATION

Preseptal (Periorbital) and Postseptal (Orbital) Cellulitis

Preseptal cellulitis is an infection of the periorbital tissues, whereas postseptal cellulitis involves the orbit. Both conditions primarily present in children <10 years old. They may present nearly identically with typical symptoms of excessive tearing, erythema, warmth, tenderness to palpation of the lids, and periorbital tissue. **In preseptal cellulitis, there is NO eye involvement**. That is, visual acuity, pupillary responses, and eye appearance are normal, and there is **no pain with extraocular movements**. If any of these characteristics are present, or if there is concern about postseptal involvement, obtain a **CT scan with contrast of the orbit** (or MRI) to rule out orbital involvement. Preseptal cellulitis in nontoxic patients may be treated as an outpatient with **amoxicillin/clavulanic acid** 20 mg/kg PO divided every 12 hours; 500 mg PO three times daily in adults or a first-generation cephalosporin, hot packs, and with 24 to 48 hours ophthalmology follow-up. In cases of preseptal cellulitis that are severe or involve high-risk patients (e.g., children <5 years or patients with significant comorbidities) or in any case of postseptal cellulitis, obtain an **emergent ophthalmology consultation** for admission for intravenous antibiotics. Empiric therapy should begin with **cefuroxime** 50 mg/kg IV every 8 hours or **ceftriaxone** 50 mg/kg every 12 hours, or **ampicillin–sulbactam** 50 mg/kg IV every 6 hours, with IV vancomycin added if methicillin-resistant *Staphylococcus aureus* (MRSA) is suspected. Use fluoroquinolones PLUS metronidazole or clindamycin in penicillin allergic adults.

Stye (External Hordeolum) and Chalazion

A **stye** is an acute infection of an oil gland at the lash line that appears as a pustule at the **lid margin**. A **chalazion** is an acute or chronic inflammation of the **eyelid** secondary to meibomian gland blockage in the tarsal plate. When it is acute, a chalazion may be painful, but is usually painless when chronic. A stye or acute chalazion is treated with warm, wet compresses four times daily and with **erythromycin** 0.5% ophthalmic ointment twice daily for 7 to 10 days. Refer persistent or recurrent lesions to an ophthalmologist for further evaluation and treatment.

Bacterial Conjunctivitis

Bacterial conjunctivitis presents as eyelash matting, mild to moderate mucopurulent discharge, and conjunctival inflammation. Fluorescein staining of the cornea should be performed in patients with suspected conjunctivitis to avoid missing abrasions, ulcers, and dendritic lesions. Prescribe **topical antibiotics** for 5 to 7 days (Table 149-1). Quinolones (ciprofloxacin or ofloxacin ophthalmic) may be used in children due to limited systemic absorption. Avoid gentamicin due to high incidence of ocular irritation. *Haemophilus influenzae* and *Moraxella catarrhalis* are considerations in children; therefore, if erythromycin ointment is being used and is ineffective, a change in antibiotics should be initiated. Contact lens wearers should receive topical antibiotic coverage for *Pseudomonas*,

TABLE 149-1 Selected Ophthalmic Medications Used in the Emergency Department

Drug	Indication	Dose
Cyclopentolate*	Short-term mydriasis and cycloplegia for examination	0.5% in children, 1 drop; 1% in adults, 1 drop; onset 30 min, duration ≤24 h
Tropicamide*	Short-term mydriasis and cycloplegia for examination	1 to 2 drops of 0.5% or 1% solution, onset 20 min; duration of action 6 h
Homatropine*	Intermediate-term pupil dilation, cycloplegia, treatment of iritis	1 to 2 drops of 2% solution; onset 30 min; duration of action 2 to 4 days; for iritis 1 to 2 drops twice a day
Naphazoline and pheniramine*	Conjunctival congestion/itching	1 drop three to four times a day
Olopatadine	Allergic conjunctivitis	0.1% solution, 1 drop twice daily, onset of action 30 to 60 min, duration 12 h
Tetracaine ophthalmic solution	Anesthetic for eye examination, foreign body removal	0.5% solution, 1 to 2 drops; onset of action 1 min, duration 30 min
Proparacaine ophthalmic solution	Anesthetic for eye examination, foreign body removal	0.5% solution, 1 to 2 drops; onset of action 20 s, duration 15 min
Erythromycin ophthalmic ointment	Conjunctivitis. Do not use for corneal abrasion if a contact lens wearer	Half inch applied to lower eyelid two to four times a day
Ciprofloxacin	Conjunctivitis, corneal abrasion if a contact lens wearer	Solution: 1 to 2 drops when awake every 2 h for 2 days; ointment, half inch applied to lower eyelid three times a day for 2 days
Tobramycin	Conjunctivitis, corneal abrasions if a contact lens wearer	0.3% solution, 1 to 2 drops every 4 h; 0.3% ointment, half inch applied to lower lid two to three times a day
Sulfacetamide sodium	Conjunctivitis. Do not use for corneal abrasion if a contact lens wearer	10% solution, 1 to 2 drops four times a day

(Continued)

TABLE 149-1 Selected Ophthalmic Medications Used in the Emergency Department (Continued)

Drug	Indication	Dose
Ofloxacin	Conjunctivitis, corneal abrasions if a contact lens wearer	Conjunctivitis: 1 to 2 drops every 2–4 h for 2 days, then 1 to 2 drops four times a day for 5 days. Corneal ulcer: 1 to 2 drops every 30 min while awake and 1 to 2 drops every 4–6 h after retiring for 2 days, then 1 to 2 drops every hour while awake for 5–7 days, then 1 to 2 drops four times a day for 2 days or until treatment completion
Trifluridine	Herpes simplex keratitis	1 drop every 2 h
Ketorolac	Allergic conjunctivitis, corneal abrasions, ultraviolet keratitis	1 drop four times/day for 3–4 days
Prednisolone acetate†	Allergic conjunctivitis, uveitis	2 drops four times a day

*Agents that affect pupillary dilation or serve as a conjunctival decongestant should be avoided in patients with glaucoma.

†Should be prescribed ONLY in conjunction with a specific recommendation from ophthalmologist.

such as **ciprofloxacin** or **tobramycin**. The lens should be discarded and not replaced until the infection has completely resolved.

A severe purulent discharge with a hyperacute onset (within 12 to 24 hours) should prompt an **emergent ophthalmology consultation** for an aggressive workup for possible gonococcal conjunctivitis. *Neisseria gonorrhoeae* infections may be confirmed by Gram stain (gram-negative intracellular diplococci). Emergency department (ED) care for *N. gonorrhoeae* infections include culture, parenteral **ceftriaxone,** and **saline solution irrigation** to remove the discharge.

If bacterial conjunctivitis is present in a neonate, suspect a sexually transmitted disease (STD) etiology. These are sight-threatening conditions which can be difficult to diagnose, and an emergent ophthalmology evaluation in the ED is warranted. If gonorrhea is suspected, an inpatient workup for disseminated disease is indicated. If chlamydia is suspected, then associated pneumonia must be ruled out prior to discharge. Herpes conjunctivitis is also a possibility. (See **Herpes Simplex Virus**.)

Viral Conjunctivitis

Viral conjunctivitis presents as watery discharge, chemosis, and conjunctival inflammation. It is often associated with viral respiratory symptoms and occasionally preauricular lymphadenopathy. Fluorescein staining should be done as in bacterial conjunctivitis, specifically in this case to rule out dendritic lesions. Treatment consists of cool compresses four times daily, **naphazoline/pheniramine** 0.025%/0.3% one drop three times daily, as needed, for conjunctival congestion or itching, **artificial tears** five or six times a day, and ophthalmology follow-up in 7 to 14 days. If a clear distinction between viral and bacterial etiologies cannot be made, consideration should be made to add topical antibiotics (Table 149-1) until reexamination by an ophthalmologist; however, **routine use of antibiotics is discouraged**. All the cases of viral conjunctivitis are extremely contagious and appropriate transmission precautions must be taken.

Allergic Conjunctivitis

Allergic conjunctivitis presents as pruritus, watery discharge, and chemosis with a history of allergies. There should be no lesions with fluorescein staining and no preauricular nodes. Conjunctival papillae are seen on slit lamp examination. Treatment consists of elimination of the inciting agent, cool compresses four times daily, **artificial tears** five or six times daily, and **naphazoline/pheniramine** 0.025%/0.3% one drop four times daily. Severe cases may require a mild topical steroid, but steroids should be only administered in consultation with an ophthalmologist.

Herpes Simplex Virus

Herpes simplex virus (HSV) infection may involve the eyelids, conjunctiva, or cornea. Corneal lesions stain brightly with fluorescein and can appear as a classic "dendrite" (a linear branching, epithelial defect with terminal bulbs) or as a "geographic ulcer" (an amoeba-like ulceration with dendrites at the edges) (Figure 149-1), but the presentation can be very variable and subtle. Corneal sensation can be decreased and should be checked. It is essential that HSV infection should not be confused with conjunctivitis, hence the necessity of a slit lamp fluorescein examination in these patients. If HSV infection is suspected, obtain an **ophthalmology consult**. If the outbreak involves only the eyelids, **acyclovir** 800 mg PO five times daily

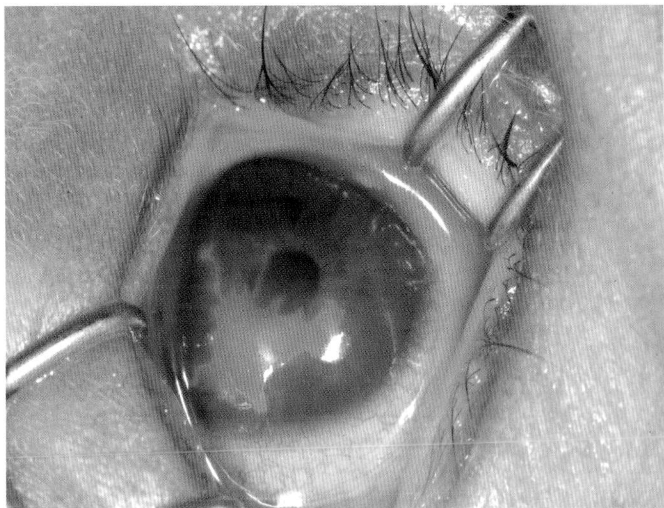

FIGURE 149-1. Herpes simplex corneal dendrite in an infant seen with fluorescein staining. Used with permission from Allen R. Katz, Department of Ophthalmology, University of Nebraska Medical Center.

for 7 to 10 days should be prescribed. If the conjunctiva is involved, prescribe **trifluorothymidine** 1% drops nine times daily. In addition, **erythromycin** ophthalmic 0.5% ointment twice daily and warm soaks three times daily to skin lesions can help prevent secondary bacterial infections. If corneal or deeper structure involvement is present, then antibiotic choice should be determined by the consulting ophthalmologist. **Topical steroids are to be strictly avoided in all cases of HSV infection**. Close follow-up from the ED and strong precautions are essential.

When conjunctivitis is present in the neonate, especially with mucocutaneous lesions, HSV also should be suspected, even in the absence of maternal infection. As with other causes of neonatal conjunctivitis, an emergent ophthalmology consult at the bedside is warranted. If HSV is diagnosed or strongly suspected, treat with **acyclovir** 20 mg/kg IV every 8 hours and topical antivirals (1% trifluridine, 0.1% iododeoxyuridine, or 3% vidarabine). Further workup for sepsis is indicated. Steroid drops should not be given.

Herpes Zoster Ophthalmicus

Shingles in a trigeminal distribution with ocular involvement is termed *herpes zoster ophthalmicus* (HZO). The presence or eventual development of HZO should be suspected in any patient whose shingles involve the tip of the nose (Hutchinson's sign). Photophobia and pain secondary to iritis are often present. Slit lamp examination may show a "pseudodendrite," a poorly staining mucus plaque without epithelial erosion. **Acyclovir** 800 mg PO five times a day, **famciclovir** 500 mg three times daily, or **valacyclovir** 1000 mg three times daily for 7 to 10 days should be prescribed if the skin lesions have been present less than 7 days. In addition, **erythromycin** 2% ointment and warm compresses should be applied to skin lesions. Ocular involvement requires **erythromycin** 0.5% ophthalmic ointment to the eye twice daily. For comfort, oral opioid analgesia, cycloplegic agents (**cyclopentolate** 1% one drop three times daily), and cool compresses are helpful. If iritis is present, **prednisolone acetate** 1% one drop every 1 to 6 hours is effective. However, because topical steroid use in patients with herpes simplex keratoconjunctivitis may be catastrophic, it is imperative that there should be no corneal lesions present on slit lamp examination before topical steroids are used. In severe cases, admission and **acyclovir** IV may be required. For this reason, all the cases of suspected HZO require **ophthalmology consultation**. All patients younger than 40 years with HZO should undergo an outpatient medical evaluation for a possible immunocompromised state.

Corneal Ulcer

A corneal ulcer is a serious infection of the corneal stroma caused by bacteria including *Pseudomonas aeruginosa*, viruses including herpes simplex and varicella zoster, and fungi. Immunocompromised patients are at risk for fungal or viral etiologies. It is commonly associated with trauma, especially in patients who use extended-wear contact lenses and those who wear lenses while sleeping. Ulcers may cause pain, redness, tearing, photophobia, and blurry vision. Slit lamp examination shows a staining corneal defect with a surrounding white hazy infiltrate, and associated iritis and sometimes a hypopyon. Topical **ofloxacin** 0.3% or **ciprofloxacin** 0.3% ophthalmic solution should be administered, one drop in the affected eye each hour. Antifungal or antiviral antibiotics may be given to immunocompromised patients in consultation with an ophthalmologist. Topical cycloplegics, such as **cyclopentolate** 1% one drop three times daily, aid in pain relief. Eye patching is strictly contraindicated because of the risk of worsening a potential *Pseudomonas* infection. **Steroid drops should be avoided** unless an ophthalmologist advises administration. It would be ideal for the patient to be seen by an ophthalmologist in the ED in order to culture the ulcer prior to starting antibiotics. However, if this is not possible, they should see the patient within 12 to 24 hours.

Iritis

Iritis is inflammation of the anterior uveal tract (iris and ciliary body) that has many causes (Table 149-2). It presents with red eye, photophobia, and decreased vision. A hallmark physical examination sign is *consensual pain* (pain in the affected eye when light is shined in the nonaffected eye). Slit lamp examination reveals WBCs in the anterior chamber, usually with associated flare, and a hypopyon can eventually occur. Perform an exam with fluorescein dye to detect corneal abrasions, ulcers, or dendritic lesions, and measure intraocular pressure (IOP), which can be elevated. Once iritis is diagnosed, undertake an appropriate ED workup for a systemic etiology and treat them, if found. Symptomatic treatment with **tropicamide** (Table 149-1) is helpful. Ophthalmology consultation is appropriate with follow-up in 24 to 48 hours. Steroid drops can be of value, but should only be given if directed by the ophthalmologist.

Endophthalmitis

Endophthalmitis is an infection involving the deep structures of the globe. Patients present with pain and visual loss. It is often seen as a complication of globe violation either from trauma or ocular surgery. Hematologic spread is possible. Pathogens include *Staphylococcus, Streptococcus, Haemophilus,* and *Bacillus* species. Emergency ophthalmology consultation

TABLE 149-2 Differential Diagnosis of Iritis

Systemic diseases	Malignancies
Juvenile rheumatoid arthritis	Leukemia
Ankylosing spondylitis	Lymphoma
Ulcerative colitis	Malignant melanoma
Reiter's syndrome	Trauma/environmental
Behçet's syndrome	Corneal foreign body
Sarcoidosis	Posttraumatic (blunt trauma)
Infectious	Ultraviolet keratitis
Tuberculosis	
Lyme disease	
Herpes simplex	
Toxoplasmosis	
Varicella zoster	
Syphilis	
Adenovirus	

and admission are warranted. Treatment may include vitreous aspiration, vitrectomy, intraocular and systemic antibiotics, and steroids.

TRAUMA

Subconjunctival Hemorrhage

This injury is a disruption of conjunctival blood vessels, typically secondary to trauma, sneezing, or the Valsalva maneuver. It requires no treatment and usually resolves within 2 weeks. Its primary clinical importance rests in the fact that it can be a sign of significant eye injury when due to trauma, and recurrent episodes should prompt an evaluation for a coagulopathy.

Corneal Abrasion and Ultraviolet Keratitis

Traumatic abrasions may cause superficial or deep epithelial defects resulting in tearing, photophobia, blepharospasm, and pain. Administration of a topical anesthetic often will facilitate the examination. **Proparacaine** 0.5% is preferred over tetracaine because it causes less pain upon administration and provides comparable anesthesia. A corneal abrasion will glow green during a fluorescein stain examination when using the cobalt blue light on the slit lamp. A careful search for an ocular foreign body (including upper lid eversion) must be done in the presence of an abrasion, especially when they are multiple and linear. Once the diagnosis of a simple abrasion is made, prescribe **ketorolac ophthalmic solution** one drop four times a day for pain control. For severe pain with large abrasions, **opioid analgesia** and/or a **cycloplegic** (e.g., **cyclopentolate** 1% one drop three times a day) may be considered. Abrasions are treated with **topical antibiotics** (Table 149-1). Most patients are treated with **erythromycin ointment**; however, abrasions associated with contact lens wear should be treated with antipseudomonal topical antibiotics (e.g., **ciprofloxacin, ofloxacin**, or **tobramycin**). Patching corneal abrasions traditionally has been recommended; however, excellent patient comfort can be achieved without it. More importantly, patching does not hasten the healing of abrasions and can greatly harm the patient if lesions prone to infection (e.g., contact lens abrasions or corneal ulcers) are patched. Prescribing topical anesthetics is absolutely contraindicated because repeated use may cause catastrophic corneal damage. All abrasions should be reexamined in 24 to 48 hours by an ophthalmologist, with those that are large or involve the visual axis seen sooner.

Exposure to ultraviolet light from welding ("arc welder's keratitis"), tanning beds, or prolonged sun exposure (especially when reflected off ice and snow-covered slopes at high altitude) can cause a diffuse burn to the cornea which appears as diffuse punctate corneal abrasions with edema. Severe pain and photophobia develop 6 to 12 hours after exposure. Treatment is similar to corneal abrasions, but more aggressive pain control is sometimes necessary. Healing typically occurs in 2 to 3 days.

Corneal Foreign Bodies

Superficial foreign bodies of the cornea are removed under slit lamp microscopy with a 25-guage needle, an eye spud, or an ophthalmic burr. Topical anesthesia (e.g., **proparacaine 0.5%**) is used and can also be instilled in the unaffected eye to depress reflex blinking. For obvious reasons, this procedure should be attempted only in a sober, cooperative patient. Any corneal foreign body deep within the corneal stroma or in the central visual axis should be removed by an ophthalmologist. Metallic foreign bodies often leave an epithelial "rust ring" that may be removed immediately with an **eye burr**; however, it is often easier to remove in 24 to 48 hours. A corneal abrasion will result from foreign body removal and is treated in the standard manner (**cycloplegics, antibiotics**). All patients should be referred to an ophthalmologist within 24 hours. The presence of either **gross or micro hyphema** should prompt further investigation for possible globe perforation. (See **Penetrating Trauma or Ruptured Globe.**)

Lid Lacerations

Many small superficial lacerations to the eye lids can be repaired by emergency physicians; however, eyelid lacerations that involve the lid margin, those within 6 to 8 mm of the medial canthus or involving the lacrimal duct or sac, those involving the inner surface of the lid, wounds associated with ptosis, and those involving the tarsal plate or levator palpebrae muscle, need repair by an oculoplastic surgeon. Due to a high chance of morbidity, lid margin lacerations >1 mm require closure by an ophthalmologist, whereas those <1 mm can heal spontaneously. For medial lid lacerations, injury to the nasolacrimal duct system should be considered. Fluorescein instilled into the tear layer that appears in an adjacent laceration confirms the injury. Nasolacrimal duct injuries, upper lid lacerations that involve the levator mechanism, and all through-and-through lid lacerations must be repaired in the operating room. **All full-thickness lid lacerations should be further investigated to rule out an associated corneal laceration and globe rupture**. If an ophthalmologist is not immediately available to evaluate a high-risk lid laceration, it is not unreasonable to prescribe **cephalexin** 500 mg PO four times daily, **erythromycin** 2% ointment four times daily, and gentle cold compresses with referral for ophthalmic evaluation within 24 hours, as long as any sight-threatening lesions have been excluded.

Blunt Eye Trauma

An eye speculum (or two bent paper clips) may be useful in visualization of the bluntly injured eye, but care should be taken to avoid any pressure on the globe. Once the eye is visualized, the integrity of the globe and visual acuity must be assessed immediately. Red flag signs such as an **abnormal anterior chamber depth**, an **irregular pupil**, or **blindness** indicate a ruptured globe until proven otherwise, and an emergent ophthalmology referral is indicated. An **eye shield** should be placed **as soon as a globe injury is suspected to protect against further injury.** If there are no hard signs of globe rupture, a complete eye exam, including slit lamp examination, should be performed to check for blowout fracture, corneal abrasions, lacerations, foreign bodies, hyphema, pupillary injury, iritis, and lens dislocation. **Postseptal hemorrhage** can also occur with blunt trauma, especially in those on anticoagulants. Pain, proptosis, impaired extraocular movements, decreased vision, possible afferent pupillary defect (APD), and elevated IOP are the hallmarks of this condition. Orbital compartment syndrome may result and may require a lateral canthotomy to alleviate sight-threatening increased IOP. A **CT of the orbit** is the ED test of choice to confirm the presence of ruptured globe, intraocular foreign body, post-septal hemorrhage, and orbital fractures, but sensitivity can be as low as 70% for occult globe injury; therefore, the involvement of an **ophthalmologist** is mandatory for possible surgical exploration in high-risk or suspicious cases. Traumatic iritis in the absence of a corneal injury can be treated with **prednisolone acetate** 1% one drop every 6 hours and **cyclopentolate** 1% one drop every 8 hours. The care of the blunt trauma eye patient should be discussed with an ophthalmologist, and the patient should follow-up with the ophthalmologist within 48 hours even if no significant injuries are initially found.

Hyphema

A hyphema is the presence of blood in the anterior chamber and often is a sign of significant trauma. It also can occur spontaneously in sickle cell patients and in patients with coagulopathies. Sight-threatening increases in IOP can occur. In all hyphemas, emergent evaluation by an ophthalmologist is indicated. **The patient should be placed either fully upright or head-of-bead (HOB) to 30° to 45°** to allow the blood to settle inferiorly, which allows faster improvement of vision and facilitates assessment of the hyphema size and posterior pole. A **protective eye shield** should be in place, except during examination and medication administration. After ruptured globe is excluded, the patient should be evaluated for other eye injuries and treated appropriately. Because of the 30% risk of rebleed in 3 to 5 days and the potential necessity of surgical intervention, any disposition decisions should be made by an ophthalmologist at the bedside, regardless of the size of the hyphema.

Orbital Blowout Fractures

Orbital blowout fractures commonly involve the inferior wall and medial wall. The resultant entrapment of the inferior rectus muscle may cause restriction of movement, with a resultant diplopia on upward gaze. Other signs include paresthesia in the distribution of the infraorbital nerve and subcutaneous emphysema, particularly when sneezing or blowing the nose. If a blowout fracture is suspected, CT of the orbit with 1.5-mm cuts should be performed, with additional studies as indicated. Because of the high incidence of associated ocular trauma (33%), make an aggressive effort to exclude associated injuries. Antibiotic prophylaxis with **cephalexin** 250 to 500 mg PO four times daily for 10 days is recommended due to sinus involvement. Refer all isolated blowout fractures, with or without entrapment, to an ophthalmologist for a formal dilated exam to rule out retinal injury.

Penetrating Trauma or Ruptured Globe

Globe penetration or rupture is a catastrophic injury that must be identified immediately. Suggestive findings include a severe subconjunctival hemorrhage, shallow or deep anterior chamber as compared with the other eye, hyphema, teardrop-shaped pupil, limitation of extraocular motility, extrusion of globe contents, or a significant reduction in visual acuity. However, it is important to note that **penetrating injury from small foreign bodies can present with a nearly normal exam**. Therefore, strongly suspect a penetrating injury when the history of a high-speed foreign body (e.g., the patient was hammering or grinding without eye protection) or a penetrating injury in proximity of the orbit is present. A bright-green streaming appearance to fluorescein instilled into the tear layer (Seidel test) is pathognomonic, although it may be absent if the wound has sealed. Therefore, **the presence of an abrasion with this mechanism does not rule out a penetrating injury**. Once a globe injury is suspected, any further manipulation or examination of the eye must be avoided. In such cases, **place a protective eye shield immediately** and place the patient upright and keep them NPO. Administer broad-spectrum antibiotics with an antiemetic to prevent increased IOP from vomiting. Update tetanus status if necessary. In unclear cases, it may be necessary to perform a CT of the orbit to confirm the presence of an orbital foreign body or a ruptured globe. However, as noted above, CT sensitivity can be low for occult globe injury; therefore, an **ophthalmologist should be called immediately if a globe rupture or a penetrating injury is strongly suspected**.

Chemical Ocular Injury

Acid and alkali burns are managed in a similar manner. The eye should be flushed immediately at the scene and sterile **normal saline** or **Ringer lactate irrigation solution** should be continued in the ED **immediately** upon arrival (even before visual acuities or patient registration) until the pH remains at or near 7.4. A **topical anesthetic** and a Morgan lens are used in this procedure. After the first 2 L of irrigation, the pH may be checked in the lower cul-de-sac with litmus paper or the pH square on a urine dipstick 5 to 10 minutes after suspending irrigation (to allow time for equilibration). Irrigation should be continued until a normal pH can be maintained **at least 30 minutes after cessation**. Irrigation volumes needed to reach normal pH may exceed 8 to 10 L, depending on the caustic substance. A persistently abnormal pH should prompt removal of any crystallized particles in the fornices with a moistened cotton-tipped applicator. Once the pH is normal, the fornices should be inspected and the eyelids everted to look for any residual particles and reswept with a moistened cotton-tipped applicator to remove them and any necrotic conjunctiva. The pH should be rechecked every 10 minutes for 30 minutes to make sure that no additional corrosive is leaching out from the tissues. A thorough slit lamp examination, with lid eversion, should be done to assess the amount of damage and any associated injuries. IOP should be measured because it can become elevated with significant burns. A cycloplegic (**cyclopentolate** 1%) one drop three times daily will alleviate ciliary spasm, and **erythromycin** 0.5% ophthalmic ointment applied every 1 to 2 hours while awake should be prescribed. Most patients will require **opioid pain medications**. Update tetanus status if necessary. If there are signs of a severe injury, such as a pronounced chemosis, conjunctival blanching, epithelial defect, corneal edema or opacification, or increased IOP, the patient should be seen in the ED by an ophthalmologist. Certain specialized burns, such as those due to hydrofluoric acid, lye, or concrete, also should be seen by an ophthalmologist immediately. Otherwise, a telephone consult with the ophthalmologist to arrange close follow-up within 24 hours should be obtained for all ocular burns.

Cyanoacrylate (Super Glue or Crazy Glue) Exposure

Cyanoacrylate glue easily adheres to the eyelids and corneal surface. Its primary morbidity stems from corneal injuries from the hard particles that form. Initial manual removal is facilitated by heavy application of **erythromycin** 0.5% ophthalmic ointment, with special care to avoid damaging underlying structures. After the easily removable pieces are removed, the patient should be discharged with **erythromycin** 0.5% ophthalmic ointment to be applied five times a day to soften the remaining glue. Complete removal of the residual glue can be accomplished by the ophthalmologist at a follow-up visit within 24 hours. Serious injury from this exposure is rare.

ACUTE VISUAL REDUCTION OR LOSS

Acute Angle Closure Glaucoma

Acute angle closure glaucoma classically presents with sudden onset of severe eye pain and/or headache, cloudy vision, colored halos around lights, and vomiting. Acute attacks in patients can be precipitated in movie theaters, while reading, and after ill-advised use of dilatory agents or inhaled anticholinergics or cocaine. Physical examination may reveal conjunctival injection, corneal clouding, a fixed mid-dilated pupil, and increased IOP of 40 to 70 mm Hg (normal range, 10 to 20 mm Hg). All cases require **immediate ophthalmologic consultation**. Simultaneous to the ophthalmology consult, attempts to decrease the IOP (Table 149-3) should begin immediately. Place the patient supine. Controlled comparative efficacy data are lacking for medical treatment, so treatment recommendations vary. However, in general, medications to administer include **timolol** 0.5%, **apraclonidine** 1.0%, and PO **acetazolamide** 500 mg in the absence of contraindications (acetazolamide is contraindicated in sickle cell and sulfa allergic patients). If IOP is greater than 50 mm Hg, if vision loss is severe, or if the patient cannot tolerate PO then **IV acetazolamide** should be given instead. If IOP remains ≥40 mm Hg 30 minutes after treatment has begun, **mannitol** should be considered. **Pilocarpine** 1% to 2% one drop every 15 minutes for two doses in the affected eye and **pilocarpine** 0.5% one drop in the contralateral eye may be given once the IOP

TABLE 149-3 Treatment of Acute Glaucoma

Treatment (Wait One Minute Between Administration of Each Eye Drop)	Effect
Topical β-blocker (timolol 0.5%), 1 drop	Blocks production of aqueous humor
Topical α-agonist (apraclonidine 1%), 1 drop	Blocks production of aqueous humor
Carbonic anhydrase inhibitor (acetazolamide), 500 mg IV or PO	Blocks production of aqueous humor
Mannitol, 1 to 2 g/kg IV	Reduces volume of aqueous humor
Recheck IOP hourly	—
Topical pilocarpine 1% to 2%, 1 drop every 15 min for two doses; once IOP is below 40 mm Hg, then four times daily	Facilitates outflow of aqueous humor

Abbreviation: IOP, intraocular pressure.

is below 40 mm Hg, although some experts recommend giving pilocarpine immediately upon diagnosis. Symptoms of pain and nausea should be treated, and the IOP should be monitored hourly. Subsequent treatment decisions and disposition of the patient should be made by an ophthalmologist at the bedside.

Optic Neuritis

Optic neuritis (ON) refers to inflammation at any point along the optic nerve and presents with acute vision loss, with a particular reduction in color vision. It is strongly associated with multiple sclerosis (MS), but many other etiologies exist (e.g., syphilis, tuberculosis, and sarcoidosis). It is often painless, but can sometimes be painful, especially with extraocular movements. The red desaturation test may be helpful in identifying optic neuropathies. This test is performed by having the patient look with one eye at a time at a dark red object. The affected eye often will see a red object as pink or lighter red. An APD often can be detected, and visual field defects may be present. In anterior ON, the optic disc appears swollen (papillitis); there are no ophthalmoscopic findings in retrobulbar cases. An ophthalmologist should direct evaluation and treatment. IV steroids, followed by oral steroids, have been shown to accelerate visual recovery and temporarily reduce the risk of developing MS, but oral steroids alone actually increase the rate of ON reoccurrence. A new diagnosis of ON should prompt a workup for MS and other causes.

Central Retinal Artery Occlusion

Central retinal artery occlusion presents as a sudden, painless, severe monocular loss of vision, often associated with a history of amaurosis fugax. Occlusion of the central retinal artery will cause complete visual loss, whereas arterial branch obstruction will cause abrupt loss of a partial visual field. Classic signs include nearly complete or complete vision loss (94% with counting fingers to light perception only), a marked APD, superficial opacification or whitening of the retina in the posterior pole, and a bright red macula "cherry red spot." Segmentation of the blood column in the arterioles ("boxcarring") sometimes can be seen. A thorough evaluation to uncover the etiology (commonly an embolic source—carotid or cardiac, vasculitis, or hypercoagulable state) is required. Giant cell arteritis must be excluded. An ophthalmologist should be contacted immediately once the diagnosis is made. In the past, digital massage, acetazolamide, and timolol have been recommended, but evidence to support these interventions is sparse. Therefore, management should be directed by an ophthalmologist per institutional protocols.

Central Retinal Vein Occlusion

Central retinal vein occlusion secondary to thrombosis causes acute, painless monocular vision loss. Examination shows optic disc edema, cotton wool spots, and retinal hemorrhages in all four quadrants. This pattern is described as "blood-and-thunder fundus." APD is often present. There is no immediate treatment for central retinal vein occlusion, but predisposing drugs (e.g., oral contraceptives or diuretics) should be discontinued. An ophthalmology consult should be obtained.

Retinal Detachment and Floaters

Patients who experience sudden change in their vision due to retinal detachment or "floaters" in their visual field usually seek medical attention in the ED. Bilateral symptoms are almost always intracranial in origin and may be due to migraine headaches. Monocular symptoms are usually due to disorders in the symptomatic eye. Retinal detachment typically presents as a sudden flashes of light, floaters, or a dark veil or curtain-like defect in the patient's visual field, affecting the symptomatic eye. Presumptive diagnosis can be made by bedside ultrasonography. Urgent ophthalmologic consultation is necessary for indirect ophthalmoscopic evaluation, and potentially laser surgery. In contrast, new "floaters" which are small particles of vitreous gel appearing to the patient as small hazy opacities need no immediate attention and can be followed up by the ophthalmologist in the office within 24 hours for a dilated exam.

Temporal Arteritis (Giant Cell Arteritis)

Temporal arteritis (TA) is a systemic vasculitis that can cause a painless ischemic optic neuropathy. Patients are typically women older than 50 years, often with a history of polymyalgia rheumatica. Associated symptoms include vision changes, headache, jaw claudication, scalp or temporal artery tenderness, fatigue, fever, sore throat, URI symptoms, and anorexia. Symptoms are usually unilateral, but may be bilateral. One-third of the cases are associated with neurologic events such as transient ischemic attacks or stroke. An APD is frequently present, and funduscopic examination may show flame hemorrhages. A sixth cranial nerve palsy may occur. When TA is suspected, an erythrocyte sedimentation rate (ESR) and C-reactive protein (CRP) should be ordered; both are elevated in TA, with the CRP the more sensitive test. Most patients with biopsy-proven cases have an ESR in the range of 70 to 110 mm/h. If TA is not treated, bilateral vision loss can develop. Therefore, if there is strong suspicion of TA or vision loss is present, the patient should be admitted for **methylprednisolone** 250 mg IV every 6 hours. For less suspicious patients with no vision loss, discharge home with **prednisone** 80 to 100 mg/d PO with close follow-up. Steroids should not be delayed pending results of a biopsy. Antiulcer medications should be prescribed to be given with systemic steroids.

OCULAR ULTRASONOGRAPHY

Ocular ultrasonography can be very useful for the emergent evaluation of the eye, especially in trauma. Ultrasonography can be useful in the emergent diagnosis of retinal detachment, retrobulbar hematoma, lens dislocation, vitreous hemorrhage, and elevated intracranial pressure. Care should be taken to avoid any pressure on the eye or eyelid if globe rupture is suspected and duration of ocular ultrasonography should be strictly limited.

FURTHER READING

For further reading in *Tintinalli's Emergency Medicine: A Comprehensive Study Guide*, 8th ed., see Chapter 241, "Eye Emergencies," by Richald A.Walker and Srikar Adhikari; Chapter 119, "Eye Emergencies in Infants and Children," by Janeva Kircher and Andrew Dixon.

CHAPTER 150

Face and Jaw Emergencies

Jeffrey G. Norvell

FACIAL INFECTIONS

Facial Cellulitis

Cellulitis is a soft tissue infection that involves the skin and subcutaneous tissues. Facial cellulitis is most commonly caused by *Streptococcus pyogenes* and *Staphylococcus aureus*, with an increasing predominance of methicillin-resistant *Staphylococcus aureus* (MRSA). Less commonly, cellulitis may represent an extension from a deeper facial infection. Cellulitis is characterized by erythema, edema, warmth, pain, and loss of function. Clinical features of a well-defined, palpable border are absent.

The diagnosis of cellulitis is clinical. Ultrasound and computed tomography (CT) may be used to evaluate for abscess or more extensive infection. In most cases, treatment involves oral antibiotics for 7 to 14 days. Antibiotic recommendations for conditions discussed in this chapter are listed in Tables 150-1 and 150-2. Consider hospitalization and parenteral antibiotics

TABLE 150-1 Antibiotic Therapy for Facial Infections

Cellulitis	Oral therapy: clindamycin, dicloxacillin, or cephalosporins Suspected MRSA: trimethoprim-sulfamethoxazole, clindamycin, doxycycline, or minocycline Parenteral therapy: vancomycin, clindamycin Total duration 7–10 days
Erysipelas	Oral therapy: penicillin Methicillin-sensitive *Staphylococcus aureus* suspected: amoxicillin/clavulanate, cephalexin, dicloxacillin Bullous erysipelas: trimethoprim-sulfamethoxazole, clindamycin, doxycycline, or minocycline Parenteral therapy: vancomycin, nafcillin, clindamycin Total duration 7–10 days
Impetigo	Topical: mupirocin or retapamulin ointment alone or with oral therapy Oral therapy: dicloxacillin, amoxicillin/clavulanate, cephalexin MRSA suspected: clindamycin or trimethoprim-sulfamethoxazole Total duration 7 days
Suppurative parotitis	Oral therapy: amoxicillin-clavulanate, clindamycin, or cephalexin and metronidazole Parenteral therapy: nafcillin, ampicillin-sulbactam, or vancomycin with metronidazole Hospital acquired or nursing home patients: include vancomycin Total duration: 10–14 days
Masticator space infection	Parenteral therapy: IV clindamycin is recommended; alternatives include ampicillin-sulbactam, cefoxitin, or the combination of penicillin with metronidazole Oral therapy: clindamycin or amoxicillin-clavulanate Total duration: 10–14 days

Abbreviation: MRSA, methicillin-resistant *Staphylococcus aureus*.

TABLE 150-2 Antibiotic Doses for Facial Infections

Antibiotic	Dosage
Topical Antibiotics	
Mupirocin ointment	2%, apply to lesions three times per day
Retapamulin ointment	1%, apply to lesions two times per day
Oral Antibiotics	
Amoxicillin/clavulanate	875/125 mg two times per day
Cephalexin	500 mg four times per day
Clindamycin	300–450mg four times per day
Dicloxacillin	500 mg four times per day
Doxycycline	100 mg two times per day
Metronidazole	500 mg every 8 hours
Minocycline	100 mg two times per day
Penicillin V	500 mg four times per day
Trimethoprim-sulfamethoxazole	1–2 double-strength tablets two times per day
Parenteral Antibiotics	
Ampicillin-sulbactam	1.5–3.0 g every 6 hours
Clindamycin	600 mg every 8 hours
Cefazolin	1 g every 8 hours
Metronidazole	1 g loading dose, then 500 mg every 8 hours
Nafcillin	1–2 g every 4 hours
Penicillin G	2–3 million units every 6 hours
Vancomycin	1 g every 12 hours

for patients with signs of systemic illness, failed outpatient therapy, or significant comorbidities.

Erysipelas

Erysipelas is a superficial form of cellulitis, involving the epidermis, upper levels of the dermis, and the lymphatic system. Most cases are caused by *S. pyogenes*; *S. aureus* is a rare etiology but is associated with bullous disease, trauma, or the presence of a foreign body. Clinical features include a red, raised, puffy appearance with a sharply defined, palpable border. The diagnosis is clinical. Most patients are treated with oral antibiotics, but hospitalization and parenteral antibiotics should be considered for patients who fail outpatient therapy, are immunocompromised, or exhibit evidence of systemic illness.

Impetigo

Impetigo is a superficial epidermal infection that can be divided into bullous and nonbullous presentations. Bullous impetigo is caused by *S. aureus* and nonbullous impetigo is caused by *S. aureus* and *S. pyogenes*. Clinical features of nonbullous impetigo include an erythematous rash with vesicles that break and form the characteristic amber crusts. Bullous impetigo presents as vesicles that enlarge to form bullae with clear yellow fluid. Topical therapy with **mupirocin** is appropriate for simple, nonbullous disease. Oral antibiotics are prescribed for more extensive or bullous lesions.

SALIVARY GLAND DISORDERS

Viral Parotitis (Mumps)

Viral parotitis is an infection that can present with unilateral or bilateral swelling of the parotid glands. It is most commonly caused by a paramyxovirus. Clinical features may include a prodrome of fever, malaise, myalgias, and headache followed by parotid gland swelling. The gland is tense and painful, but lacks erythema and warmth. Pus cannot be expressed from Stensen's duct.

The diagnosis is clinical and treatment is supportive. Swelling may persist for 5 days. The patient is contagious for approximately 9 days after the onset of parotid swelling. Extrasalivary gland involvement includes orchitis in 20% to 30% of males and oophoritis in 5% of females. Other systemic complications include pancreatitis, aseptic meningitis, hearing loss, myocarditis, arthritis, hemolytic anemia, and thrombocytopenia. Consider hospitalization for patients with systemic complications.

Suppurative Parotitis

Suppurative parotitis is a serious bacterial infection that occurs in patients with diminished salivary flow. Retrograde transmission of bacteria leads to infection. Factors that lead to decreased salivary flow include recent anesthesia, dehydration, prematurity, advanced age, medications (e.g., diuretics, β-blockers, antihistamines, phenothiazines, and tricyclic antidepressants), and certain disorders (Sjögren's syndrome, diabetes, hypothyroidism, cystic fibrosis, and human immunodeficiency virus). Clinical features may include fever, trismus, erythema, and pain over the parotid gland. Pus may be expressed from Stensen's duct.

The diagnosis is clinical. Ultrasound or CT may be ordered if an abscess is suspected. Treatment should optimize salivary flow by using sialogogues such as lemon drops and stopping any medications that cause dry mouth. Oral antibiotics are appropriate for those tolerating oral intake and are without trismus. Hospitalization is appropriate for patients with signs of systemic illness, immunocompromise, inability to tolerate oral intake, or those that have failed outpatient therapy. Close follow-up should be arranged.

Sialolithiasis

Sialolithiasis is the development of stones in a stagnant salivary duct. Eighty percent of stones occur in the submandibular duct. Sialolithiasis is typically unilateral and presents with pain, swelling, and tenderness that may be exacerbated with eating. The diagnosis is clinical. A stone may be palpated within the duct and the gland is firm. Treatment includes analgesics, massage, sialogogues such as lemon drops, and antibiotics if a concurrent infection is suspected. Palpable stones may be milked from the duct. Persistent retained calculi may be removed by an otolaryngologist.

Masticator Space Abscess

The masticator space consists of potential spaces bounded by the muscles of mastication. Infection is usually polymicrobial and is commonly associated with an odontogenic source. Clinical features include facial swelling, pain, erythema, and trismus. In advanced cases, signs of sepsis may be present. The diagnosis is made with contrast-enhanced CT scan. Because the masticator spaces ultimately communicate with tissue planes that extend into the mediastinum, early treatment is imperative. ED treatment includes stabilization, antibiotics, otolaryngology consult, and hospitalization.

MANDIBLE DISORDERS

Temporomandibular Joint Dysfunction

The temporomandibular joint (TMJ) combines a hinge and a gliding action. Anatomic derangements or systemic disease can cause dysfunction of this joint. Clinical features include pain over the muscles of mastication or in the region of the TMJ and there may be a limited range of motion. The diagnosis is usually clinical. For patients with acute trauma, imaging with CT or panoramic x-ray may be warranted. Treatment for nontraumatic conditions consists of analgesics, soft diet, and referral to a dental specialist. An oral and maxillofacial surgeon manages fractures.

Trigeminal Neuralgia

Trigeminal neuralgia presents with facial pain in the distribution of the fifth cranial nerve. It is characterized by paroxysms of severe pain lasting seconds, with normal findings on physical exam. **Carbamazepine**, starting at 100 mg PO twice a day and then increasing dosage as needed, is an effective treatment.

Bell's Palsy

Bell's palsy is characterized by an acute onset of unilateral upper and lower facial paralysis. A detailed neurologic exam is useful in ruling out other conditions, such as stroke. Sparing of the forehead muscles on the affected side is suggestive of a central process. Examine the ear for presence of cranial herpes zoster. Treatment with **steroids** within the first 72 hours of symptom onset is thought to improve chances of a full recovery. The recommended dosing is 1 mg/kg of prednisone or equivalent, up to 60 mg/d, for 6 days followed by a 10-day taper. The use of antivirals is controversial and benefit modest at best. Ocular lubricants should be used to prevent dry eyes.

Dislocation of the Mandible

The mandible can be dislocated in an anterior, posterior, lateral, or superior position. Anterior dislocation is the most common. Patients with an acute jaw dislocation present with pain, difficulty swallowing, and malocclusion. In anterior dislocations, a history of extreme mouth opening is typical and there is difficulty with jaw movement. Other dislocations usually require significant trauma.

The diagnosis of atraumatic anterior dislocations is clinical. Imaging with panoramic x-ray or CT is indicated for all other dislocations. Treatment of anterior dislocations without fracture is closed reduction and this is made easier with analgesia, muscle relaxants, or procedural sedation. Reduction is most commonly done in a seated patient. The thumbs are padded with gauze, placed over the molars, and pressure is applied downward and backward. Patients with open or nonreducible dislocations, fractures, or nerve injury should be referred emergently to an oral and maxillofacial surgeon. After reduction, patients should be instructed to not open their mouth more than 2 cm for 2 weeks. Elective referral to an oral and maxillofacial surgeon is recommended.

FURTHER READING

For further reading in *Tintinalli's Emergency Medicine: A Comprehensive Study Guide*, 8th ed., see Chapter 243, "Face and Jaw Emergencies," by Stephanie A. Lareau and Corey R. Heitz.

CHAPTER 151 Ear, Nose, and Sinus Emergencies

Michael E. Vrablik

OTOLOGIC EMERGENCIES

Otitis Externa

Otitis externa, or "swimmer's ear," is characterized by pruritus, pain, and tenderness of the external ear. Erythema and edema of the external auditory canal, otorrhea, crusting, and hearing impairment may also be present. Pain is elicited with movement of the pinna or tragus. Risk factors for development of otitis externa include swimming, trauma of the external canal, and any process that elevates the pH of the canal.

The most common organisms implicated in otitis externa are *Pseudomonas aeruginosa, Enterobacteriaceae* and *Proteus species*, and *Staphylococcus aureus*, with *P. aeruginosa* being the most common organism causing malignant otitis externa. Otomycosis, or fungal otitis externa, is found in tropical climates and in the immunocompromised or subsequent to long-term antibiotic therapy. *Aspergillus* and *Candida* are the most common fungal pathogens.

The treatment of otitis externa includes analgesics, cleaning the external auditory canal, acidifying agents, topical antimicrobials, and occasionally topical steroid preparations. Cleansing can be performed with irrigation of the canal using **hydrogen peroxide** in a 1:1 dilution with warm saline or water or with gentle suction under visualization. **Ofloxacin** otic 5 drops two times daily, **acetic acid/hydrocortisone** otic 5 drops three times daily (do not use with perforated TM), and **ciprofloxacin/hydrocortisone** otic 3 drops two times daily are commonly used for 7 days to treat otitis externa. If significant swelling of the external canal is present, a wick or piece of gauze may be inserted into the canal to allow passage of topical medications. Oral antibiotics are not indicated as first-line agents unless fever or periauricular spread is present.

Malignant otitis externa is a potentially life-threatening infection of the external auditory canal with variable extension to the skull base (osteomyelitis). Historically, greater than 90% of cases were caused by *Pseudomonas aeruginosa*; however, 15% are now caused by methicillin-resistant *Staphylococcus aureus* (MRSA). Elderly, diabetic, and immunocompromised patients are most commonly affected. Diagnosis of malignant otitis externa requires a high index of suspicion. Computed tomography (CT) is necessary to determine the extent and stage of the disease. Emergent otolaryngology (ENT) consultation, **tobramycin** 2 mg/kg IV and **piperacillin** 3.375 to 4.5 g IV, or **ceftriaxone** 1 g IV, or **ciprofloxacin** 400 mg IV, and admission to the hospital are needed.

Otitis Media

The incidence and prevalence of otitis media (OM) peak in the preschool years and decline with advancing age. The most common bacterial pathogens in acute OM are *Streptococcus pneumoniae, Haemophilus influenzae,* and *Moraxella catarrhalis*. The predominant organisms involved in chronic OM are *Staphylococcus aureus*, *Pseudomonas aeruginosa*, and anaerobic bacteria.

Patients with OM present with otalgia, with or without fever; occasionally, hearing loss and otorrhea are present. The tympanic membrane (TM) may be retracted or bulging and will have impaired mobility on pneumatic otoscopy. The TM may appear red as a result of inflammation or may be yellow or white due to middle-ear secretions. Additionally, assessment of the facial nerve should be performed.

In the pediatric population the "wait-and-see" method can be used; however, this treatment plan has not been studied in adults. For adults, a 10-day course of **amoxicillin** 250 to 500 mg PO three times daily for 7 to 10 days is the preferred initial treatment for OM. Alternative agents include **azithromycin** 500 mg PO daily for 1 day then 250 mg PO daily for 4 days, or **cefuroxime** 500 mg PO two times daily for 10 days. **Cefuroxime** or **amoxicillin/clavulanate** may be given for OM unresponsive to first-line therapy after 72 hours. Antibiotic coverage should be extended to 3 weeks for patients with OM with effusion. Analgesics should be prescribed for patients with any degree of pain. Patients should follow-up with a primary care physician for reexamination and to assess the effectiveness of therapy.

Complications of OM include TM perforation, conductive hearing loss, acute serous labyrinthitis, facial nerve paralysis, acute mastoiditis, lateral sinus thrombosis, cholesteatoma, and intracranial complications. TM perforation and conductive hearing loss are most often self-limiting and often require no specific intervention. Facial nerve paralysis is uncommon but requires emergent ENT consultation.

Acute Mastoiditis

Acute mastoiditis occurs as infection spreads from the middle ear to the mastoid air cells. Patients present with otalgia, fever, and postauricular erythema, swelling, and tenderness. Protrusion of the auricle with obliteration of the postauricular crease may be present. CT will delineate the extent of bony involvement. Emergent ENT consultation, **vancomycin** 1 to 2 g IV or **ceftriaxone** 1 g IV, and admission to the hospital are necessary. Surgical drainage ultimately may be required.

Lateral Sinus Thrombosis

This condition arises from extension of infection and inflammation into the lateral and sigmoid sinuses. Headache is common and papilledema, sixth nerve palsy, and vertigo may be present. Diagnosis may be made with CT, although magnetic resonance imaging or angiography is more sensitive and may be necessary. Therapy consists of emergent ENT consultation, combination therapy with **nafcillin** 2 g IV, **ceftriaxone** 1 g IV, and **metronidazole** 500 mg IV, and hospital admission.

Bullous Myringitis

Bullous myringitis is a painful condition of the ear characterized by bulla on the TM and deep external auditory canal (EAC). Numerous pathogens have been implicated including viruses, *Mycoplasma pneumoniae*, and *Chlamydia psittaci*. The diagnosis is made by clinical examination. The treatment consists of pain control and warm compresses. Antibiotics can be given for concomitant OM.

Trauma to the Ear

A hematoma can develop from any type of trauma to the ear. Improper treatment of ear hematomas can result in stimulation of the perichondrium and development of asymmetric cartilage formation. The resultant deformed auricle has been termed "cauliflower ear." Immediate incision and drainage of the hematoma with a compressive dressing is necessary to prevent reaccumulation of the hematoma. Antibiotic coverage for *P. aeruginosa and S. aureus* should be given to immunocompromised patients.

Thermal injury to the auricle may be caused by excessive heat or cold. Superficial injury of either type is treated with cleaning, topical nonsulfa-containing antibiotic ointment, and a light dressing. Frostbite is treated with rapid rewarming by using saline soaked gauze at 38°C to 40°C. The rewarming process may be very painful and analgesics will be necessary. Any second- or third-degree burn requires immediate ENT or burn center consultation.

Foreign Bodies in the Ear

On examination, the foreign body is usually visualized and signs of infection or TM perforation should be sought. Live insects should be immobilized with 2% **lidocaine** solution distilled into the ear canal before removal. Foreign bodies may be removed with forceps and direct visualization or with the aid of a hooked probe or suction catheter. Irrigation is often useful for small objects; however, organic material may absorb water and swell. ENT consultation is required for cases of foreign body with TM perforation or if the object cannot be safely removed.

Cerumen Impaction

Cerumen impaction can cause symptoms of hearing loss, pressure, dizziness, tinnitus and otalgia. Impaction is often precipitated by the use of cotton swabs in the ear canal. Cerumen scoops/loops can be used to remove the impaction. If significant amounts of cerumen are in the canal then half-strength **hydrogen peroxide, sodium bicarbonate, mineral oil, or carbamide peroxide otic** can be instilled in the canal to soften the cerumen and help with removal. Additionally cerumen impactions can be removed with irrigation of the EAC using body-temperature fluid via an 18ga IV catheter or ear syringe making sure that the irrigation is directed to the EAC wall not the TM. Cerumen removal in the emergency department (ED) is often not required; asymptomatic or minimally symptomatic patients with cerumen impaction may be safely discharged home with a cerumen-softening otic and follow-up.

Tympanic Membrane Perforation

TM perforations can result from middle-ear infections, barotrauma, blunt/penetrating/acoustic trauma, and, rarely, lightning strikes. Acute pain and hearing loss are usually noted, with or without bloody otorrhea. Vertigo and tinnitus, when present, are usually transient. As most TM perforations heal spontaneously, antibiotics are not necessary unless there is persistent foreign material in the canal or middle ear. Patients with perforations from isolated blunt or noise trauma can be discharged with expedited specialty referral and should be instructed not to allow water to enter the ear canal.

Tinnitus

Tinnitus is the perception of sound without external stimuli. It may be constant, pulsatile, high or low pitched, hissing, clicking, or ringing in nature. Objective tinnitus can be heard by the examiner, whereas the more common subjective tinnitus cannot. Causes of tinnitus include vascular, mechanical, neurologic, Ménière's disease, and others. Common medications resulting in tinnitus include aspirin, nonsteroidal anti-inflammatory drugs, aminoglycosides, loop diuretics, and chemotherapeutics. If the patient's condition allows, potentially offending drugs should be stopped. Accurate diagnosis usually requires referral to an otolaryngologist.

Hearing Loss

Causes of sudden hearing loss are varied and may be idiopathic (most common), infectious, vascular or hematologic, metabolic, rheumatologic, or conductive. Other causes include Ménière's disease, Cogan's syndrome, acoustic neuroma, cochlear rupture, and ototoxic medications. Indicators of poor prognosis include severe hearing loss on presentation and the presence of vertigo. If the cause is not readily determined by history and physical examination, otolaryngologic consultation is necessary.

NASAL EMERGENCIES AND SINUSITIS

Epistaxis

Epistaxis is classified as anterior or posterior. Posterior epistaxis is suggested if an anterior source is not visualized, if bleeding occurs from both nares, or if blood is seen draining into the posterior pharynx after anterior sources have been controlled.

1. Perform a quick history to determine the duration and severity of the hemorrhage and the contributing factors (trauma, anticoagulant use, infection, bleeding diathesis, etc.).
2. Have the patient blow his or her nose to dislodge any clots. Instill 0.05% **oxymetazoline** 2 sprays/nostril or 0.25% **phenylephrine** 2 sprays/nostril.
3. Inspect for anterior bleeding using a good light source, a nasal speculum, and a suction catheter.
4. Apply direct external pressure to the cartilage just distal to the nasal bones for 15 minutes while leaning forward in the "sniffing" position. Reexamine the patient. Repeat once if necessary.
5. If bleeding continues, and an anterior source of bleeding is visualized, proceed to chemical cautery. If no source is identified, proceed to packing.
6. Chemical cautery with **silver nitrate** is the standard of care for ED treatment of anterior epistaxis. Insert cotton swabs or pledgets soaked in a 1:1 mixture of a 4% **lidocaine** and 0.05% **oxymetazoline** into the nasal cavity with bayonet forceps. After hemostasis is achieved, the mucosa is cauterized by firmly rolling the tip of a **silver nitrate** applicator over the

area until it turns silvery-black. A small surrounding area also should be cauterized to control local arterioles. Overzealous use of cautery and bilateral septal cautery is discouraged because they may cause septal perforation and unintended local tissue necrosis.

7. Anterior nasal packing may be performed with thrombogenic foams and gels, commercial devices, or gauze. Dehydrated nasal sponges are available in several lengths to control anterior and posterior epistaxis. A film of antibiotic ointment is applied, then the sponge is rapidly inserted along the floor of the nasal cavity where it expands upon contact with blood or secretions. Expansion can be hastened by rehydrating the sponge with sterile water from a catheter-tipped syringe. The longer sponges used to control posterior hemorrhages have been associated with some morbidity and should be used only for posterior epistaxis. Inflatable epistaxis tamponade balloons can also be used to control anterior and/or posterior hemorrhage, are easy to use, and are generally more comfortable than nasal sponges. Thrombogenic foams and gels are bioabsorbable, do not require removal, and are generally well tolerated. All nonabsorbable nasal packs should be removed in 2 to 3 days by an ENT physician. **Tranexamic acid** 5 mL (500 mg) applied to the nasal mucosa via a 15-cm cotton pledget can also be used to stop epistaxis. If packing or local cautery fails to control anterior bleeding, ENT consultation is necessary.
8. Posterior epistaxis may be treated with a dehydrated posterior sponge pack, as outlined above, or an inflatable balloon tamponade device. The balloon devices use independently inflatable anterior and posterior balloons to quickly control refractory epistaxis at these sites; the instructions for insertion are included in the balloon kit. To protect against potentially serious complications, all patients with posterior packs require ENT consultation for possible hospital admission. Posterior packs are removed 2 to 3 days after placement.
9. All patients with nasal packs should be started on antibiotic prophylaxis with **amoxicillin/clavulanate** 500/125 mg PO three times daily.

Complications of nasal packing include vasovagal syncope, dislodgment of the pack, recurrent bleeding, sinusitis, and toxic shock syndrome. Treatment of elevated blood pressure during an acute episode of epistaxis is generally not advised except in consultation with an otolaryngologist for cases of persistent epistaxis not controlled by the above measures.

Nasal Fractures

Nasal fracture is a clinical diagnosis suggested by the injury mechanism, swelling, tenderness, crepitance, gross deformity, and periorbital ecchymosis. Radiographic diagnosis usually is not necessary in the ED. Intermittent ice application, analgesics, and over-the-counter decongestants are the normal treatment. ENT follow-up within 6 to 10 days for reexamination and possible fracture reduction is prudent.

A fracture of the cribriform plate may violate the subarachnoid space and cause cerebrospinal fluid rhinorrhea. Symptoms may be delayed for several weeks. If a cribriform plate injury is suspected, CT and immediate neurosurgical consultation should be obtained.

Nasal Septal Hematoma

A nasal septal hematoma should be suspected whenever there is trauma to the nose. A thorough evaluation of the nasal septum, with good lighting, should be performed. The septum should be visualized and palpated to assess for a hematoma. A nasal septal hematoma elevates the vascular perichondrium off of the cartilage thus disrupting the blood supply. It is important to remove the hematoma to return blood supply and prevent ischemic necrosis of the septum. If a nasal septal hematoma is identified then evacuation of the hematoma is necessary.

1. Place patient in "sniffing position" and examine the anterior nares with a nasal speculum under good lighting. Have suction, irrigation, and nasal packing materials ready.
2. Anesthetize the nasal mucosa by placing cotton pledgets soaked in 4% **lidocaine** into the affected nare. Infiltrative anesthesia of **lidocaine without epinephrine** can be administered if needed.
3. Visualize the hematoma and make a horizontal incision through the mucosa, avoid incising the cartilage.
4. Remove the hematoma.
5. Insert bilateral anterior nasal packing coated in antibiotic ointment.
6. Prescribe prophylactic antibiotics (**amoxicillin/clavulanate** 500/125 mg PO three times daily) if the nasal packing will be in for greater than 24 hours.
7. Patients should follow up with ENT.

Nasal Foreign Bodies

Nasal foreign bodies should be suspected in patients with unilateral nasal obstruction, foul rhinorrhea, or persistent unilateral epistaxis. After topical vasoconstriction with 0.05% **oxymetazoline** and possibly local anesthesia with 4% nebulized **lidocaine**, the foreign body should be removed under direct visualization. Tools for removal include forceps, suction catheters, hooked probes, and balloon-tipped catheters. Consult ENT if removal is unsuccessful.

Sinusitis and Rhinosinusitis

Sinusitis is inflammation of the mucosal lining of the paranasal sinuses (maxillary, frontal, ethmoid). Rhinosinusitis is sinusitis also involving the nasal cavity, almost always involves rhinitis, and is extremely common. It can be classified as acute, subacute, or chronic.

Symptoms include nasal congestion or blockage, facial pain or pressure, hyposmia, nasal discharge, tooth pain, fever, and sinus pressure with head/body movement. There may be pain and tenderness with sinus percussion, mucosal swelling, facial swelling, and redness.

Complications include meningitis, cavernous sinus thrombosis, intracranial abscess and empyema, orbital cellulitis, and osteomyelitis. Patients with these deeper complications usually appear systemically ill or have focal neurologic findings.

The diagnosis of uncomplicated acute rhinosinusitis is clinical, and imaging is not necessary. CT scans are helpful in evaluating toxic patients and possible intracranial extension. Patients with chronic rhinosinusitis or recurrent acute rhinosinusitis warrant bacterial cultures and a sinus CT, preferably as an outpatient.

Treatment for acute uncomplicated disease is generally supportive. Nasal irrigation with or without nasal decongestants (0.05% **oxymetazoline** 2 sprays/nostril two times daily or 0.25% **phenylephrine** 2 sprays/nostril four times daily) is first-line therapy. Decongestant's use is to be limited to less than or equal to 3 days. Oral antibiotics should be reserved for patients with purulent nasal secretions and severe symptoms for more than 10 days. If prescribed, choices for a 10-day antibiotic regimen include **amoxicillin** 500 mg PO three times daily (first-line), **trimethoprim/sulfamethoxazole** 160/800 mg two times daily or **erythromycin** 250 to 500 mg two times daily (if penicillin allergic), and **levofloxacin** 500 mg daily (if antibiotics in prior 6 weeks).

FURTHER READING

For further reading in *Tintinalli's Emergency Medicine: A Comprehensive Study Guide*, 8th ed., see Chapter 242, "Ear Disorders," by Kathleen Hosmer; Chapter 244, "Nose and Sinuses," by Henderson D.McGinnis.

CHAPTER 152 Oral and Dental Emergencies

Steven Go

DENTAL ANATOMY

The relevant dental anatomy is shown in Figure 152-1.

OROFACIAL PAIN

Tooth Eruption and Pericoronitis

Eruption of the primary teeth ("teething") in children may be the primary cause of pain, irritability, and drooling, but NOT fever and diarrhea; therefore, other causes of these latter symptoms must be excluded. Give the child a **frozen, damp towel** to suck on and **acetaminophen** 15 mg/kg orally (PO) every 6 hours to control symptoms. Topical anesthetics should

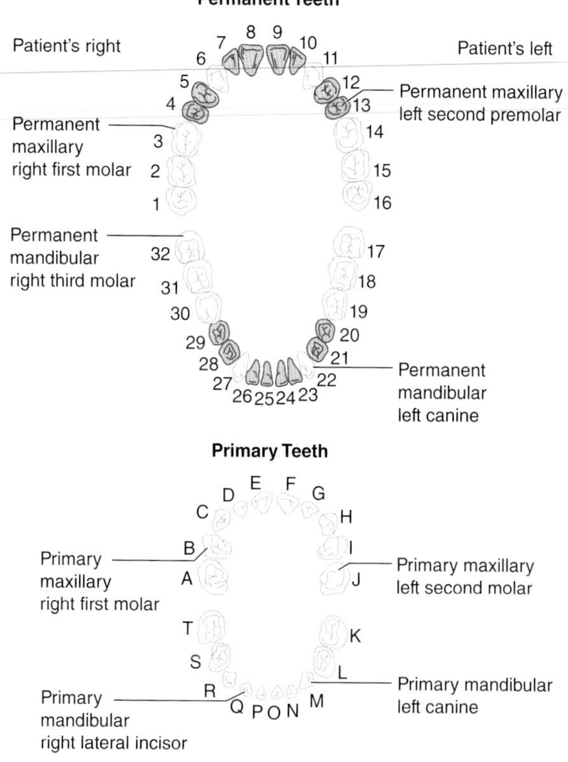

FIGURE 152-1. Identification of teeth.

be used with great caution in young infants due to its potential to depress the gag reflex.

Adults and teens may experience *pericoronitis* (pain and local inflammation) with the eruption of the third molars ("wisdom teeth"). Prescribe **penicillin VK** 500 mg PO four times daily or **clindamycin** 300 mg PO four times daily, **ibuprofen** 400 to 800 mg PO three times daily (with or without **hydrocodone** 5 mg/**acetaminophen** 325 mg one to two tablets PO four times daily), and **warm saline mouth rinses**. Refer the patient to an oral surgeon or a general dentist for consideration of **third molar extraction**.

Dental Caries and Pulpitis

Dental caries are caused by bacteriogenic acid eroding through the enamel. Examination may reveal a grossly decayed tooth, although occasionally there is no visible pathology—in these cases, localization may be accomplished by percussing individual teeth with a metallic object. If dental caries are not treated, pulpitis is the result. *Reversible pulpitis* is characterized by sudden, transient pain lasting seconds, often triggered by heat or cold. In contrast *irreversible pulpitis* pain lasts minutes to hours. Although antibiotics such as **penicillin VK** 500 mg PO four times daily or **clindamycin** 300 mg PO four times daily are commonly prescribed for pulpitis, their efficacy is controversial. Treat with **ibuprofen** 400 to 800 mg PO three times daily, **hydrocodone** 5 mg/**acetaminophen** 325 mg one to two tablets PO four times daily, and **warm saline mouth rinses**. A **dental block** may also be performed for short-term pain relief. Refer to a dentist for definitive management. If an abscess is present, antibiotics and incision and drainage should be considered.

Facial Space Infections

Odontogenic infections can spread readily to the facial spaces. Therefore, it is imperative to exclude deep-space involvement whenever a dental infection is encountered. *Ludwig's angina* is a cellulitis involving both submandibular spaces and the sublingual space that can spread to the neck and mediastinum, causing airway compromise, overwhelming infection, and even death. If dental infections spread to the infraorbital space, a *cavernous sinus thrombosis* may result. This condition may present with limitation of lateral gaze, meningeal signs, sepsis, and coma. Administer intravenous antibiotics and obtain emergent surgical consultation for both conditions, with anticoagulation added for cavernous sinus thrombosis.

Postextraction Pain and Postextraction Alveolar Osteitis (Dry Socket)

Pain experienced within 24 to 48 hours after a tooth extraction responds well to icepacks, head elevation, and analgesics. *Postextraction alveolar osteitis* ("dry socket") occurs 48 to 72 hours postoperatively when the clot from the socket is displaced. It is associated with smoking, carbonated beverage consumption, and drinking with straws. It presents with severe pain along with foul odor and taste. Perform gentle **saline or 0.12% chlorhexidine irrigation** of the socket, followed by packing the socket with **eugenol-impregnated gauze**, which will relieve the pain. Prescribe **penicillin VK** 500 mg PO four times daily or **clindamycin** 300 mg PO four times daily in severe cases, along with analgesia, daily packing changes, gentle **0.12% chlorhexidine mouth rinses** twice daily, and dental follow-up in 24 hours.

Postextraction Bleeding

Control bleeding after dental extraction by instructing the patient to bite on gauze positioned over the bleeding site for 20 minutes. If bleeding persists, pack the socket with **Gelfoam®, Avitene®, or Surgicel®**. Loosely approximating sutures can be used to hold these packing agents in place. Other emergency department (ED) treatments may include local injection of **1% lidocaine with epinephrine** or careful **silver nitrate** application. Failure of these measures warrants a screening coagulation profile and consultation with an oral surgeon.

Periodontal Abscess

A *periodontal abscess* results from plaque and debris entrapped between the tooth and gingiva. For small abscesses, administer **penicillin VK** 500 mg PO four times daily or **clindamycin** 300 mg PO four times daily, **analgesics**, and short-term **0.12% chlorhexidine mouth rinses** twice daily. Larger abscesses require **incision and drainage**. All patients need prompt **dental referral**.

Acute Necrotizing Ulcerative Gingivitis

Acute necrotizing ulcerative gingivitis (ANUG) presents with pain, ulcerated or "punched out" interdental papillae, gingival bleeding, foul taste, lymphadenopathy, and fever. The associated putrid breath gives this disorder its nickname of "trench mouth." It occurs mainly in young patients with compromised resistance to infection due to HIV, stress, malnourishment, substance abuse, and various infections. Prescribe **metronidazole** 500 mg PO three times daily and **0.12% chlorhexidine mouth rinses** twice daily, along with a protein-rich soft diet, multivitamins, and PO fluids. Symptomatic improvement is typically dramatic within 24 hours, and the patient should be referred for dental debridement, scaling, and workup of predisposing factors.

Peri-implantitis

Dental implants are being increasingly used to replace teeth. If they become infected, they present similarly to a periodontal abscess. Irrigate around the implant with 0.12% chlorhexidine solution and administer **metronidazole** 500 mg PO three times daily or **amoxicillin** 500 mg PO three times daily for 10 days. Prescribe **analgesics** and refer the patient to a dentist for definitive management.

SOFT TISSUE LESIONS OF THE ORAL CAVITY

Aphthous Stomatitis

Aphthous stomatitis, or aphthous ulcer, presents with painful lesions, which are frequently multiple, involve the labial and buccal mucosa, and measure from 2 mm to several centimeters in diameter. Treat with **0.1% triamcinolone acetonide dental paste** (Kenalog® in Orobase®) applied topically to lesions two to three times a day or **0.12% chlorhexidine** applied topically twice a day. The lesions often heal within 7 to 10 days.

Oral Cancer

Emergency physicians should be vigilant for oral cancers and their precursors because early diagnosis is associated with improved outcomes. Cancers can present early as *leukoplakia* (nonremovable white mucosal patches) and *erythroplakia* (red patch that cannot be classified as any other disease). The most common site for oral cancer to develop is the posterolateral border of the tongue. Symptoms and signs of oral cancer include pain, paresthesias, persistent ulcers, bleeding, lesion rigidity, induration, lymphadenopathy, and functional impairment. Refer all suspicious lesions or lesions that persist >14 days despite treatment for urgent follow-up with an oral surgeon for biopsy.

OROFACIAL TRAUMA

Dental Fractures

The Ellis system is used to classify the anatomy of fractured teeth. *Ellis class 1* fractures solely involve the enamel. These injuries may be smoothed with an emery board or referred to a dentist for cosmetic repair. *Ellis class 2* fractures reveal the creamy yellow dentin underneath the white enamel. The patient complains of air and temperature sensitivities. To decrease pulpal contamination, dry the dentin and promptly cover the lesion with **calcium hydroxide paste** or **glass ionomer cement**. All patients should see a dentist within 24 hours. *Ellis class 3* fractures are tooth-threatening fractures that involve the pulp and can be identified by a red blush in the exposed dentin or a visible drop of blood after wiping the tooth. Apply a thin layer of **calcium hydroxide paste** to cover the pulp, followed by an overlying layer of **glass ionomer cement** to completely cover the patch and dentin as well. Ideally, a dentist should evaluate the patient in the ED, but if the amount of exposed pulp is very small, the patched lesion can be evaluated by a dentist within 24 hours. Oral **analgesics** may be needed, but topical anesthetics are contraindicated. The use of prophylactic antibiotics is controversial.

Concussions, Luxations, and Avulsions

Concussion injuries involve posttraumatic tenderness to percussion with no mobility. Posttraumatic mobility without evidence of dislodgment is called *subluxation*, which has a higher incidence of future pulp necrosis. Prescribe **nonsteroidal anti-inflammatory drugs (NSAIDs)** and soft diet, and refer urgently to a dentist to rule out a more severe injury.

Extrusive luxation occurs when a tooth is partly avulsed out from the alveolar bone. Treatment involves gentle repositioning of the tooth to its original location (often with the aid of a dental block) and splinting with **zinc oxide** periodontal dressing. A dentist should evaluate these patients within 24 hours. When the tooth is laterally displaced with a fracture of the alveolar bone, the condition is called *lateral luxation*. Although manual relocation is possible, the treatment of such injuries is best done in consultation with a dentist. If the alveolar bone fracture is significant, splinting by a dentist in the ED is required. An *intrusive luxation* occurs when the tooth is forced below the gingiva and often has a poor outcome. For all luxations, prescribe a soft diet, meticulous oral hygiene, and **0.12% chlorhexidine mouth rinses** twice daily, and refer to a dentist to be seen within 24 hours.

Dental *avulsion* is a bona fide dental emergency in which a tooth has been completely removed from the socket. *Primary teeth* in children are **NOT** replaced because of potential damage to the permanent teeth (Fig. 152-2).

Replant *permanent teeth* that have been avulsed for less than 3 hours **immediately** to attempt to save the periodontal ligament fibers. At the scene, handle an avulsed tooth by the crown only, **rinse** with water <10 seconds, and **replant immediately**. If replantation at the scene is not possible due to risk of aspiration, rinse the tooth and place in a nutrient solution, such as **Hank's balanced salt solution** (preserves cell viability for up to 4 to 6 hours), cold milk, saliva, or sterile saline. Transport the tooth immediately with the patient to the ED. An effective, but somewhat unsettling, way to safely transport the avulsed tooth is underneath the tongue of an alert, sober, cooperative patient or parent (if the patient is a child). Upon arrival in the ED, if the tooth has not already been replanted, gently rinse the tooth with **Hank's solution or sterile saline** and soak in either fluid. Remove the clot in the empty socket and gently irrigate with **sterile normal saline**. Examine the tooth to determine whether the apex at the root tip is open, then proceed with the appropriate tooth replantation procedure if indicated. (See Table 152-1 for specific recommendations for tooth replantation.)

Early consultation with a dentist is imperative, but **do not delay replantation** while awaiting the arrival of the specialist. After replantation, adults should receive **doxycycline** 100 mg PO BID for 7 days. Children <12 years old should receive **penicillin VK** 12.5 mg/kg/dose four times a day

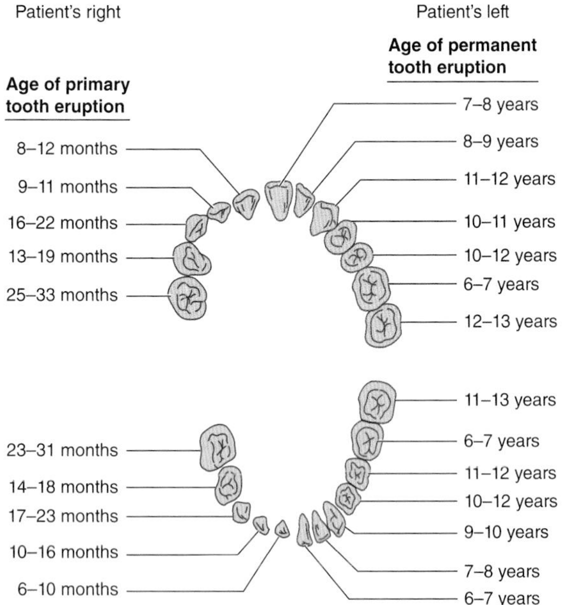

FIGURE 152-2. Normal eruptive patterns of the primary and permanent dentition.

TABLE 152-1 Specific Recommendations for Replantation of Avulsed Teeth

Clinical Scenario	Treatment
Moist tooth with OPEN apex stored in acceptable media and/or <60 min extra oral dry time	1. Gently irrigate the tooth root clean with sterile saline. 2. If available, cover root with minocycline hydrochloride microspheres (Arestin™, OraPharma, Inc.) or soak for 5 min in doxycycline solution (doxycycline, 1 mg/20 mL saline) 3. Administer local anesthesia 4. Remove coagulum from the socket with a stream of saline. Examine the socket. If there is a fracture of the socket wall, reposition it with an appropriate instrument 5. Firmly replant tooth and verify the tooth position clinically and radiographically, if possible 6. Flexible splint for up to 2 weeks
Moist tooth with CLOSED apex stored in acceptable media and/or <60 min extra oral dry time	1. Gently irrigate the tooth root clean with sterile saline 2. Administer local anesthesia 3. Remove coagulum from the socket with a stream of saline. Examine the socket. If there is a fracture of the socket wall, reposition it with an appropriate instrument 4. Firmly replant tooth and verify the tooth's position clinically and radiographically, if possible 5. Flexible splint for up to 2 weeks
Tooth (with OPEN or CLOSED apex) and extra oral dry time >60 min or other reason suggesting nonviable cells	1. Remove necrotic soft tissue from tooth carefully with gauze 2. If available, immerse tooth in 2% stannous fluoride solution for 20 min 3. Administer local anesthesia 4. Remove coagulum from the socket with a stream of saline. Examine the socket. If there is a fracture of the socket wall, reposition it with an appropriate instrument 5. Firmly replant tooth and verify the tooth's position clinically and radiographically, if possible 6. Flexible splint for up to 4 weeks

for 7 days. If a patient arrives with an empty socket and the tooth cannot be located, search adjacent tissue for the tooth. If a missing tooth cannot be found or if a partial tooth is found, order **face, neck, or chest radiographs** to exclude a displaced or aspirated tooth.

All types of dental trauma may be associated with alveolar ridge, maxillary, or mandible fractures; therefore, **order appropriate imaging studies** to exclude these fractures if clinical suspicion warrants. Even with proper treatment, the prognosis of luxated or avulsed teeth can be rather poor (e.g., 50% pulp necrosis within 1.5 years in extrusive luxation); therefore, be certain to **inform the patient** of potential suboptimal outcomes and stress the importance of **prompt dental follow-up**.

Soft Tissue Trauma

Stabilize dental trauma before repairing soft tissue trauma. In addition, perform a thorough search for retained foreign bodies before repair and update tetanus status if necessary. **When a child presents with oral trauma, consider the possibility of abuse**.

Laceration of the *maxillary labial frenulum* usually does not require repair. The *lingual frenulum* is very vascular and usually should be repaired with **4-0 absorbable sutures**.

Tongue lacerations pose a special challenge due to the organ's vascularity. While massive bleeding or delayed venous swelling from tongue trauma can both obstruct the airway, the more common ED presentation involves localized injuries. The indications for closure of tongue lacerations remain controversial. Some authors recommend all lacerations be repaired while others allow nearly any wound to heal by secondary intention. Published indications for primary closure include bisection of the tongue, widely gaping wounds at rest, active bleeding, flap or U-shaped wounds, involvement of the tongue edge, and lacerations >1 cm. There is general agreement that non-gaping, superficial, linear lacerations <1 cm located on the central aspect of the dorsal tongue require no repair. An assistant may be required to hold the tongue with gauze to allow repair. Obtain local anesthesia with gauze soaked with **4% lidocaine** applied topically for 5 minutes. In some cases, local infiltration with **1% lidocaine with epinephrine** or a bilateral lingual nerve block (for lesions located within the anterior two-thirds of the tongue) may be necessary. If greater control is required, an anesthetized tip of the tongue may be grasped with a towel clamp or a temporary silk suture may be placed. A dental bite block may be useful to prevent bites to health care providers during repair. Repair lacerations with **4-0 or 5-0 absorbable sutures**. Keep sutures *loose* (to avoid necrosis in case the tongue swells significantly within the first 2 days), wide, and deep. Approximate all of the involved tongue layers at once with single-interrupted sutures. Alternatively, a two- or three-layer closure technique may be used. Sometimes in children it is desirable to only close the deep muscle layer while eschewing surface layer closure. This avoids surface knots which can trouble children. Align wound edges as precisely as possible to avoid subsequent formation of clefts, which can have cosmetic and functional consequences. Complete every exposed stitch **with at least four knots** to avoid the suture becoming undone by subsequent tongue movement. In approximately 7 days, sutures will fall out by themselves or will be absorbed. Aftercare is similar to that of other intraoral lacerations. Obtain emergent specialty consultation for tongue lacerations in patients who require procedural sedation, large or complex lacerations, full or partial amputations, and difficulties with hemostasis.

FURTHER READING

For further reading in *Tintinalli's Emergency Medicine: A Comprehensive Study Guide* 8th ed., see Chapter 245, "Oral and Dental Emergencies," by Ronald W. Beaudreau.

CHAPTER 153

Neck and Upper Airway Disorders

Rebecca Kornas

PHARYNGITIS AND TONSILLITIS

Clinical Features

Viral pharyngitis/tonsillitis may present with fever, odynophagia, and petechial or vesicular lesions on the soft palate and tonsils. Compared to bacterial pharyngitis, viral pharyngitis is more often associated with cough, rhinorrhea, and congestion. Viral infections typically lack tonsillar exudates and cervical adenopathy. Bacterial pharyngitis, particularly group A β-hemolytic streptococcus (GABHS) pharyngitis, presents with acute onset of fever, sore throat, odynophagia, and often headache. Patients often display tonsillar erythema, exudates, and tender anterior cervical adenopathy. Cough, conjunctivitis, and rhinorrhea are typically lacking.

Diagnosis and Differential

The Centor criteria for GABHS pharyngitis are (1) tonsillar exudates, (2) tender anterior cervical adenopathy, (3) absence of cough, and (4) fever. Perform a rapid antigen test on patients with two or more criteria and treat based on the results on the rapid test. Additional diagnostic testing should be performed if mononucleosis, influenza, or acute retroviral syndrome is suspected.

Emergency Department Care and Disposition

1. Nonbacterial causes are treated with supportive care: **antipyretics, analgesics**, and **IV fluids**, if the patient is dehydrated.
2. Treat GABHS pharyngitis with a single dose of **benzathine penicillin G** 1.2 million units IM, **penicillin VK** 500 mg PO twice daily for 10 days, or **amoxicillin** 500 mg twice daily or 1000 mg per day. Treat penicillin-allergic patients with a first-generation **cephalosporin** or **clindamycin**.

PERITONSILLAR ABSCESS

Clinical Features

Patients appear ill and often complain of sore throat, fever, odynophagia, trismus, and dysphagia. A muffled voice may be noted. The infected tonsil is typically displaced medially, causing contralateral deflection of the uvula.

Diagnosis and Differential

Additional conditions to consider include peritonsillar cellulitis, infectious mononucleosis, retropharyngeal abscess, herpes simplex tonsillitis, neoplasm, and internal carotid artery aneurysm. Diagnosis is typically made through the history and physical exam. If diagnosis is in question, intraoral ultrasound is very sensitive and specific. CT scan with contrast can be employed if there is concern for extension of infection beyond the peritonsillar space.

Emergency Department Care and Disposition

1. Peritonsillar abscess is treated with needle aspiration with an 18-G needle or incision and drainage (I&D) after local anesthesia. **Cut the plastic needle sheath at about 1 cm from its tip to deter from penetrating to the level of the internal carotid artery.**
2. After adequate aspiration or drainage, patients able to tolerate PO may be discharged home on antibiotics. Give **Penicillin VK** PLUS **metronidazole** for 10 days. Choose **clindamycin** for penicillin-allergic patients. Toxic patients should receive **piperacillin-tazobactam** 3.375 g IV and admitted for observation.

ADULT EPIGLOTTITIS (SUPRAGLOTTITIS)

Clinical Features

Patients typically present with a 1- to 2-day history of worsening dysphagia, odynophagia, and dyspnea, worse when supine, and often will have anterior neck tenderness with pain on gentle palpation of the larynx and upper trachea. They classically position themselves in the upright position, leaning forward, mouth open, and neck extended, and may display drooling and inspiratory stridor.

Diagnosis and Differential

Diagnosis is made through history and physical, lateral cervical soft tissue radiograph with obliteration of the vallecula and a "thumb print sign", and/or transnasal fiberoptic laryngoscopy.

Emergency Department Care and Disposition

1. Suspected epiglottitis requires immediate otolaryngology consultation, and the emergency physician must be prepared to establish a surgical airway.
2. Patients should remain in the upright position. Initial airway management consists of humidified oxygen, IV hydration, cardiac monitoring, and pulse oximetry.
3. **Cefotaxime 50 mg/kg** plus **vancomycin** 15 mg/kg IV are first-line antibiotics. Penicillin allergic patients should receive **a respiratory fluoroquinolone**. **Methylprednisolone** 125 mg IV may reduce airway inflammation and edema.
4. **Endotracheal intubation** is generally performed in the operating room via the "awake" fiberoptic method, although with sufficient expertise and equipment, intubation can be performed in the emergency department.

RETROPHARYNGEAL ABSCESS

Clinical Features

Common symptoms include sore throat, neck pain, torticollis, and dysphagia. Additionally, patients may have a muffled voice, cervical adenopathy, and respiratory distress. Stridor is more common in children.

Diagnosis and Differential

A CT of the neck with IV contrast is the gold standard diagnostic exam and differentiates cellulitis from an abscess.

Emergency Department Care and Disposition

1. Prepare for emergent airway management as needed.
2. Consult with otolaryngology early.
3. Administer IV fluids, **clindamycin,** or **cefoxitin** IV.

ODONTOGENIC ABSCESS

Clinical Features

Most deep space neck infections are odontogenic, usually from the mandibular teeth. Patients may present with trismus, fever, neck mass, dysphagia, and dyspnea. Infection can range from diffuse cellulitis to abscesses in the labial or buccal gingiva. Infections can spread through many fascial layers into potential spaces in the face, neck, and mouth.

Diagnosis and Differential

Bedside ultrasound can detect superficial odontogenic abscesses, but if deep space infection is suspected, CT of the neck with IV contrast is recommended.

Emergency Department Care and Disposition

1. Perform surgical drainage of the abscess, either with I&D in the emergency department or in the operating room.
2. Prescribe **Penicillin VK** or **amoxicillin** for patients who can be discharged after drainage. Penicillin allergic patients may be treated with **clindamycin** or **levofloxacin**.
3. In patients with deep space neck infections, administer IV **ampicillin/sulbactam** along with **clindamycin** and **ciprofloxacin**.

Complications

Ludwig's angina is an infection of the submental, sublingual, and submandibular spaces. Clinical exam reveals trismus and edema of the entire upper neck and floor of the mouth. Critically ill patients may have a **necrotizing infection.** These are associated with skin discoloration, crepitus of the subcutaneous tissue, and systemic signs of illness including fever, tachycardia, hypotension, and confusion. **Immediate surgical consultation** is required, as these patients need **fasciotomy** with wide local debridement and broad-spectrum IV antibiotics.

NECK AND UPPER AIRWAY MASSES

Clinical Features

Neck masses can be congenital, infectious, glandular, or neoplastic. In adults >40 years old, up to 80% of lateral neck masses persistent for >6 weeks are malignant.

Diagnosis and Differential

Patients with airway compromise or significant dysphagia or odynophagia should be evaluated using **flexible nasopharyngolaryngoscopy***before* CT scan. **CT scan** is often required for planning surgical intervention and will help to delineate the extent of the mass (Table 153-1).

Emergency Department Care and Disposition

1. Inflammatory lymph nodes should be treated with empiric antibiotics such as **cephalexin** 500 mg PO three to four times daily or **amoxicillin** 500 mg three to four times daily or **clindamycin** 300 mg three to four times daily.
2. Empiric therapy for sialoadenitis should cover staphylococcal infection with an antibiotic such as **clindamycin**.

POSTTONSILLECTOMY BLEEDING

Clinical Features

Postoperative bleeding is a well-known complication of tonsillectomy and can cause death from airway obstruction or hemorrhagic shock. Incidence ranges from 1% to 8.8% with about half of patients requiring surgical intervention to control bleeding. Most significant hemorrhage occurs between postoperative days 5 and 10, but bleeding can be seen within 24 hours of surgery.

Emergency Department Care and Disposition

1. Keep the patient NPO and sitting upright.
2. Consult otolaryngology early.
3. Apply direct pressure to the bleeding tonsillar bed using a tonsillar pack or 4 × 4 gauze on a long clamp moistened with either thrombin or lidocaine and epinephrine.

TABLE 153-1 Neck Masses in Young and Older Adults

Young Adult	Adult
Reactive lymphadenopathy	Metastatic aerodigestive tract carcinoma
Mononucleosis	Salivary gland infection or neoplasm
Lymphoma	
Branchial cleft cyst	Lymphoma
Thyroglossal duct cyst	Thyroid disorder Tuberculosis

4. Alternatively, if the bleeding site is visualized, locally infiltrate with lidocaine and epinephrine then cauterize with silver nitrate.
5. Massive bleeding is rare but when it occurs the only means of protecting the airway is intubation. Plan for emergent cricothyrotomy prior to attempting intubation.

COMPLICATIONS OF AIRWAY DEVICES

Tracheostomy Tubes and Cannulas

Early complications include bleeding, obstruction, dislodgement, and infection. These typically occur within the first postoperative week. Late complications like granulation, tracheal stenosis, and fistula formation occur after the first postoperative week. Emergency medicine providers must be proficient in replacing uncuffed with cuffed tracheostomy tubes for mechanical ventilation, replacement of tracheostomy tubes after accidental decannulation, correction of tube obstruction, and control of bleeding or infection at the tracheostomy site.

Tracheostomy Tube with Airway Obstruction

If the tracheostomy tube is patent, leave it in place. Consider mucus plugging of the trachea or mainstem bronchi distal to the tube and attempt to suction. Preoxygenation and placement of sterile saline into the trachea will aid in suctioning. You may have to remove the inner cannula and occasionally the entire tracheostomy tube if suctioning fails.

Tracheostomy Dislodgement

If a suction catheter cannot be passed through the tube and on x-ray the tracheostomy tube is seen extrinsically compressing the trachea, the tube is likely dislodged. Remove the entire tracheostomy tube. Insert a nasopharyngoscope or flexible bronchoscope into the visible stoma to identify the true tracheal opening. If the opening cannot be identified obtain otolaryngology or general surgery consultation. If the patient cannot maintain his or her airway, you should orally intubate.

Tracheostomy Site Infection

Stomal skin infection, tracheitis, and bronchitis can be recurring problems. Treat polymicrobial infections in stable patients with **amoxicillin-clavulanate** 875 mg PO twice daily. Unstable or systemically ill patients should receive **piperacillin-tazobactam** 3.375 g IV plus **vancomycin** 1 g IV. Add a fluoroquinolone for *Pseudomonas*. Local wound infections can be treated with **gauze soaked in 0.25% acetic acid**.

Tracheostomy Site Bleeding

Sources of hemorrhage include granulation tissue in the stoma, trachea, or thyroid or erosion of the thyroid vessels, the tracheal wall, or the innominate artery. Packing with saline soaked gauze can control slow bleeding from the stoma. If this is ineffective remove the tube and examine the stoma and tracheal wall. Local bleeding can be controlled with **silver nitrate**. If bleeding is brisk, replace the tracheostomy tube with a cuffed endotracheal tube with the cuff below the bleeding site.

Tracheoinnominate artery fistula is a rare but life-threatening complication of tracheostomy. This is typically seen during the first 3 weeks after tracheostomy and is due to vessel erosion from high (>25 mm Hg) cuff pressures or direct pressure from the tip of the tracheal cannula against the innominate artery. Some patients present with hemoptysis or a sentinel arterial bleed. Immediate orolaryngologic or thoracic surgery consultation is required.

If the patient presents with massive bleeding, the first maneuver is to hyperinflate the cuff to control brisk bleeding while planning operative intervention. If bleeding persists, slowly withdraw the tube while exerting anterior pressure on the anterior trachea. If these interventions fail to control bleeding, place an endotracheal tube from above the tracheoinnominate fistula, using direct visualization with a flexible intubating scope while an assistant removes the tracheostomy tube allowing the endotracheal tube to pass. Then use digital pressure of the innominate artery against the manubrium to control stomal hemorrhage.

Tracheal Stenosis

Weeks to months after decannulation, mucosal necrosis, and subsequent scarring can cause tracheal stenosis. Patients with stenosis have dyspnea, wheezing, stridor, and inability to clear secretions. Treatment in the emergency department includes **humidified oxygen, nebulized racemic epinephrine, and steroids**. Further treatment may include rigid bronchoscopy laser excision of scar bands, stenting, or tracheal reconstruction.

Changing a Tracheostomy Tube

If the tracheostomy is less than 7 days old and the situation is not emergent, tracheostomy tubes should be changed by a surgeon familiar with the procedure, as tracts are not yet mature and manipulation may easily create a false passage. Tracts can also easily collapse in patients with obesity or neck masses.

LARYNGECTOMY PATIENTS

It is impossible to orally intubate patients after laryngectomy. Laryngectomy patients can be emergently intubated by placing an endobronchial tube into the tracheostoma. Do not advance the tube too far, as the carina can be only 4 to 6 cm from the tracheostoma.

Speech Devices

A Passy-Muir valve is a one-way valve that fits directly over the opening of an uncuffed tracheostomy tube, allowing for hands free speech. Because patients exhale around the tracheostomy tube, a Passy Muir valve should not be used with a cuffed tube. **If a patient with a Passy-Muir valve develops respiratory distress or an inability to speak, your first intervention should be to remove the speech valve. Then check the tracheostomy tube for obstruction**.

FURTHER READING

For further reading in *Tintinalli's Emergency Medicine: A Comprehensive Study Guide*, 8th ed., see Chapter 246, "Neck and Upper Airway," by Nicholas D. Hartman; Chapter 247 "Complications of Airway Devices," by John P. Gaillard.

SECTION 17

Disorders of the Skin

CHAPTER 154 Dermatologic Emergencies

Jason P. Stopyra

ERYTHEMA MULTIFORME AND STEVENS–JOHNSON SYNDROME

Clinical Features

Erythema multiforme (EM) strikes all ages, with the highest incidence in young adults (20 to 40 years of age). It affects males twice as often as females, and occurs more commonly in the spring and fall. EM is an acute inflammatory skin disease with presentations that range from a mild papular eruption (EM minor) to diffuse vesiculobullous lesions with mucous membrane involvement and systemic toxicity (Stevens–Johnson syndrome). Precipitating factors include infection (mycoplasma and herpes simplex), drugs (antibiotics and anticonvulsants), and malignancy. No specific cause is found in about half of the cases.

Malaise, arthralgias, myalgias, fever, a generalized burning sensation, and diffuse pruritus may precede the development of skin lesions. Skin lesions begin as erythematous papules and macular lesions followed by the development of target lesions in 24 to 48 hours. Lesions can be diffuse and may be located on the palms and soles. Urticarial plaques, vesicles, bullae, vesiculobullous lesions, and mucosal (oral, conjunctival, respiratory, and genitourinary) erosions may also develop (Fig. 154-1). Systemic toxicity along with significant fluid and electrolyte deficiencies and secondary infections may be seen in severe disease.

Diagnosis and Differential

Target lesions are highly suggestive of EM. The presence of mucosal involvement suggests Stevens–Johnson syndrome. The differential diagnosis includes herpetic infections, vasculitis, toxic epidermal necrolysis, primary blistering disorders, Kawasaki disease, and the toxic and infectious erythemas.

Emergency Department Care and Disposition

1. Patients without systemic manifestation or mucous membrane involvement may be managed as outpatients with dermatologic consultation.

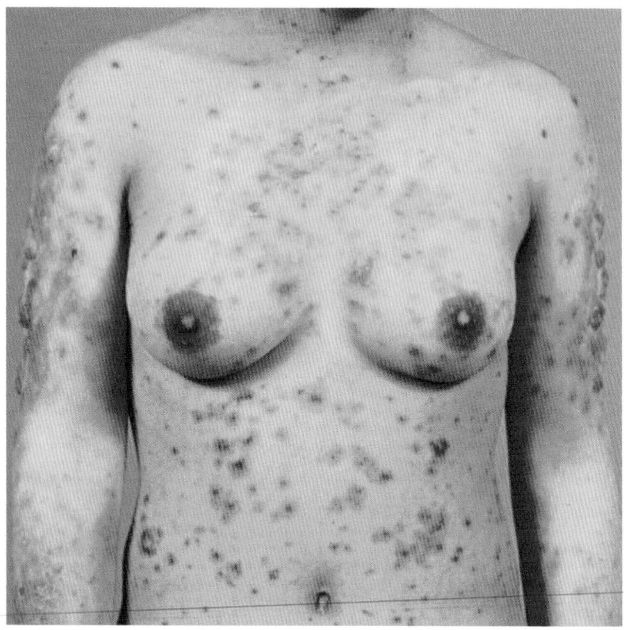

FIGURE 154-1. Erythema multiforme.

Prednisone 60 to 80 mg PO daily for 3 to 5 days are often prescribed for mild disease but are unproven to change duration and outcomes. Acyclovir may reduce recurrent HSV-related EM.

2. Admit patients with extensive disease or systemic toxicity for critical care and consultation with a dermatologist and ophthalmologist. Intensively manage fluid, electrolyte, infectious, nutritional, and thermoregulatory issues. **Diphenhydramine** and **lidocaine rinses** provide symptomatic relief for stomatitis. Cool **Burrow's solution** (5% aluminum acetate) compresses can be applied to blistered regions.

TOXIC EPIDERMAL NECROLYSIS

Toxic epidermal necrolysis (TEN) is a severe inflammatory skin disease that strikes all ages and both sexes equally. Some authorities consider TEN to be a variant of Stevens–Johnson syndrome.

Clinical Features

Potential etiologies include chemicals, infections, and malignancy, but medications are the most common causes of TEN. Malaise, anorexia, myalgias, arthralgias, fever, and upper respiratory infection symptoms may precede skin findings by 1 to 2 weeks. Skin findings progress from tender erythematous areas that become confluent within hours to flaccid bullae and erosions with exfoliation (Fig. 154-2). A positive Nikolsky sign is slippage of the epidermis from the dermis when slight tangential pressure is applied

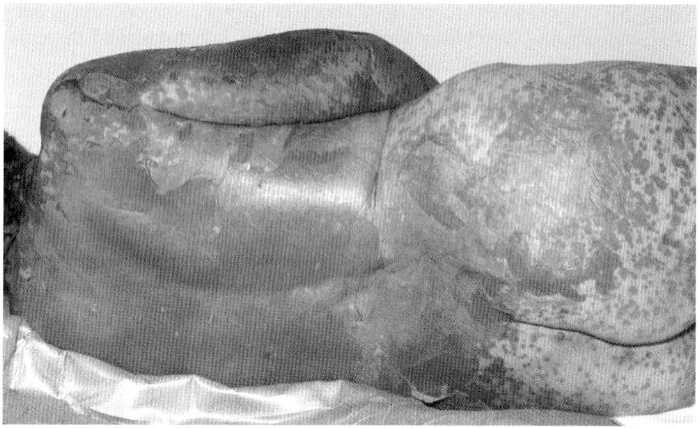

FIGURE 154-2. Toxic epidermal necrolysis.

to the skin. Systemic toxicity as well as oral, ocular, and anogenital mucosal lesions are common. TEN has a mortality rate of 25% to 35%, and poor prognostic indicators include advanced age, extensive disease, multiple medication use, leukopenia, azotemia, and thrombocytopenia.

Diagnosis and Differential

Initial diagnosis is based on the clinical features, while skin biopsy results can confirm the diagnosis. The differential diagnosis includes erythema multiforme, exfoliative dermatitis, primary blistering disorders, Kawasaki disease, and toxic infectious erythemas.

Emergency Department Care and Disposition

1. Admit patients with TEN to a critical care setting, preferably a burn unit with expertise managing appropriate cardiopulmonary, fluid, electrolyte, and sepsis resuscitation.
2. Emergent dermatologic consultation is recommended.

MENINGOCOCCEMIA

Clinical Features

Meningococcemia is a serious and potentially fatal systemic infection caused by *Neisseria meningitides*. Clinical disease usually develops within 3 to 4 days after exposure and can present with a fulminant course. Possible presenting features can include headache, fever, altered mental status, nausea, vomiting, myalgias, arthralgia, and neck stiffness. Dermatologic manifestations of this infection include petechia, urticaria, hemorrhagic vesicles, and macules that evolve into palpable purpura with grey necrotic centers.

Diagnosis and Differential

Consider meningococcemia in ill-appearing patients with a petechial rash and associated symptoms of infection. The differential diagnosis includes

Rocky Mountain spotted fever, toxic shock syndrome, gonococcemia, bacterial endocarditis, vasculitis, viral and bacterial infections, and disseminated intravascular coagulation.

Emergency Department Care and Disposition

1. Treat meningococcemia in adult patients with an IV third-generation cephalosporin such as **ceftriaxone** or **cefotaxime**. Consider additional empiric antibiotic coverage for patients with suspected bacteremia when the pathogen is uncertain.
2. Admit patients with meningococcal infection for close monitoring, supportive care, and continued antibiotic treatment.

PEMPHIGUS VULGARIS

Clinical Features

Pemphigus vulgaris is a generalized, mucocutaneous, autoimmune, blistering eruption with a grave prognosis. Primary lesions are clear, tense vesicles or bullae that vary in diameter, and are first noted on the head, trunk, and mucous membranes. Within 2 to 3 days, the bullae become turbid and flaccid then rupture, producing painful, denuded areas that are slow to heal and prone to secondary infection (Fig. 154-3).

Diagnosis and Differential

Pemphigus vulgaris is suspected by the appearance of lesions and confirmed by skin biopsy and immunofluorescence testing. The differential diagnosis includes bullous pemphigoid, TEN, EM major, dermatitis herpetiformis, and other blistering skin diseases. Bullous pemphigoid is a mucocutaneous blistering disease typically found in the elderly.

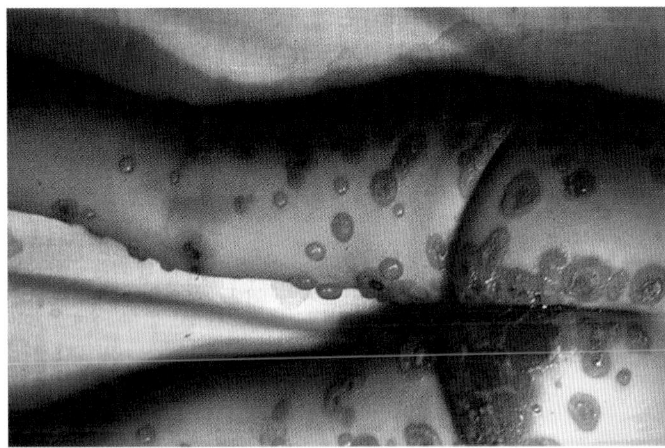

FIGURE 154-3. Scattered bullous lesions intermixed with erosions and painful inflammatory plaques in a patient with pemphigus vulgaris.

Emergency Department Care and Disposition

1. Treat fluid and electrolyte disturbances aggressively.
2. Consult with a dermatologist for management of pemphigus vulgaris. Corticosteroids and immunosuppressives are the mainstays of therapy. Plasmaphoresis and IV immunoglobins may also be needed.

FURTHER READING

For further reading in *Tintinalli's Emergency Medicine: A Comprehensive Study Guide*, 8th ed., see Chapter 141, "Rashes in Infants and Children," by Gary Bonfante and Amy Dunn; Chapter 249, "Generalized Skin Disorders," by Mark Sochor, Amit Pandit, and William J. Brady.

CHAPTER 155

Other Dermatologic Disorders

Jason P. Stopyra

HERPES ZOSTER

Clinical Features

Herpes zoster results from cutaneous activation of latent varicella zoster virus along a sensory nerve root dermatome. Pain or dysesthesia in an involved dermatome begins 3 to 5 days before lesions emerge. Erythematous papules develop first, progress to vesicular clusters, and these lesions crust after about a week. Herpes zoster of the ophthalmic branch of the trigeminal nerve, especially if accompanied by lesions on the nose, are concerning for possible eye involvement that can lead to keratitis or corneal ulceration (Fig. 155-1). A thorough eye exam should be performed (see Chapter 149, "Ocular Emergencies"). Generalized eruptions involving more than one dermatome may occur in immunocompromised patients.

Diagnosis and Differential

The differential diagnosis for these kinds of skin eruptions includes herpes simplex, impetigo, and contact dermatitis. The characteristic skin rash of herpes zoster presents in a unilateral distribution along a single sensory dermatome and is accompanied by localized pain at the site. A swab of the

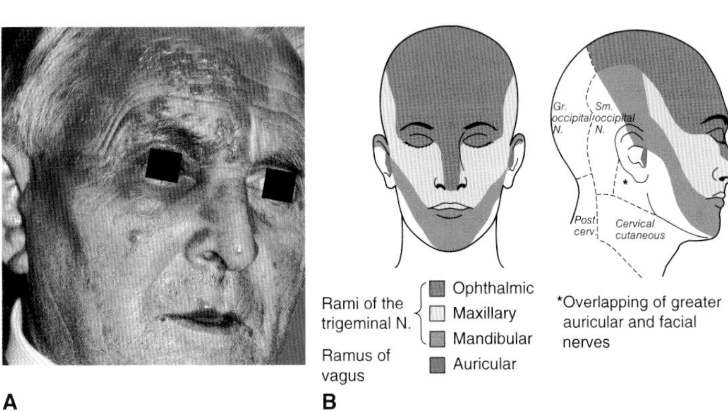

FIGURE 155-1. A. Herpes zoster in trigeminal nerve distribution. Note lesion on the tip of the nose, which suggests nasociliary branch involvement. **B.** Dermatomes of the head and neck. cerv. = cervical; Gr. = greater; N. = nerve; Sm. = smaller. A. Reproduced with permission from Fleischer A Jr, Feldman S, McConnell C, et al. *Emergency Dermatology: A Rapid Treatment Guide*. New York, NY: McGraw-Hill; 2002. B. Reproduced with permission from Wolff K, Johnson R, Saavedra AP. *Fitzpatrick's Color Atlas & Synopsis of Clinical Dermatology*, 7th ed. New York: McGraw-Hill; 2013.

base of the vesicle can be sent for viral PCR to confirm the clinical diagnosis when uncertainty exists.

Emergency Department Care and Disposition

1. Antiviral medications started in the first 72 hours of illness shorten healing time, decrease formation of new lesions, and help prevent postherpetic neuralgia. Antiviral choices include **acyclovir** 800 mg PO five times per day for 7 to 10 days or **valacyclovir** 1000 mg PO three times a day for 7 days. Immunocompromised patients with severe disease can be treated with **acyclovir**, 10 mg/kg IV every 8 hours for 7 to 10 days.
2. Aluminum acetate compressions three times daily and analgesics provide symptomatic relief.
3. Advise patients that herpes zoster is contagious to anyone who has not had chicken pox or the varicella zoster vaccine.
4. Consult with an ophthalmologist if eye involvement is suspected.

HERPES SIMPLEX VIRUS INFECTIONS

Herpes simplex virus (HSV) lesions are painful grouped vesicles with an erythematous base. Primary disease may be preceded with or accompanied by constitutional symptoms. Tingling or burning precedes recurrent lesions. Oral lesions ("cold sores") are usually caused by HSV1, but may also be caused by HSV2. The diagnosis can be confirmed with an HSV PCR test if necessary. Treatment (Table 155-1) is most effective when started within 24 hours of symptom onset. See Chapter 87, "Sexually Transmitted Infections," for discussion and treatment of genital herpes.

TINEA INFECTIONS

Clinical Features

Tinea refers to skin infections caused by dermatophytes (fungi). *Tinea capitis* is characterized by patchy areas of alopecia with broken off hairs and scales at the periphery. *Tinea barbae* presents with severe inflammatory plaques and follicular pustules in the beard area. Interdigital scaling, maceration, plantar or palmar erythema or scaling, and pruritis are seen in

TABLE 155-1 Treatment of Herpes Simplex Virus (HSV) Gingivostomatitis (Herpes Labialis)

Condition	Acyclovir Treatment	Valacyclovir Treatment
First episode	400 mg PO three times a day for 7 days *or* 200 mg PO five times a day for 7 days	1 g PO twice a day for 7 days
Recurrent episode	400 mg PO three times a day for 5 days *or* 800 mg PO three a day for 2–5 days	500 mg PO twice a day for 3 days
Suppression	400 mg PO twice a day	1 g PO a day, may decrease to 500 mg PO a day if <10 outbreaks/year

Tinea pedis (also known as athlete's foot) and *Tinea manuum* (hand). Onchomycosis may occur. Findings in *Tinea cruris* (commonly called jock itch) include erythema with a peripheral annular scaly edge that extends onto the thighs and buttocks but spares the penis and scrotum. *Candida intertrigo* involves the skinfolds. *Tinea Corporus* (trunk, neck, arms, and legs lesions) are typically circular, covered with scales and surrounded by a raised border.

Diagnosis and Differential

Identification of fungal elements on a potassium hydroxide preparation or with fungal culture may be completed if the diagnosis is uncertain. The differential diagnosis includes psoriasis, atopic, seborrheic, and chronic dermatitis (Table 155-2).

TABLE 155-2 Comparison Features of Common Papulosquamous Eruptions

Condition	Distinguishing Clinical Features	Location	Special Signs	Comments
Psoriasis	Erythematous, well-marginated papules and plaques with silvery scale	Trunk, extensor surfaces, scalp	Auspitz sign; Koebner phenomenon, nail pitting	Hereditary predilection; onset in early 20s
Seborrheic dermatitis	Greasy, yellow scales	Midchest, suprapubic, scalp, facial creases	Can overlap with psoriasis, "sebopsoriasis"	Debilitated, elderly, or infants (cradle cap)
Atopic dermatitis	Ill-defined vesicles forming plaques with scale; chronic lesions lichenified	Flexures > trunk	Spares the nose	Pruritus "itch that rashes"; atopic individuals
Lichen planus	5 P's: purple, pruritic, polygonal, planar papules	Any skin, mucous membranes, hair follicles	Wickham striae; Koebner phenomenon	Age 20–60 years old
Pityriasis rosea	Lines of skin tension, collarette of scale	Trunk, in Christmas tree pattern following skin lines	Herald patch 1–2 weeks before general eruption	Spring and fall, age 15–40 years old; viral exanthem, herpes 6 and 7
Tinea corporis	Sharply demarcated, erythematous, scaly annular plaques; may coalesce into gyrate patterns	Trunk, legs, arm, neck	May need KOH/culture to diagnose; septate branching hyphae on KOH	All ages; from pets, soil, or autoinoculation from hands/feet; incubation days or months
Pityriasis (tinea) versicolor	Versicolored—red, salmon, light brown, dark brown, hypopigmented; well-demarcated scaly patches	Central upper chest and back	Spaghetti and meatballs on KOH; nonseptate pseudohyphae and budding yeast	Young adults, summer, hot humid environments

(Continued)

TABLE 155-2 Comparison Features of Common Papulosquamous Eruptions (Continued)

Condition	Distinguishing Clinical Features	Location	Special Signs	Comments
Secondary syphilis	At 2–10 weeks, macular erythema on trunk, abdomen, inner extremities; followed by papular or papulosquamous lesions	Palms, soles, trunk	Serology	Great masquerader—can take any form; can be confused with pityriasis rosea
Scabies	Pruritic papules and burrows with crusting	Finger webs, wrists, axillae, areolae, umbilicus, abdomen, waistband, genitals	Scrapings show mites, feces, eggs	Can be chronic "7-year itch"; intensely pruritic, especially at night

Abbreviation: KOH = potassium hydroxide.

Emergency Department Care and Disposition

1. Treat *Tinea capitis* with liquid **microsize griseofulvin** 20 to 25 mg/kg PO daily (maximum, 1 g/d) for 8 weeks, **ultramicrosize griseofulvin** (tablets only), 10 to 15 mg/kg/d (maximum, 750 mg/d) for 8 weeks, or **terbinafine granules** 125 mg PO daily for patients weighing <25 kg, 187.5 mg/d for patients weighing 25 to 35 kg, and 250 mg/d for patients weighing >35 kg for 6 weeks. Consider baseline liver function tests as oral antifungal treatment in patients with abnormal hepatic function is not recommended. Advise patients to wash hair with **selenium sulfide 2.5% shampoo** or **ketoconazole 2% shampoo** three times per week for the first 2 weeks of therapy.
2. Treat *Tinea barbae* with **microsize griseofulvin**, 500 mg PO daily or **ultramicrosize griseofulvin**, 375 mg PO daily, for 4 to 6 weeks. **Tervinafine** can also be used. Consider baseline liver function tests. Shaving or depilating the hair along with warm compresses is recommended.
3. Treat nonbullous *tinea pedis* and *manuum, intertrigo, tinea corpora, and tinea cruris,* with topical antifungal agents such as **clotrimazole**, **miconazole**, **ketoconazole**, or **econazole** twice daily for 4 weeks. Continue treatment 1 week after clearing has occurred. Antifungal powders used on a daily basis help prevent recurrences of *tinea cruris*.
4. Onchomycosis usually requires long-term oral treatment.
5. Follow-up with a primary care physician or dermatologist is recommended, especially if the lesions are not resolved in 4 to 6 weeks.

ALLERGIC CONTACT DERMATITIS

Clinical Features

Contact dermatitis occurs after direct contact with an irritant or allergen. Reactions occasionally occur after exposure to aerosolized particles, such as burned poison ivy or oak. Detergents and soaps are common irritants, while nickel, plants, cosmetic preservatives, contact lens solutions, and skin tape are common allergens. Physical findings include erythema, papules, vesicles, and bullae. Scaling and fissuring are seen with chronic contact dermatitis.

Emergency Department Care and Disposition

1. Begin treatment by identifying and removing the likely offending agent.
2. **Aluminum acetate** (Burow's solution) compresses two or three times per day may ease acute irritation.
3. Depending on severity, topical or oral corticosteroids and oral antihistamines can be used in medical management. Patients with extensive, severe allergic contact dermatitis may benefit from a short course of systemic corticosteroids.

SUNBURN AND PHOTOSENSITIVITY

Clinical Features

Patients with sunburn have an inflammatory response to ultraviolet (UV) radiation and may present with minimal discomfort in mild cases or extreme pain with extensive blistering for more severe exposures. Tender and warm areas of erythema in sun-exposed areas are characteristic of sunburn. Sunburn reactions develop 2 to 6 hours after exposure and peak in 1 to 3 days.

Exogenous photosensitivity disorders result from topical application or ingestion of an agent that increases the skin's sensitivity when exposed to UV light. Photosensitivity disorders may be phototoxic (occur quickly with characteristics similar to sunburn) or photoallergic (delayed onset characterized by eczema-like changes with vesiculation). Photosensitivity eruptions occur on sun-exposed skin and are associated with topically applied furocoumarins (lime juice, various fragrances, figs, celery, parsnips), and numerous medications, including sulfonamides, thiazides, furosemide, fluoroquinolones, and tetracyclines.

Emergency Department Care and Disposition

1. Sunburns are treated symptomatically with tepid baths, NSAIDs, and local wound care including topical antibiotics to blistered areas.
2. Initial management of exogenous photosensitivity is similar to the sunburn reaction, including the avoidance of the sun until the eruption has cleared. Identify and discontinue the causative agent, if possible.

SECONDARY SYPHILIS

Clinical Features

Early secondary syphilis eruptions emerge 2 to 10 weeks after the appearance of the primary chancre (see Chapter 87, "Sexually Transmitted Infections"). This evanescent macular rash on the trunk and inner extremities may last only a few hours or days. Subsequent rash, often referred to as the "great imitator" because of the varied clinical appearance, lasts 2 to 6 weeks and may present in a variety of forms. These eruptions are often papular lesions 2 to 5 mm in size, generalized, and reddish to copper in color. Involvement of the palms and soles is a helpful diagnostic finding. Consider risk factors and the possibility of secondary syphilis rash when

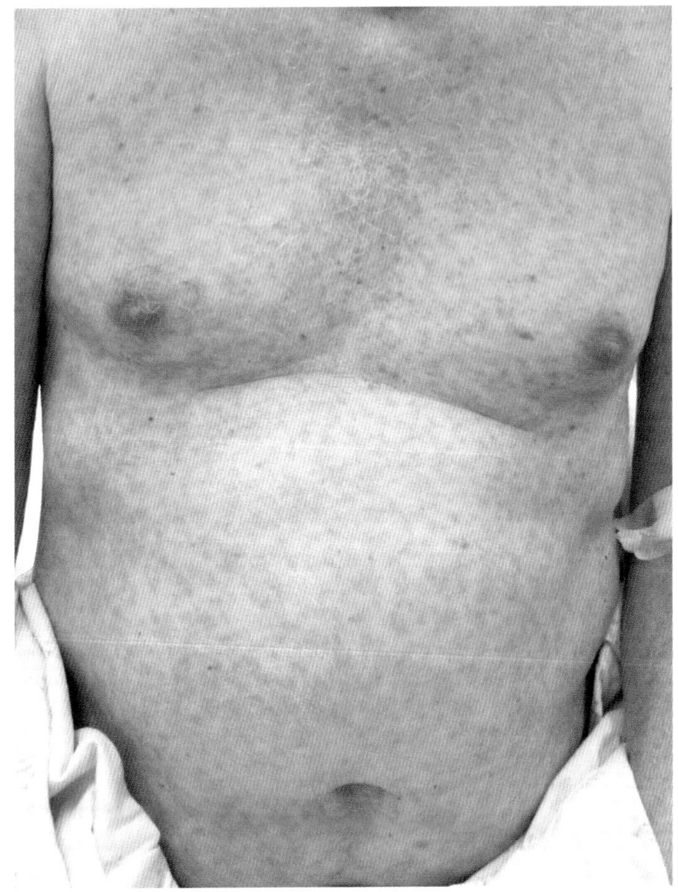

FIGURE 155-2. Secondary syphilis. Papulosquamous eruption. Used with permission from University of Carolina Department of Dermatology.

evaluating patients with papulosquamous conditions (Fig. 155-2). The nontreponemal serologic tests are frequently strongly reactive in secondary syphilis and can be helpful for diagnosis.

Emergency Department Care and Disposition

Treat secondary syphilis with **benzathine penicillin G** (single dose of 2.4 million IM, 1.2 million units in each buttock). **Doxycycline**, 100 mg PO twice a day for 2 weeks, can be used in patients with penicillin allergy.

MOLLUSCUM CONTAGIOSUM

Molluscum contagiosum is a common viral infection of the epidermis occurring in children, sexually active adults, and immunosuppressed individuals (especially patients with human immunodeficiency virus).

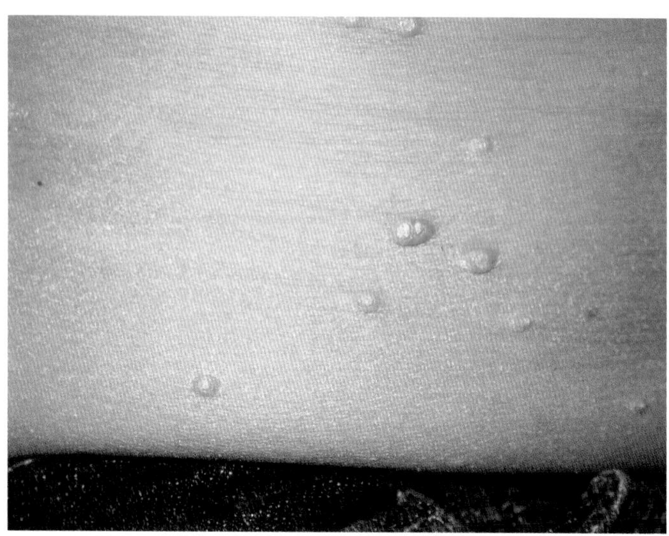

FIGURE 155-3. Molluscum contagiosum. Centrally umbilicated papules. Used with permission from University of Carolina Department of Dermatology.

Transmission is by direct skin-to-skin contact. These lesions can present as a single skin-colored, pearly, umbilicated papule (1 to 2 mm) or as multiple, scattered papules or nodules and plaques (5 to 10 mm) (Fig. 155-3). Autoinoculation may lead to clustering of lesions by scratching. Most patients do not require specific treatment for this condition and it typically resolves within 6 months to 4 years. Options for treatment in appropriate circumstances include curettage, cryotherapy, or electrodesiccation. In individuals with human immunodeficiency virus, treatment of the underlying human immunodeficiency virus infection may lead to resolution.

HIDRADENITIS SUPPURATIVA

Hidradenitis suppurativa is an inflammatory condition, typically affecting the apocrine gland-bearing areas of the skin with recurrent, painful, and draining nodules. The inciting event is follicular occlusion, prompting rupture of the follicular contents, and resulting intense inflammation. Axillary and inguinal skin demonstrates varying numbers of inflammatory nodules, many of which may form connecting tracts, with resultant drainage onto the skin surface (Fig. 155-4). See Chapter 90, "Soft Tissue Infections."

Emergency Department Care and Disposition

1. Recommend clindamycin 1% lotion twice daily and use antibacterial soaps once to twice weekly for patients without discrete areas of abscess.
2. Acute abscesses can be treated with incision and drainage, although minimizing this approach when possible may be appropriate due to the recurrent nature of this disease. In severe and recurrent cases, outpatient surgical referral may be indicated.

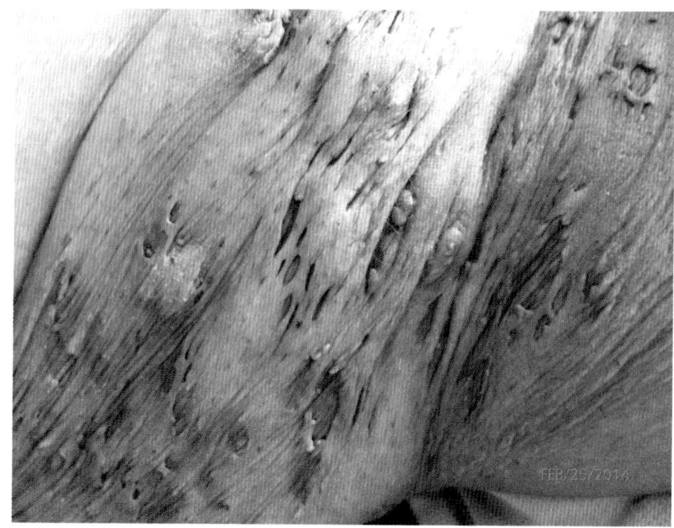

FIGURE 155-4. Hidradenitis suppurativa involving the buttock region. Used with permission from University of Carolina Department of Dermatology.

FURTHER READING

For further reading in *Tintinalli's Emergency Medicine: A Comprehensive Study Guide*, 8th ed., see Chapter 250, "Skin Disorders: Face and Scalp," by Dean S. Morrell and Kevin W. Dahle; Chapter 251, "Skin Disorders: Trunk," by Dean S. Morrell and Kara Luersen Brooks; Chapter 252, "Skin Disorders: Groin and Skinfolds," by Dean S. Morrell and Edith V. Bowers; Chapter 253, "Skin Disorders: Extremities," by Rachna A. Bhandari and Dean S. Morrell.

SECTION 18 Trauma

CHAPTER 156 Trauma in Adults

Rita K. Cydulka

Trauma care is guided by the concepts of rapid assessment, triage, resuscitation, serial reassessment, diagnosis, and therapeutic intervention.

CLINICAL FEATURES

Trauma patients can sustain a multitude of injuries. Many people will present with abnormal vital signs, neurologic deficits, or other gross evidence of injury. These signs should prompt both a thorough search for the specific underlying injuries and rapid interventions to correct the abnormalities. Nonspecific signs such as tachycardia, tachypnea, or mild alterations in consciousness should similarly be presumed to signify serious injury until proven otherwise. Further, without signs of significant trauma, the mechanism of injury may suggest potential problems, which should be pursued diligently.

DIAGNOSIS AND DIFFERENTIAL

The assessment of trauma patients begins with a focused history from the patient, family members, witnesses, or prehospital providers. Patterns of injuries, and expected physiologic responses to these injuries, can be ascertained by collecting history regarding the circumstances of the event (e.g., single vehicle crash, fall from height, smoke inhalation, or environmental exposures), ingestion of intoxicants, preexisting medical conditions, and medications.

To facilitate an organized approach to the trauma patient, the examination is divided into primary and secondary surveys (Table 156-1). The goal of the primary survey is to identify and immediately treat life-threatening conditions. To do so, the acronym ABCDE encourages the clinician to examine the patient's airway, breathing, circulation, and disability (mental status, Glasgow Coma Scale (GCS), and neurologic examination), and to completely expose each patient so that occult injuries or exposures are visualized. After this initial primary survey, perform a thorough head-to-toe examination (the secondary survey, Table 156-1), then proceed with appropriate diagnostic testing and further therapeutic interventions.

TABLE 156-1 Primary and Secondary Surveys in Trauma Resuscitation

Primary Survey (rapid identification and management of immediately life-threatening injuries)

A. Airway and cervical spine

Assess, clear, and protect airway: jaw thrust/chin lift, suctioning.
Perform endotracheal intubation with in-line stabilization for patient with depressed level of consciousness or inability to protect airway.
Create surgical airway if there is significant bleeding or obstruction or laryngoscopy cannot be performed.

B. Breathing

Ventilate with 100% oxygen; monitor oxygen saturation.
Auscultate for breath sounds.
Inspect thorax and neck for deviated trachea, open chest wounds, abnormal chest wall motion, and crepitus at neck or chest.
Consider immediate needle thoracostomy for suspected tension pneumothorax.
Consider tube thoracostomy for suspected hemopneumothorax.

C. Circulation

Assess for blood volume status: skin color, capillary refill, radial/femoral/carotid pulse, and blood pressure.
Place two large-bore peripheral IV catheters.
Begin rapid infusion of warm crystalloid solution, if indicated.
Apply direct pressure to sites of brisk external bleeding.
Consider central venous or interosseous access if peripheral sites are unavailable.
Consider pericardiocentesis for suspected pericardial tamponade.
Consider left lateral decubitus position in late-trimester pregnancy.

D. Disability

Perform screening neurologic and mental status examination, assessing:
– Pupil size and reactivity
– Limb strength and movement, grip strength
– Orientation, Glasgow Coma Scale score
Consider measurement of capillary blood glucose level in patients with altered mental status.

E. Exposure

Completely disrobe the patient, and inspect for burns and toxic exposures.
Logroll patient, maintaining neutral position and in-line neck stabilization, to inspect and palpate thoracic spine, flank, back, and buttocks.

Secondary Survey (head-to-toe examination for rapid identification and control of injuries or potential instability)

Identify and control scalp wound bleeding with direct pressure, sutures, or surgical clips.
Identify facial instability and potential for airway instability.
Identify hemotympanum.
Identify epistaxis or septal hematoma; consider tamponade or airway control if bleeding is profuse.
Identify avulsed teeth or jaw instability.
Evaluate for abdominal distention and tenderness.
Identify penetrating chest, back, flank, or abdominal injuries.
Assess for pelvic stability; consider pelvic wrap or sling.
Inspect perineum for laceration or hematoma.
Inspect urethral meatus for blood.
Consider rectal examination for sphincter tone and gross blood.
Assess peripheral pulses for vascular compromise.
Identify extremity deformities, and immobilize open and closed fractures and dislocations.

EMERGENCY DEPARTMENT CARE AND DISPOSITION

1. The ED management of trauma patients begins prior to the patient's arrival. Emergency medical service providers inform the receiving ED about the mechanism of trauma, vital sign values, suspected injuries, and treatments provided.
2. Airway patency is confirmed at the outset of the primary survey. In patients making inadequate respiratory efforts, perform a jaw thrust, and then insert an oral or nasal airway. Avoid nasal airway placement in patients with suspected basilar skull fractures. Endotracheal intubation is indicated in comatose patients (GCS < 8) to protect the airway and prevent secondary brain injury from hypoxemia. Agitated trauma patients who need further diagnostic or therapeutic interventions or patients whose expected course necessitates immediate operative management are also candidates for intubation. Whenever possible, use a two-person spinal stabilization technique in which one caregiver provides in-line immobilization of the cervical spine while the other manages the airway. Trauma patients are often difficult to intubate due to associated facial trauma, cervical spine immobilization, or the presence of blood or vomitus. In virtually all trauma patients requiring urgent intubation, a rapid sequence intubation technique should be used. In cases of extensive facial trauma or when endotracheal intubation is not possible, cricothyrotomy or another advanced airway technique may be used to secure the airway.
3. Once the airway is secured, examine the neck and thorax to detect abnormalities such as a deviated trachea (tension pneumothorax), crepitus (pneumothorax), paradoxical movement of a chest wall segment (flail chest), sucking chest wound, fractured sternum, or the absence of breath sounds on either side of the chest (simple or tension pneumothorax, massive hemothorax, or right mainstem intubation). Treat tension pneumothorax immediately with needle decompression followed by tube thoracostomy.
4. Rapidly assess the patient's hemodynamic status during the primary survey by noting the level of consciousness, skin color, and the presence and magnitude of peripheral pulses. Note the heart rate, blood pressure, and pulse pressure (systolic minus diastolic blood pressure). Hemorrhage of up to 30% of total blood volume may be associated with only mild tachycardia and a decrease in pulse pressure, but may quickly progress to shock if not recognized early. Establish two large-bore peripheral IV lines, and obtain blood samples for laboratory studies, particularly the blood type and screen. Establish a central line in patients who are unstable or in whom upper extremity peripheral veins are not easily cannulated. Current evidence indicates that early administration of tranexamic acid may reduce mortality.
5. Reassess hemodynamically unstable patients without an obvious indication for surgery after infusion of 2 L of warm crystalloid solution. If there is no marked improvement, consider the need to transfuse type O blood (O-negative for females of childbearing age). An extended focused assessment with sonography for trauma (eFAST) examination screens for causes of shock immediately after the primary survey. If a patient is hemodynamically stable, definitive imaging can be performed

with a CT scan of the abdomen and pelvis with IV contrast. Patients with penetrating abdominal trauma who are in shock should undergo early operative intervention.

6. Patients who sustain major trauma may develop a bleeding diathesis, which results in defective clotting and platelet function. If patients require >10 units of packed red blood cells (PRBC), patients should receive PRBC in a 1:1 ratio with fresh frozen plasma. Both acidosis and hypothermia contribute to the coagulopathy and should be corrected as soon as possible.
7. After the primary survey and stabilization, perform an abbreviated neurologic examination, including an assessment of the patient's level of consciousness, GCS, pupillary size and reactivity, and motor function. A search for the cause of depressed level of consciousness includes the measurement of capillary blood glucose levels and the consideration of possible intoxicants, though one should begin with the assumption this is due to significant traumatic brain injury (TBI). In order to quickly identify potentially operative intracranial injuries among patients with suspected traumatic brain injury and coma (GCS of 3 to 8), defer any procedures that do not correct a specific problem during the primary survey until after the CT scan of the head is performed. Intubated patients should undergo continuous capnography. GCS assessment can be insensitive in patients with normal or near-normal scores, and a GCS score of 15 does not exclude the presence of TBI.
8. Once the patient is hemodynamically stable and the airway is secured, log-roll the patient with one team member assigned to maintain in-line cervical stabilization. Palpate the spinous processes of the thoracic and lumbar spine for tenderness or deformity. Consider performing a rectal examination to assess for gross blood, displaced prostate, or determining rectal tone in the setting of a suspected spinal injury.
9. Certain conditions, such as injuries to the esophagus, diaphragm, and small bowel, often remain undiagnosed even with diligent examination, and further imaging and hospital observation for delayed presentation may be required. The most frequently missed injuries are orthopedic.
10. Expeditiously transport patients with hemodynamic instability and ongoing bleeding to the operating room or transfer them to another facility with appropriate surgical or critical care resources. Serial examinations are essential in patients without obvious indications for surgery identified on the initial assessment. These examinations may be performed in the inpatient or, in some cases, the ED observation unit settings.

FURTHER READING

For further reading in *Tintinalli's Emergency Medicine: A Comprehensive Study Guide*, 8th ed., see Chapter 254, "Trauma in Adults," by Peter Cameron and Barry J. Knapp.

CHAPTER 157 Trauma in Children

Matthew Hansen

Trauma is the most common cause of death in children older than 1 year. Differences in anatomy and physiology mandate modifications to trauma evaluation and management in children.

CLINICAL FEATURES

Head trauma is the most frequent pediatric injury resulting in death. Overall, motor vehicle crash is the most common mechanism, and it is the leading mechanism of traumatic death in children older than 1 year.

Airway: Airway management in children can be challenging. Anatomic differences include a large occiput, large tongue, and cephalad location of the larynx.

Breathing: Observe the rate, depth, pattern, and work of breathing as well as symmetry of rise and fall of the chest wall. Agitation or somnolence could be a result of hypoxia or hypercapnea, respectively. Children experience oxygen desaturation more quickly due to high oxygen demand and small lungs.

Circulation: Recognize early signs of circulatory shock including tachycardia, mental status changes, and color and perfusion abnormalities, because hypotension is typically a terminal event in children. Estimate normal systolic blood pressure in children 1 to 10 years of age using the following formula: $90 + (2 \times \text{age})$ mm Hg; hypotension can be estimated as systolic blood pressure less than $70 + (2 \times \text{age})$ mm Hg.

Disability: In younger children, the Modified Pediatric Glasgow Coma Scale (Table 157-1) should be used. This mirrors the Glasgow Coma Scale for eye opening and motor responses, but incorporates age-appropriate modifications for verbal responses. Perform a pupillary examination and basic assessment of tone and strength.

Exposure: Disrobe and expose the child to completely assess for injuries. However, the ratio of surface area to mass is greater in children, putting them at greater risk for hypothermia. Care should be taken to maintain normothermia.

DIAGNOSIS AND DIFFERENTIAL

Head Injury

Infants and neonates are at the highest risk of significant intracranial injury. Mental status assessment should account for developmental stage and patient anxiety. Parietal and occipital skull fractures are frequently

TABLE 157-1 Modified Pediatric Glasgow Coma Scale

Coos or babbles = 5
Irritable cry = 4
Cries to pain = 3
Moans to pain = 2
No response = 1

associated with intracranial bleeding. Noncontrast CT is the imaging modality of choice for intracranial injury in children. Scalp injuries, particularly in neonates, may result in significant blood loss and shock. Please see Chapter 160 for a discussion on CT imaging in head trauma.

Spine Injuries

Young children with spinal cord injuries often do not have associated fractures since the ligaments are relatively elastic. "Clearing the cervical spine" in children is challenging as there is little evidence to guide practice. Multisystem trauma and head trauma are general indications for neck immobilization and cervical spine imaging. Please see Chapter 161 for a detailed discussion on the management of spine and spinal cord injuries. Due to the nature of spine injuries and the need to lower ionizing radiation, plain films of the spine remain a useful tool.

Chest Trauma

The chest radiograph is an essential tool in the evaluation of any child with chest trauma and CT imaging of the chest rarely changes management. Pulmonary contusions are the most common thoracic injury in children. The relatively compliant chest wall of the child means that serious injuries to intrathoracic structures can be present without significant external signs. Rib fractures are less common in children and generally require a significant mechanism of injury.

Abdominal and Genitourinary Trauma

Indications for CT include suspicious mechanism of injury, tenderness on exam, seatbelt sign, distention, and vomiting. A study of over 12,000 pediatric patients with blunt abdominal trauma recently found the following factors predicted very low risk for significant intraabdominal injury: (1) no evidence of abdominal wall trauma/seat belt sign nor Glasgow Coma Scale <14 with blunt abdominal trauma; (2) no abdominal tenderness on examination; and (3) no thoracic wall trauma, and no complaints of abdominal pain, decreased bowel sounds, or vomiting. Identification of a pelvic fracture, particularly an anterior ring fracture, should prompt investigation for associated urethral or bladder injury. The role of ultrasound for pediatric abdominal trauma, especially in stable patients, is not well established.

EMERGENCY DEPARTMENT CARE AND DISPOSITION

1. Perform basic airway maneuvers such as jaw thrust and oropharyngeal suctioning and maintain a sniffing position to align the airway axes, often by placing a towel roll under the shoulders, which is especially helpful in younger children to align the airway.
2. **Orotracheal intubation** is indicated for definitive airway management. The following formula is used to estimate the endotracheal tube size: size = 4 + (age/4), subtract ½ size for cuffed tubes which are often preferred. Maintain in-line cervical spine stabilization at all times. Rapid sequence intubation is the safest method of intubating a trauma patient with a full stomach. When possible, limit positive-pressure ventilation before intubation to avoid gastric insufflation and vomiting.

3. Vascular access can be challenging. Place two proximal IVs in critically ill patients. Obtain **intraosseous access** early, as needed. If central venous access is needed, the femoral vein is the most easily accessed site. Administer fluids in **20 mL/kg boluses of crystalloid;** if there is no response to two boluses, then administer **10 mL/kg boluses of packed red blood cells**. Permissive hypotension is not an evidence-based practice in children and may be harmful. Consider using a massive transfusion protocol if large volume resuscitation is anticipated.
4. For pain control, **fentanyl 1 μg/kg** or **morphine 0.05 to 0.1 mg/kg** are appropriate.
5. If a head injured patient has clinical signs of impending herniation, maintain the $PaCO_2$ at 35 to 40 mm Hg, optimize blood pressure with IV fluids, and elevate the head of the bed 20° to 30°. See Table 157-2 for head injury management suggestions.

TABLE 157-2 Management of Serious Traumatic Brain Injury in Children

Considerations	Primary Goals	Comments
Cervical spine	Maintain spinal precautions	
Airway	Maintain airway, intubate for GCS <8 or as needed for oxygenation and ventilation	
Oxygenation and ventilation	Oxygen saturation >90%; PCO_2 35–40 mm Hg	No prophylactic hyperventilation
Blood pressure	SBP > 70 + (2 × age)	No permissive hypotension
Cerebral perfusion pressure (CPP)	CPP = 40–65 mm Hg	
Intracranial pressure (ICP) monitoring	ICP ≤20 mm Hg	Consultation with neurosurgeon
GCS	GCS before paralytics if possible	Serial GCS to document changes
Sedation and pain management	Midazolam Fentanyl	Consider paralytics once thorough neurologic examination is completed
Neuroimaging (noncontrast head CT and cervical spine CT when indicated)	Identify intracranial injury and signs of increased intracranial pressure or herniation	Transcranial Doppler may be useful in infants with open fontanelles but requires an experienced pediatric radiologist
Glucose	Treat hypoglycemia and hyperglycemia	Maintain normal blood glucose
Increased ICP/impending herniation	Elevate head of bed 30 degrees	3% normal saline 5 mL/kg bolus over 10 min followed by infusion of 0.1 mL/kg/h to maintain serum Na within 155–165 mEq/L *or* Mannitol 0.5–1 g/kg if normotensive (response is not dose-dependent)
Core temperature	Maintain temperature 36–38°C	Hypothermia in children not recommended; avoid hyperthermia

(Continued)

TABLE 157-2 Management of Serious Traumatic Brain Injury in Children (Continued)

Considerations	Primary Goals	Comments
Seizure prophylaxis	Optional: consider for children with witnessed posttraumatic seizures and intracranial blood	Phenytoin 20 mg/kg (or fosphenytoin 20 PE/kg) *or* Levetiracetam 10–20 mg/kg (maximum, 500 mg/dose) for first week following severe traumatic brain injury
Anemia	Transfuse for hemoglobin <7 g/dL	
Neurosurgery/transfer	ICP monitoring, evacuation of intracranial blood, or cerebrospinal fluid shunt for refractory intracranial hypertension	

Abbreviations: GCS, Glasgow Coma Scale; PCO_2, partial pressure of carbon dioxide; PE, phenytoin equivalent; SBP, systolic blood pressure.

6. Admit children with intracranial hemorrhage, spinal trauma, significant chest trauma, abdominal trauma with internal organ injury, significant burns, or other concerning injuries. Indications for referral to a pediatric trauma center are listed in Table 157-3.

TABLE 157-3 Indications for Transfer to a Pediatric Trauma Center

Mechanism of injury	Ejection from motor vehicle Fall from a significant height Motor vehicle collision with prolonged extrication Motor vehicle collision with death of another vehicle occupant
Anatomic injury	Multiple severe trauma More than three long-bone fractures Spinal fractures or spinal cord injury Amputations Severe head or facial trauma Penetrating head, chest, or abdominal trauma

Source: Reproduced with permission from Harris BH, Barlow BA, Ballantine TV, et al: American Pediatric Surgical Association principles of pediatric trauma care. *J Pediatr Surg.* 1992;27:423. Copyright Elsevier.

FURTHER READING

For further reading in *Tintinalli's Emergency Medicine: A Comprehensive Study Guide*, 8th ed., see Chapter 110, "Pediatric Trauma," by Camilo E. Gutiérrez.

CHAPTER 158

Trauma in the Elderly

O. John Ma

Emergency physicians need to be aware of the many unique mechanisms of injury and clinical features associated with geriatric trauma patients and apply special management principles when caring for them.

CLINICAL FEATURES

Falls are the most common cause of fatal and non-fatal injury in people ≥65 years of age. Syncope, which has been implicated in many cases, may be secondary to dysrhythmias, venous pooling, autonomic derangement, hypoxia, anemia, or hypoglycemia. Motor vehicle crashes are the second most common cause of injury in the elderly and are the leading cause of death. Elderly pedestrians struck by a motor vehicle are much more likely to die than younger pedestrians. Intentional injuries and those caused by neglect should also be considered.

Evaluate the geriatric trauma patient as both a medical and a trauma patient. Since elderly patients may have a significant past medical history that impacts their trauma care, obtaining a precise history is vital. Family members, medical records, and the patient's primary physician may be helpful in gathering information regarding the traumatic event and the patient's previous level of function. Document medications, such as cardiac agents, diuretics, psychotropic agents, and anticoagulants. Investigating the cause of a fall may uncover serious underlying medical causes or prevent future trauma.

On physical examination, frequent monitoring of vital signs is essential. Avoid feeling reassured by "normal" vital signs. A normal tachycardic response to pain, hypovolemia, or anxiety may be absent or blunted in the elderly trauma patient. Medications such as β-blockers may mask tachycardia and delay appropriate resuscitation. Blood pressures are also misleading in the elderly patient. Because of the high incidence of underlying hypertension, consider using a higher cutoff for hypotension than in younger patients. In blunt trauma patients ≥65 years, mortality increases when systolic blood pressure dips below 110 mm Hg and heart rates exceed 90 beats per minute.

Pay special attention to anatomical variations that may make airway management more difficult. These include the presence of dentures, cervical arthritis, or temporomandibular joint arthritis. A thorough secondary survey is essential to uncover less serious injuries. These "minor" injuries may not be severe enough to cause problems during the initial resuscitation, but cumulatively may cause significant morbidity and mortality. Seemingly stable geriatric trauma patients can deteriorate rapidly and without warning.

DIAGNOSIS AND DIFFERENTIAL

Head Injury

Never assume that alterations in mental status are due solely to any underlying dementia or senility when evaluating the elderly patient's mental status. Elderly persons suffer a much lower incidence of epidural hematomas than the general population; however, there is a higher incidence of subdural and intraparenchymal hematomas in the elderly than in younger patients. The rate of intracranial hemorrhage approaches 7% to 14% in anticoagulated patients with blunt head injury who are experiencing no or minimal symptoms. Order non-contrast head CT for patients who take warfarin and have a mechanism of injury concerning for even a minor head injury.

Cervical Spine Injuries

The pattern of cervical spine injuries in the elderly is different than in younger patients, as there is an increased incidence of C1 and C2 fractures with the elderly. Place special emphasis on maintaining cervical immobilization until the cervical spine is properly assessed. Because of the higher pre-test probability of injury, as well as the difficulties in interpreting plain radiographs in a patient with age-related degeneration, CT scan is the preferred initial modality for assessing the geriatric cervical spine.

Chest Trauma

Rib fractures are more common after blunt trauma due to osteoporotic changes. The pain associated with rib fractures, along with any decreased physiologic reserve, may predispose patients to respiratory complications. More severe thoracic injuries, such as hemopneumothorax, pulmonary contusion, flail chest, and cardiac contusion, can quickly lead to decompensation in elderly individuals whose baseline oxygenation status may already be diminished.

Abdominal Trauma

The abdominal examination in elderly patients is notoriously unreliable. The focused assessment with sonography for trauma (FAST) examination assists in evaluating for hemoperitoneum and the need for exploratory laparotomy in hemodynamically unstable patients. The FAST examination has largely replaced diagnostic peritoneal lavage. Use CT with contrast for patients who are hemodynamically stable. Ensure adequate hydration and baseline assessment of renal function prior to the contrast load for the CT scan. Some patients may be volume-depleted due to medications, such as diuretics. This hypovolemia coupled with contrast administration may exacerbate any underlying renal pathology.

Orthopedic Injuries

Hip fractures occur primarily in four areas: intertrochanteric, transcervical, subcapital, and subtrochanteric. Intertrochanteric fractures are the most common, followed by transcervical fractures. Be aware that pelvic and long bone fractures are not infrequently the sole etiology for hypovolemia in elderly patients. Coordinate timely orthopedic consultation, evaluation, and treatment with open reduction and internal fixation with the diagnosis and management of other injuries. Consider ordering CT of the pelvis in stable patients with pelvic tenderness after an injury if plain radiographs are negative.

Long bone fractures of the femur, tibia, and humerus may produce a loss of mobility with a resulting decrease in the independent lifestyle of elderly patients. Early orthopedic consultation for intramedullary rodding of these fractures may result in increased early mobilization.

The incidence of Colles fractures and humeral head and surgical neck fractures in elderly patients is increased by falls on the outstretched hand or elbow. Localized tenderness, swelling, and ecchymosis to the proximal humerus are characteristic of these injuries. Arrange for early orthopedic referral.

EMERGENCY DEPARTMENT CARE AND DISPOSITION

As in all trauma patients, perform the primary and secondary surveys expeditiously.

1. The main therapeutic goal is maintaining adequate oxygen delivery. **Consider prompt tracheal intubation** and use of mechanical ventilation in patients with more severe injuries, respiratory rates > 40 breaths/min, or when the PaO_2 is < 60 mm Hg or $PaCO_2$ > 50 mm Hg. While nonventilatory therapy helps prevent respiratory infections and is always desirable, early mechanical ventilation may avert the disastrous results associated with hypoxia.
2. Geriatric trauma patients can decompensate with over-resuscitation just as quickly as they can with inadequate resuscitation. During the initial resuscitative phase, administer crystalloid judiciously since elderly patients with diminished cardiac compliance are more susceptible to volume overload. Consider early and more liberal use of **packed red blood cell transfusion**. This practice early in the resuscitation enhances oxygen delivery and helps minimize tissue ischemia.
3. **Base deficit and lactate levels are useful initial indicators of shock, and serial measurements can guide resuscitation progress.**
4. Early invasive monitoring has been advocated to help physicians assess the elderly's hemodynamic status. One study found that urgent invasive monitoring provides important hemodynamic information early, aids in identifying occult shock, limits hypoperfusion, helps prevent multiple organ failure, and improves survival. Given the complications associated with pulmonary-artery catheters, research on the assessment of shock by serum lactate and central or mixed venous oxygen saturation, and ongoing advances in less invasive hemodynamic monitoring and echocardiography, the optimal approach to recognizing and treating occult hypoperfusion is uncertain. A general strategy is to perform the initial imaging necessary to identify life-threatening injuries (e.g., CT of the head, spine, chest, abdomen, and pelvis) and then transport to the ICU for aggressive optimization of hemodynamics, after which nonessential imaging and interventions (e.g., extremity radiographs and suturing) can be performed.
5. Rapidly reverse anticoagulation in patients taking warfarin with intracranial bleeding on CT scan. Lacking sufficient evidence for or against, it is reasonable to reverse other forms of anticoagulation (e.g., aspirin, clopidogrel, heparin) in patients with diagnosed intracranial hemorrhage.

6. Maintain a low threshold for admitting elderly patients with rib fractures for a period of observation until good pain control and pulmonary toilet is assured.
7. Admit elderly patients with polytrauma, significant chest wall injuries, abnormal vital signs, or evidence of overt or occult hypoperfusion to the ICU.

FURTHER READING

For further reading in *Tintinalli's Emergency Medicine: A Comprehensive Study Guide*, 8th ed., see Chapter 255, "Trauma in the Elderly," by Ross J. Fleischman and O. John Ma.

CHAPTER 159

Trauma in Pregnancy

John Ashurst

Trauma is the leading cause of nonobstetric morbidity and mortality in pregnant women. Motor vehicle collisions followed by falls and domestic violence are the most common causes of trauma in pregnancy and fetal survival is highly dependent on maternal stabilization.

CLINICAL FEATURES

Physiologic changes of pregnancy make it difficult to determine the severity of injury. Heart rate increases 10 to 20 beats per minute in the second trimester while systolic and diastolic blood pressures drop 10 to 15 mm Hg. Blood volume can increase by 45%, but red cell mass increases to a lesser extent, leading to a physiologic anemia of pregnancy. It may be difficult to determine whether tachycardia, hypotension, or anemia is due to blood loss or normal physiologic changes. Due to the relative hypervolemic state, the patient may lose 30% to 35% of blood volume before manifesting signs of shock. Pulmonary changes in pregnancy include elevation of the diaphragm and a decrease in residual volume and function residual capacity. Tidal volume increases, resulting in hyperventilation with associated respiratory alkalosis. However, renal compensation causes the serum pH to remain unchanged. Gastric emptying is also delayed, which places the pregnant trauma patient at a higher risk of aspiration.

The anatomic changes in pregnancy affect the types of injuries that are typically seen in the mother. Splenic injury remains the most common cause of abdominal hemorrhage in the pregnant trauma patient. After the 12th week of gestation, the enlarging uterus emerges from the pelvis and by 20 weeks reaches the level of the umbilicus. Uterine blood flow increases, making severe maternal hemorrhage from uterine trauma more likely. The uterus also can compress the inferior vena cava when the patient is supine, leading to the "supine hypotension syndrome." As pregnancy progresses, the small intestines are pushed cephalad, which causes an increased likelihood of injury in penetrating trauma to the upper abdomen. The bladder moves into the abdomen in the third trimester, thereby increasing its susceptibility to injury.

Abdominal trauma affects not only the mother but also the fetus. Fetal injuries are more likely to be seen in the third trimester and are often associated with pelvic fractures or penetrating trauma in the mother. Uterine rupture is rare but is associated with a very high fetal mortality rate. More common complications of trauma include uterine irritability, preterm labor, and placental abruption. Classically, the mother will demonstrate abdominal pain, vaginal bleeding, and uterine contractions. Fetal–maternal hemorrhage occurs in more than 30% of cases of significant trauma and may result in rhesus (Rh) isoimmunization of Rh-negative women.

DIAGNOSIS AND DIFFERENTIAL

Maternal stability and survival offer the best chance for fetal well-being, and no critical interventions or diagnostic procedures should be withheld out of concern for potential adverse effects to the fetus. The initial sequence of trauma resuscitation is unchanged. Special attention should be directed to the gravid abdomen, examining for evidence of injury, tenderness, or uterine contractions. If abdominal or pelvic trauma is suspected, perform a sterile pelvic examination to assess for genital trauma, vaginal bleeding, or ruptured amniotic membranes after pelvic ultrasound to determine placental location. Fluid with a pH of 7 in the vaginal canal suggests amniotic rupture, as does "ferning," a branch-like pattern on drying of vaginal fluid on a microscope slide.

Initial laboratory studies include a complete blood count, serum chemistries, blood type, Rh status, and coagulation studies including fibrin split products and fibrinogen to determine the presence of disseminated intravascular coagulation. The Apt test or Kleihauer–Betke test should be obtained to assess for the presence of fetal hemoglobin in the maternal blood.

Obtain radiographs based on fundamental principles of trauma management. Adverse fetal effects from radiation are negligible from doses <5 rad, which is an exposure far greater than that received from most plain radiographs. Reducing the number of imaging CT cuts and shielding of the abdomen and pelvis when possible may decrease radiation exposure from medical imaging. Bedside ultrasonography is a highly sensitive, specific, and radiation-free alternative for imaging the abdomen. In addition to evaluating fetal heart rate, ultrasonography can assess gestational age, fetal activity or demise, placental location, and amniotic fluid volume. Diagnostic peritoneal lavage has largely been replaced by ultrasonography. If it is indicated, use the open supraumbilical technique.

Auscultate fetal heart tones to determine fetal viability and identify fetal distress early in the evaluation. A Doppler stethoscope or ultrasound facilitates this assessment. A normal fetal heart rate ranges between 120 and 160 beats per minute. Fetal bradycardia is most likely a result of hypoxia due to maternal hypotension, respiratory compromise, or placental abruption. Fetal tachycardia is most likely due to hypoxia or hypovolemia. In the setting of blunt abdominal trauma, external fetal monitoring is indicated for at least 4 to 6 hours for all patients beyond week 20 of gestation. Fetal tachycardia, lack of beat-to-beat or long-term variability, or late decelerations on tocodynamometry are diagnostic of fetal distress and may be indications for emergent cesarean section if beyond the viable gestational age.

EMERGENCY DEPARTMENT CARE AND DISPOSITION

As is the case of all trauma patients, initial priorities are the primary and secondary surveys directed at the pregnant trauma patient. Coordinate care with surgical and obstetric consultants.

1. Aggressive maternal resuscitation generally leads to the best possible fetal resuscitation.
2. Initiate supplemental oxygen and crystalloid infusions at 50% above that given to nonpregnant patients. For patients beyond week 20 of gestation who must remain supine, place a wedge under the right hip,

tilting the patient 30° to the left, thus reducing the likelihood of supine hypotension syndrome. Otherwise, keep the patient in a left lateral decubitus position.

3. Avoid **vasopressors** if possible as they can have deleterious effects on uterine perfusion.
4. Administer **tetanus prophylaxis** when indicated.
5. Give **Rho (D) immunoglobulin** for all Rh-negative pregnant patients if indicated.
6. Institute cardiotocodynamometry as soon as possible to monitor for fetal distress and uterine irritability.
7. **Tocolytics** have a variety of side effects, including fetal and maternal tachycardia. Administer only in consultation with an obstetrician.
8. Indications for emergent laparotomy in the pregnant patient remain the same as those in the nonpregnant patient.
9. The decision to admit or discharge a pregnant trauma patient is first based on the nature and severity of the presenting injuries. Women at 20 weeks of gestation require observation or admission for a minimum of 4 to 6 hours for external tocodynamometric monitoring.
10. Screen for potential intimate partner violence.
11. Instruct discharged patients to seek medical attention immediately if they develop abdominal pain or cramps, vaginal bleeding, leakage of fluid, or perception of decreased fetal activity.

FURTHER READING

For further reading in *Tintinalli's Emergency Medicine: A Comprehensive Study Guide*, 8th ed., see Chapter 256, "Trauma in Pregnancy," by Nicole M. Deiorio.

CHAPTER 160

Head Trauma

O. John Ma

CLINICAL FEATURES

Traumatic brain injury (TBI) is the impairment in brain function after direct or indirect forces to the brain. The force of an object striking the head or a penetrating injury causes direct injury. Indirect injuries occur from acceleration/deceleration forces that result in the movement of the brain within the skull.

Traumatic brain injury can be classified as mild, moderate, and severe. Mild TBI includes patients with a Glasgow Coma Scale (GCS, see Table 160-1) score ≥14. Patients may be asymptomatic with only a history of head trauma, or may be confused and amnestic of the event. They may have experienced a brief loss of consciousness and complain

TABLE 160-1 Glasgow Coma Scale for All Age Groups

	4 Years to Adult	Child <4 Years	Infant
Eye opening			
4	Spontaneous	Spontaneous	Spontaneous
3	To speech	To speech	To speech
2	To pain	To pain	To pain
1	No response	No response	No response
Verbal response			
5	Alert and oriented	Oriented, social, speaks, interacts	Coos, babbles
4	Disoriented conversation	Confused speech, disoriented, consolable, aware	Irritable cry
3	Speaking but nonsensical	Inappropriate words, inconsolable, unaware	Cries to pain
2	Moans or unintelligible sounds	Incomprehensible, agitated, restless, unaware	Moans to pain
1	No response	No response	No response
Motor response			
6	Follows commands	Normal, spontaneous movements	Normal, spontaneous movements
5	Localizes pain	Localizes pain	Withdraws to touch
4	Moves or withdraws to pain	Withdraws to pain	Withdraws to pain
3	Decorticate flexion	Decorticate flexion	Decorticate flexion
2	Decerebrate extension	Decerebrate extension	Decerebrate extension
1	No response	No response	No response
3–15			

Note: In intubated patients, the Glasgow Coma Scale verbal component is scored as a 1, and the total score is marked with a "T" (or tube) denoting intubation (e.g., 8T).

of a diffuse headache, nausea, and vomiting. Patients at high risk in this subgroup include those with a skull fracture, large subgaleal swelling, focal neurologic findings, coagulopathy, age >60 years, or drug/alcohol intoxication.

Moderate TBI includes patients with a GCS score of 9 to 13. Overall, 40% of these patients have an abnormality on CT scan and 8% require neurosurgical intervention.

The mortality of severe TBI (GCS score <9) approaches 40%. The immediate clinical priority in these patients is to prevent secondary brain injury, identify other life-threatening injuries, and identify treatable neurosurgical conditions.

Prehospital medical personnel often provide critical parts of the history, including mechanism and time of injury, presence and length of unconsciousness, initial mental status, seizure activity, vomiting, verbalization, and movement of extremities. For an unresponsive patient, contact family and friends to gather key information including past medical history, medications (especially anticoagulants), and recent use of alcohol or drugs.

Perform a detailed neurologic examination that includes assessing the mental status and GCS, pupils for size, reactivity, and anisocoria, cranial nerve function, motor and sensory function, and any development of decorticate or decerebrate posturing.

Specific Injuries

Skull Fractures

Depressed skull fractures are classified as open or closed, depending on the integrity of the overlying scalp. Although basilar skull fractures can occur at any point in the base of the skull, the typical location is in the petrous portion of the temporal bone. Findings associated with a basilar skull fracture include hemotympanum, cerebrospinal fluid (CSF) otorrhea or rhinorrhea, periorbital ecchymosis ("raccoon eyes"), and retroauricular ecchymosis (Battle's sign).

Cerebral Contusion and Intracerebral Hemorrhage

Common locations for contusions are the frontal poles, the subfrontal cortex, and the temporal lobes. Contusions may occur directly under the site of impact or on the contralateral side (contrecoup lesion). The contused area is usually hemorrhagic with surrounding edema, and occasionally associated with subarachnoid hemorrhage. Neurologic dysfunction may be profound and prolonged, with patients demonstrating mental confusion, obtundation, or coma. Focal neurologic deficits are usually present.

Traumatic Subarachnoid Hemorrhage

This condition results from the disruption of subarachnoid vessels and presents with blood in the CSF. Patients may complain of diffuse headache, nausea, or photophobia. Traumatic subarachnoid hemorrhage may be the most common CT abnormality in patients with moderate or severe TBI. Some cases may be missed if the CT scan is obtained less than 6 hours after injury.

Epidural Hematoma

An epidural hematoma results from an acute collection of blood between the inner table of the skull and the dura mater. It is typically associated with a skull fracture that lacerates a meningeal artery, most commonly the middle meningeal artery. Underlying injury to the brain may not necessarily be severe. In the classic scenario, the patient experiences loss of consciousness after a head injury. The patient may present to the ED with clear mentation, signifying the "lucid interval," and then begin to develop mental status deterioration in the ED. A fixed and dilated pupil on the side of the lesion with contralateral hemiparesis is a classic late finding. The high-pressure arterial bleeding of an epidural hematoma can lead to herniation within hours of injury. An epidural hematoma appears biconvex on CT scan.

Subdural Hematoma

A subdural hematoma (SDH), which is a collection of venous blood between the dura matter and the arachnoid, results from tears of the bridging veins that extend from the subarachnoid space to the dural venous sinuses. A common mechanism is sudden acceleration–deceleration. Patients with brain atrophy, such as in alcoholics or the elderly, are more susceptible to a SDH. In acute SDH, patients present within 14 days of the injury, and most become symptomatic within 24 hours of injury. After 2 weeks, patients are defined as having a chronic SDH. Symptoms may range from a headache to lethargy or coma. It is important to distinguish between acute and chronic SDHs by history, physical examination, and CT scan. An acute SDH appears as a hyperdense, crescent-shaped lesion that crosses suture lines.

Herniation

Diffusely or focally increased intracranial pressure (ICP) can result in herniation of the brain at several locations. *Transtentorial (uncal) herniation* occurs when a SDH or temporal lobe mass forces the ipsilateral uncus of the temporal lobe through the tentorial hiatus into the space between the cerebral peduncle and the tentorium. This results in compression of the oculomotor nerve and parasympathetic paralysis of the ipsilateral pupil, causing it to become fixed and dilated. When the cerebral peduncle is further compressed, it results in contralateral motor paralysis. The increased ICP and brainstem compression result in progressive deterioration in the level of consciousness. Occasionally, the contralateral cerebral peduncle is forced against the free edge of the tentorium on the opposite side, resulting in paralysis ipsilateral to the lesion—a false localizing sign. *Central transtentorial herniation* occurs with midline lesions in the frontal or occipital lobes, or in the vertex. Bilateral pinpoint pupils, bilateral Babinski signs, and increased muscle tone are found initially, which eventually develop into fixed midpoint pupils, prolonged hyperventilation, and decorticate posturing. *Cerebellotonsillar herniation* through the foramen magnum occurs much less frequently. Medullary compression causes flaccid paralysis, bradycardia, respiratory arrest, and sudden death.

Penetrating Injuries

Gunshot wounds and penetrating sharp objects can result in penetrating injury to the brain. The degree of neurologic injury will depend on the energy of the missile, whether the trajectory involves a single or multiple lobes or hemispheres of the brain, the amount of scatter of bone and metallic fragments, and whether a mass lesion is present.

DIAGNOSIS AND DIFFERENTIAL

Tables 160-2 and 160-3 provide evidence-based indications for obtaining a CT scan of the head after injury.

TABLE 160-2 New Orleans Criteria and Canadian CT Head Rule Clinical Decision Rules

New Orleans Criteria—GCS 15*	Canadian CT Head Rule—GCS 13–15*
Headache	GCS <15 at 2 h
Vomiting	Suspected open or depressed skull fracture
Age >60 years	Age ≥65 years
Intoxication	More than one episode of vomiting
Persistent antegrade amnesia	Retrograde amnesia >30 min
Evidence of trauma above the clavicles	Dangerous mechanism (fall >3 ft or struck as pedestrian)
Seizure	Any sign of basal skull fracture
Identification of patients who have an intracranial lesion on CT	
100% sensitive, 5% specific	83% sensitive, 38% specific
Identification of patients who will need neurosurgical intervention	
100% sensitive, 5% specific	100% sensitive, 37% specific

*Presence of any one finding indicates need for CT scan.

Abbreviation: GCS, Glasgow Coma Scale.

TABLE 160-3 CT Scanning for Adults with Brain Injury (American College of Emergency Physicians Guidelines)

Adults with a Glasgow Coma Scale score of <15 at the time of evaluation should undergo CT imaging

Mild traumatic brain injury with or without loss of consciousness: if one or more of the following is present:

- Glasgow Coma Scale score <15
- Focal neurologic findings
- Vomiting more than two times
- Moderate to severe headache
- Age >65 years
- Physical signs of basilar skull fracture
- Coagulopathy
- Dangerous mechanism of injury (e.g., fall >4 ft)

Mild traumatic brain injury with loss of consciousness or amnesia: if one or more of the following is present:

- Drug or alcohol intoxication
- Physical evidence above the clavicles
- Persistent amnesia
- Posttraumatic seizures

Approximately 8% of patients suffering a severe TBI will have an associated cervical spine fracture. Obtain imaging studies of the cervical spine on all trauma patients who present with altered mental status, neck pain, intoxication, neurologic deficit, severe distracting injury, or if the mechanism of injury is deemed serious enough to potentially produce cervical spine injury.

Laboratory work should include type and crossmatching, complete blood count, basic metabolic panel, arterial blood gas analysis, directed toxicologic studies, and coagulation studies.

EMERGENCY DEPARTMENT CARE AND DISPOSITION

1. Initiate standard protocols for evaluation and stabilization of trauma patients (see Chapter 156). Diligently assess for other significant injuries.
2. Administer oxygen, and secure cardiac monitoring and two IV lines. For patients with severe TBI, **endotracheal intubation** (via rapid sequence intubation) to protect the airway and prevent hypoxemia is the top priority. Provide cervical spine immobilization, and use an adequate sedation/induction agent when securing the airway.
3. Hypotension is associated with increased mortality rates. Restoration of an adequate blood pressure is vital to maintain cerebral perfusion. Resuscitation with **IV crystalloid fluid** to a mean arterial pressure (MAP) of 80 mm Hg is indicated; if aggressive fluid resuscitation is not effective, then add **vasopressors** to maintain a MAP of 80 mm Hg.
4. Obtain immediate **neurosurgical consultation** after a head CT scan demonstrating intracranial injury has been identified. Patients with new neurologic deficits from an acute epidural or SDH require emergent neurosurgical treatment.
5. All patients who demonstrate signs of increased ICP should have the **head of their bed elevated to 30°** (provided that the patient is not hypotensive), adequate sedation, and maintenance of adequate arterial oxygenation. If the patient is not hypotensive, consider administering **mannitol** 0.25 to 1.0 g/kg IV in repetitive boluses. If the patient is hypotensive or inadequately fluid resuscitated, consider administering **hypertonic saline** as an alternative to mannitol. The adult dose of 3% NaCl is 250 mL over 30 minutes.
6. Hyperventilation is not recommended as a prophylactic intervention to lower ICP because of its potential to cause cerebral ischemia. Reserve hyperventilation as a last resort for decreasing ICP; if used, implement it as a temporary measure and monitor the PCO_2 closely to maintain a range of 30 to 35 mm Hg.
7. Patients with signs of impending brain herniation may need emergency decompression by trephination ("burr holes") when all other methods to control the elevated ICP have failed. CT scan prior to attempting trephination is recommended to localize the lesion and direct the decompression site.
8. Treat seizures immediately with **benzodiazepines**, such as lorazepam, and **fosphenytoin** at a loading dose of 18 to 20 mg PE per kilogram IV.
9. Use of prophylactic anticonvulsants remains controversial, and its administration should be in consultation with the neurosurgeon.

10. Admit patients with a basilar skull fracture or penetrating injuries (gunshot wound or stab wound) to the neurosurgical service, and start them on prophylactic antibiotic therapy (e.g., ceftriaxone 2 g IV and vancomycin 1 g IV).
11. Discharge patients who have an initial GCS score of 15 that is maintained during an observation period and who have normal serial neurologic examinations and a normal CT scan. Those who have an abnormal CT scan require neurosurgical consultation and admission. Patients who have an initial GCS score of 14 and a normal CT scan should be observed in the ED. If their GCS score improves to 15 and they remain symptom free and neurologically intact after serial examinations, they can be discharged home. Discharge patients home with a reliable companion who can observe them for at least 24 hours, and carry out appropriate discharge instructions.

FURTHER READING

For further reading in *Tintinalli's Emergency Medicine: A Comprehensive Study Guide*, 8th ed., see Chapter 257, "Head Trauma" by David W. Wright and Lisa H. Merck.

CHAPTER 161 Spine Trauma

Jeffrey Dan

Spine and spinal cord injuries (SCIs) can be devastating, life-changing events that include injury to the bony elements (vertebral fracture), the neural elements (spinal cord and nerve root injury), or both.

CLINICAL FEATURES

The spinal cord is most commonly injured by a direct mechanical cause, with resultant hemorrhage, edema, and ischemia. Patients may complain of neck and back pain, and close examination may note pain or bony abnormalities with palpation. Unstable spinal fractures may present without obvious spinal cord or nerve root trauma. Symptomatic patients may complain of paresthesias, dysesthesias, weakness, bowel or bladder incontinence, urinary retention, or other sensory disturbances with or without specific physical examination findings. More severely injured patients may have obvious neurologic deficits.

Complete spinal cord lesions are characterized by the absence of sensory and motor function below the level of injury (Figs. 161-1 and 161-2). **Incomplete** lesions have a better prognosis, and denote some degree of neurologic activity below the injury, but their initial diagnosis may be obscured because of spinal shock. **Spinal shock** is the temporary loss or depression of spinal reflex activity below the level of injury to the spinal cord. Spinal shock can persist for days to weeks and prohibit the differentiation of an incomplete and complete lesion (Table 161-1).

Neurogenic shock refers to the loss of sympathetic innervation leading to relative bradycardia and hypotension. Hemorrhage must be excluded as the explanation for hypotension before neurogenic shock is considered. The presence of neurogenic shock may necessitate inotropic support.

Spinal cord injury without radiographic abnormality (SCIWORA) is an entity seen most often in the pediatric population. Numbness, paresthesias, or other neurologic complaints with normal plain radiographs or CT should prompt further evaluation with MRI.

DIAGNOSIS AND DIFFERENTIAL

Consider an injury to the spine or spinal cord in any patient with an appropriate traumatic mechanism. Suspect SCI with any neurologic complaints, even if transitory. A complete neurologic examination should include motor strength and tone (corticospinal tract), pain and temperature sensation (spinothalamic tract), proprioception and vibration sensation (dorsal columns), reflexes, perianal sensation and wink, and bulbocavernosus reflex. "Sacral sparing" denotes preservation of reflexes and an incomplete SCI.

Validated clinical guidelines exist to identify patients who may benefit from cervical spine imaging. The NEXUS (Tables 161-2) and the Canadian Cervical Spine Rule for Radiography (Table 161-3) are intended for alert, stable adult patients.

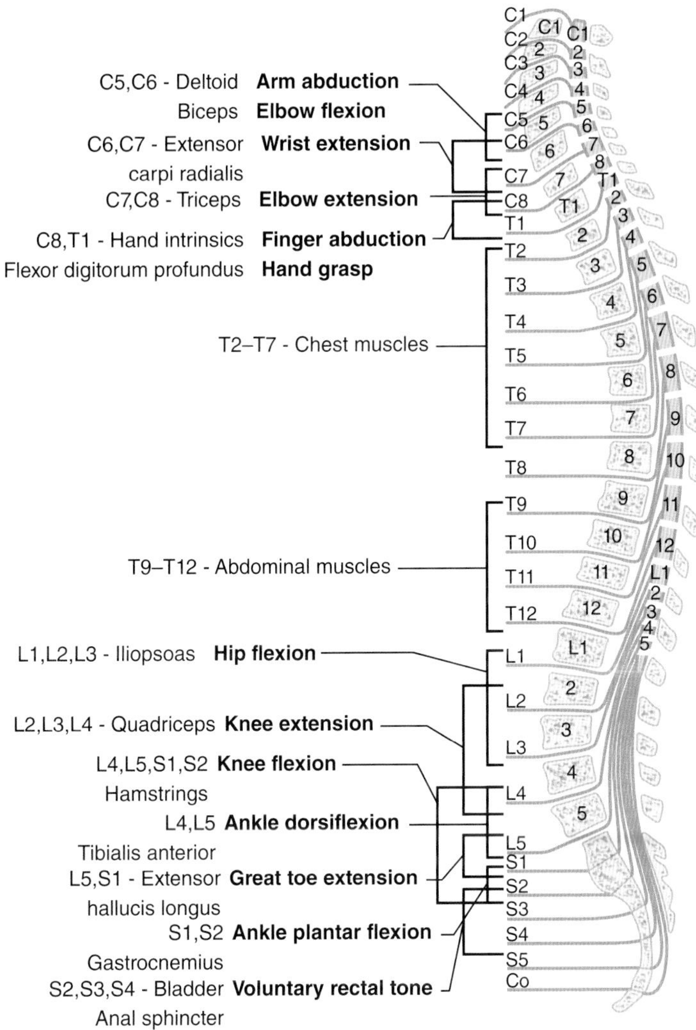

FIGURE 161-1. Spinal cord level. The spinal cord level of injury can be delineated by physical examination, including a detailed neurologic examination.

High-resolution CT is more sensitive and specific for cervical spine fractures than plain films, and is the modality of choice at most trauma centers for suspected cervical spine injuries. For plain radiography of the cervical spine, at least three views (lateral, odontoid, and anteroposterior) are necessary.

Both CT and plain radiography can miss purely ligamentous injuries. Sensitivity is not high enough to rely on flexion-extension films. When ligamentous injury is suspected, reliable patients can be discharged with a firm foam collar for follow-up in 3 to 5 days with a spine surgeon.

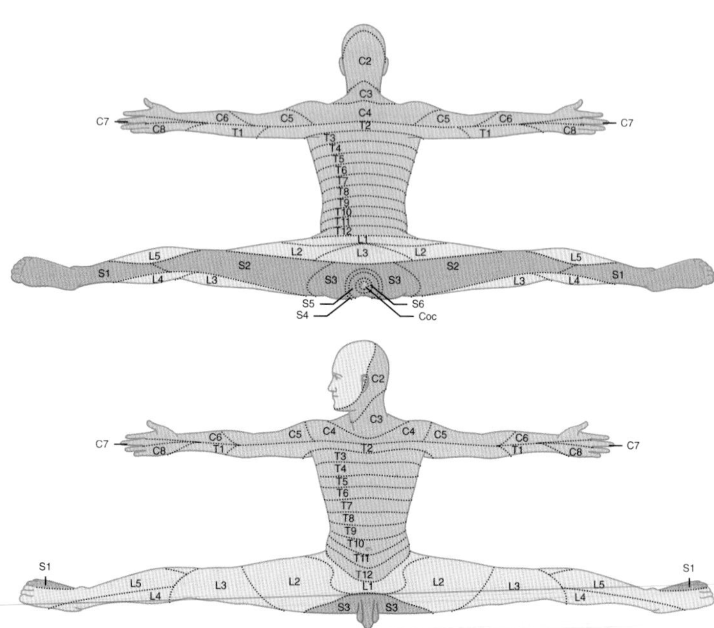

FIGURE 161-2. Dermatomes for sensory examination.

Alternatively, MRI provides the most sensitive and specific view of the ligaments and neural structures. The mechanisms, characteristics, and stability of common cervical spine fractures are summarized in Table 161-4.

TABLE 161-1 Four Major Incomplete Spinal Cord Syndromes

Syndrome	Mechanisms	Symptoms	General Prognosis*
Anterior cord	Direct anterior cord compression Flexion of cervical spine Thrombosis of anterior spinal artery	Complete paralysis below the lesion with loss of pain and temperature sensation Preservation of proprioception and vibratory function	Poor
Central cord	Hyperextension injuries Disruption of blood flow to the spinal cord Cervical spinal stenosis	Quadriparesis—greater in the upper extremities than the lower extremities. Some loss of pain and temperature sensation, also greater in the upper extremities	Good
Brown- Séquard	Transverse hemisection of the spinal cord Unilateral cord compression	Ipsilateral spastic paresis, loss of proprioception and vibratory sensation, and contralateral loss of pain and temperature sensation	Good

*Outcome improves when the effects of secondary injury are prevented or reversed.

TABLE 161-2 NEXUS Criteria

Absence of midline cervical tenderness
Normal level of alertness and consciousness*
No evidence of intoxication
Absence of focal neurologic deficit
Absence of painful distracting injury†

*Abnormal defined as Glasgow coma scale score <15; disorientation to person, place, time, or events; inability to remember three objects at 5 minutes; delayed or inappropriate response to external stimuli.

†Any injury thought "to have the potential to impair the patient's ability to appreciate other injuries."

With regard to the thoracic and lumbar spine, plain radiography may still have a role in the mildly injured patient, but CT imaging is the standard at most trauma centers as it is more sensitive than plain radiography and CT is better at defining the extent and stability of spinal fractures.

EMERGENCY DEPARTMENT CARE AND DISPOSITION

Treat blunt and penetrating injuries to the spine with identification and stabilization of identified injuries, and prevention of secondary injuries.

1. Airway and breathing should be assessed with a low threshold for endotracheal intubation for patients with cervical spine injury at C5 and above since the diaphragm is innervated by C3 through C5. Airway compromise can also occur due to soft tissue swelling associated with high cervical spine fractures.
2. Hypotension should be assumed to be from hypovolemic shock until proven otherwise. Hypotensive neurogenic shock should be considered if the patient has a probable spinal cord injury, does not have acute blood loss, and is warm and relatively bradycardic.
3. Collars and long boards should be removed as soon as clinically appropriate. In patients with penetrating neck injuries who are neurologically

TABLE 161-3 Canadian Cervical Spine Rule for Radiography: Cervical Spine Imaging Unnecessary in Patients Meeting These Three Criteria

Assessment	Definitions
Assessment #1: There are no high-risk factors that mandate radiography.	High-risk factors include: Age 65 years or older A dangerous mechanism of injury* The presence of paresthesias in the extremities
Assessment #2: There are low-risk factors that allow a safe assessment of range of motion.	Low-risk factors include: Simple rear-end motor vehicle crashes Patient able to sit up in the ED Patient ambulatory at any time Delayed onset of neck pain Absence of midline cervical tenderness
Assessment #3: The patient is able to actively rotate his/her neck (regardless of pain).	Can rotate neck 45 degrees to the left and to the right

*Defined as fall from a height of >3 feet; an axial loading injury; high-speed motor vehicle crash, rollover, or ejection; motorized recreational vehicle or bicycle collision.

TABLE 161-4 Cervical Spine Injuries
Flexion
Anterior subluxation (hyperflexion sprain) (stable)*
Bilateral interfacetal dislocation (unstable)
Simple wedge (compression) fracture (usually stable)
Spinous process avulsion (clay-shoveler's fracture) (stable)
Flexion teardrop fracture (unstable)
Flexion-rotation
Unilateral interfacetal dislocation (stable)
Pillar fracture
Fracture of lateral mass (can be unstable)
Vertical compression
Jefferson burst fracture of atlas (potentially unstable)
Burst (bursting, dispersion, axial-loading) fracture (unstable)
Hyperextension
Hyperextension dislocation (unstable)
Avulsion fracture of anterior arch of atlas (stable)
Extension teardrop fracture (unstable)
Fracture of posterior arch of atlas (stable)
Laminar fracture (usually stable)
Traumatic spondylolisthesis (hangman's fracture) (unstable)
Lateral flexion
Uncinate process fracture (usually stable)
Injuries caused by diverse or poorly understood mechanisms
Occipital condyle fractures (can be unstable)
Occipitoatlantal dissociation (highly unstable)
Dens fractures (type II and III are unstable)

*Usual occurrence. Overall stability is dependent on integrity of the other ligamentous structures.

intact and fully conscious, spinal immobilization is no longer recommended. Log rolling and maintenance of inline immobilization should be used while removing the board.

4. Patients with cervical fractures will typically require admission. Spine precautions should be maintained and assessment and stabilization of other injuries should be performed.
5. Thoracic and lumbar fractures are high-energy fractures and patients are at risk for other injuries, such as injuries to the aorta, spinal cord, intraabdominal or thoracic organs. Most patients with acute fractures should be admitted to or managed by a spine surgeon. Patients with compression or wedge fractures with <40% vertebral height loss may, in consultation with a spine surgeon, be treated as an outpatient, but patients with burst fractures and chance fractures should be admitted. Imaging with CT should be considered.
6. Injuries to the sacral spine and nerve roots are unusual, and are usually found in association with pelvic fractures. Bladder and bowel dysfunction, radiculopathy and damage to the cauda equina can all result from sacral fractures. Isolated coccyx fractures usually require pain control and a rubber doughnut pillow.
7. High-dose steroids (methylprednisolone) are no longer routinely recommended for spinal cord injuries as a result of blunt trauma due to

potentially harmful side effects. If high-dose steroids are considered, consultation with the spinal surgeon is recommended prior to administration.

8. Discharge patients who are adequately evaluated and found to have no indications for admission with appropriate follow-up in 3 to 5 days. Provide these patients with analgesics and specific return precautions.

FURTHER READING

For further reading in *Tintinalli's Emergency Medicine: A Comprehensive Study Guide*, 8th ed., see Chapter 258, "Spine Trauma," by Go Steven.

CHAPTER 162 Facial Injuries

Gerald (Wook) Beltran

Severe facial injuries are associated with injuries to the brain, orbit, cervical spine, and lungs. After stabilization of life-threatening injuries during the primary survey, a thorough secondary survey should identify facial injuries that could affect the patient's normal appearance, vision, smell, mastication, and sensation.

CLINICAL FEATURES

A thorough history should begin with questions directed toward whether the patient has vision changes, malocclusion, or facial numbness (Table 162-1). The physical examination begins with inspection, noting facial asymmetry, facial elongation, exophthalmos or enophthalmos, and periorbital or mastoid ecchymosis. Next, palpate the entire face, noting step-offs and tenderness that suggest fractures, and crepitus that suggests a sinus fracture. Finally, perform a focused and thorough examination of the eyes, nose, ears, and mouth, as described in Table 162-1.

TABLE 162-1 Important Clinical Issues in Facial Trauma

- History
  - How is your vision?
    - Binocular diplopia suggests entrapment of the extraocular muscles; monocular diplopia suggests a lens dislocation.
  - Do any parts of your face feel numb?
    - Anesthesia suggests damage to the supraorbital, infraorbital, or mental nerves.
  - Does your bite feel normal?
    - Malocclusion typically occurs with mandibular or maxillary fractures.
- Inspection
  - Lateral view for dish face with Le Fort III fractures.
  - Frontal view for donkey face with Le Fort II or III fractures.
  - Bird's eye view for exophthalmos with retrobulbar hematoma.
  - Worm's view for endophthalmos with blow-out fractures or flattening of malar prominence with zygomatic arch fractures.
  - Raccoon's eyes (bilateral periorbital ecchymosis) and Battle sign (mastoid ecchymosis) typically develop over several hours, suggesting basilar skull fracture.
- Palpation
  - Palpating the entire face will detect the majority of fractures.
  - Intraoral palpation of the zygomatic arch, palpating lateral to posterior maxillary molars to distinguish bony from soft tissue injury.
  - Assess for Le Fort fractures by gently rocking the hard palate with one hand while stabilizing the forehead with the other.

(Continued)

TABLE 162-1 Important Clinical Issues in Facial Trauma (Continued)

Eye Examine early before swelling of lids, or use retractors. Document visual acuity. Fat through eyelid wound indicates an orbital septum perforation. Widening of the distance between the medial canthi, or telecanthus, suggests serious nasoethmoidal-orbital complex trauma. Widening of the distance between the pupils, or hypertelorism, results from orbital dislocation and often is associated with blindness. Examine extraocular muscle movements. Limited upward gaze occurs with entrapment of the inferior rectus or inferior oblique muscles, or damage to the oculomotor nerve. Systematically examine the eye. Specifically, the pupil for teardrop sign pointing to globe rupture, the anterior chamber for hyphema, and swinging flashlight test for afferent papillary defect. Perform a fluoroscein test for corneal abrasions or ulcers. Check intraocular pressure for evidence of orbital compartment syndrome only in absence of globe injury.
Nose Crepitus over any facial sinus suggests sinus fracture. Septal hematoma appears as blue, boggy swelling on nasal septum. Should be incised and drained to avoid a saddle nose deformity.
Ears Auricular hematomas should be incised and drained to avoid a cauliflower deformity. Cerebrospinal fluid leak, auditory canal lacerations, and hemotympanum suggest basilar skull fracture.
Oral Jaw deviation due to mandible dislocation or condyle fracture. Malocclusion occurs in mandible, zygomatic, and Le Fort fractures. Assess for missing or injured teeth. Lacerations and mucosal ecchymosis suggest mandible fracture. Place finger in external ear while the patient gently opens and closes jaw to detect condyle fractures. Tongue blade test: Patient without fracture can bite down on a tongue blade enough to break blade twisted by examiner.

DIAGNOSIS AND DIFFERENTIAL

Diagnosis of many maxillofacial injuries is made clinically and with radiographs. Plain films are helpful if CT is not available or to screen for injuries in low-risk patients. Facial CT is frequently required to make the definitive diagnosis and guide surgical management. Imaging recommendations based on suspected injury sites and pretest clinical suspicion are summarized in Table 162-2.

EMERGENCY DEPARTMENT CARE AND DISPOSITION

During the primary survey of facial trauma patients, the airway must be secured and stabilized as clinically indicated. When endotracheal intubation is required, the orotracheal route is preferred over the nasotracheal route because of concern for nasocranial intubation, worsening of injury, and severe epistaxis. While rapid sequence intubation is the preferred method of airway management in trauma, always plan for a difficult airway in patients with facial trauma. To prevent the "can't intubate/can't oxygenate" failed airway, do not administer paralytics unless a patient can be bagged effectively or alternative airway devices or plans are in place.

TABLE 162-2 Recommendations for Imaging Based on Level of Injury and Clinical Findings

Level	Low Suspicion	Significant Clinical Findings	Additional Considerations
Frontal bone	Head CT	Head CT (skull windows)	Facial CT with orbital involvement. Cervical spine CT with significant clinical findings
Midface	Waters' view	Face CT with coronal and axial sections	Coronal face sections require cervical spine clearance for positioning. Computer-generated, three-dimensional reconstructions with complex injuries Head CT can replace Waters' view
Mandible	Panorex	Mandible CT	Facial CT detects mandible fractures

Awake intubation with sedation and local airway anesthesia may allow the emergency physician to determine the feasibility of orotracheal intubation while still preserving a patient's airway reflexes. When endotracheal intubation appears impossible or is unsuccessful, perform emergent cricothyroidotomy to secure the airway. The laryngeal mask airway may be used as a temporizing measure, but it does not protect the airway from aspiration of stomach contents and may not be possible with injuries involving the pharynx.

Severe midfacial and mandibular injuries can result in substantial hemorrhage from the sphenopalatine and greater palatine branches of the external carotid artery. Posterior nasal epistaxis can be controlled with nasal tampons, dual balloon devices, or Foley catheter placement with layered gauze packing anteriorly, again being careful to avoid intracranial placement in severe midfacial fractures. Rarely, reduction of significantly displaced nasal fractures and Le Fort injuries is needed to stop arterial bleeding. If bleeding persists, immediate operative intervention may be required to ligate injured vessels. Alternatively, arterial embolization may be pursued to control bleeding from branches of the external carotid artery.

Management decisions will be dictated by the location and severity of the facial fractures, as well as concurrent injuries. Typically patients with sinus fractures should receive oral or intravenous antibiotics, such as first-generation cephalosporins, clindamycin, or amoxicillin-clavulanate.

Frontal sinus fractures are uncommon, and increase the immediate risk of traumatic brain injury, additional facial fractures, and cervical spine injury due to the amount of force needed to fracture the thick frontal bone. Because the dura is adherent to the posterior table of the frontal sinus, operative repair of through-and-through frontal sinus fractures is necessary to prevent pneumocephalus, cerebrospinal fluid (CSF) leak, and infection. Patients with depressed fractures also require admission for IV antibiotics and operative repair. Patients with isolated anterior table fractures of the frontal sinus may be discharged with appropriate follow-up with a facial surgeon.

Naso-orbito-ethmoid fractures result from significant trauma to the nasal bridge, and often have associated injury to the lacrimal duct, dural tears, and traumatic brain injury. Patients with these fractures require admission for specialty consultation with facial surgery and neurosurgery.

Orbital blowout fractures occur when a blunt object strikes the globe, transmitting force through the fluid-filled eye, and fracturing the medial or inferior orbital wall. Surgery may be required if these injuries result in extraocular muscle or oculomotor nerve entrapment, or significant enophthalmos. A fracture involving the superior orbital fissure can damage the oculomotor and ophthalmic divisions of the trigeminal nerve (the "orbital fissure syndrome"), and can involve the optic nerve as well (the "orbital apex syndrome"). Patients with either of these syndromes require emergent ophthalmologic consultation. All other patients with isolated orbital fractures can be managed expediently as an outpatient with oral **amoxicillin-clavulanate**, decongestants, and instructions to avoid nose blowing until the defect has been repaired. Emergent ophthalmological consultation should be requested for ocular injury associated with orbital fractures. An ocular compartment syndrome may occur with a retrobulbar hematoma or malignant orbital emphysema which can cause an acute ischemic optic neuropathy.

Zygoma fractures occur in two major patterns: tripod fractures and isolated zygomatic arch fractures. **Tripod fractures** involve disruption of the infraorbital rim, the zygomaticofrontal suture, and the zygomaticotemporal junction. These fractures require admission for IV antibiotics and surgical repair. Patients with isolated fractures of the zygomatic arch may have elective outpatient repair.

Midfacial fractures are high-energy injuries and are often seen in victims of multisystem trauma. Patients frequently require endotracheal intubation for airway control. Oral packing is often required for hemorrhage control with fractures of the hard palate. **Le Fort injury** patterns are illustrated in Figure 162-1. Visual acuity should be tested, especially with Le Fort III and IV fractures, in which the incidence of blindness is around

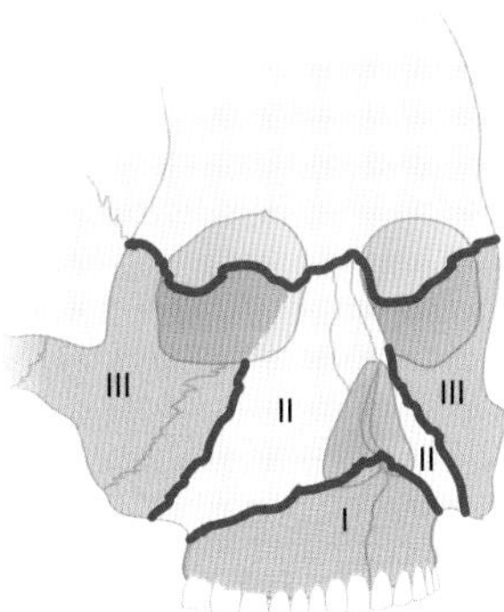

FIGURE 162-1. Le Fort injury patterns. Illustration of the fracture lines of Le Fort I (alveolar), Le Fort II (zygomatic maxillary complex), and Le Fort III (craniofacial dysfunction) fractures. Reproduced with permission from Tintinalli JE, Stapczynski JS, Ma OJ, et al: *Tintinalli's Emergency Medicine: A Comprehensive Study Guide*, 8th ed. New York: McGraw-Hill; 2015.

3% most commonly secondary to injury of the optic nerve. Both Le Fort II and III injuries can result in CSF leaks. Le Fort injuries require admission for management of significant associated injuries, IV antibiotics, and surgical repair.

Mandible fractures are often diagnosed in the setting of malocclusion and pain with attempted movement. Always look for multiple mandibular fractures, with one injury at the site of impact and a second subtle injury on the opposite side of the ring. A careful intraoral examination is important to exclude small breaks in the mucosa seen with open fractures, sublingual hematomas, and dental or alveolar ridge fractures. Patients with closed fractures may be given urgent outpatient follow-up, while open fractures require admission for IV antibiotics and operative repair. In the patient with a stable airway, a Barton bandage, an ace wrap over the top of the head and underneath the mandible, will stabilize the fracture and help relieve pain.

FURTHER READING

For further reading in *Tintinalli's Emergency Medicine: A Comprehensive Study Guide*, 8th ed., see Chapter 259, "Trauma to the Face," by John Bailitz and Tarlan Hedayati.

CHAPTER 163

Neck Injuries

Steven Go

Neck trauma causes a diverse combination of injuries because of the high concentration of critical structures in the neck. Presenting signs of neck injury may be obvious, subtle, or obscured by trauma to other body regions. Missed injuries and delays in diagnosis lead to increased patient morbidity and mortality.

CLINICAL FEATURES

Historical and physical examination findings of vascular, laryngotracheal, or pharynoesophageal injury of the neck are characterized as hard or soft signs (Table 163-1), with 90% of patients with hard signs having an injury requiring emergent repair.

Vascular injuries are the most common cervical injury and cause of death from penetrating neck trauma. Symptoms include frank exsanguination and expanding hematomas, which may cause airway obstruction. Cervical artery injury can also cause various vascular and neurological signs and symptoms (Table 163-2).

TABLE 163-1 Signs and Symptoms of Neck Injury

Hard	Soft
Vascular injury	
Shock unresponsive to initial fluid therapy	Hypotension in field
Active arterial bleeding	History of arterial bleeding
Pulse deficit	Nonpulsatile or nonexpanding hematoma
Pulsatile or expanding hematoma	Proximity wounds
Thrill or bruit	
Laryngotracheal injury	
Stridor	Hoarseness
Hemoptysis	Neck tenderness
Dysphonia	Subcutaneous emphysema
Air or bubbling in wound	Cervical ecchymosis or hematoma
Airway obstruction	Tracheal deviation or cartilaginous step-off
	Laryngeal edema or hematoma
	Restricted vocal cord mobility
Pharyngoesophageal injury	
	Odynophagia
	Subcutaneous emphysema
	Dysphagia
	Hematemesis
	Blood in the mouth
	Saliva draining from wound
	Severe neck tenderness
	Prevertebral air
	Transmidline trajectory

TABLE 163-2 Compiled Screening Criteria for Blunt Cerebral Vascular Injury

- Signs and symptoms
  - Arterial hemorrhage from nose, neck, or mouth
  - Cervical bruit in patients <50 years old
  - Expanding cervical hematoma
  - Focal neurologic deficit: transient ischemic attack, hemiparesis, vertebrobasilar symptoms, Horner's syndrome
  - Stroke on secondary CT
  - Neurologic deficit unexplained by head CT
- Risk factors for blunt cerebral vascular injury
  - High-energy transfer mechanism and one of the following:
    - Facial fractures: Le Fort II or III fracture, mandible fracture, frontal skull fracture, orbital fracture
    - Cervical spine fracture patterns: subluxation, fractures extending into the transverse foramen, fractures of C1–C3
    - Any basilar skull fracture or occipital condyle fracture
    - Petrous bone fracture
    - Diffuse axonal injury with Glasgow Coma Scale score ≤8
    - Concurrent traumatic brain and thoracic injuries
    - Neck hanging with anoxic brain injury
    - Clothesline type injury with significant swelling, pain, or altered mental status

Laryngotracheal injuries can present with immediate signs of impending airway obstruction (Table 163-3) or have an insidious onset of airway compromise after a quiescent phase.

Pharyngeal and esophageal injuries have no hard signs of injury and may initially present with few symptoms.

Neurologic injuries can result from injury to the cervical spine, spinal cord, lower cranial nerves, or brachial plexus. Symptoms can range from sensory complaints to quadriplegia.

Strangulation is a type of blunt neck injury whose presentation largely depends on the duration and degree of vascular compression rather than on airway obstruction. Cerebral anoxia, laryngotracheal fractures, cervical spine fractures, pharyngeal lacerations, and carotid artery injuries are possible. The most common symptoms are neck pain, voice changes, trouble swallowing, and difficulty breathing, while common signs are petechiae and neck contusions. However, 50% of patients have no signs of trauma and 67% are asymptomatic. Some patients with ultimately life-threatening injuries are asymptomatic at presentation.

TABLE 163-3 Clinical Factors Indicating Need for Aggressive Airway Management

- Stridor
- Acute respiratory distress
- Airway obstruction from blood or secretions
- Expanding neck hematoma
- Profound shock
- Extensive subcutaneous emphysema
- Alteration in mental status
- Tracheal shift

DIAGNOSIS AND DIFFERENTIAL

The zone classification summarizes structures placed at risk for injury in penetrating neck trauma (Fig. 163-1). Zone I structures include the lung apices, thoracic vessels, distal trachea, esophagus, cervical spine, and vertebral and carotid arteries. Zone II structures include the mid-carotid and vertebral arteries, jugular veins, esophagus, cervical spine, larynx, and trachea. Zone III structures include the proximal carotid and vertebral arteries, oropharynx, and cervical spine.

In penetrating neck trauma, a careful, structured physical exam is >95% sensitive for clinically significant vascular and aerodigestive injuries. Particular attention should be paid to whether the platysma has been violated. If violation has occurred, the presence of deep structure injury is assumed until proven otherwise. The combination of physical examination with multidetector CT angiography (MDCTA) (100% sensitive and 97.5% specific for significant vascular or aerodigestive injury) has been recommended over mandatory operative exploration and selective management strategies for diagnosis in stable patients. Additional studies may be required if MDCTA detects a penetrating injury, but these are typically ordered in conjunction with the specialist who will be repairing the suspected injury. An algorithm for the diagnosis and management of penetrating neck injuries is shown in Fig. 163-2.

Safely managing blunt neck trauma victims requires a heightened level of suspicion and an aggressive approach to diagnosis because catastrophic injuries can present subtly. Therefore, MDCTA should be used liberally. If the MDCTA is negative, but significant suspicion of vascular injury remains, formal cerebral angiography may be required. Likewise, if a strong suspicion of blunt laryngotracheal or esophageal injury remains after

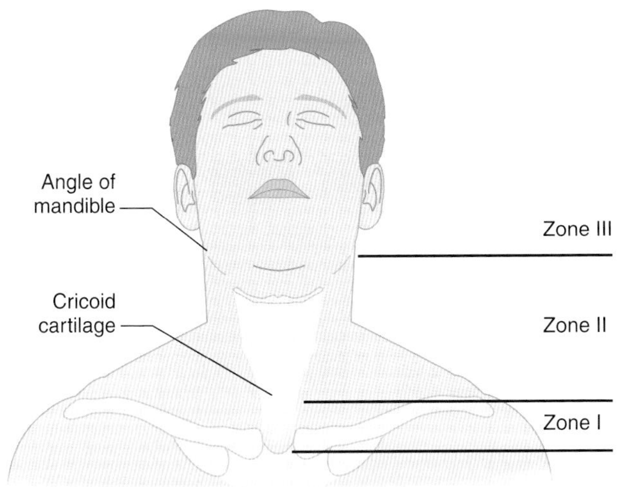

FIGURE 163-1. Zones of the neck.

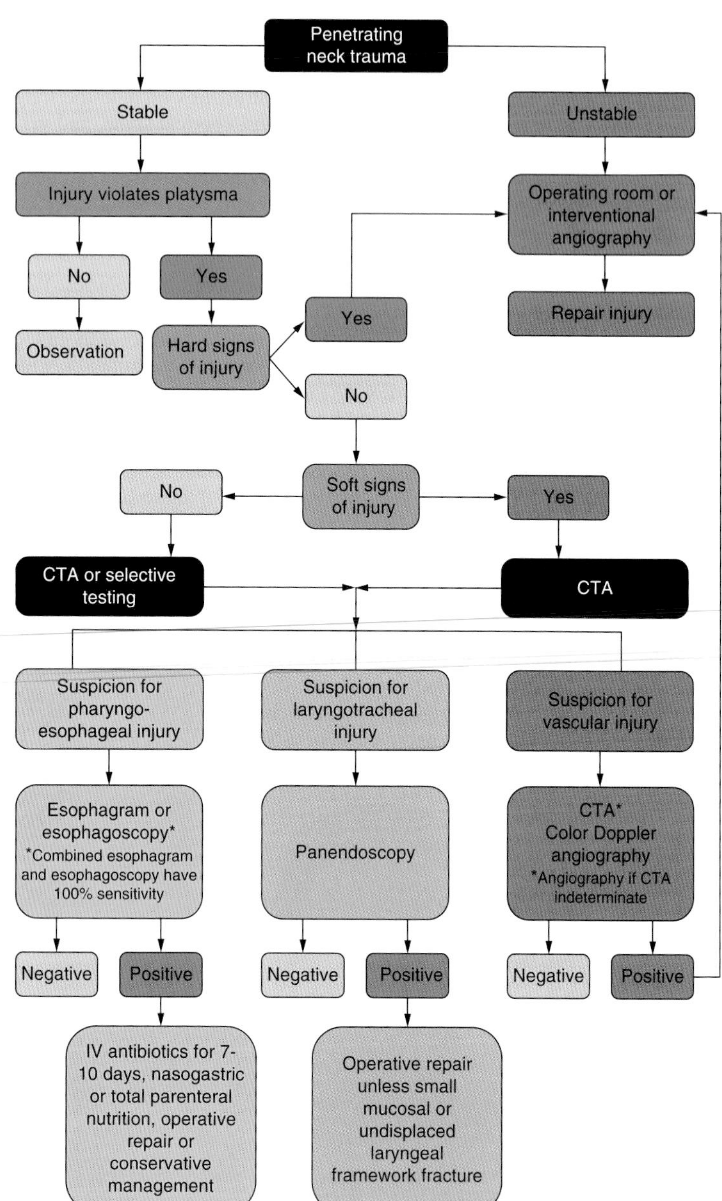

FIGURE 163-2. Penetrating neck trauma protocol.

a negative MDCTA, laryngobronchoscopy, endoscopy, or swallowing studies may be necessary.

EMERGENCY DEPARTMENT CARE AND DISPOSITION

1. Initiate standard ATLS protocol for the stabilization of trauma patients. Establish IV access, administer oxygen, and begin cardiac and respiratory monitoring.
2. Emergent airway control is indicated for patients with the clinical factors listed in Table 163-3. **Have adjunct airway devices at hand and use paralytics with extreme caution, as these airways can be extremely difficult to secure.** If oral intubation is not possible or is contraindicated, a surgical airway is indicated.
3. Penetrating neck trauma is associated with pneumothorax and hemothorax 20% of the time. Diagnose tension pneumothorax clinically and perform immediate needle thoracostomy. Otherwise, pneumothorax and hemothorax may be detected by bedside ultrasound or chest radiograph, and tube thoracostomy is indicated.
4. Apply direct pressure with hemostatic dressings to control active hemorrhage without occluding carotid arteries or the airway. **Blind clamping of blood vessels is contraindicated due to a risk of subsequent neurovascular injury.** Topical hemostatic agents may be used along with direct pressure. If direct pressure fails, inflating a Foley catheter in the wound tract may help control hemorrhage. Administration of **tranexamic acid** 1 g intravenously over 10 minutes then 1 g intravenously over 8 hours should be considered in exsanguinating patients with wounds less than 3 hours old. Uncontrolled hemorrhage despite these measures requires emergent surgery.
5. Immobilize the cervical spine in patients with altered level of consciousness, blunt trauma, or penetrating trauma with neurologic deficits after careful examination for penetrating injury, bleeding, hematoma, or bruits/thrills. Cervical collars should not be placed at the expense of monitoring injuries or the ability to perform life-saving procedures.
6. All penetrating wounds that violate the platysma muscle mandate surgical consultation. Unstable patients with penetrating neck trauma require an emergent surgical or interventional radiologic procedure. Therefore, egress from the ED should not be delayed for unnecessary procedures or tests. Stable patients should undergo diagnostic evaluation for deep structure injuries (Fig. 163-2).
7. Penetrating wounds that do not violate the platysma require standard wound care and closure and the patient may be discharged if they are asymptomatic.
8. Patients with blunt neck trauma and hard signs of injury require emergent surgical consultation (Table 163-1). Patients with stable, symptomatic blunt neck trauma should be aggressively evaluated for injuries to deep structures utilizing MDCTA and other modalities. Surgical consultation and admission for these symptomatic patients are advised even if no injury is seen on the initial study.
9. The optimal management of asymptomatic blunt neck trauma patients remains unclear. Consider liberal use of MDCTA (and other adjunctive tests as necessary) and extended observation (4 to 6 hours) to detect

delayed respiratory and neurological dysfunction. This is especially recommended for patients with risk factors for blunt cerebral vascular injury (Table 163-2).

10. Address the associated psychosocial issues of strangulation victims.

FURTHER READING

For further reading in *Tintinalli's Emergency Medicine: A Comprehensive Study Guide*, 8th ed., see Chapter 260, "Trauma to the Neck" by Ashley S. Bean.

CHAPTER 164

Cardiothoracic Injuries

Paul Nystrom

Bedside diagnosis and immediate intervention by the emergency provider may be lifesaving for significant injuries associated with severe chest trauma such as tension pneumothorax, hemothorax, and cardiac tamponade. Initial resuscitation and airway management should follow established principles, as discussed in Chapter 156, "Trauma in Adults." It is important to **avoid hypoxia and hypotension** to prevent secondary injury in head-injured patients. In the hemodynamically unstable, polytrauma patient who requires emergency surgery without CT imaging, **exclude immediate life threats rapidly at the bedside using ultrasound**, radiographs, and physical examination.

Physical examination should include assessment for visible trauma to the chest wall including any "seat belt sign," focal areas of tenderness, subcutaneous emphysema, and open chest wounds. Tracheal deviation, unequal chest rise, abnormal breath sounds, and bowel sounds in the chest are less frequent but also important to note. **Consider endotracheal intubation for patients in respiratory distress** (Table 164-1).

LUNG INJURIES

Tension pneumothorax occurs when air enters the pleural space, either by escaping from damaged lung, tracheobronchial tissue, or an open chest wound. The pneumothorax may become pressurized during respiration causing tension with resultant respiratory and circulatory compromise. Patients may have dyspnea, tachycardia, hypotension, distended neck veins, tracheal deviation, and unequal breath sounds. Recognize and **treat tension pneumothorax immediately with needle decompression** without waiting for radiographs. Insert a 14-G, 4.5-cm over-the-needle catheter in the second intercostal space at the midclavicular line (a standard 14-G IV catheter may not reach the pleural space in many patients). A rush of air through the catheter is confirmatory. Leave the catheter in until a chest tube can be inserted, as the catheter converts the tension pneumothorax to an open pneumothorax.

Treat a small pneumothorax with inpatient observation; tube thoracostomy may not be necessary. **Treat a large pneumothorax with tube thoracostomy** (24 to 28 F (8.0 to 9.3 mm)). Patients with pneumothoraces

TABLE 164-1 Considerations for Early Ventilatory Assistance after Thoracic Trauma

Altered mental status
Hypovolemic shock
Multiple injuries
Multiple blood transfusions
Elderly patients
Preexisting pulmonary disease
Respiratory distress
Poor oxygen saturation
Severe pulmonary contusions

TABLE 164-2 Causes for Failure of Complete Lung Expansion or Evacuation of a Pneumothorax
Improper connections or leaks in the external tubing or water-seal collection apparatus
Improper positioning of the chest tube
Occlusion of bronchi or bronchioles by secretions or foreign body
Tear of one of the large bronchi
Large tear of the lung parenchyma

of any size and those with subcutaneous emphysema (requiring presumption of an occult pneumothorax) who will be intubated or who will be transported by air should receive a tube thoracostomy, as positive pressure ventilation and decreased barometric pressure can cause expansion of trapped air and progression to a tension pneumothorax. Never clamp a chest tube, but always place it on water seal when taken off suction. See Table 164-2 for causes of failure of the lung to fully reinflate after tube thoracostomy.

Treat a hemothorax with tube thoracostomy. A 32- to 40-F (10.7 to 13.4 mm) chest tube has historically been used but the larger size may not be necessary. Indications for surgery include an immediate return of 1 L of blood or ongoing bleeding of 150 to 200 mL/h for 2 to 4 hours. Consider using a heparinized autotransfusion device if massive hemothorax is suspected but do not delay tube thoracostomy.

Pulmonary contusions are direct injuries to the lung parenchyma without laceration. Hypoxia develops as bleeding and edema compromise contused lung tissue. Seventy percent of pulmonary contusions are not immediately visible on initial chest radiograph, but may appear as patchy opacities, typically within 6 hours. CT scan is much more sensitive. **Initial management should include pain control to prevent hypoventilation, avoidance of unnecessary IV fluids to prevent pulmonary edema, and strict pulmonary toilet.** Administer crystalloids judiciously to maintain perfusion and use blood products early in resuscitation. A trial of positive pressure ventilation by mask is reasonable in a patient with normal mental status who requires limited respiratory support. Patients with involvement of >25% of lung tissue will likely require intubation, but should not be intubated preemptively. If intubated, use positive-end expiratory pressure. Use diuretics if the patient is thought to have volume overload.

CHEST WALL INJURIES

A small open chest wound can progress to a tension pneumothorax through a one-way valve effect. Cover the wound with sterile petroleum gauze taped on three sides to allow air to exit but not enter. **Perform tube thoracostomy** but not through the wound.

Flail chest occurs when a section of ribs fractures in multiple locations, causing instability of a segment of the chest wall. Intubation and positive pressure ventilation will stabilize the flail segment. Surgical fixation may be needed, although the greater danger is the underlying lung contusion that compromises respiration.

Rib fractures may suggest other injuries or cause morbidity independently. Fractures of the first and second ribs require great force and should therefore cause high suspicion for other major thoracic injuries including myocardial, vascular, and bronchial injuries. Multiple lower rib fractures should raise suspicion for liver or splenic injuries. The focus of diagnostic imaging is to exclude other injuries such as pneumothorax, pulmonary contusion, and intraabdominal injury.

Even in the absence of coexisting injury, the pain of rib fractures may eventually lead to splinting, ventilatory compromise, and pneumonia. Consider intercostal nerve blocks and epidural anesthesia for pain control. Patients being discharged should generally receive nonsteroidal anti-inflammatory drugs (NSAIDs) and opioid analgesics. Remind them to breathe deeply or perform incentive spirometry exercises. Admit patients with multiple fractures, medical comorbidities, or older age for a period of observation until they are stabilized on a regimen of pain control and pulmonary toilet. Do not attempt to stabilize the chest wall with tape or binding. Assess patients with a sternal fracture for cardiac injury by ECG, serial troponin measurements, and cardiac monitoring.

Assume patients with subcutaneous emphysema have a pneumothorax even if not seen on the initial chest radiograph. Supine chest radiograph is a relatively insensitive screening tool for pneumothorax and for hemothoraces of <200 mL. Up to 1000 mL may appear as only diffuse haziness. Lung collapse from intubation of a mainstem bronchus can have a similar appearance. If the patient can safely sit up, upright and expiratory views can increase sensitivity. **Ultrasound has been shown to have good sensitivity for pneumothorax, with loss of the sliding pleura sign while a hemothorax will show fluid in the dependent portion of the chest.** CT scan is highly sensitive for both of these conditions. If subclavian venous cannulation is attempted, it should be done on the side of the suspected injury so that an iatrogenic pneumothorax does not result in bilateral pneumothoraces.

Penetrating wounds should never be deeply probed. A small stab wound may develop into a delayed pneumothorax; repeat the ultrasound or chest radiograph at 4 to 6 hours after the initial presentation.

PNEUMOMEDIASTINUM AND TRACHEOBRONCHIAL INJURIES

Pneumomediastinum is most often caused by ruptured alveoli with dissection of air to the mediastinum and does not require treatment in the asymptomatic patient. Coughing, heavy breathing (such as seen in drug inhalation), or exertion can rupture alveoli and release air into the mediastinum. However, pneumomediastinum can also be the result of injuries to the trachea and large airways from high energy or major deceleration. Dyspnea, hemoptysis, subcutaneous emphysema in the neck, a crunching sound with the cardiac cycle, and a massive continued air leak through a chest tube suggest tracheobronchial injury.

DIAPHRAGMATIC INJURIES

All penetrating injuries from the level of the nipples to the umbilicus have the potential to injure the diaphragm. Small lacerations can be asymptomatic and then progress to the rupture of abdominal contents into the chest weeks to months later. The diagnosis is obvious if imaging shows herniation of abdominal contents into the chest or coiling of a gastric tube within the chest. Subtle abnormalities may also be seen on chest radiograph, CT, or upper GI series with contrast. Laparotomy and laparoscopy remain the gold standards to exclude diaphragmatic injuries. All diaphragmatic lacerations require surgical repair.

PENETRATING CARDIAC INJURIES

The right ventricle is the most commonly injured portion of the heart because of its large anterior exposure. Accumulation of blood in the pericardial space compresses the heart, which prevents diastolic filling. The diagnosis is typically made by bedside ultrasound. Pericardiocentesis should only be attempted for a patient in shock with confirmed cardiac tamponade since it is technically difficult and may result in laceration of a coronary artery or injury to the myocardium. Stable patients should have a pericardial window or thoracotomy performed in the operating room.

Patients with penetrating chest injuries with signs of life in the field but who subsequently become pulseless may be candidates for ED thoracotomy. Relieving cardiac tamponade, controlling hilar bleeding, cross clamping the descending aorta, or repairing a myocardial laceration may be lifesaving. Stab wounds to the heart are more likely to be amenable to repair than injuries from gunshot wounds. Once the chest is opened, the heart is delivered from the pericardium so that potential injuries can be visualized. Direct digital pressure, staples, sutures, or a Foley catheter with inflated balloon may be used to temporize bleeding lacerations on the way to the operating room for definitive repair.

BLUNT INJURIES TO THE HEART

Blunt cardiac injury can lead to death from damage to cardiac structures, coronary artery injury and thrombosis, and contusion of the myocardium resulting in impaired contractility and arrhythmias. ECG changes consistent with ischemia suggest coronary artery dissection or thrombosis, which are evaluated and treated by cardiac catheterization and stenting. A direct blow to the chest such as when a young athlete is struck by a hard ball can induce ventricular fibrillation cardiac arrest even without myocardial injury (commotio cordis). **Treat according to advanced cardiac life support (ACLS) algorithms** because there is usually no structural damage to the heart.

A patient with cardiac injury may present with chest pain, tachycardia unexplained by hemorrhage, and arrhythmias. Bedside echocardiography by the emergency provider should be performed as a first screen for cardiac tamponade and grossly impaired contractility. **Treat tamponade the same as tamponade from penetrating cardiac injury**. Patients with hypotension not explained by another cause, arrhythmias, and impaired contractility should undergo further evaluation by formal echocardiography and cardiac enzymes, with transesophageal echocardiogram being three times more sensitive than transthoracic echocardiogram for blunt myocardial injury. Give antiarrhythmic and inotropic medications according to ACLS algorithms. Indications for admission include abnormalities on echocardiogram, ECG, or cardiac enzymes. Discharge patients with normal vital signs, normal initial ECG, no underlying cardiac disease, and age <55 years after 4 to 6 hours of normal cardiac monitoring.

TRAUMA TO THE GREAT VESSELS

Trauma to the major thoracic vessels is often lethal, with 90% of those sustaining blunt aortic injury dying at the scene. The most common site of blunt aortic injury is at the proximal descending aorta between the left subclavian artery and the ligamentum arteriosum. Injury to the subclavian and innominate arteries can be related to shoulder belts, fractures of the first and second ribs, and proximal clavicle. Half of patients present without external physical findings, so suspicion for this injury needs to be high with mechanisms involving high-speed deceleration.

Table 164-3 shows radiographic findings of thoracic aortic injury, although a normal chest radiograph does not exclude major vascular injury. All the patients with a mechanism highly concerning for great vessel injury should undergo CT angiogram with IV contrast. Conventional aortography is still used in some cases to assess injuries and guide operative planning. Transesophageal echocardiogram is useful for diagnosing aortic intimal lesions, but is contraindicated in airway compromise or suspected cervical spinal injury.

Indications for immediate operation for vascular injury are hemodynamic instability, radiographic evidence of a rapidly expanding hematoma, or large-volume chest tube output. Control hypertension in order to decrease shear stress on the vessel wall by titration of narcotic pain medications and sedatives. A short-acting β-blocker, such as **esmolol**, may be titrated to a systolic blood pressure of 100 to 120 mm Hg and a heart rate above 60 beats/min. If bradycardia prevents further dosing of a β-blocker, infuse an arterial dilator such as **sodium nitroprusside**. Do not use sodium nitroprusside without a β-blocker secondary to the reflex tachycardia that may develop.

TABLE 164-3 Radiographic Findings Suggestive of a Great Vessel Injury
Fractures
Sternum
Scapula
Multiple ribs
Clavicle in multisystem-injured patients
First and second rib
Mediastinal Clues
Obliteration of the aortic knob contour
Widening of the mediastinum
Depression of the left mainstem bronchus
Loss of paravertebral pleural stripe
Calcium layering at aortic knob
Abnormal general appearance of mediastinum
Deviation of nasogastric tube to the right
Lateral displacement of the trachea
Other Findings
Apical pleural hematoma (cap)
Massive left hemothorax
Obvious diaphragmatic injury

Source: Reproduced with permission from Mattox KL, Moore EE, Feliciano DV: *Trauma*, 7th ed. New York, NY: McGraw-Hill; 2013.

ESOPHAGEAL AND THORACIC DUCT INJURIES

Penetrating and occasionally blunt trauma may cause injury to the thoracic esophagus. If suspected, evaluate the patient by esophagram with water-soluble contrast, which is less likely to cause mediastinitis. A negative study with water-soluble contrast should be followed by the use of barium contrast, which has a higher sensitivity for injury. Flexible esophagoscopy is an alternative modality for assessing injury. Delayed diagnosis of esophageal injury has a high mortality if mediastinitis ensues. Injuries to the area of the left proximal subclavian vein may result in chylothorax, causing delayed pleural effusion with a mortality rate of approximately 50%. **Initial treatment is chest tube insertion**.

PERICARDITIS

Patients may develop chest pain, fever, and a friction rub 2 to 4 weeks after cardiac trauma or surgery which may indicate pericarditis. ECG may show diffuse ST-segment elevation consistent with pericarditis. Pericardial and pleural effusions may be seen on echocardiography and chest radiograph, respectively. **Treatment is with nonsteroidal anti-inflammatory medications**.

FURTHER READING

For further reading in *Tintinalli's Emergency Medicine: A Comprehensive Study Guide*, 8th ed., see Chapter 254, "Trauma in Adults," by Peter Cameron and Barry J. Knapp; Chapter 261, "Pulmonary Trauma," by David Jones, Anna Nelson, O. John Ma; Chapter 262, "Cardiac Trauma," by Christopher Ross and Theresa Schwab.

Abdominal Injuries

O. John Ma

The primary goal in the evaluation of abdominal trauma is to promptly recognize conditions that require immediate surgical exploration. The most critical error is to delay operative intervention when it is needed.

CLINICAL FEATURES

Solid Organ Injuries

Injury to the solid organs causes morbidity and mortality, primarily as a result of acute blood loss. An increase in pulse pressure may be the only clue to loss of ≤15% of total blood volume. As blood loss continues, heart and respiratory rate increase. Hypotension may not occur until a 30% decrease in circulating volume occurs. The spleen is the most frequently injured organ in blunt abdominal trauma and is commonly associated with other intra-abdominal injuries. The liver also is commonly injured in blunt and penetrating injuries. Kehr sign, representing referred left shoulder pain, is a classic finding in splenic rupture. Lower left rib fractures should heighten clinical suspicion for splenic injury. Some patients with solid organ injury occasionally present with minimal symptoms and nonspecific findings on physical examination. This is commonly seen in younger patients and those with distracting injuries, head injury, or intoxication. Serial physical examinations on an awake, alert, and reliable patient are important for identifying intra-abdominal injuries.

Hollow Visceral Injuries

These injuries produce symptoms by the combination of blood loss and peritoneal contamination. Perforation of the stomach, small bowel, or colon is accompanied by blood loss from a concomitant mesenteric injury. Gastrointestinal contamination will produce peritoneal signs over time. Patients with head injury, distracting injuries, or intoxication may not exhibit peritoneal signs initially.

Small bowel and colon injuries are most frequently the result of penetrating trauma. However, a deceleration injury can cause a bucket-handle tear of the mesentery or a blow-out injury of the antimesenteric border. Suppurative peritonitis may develop from small bowel and colonic injuries. Inflammation may take 6 to 8 hours to develop.

Retroperitoneal Injuries

The diagnosis of retroperitoneal injuries can be challenging. Signs and symptoms may be subtle or absent at initial presentation. Duodenal injuries most often are associated with high-speed vertical or horizontal decelerating trauma. These injuries may range in severity from an intramural hematoma to an extensive crush or laceration. Duodenal ruptures are usually contained within the retroperitoneum. Clinical signs of duodenal injury are often slow to develop. Patients may present with abdominal pain, fever, nausea, and vomiting, although these symptoms may take hours to become clinically apparent.

Pancreatic injury often accompanies rapid deceleration injury or a severe crush injury. Unrestrained drivers who hit the steering column or bicyclists who fall against a handlebar are at risk for pancreatic injuries. Pancreatic injuries can present with subtle signs and symptoms, making the diagnosis elusive.

Diaphragmatic Injuries

Presentation of diaphragm injuries is often insidious. Only occasionally is the diagnosis obvious when bowel sounds can be auscultated in the thoracic cavity. Herniation of abdominal contents into the thoracic cavity or a nasogastric tube coiled in the thorax confirms the diagnosis on chest radiograph. In most cases, however, the only finding on chest radiograph is blurring of the diaphragm or an effusion.

DIAGNOSIS AND DIFFERENTIAL

Plain Radiographs

A chest radiograph is helpful in evaluating for herniated abdominal contents in the thoracic cavity and for evidence of free air under the diaphragm. An anteroposterior pelvis radiograph is important for identifying pelvic fractures, which can produce significant blood loss and be associated with intra-abdominal injury.

Ultrasonography

The focused assessment with sonography for trauma (FAST) examination (Table 165-1) is a widely accepted primary diagnostic study. The underlying premise of the FAST exam is that many clinically significant injuries will be associated with free intraperitoneal fluid. The greatest benefit of

TABLE 165-1 Advantages and Disadvantages of the Focused Assessment with Sonography for Trauma Examination

Advantages	Disadvantages
Accurate, sensitive, and specific for detecting free intraperitoneal fluid	Inability to determine the exact etiology of the free intraperitoneal fluid
Rapid (<4 min)	Operator-dependent
Noninvasive Repeatable Portable	Difficulty in interpreting the images in patients who are obese or have subcutaneous air or excessive bowel gas
No nephrotoxic contrast material needed	Inability to distinguish intraperitoneal hemorrhage from ascites
No radiation exposure Can evaluate for free pericardial and pleural fluid	Cannot evaluate the retroperitoneum as well as CT scan
Can evaluate for pneumothorax	
No risk for patients who are pregnant, coagulopathic, or have had previous abdominal surgery	

FAST is the rapid identification of free intraperitoneal fluid in the hypotensive patient with blunt abdominal trauma. Since the FAST examination can reliably detect small amounts of free intraperitoneal fluid and can estimate the rate of hemorrhage through serial examinations, it has essentially replaced diagnostic peritoneal lavage (DPL) for blunt abdominal trauma in the majority of North American trauma centers.

Computed Tomography

Abdominopelvic CT with IV contrast (Table 165-2) is the noninvasive gold standard study for the diagnosis of abdominal injury (unless the patient has an allergy to iodinated contrast). The addition of PO contrast is too time-consuming to be practical in trauma management. The major advantage of IV contrast CT over other diagnostic modalities is that the precise location(s) and grade of injury can be identified. CT can quantify and differentiate the amount and type of free fluid in the abdomen. Because CT can evaluate for retroperitoneal injuries, it is the ideal study for assessment of the duodenum and pancreas. The use of multiphasic CT (arterial, portal, and equilibrium phases) accurately identifies life-threatening mesenteric hemorrhage and transmural bowel injuries.

Diagnostic Peritoneal Lavage

The wide availability of CT and ED ultrasound has relegated DPL (Table 165-3) to a second-line screening test for evaluating abdominal

TABLE 165-2 Advantages and Disadvantages of CT in Abdominal Trauma

Advantages	Disadvantages
Ability to precisely locate intra-abdominal lesions	Expense
Ability to evaluate the retroperitoneum	Need to transport the trauma patient to the radiology suite
Ability to identify injuries that may be managed nonoperatively	Need for contrast materials
Noninvasive	Radiation exposure

TABLE 165-3 Advantages and Disadvantages of Diagnostic Peritoneal Lavage in Abdominal Trauma

Advantages	Disadvantages
Sensitivity	Invasive
Availability	Potential for iatrogenic injury
Relative speed with which it can be performed	Lack of specificity
Low complication rate	Inability to identify injuries that may be managed nonoperatively
Ability to detect early evidence of bowel perforation	Misapplication for evaluation of retroperitoneal injuries
No nephrotoxic contrast material needed	
No radiation exposure	

trauma. For blunt trauma, indications for DPL include (a) patients who are too hemodynamically unstable to leave the ED for CT and (b) unexplained hypotension in patients with an equivocal physical examination. DPL is considered positive if more than 10 mL of gross blood is aspirated immediately, the red blood cell count is higher than 100,000 cells/mm^3, the white blood cell count is higher than 500 cells/mm^3, bile is present, or if vegetable matter is present.

The only absolute contraindication to DPL is when surgical management is clearly indicated, in which case the DPL would delay patient transport to the operating room. Relative contraindications include patients with advanced hepatic dysfunction, severe coagulopathies, previous abdominal surgeries, or a gravid uterus.

EMERGENCY DEPARTMENT CARE AND DISPOSITION

1. Initiate standard protocols for evaluation and stabilization of trauma patients. See Chapter 156.
2. Administer oxygen as needed, attach cardiac monitoring, and secure two large-bore IV lines.
3. Administer **IV crystalloid fluid** to hypotensive abdominal trauma patients. Transfuse with O-negative or type-specific packed red blood cells as indicated.
4. Order laboratory work for abdominal trauma patients based on the mechanism of injury (blunt vs penetrating); labs may include type and crossmatching, complete blood count, electrolytes, lactate level, directed toxicologic studies, coagulation studies, hepatic enzymes, and lipase.
5. Table 165-4 lists the **indications for exploratory laparotomy**. When a patient presents to the ED with an obvious high-velocity gunshot wound to the abdomen, do not delay transport of the patient to the operating room by performing a FAST examination unless there is a suspicion for

TABLE 165-4 Indications for Laparotomy

	Blunt	Penetrating
Absolute	Anterior abdominal injury with hypotension Abdominal wall disruption Peritonitis Free air under diaphragm on chest radiograph Positive FAST or DPL in hemodynamically unstable patient CT-diagnosed injury requiring surgery (i.e., pancreatic transection, duodenal rupture, diaphragm injury)	Injury to abdomen, back, and flank with hypotension Abdominal tenderness GI evisceration High suspicion for transabdominal trajectory after gunshot wound CT-diagnosed injury requiring surgery (i.e., ureter or pancreas)
Relative	Positive FAST or DPL in hemodynamically stable patient Solid visceral injury in stable patient Hemoperitoneum on CT without clear source	Positive local wound exploration after stab wound

Abbreviations: DPL, diagnostic peritoneal lavage; FAST, focused assessment with sonography for trauma.

cardiac injury. If organ evisceration is present, cover the wound with a moist, sterile dressing before surgery.

6. For an equivocal stab wound to the abdomen, obtain surgical consultation for local wound exploration. If the local wound exploration demonstrates no violation of the anterior fascia, the patient can be discharged home.
7. For the hemodynamically stable, blunt trauma patient with a positive FAST examination, further evaluation with CT may be warranted before admission to the surgical service.

FURTHER READING

For further reading in *Tintinalli's Emergency Medicine: A Comprehensive Study Guide*, 8th ed., see Chapter 263, "Abdominal Trauma," by L. Keith French, Stephanie Gordy, and O. John Ma.

Penetrating Trauma to The Flank and Buttocks

Sum Ambur

Challenges in evaluating penetrating trauma to the flank and buttocks include recognizing peritoneal and retroperitoneal injuries and determining which patients need immediate surgery and which can be managed more conservatively. Trajectories and resultant severity and pattern of injury can vary widely with both stab and gunshot wounds. Hemodynamically unstable patients need immediate operative intervention. Mechanism and time of injury, weapon characteristics, and determining the bullet path or stab wound depth may also assist in determining the initial diagnostic approach if the patient is otherwise stable.

PENETRATING FLANK TRAUMA

Clinical Features

Presentation may vary from stable vital signs with an innocuous-appearing wound to hemodynamic shock and peritonitis. Gross blood on rectal examination suggests bowel injury. Blood at the urethral meatus or hematuria suggests genitourinary injury.

Diagnosis and Differential

CT imaging is the diagnostic modality of choice for hemodynamically stable patients. Protocols vary by institution, but may include PO or rectal contrast if there is suspicion for hollow viscous injury. Contrast-enhanced CT can also often help determine stab wound depth. Bedside ultrasound (eFAST exam) can be used to assess for intraabdominal free fluid and thus help predict the need for surgical intervention.

Emergency Department Care and Disposition

1. Follow standard trauma resuscitation protocols. Patients who require emergent exploratory laparotomy include those who are hemodynamically unstable, display peritonitis, and have sustained gunshot wounds to the flank.
2. If there is concern that the peritoneum is violated or the patient displays signs of peritonitis, administer broad-spectrum antibiotics, such as **pipercillin/tazobactam** 3.375 g IV.
3. Many patients with stab wounds can be managed conservatively. High-risk patients (stab wounds with penetration beyond deep fascia) require surgical consultation and admission. Low-risk patients (stab wounds superficial to deep fascia) may be discharged if serial examinations are unremarkable and the patient remains stable throughout an observation period.

PENETRATING BUTTOCK TRAUMA

Clinical Features

Gunshot wounds are much more likely to require laparotomy than stab wounds. Gunshot wounds above the level of the greater trochanter and gross hematuria predict the need for surgery. Rectal examination to assess for gross blood, evaluation of lower extremity pulses, and neurologic examination to assess for sciatic and femoral nerve injury should be performed.

Diagnosis and Differential

Hemodynamically stable patients should undergo CT with oral, IV, and rectal contrast (to avoid missed colon and rectal injuries). Cystourethrogram should be performed on patients with findings of hematuria or wounds near the genitourinary tract. CT angiography or traditional angiography and venography may be indicated if a pelvic hematoma is found on CT. Bedside ultrasound (eFAST exam) can also be used to assess for intraabdominal free fluid and thus help predict the need for surgical intervention.

Emergency Department Care and Disposition

1. Follow standard trauma resuscitation protocols. Patients who are hemodynamically unstable, display peritonitis, or are likely to have intrapelvic or transabdominal bullet paths require **exploratory laparotomy**.
2. If the patient displays signs of peritonitis or there is high suspicion for peritoneal violation, administer antibiotics, such as **pipercillin/tazobactam** 3.375 g IV.
3. **Interventional angiography** may be required to treat extensive intrapelvic bleeding.
4. Wound exploration is of limited value. Only very superficial stab wounds may be managed and discharged from the ED. Most patients with penetrating trauma to the buttocks require **admission and observation** due to the risk of occult injuries.

FURTHER READING

For further reading in *Tintinalli's Emergency Medicine: A Comprehensive Study Guide*, 8th ed., see Chapter 264, "Trauma to the Flank and Buttocks," by Alicia Devine.

CHAPTER 167

Genitourinary Injuries

Thomas Dalton

Genitourinary (GU) injuries frequently occur in the setting of polytrauma, so a thorough evaluation is necessary to avoid missing significant injuries.

CLINICAL FEATURES

Injuries should be suspected with any blunt or penetrating trauma near the GU tract, including any rapid deceleration, which can cause major vascular or parenchymal injury even without specific signs or symptoms. Hematuria of any amount raises the index of suspicion for GU injury, and difficulty with urination can be due to bladder or urethral injury or associated concomitant spinal cord injury. Flank contusions or hematomas, evidence of lower rib fractures, or penetrating flank injuries raise concern for renal injury. Lower abdominal pain, tenderness, ecchymosis, or evidence of a pelvic fracture as well as perineal or scrotal edema are consistent with possible bladder injury. Vaginal bleeding, a high-riding prostate, a perineal hematoma, and/or blood at the urethral meatus are concerning for urethral disruption.

DIAGNOSIS AND DIFFERENTIAL

There is no direct relationship between the degree of hematuria and the severity of renal injury. There is some evidence that microscopic hematuria in patients with a blood pressure <90 mm Hg or any gross hematuria is associated with a more significant renal injury. In children where renal trauma is being considered, isolated microscopic hematuria with <50 red blood cells per high-powered field makes a significant renal injury less likely. An IV contrast-enhanced abdominal/pelvic CT scan is the imaging "gold standard" for the stable trauma patient with a suspected kidney injury. A 10-minute delayed image is needed to ascertain whether there is any urine extravasation but can be omitted if the kidney is normal and there are no fluid collections. A retrograde cystogram (plain film or CT) is the "gold standard" for demonstrating bladder injury, and a retrograde urethrogram is indicated for demonstrating urethral injuries. Color Doppler ultrasonography is the preferred imaging technique for investigating closed scrotal and testicular injuries. A focused assessment with sonography in trauma (FAST) exam can detect intra-abdominal fluid collections but cannot reliably evaluate renal, bladder, or ureteral injuries Table 167-1.

EMERGENCY DEPARTMENT CARE AND DISPOSITION

Take a standardized approach to all multiple trauma patients to identify and treat life-threatening injuries (primary survey) and then perform a thorough secondary survey, including a GU examination, to diagnose all injuries. Obtain appropriate diagnostic imaging and laboratory testing as indicated by the initial history and examination.

TABLE 167-1 Imaging for Genitourinary Trauma

Injury	Imaging	Comments
Multisystem trauma or suspected renal parenchymal or vascular injury	Abdominal-pelvic IV contrast CT scan	Include pelvis to view entire GU tract Delayed films needed to identify urinary extravasation
Any visceral injury resulting in free intraperitoneal fluid	FAST	Identifies free fluid, but does not specify type of visceral injury and does not identify renal vascular injury
Renal artery injury	Renal angiography	Details vascular injuries
Ureteral injury	Abdominal-pelvic IV contrast CT scan	Delayed films needed to identify extravasation; obtain IV pyelogram or retrograde pyelogram if still suspicious with negative CT
Bladder injury	Retrograde cystogram	Can use plain radiographs or CT scan
Urethral injury	Retrograde urethrogram	Discuss sequencing with radiologist, because if performed prior to abdominal-pelvic contrast CT scan, can interfere with diagnosis
Scrotal/testicular injury	Color Doppler US	Contrast-enhanced US or MRI if suspicion is high and initial US is negative

MANAGEMENT OF SPECIFIC INJURIES

Kidney

Kidney injuries include contusions, hematomas, lacerations, and completely shattered kidneys with or without vascular injuries. Eighty percent of patients with kidney injury have additional visceral or skeletal injuries that complicate their management. Most renal injuries are handled nonoperatively, but indications for operative treatment include life-threatening bleeding from the kidney; expanding, pulsatile, or non-contained hematoma (thought to be from an avulsion injury); renal avulsion injury; and extravasation from the renal pelvis or from a ureteral injury. There are little data to support specific treatment recommendations for patients with isolated renal trauma. Patients with microscopic hematuria and no indication for imaging can be discharged home with instructions for no strenuous activity and follow-up in 1 to 2 weeks for repeat urinalysis. Those with a contusion (normal imaging and microscopic hematuria) can be discharged as above. Those with a higher-grade injury and/or gross hematuria should be admitted for observation (to include repeat hematocrit and urinalysis), hydration, and rest until gross hematuria clears, or general improvement ensues.

Ureter

Ureteral injuries are almost always due to iatrogenic complications of instrumentation or penetrating trauma. Notably the absence of hematuria does not exclude an injury. In a stable patient a delayed CT scan of the abdomen and pelvis with IV contrast can identify ureteral injuries. If the CT scan is non-diagnostic and there is a high concern for an injury then an IV pyelogram or retrograde pyelogram is indicated. Treatment is operative, including stenting in some cases.

Bladder

Bladder injuries occur in about 2% of blunt abdominal trauma patients and 80% are associated with pelvic fractures. Gross hematuria is present in about 95% of patients with significant injury and warrants a retrograde cystogram. Bladder injuries can also be present in pelvic fractures with only the presence of microscopic hematuria but the degree of microscopic hematuria warranting a cystogram is unclear. Extraperitoneal rupture is most common and can usually be treated by bladder catheter drainage alone. Intraperitoneal rupture always requires surgical exploration and repair. A retrograde cystogram can be performed by infusing ~350 ml of contrast material to distend the bladder. Passive bladder filling is not sensitive enough to exclude a bladder rupture. Sonographic diagnosis of a bladder injury is not accurate.

Urethra

Posterior urethral injuries (membranous and prostatic urethra) are typically related to major blunt force trauma and are associated with pelvic fractures. Treatment is via suprapubic bladder drainage followed by surgical repair in several weeks. Because a urinary catheter can disrupt a partial posterior urethral injury, one should not be placed if there is suspicion of injury without first obtaining a retrograde urethrogram. Anterior urethral injuries usually occur due to direct trauma such as from a straddle injury or a direct blow to the bulbar or penile urethra. The absence of hematuria does not rule-out a urethral injury. If there is concern for an injury, then avoid placing a foley catheter and obtain a retrograde urethrogram by injecting 20 to 30 mL of contrast into the urethra and obtain a radiograph. If a foley catheter has already been placed, then a 16-gauge angiocatheter can be used to inject contrast between the catheter and urethra. Treatment is supportive, which may include a urinary catheter. Penetrating trauma to the anterior urethra generally requires operative repair.

Testicles and Scrotum

Evaluate blunt testicular trauma with an ultrasound examination. If testicular rupture is present, exploration and repair is indicated. If the testicle is intact, conservative treatment with ice, elevation, scrotal support, and pain medication is appropriate. Hematomas and hematoceles are managed on a case-by-case basis. Penetrating testicular trauma warrants surgical exploration and repair. Scrotal lacerations can be directly repaired and scrotal avulsions require surgical repair with the testicle covered in the remaining scrotum.

Penis

Simple contusions are managed conservatively with cold packs, rest, and pain medications. Simple lacerations involving skin only can be directly repaired, but deeper lacerations and/or penetrating injuries require operative exploration and repair. Amputation requires microsurgical reimplantation if the amputated segment is viable. Penile fractures require exploration and repair.

FURTHER READING

For further reading in *Tintinalli's Emergency Medicine: A Comprehensive Study Guide*, 8th ed., see Chapter 265, "Genitourinary Trauma," by Matthew C. Gratton and French L. Keith.

CHAPTER 168

Trauma to The Extremities

Amy M. Stubbs

Isolated penetrating trauma to the extremities that is associated with vascular injury has a nearly 10% incidence of mortality or limb loss. Early identification of injuries requiring imaging and/or surgical intervention has reduced the rates of limb loss and disability.

CLINICAL FEATURES

As with all traumatic injuries, a thorough primary survey with attention to life-threatening injuries should be accomplished prior to a detailed extremity exam. Direct pressure or a tourniquet should be applied to actively bleeding injuries. Once an extremity injury is identified, a meticulous vascular and neuromuscular exam should then be performed.

Note pulses distal to the injury, capillary refill, and the color and temperature of the limb. Use a Doppler to detect a signal in the absence of a pulse. Any "hard" signs of arterial injury should prompt immediate surgical consultation and intervention. Soft signs of arterial injury should also be noted and require further evaluation, typically imaging and observation (Table 168-1).

Document the size and shape of each wound, as well as any bony deformities or soft tissue defects. Evaluate the surrounding area for pain with palpation or range of motion. Carefully evaluate joints in the proximity of the wound for the possibility of an open joint. Perform detailed strength and sensory exams on the affected limb to check for peripheral nerve injury. Consult the appropriate surgical specialist for signs of injury to an artery, nerve, joint, or bone, or suspicion of compartment syndrome (see Fig. 168-1).

TABLE 168-1 Clinical Manifestations of Extremity Vascular Trauma

Hard signs
Absent or diminished distal pulses
Obvious arterial bleeding
Large expanding or pulsatile hematoma
Audible bruit
Palpable thrill
Distal ischemia (pain, pallor, paralysis, paresthesias, coolness)
Soft signs
Small, stable hematoma
Injury to anatomically related nerve
Unexplained hypotension
History of hemorrhage
Proximity of injury to major vascular structures
Complex fracture

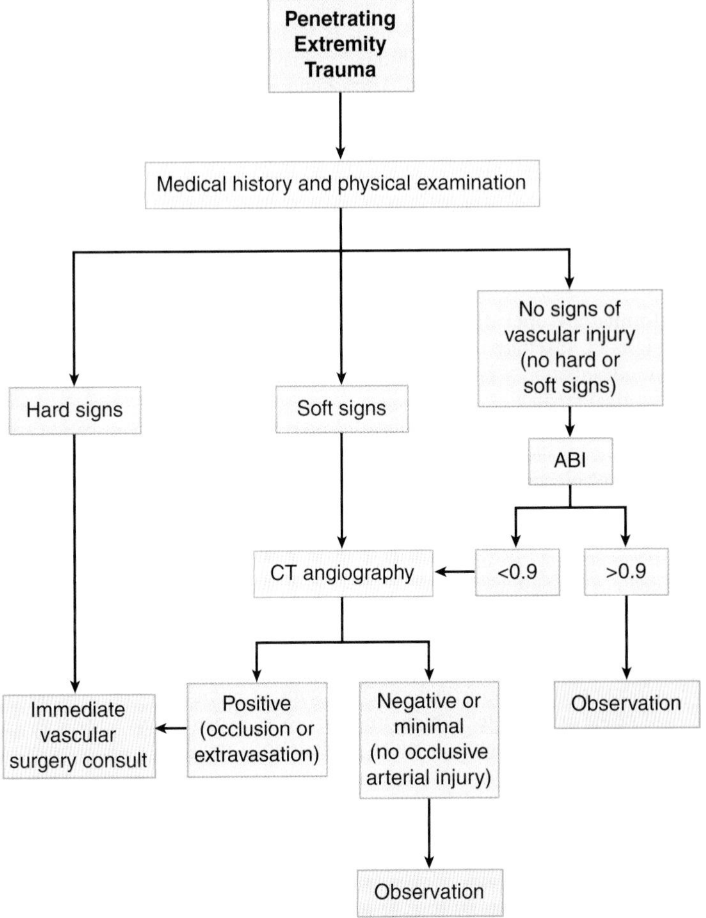

FIGURE 168-1. Algorithm for penetrating extremity trauma. ABI, ankle-brachial index.

DIAGNOSIS AND DIFFERENTIAL

Obtain ankle-brachial indexes (ABIs) on the affected and unaffected limb using a Doppler and manual blood pressure cuff. Though they have variable sensitivity and specificity for arterial injury and do not reliably detect nonocclusive injuries such as intimal flaps or pseudoaneurysms, a result of <0.9 is concerning for arterial injury. Soft signs of vascular injury or an abnormal ABI requires further imaging.

At minimum, AP and lateral films of the affected limb are necessary to evaluate for bone or joint injuries. Retained foreign bodies or embolized bullet fragments may also be seen. Image the joint above and below the injury site.

CT angiography has largely supplanted conventional angiography in the evaluation of vascular injuries as it is widely available, rapid, relatively noninvasive, and provides high-quality images that may also be useful in evaluating concurrent injuries. Ultrasound is neither as sensitive nor as specific as angiography and cannot reliably rule out a vascular injury.

Laboratory testing is not required, though a CBC, type and screen, or creatinine may be indicated in certain settings, such as when there is profuse bleeding or concern exists for renal insufficiency when angiography is a consideration.

EMERGENCY DEPARTMENT CARE AND DISPOSITION

1. **Immediate operative intervention is typically indicated when hard signs of vascular injury are identified**. For certain injuries, imaging, in consultation with the vascular surgeon, may be appropriate prior to surgical repair.
2. In the absence of arterial injury, 24-hour admission for observation and serial exams may be reasonable.
3. Control bleeding with direct pressure, pressure dressings, or a tourniquet. Vessels should not be clamped or ligated to avoid injury to adjacent nerves.
4. Bone or joint capsule injuries should be evaluated by an orthopedic surgeon as patients are at risk for infection, posttraumatic arthritis, and loss of function. Fractures due to penetrating injuries should be treated as open fractures, requiring surgical debridement and admission for **intravenous antibiotics**, such as a cephalosporin plus gentamycin.
5. Update tetanus and irrigate wounds with, at minimum, 500 to 1000 cc of saline or tap water at high pressure (15 to 20 pounds per square inch). Grossly contaminated or older wounds may require gentle scrubbing and/or debridement.
6. Closure of the wound depends on the timing of presentation and amount of contamination. Repair low-risk wounds and arrange follow-up in 24 to 48 hours. Wounds with tissue destruction, gross contamination, or retained foreign bodies should be repaired via delayed primary closure after 72 to 96 hours. If there is no fracture, antibiotics are generally not indicated for low risk injuries, but should be considered for high-risk cases such as hand injuries, gross contamination, or immunocompromised patients.
7. The decision to remove foreign bodies such as bullet fragments depends on the size, location, and composition of the object. As aggressive exploration may cause further tissue damage and increase infection risk; the risk/benefit ratio should be carefully considered.

FURTHER READING

For further reading in *Tintinalli's Emergency Medicine: A Comprehensive Study Guide*, 8th ed., see Chapter 266, "Trauma to the Extremities," by James Heilman.

SECTION 19

Injuries to the Bones, Joints, and Soft Tissue

CHAPTER 169 Initial Evaluation and Management of Orthopedic Injuries

Gregory M. Johnston

Orthopedic injuries have implications beyond localized pain and swelling at the site of injury. The clinician must methodically evaluate the patient to prevent missing an occult or concomitant injury. Prompt recognition and appropriate treatment are needed to prevent prolonged pain, temporary or permanent disability, or even death.

CLINICAL FEATURES

Key to any emergency department encounter is obtaining a concise history from the patient and, when this is not feasible, from pre-hospital personnel or family members, and performing a meticulous physical examination. For instance, a patient may present with a deformed lower extremity, but a history of a fall from height will cue the clinician to consider the possibility of a concomitant spinal injury, or the spontaneous occurrence of a fracture in a patient with a history of malignancy may indicate a pathologic fracture. The clinician should conduct systematic palpation, since it is not uncommon for the pain of a fracture or dislocation to be referred to another area. Other essential aspects of the physical examination include inspection for swelling, discoloration, and deformity, documentation of both active and passive range of motion proximal and distal to the reported injury, and assessment of neurovascular status to include sensorimotor testing of peripheral nerve function. Vascular status should be assessed as soon as possible, since rapid correction of circulatory compromise can prevent ischemia, tissue loss, or amputation.

Diagnostic imaging should not be used as a substitute for physical examination, since it is possible for an occult fracture to escape detection on initial radiographic imaging. In addition, some fractures may only be detected on specialized radiographic views. If a patient has significant tenderness to palpation, pain with weight bearing, or with passive range of motion, then the possibility of an occult fracture should be considered. A negative plain film report does not exclude a significant injury. In such instances the fracture may only be detected by more advanced imaging modalities such as CT, bone scan, or MRI.

DIAGNOSIS AND DIFFERENTIAL

Consider obtaining studies of joints above and below the suspected fracture site, since additional injuries may be present. Pediatric patients present a special challenge due to the presence of ossifying growth centers. If a fracture is suspected, it is often helpful to obtain comparison films of the unaffected side. While many injuries may be treated in the emergency department and then routinely referred for outpatient follow-up, more significant injuries mandate immediate discussion with the orthopedic surgeon. Digital imaging is becoming more common, so it is often possible for the consulting orthopedist to conduct a contemporaneous review of the diagnostic studies when consulted by the emergency physician. This is not always feasible in rural medical facilities or military environments; therefore, overreliance on technology should not supplant the fundamental skill of describing radiographs. The following is a recommended way to verbally describe the fracture to the consultant in order to best communicate the findings of the radiograph:

- Open (overlying skin disrupted) versus closed (overlying skin intact): Open injuries frequently require urgent operative intervention, and mandate thorough irrigation and prophylactic antibiotics to prevent the morbid sequelae of osteomyelitis and sepsis. Tetanus prophylaxis, administration of first-generation cephalosporin, i.e., Cefazolin, and the inclusion of an aminoglycoside for contaminated wounds, i.e., Gentamicin, are recommended.
- Location of the fracture: Orthopedic conventions include midshaft, junction of the proximal and middle thirds, junction of middle and distal thirds, anatomic boney reference points, e.g., supracondylar or intertrochanteric, and intra-articular. The later has operative implications due to the association of traumatic arthritis in cases not operatively managed.
- Orientation of the fracture: (see Fig. 169-1).
- Displacement and separation: Amount (in millimeters or percentage) and direction the distal fragment is detached and deviated from the proximal fragment. A separated fragment is maintained in anatomic alignment, but is offset from normal anatomic position.
- Shortening: reduction (in millimeters or centimeters) in bone length due to impaction or overriding fragments. Frequently requires surgical intervention.
- Angulation: Degree and direction of the angle formed by the distal fragment.
- Rotational deformity: Degree distal fragment is twisted on axis relative to the proximal fragment. Found on physical examination, and is not typically discernable by radiographs.
- Concomitant dislocation or subluxation: Complete loss of proper joint alignment (dislocation) compared to partial loss of joint surface contact (subluxation). Frequently requires surgical intervention.
- Salter-Harris fractures: Injuries to the epiphyseal plate of a growing child (see Fig. 169-2 and Table 169-1). Types I and V may not be noted on radiographs, and should be suspected clinically, immobilized and referred for follow-up. Unlike type I, type V injuries are associated with an axial loading force.

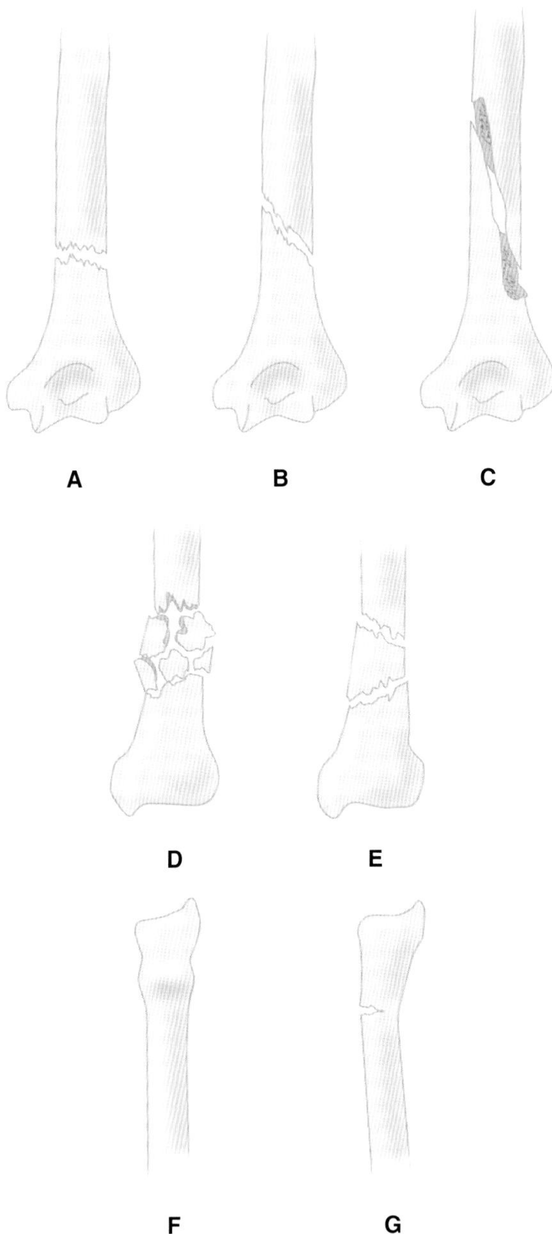

FIGURE 169-1. Fracture Line Orientation. **A**. Transverse. **B**. Oblique. **C**. Spiral. **D**. Comminuted. **E**. Segmental. **F**. Torus. **G**. Greenstick.

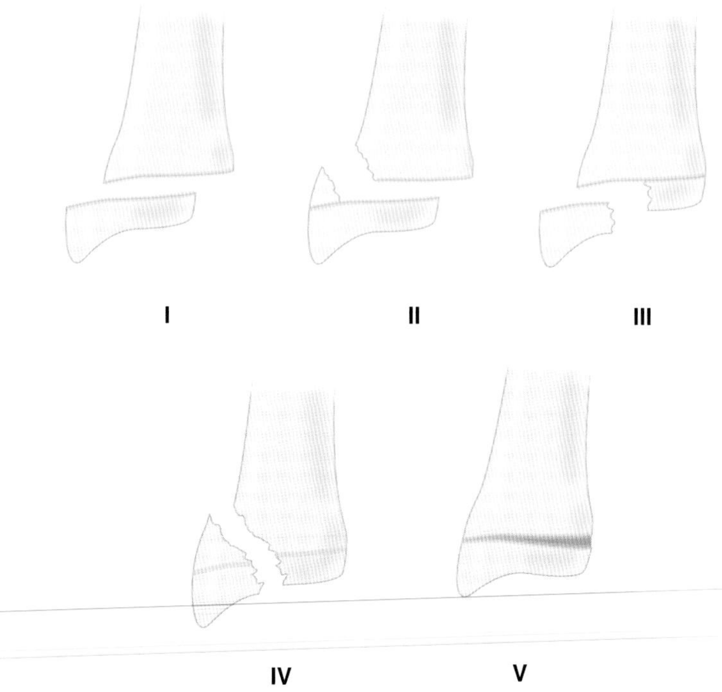

FIGURE 169-2. Epiphyseal plate fractures based on the classification of Salter and Harris.

EMERGENCY DEPARTMENT CARE AND DISPOSITION

1. Control pain and swelling: Swelling intensifies pain and when unchecked can result in neurovascular compromise. Administer narcotic analgesics. Avoid use of oral analgesics in individuals with possible operative lesions.
2. Remove constricting items such as jewelry, watches, and rings as soon as possible.
3. Apply cold packs to reduce swelling and also to reduce pain.
4. Elevate the affected extremity.

TABLE 169-1 Description of Salter-Harris Fractures

Salter Type	What Is Broken Off
I	The entire epiphysis
II	The entire epiphysis *along with* a portion of the metaphysis
III	A portion of the epiphysis
IV	A portion of the epiphysis *along with* a portion of the metaphysis
V	Compression injury of the epiphyseal plate (nothing is "broken off")

5. Withhold oral intake: Pending complete evaluation and treatment. A patient who does not require an operation may still require procedural sedation.
6. Reduce fracture deformity and dislocations: Application of gradual and steady longitudinal traction is sufficient to reduce most fractures. Reduction will decrease swelling and pain, relieve tension on neurovascular structures adjacent to the deformity, reduce the risk of converting a closed fracture to an open one, and restore circulation to a pulseless extremity. Techniques for dislocation reduction vary based upon the site of injury. The best results are achieved when the patient is relaxed and sedated.
7. Recognize injuries that require orthopedic consultation: Many orthopedic injuries can be treated in the ED and discharged to home with outpatient follow-up. Some injuries require inpatient management due to co-morbid health conditions or issues related to pain control or ambulatory dysfunction, such as hip fractures. Other injuries, such as open fractures, compartment syndrome, irreducible dislocations, circulatory compromise, and injuries needing surgical intervention, require direct communication and urgent consultation in the ED with the on-call orthopedic surgeon.
8. Splinting and immobilization: Reduces pain, facilitates healing, and helps to prevent re-injury of the affected extremity (see Table 169-2).

TABLE 169-2 Immobilization Devices and Uses

Immobilization Technique	Clinical Application
Shoulder immobilizer	Clavicle fracture Acromioclavicular separation Shoulder dislocation (postreduction) Humeral neck fracture
Sling	A variety of upper-extremity injuries, in conjunction with other immobilization techniques; may be used alone for nondisplaced or clinically suspected fracture of the radial head
Long-arm gutter	Elbow fracture other than nondisplaced radial head fracture Reduced elbow dislocation
Sugar-tong	Wrist or forearm fracture
Short-arm gutter	Metacarpal or proximal phalanx fracture. (Ulnar gutter for fourth or fifth ray; radial gutter for second [index] or third [middle] ray)
Thumb spica	Scaphoid fracture (proven or suspected) Thumb metacarpal or proximal thumb phalanx fracture
Knee immobilizer	Fracture or reduced subluxation of patella Knee dislocation, postreduction (temporary) Tibial plateau fracture Knee ligament injury Suspected meniscal tear (provided the knee can be fully extended)

(Continued)

TABLE 169-2 Immobilization Devices and Uses (Continued)

Immobilization Technique	Clinical Application
Posterior ankle mold (consider above-the-knee extension and/or adjunctive use of ankle sugar-tong for unstable ankle injuries)	Ankle dislocation or fracture-dislocation Unstable ankle fracture (high distal fibular fracture or medial and/or posterior malleolar fracture) Widened medial mortise (indicates disruption of stabilizing medial structures) Metatarsal fracture (alternative immobilization dressings may be used)
Ankle stirrup	Simple ankle sprain Stable lateral malleolus fracture (below the superior border of the talus) without other ankle involvement (no medial swelling or tenderness, posterior malleolus intact)
Hard-soled shoe	Toe fracture Some metatarsal fractures
Short-leg walking boot	Some toe or foot contusions or fractures where weightbearing is allowed

FURTHER READING

For Further reading in *Tintinalli's Emergency Medicine: A Comprehensive Study Guide*, 8th ed., see Chapter 267, "Initial Evaluation and Management of Orthopedic Injuries," by Jeffrey S. Menkes.

CHAPTER 170

Hand and Wrist Injuries

Robert R. Cooney

HAND INJURIES

The hand is innervated by the median, ulnar, and radial nerves. Motor function of the median nerve can be screened by flexing the thumb distal phalanx against resistance, the ulnar nerve by spreading the fingers against resistance, and the radial nerve by maintaining extension of the finger MCP joints against resistance. Sensory innervation (Fig. 170-1) is best screened by the presence of normal two-point discrimination (<5 mm). Injuries requiring hand surgery consultation are listed in Tables 170-1 and 170-2.

Tendon injuries can be easily missed. Up to 90% of a tendon can be lacerated with preserved range of motion without resistance, so test function against resistance and compare to the uninjured side. Pain along the course of the tendon suggests a partial laceration even if strength is normal. Although extensor tendon repair has often been performed by the emergency physician, there is a movement toward operative repair. Flexor tendon repair should be performed by the hand surgeon. It is acceptable to stabilize the injury by closing the skin and splinting until definitive repair by the hand surgeon. Follow-up and rehabilitation of all tendon injuries are necessary, even those not requiring repair.

Mallet finger results when complete rupture of the extensor tendon occurs at the level of the distal phalanx. On examination, the distal interphalangeal (DIP) joint is flexed at 40°. Splint the DIP joint in slight hyperextension.

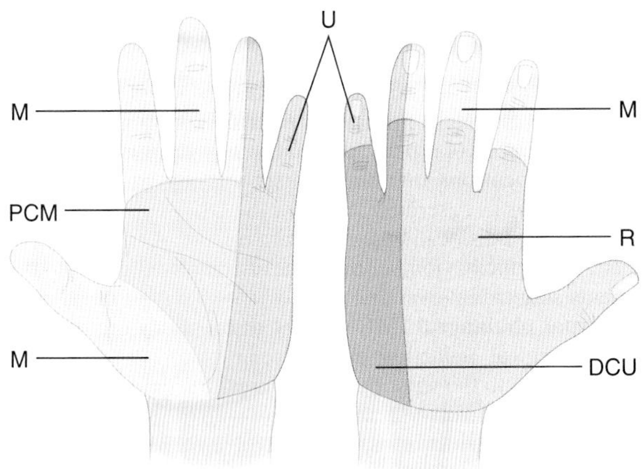

FIGURE 170-1. The cutaneous nerve supply in the hand. DCU, dorsal cutaneous branch of ulnar nerve; M, median nerve; PCM, palmar cutaneous branch of median nerve; R, superficial radial nerve; U, ulnar nerve.

TABLE 170-1 Immediate Hand Surgery Consultation Guidelines
Vascular injury with signs of tissue ischemia or poorly controlled hemorrhage
Irreducible dislocations
Grossly contaminated wounds
Severe crush injury
Open fracture
Compartment syndrome
High-pressure injection injury
Hand/finger amputation

TABLE 170-2 Delayed Hand Surgery Consultation Guidelines
Extensor/flexor tendon laceration
Flexor digitorum profundus rupture (Jersey finger)
Extensor digitorum rupture (mallet finger)
Nerve injury (proximal to mid middle phalanx)
Closed fractures
Dislocations
Ligamentous injuries with instability

Boutonniere deformity results from an injury at the dorsal surface of the proximal interphalangeal (PIP) joint that disrupts the extensor hood apparatus. Lateral bands of the extensor mechanism become flexors of the PIP joint and hyperextensors of the DIP joint. Splint the PIP joint in extension.

DIP joint dislocations are uncommon because of the firm attachment of skin and fibrous tissue to underlying bone. Dislocations are usually dorsal. Reduction is performed under digital block anesthesia. The dislocated phalanx is distracted using longitudinal traction, slightly hyperextended, then repositioned. Splint the joint in full extension. An irreducible joint may be from an entrapped volar plate, profundus tendon, or avulsion fracture.

PIP joint dislocations are usually dorsal with rupture of the volar plate. Closed reduction is as described above for the DIP joint. Splint the joint in 30° flexion. Lateral dislocation results from rupture of one of the collateral ligaments. An irreducible joint or evidence of complete ligamentous disruption warrants surgical intervention.

Metacarpal phalangeal (MCP) joint dislocations are usually dorsal and require surgical reduction due to volar plate entrapment. Attempt closed reduction with the wrist flexed and pressure applied to the proximal phalanx in a distal and volar direction. Splint with the MCP joint in flexion.

Thumb IP joint dislocations usually involve volar plate rupture and are often open. Closed reduction is as described above for the DIP joint. Place in a splint with 15° to 20° of flexion.

Thumb MCP dislocations are usually dorsal and involve volar plate rupture. Reduce by flexing and abducting the metacarpal and apply pressure directed distally to the base of the proximal phalanx. Place in a thumb spica splint.

Thumb MCP ulnar collateral ligament rupture (gamekeeper's or skier's thumb) results from forced radial abduction at the MCP joint, with the rupture occurring at the insertion on the proximal phalanx. The joint capsule and volar plate are usually involved. A complete tear is diagnosed when abduction stress on the proximal phalanx causes more than 30° to 35° of radial angulation relative to the metacarpal. Place in a thumb spica splint. Complete tears mandate surgical referral.

Distal phalanx fractures most commonly involve the tuft. These are associated with nail bed laceration. Place a volar or hairpin splint to the DIP joint. Avulsion fractures of the base often represent associated tendon involvement.

Proximal and middle phalanx fractures of the base and neck that are nondisplaced and stable can be treated with buddy taping. Transverse or spiral midshaft fractures or intraarticular fractures often require surgical fixation. Place a gutter splint with the MCP joint flexed at 70°, the IP joints in extension.

Metacarpal (MC) fractures most commonly involve the fourth or fifth MC neck (boxer's fracture). Skin lacerations over the fracture should raise concern for a "fight bite." Angulation more than 20° in the fourth MC, 40° in the fifth MC, or 15° in the second or third MC should be reduced. Place an ulnar gutter splint for fractures of the fourth or fifth MC and a radial gutter splint for fractures of the second or third MC with the wrist extended at 20° and the MCP joint flexed at 70°. Thumb MC fractures usually involve the base with intraarticular involvement (Bennett and Rolando fractures). Place in a thumb spica splint.

Compartment syndrome of the hand may result from crush injury or extravasation of IV fluids or radiocontrast media. The patient will complain of pain that is out of proportion to exam findings. On examination, the hand, at a resting position, is extended at the MCP joint and slightly flexed at the PIP joint. There is tense edema and pain with passive stretch of the involved compartment. This is an orthopedic emergency and the diagnosis is made clinically due to the difficulty in obtaining accurate compartment pressures.

High-pressure injection injury occurs when substances in a high pressure device (>2000 psi), such as grease, paint, or hydraulic fluid, are injected into the hand. Oil-based paint causes a severe tissue reaction that can result in ischemia and eventual need for amputation. Obtain hand and forearm radiographs searching for radiopaque substances and subcutaneous air. While it appears benign, this injury requires emergent surgical evaluation.

WRIST INJURIES

Scapholunate dissociation presents with wrist tenderness and swelling at the scapholunate joint. The PA radiograph demonstrates a space between the scaphoid and lunate that is >3 mm. Treat with a radial gutter splint and prompt referral.

Perilunate and lunate dislocations are best noted on lateral wrist radiograph. In both injuries, the normal alignment of the radius-lunate-capitate (the "3 C's" sign) is lost. With a perilunate dislocation, the lunate remains aligned with the radius, but the carpals are dislocated, usually dorsal to the lunate. With a lunate dislocation, the lunate dislocates volar to

TABLE 170-3 Summary of Carpal Bone Fractures and ED Management

Carpal Bone	Mechanism of Injury	Examination	Initial ED Management
Scaphoid	Fall on outstretched hand	Snuffbox tenderness. Pain with radial deviation and flexion	Short arm, thumb spica, in dorsiflexion with radial deviation
Triquetrum	Avulsion fracture—twisting of hand against resistance or hyperextension Body fracture—direct trauma	Tenderness at the dorsum of the wrist, distal to the ulnar styloid	Short arm, sugar-tong splint
Lunate	Fall on outstretched hand	Tenderness at shallow indentation of the middorsum of the wrist, ulnar and distal to Lister tubercle	Short arm, thumb spica splint
Trapezium	Direct blow to thumb; force to wrist while dorsiflexed and radially deviated	Painful thumb movement and weak pinch strength Snuffbox tenderness	Short arm, thumb spica splint
Pisiform	Fall directed on the hypothenar eminence	Tender pisiform, prominent at the base of the hypothenar eminence	Short arm, volar splint in 30° of flexion and ulnar deviation
Hamate	Interrupted swing of a golf club, bat, or racquet	Tenderness at the hook of the hamate, just distal and radial to the pisiform	Short arm, volar wrist splint with fourth and fifth metacarpal joints in flexion
Capitate	Forceful dorsiflexion of the hand with radial impact	Tenderness over the capitate just proximal to the third metacarpal	Short arm, volar wrist splint
Trapezoid	Axial load onto the index metacarpal	Tenderness over the radial aspect of the base of the index metacarpal	Short arm, thumb spica splint

the radius, but the remainder of the carpus aligns with the radius. Lunate dislocation on PA radiograph has a triangular shape, the "piece of pie" sign, and on lateral view, the "spilled teacup" sign. Emergent consult for closed reduction or surgical repair is indicated.

Carpal bone fractures are managed as summarized in Table 170-3. The scaphoid is the most common carpal bone fractured. Fracture of the scaphoid, lunate, or capitate can cause avascular necrosis of the bone. Scaphoid and lunate fractures are often not detected on plain radiographs, so ED diagnosis and treatment should be based on clinical findings alone.

Colles, Smith, and Barton fractures involve the distal radius at the metaphysis (Table 170-4). Most of these fractures can be treated with closed reduction and a sugar-tong splint.

Radial styloid fracture can produce carpal instability with scapholunate dissociation as major carpal ligaments insert here. Splint the wrist in mild flexion and ulnar deviation.

TABLE 170-4 Radiographic Appearance of Distal Radius Fractures

Colles' fracture Dorsal angulation of the plane of the distal radius Distal radius fragment is displaced proximally and dorsally Radial displacement of the carpus Ulnar styloid may be fractured
Smith's fracture Volar angulation of the plane of the distal radius Distal radius fragment is displaced proximally and volarly Radial displacement of the carpus The fracture line extends obliquely from the dorsal surface to the volar surface 1 to 2 cm proximal to the articular surface
Barton's fracture Volar and proximal displacement of a large fragment of radial articular surface Volar displacement of the carpus Radial styloid may be fractured

Ulnar styloid fracture may result in radioulnar joint instability. Place an ulnar gutter splint with the wrist in neutral position and slight ulnar deviation.

FURTHER READING

For further reading in *Tintinalli's Emergency Medicine: A Comprehensive Study Guide*, 8th ed., see Chapter 268, "Injuries to the Hand and Digits," by Moira Davenport and Peter Tang; Chapter 269, "Wrist Injuries," by Robert Escarza, Maurice F. Loeffel ,III, and Dennis T. Uehara.

CHAPTER 171 Forearm and Elbow Injuries

Sandra L. Najarian

SOFT TISSUE INJURIES

Biceps and Triceps Tendon Ruptures

Clinical Features

Patients with proximal long-head biceps tendon ruptures typically describe a "snap" or "pop" and complain of pain in the anterior shoulder. Examination reveals tenderness, swelling, and crepitus over the bicipital groove in the anterior shoulder. A mid-arm "ball" (the distally retracted biceps) appears when the elbow is flexed. Elbow flexion strength is maintained due to the preserved action of the brachialis and supinators. This is in contrast to distal biceps tendon rupture where elbow flexion and supination is weak. Examination of distal biceps rupture reveals swelling, ecchymosis, tenderness, and inability to palpate the tendon in the antecubital fossa. With the patient seated, the elbow flexed 60 to 80 degrees, and forearm resting on the patient's lap, the examiner squeezes the muscle belly of the biceps causing the forearm to supinate (biceps squeeze test). If no supination is noted, then this is a positive test indicating a distal biceps tendon rupture. Triceps tendon ruptures are rare, and the majority occur distally. Patients present with pain, swelling, and tenderness proximal to the olecranon; a sulcus with a proximal mass (the proximally retracted triceps tendon) may be palpable. Forearm extension is weak. A modified Thompson test can be used to assess triceps function. With the arm supported, elbow flexed at 90 degrees, and forearm hanging in a relaxed position, squeezing the triceps muscle should produce extension of the forearm unless a complete tear is present.

Diagnosis and Differential

Diagnosis is clinical. Obtain radiographs to exclude an associated avulsion fracture.

Emergency Department Care and Disposition

Treatment includes sling, ice, analgesics, and referral to an orthopedic surgeon for definitive management. Complete tendon tears in young active individuals often require surgical repair.

Overuse Syndromes

Clinical Features

Lateral epicondylitis or "tennis elbow" is more common than medial epicondylitis or "golfer's elbow." Lateral epicondylitis affects the forearm and wrist extensors, and medial epicondylitis affects the forearm and wrist flexors. Patients with medial epicondylitis may develop an ulnar neuropathy. Both syndromes result from repetitive activity involving these muscle groups.

Diagnosis and Differential

Diagnosis is clinical. Radiographs may help in ruling out an associated avulsion fracture of the lateral or medial epicondyle.

Emergency Department Care and Disposition

Management is conservative including rest, ice, anti-inflammatory medications, and bracing. Occupational therapy can be useful in treating these syndromes. Surgery is reserved for refractory cases.

ELBOW DISLOCATIONS

Clinical Features

The majority of elbow dislocations are posterolateral and often occur as a result of a fall on an outstretched hand. On examination, the patient holds the elbow in 45 degrees of flexion. Significant swelling of the elbow often obscures the olecranon, which is directed posteriorly. Neurovascular assessment is essential (Table 171-1). An open dislocation, absence of radial pulse before reduction, and presence of systemic injuries are all factors associated with arterial injury.

Diagnosis and Differential

Radiographs confirm the diagnosis. The lateral view reveals both the ulna and radius displaced posterior. The AP view reveals either medial or lateral displacement of the ulna and radius with maintenance of their normal relationship to each other. The presence of associated fractures, especially to the radial head and coronoid process, can render the elbow joint unstable and complicate treatment.

Emergency Department Care and Disposition

The goals of treatment are reduction with procedural sedation and recognition of neurovascular complications, associated fractures, and postreduction instability. Intra-articular lidocaine may provide analgesia for closed reduction.

1. Several methods can be used for reduction. With the first two-person method (Fig. 171-1), start by placing the patient supine, and apply gentle longitudinal traction on the wrist and forearm while an assistant applies countertraction on the arm. Correct any medial or lateral

TABLE 171-1 Sensory and Motor Function Testing of the Radial, Median, and Ulnar Nerves

	Radial	Median	Ulnar
Test for sensory function	Dorsum of the thumb and index web space	Two-point discrimination over the tip of the index finger	Two-point discrimination over the little finger
Test for motor function	Extend both wrist and fingers against resistance	"OK" sign with thumb and index finger; abduction of the thumb (recurrent branch)	Abduct index finger against resistance

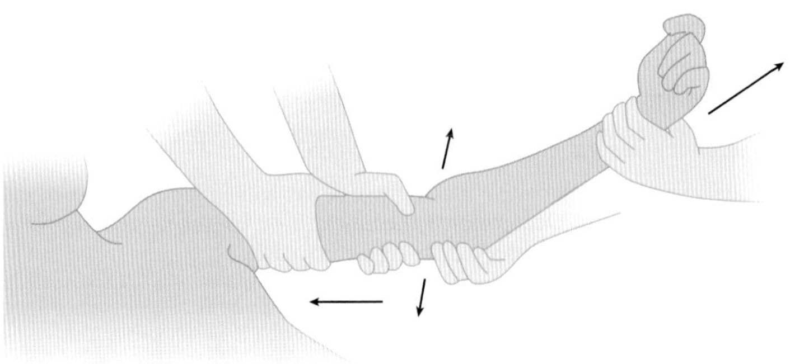

A

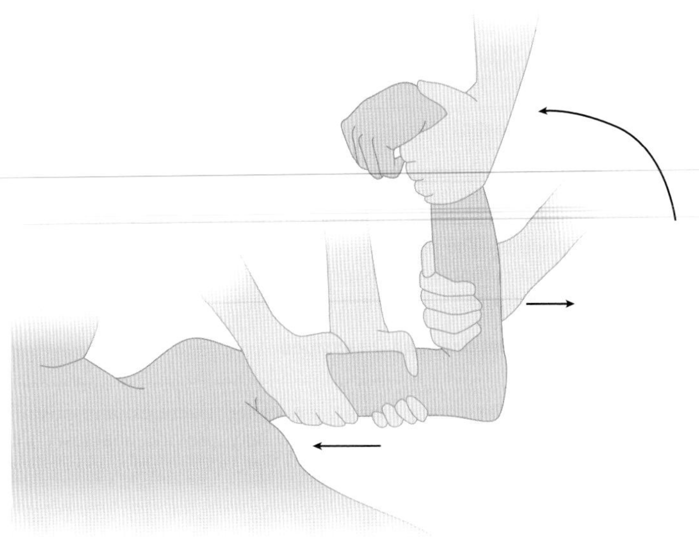

B

FIGURE 171-1. Traction and flexion method of reducing a posterior elbow dislocation. **A.** Side-to-side manipulation is used to correct medial or lateral displacement. **B.** The elbow is then flexed while maintaining longitudinal traction.

displacement with the other hand. Then, apply downward pressure on the proximal forearm to disengage the coronoid process from the olecranon. A palpable clunk indicates a successful reduction. With the second two-person method (Fig. 171-2), start with the patient supine with the arm adducted across the torso and elbow slightly flexed. The patient may also be positioned prone with the affected arm abducted and the elbow slightly flexed. The assistant applies longitudinal traction

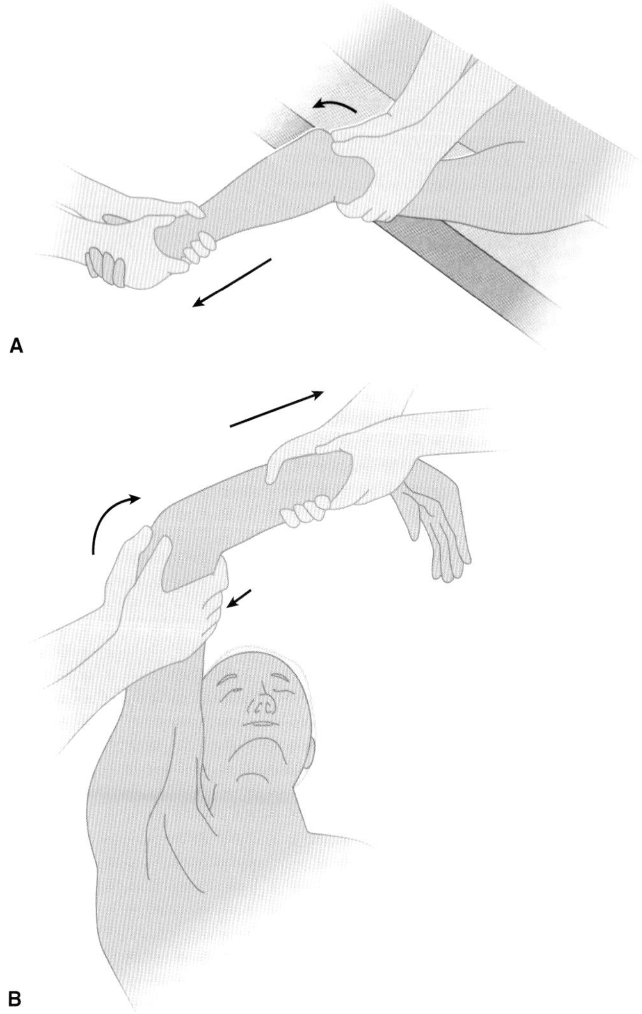

FIGURE 171-2. Olecranon manipulation method of reducing a posterior elbow dislocation with the patient positioned prone **(A)** or supine **(B)**.

on the wrist and forearm, while the operator holds the elbow with both thumbs behind the olecranon. Apply firm pressure with thumbs to push the olecranon over the trochlea and back into position. The single-person method (Fig. 171-3) starts with the patient prone and the affected arm on the stretcher with the elbow flexed over the edge of the stretcher. Place a pillow or folded blanket under the humerus and hang a 5-lb weight to the wrist. The elbow should spontaneously reduce over several minutes. Gentle pressure to the olecranon can aid the reduction.

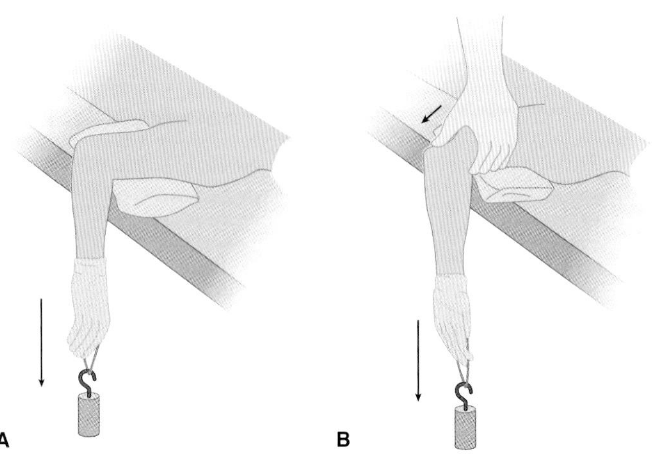

FIGURE 171-3. **A**. Hanging arm method of reducing a posterior elbow dislocation. **B**. Gentle manipulation can be applied to the olecranon, if necessary.

2. After the reduction, range the elbow fully to assess stability.
3. Assess neurovascular status after reduction and over a period of observation.
4. Obtain post reduction films.
5. Immobilize the elbow in a long arm posterior splint with the elbow in slightly less than 90 degrees of flexion and the forearm in mild pronation. Arrange for close orthopedic follow-up.
6. Immediate orthopedic consultation is necessary for patients with instability, neurovascular compromise, or open dislocations. Admission may be necessary to monitor neurovascular status.

ELBOW FRACTURES

Clinical Features

Radial head fractures present with pain, swelling, and tenderness over the lateral elbow, and inability to fully extend the elbow. Supracondylar and intercondylar fractures present with significant swelling, tenderness, and limited range of motion at the elbow. Supracondylar fractures may resemble a posterior elbow dislocation. Olecranon fractures present with pain, swelling, and crepitus over the posterior elbow. Epicondyle, condyle, trochlear, capitellum, and coronoid fractures are uncommon and can occur in association with other elbow injuries such as dislocations. An Essex–Lopresti lesion, a radial head fracture with associated distal radioulnar joint dissociation, presents with wrist and forearm pain in addition to lateral elbow pain. A neurovascular assessment is essential in all elbow fractures. Potential complications of supracondylar fractures are numerous (Table 171-2). A decreased or absent radial pulse is common in children and often secondary to brachial artery injury, even if the hand appears warm and perfused. Signs of Volkmann ischemic contracture

TABLE 171-2 Complications of Supracondylar Fractures

Early complications	**Neurologic** Radial nerve injury Median nerve (anterior interosseous branch) injury Ulnar nerve injury **Vascular** Volkmann's ischemic contracture (compartment syndrome of the forearm)
Late complications	Nonunion Malunion Myositis ossificans Loss of motion

(compartment syndrome of the forearm) include refusal to open the hand, pain with passive extension of the fingers, and forearm tenderness. Absence of radial pulse alone does not constitute ischemia unless accompanied by these other signs.

Diagnosis and Differential

Fracture lines may not be visible on standard AP and lateral radiographs of the elbow. Abnormal fat pads, a visible posterior fat pad, or a prominent anterior fat pad ("sail sign") may be the only evidence of injury. Disruption of the radiocapitellar line may be another clue to injury. A line drawn from the center of the radial shaft should transect the radial head and capitellum in all views. On the lateral view, a line drawn along the anterior cortex of the humerus (anterior humeral line) should transect the posterior two-thirds of the capitellum. If the anterior humeral line transects the anterior one-third of the capitellum, then this is suggestive of a distal humerus or supracondylar fracture. CT imaging can be considered for certain elbow fractures, such as coronoid or comminuted intra-articular fractures.

Emergency Department Care and Disposition

Immobilization in a splint and orthopedic referral are appropriate for nondisplaced fractures. Nondisplaced radial head fractures with no mobility restrictions are treated with sling immobilization. Immediate orthopedic consultation is warranted for all displaced fractures, open fractures, and evidence of neurovascular compromise. Admit patients who have displaced fractures with significant swelling for observation of neurovascular status.

FOREARM FRACTURES

Clinical Features

Both bone forearm fractures present with swelling, tenderness, and deformity of the forearm. Isolated ulna or radius fractures present with localized swelling and tenderness. Monteggia fracture-dislocation, a fracture of the proximal third of the ulna with a radial head dislocation, presents with significant pain and swelling over the elbow. Galeazzi fracture-dislocation, a fracture of the distal radius with an associated distal radioulnar joint dislocation, presents with localized tenderness and swelling over the distal radius and wrist.

Diagnosis and Differential

AP and lateral radiographs confirm the diagnosis. In a Monteggia fracture, the radiocapitellar line is disrupted, and the apex of the ulna fracture points in the direction of the radial head dislocation. In a Galeazzi fracture, the distal radioulnar joint space is widened on the AP view, and the ulna is displaced dorsally on the lateral view.

Emergency Department Care and Disposition

Treat nondisplaced fractures, torus or greenstick fractures with less than 15 degrees angulation with long arm splint immobilization and referral to orthopedics. Immediate orthopedic consultation is necessary for all displaced fractures. Closed reduction is often adequate for both bone fractures in children. Open reduction and internal fixation are usually required for displaced fractures in adults and for Monteggia and Galeazzi fracture-dislocations (Table 171-3).

TABLE 171-3 Immobilization and Follow-Up Guidelines

Injury	Splint	Referral
Soft tissue injuries		
Biceps tendon rupture	Sling immobilization	1 week
Triceps tendon rupture	Sling immobilization	1 week
Lateral/medial epicondylitis	Forearm counterforce brace	2–4 week PRN
Elbow dislocation		
Stable/postreduction	Long arm posterior splint, forearm in pronation	1 day
Unstable/postreduction	Long arm posterior splint (presurgical stabilization)	Immediate
Irreducible	Long arm posterior splint (presurgical stabilization)	Immediate
Elbow fractures		
Distal humerus nondisplaced	Long arm posterior splint, forearm neutral	1 week
Supracondylar	Long arm posterior splint (presurgical stabilization)	Immediate
Intercondylar	Long arm posterior splint, forearm neutral	1–2 days
Lateral condyle/epicondyle		
Nondisplaced	Long arm posterior splint, forearm in supination, wrist extended	1–2 days
Displaced	Long arm posterior splint (presurgical stabilization)	Immediate
Medial condyle/epicondyle		
Nondisplaced	Long arm posterior splint, forearm in pronation, wrist flexed	1-2 days
Displaced	Long arm posterior splint (presurgical stabilization)	Immediate
Articular surface	Long arm posterior splint, forearm neutral	1-2 days

(Continued)

TABLE 171-3 Immobilization and Follow-Up Guidelines (Continued)

Injury	Splint	Referral
Coronoid		
Nondisplaced or minimally displaced	Long arm posterior splint, elbow past 90 degrees, forearm in supination	1–2 days
Markedly displaced or unstable	Long arm posterior splint (presurgical stabilization)	Immediate
Olecranon	Long arm posterior splint, forearm neutral	<24 h
Radial head		
Nondisplaced	Sling immobilization with early range of motion	1 week
Displaced or range of motion block	Long arm posterior splint	<24 h
Forearm fractures		
Both bones		
Pediatric		
Greenstick	Long arm posterior splint	1 week
Displaced	Long arm posterior splint (prereduction stabilization)	Immediate
Adult		
Nondisplaced	Anteroposterior long arm splint	1 week
Displaced	Long arm posterior splint (presurgical stabilization)	<24 h
Isolated ulna shaft	Long arm posterior splint, forearm neutral *or* sugar tong splint if stable and nondisplaced	1 week
Proximal two thirds of radius	Long arm posterior splint, forearm neutral	1 week
Monteggia's	Long arm posterior splint (presurgical stabilization)	Immediate
Galeazzi's	Long arm posterior splint (presurgical stabilization)	Immediate

FURTHER READING

For further reading in *Tintinalli's Emergency Medicine: A Comprehensive Study Guide*, 8th ed., see Chapter 270, "Elbow and Forearm Injuries," by Yvonne C. Chow

CHAPTER 172

Shoulder and Humerus Injuries

Sandra L. Najarian

STERNOCLAVICULAR SPRAINS AND DISLOCATIONS

Clinical Features

Patients with simple sprains have pain and tenderness localized to the joint, whereas patients with dislocations have severe pain, which is exacerbated by arm motion and lying supine. In anterior dislocations, the medial clavicle is visibly prominent and palpable anterior to the sternum. In posterior dislocations, the medial clavicle is less visible and often not palpable. Symptoms of hoarseness, dysphagia, dyspnea, upper extremity paresthesia, or weakness may indicate life-threatening injuries to mediastinal structures, such as pneumothorax or compression or laceration of surrounding great vessels, trachea, and esophagus.

Diagnosis and Differential

Computed tomography (CT) is the imaging test of choice. However, the contrast may be needed to detect injury to adjacent mediastinal structures. Consider septic arthritis in the nontraumatic patient, especially in injection drug users.

Emergency Department Care and Disposition

Treatment for sternoclavicular sprains and uncomplicated anterior dislocations includes ice, analgesics, and sling immobilization. Attempted closed reduction is not necessary as this injury is often unstable. Posterior dislocations require immediate orthopedic consultation for open reduction and internal fixation.

CLAVICLE AND SCAPULA FRACTURES

Clinical Features

Patients with clavicle fractures present with pain, swelling, and tenderness over the clavicle. The scapula is a well-protected bone; therefore, fractures usually occur in association with injuries to the ipsilateral lung, thorax, and shoulder girdle. Patients have pain and localized tenderness over the scapula, hold their arm in adduction, and resist any arm movement.

Diagnosis and Differential

Routine radiographs may miss some clavicle and scapular fractures. CT can confirm the diagnosis as well as identify any associated pathology.

Emergency Department and Disposition

The majority of clavicle and scapula fractures can be managed conservatively with sling immobilization, ice, and analgesics. Early range-of-motion exercises are important. Orthopedic consultation is warranted for clavicle fractures that are open, have neurovascular compromise, or have persistent skin tenting. Clavicle fractures that are severely comminuted or displaced may benefit from operative intervention so consider early referral to orthopedics in those instances. Presence of a scapula fracture mandates investigation for associated intrathoracic injuries. Displaced glenoid articular fractures, angulated glenoid neck fractures, and certain acromial and coracoid fractures may require surgical intervention.

ACROMIOCLAVICULAR JOINT INJURIES

Clinical Features

Acromioclavicular joint injuries range from mild sprain to complete disruption of all ligaments that attach the scapula and clavicle. AC joint injuries occur from a direct force to the joint with the arm adducted or from a fall on the outstretched hand with an indirect force transmitted to the joint. Classification of these injuries and their physical findings are described in Table 172-1.

Diagnosis and Differential

Diagnosis is clinical. Acromioclavicular radiographs can help determine the severity of the injury and identify any associated fractures.

TABLE 172-1 Classification and Physical Findings in Acromioclavicular Joint Injuries

Type	Injury	Mechanism	Radiograph/Exam
I	Sprained acromioclavicular ligaments	Type I	Radiograph: Normal Exam: Tenderness over acromioclavicular joint
II	Acromioclavicular ligaments ruptured; coracoclavicular ligaments sprained	Type II	Radiograph: Slight widening of acromioclavicular joint; clavicle elevated 25%–50% above acromion; may be slight widening of the coracoclavicular interspace Exam: Tenderness and mild step-off deformity of acromioclavicular joint
III	Acromioclavicular ligaments ruptured; coracoclavicular ligaments ruptured; deltoid trapezius muscles detached	Type III	Clavicle elevated 100% above acromion; coracoclavicular interspace widened 25%–100% Exam: Distal end of clavicle prominent; shoulder droops

(Continued)

TABLE 172-1 Classification and Physical Findings in Acromioclavicular Joint Injuries (Continued)

Type	Injury	Mechanism	Radiograph/Exam
IV	Rupture of all supporting structures; clavicle displaced posteriorly in or through the trapezius	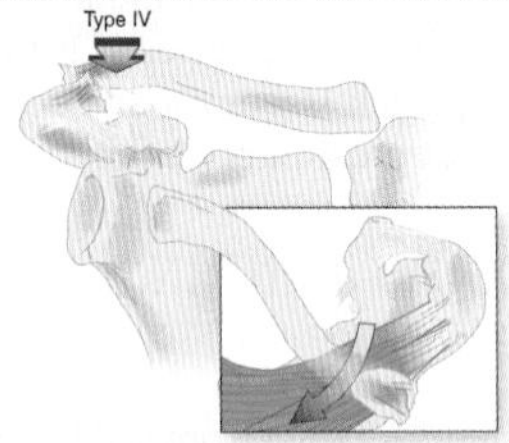	Radiograph: May appear similar to type II and III; axillary radiograph required to visualize posterior dislocation Exam: Possible posterior displacement of clavicle
V	Rupture of all supporting structures (more severe form of type III injury)	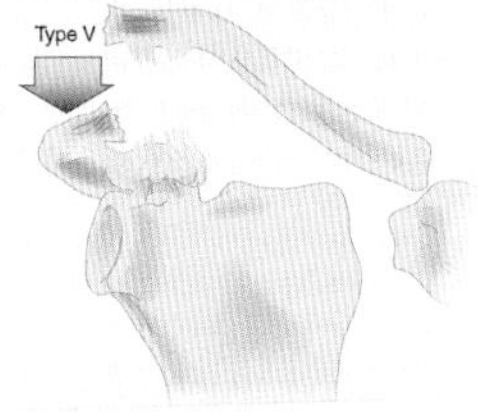	Radiograph: Acromioclavicular joint dislocated; generally 200%–300% disparity of coracoclavicular interspace compared to normal shoulder Exam: More pain; gross deformity of clavicle
VI	Acromioclavicular ligaments disrupted; coracoclavicular ligaments may be disrupted; deltoid and trapezius muscles disrupted	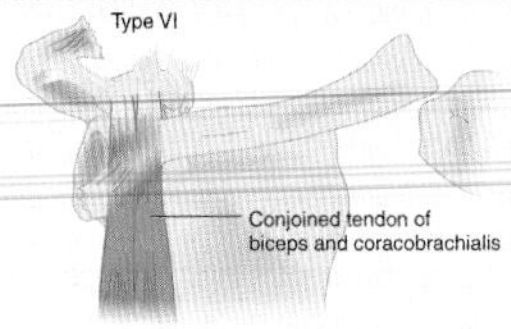	Radiograph: Acromioclavicular joint dislocated; clavicle displaced inferiorly Exam: Severe swelling; multiple associated injuries

Emergency Department Care and Disposition

Treatment for type I and II injuries includes sling immobilization, rest, ice, and analgesics. Early range-of-motion exercises are recommended at 7 to 14 days post injury. Treatment for type III is controversial, but the trend favors conservative management with sling immobilization rather than operative management. Treatment for type IV through VI is operative and warrants orthopedic consultation.

GLENOHUMERAL JOINT DISLOCATION

Clinical Features

Anterior shoulder dislocations, the most common type of shoulder dislocations, are generally the result of an abduction, extension, and external rotation force on the arm. Patients present with pain, holding their arm in slight abduction and external rotation. The affected shoulder loses its normal contour. Patients resist any adduction or internal rotation. The humeral head is sometimes palpable anteriorly. Decreased pinprick sensation over the skin of the lateral deltoid is a sign of axillary nerve injury. Posterior shoulder dislocations often result from an indirect, abduction and internal rotational force or from a direct blow to the anterior shoulder. Patients present with pain, anterior flattening of the normal shoulder contour, and prominence of the posterior shoulder. Patients are unable to externally rotate or abduct the affected arm. Inferior shoulder dislocations (luxatio erecta) result from a hyper abduction force. Patients present with their arm completely abducted, elbow flexed, and hand resting on or behind their head. The humeral head is palpable on the lateral chest wall. Superior shoulder dislocations are very rare.

Diagnosis and Differential

Anteroposterior and scapular "Y" view radiographs confirm the type of dislocation and identify any associated fractures. The presence of minor fractures, such as Hill–Sachs lesions (humeral head defects) or Bankart lesions (glenoid labral defects), does not change ED management. Consider omitting prereduction radiographs in patients, who have a history of recurrent shoulder dislocation, presenting with signs and symptoms of a recurrence in the absence of trauma.

Emergency Department Care and Disposition

Reduction techniques include traction, leverage, and scapular manipulation. Be familiar with at least two or three techniques. The most common techniques are detailed below. Procedural sedation is recommended; however, an intraarticular injection of 10 to 20 mL of 1% lidocaine can facilitate reduction and may obviate the need for sedation.

1. **Modified Hippocratic technique.** This method uses traction-countertraction. Place the patient supine with their arm abducted and the elbow flexed 90°. A sheet is placed across the thorax of the patient and tied around the waist of the assistant. Another sheet is placed around the patient's flexed elbow and the clinician's waist. Gradually apply traction to the patient's proximal forearm while the assistant provides countertraction. Gentle internal and external rotation may help the reduction.
2. **Snowbird technique.** This is another version of the traction-countertraction technique where the patient is sitting and the elbow is flexed to 90°. A belt or strap is placed around the proximal forearm with the loop of the belt hanging. The clinician can step on the belt loop to provide traction using downward pressure while an assistant uses a sheet around the patient's torso to provide countertraction. Gentle external rotation of the arm can aid the reduction.
3. **Stimson technique.** Place the patient prone with the affected arm hanging over the side of the stretcher. Attach at 10-lb weight to the wrist. Inject intraarticular lidocaine. Reduction generally occurs in 20 to 30 minutes after the muscles have completely relaxed.
4. **Scapular manipulation technique.** Scapular manipulation accomplishes reduction by repositioning the glenoid fossa rather than the humeral head. The first step is to apply traction to the patient's arm held in 90° of forward flexion. This can be accomplished in the prone position or in a seated position with an assistant applying traction. Position the arm in slight external rotation. Push the scapular tip as far medially

as possible while stabilizing the superior aspect of the scapula with the other hand. A small amount of dorsal displacement of the scapula tip is recommended.

5. **External rotation (Kocher's) technique.** Place the patient supine with the arm adducted to the side. With the patient's elbow flexed to 90°, slowly and gently externally rotate the arm. No traction is applied. Reduction is subtle and usually occurs before reaching the coronal plane.
6. **Milch technique.** With the patient supine, slowly abduct and externally rotate the arm to the overhead position. Apply gentle traction with the elbow fully extended. If reduction is not achieved, attempt to manipulate the humeral head into the glenoid fossa with the free hand.
7. **Cunningham technique.** With the patient seated and the clinician sitting to the side of the patient, have the patient rest their hand of the affected extremity on the clinician's shoulder. The affected arm should be fully adducted with the elbow flexed. The clinician then gently massages the trapezius and deltoid, which helps relax the patient. It is important for the patient to remain seated in an upright position with their scapula and shoulders retracted as much as possible. Continue to massage the biceps at mid-humeral level as the patient elevates and shrugs or retracts their shoulders. Once the patient is relaxed, the humerus will reduce back into place.

Once reduced, assess neurovascular status and provide sling immobilization in order to maintain the shoulder in adduction and internal rotation. Post reduction radiographs are useful for confirmation and documentation of successful reduction. Urgent orthopedic follow-up is necessary. Complications include recurrence, rotator cuff tears, humeral head defects, glenoid labral defects, and neurovascular injuries. Early operative repair may decrease the incidence of recurrence.

HUMERUS FRACTURES

Clinical Features

Patients with proximal humeral fractures have pain, swelling, tenderness, ecchymosis, and crepitus about the shoulder. Range of motion is severely limited; patients hold their arm closely against the chest wall. Patients with humeral shaft fractures present with pain, swelling, localized tenderness, limited mobility, and crepitus on palpation. Shortening of the arm can be seen in displaced fractures. A careful neurovascular exam is essential. Injuries to the axillary nerve and artery are common in proximal humerus fractures. The radial nerve is most frequently injured in humeral shaft fractures and manifests as weak wrist extension, wrist drop, or altered sensation in the dorsal web space of the thumb index web space.

Diagnosis and Differential

Radiographs confirm the diagnosis. The Neer classification system divides the proximal humerus into four parts (articular surface of the humeral head, greater tubercle, lesser tubercle, and diaphysis of the humerus) and is used to guide treatment.

Emergency Department Care and Disposition

Proximal humerus fractures that are nondisplaced or one-part fractures (displaced <1 cm or angulated <45°) require sling immobilization, ice, analgesics, and orthopedic referral. Humeral shaft fractures that are nondisplaced require a coaptation splint (sugar tong), hanging cast, or functional bracing. In addition, humeral shaft fractures that have less than 20° angulation in the sagittal plan, less than 30° of varus or valgus deformity, and are shortened less than 2 cm can be managed conservatively. Multipart proximal humeral fractures, significantly displaced or angulated shaft fractures, open fractures, or fractures with neurovascular injuries require immediate orthopedic consultation.

BRACHIAL PLEXUS INJURIES

Clinical Features

Traumatic brachial plexus injuries are the most common form of plexus injuries, often resulting from penetrating, compression, or closed traction mechanisms. Injuries can be classified into supraclavicular (roots and trunks) or infraclavicular (cords and terminal nerve) injuries. Patients complain of constant, burning arm pain and will have sensory and motor deficits. Patients may have significant swelling and soft tissue injury to the neck and shoulder girdle. Horner's syndrome may be present if the adjacent ganglions are damaged. Unless the patient is responsive, the neurologic impairment is often not appreciated clinically until after the initial stabilization and treatment. Figure 172-1 demonstrates the sensory distributions of the cervical roots and peripheral nerves.

Diagnosis

Diagnosis is largely clinical. MRI and CT myelography are frequently obtained. Electromyography and nerve conduction velocity studies can aid in the diagnosis. Sometimes surgical exploration is necessary.

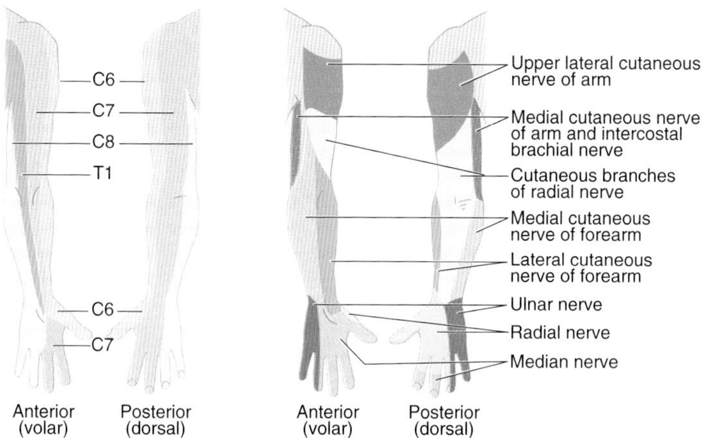

FIGURE 172-1. Sensory distribution of the brachial plexus.

Emergency Department Care and Disposition

The location and extent of nerve damage guides treatment and determines prognosis. It is important to be able to recognize this injury and refer appropriately.

FURTHER READING

For further reading in *Tintinalli's Emergency Medicine: A Comprehensive Study Guide*, 8th ed., see Chapter 271, "Shoulder and Humerus Injuries," by Lars Petter Bjoernsen and Alexander Ebinger.

CHAPTER 173

Pelvis, Hip, and Femur Injuries

Jeffrey G. Norvell

PELVIC INJURIES

Clinical Features

Signs and symptoms of pelvic injuries vary from local pain and tenderness to pelvic instability and severe shock. Examine the patient for pain, pelvic instability, deformities, lacerations, ecchymoses, and hematomas. Avoid excessive movement of unstable fractures as this could produce further injury and cause additional blood loss. Rectal examination may reveal displacement of the prostate or rectal injury. Blood at the urethral meatus suggests urethral injury. A vaginal speculum examination may be indicated to detect lacerations that would suggest an open fracture. If a pelvic fracture is found, assume associated intraabdominal, retroperitoneal, gynecologic, or urologic injuries exist until proven otherwise.

Diagnosis and Differential

In patients with a suspected pelvic fracture, obtain a standard anteroposterior (AP) pelvis radiograph to evaluate for bony injury. Other radiographic views include lateral views, AP views of the hemipelvis, internal and external oblique views of the hemipelvis, or inlet and outlet views of the pelvis. CT is superior to pelvic radiographs for identifying pelvic fractures and evaluating pelvic ring instability. Therefore, consider CT if there is a high suspicion for fracture but negative pelvic radiographs. In an unstable blunt trauma patient, use an AP pelvic radiograph to identify a pelvic fracture quickly, allowing for emergent stabilization maneuvers and therapeutic interventions. Routine pelvic radiographs are not needed in stable trauma patients who will undergo an emergent CT of the abdomen and pelvis.

Pelvic fractures include those that involve a break in the pelvic ring, fractures of a single bone without a break in the pelvic ring, and acetabular fractures. Single bone fractures are described in Table 173-1.

Acetabular fractures are commonly associated with lateral compression forces or hip dislocations and can be diagnosed with pelvis radiographs and Judet views. CT is more sensitive than radiography in detecting acetabular injury and is helpful in preoperative planning.

Emergency Department Care and Disposition

1. Due to associated hemorrhage and other injuries, patients with pelvic fractures may need resuscitation with crystalloid and blood products.
2. Stabilize an unstable pelvic fracture with a pelvic binding device or bedsheet to stabilize fracture ends.
3. In hemodynamically unstable patients, evaluate for other locations of bleeding such as the thorax and the peritoneal cavity using a chest radiograph and the focused abdominal sonogram for trauma (FAST) examination.

TABLE 173-1 Avulsion and Single Bone Fractures

Fracture	Description/ Mechanism of Injury	Clinical Findings/ Associated Injuries	Treatment	Disposition and Follow-Up
Iliac wing (Duverney) fracture	Direct trauma, usually lateral to medial	Swelling, tenderness over iliac wing; abdominal pain; ileus; acetabular fractures; serious injury infrequent	Analgesics, non-weight-bearing until hip abductors pain-free, usually nonoperative	Discharge with orthopedic follow-up in 1–2 weeks; admit for open fracture or concerning abdominal examination
Single ramus of pubis or ischium	Fall or direct trauma in elderly; exercise-induced stress fracture in young or in pregnant women	Local pain and tenderness; may have inability to ambulate	Analgesics, crutches	Discharge with PCP or orthopedic follow-up in 1–2 weeks
Ischium body	External trauma or from fall in sitting position; least common pelvic fracture	Local pain and tenderness; pain with hamstring movement	Analgesics, bed rest, donut-ring cushion, crutches	Discharge with orthopedic follow-up in 1–2 weeks
Sacral fracture	Transverse fractures from direct anteroposterior trauma; upper transverse fractures from fall in flexed position	Pain on rectal examination; sacral root injury with upper transverse fractures; vertical fractures may transect the pelvic ring	Analgesics, bed rest, surgery may be needed for displaced fractures or neurologic injury	Discharge with orthopedic follow-up in 1–2 weeks; orthopedic consultation for displaced fractures or neurologic deficits
Coccyx fracture	Fall in sitting position; more common in women	Pain, tenderness over sacral region; pain on compression during rectal examination	Analgesics, bed rest, stool softeners, sitz baths, donut-ring cushion	PCP or orthopedic follow-up in 2–3 weeks; surgical excision of fracture fragment if chronic pain
Anterior-superior iliac spine	Forceful sartorius muscle contraction (e.g., adolescent sprinters)	Pain with hip flexion and abduction	Analgesics, bed rest for 3–4 weeks with hip flexed and abducted, crutches	Discharge with orthopedic follow-up in 1–2 weeks
Anterior-inferior iliac spine	Forceful rectus femoris muscle contraction (e.g., adolescent soccer players)	Pain in groin; pain with hip flexion	Analgesics, bed rest for 3–4 weeks with hip flexed, crutches	Discharge with orthopedic follow-up in 1–2 weeks
Ischial tuberosity	Forceful contraction of hamstrings	Pain with sitting or flexing the thigh	Analgesics, bed rest for 3–4 weeks in extension, external rotation, crutches	Discharge with orthopedic follow-up in 1–2 weeks

Abbreviation: PCP, primary care physician.

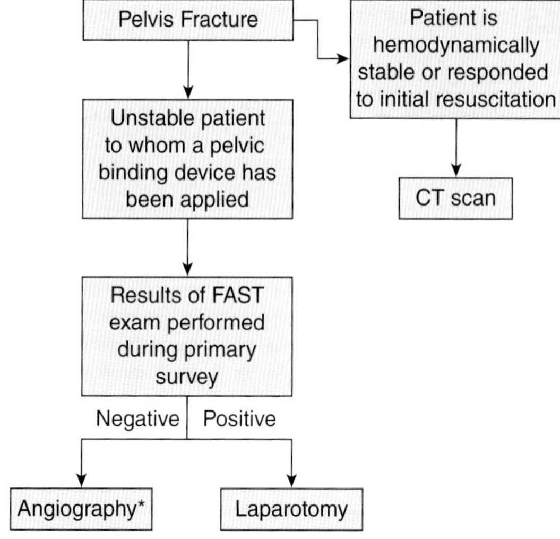

FIGURE 173-1. Suggested algorithm for pelvic fracture treatment. FAST, focused abdominal sonogram for trauma; OR, operating room.

4. After excluding other sources of hemorrhage, treatment for ongoing hemodynamic instability in patients with pelvic fractures includes angiography with embolization and external fixation.
5. An algorithm for treating severe pelvic fractures is listed in Figure 173-1.
6. With the exception of lateral compression type I and AP compression type I injuries, all other pelvic ring fractures require open reduction and internal fixation (ORIF).
7. Acetabular fractures require orthopedic consultation and hospital admission. Nondisplaced fractures may be treated with analgesia and bed rest. Displaced fractures are treated with early ORIF.
8. The treatment and disposition of single bone fractures are listed in Table 173-1.

HIP FRACTURES

Clinical Features

The vast majority of hip fractures occur in elderly patients with osteoporosis or other bony pathology who present after a fall (Table 173-2). The affected leg is classically shortened and externally rotated. Patients with hip fractures may complain of pain at the site of injury or in the groin and knee. After performing a primary survey and stabilizing the patient, examine the patient for pain, shortening, rotation, deformities, pelvic or sacral tenderness, and neurovascular status. If no significant abnormalities are found, carefully evaluate range of motion. A history of fall or significant trauma should prompt the examiner to evaluate for other injuries.

TABLE 173-2 Proximal Femur Fractures: Demographics and Clinical Features

Fracture	Incidence/ Demographics	Mechanism	Clinical Findings	Concomitant Injuries
Femoral head	Isolated fracture rare; seen in 6–16% of hip dislocations	Usually result of high-energy trauma; dashboard to flexed knee most common	Limb shortened and externally rotated (anterior dislocation); shortened, flexed, and internally rotated (posterior dislocation)	Closed head injury; intrathoracic and/or intraabdominal injuries; pelvic fracture, knee injuries
Femoral neck	Common in older patients with osteoporosis; rarely seen in younger patients	Low-impact falls or torsion in elderly; high-energy trauma or stress fractures in young	Ranges from pain with weight-bearing to inability to ambulate; limb may be shortened and externally rotated	Ipsilateral femoral shaft fracture
Greater trochanteric	Uncommon; older patients or adolescents	Direct trauma (older patients); avulsion due to contraction of gluteus medius (young patients)	Ambulatory; pain with palpation or abduction	—
Lesser trochanteric	Uncommon; adolescents (85%) > adults	Avulsion due to forceful contraction of iliopsoas (adolescents); avulsion of pathologic bone (older adults)	Usually ambulatory; pain with flexion or rotation	—
Intertrochanteric	Common in older patients with osteoporosis; rare in younger patients	Falls; high-energy trauma	Severe pain; swelling; limb shortened and externally rotated	Anemia from blood loss into thigh; concomitant traumatic injuries
Subtrochanteric	Similar to intertrochanteric; 15% of hip fractures	Falls; high-energy trauma; may also be pathologic	Severe pain; ecchymosis; limb shortened, abducted, and externally rotated	Vascular injuries, anemia/ hypovolemic shock from fracture itself or other traumatic injuries

Diagnosis and Differential

Radiographic evaluation of the hip includes AP and lateral views. Other radiographic views that may be helpful include an AP pelvis, which allows a comparison of both sides, and Judet views. Radiographs of the femur and knee may also be indicated. Significant pain with weight-bearing or inability

TABLE 173-3 Proximal Femur Fractures: Treatment Issues

Fracture	ED Management	Disposition and Follow-Up	Complications
Femoral head	Immediate orthopedic consultation; emergent closed reduction of dislocation; ORIF if closed reduction is unsuccessful	Admission to orthopedic or trauma service	AVN; posttraumatic arthritis; sciatic nerve injury; heterotopic ossification
Femoral neck	Orthopedic consultation; ranges from nonoperative to total hip arthroplasty	Admission to orthopedic service	AVN; infection; DVT and/or pulmonary embolus
Greater trochanteric	Analgesics; protected weight-bearing	Orthopedic follow-up 1–2 weeks; possible ORIF if displacement >1 cm	Nonunion rare
Lesser trochanteric	Analgesics; weight-bearing as tolerated; evaluate for possible pathologic fracture	Orthopedic or PCP follow-up in 1–2 weeks; admit or urgent follow-up for pathologic fracture	Nonunion rare
Intertrochanteric	Orthopedic consultation	Admit for eventual ORIF; may need preoperative testing and clearance by PCP or hospitalist	DVT and/or pulmonary embolism; infection
Subtrochanteric	Orthopedic consultation; consider Hare® or Sager® splint	Admit for ORIF	DVT and/or pulmonary embolism; infection; malunion (shortened limb); nonunion

Abbreviations: AVN, avascular necrosis; DVT, deep venous thrombosis; ORIF, open reduction and internal fixation; PCP, primary care physician.

to bear weight in patients with normal radiographs should raise suspicion for occult fracture, especially at the femoral neck or acetabulum. MRI is very sensitive (nearly 100%) for identifying occult hip fractures and may identify other sources of pain. CT may be useful in identifying fractures not seen on radiographs, but it is not as sensitive as MRI. The differential diagnosis includes pelvic fracture, hip dislocation, femur fracture, sprains, and strains.

Emergency Department Care and Disposition

1. The treatment of hip fractures is listed in Table 173-3.
2. If clinical suspicion of an occult fracture is high, obtain an MRI scan in the ED. Alternatively, arrange follow-up MRI within 24 to 48 hours and have the patient remain non-weight-bearing.
3. Traction devices may be used for immobilization of subtrochanteric fractures; however, they are contraindicated in femoral neck fractures.

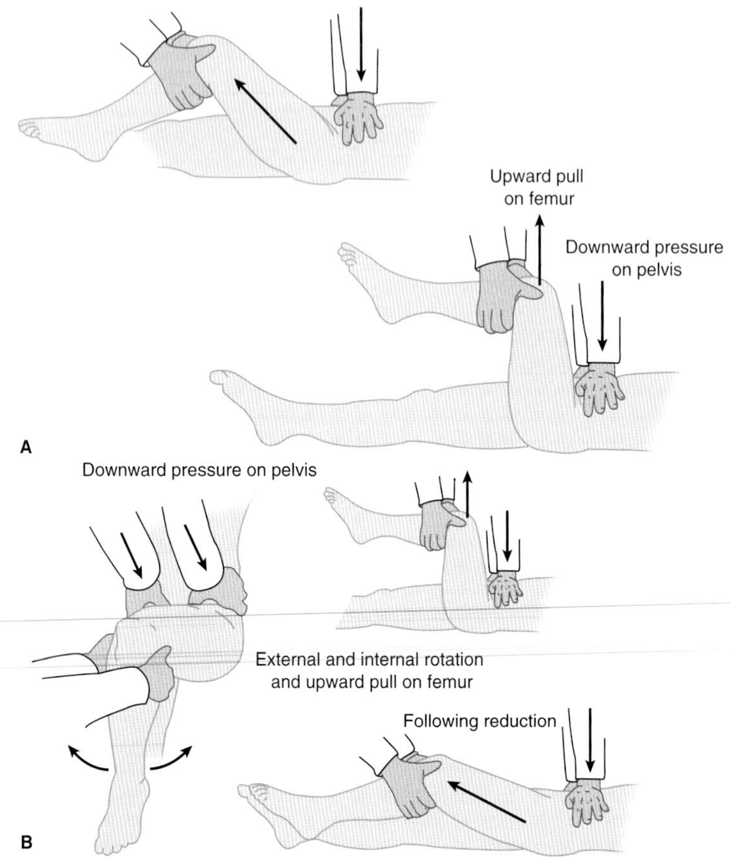

FIGURE 173-2. A and B. Allis maneuver for reduction of posterior hip dislocation.

HIP DISLOCATIONS

Hip dislocations may be anterior or posterior, and commonly result from a high-speed motor vehicle crash. Ninety percent of hip dislocations are posterior, and they may be associated with acetabular fractures. On examination, the extremity is shortened, internally rotated, and adducted. With anterior dislocations the extremity is held in abduction and external rotation. Assess the patient's neurovascular status. Obtain radiographs of the hip and pelvis to evaluate for hip dislocation. Further assessment of the acetabulum and femur may be done with Judet views or CT.

Hip dislocations are true orthopedic emergencies and should be reduced within 6 hours because delays in reduction are associated with a higher incidence of avascular necrosis. One of the most common methods for hip reduction is described in Figure 173-2. After reduction, gently test range of motion and repeat the neurovascular exam. Order post-reduction radiographs or CT to confirm reduction and evaluate for injuries not apparent on initial radiographs. Coordinate post-reduction care with the orthopedist.

Prosthetic hips may dislocate relatively easily from minor trauma or movements that flex the hip past 90 degrees. It is advisable to discuss the treatment plan with the consulting orthopedist prior to any reduction maneuvers. Most dislocations of prosthetic hips are posterior and can be reduced using the techniques described here.

FEMORAL SHAFT FRACTURES

Fractures of the femoral shaft occur most commonly in younger patients secondary to high-energy trauma. Pathologic fractures can occur due to malignancies. Clinical features include shortening, pain, swelling, and deformity. Assess the patient for neurovascular status, signs of an open fracture, and other injuries. ED treatment includes splinting the extremity with a traction splint unless the patient has a sciatic nerve injury, knee injury, vascular injury, or open fracture. Splint without traction if these conditions exist. Open femur fractures require broad-spectrum antibiotics and copious irrigation. Obtain early orthopedic consultation for definitive management.

FURTHER READING

For further reading in *Tintinalli's Emergency Medicine: A Comprehensive Study Guide*, 8th ed., see Chapter 272, "Pelvis Injuries," by Melissa A. Barton, H. Scott Derstine, and Ciara J. Barclay-Buchanan; and Chapter 273, "Hip and Femur Injuries," by Mark Steele and Amy M. Stubbs.

CHAPTER 174

Knee and Leg Injuries

Sandra L. Najarian

FRACTURES

Clinical Features

Patients with patellar fractures present with focal tenderness, swelling, and often a loss of the extensor mechanism. Patients with femoral condyle fractures present with pain, swelling, deformity, rotation, shortening, and an inability to ambulate. Popliteal artery injury, deep peroneal nerve injury, ipsilateral hip dislocation or fracture, and quadriceps mechanism injury can be associated with femoral condyle fractures. Tibial spine fractures present with tenderness, swelling, inability to extend the knee, and a positive Lachman's test. Patients with tibial plateau fractures have pain, swelling, and limited range of motion. Ligamentous instability is present in about one-third of these fractures. Patients with tibial shaft fractures present with pain, swelling, and crepitance about the knee. Distal tibial fractures involving the articular surface (tibial plafond or Pilon fracture) present with pain, swelling, and tenderness about the ankle. The risk of compartment syndrome is high with tibial fractures and mandates a thorough neurovascular exam. Proximal fibular fractures may be associated with ankle injuries. Patients with isolated fibular shaft fractures may be able to bear weight.

Diagnosis and Differential

The Pittsburgh Knee Rules (Fig. 174-1) or the Ottawa Knee Rules (Table 174-1) should be used to determine if radiography is needed. These rules have been validated in both children and adults. In suspected tibial and fibular injuries, radiographs of the ankle and knee may be necessary to exclude associated fractures. CT scanning may be considered if x-rays are negative, and the patient is unable to bear weight.

Emergency Department Care and Disposition

Table 174-2 describes the mechanism and treatment for the various knee fractures. Most tibial fractures require emergent orthopedic consultation. Indications for emergent operative repair include open fractures, vascular compromise, or compartment syndrome. Patients may be placed in long-leg immobilization and discharged home if they have a low-energy mechanism, have their pain well controlled, and are not at risk for compartment syndrome. Treatment for isolated fibular shaft fractures includes splinting, ice, elevation, and orthopedic or primary care physician follow-up. Proximal fibular fractures associated with ankle injuries require surgical intervention and urgent orthopedic consult.

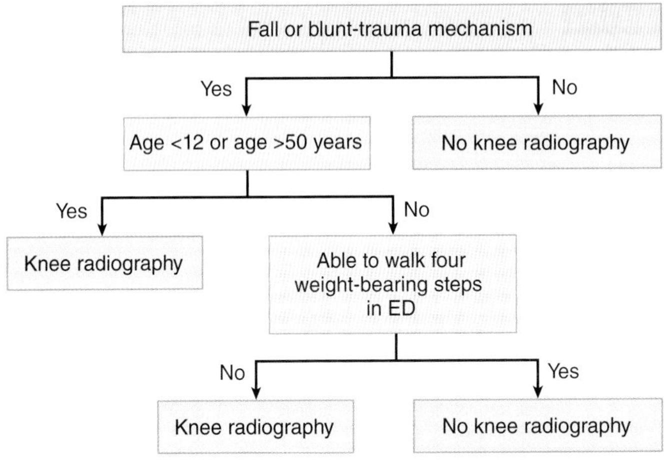

FIGURE 174-1. Pittsburgh Knee Rules for radiography. Reproduced with permission from Seaberg DC, Yealy DM, Lukens T, et al: Multicenter comparison of two clinical decision rules for the use of radiography in acute, high-risk knee injuries, *Ann Emerg Med.* 1998;Jul;32(1):8-13.

TABLE 174-1 Ottawa Knee Rules: Radiograph If One Criterion Is Met

Patient age >55 years (rules have been validated for children 2–16 years of age)
Tenderness at the head of the fibula
Isolated tenderness of the patella
Inability to flex knee to 90 degrees
Inability to transfer weight for four steps both immediately after the injury and in the ED

TABLE 174-2 Mechanism of Knee Injury and Treatment

Fracture	Mechanism	Treatment
Patella	Direct blow (i.e., fall, motor vehicle crash) or forceful contraction of quadriceps muscle	Nondisplaced fracture with intact extensor mechanism: knee immobilizer, rest, ice, analgesia. Follow-up for serial radiographs Displaced >3 mm, articular incongruity >2 mm, or with disruption of extensor mechanism: above treatment plus early referral for ORIF Severely comminuted fracture: surgical debridement of small fragments and suturing of quadriceps and patellar tendons Open fracture: irrigation and antistaphylococcal antibiotics in the ED; debridement and irrigation in the operating room
Femoral condyles	Fall with axial load with valgus/varus/rotational forces, or a blow to the distal femur	Incomplete or nondisplaced fractures in any age group or stable impacted fractures in the elderly: long leg splinting and orthopedic referral Displaced fractures or fractures with any degree of joint incongruity: splinting and orthopedic consult for ORIF

(Continued)

TABLE 174-2 Mechanism of Knee Injury and Treatment (Continued)

Fracture	Mechanism	Treatment
Tibial spines and tuberosity	Force directed against flexed proximal tibia in an anterior or posterior direction (i.e., motor vehicle crash, sporting injury)	Incomplete or nondisplaced fractures: immobilization in full extension (knee immobilizer) and orthopedic referral in 2–7 days Complete or displaced fracture: early orthopedic referral, often requires ORIF
Tibial tuberosity	Sudden force to flexed knee with quadriceps contracted	Incomplete or small avulsion fracture: immobilization Complete avulsion: ORIF
Tibial plateau	Valgus or varus forces combined with axial load that drives the femoral condyle into the tibia (i.e., fall, leg hit by car bumper)	Nondisplaced, lateral fracture: knee immobilizer with non-weight-bearing and orthopedic referral in 2–7 days Depression of articular surface: early orthopedic consult for ORIF

Abbreviation: ORIF, open reduction internal fixation.

DISLOCATIONS

Clinical Features

Patella dislocation results in pain and deformity of the knee. Tearing of the medial knee joint capsule can occur. Knee dislocation results in significant ligamentous and capsular disruption. Spontaneous reduction occurs in 50% of patients. Multidirectional instability of the knee should raise the suspicion for a spontaneously reduced knee dislocation. Knee dislocations have a high incidence of associated injures, such as popliteal artery injury and peroneal nerve injury.

Diagnosis and Differential

Radiographs may help exclude associated fractures. Some authors recommend arteriography for all patients with confirmed knee dislocations. Others advocate for Doppler pressure indices (ankle-brachial index) and serial vascular exams if distal pulses are present, and there are no other signs of vascular injury (including ischemia, hemorrhage, or an expanding hematoma).

Emergency Department Care and Disposition

Procedural sedation is recommended to facilitate otherwise painful reductions. For patellar dislocation, flexing the hip and hyperextending the knee help slide the patella back into place. Knee immobilization and orthopedic or primary care physician follow-up are necessary. For knee dislocation, early reduction is essential along with documentation of pre-and post-reduction neurovascular status. Splinting the affected knee in 20 degrees of flexion is essential. Immediate orthopedic and vascular surgery consultation is warranted for all knee dislocations, and admission is mandatory for observation of neurovascular status.

TENDON, LIGAMENTOUS, AND MENISCAL INJURIES

Clinical Features

Patients with quadriceps or patellar tendon rupture have pain and swelling about the knee and will not be able to extend the knee against resistance. A palpable defect is present above or below the knee depending on which tendon is involved. Patients with Achilles tendon rupture have severe pain in the calf and are unable to perform toe walk, run, or climb stairs. A palpable defect is often present in the Achilles tendon 2 to 6 cm above the calcaneus. A positive Thompson test is diagnostic; with the patient lying prone and knee flexed at 90 degrees, the foot fails to plantar flex when the calf is squeezed. Most ligamentous injuries present with hemarthroses, though serious ligamentous injuries may present with little pain and no hemarthrosis due to complete disruption of the capsule. Patients with anterior cruciate ligament (ACL) tears often describe a "pop" and significant swelling over the next several hours after injury. Lachman's test is the most sensitive test for ACL injuries. The anterior drawer and pivot shift test are also useful for diagnosis. Posterior cruciate ligament (PCL) injuries may result in a positive posterior drawer test; the composite history and exam findings, however, are more accurate for diagnosis of PCL injury. Medial and lateral collateral ligament injuries are diagnosed with abduction (valgus) and adduction (varus) stress testing in 30 degrees flexion. Laxity greater than 1 cm without a firm end point compared with the other knee is diagnostic for a complete torn medial or lateral collateral ligament. Stress testing should be repeated in extension. If laxity is present in extension, then this indicates injury to the cruciate ligament and posterior or posterolateral capsule. Peroneal nerve injury may occur with lateral injuries. Symptoms of meniscal injury include painful locking of the knee, a popping, clicking or snapping sensation, or a sense of instability with activity or joint swelling after activity. McMurray's test and other tests for meniscal injury are not sensitive. Ligamentous injuries may be present as well. A patient with a "locked knee" from a torn meniscus will not be able to actively or passively range the affected knee and will have significant pain.

Diagnosis and Differential

The diagnosis is largely clinical. A high-riding patella may be seen on the lateral radiograph of the knee with patellar tendon rupture. Ultrasound or MRI can help identify Achilles tendon rupture when the diagnosis is not clear. Radiographs are usually normal or show a joint effusion in ligamentous or meniscal injuries. An avulsion fracture at the site of the lateral capsular ligament on the lateral tibial condyle (Segond fracture) is associated with ACL rupture. Outpatient MRI or arthroscopy provides definitive diagnosis.

Emergency Department Care and Disposition

Treatment of patellar or quadriceps tendon rupture includes knee immobilization and orthopedic consultation for surgical repair, usually within the first 7 to 10 days after the injury. Treatment of Achilles tendon rupture includes splinting in plantar flexion, non-weight-bearing, and referral to orthopedics for possible surgical repair. Treatment for ligamentous and meniscal injuries includes knee immobilization, ice, elevation, analgesics, and orthopedic referral. Treatment for a "locked knee" includes analgesia and closed reduction. Procedural sedation may be necessary. Place the patient supine with the knee flexed 90 degrees over the side of the bed. Apply longitudinal traction to the knee, and at the same time, apply internal and external rotation to the knee to unlock the joint. Consult orthopedics if the reduction is not successful.

OVERUSE INJURIES

Patellar tendonitis or "jumper's knee" presents with pain over the patellar tendon worsened by running up hills, jumping, or standing from a seated position. Treatment includes heat, nonsteroidal anti-inflammatory drugs (NSAIDs), and quadriceps-strengthening exercises. Steroid injections should be avoided. Shin splints and stress fractures can present with pain over the anterior leg. Patients typically describe a change or sudden increase in their training pattern. Patients present with activity-induced pain relieved by rest, which can progress to constant pain. Radiographs are often normal. Discontinuation of the activity for several weeks is the treatment for both shin splints and stress fractures. If a stress fracture is suspected, an outpatient bone scan or MRI can confirm the diagnosis.

FURTHER READING

For further reading in *Tintinalli's Emergency Medicine: A Comprehensive Study Guide*, 8th ed., see Chapter 274, "Knee Injuries" by Rachel R. Bengtzen, Jeffrey N. Glaspy and Mark T. Steele; Chapter 275, "Leg Injuries" by Paul R. Heller.

CHAPTER 175 Ankle and Foot Injuries

Sarah Elisabeth Frasure

ANKLE INJURIES

Tendon and Ligament Injuries

Clinical Features

Tendon injuries typically result from *hyperdorsiflexion* (peroneal tendon injury) or sudden *plantarflexion* (Achilles tendon injury). Patients with an Achilles tendon rupture complain of severe pain and are unable to walk on their toes, run, or climb stairs. Ligamentous sprains are caused by *inversion* and *eversion* injuries. The most common ankle sprain involves the anterior talofibular ligament. Though an isolated sprain of the medial deltoid ligament is rare, it is occasionally associated with a fibular fracture (Maisonneuve fracture) or syndesmotic ligament injury. Any injury with signs of neurovascular compromise requires immediate attention.

Diagnosis and Differential

Evaluate the ankle as well as the joints above and below the injury. A positive Thompson test (with the patient lying prone and knee flexed at 90°, the foot fails to plantarflex when the calf is squeezed) is diagnostic of Achilles tendon rupture. Palpate the proximal fibula for tenderness resulting from a fracture or fibulotibialis ligament tear. Squeeze the fibula toward the tibia to evaluate for syndesmotic ligament injury. If tenderness is isolated to the posterior aspect of the lateral malleolus, then a peroneal tendon subluxation may be present.

The Ottawa Ankle Rules were developed to help clinicians determine when imaging studies are necessary for patients with ankle injuries (see Fig. 175-1).

Joint stability dictates the treatment plan for an ankle sprain. Instability is usually suspected based on the physical examination and imaging studies. The examiner may perform the anterior drawer and talar tilt tests to assess stability. If the examiner is unable to perform reliable stress testing, the injury is considered potentially unstable. Asymmetry of the gap between the talar dome and the malleoli on the talus x-ray view also suggests joint instability.

Emergency Department Care and Disposition

1. If the patient has a stable joint and is able to bear weight, then **protection** with an elastic bandage or ankle brace, **rest, ice, compression, and elevation (PRICE)** for up to 72 hours is indicated. Prescribe analgesics, and add motion and strength exercises within 48 to 72 hours. If pain persists beyond one week, the patient should follow up with an orthopedist for a repeat evaluation.
2. A patient with a stable joint who is *unable* to bear weight requires an **ankle brace**, crutches, and orthopedic follow-up.

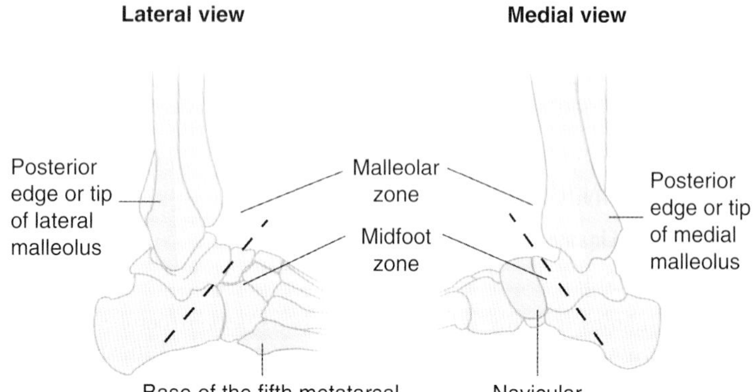

FIGURE 175-1. Ottawa ankle rules for ankle and midfoot injuries. Ankle radiographs are required only if there is any pain in the malleolar zone or midfoot zone along with bony tenderness in any of these four locations or the inability to bear weight both immediately after the injury *and* in the ED.

3. A patient with an *unstable* joint requires a **posterior splint, crutches,** and timely referral to an orthopedist for definitive care.
4. Treatment of Achilles tendon rupture includes splinting in plantar flexion, crutches to ensure nonweightbearing, and early referral to an orthopedist for possible operative repair.

Dislocations Posterior dislocations, the most common type of ankle dislocations, occur with a backward force on the plantarflexed foot. This injury usually results in the rupture of the tibiofibular ligaments or a lateral malleolus fracture. Reduce ankle dislocations immediately if vascular compromise (absent pulses or a dusky foot) or skin tenting are present. First, provide analgesia and sedation as needed. Grasp the heel and foot with both hands and apply axial traction while reducing the ankle into anatomical alignment. Following successful reduction, assess post-reduction neurovascular status, apply a splint, obtain post-reduction radiographs, and immediately consult orthopedics.

Fractures Ankle fractures are classified as unimalleolar, bimalleolar, and trimalleolar. Bimalleolar and trimalleolar fractures require definitive open reduction and internal fixation (ORIF) by an orthopedist. ED care includes initial reduction as needed, posterior splinting, elevation, ice application, and orthopedic consultation. Treat unimalleolar fractures with nonweightbearing status and posterior splinting. Manage minimally displaced avulsion fractures of the fibula (<3 mm in diameter) like ankle sprains. Ankle fractures may be occult and are occasionally associated with injuries to other parts of the lower extremity (Table 175-1). Patients with open fractures require initial reduction as needed, wet sterile dressing, splinting, tetanus toxoid as necessary, a first generation cephalosporin such as **cefazolin** 1 g IV, and immediate orthopedic consultation.

TABLE 175-1 Associated and Occult Injuries of the Ankle

Injury	Clinical Suspicion	Confirmatory Test
Important to identify in the ED		
Maisonneuve fracture	Examine proximal fibula and shaft, tenderness to palpation; proximal fracture and syndesmosis tear indicate unstable fracture	Fibula radiograph
Peroneal tendon dislocation	Palpable anterior tendon dislocation or subluxation	Clinical examination
Usually identified in follow-up of ankle sprains		
Osteochondral injuries	Diffuse ankle swelling, passive plantarflexion	Ankle mortise view/CT
Syndesmosis tear	Significant ankle pain, positive squeeze test	Widened mortise with weight bearing
Anterior calcaneal process fracture	Tenderness more inferoanterior than a typical ankle sprain	Lateral ankle radiograph/CT
Lateral talar process fracture	Tenderness just distal to the tip of fibula	Ankle mortise view/CT
Os trigonum	Tenderness anterior to Achilles tendon	Lateral ankle radiograph

FOOT INJURIES

Clinical Features

The foot is divided into the hindfoot, midfoot, and forefoot. The Chopart joint separates the hindfoot from the midfoot. The Lisfranc joint separates the midfoot from the forefoot.

Diagnosis and Differential

Pay special attention on physical examination to the base of the *fifth* metatarsal and the base of the *second* metatarsal. If plain radiographs are nondiagnostic, CT is indicated for suspected Lisfranc joint injuries.

Hindfoot Injuries

Calcaneal injuries require a large force, and associated injuries are common. Measure Boehler's angle on a lateral radiograph view (formed by the intersection of a line connecting the posterior tuberosity and apex of the posterior facet, and a line from the posterior facet to the apex of the anterior facet) if concerned for a calcaneal compression fracture. An angle $<20°$ is suggestive of a fracture. Treat with a posterior splint, elevation, analgesics, and orthopedic consultation. Manage small avulsion fractures of the talus with posterior splinting and timely orthopedic follow-up. Subtalar dislocations, as well as major fractures of the talar neck or body, require immediate orthopedic consultation.

Midfoot Injuries

Injuries of the tarsometatarsal joint combined with pain with midfoot torsion are suspicious for a Lisfranc injury. Lisfranc joint injuries are often

TABLE 175-2 Summary of Emergent Care of Bony Foot Injuries

Fracture or Injury Type	ED Imaging	ED Care*	Orthopedic Referral (immediate: within 24 h; early: within 2 wk)	Home Care/ Weight-Bearing Status	Advice on Long-Term Care and Management	Special Considerations
Calcaneal, intra- and extra-articular	Plain films, Boehler angle; CT for subtle findings	Posterior splint	Intra-articular: immediate; extra-articular: early	NWBS; RICE	Possible surgery	
Talus fracture	CT	Posterior splint	Major: immediate; minor: early	NWBS; RICE	Possible surgery	Risk of avascular necrosis
Lisfranc	CT	Splint	Displaced: ortho consult in ED; nondisplaced: early	NWBS; RICE	Possible surgery	Risk of compartment syndrome; arthritis
Navicular fracture	Plain films or CT	Splint	Nondisplaced: early; displaced: immediate	NWBS; RICE	Possible surgery	Risk of avascular necrosis; non-union
Cuboid fracture	Plain films or CT	Splint	Early	NWBS; RICE	Comminuted: possible surgery	
Cuneiform fracture	Plain films or CT	Splint	Early	NWBS; RICE	Medial: possible surgery	
Jones	Plain films; CT for athletes	Splint	Early	NWBS; RICE	Athletes: possible surgery	
Metatarsal fracture	Plain films	Posterior splint	Within a week for a cast	NWBS; RICE	Surgery not likely	
Stress fracture	Clinical			Cessation of causative activity		
Phalange fracture	Plain films	Buddy taping		Hard-soled shoe and weight bearing as tolerated		
Open fractures of any kind	Consider antibiotics, Td	Pain control	Ortho consult in ED			

*All patients with fractures should receive adequate analgesia, and splints should be well padded.

Abbreviations: NWBS, nonweightbearing status; ortho, orthopedist; RICE, rest, ice, compression, elevation; Td, Tetanus booster.

associated with a fracture, most frequently noted at the base of the second metatarsal. A gap of >1 mm between the bases of the first and second metatarsal bones on plain film is considered unstable. If standard radiographs are nondiagnostic, complete workup may require CT imaging. Isolated navicular, cuboid, and cuneiform injuries are rare and treated conservatively.

Forefoot

Treat nondisplaced metatarsal shaft fractures with a posterior splint or orthopedic shoe. Fractures with greater than 3 to 4 mm displacement on plain films, however, require surgical reduction. Treat pseudo Jones fractures (nondisplaced avulsion fractures of the tuberosity of the fifth metatarsal) with a walking cast. Manage true Jones fractures (metaphyseal-diaphyseal junction fracture of the fifth metatarsal) with a nonweightbearing cast and timely orthopedic follow-up for potential surgery. Nondisplaced phalangeal fractures require buddy taping and a stiff-sole (orthopedic) shoe. Treat displaced phalangeal fractures and dislocations with a digital block, reduction by manual traction, and buddy taping. Recommended imaging and care for foot injuries can be found in Table 175-2.

FURTHER READING

For further reading in *Tintinalli's Emergency Medicine: A Comprehensive Study Guide*, 8th ed., see Chapter 276, "Ankle Injuries," by Daniel A. Handel and Sarah Andrus Gaines; and Chapter 277, "Foot Injuries," by Sarah Andrus Gaines and Daniel A. Handel.

CHAPTER 176 Compartment Syndrome

Sandra L. Najarian

Elevated pressures within a confined muscle compartment can lead to functional and circulatory impairment of that limb. The most common compartments affected are in the lower leg and forearm. This syndrome develops as a result of external compressive forces on a limb or from any mechanism that increases the compartmental size and pressure (Table 176-1).

CLINICAL FEATURES

Severe and difficult-to-control pain, pain out of proportion to examination, and pain with passive stretch of the limb are the hallmark symptoms of this disease. Nerve dysfunction often accompanies the pain and causes burning or dysesthesias in the sensory distribution of the nerve. Motor function can be impaired as well. On exam, the compartment is often swollen, firm, and tender to palpation. Since tissue pressure does not typically exceed arterial pressure, the affected limb often has normal distal pulse, temperature, and color. Symptoms can begin within a few hours after the injury or up to 48 hours after the inciting event.

DIAGNOSIS AND DIFFERENTIAL

Diagnosis is largely clinical. Direct measurement of the compartment is necessary when the diagnosis is in question or in patients who are obtunded or sedated. Several commercial devices are available to measure compartment pressures. Normal compartment pressure is < 10 mm Hg. The exact pressure elevation at which cell death occurs is unclear. Pressures between 30 to 50 mm Hg are felt to be detrimental if left untreated for several hours. The diastolic blood pressure minus the measured tissue pressure, or "delta pressure," better predicts the potential for irreversible muscle damage. A delta pressure of 30 mm Hg is most commonly used to diagnose acute

TABLE 176-1 Causes of Compartment Syndrome

Orthopedic	Tibial fractures Forearm fractures
Vascular	Ischemic-reperfusion injury Hemorrhage
Iatrogenic	Vascular puncture in anticoagulated patients IV/intra-arterial drug injection Constrictive casts
Soft tissue injury	Prolonged limb compression Crush injury Burns
Hematologic	Hemophilia Adverse effects of anticoagulants (warfarin)

compartment syndrome. Hypotensive patients do not tolerate elevated compartment pressures as well as normotensive patients. The differential diagnosis for compartment syndrome includes other causes of pain, such as fracture, hematoma, or infection, and other causes of neurologic or vascular compromise.

EMERGENCY DEPARTMENT CARE AND DISPOSITION

Once the diagnosis is confirmed, surgical fasciotomy is necessary. Admit all patients to the operating room or appropriate inpatient service for observation and serial examinations.

1. While definitive management is being arranged, administer supplemental oxygen, correct hypotension, remove constrictive casts or dressings, and place the affected limb at the level of the heart.
2. Reverse anticoagulation in anticoagulated patients, and replace factor levels in hemophiliacs.
3. Functional outcomes are favorable when diagnosis and treatment of compartment syndrome occurs within 6 hours of its onset. Fasciotomy may be futile if tissue pressures have been elevated to 24 to 48 hours as permanent dysfunction may already be present.

FURTHER READING

For further reading in *Tintinalli's Emergency Medicine: A Comprehensive Study Guide*, 8th ed., see Chapter 278, "Compartment Syndrome" by Paul R. Haller.

SECTION

20

Nontraumatic Musculoskeletal Disorders

Neck and Back Pain

Amy M. Stubbs

Neck and back pain are major causes of disability in the United States and are commonly seen in the ED. While the majority of cases have nonspecific or benign etiologies, serious underlying pathology may exist. Clinicians must be vigilant in obtaining a thorough history, focusing on risk factors for pathology, and physical examination that includes a detailed neurologic examination.

CLINICAL FEATURES

Neck and back pain have myriad causes, but can often be classified into two groups: uncomplicated musculoskeletal pain and those with pain attributable to radiculopathy (spinal nerve root compression) or myelopathy (spinal cord compression) (see Tables 177-1, 177-2, and 177-3). Thoracolumbar pain may also be categorized by symptom duration: acute (<6 weeks), subacute (6 to 12 weeks), or chronic (>12 weeks).

The history should include the onset, circumstances, location, radiation, duration, and exacerbating/alleviating factors of the pain. Historical risk factors or symptoms concerning for serious pathology should be sought (see Table 177-4).

Examination should include evaluation of mobility and range of motion. The patient should be exposed, observing and palpating the neck and back for point tenderness, deformity, lymphadenopathy, or signs of infection. A thorough neurologic examination, including assessment of specific nerve roots' strength, sensation, and reflexes, is essential (see Tables 177-2 and 177-3). Specific examination maneuvers should be performed as indicated for the complaint (see Table 177-5).

A rectal examination evaluating for tone, sensation, and masses is requisite if concern exists for spinal cord compression or other serious pathology.

DIAGNOSIS AND DIFFERENTIAL

The differentials for neck and back pain are broad but can generally be guided by the history and physical examination. The majority of patients with neck and back pain will not require emergent imaging or diagnostic testing.

TABLE 177-1 Differentiating Cervical Radiculopathy from Uncomplicated Musculoskeletal Neck Pain

Factors Favoring Cervical Radiculopathy or Myelopathy*	Factors Favoring Uncomplicated Musculoskeletal Neck Pain*
Pain from the neck radiates down the arm in dermatome pattern.	Tenderness of involved muscles; examiner may find a focal point of tenderness.
Sensory changes along dermatome distribution.	Atrophy or thinning of shoulder muscles may occur after rotator cuff injury.
Pushing down on top of head, with neck in extension (chin up) and head leaning toward symptomatic side elicits pain, typically toward or down the arm (positive **Spurling's sign**); 90% specific, 45% sensitive.	Pain increases with shoulder abduction on the side of neck pain (increased pain could derive from rotator cuff-related pain; radicular pain may decrease with this maneuver).
Pain may worsen with Valsalva, which increases intrathecal pressure.	Repetitive movement of arm or shoulder at work or play; may be new activity.
Flex neck forward until chin meets chest or pain stops movement. An electric shock sensation radiating down spine into both arms is a positive result (**Lhermitte's sign**). Occasionally, paresthesias occur.	History of recent injury or recent event of awkward position (such as neck or head position during sleep in an unfamiliar setting) or awkward standing posture to accommodate a special situation.
Depressed reflexes or, uncommonly, increased reflexes (see also Table 177-2).	Pain is accompanied by "stiffness" of involved muscle group.

*Patient in either pain category is not expected to have all, or majority, of listed signs.

TABLE 177-2 Signs and Symptoms of Cervical Radiculopathy

Disk Space	Cervical Root	Pain Complaint	Sensory Abnormality	Motor Weakness	Altered Reflex
C1–C2	C2	Neck, scalp	Scalp		
C4–C5	C5	Neck, shoulder, upper arm	Shoulder	Infraspinatus, deltoid, biceps	Reduced biceps reflex
C5–C6	C6	Neck, shoulder, upper medial, scapular area, proximal forearm, thumb, index finger	Thumb and index finger, lateral forearm	Deltoid, biceps, pronator teres, wrist extensors	Reduced biceps and brachioradialis reflex
C6–C7	C7	Neck, posterior arm, dorsum proximal forearm, chest, medial third of scapula, middle finger	Middle finger, forearm	Triceps, pronator teres	Reduced triceps reflex
C7–T1	C8	Neck, posterior arm, ulnar side of forearm, medial inferior scapular border, medial hand, ring, and little fingers	Ring and little fingers	Triceps, flexor carpi ulnaris, hand intrinsics	Reduced triceps reflex

TABLE 177-3 Symptoms and Signs of Lumbar Radiculopathies

Disk Space	Nerve Root	Pain Complaint	Sensory Change	Motor Weakness	Altered Reflex
L2–3	L3	Medial thigh, knee	Medial thigh, knee	Hip flexors	None
L3–4	L4	Medial lower leg	Medial lower leg	Quadriceps	Knee jerk
L4–5	L5	Anterior tibia, great toe	Medial foot	Extensor hallicus longus	Biceps femoris
L5–S1	S1	Calf, little toe	Lateral foot	Foot plantar flexors	Achilles

TABLE 177-4 Risk Factors for Serious Causes of Neck and Back Pain

Risk Factors	Concern
Historical Risk Factors	
Pain >6 weeks	Tumor, infection
Age <18, >50	Congenital anomaly, tumor, infection
Major trauma	Fracture
Minor trauma in elderly or rheumatologic disease	Fracture
History of cancer	Tumor
Fever and rigors	Infection
Weight loss	Tumor, infection
Injection drug use	Infection
Immunocompromised	Infection
Night pain	Tumor, infection
Unremitting pain, even when supine	Tumor, infection
Incontinence	Epidural compression
Saddle anesthesia	Epidural compression
Severe/progressive neurologic deficit	Epidural compression
Anticoagulants and coagulopathy	Epidural compression
Physical Risk Factors	
Fever	Infection
Patient writhing in pain	Infection, vascular cause
Unexpected anal sphincter laxity	Epidural compression
Perianal/perineal sensory loss	Epidural compression
Major motor weakness/gait disturbance	Nerve root or epidural compression
Positive straight leg raise test	Herniated disk

TABLE 177-5 Diagnostic Maneuvers for Neck and Back Pain

Exam Finding/Maneuver	Significance
Spurling's sign: Downward pressure with head in extension and leaning toward symptomatic sign produces pain	Cervical radiculopathy
Abduction relief sign: Relief placing hand of affected arm on top of head	Disc protrusion/radiculopathy
Lhermitte's sign: Forward neck flexion causes electric shock like pain in spine/arms	Cord compression
Hoffman's sign: Flexion of thumb and index finger when flicking tip of middle finger with hand in relaxed position	Upper motor neuron lesion
Straight leg test: Hip flexion to ~70 with knee in extension produces pain in affected leg below knee	L4/L5 or L5/S1 disc herniation
Crossed leg test: Hip flexion to ~70 with knee in extension in opposing leg produces pain in affected leg below knee	L4/L5 or L5/S1 disc herniation

Imaging is usually not indicated in cases of acute, nontraumatic neck or back pain without concerning historical features or exam findings. Plain films of the spine have low sensitivity but may be considered as an initial imaging step if clinical suspicions include tumor, fracture, or infection. **For patients with pain and neurologic deficits, MRI is the definitive test**. CT scan is helpful for identification of disorders of the bony skeleton, but its sensitivity for nerve root or spinal cord disorders is poor. CT myelography can serve as an alternative to MRI, if the latter is contraindicated or unattainable.

Plain films or CT scan of the cervical spine should be considered in patients with chronic neck pain not previously imaged or those with a history or trauma, surgery, malignancy, or rheumatologic disease. Flexion-extension films or MRI may be considered if instability or ligamentous injury is suspected. If radiographs are normal, or show only degenerative disease, and the patient has a benign examination, no further imaging is required. For patients with back pain, in whom plain thoracic and/or lumbar radiographs are indicated (as discussed above), anteroposterior and lateral views suffice. Careful attention should be paid to end plate erosions, disc space narrowing, or lytic lesions, which are worrisome for infection or neoplasm. Advanced imaging is necessitated by the presence of neurological deficits or abnormal plain radiographs.

Laboratory testing will not be useful in the majority of patients with neck and back pain. If serious pathology is suspected, a complete blood count, erythrocyte sedimentation rate (ESR), and urinalysis should be ordered. ESR has a sensitivity of 90% to 98% for infectious causes of back pain. Urinalysis is useful to rule out urinary or renal pathology as a pain source. Postvoid residual (PVR) assessment, with ultrasound or catheterization, should be performed on patients with complaints or exam findings concerning for epidural compression. Urinary retention is the most common finding in cauda equina syndrome, and PVR volume exceeding 500 mL, alone or in combination with other concerning findings, is an important predictor of MRI-proven cauda equina compression.

Mechanical disorders, such as strain caused by trauma, are often characterized by delayed pain and paraspinous pain and stiffness. See Chapters 161 and 163 for further discussion of traumatic neck and back injuries.

Cervical disc herniation, spondylosis, or stenosis can lead to radiculopathy or myelopathy. Signs and symptoms of radiculopathy include pain and weakness in a dermatomal distribution. Lower extremity hyperreflexia, a positive Babinski sign, and loss of sphincter tone are suspicious for myelopathy; any of these findings necessitate MRI. Metastatic cancer may cause a radiculopathy or myelopathy and should be included in the differential for chronic pain. Osteomyelitis, epidural abscess, hematoma, and transverse myelitis may cause neck pain with neurologic deficits, although these disorders are more commonly observed in the thoracic or lumbar spine.

Neck pain can be caused by a variety of other disorders such as myofascial pain syndrome, lymphadenopathy, temporal arteritis, ischemic heart disease, and neurodegenerative disorders. The distribution of symptoms in these disorders will typically not be dermatomal, and other historical features will usually distinguish them.

The majority of patients with back pain have nonspecific back pain; they have no radiculopathy or myelopathy and no specific etiology is found.

These patients typically have benign examinations and movement often exacerbates their pain. Diagnostic evaluation is negative.

As with neck pain, disc herniation and degenerative changes of the thoracic or lumbar spine can be a cause of acute or chronic back pain. More than 95% of disc herniations are at the L4–L5 or L5–S1 nerve roots, compression of which can cause sciatica. These patients may have leg pain, neurologic deficits localized to a unilateral nerve root, and a positive straight-leg test. Spinal nerve root compression can occur at any level in the thoracic or lumbar spine, with associated radicular symptoms. Epidural compression syndromes, which include spinal cord compression, cauda equina syndrome, and conus medullaris syndrome, may cause pain, neurologic deficits, or autonomic dysfunction at any cord level. The thoracic spine is the most common site of compression due to neoplasm; however, if suspected, the entire spinal cord should be imaged, as 10% of patients will have additional metastatic lesions.

Infectious causes of back pain, including osteomyelitis, discitis, and epidural abscess, are often missed on initial presentation. A high level of suspicion should be maintained in patients with risk factors such as immunocompromise, recent back surgery, retained hardware, or intravenous drug use. Plain films may show bony destruction in patients with osteomyelitis, but x-rays are often initially normal in cases of infectious back pain. MRI is typically required for diagnosis. The ESR will be elevated in the majority of cases.

Other causes of back pain may originate from the spine itself or from nonspinal causes. Spinal stenosis can cause low back and leg pain that mimics claudication, worsening with walking and improving with rest. Ankylosing spondylitis, an autoimmune arthritis, causes chronic back pain and is identifiable by a characteristic squaring of vertebral bodies on radiography. Transverse myelitis, an inflammatory disorder of the spinal cord, may mimic a compression syndrome. Ruptured abdominal aneurysm, pyelonephritis, pancreatitis, or renal infarction should be considered in patients with nonspecific back pain accompanied by concerning history or exam findings.

EMERGENCY DEPARTMENT CARE AND DISPOSITION

1. Patients with neck and back pain that have progressive neurologic deficits, myelopathy, or intractable pain should be imaged as indicated (typically MRI) and admitted to the appropriate service for further management. **Dexamethasone 10 mg IV should be given prior to imaging for suspected epidural compression**.
2. Suspected or proven spinal infections require emergent consultation with a spinal surgeon. Empiric broad-spectrum antibiotics, such as **vancomycin** 1 g IV and **piperacillin-tazobactam** 3.375 g IV, should be given unless explicit instructions to withhold are given by the consultant.
3. Patients with a stable or mild radiculopathy may be managed conservatively with pain medication, routine activity as tolerated, and strict return precautions for worsening symptoms. Outpatient MRI and neurosurgical follow-up should be considered for patients who have failed conservative treatment.

4. Pain management may include NSAIDs, acetaminophen, or muscle relaxants used alone or in combination; all have been shown to be effective. A short course of oral opioids may be prescribed for patients with moderate to severe pain, but long-term use is discouraged. The evidence for manipulation, soft-collars, corticosteroids, or other alternative treatments is limited and should generally not be prescribed from the ED. Chronic pain often requires a multidisciplinary approach.
5. The majority of patients with neck or back pain will have a benign course and improve with time. Patients may be prescribed pain medicine as appropriate and activity as tolerated. Return precautions and instruction for follow-up should be provided.

FURTHER READING

For further reading in *Tintinalli's Emergency Medicine: A Comprehensive Study Guide*, 8th ed., see Chapter 279, "Neck and Back Pain," by David Della-Giustina, Jeffrey S. Dubin, and William Frohna.

CHAPTER 178

Shoulder Pain

Andrew D. Perron

Shoulder pain is a common musculoskeletal complaint, especially in patients older than 40 years. Occupational, recreational, and normal daily activities stress the shoulder joint and may result in pain from acute injury or, more commonly, chronic overuse conditions. Complicating the evaluation of shoulder pain is that the origin of pain may be from pathology intrinsic to the shoulder joint or from extrinsic disorders causing referred pain.

CLINICAL FEATURES

The pain of musculoskeletal shoulder pathology often is described by patients as an aching sensation, particularly in the setting of a more chronic process. Nighttime pain is a common feature of intrinsic shoulder pathology. Specific motions may exacerbate it, and this history is helpful in making a specific diagnosis. Decreased range of motion, crepitus, weakness, or muscular atrophy may be associated with certain conditions. Any systemic symptoms such as shortness of breath, fever, or radiation of pain from the chest or abdomen should raise suspicion for extrinsic and potentially life-threatening problems.

DIAGNOSIS AND DIFFERENTIAL

The primary diagnostic maneuver is a thorough history and physical examination. Knowledge of shoulder anatomy aids in identifying specific injuries (Figs. 178-1 and 178-2). Examination of the shoulder joint

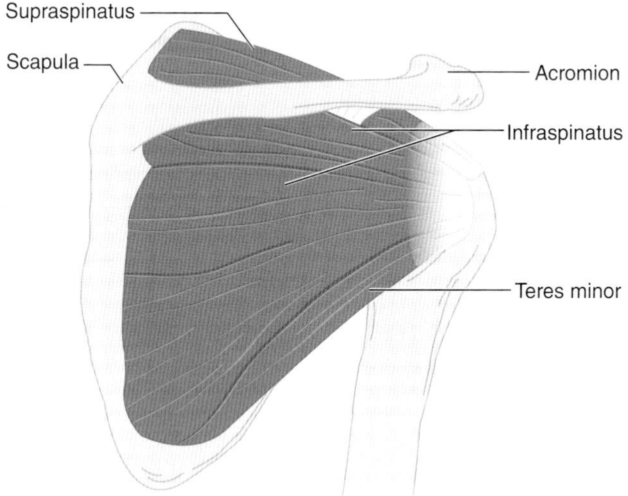

FIGURE 178-1. Posterior view of the shoulder illustrating rotator cuff muscles.

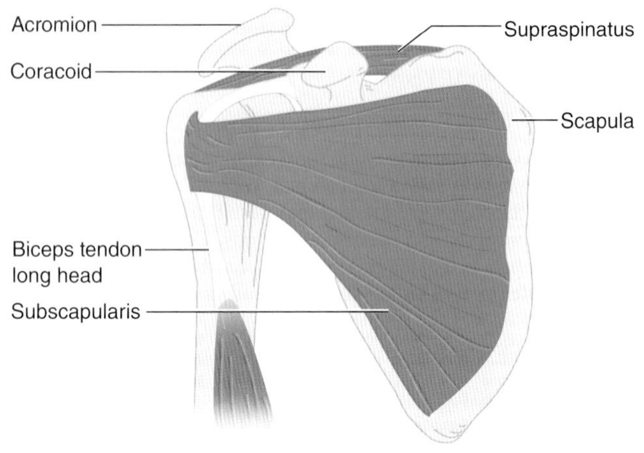

FIGURE 178-2. Anterior view of the shoulder illustrating the supraspinatus muscle and the long head of the biceps.

should include range of motion and muscle strength testing, palpation for local tenderness or other abnormality, and identification of any neurovascular deficit. Specific tests for impingement and individual tests of rotator cuff muscle function are often helpful in intrinsic disease. Absent significant trauma, plain radiographic studies of the shoulder joint are rarely diagnostic but may be helpful to exclude bony abnormalities in selected patients or to evaluate for abnormal calcifications. In patients in whom extrinsic causes of shoulder pain are suspected, further diagnostic testing may be indicated, such as laboratory studies, additional radiographs, and an electrocardiogram.

The differential diagnosis includes a variety of intrinsic musculoskeletal disorders, and individual patients may exhibit considerable overlap in their symptoms manifesting a combination of specific conditions. *Impingement syndrome* is a term that has been adopted to encompass many painful shoulder syndromes that result most frequently from repetitive overhead use of the arm. The pathologic entities included in this syndrome are subacromial tendonitis and bursitis, supraspinatus tendonitis, rotator cuff tendonitis, and the painful arc syndrome. Impingement syndrome is a painful overuse condition characterized by positive findings with impingement testing and relief of pain with anesthetic injection of the subacromial space. *Subacromial bursitis* is generally seen in patients younger than 25 years and will present with positive impingement tests with different degrees of tenderness at the lateral proximal humerus or in the subacromial space. *Rotator cuff tendonitis* is distinguished by an incidence primarily in individuals 25 to 40 years of age and findings of tenderness of the rotator cuff with mild to moderate muscular weakness. In more chronic disease, crepitus, decreased range of motion, and osteophyte formation visible on plain radiograph also may be apparent. *Rotator cuff tears* occur primarily in patients older than 40 years and are associated with muscular weakness (especially with abduction and external rotation) and cuff tenderness. Ninety percent will be chronic tears with a history of minimal or no trauma; in severe disease, muscular atrophy may be present. Acute tears may occur in patients of any age and result from significant force producing a tearing sensation with immediate pain and disability. In patients between the ages of 30 and 50 years, abnormal calcifications on radiograph in the clinical setting of a painful shoulder with rotator cuff tenderness and often crepitus suggest the diagnosis of calcific tendonitis. *Osteoarthritis* is characteristically associated with degenerative disease in other joints (primary) or previous fracture or other underlying disorder (secondary). The hallmark of *adhesive capsulitis* is significantly painful and limited range of motion often, but not always, associated with a period of immobilization. Radiographs should be obtained to exclude posterior glenohumeral dislocation. Biceps tendon pathology can also manifest as shoulder pain. The proximal long head of the biceps inserts on the superior aspect of the shoulder. Tendinopathy, subluxation, dislocation, and partial or complete tears can produce pain. Biceps tendinopathy can arise due to inflammation (tendonitis) or collagen tears around the tendon (tendinosis) and may be acute or chronic. Diagnosis is made by palpating the proximal tendon along the bicipital groove or resisted forearm supination. Reproduction of pain by these maneuvers suggests biceps pathology. Tendinitis and subluxation can be managed with sling immobilization, analgesics, anti-inflammatory agents, and frequent ice application, followed by early mobilization.

Other causes of shoulder pain that should be considered are a number of extrinsic conditions. *Pancoast tumor* may compress the brachial plexus and manifest as shoulder pain. *Degenerative disease of the cervical spine, brachial plexus disorders, and suprascapular nerve compression* are neurologic processes that should be sought in patient evaluation. Vascular pathology, notably *axillary artery thrombosis*, also may cause shoulder pain. Acute cardiac, aortic, pulmonary, and abdominal pathology may cause pain referred to the shoulder, and the clinician must remain alert to this possibility.

EMERGENCY DEPARTMENT CARE AND DISPOSITION

1. For intrinsic disease, the primary goals of emergency department care are to reduce pain and inflammation and prevent progression of disease. For most conditions, this translates to relative rest of the joint assisted by use of a sling as full immobilization is not suggested. Treatment also includes **nonsteroidal anti-inflammatory drugs**, opioid analgesics as needed, and the application of cold packs. Range-of-motion exercises should be encouraged as soon as pain allows to prevent loss of flexibility and to maintain strength.
2. **Joint space injection** with glucocorticoids such as **triamcinolone** 20 to 40 mg with or without a local anesthetic such as lidocaine should be used judiciously in view of the potential deleterious effects on soft tissues, tendon rupture with direct injection, and a recommended limitation of three injections into a single area. For all intrinsic disorders, follow-up with a primary care physician with expertise in joint disease

or orthopedic referral is suggested within 7 to 14 days. Physical therapy referral for stretching and strengthening also may be valuable.

3. In extrinsic disease, the treatment and referral pattern will depend on the diagnosis. Neurologic problems will require analgesia and anti-inflammatory medications and may require neurology or neurosurgical follow-up. Vascular causes of shoulder pain must be evaluated carefully and, with axillary artery thrombosis, immediate consultation made to initiate thrombolysis. Treatment of other extrinsic conditions depends on the specific diagnosis.

FURTHER READING

For further reading in *Tintinalli's Emergency Medicine: A Comprehensive Study Guide*, 8th ed., see Chapter 280, "Shoulder Pain," by David Della-Giustina and David Hile.

CHAPTER 179

Hip and Knee Pain

Augusta Czysz

Hip and knee pain are common complaints, especially among athletes and the obese due to increased forces on their joints. Knee pain is usually due to local pathology, whereas hip pathology commonly causes referred pain in the buttocks and lower extremity and may be due to extraarticular pathology. Each pain has a broad differential diagnosis, but a focused history and physical examination will often lead to the diagnosis (Table 179-1).

PSOAS ABSCESS

Abscess of the psoas muscle usually occurs through hematogenous spread and may present with abdominal pain radiating to the hip or flank, fever, and limp, or other constitutional symptoms. Eighty percent of the time, it is caused by *Staphylococcus aureus*. The diagnosis is made by CT. Treatment includes **organism-specific antibiotics** and **surgical drainage**.

REGIONAL NERVE ENTRAPMENT SYNDROMES

Meralgia paresthetica, a compressive inflammation of the lateral femoral cutaneous nerve, causes pain in the hip, thigh, or groin, along with burning or tingling paresthesias, and hypersensitivity to light touch. **Address the source** of nerve irritation (e.g., obesity, pregnancy, tight pants, belt) and provide **nonsteroidal anti-inflammatory drugs (NSAIDs)** to treat in the ED. Obturator nerve entrapment usually occurs after pelvic fractures, with masses, or in athletes with a fascial band at the distal obturator canal, which causes pain in the groin and down the inner thigh. **Surgery** may be needed for pain relief. Ilioinguinal nerve entrapment is associated with pregnancy or hypertrophy of the abdominal wall musculature and causes groin pain. Piriformis syndrome, irritation of the sciatic nerve from the piriformis muscle, manifests as pain in the buttocks and hamstring muscles that worsens with sitting, climbing stairs, or squatting. ED treatment is **conservative** for all of these nerve entrapment syndromes (Table 179-2).

TABLE 179-1 Suggested Clues for the Differential Diagnosis of Hip and Knee Pain
Determine the location of the pain to narrow down the potential diagnosis.
Determine the activities that bring on the pain.
Complaints that the joint "gives out" or "buckles" generally are due to pain and reflex muscle inhibition rather than an acute neurologic emergency. This complaint may also represent patellar subluxation or ligamentous injury and joint instability.
Poor conditioning or quadriceps weakness generally causes anterior knee pain of the patellofemoral syndrome; therapy should address this weakness.
Locking of the knee suggests a meniscal injury, which may be chronic.
A popping sensation or sound at the onset of pain is reliable for a ligamentous injury.
A recurrent knee effusion after activity suggests a meniscal injury.
Pain at the joint line of the knee (palpable indentation between distal femur and proximal tibia) suggests a meniscal injury.

TABLE 179-2 Selected Syndromes by Location

Diagnosis Category	Diagnosis	Pain Location
Nerve entrapment	Meralgia paresthetica	Anterolateral thigh pain or paresthesias
	Obturator nerve entrapment	Groin and inner thigh pain
	Ilioinguinal nerve entrapment	Groin pain
	Piriformis syndrome (sciatic nerve compression by piriformis muscle)	Buttocks and hamstrings pain
Hip bursitis	Trochanteric bursitis	Hip pain when lying on side or with hip abduction and adduction
	Ischiogluteal bursitis	Ischial pain
	Iliopectineal and iliopsoas bursitis	Anterior pelvis and groin, hip extension
Knee bursitis	Pes anserine bursitis	Anterior medial knee pain
	Prepatellar bursitis	Pain anterior to patella
Hip overuse syndromes	External snapping hip syndrome (coxa saltans)	Posterior lateral hip pain
	Fascia lata syndrome	Lateral thigh pain
Knee overuse syndromes	Patellofemoral syndrome (runner's knee)	Anterior knee pain, worse with prolonged knee flexion
	Medial plica syndrome	Anterior medial knee pain, knee snapping during repeated flexion/extension
	Iliotibial band syndrome or snapping knee syndrome	Pain over lateral epicondyles, or snapping when iliotibial band passes over femoral condyle
	Popliteus tendinitis	Posterior lateral knee pain, worse on downhill exercise
	Patellar tendinitis (jumper's knee)	Inferior patellar or proximal patellar tendon pain
	Quadriceps tendinitis	Proximal patellar pain
	Popliteal (Baker) cyst	Posterior knee pain

BURSAL SYNDROMES OF THE HIP AND KNEE

Inflamed or infected hip and knee bursae may cause localized pain. Inflammatory changes may be due to repetitive minor trauma, rheumatologic disorders such as psoriatic arthritis, rheumatoid arthritis or ankylosing spondylitis and crystalline disease including gout and pseudogout. Infection may be difficult to distinguish clinically from more benign disorders; analysis of bursal aspirate will help. Treatment is directed at the underlying cause. **NSAIDs**, **rest**, **heat**, and **time** are the basis of treatment for inflammatory conditions. **Steroid injections** into readily accessible bursae may be useful if infection has been excluded. Avoid injecting tendons with steroids. Treat infections with **antibiotics** (see Chapter 180, "Acute Disorders of the Joints and Bursae," for specific recommendations). Admit immunocompromised patients with suspected infections for IV antibiotics and orthopedic surgery consultation (Table 179-2).

MYOFASCIAL SYNDROMES/OVERUSE SYNDROMES

Repetitive microtrauma that outpaces the body's ability to heal results in overuse syndromes. Treatment generally consists of **NSAIDs**, **heat**, and **rest**, followed by gradual resumption of activities, physical therapy, and strengthening where appropriate (Table 179-2).

BONE/ARTICULAR DERANGEMENTS

Osteonecrosis (also called aseptic necrosis, ischemic necrosis, or avascular necrosis) is bone infarction caused by a lack of blood supply. It may be an idiopathic or a primary disorder, secondary to a systemic condition, or due to trauma. Conditions associated with osteonecrosis of the femoral head include femoral neck fracture, hip dislocation, occult or minor trauma, sickle cell disease, collagen vascular diseases, alcohol abuse, renal transplant, systemic lupus erythematosus, dysbarism, chronic pancreatitis, exogenous steroid administration, Cushing disease, decompression sickness, Gaucher disease, and renal osteodystrophy. Osteonecrosis of the hip may cause pain anywhere from the buttock to the knee. X-ray, CT, or MRI may aid in diagnosis. **Joint replacement** may be needed.

Osteomyelitis is an infection of the bone that results in bony destruction commonly caused by *Staphylococcus aureus*. Patients have local pain and may have associated warmth, swelling, and erythema. Imaging may be normal. MRI is the preferred imaging study but bone biopsy is required for confirmation. The acutely ill patient should receive **high-dose, broad-spectrum, parenteral antibiotics** based on the patient's risk factors and most likely organisms (Table 179-3).

TABLE 179-3 Risk Factors, Likely Infecting Organism, and Recommended Initial Empiric Antibiotic Therapy for Osteomyelitis

Risk Factor	Likely Infecting Organism	Recommended Initial Empiric Antibiotic Therapy*
Elderly, hematogenous spread	*Staphylococcus aureus*, including MRSA, gram-negative bacteria	Vancomycin *plus* piperacillin-tazobactam, or imipenem
Sickle cell disease	*Salmonella*, gram-negative bacteria (*S. aureus* becoming more common)	Ciprofloxacin; consider vancomycin
Diabetes mellitus, or vascular insufficiency	Polymicrobial: *S. aureus, Streptococcus agalactiae*, and *Streptococcus pyogenes* plus coliforms and anaerobes	Vancomycin *plus* piperacillin-tazobactam, or imipenem
Injection drug user	*S. aureus*, including MRSA, and *Pseudomonas*	Vancomycin
Developing nations	*Mycobacterium tuberculosis*	See Chapter 31, "Tuberculosis"
Newborn	*S. aureus* including MRSA, gram-negative bacteria, group B *Streptococcus*	Vancomycin *plus* ceftazidime
Children	*S. aureus* including MRSA	Vancomycin *plus* ceftazidime

(Continued)

TABLE 179-3 Risk Factors, Likely Infecting Organism, and Recommended Initial Empiric Antibiotic Therapy for Osteomyelitis (Continued)

Risk Factor	Likely Infecting Organism	Recommended Initial Empiric Antibiotic Therapy*
Postoperative with or without retained orthopedic hardware	*S. aureus* and coagulase-negative staphylococci	Vancomycin
Human bite	Streptococci or anaerobic bacteria	Piperacillin-tazobactam or imipenem
Animal bite	*Pasteurella multocida, Eikenella corrodens*	Cefuroxime if known *P. multocida*, piperacillin-tazobactam or imipenem

Abbreviation: MRSA, methicillin-resistant *Staphylococcus aureus*.

*All patients require bone biopsy and debridement of infected/dead bone.

Osteitis pubis occurs following pregnancy, in athletes due to overuse of the adductors and gracilis muscles, and after bladder and prostate surgery. It causes pain in the region of the pubis and generally resolves over a period of months with **rest** and **NSAIDs**. Myositis ossificans (also known as heterotopic calcification) is the deposition of bone in abnormal sites after direct trauma. Pain and a palpable mass will be present. Pain or physical obstruction may limit motion in the affected muscle or joint. **Surgery** may be required.

FURTHER READING

For further reading in *Tintinalli's Emergency Medicine: A Comprehensive Study Guide*, 8th ed., see Chapter 281, "Hip and Knee Pain," by Kelly P. O'Keefe and Tracy G. Sanson.

CHAPTER 180

Acute Disorders of The Joints and Bursae

Andrew D. Perron

Acute disorders of the joints and bursae are common emergency conditions that involve a wide spectrum of ages, acuities, and etiologies. Mismanagement of certain pathologic entities can lead to significant morbidity for the patient.

CLINICAL FEATURES

Multiple pathways can cause disruption of the normal joint milieu leading to acute joint complaints. These pathways include degeneration of articular cartilage with osteoarthritis, deposition of immune complexes as in rheumatoid arthritis, crystal-induced inflammation in gout and pseudogout, seronegative spondyloarthropathies such as ankylosing spondylitis and Reiter's syndrome, and the bacterial or viral invasion of septic arthritis. These pathologic events invariably lead to pain, the most common complaint of patients with a joint problem. Important historical factors to elicit include a determination of previous joint or bursal disease, presence of constitutional symptoms and whether the pain is acute, chronic, or acute on chronic. Determining the number and distribution of joints affected can help narrow the differential diagnosis (Table 180-1). A migratory pattern of

TABLE 180-1 Differential Diagnosis of Arthritis by Number of Affected Joints

Number of Joints	Differential Considerations for Typical Presentations
1 = Monoarthritis	85% of nongonococcal septic arthritis* Crystal-induced (gout, pseudogout) Gonococcal septic arthritis Trauma-induced arthritis Osteoarthritis (acute) Lyme disease Avascular necrosis Tumor
2–3 = Oligoarthritis†	15% of nongonococcal septic arthritis, more common with *Staphylococcus aureus* and *Streptococcus pneumonia* Lyme disease Reactive arthritis (Reiter's syndrome) Gonococcal arthritis Rheumatic fever
>3 = Polyarthritis†	Rheumatoid arthritis Systemic lupus erythematosus Viral arthritis Osteoarthritis (chronic) Serum sickness Serum sickness-like reactions

*Involvement of more than one joint does not rule out septic arthritis.

†The distinction between oligoarthritis and polyarthritis varies in the literature with a cut point of either three or four joints.

joint pain can be seen with systemic lupus erythematosus and in many infectious etiologies such as gonococcal arthritis, acute rheumatic fever, Lyme disease, and viral arthritis.

On physical examination, arthritis should be distinguished from more focal periarticular inflammatory processes such as cellulitis, bursitis, and tendonitis. True arthritis produces joint pain exacerbated by active and passive motions. Skin erythema and warmth overlying a joint should be noted, although it is nonspecific regarding etiology of joint pathology.

DIAGNOSIS AND DIFFERENTIAL

With the exception of recent joint surgery or cellulitis overlying a prosthetic knee or hip, history, physical examination, and routine blood tests do not distinguish acute septic arthritis from other forms of arthritis. Clinicians who suspect septic arthritis based on the patient's presentation should perform arthrocentesis. Synovial fluid should be sent for culture, Gram stain, cell count, and crystal evaluation (Table 180-2). Except in pediatric septic arthritis, where the erythrocyte sedimentation rate has been shown to have 90% sensitivity, the serum white blood cell count and erythrocyte sedimentation rate lack the sensitivity and specificity to be reliable discriminators in disorders of the joints and bursae. Adults with risk factors for sexually transmitted disease and migratory symptoms or tenosynovitis should be evaluated for gonococcal arthritis.

Radiographs should be obtained when the differential diagnosis includes trauma, tumor, osteomyelitis, ankylosing spondylitis, or avascular necrosis. More sophisticated modalities such as computed tomography, magnetic resonance imaging, and radioisotope scanning are used in isolated cases.

TABLE 180-2 Examination of Synovial Fluid

	Normal	Noninflammatory	Inflammatory	Septic
Clarity	Transparent	Transparent	Cloudy	Cloudy
Color	Clear	Yellow	Yellow	Yellow
WBC/μL	<200	<200 to 2000	200 to 50 000	>50 000
PMNs (%)*	<25	<25	>50%	>50%
Culture	Negative	Negative	Negative	>50% positive†
Crystals	None	None	Multiple or none	None
Associated conditions		Osteoarthritis, trauma, rheumatic fever	Gout, pseudogout, RA, Lyme disease, SLE	Septic arthritis

*The WBC and PMNs are affected by a number of factors, including disease progression, affecting organism, and host immune status. The joint aspirate WBC and %PMNs should be considered part of a continuum for each disease, particularly septic arthritis, and should be correlated with other clinical information.

†Gonococcal arthritis is frequently culture negative.

Abbreviations: RA, rheumatoid arthritis, SLE, systemic lupus erythematosus, PMNs, polymorphonuclear neutrophils.

EMERGENCY DEPARTMENT CARE AND DISPOSITION

Septic arthritis is a condition that can rapidly lead to irreversible joint destruction if inadequately treated. It typically presents as a monoarticular arthritis and may be associated with fever, chills, or malaise, although absence of these symptoms does not exclude the diagnosis. The synovial fluid may help confirm the diagnosis, although there is significant overlap in fluid findings between a number of pathological entities that can affect a joint. Therapy requires admission for parenteral antibiotics and repeated needle aspiration, arthroscopy, or open surgical drainage. Specific patient demographics can help guide empiric antibiotic therapy in septic arthritis (Table 180-3). For most of these conditions, arthrocentesis will guide diagnosis, therapy, and disposition. As a general rule, skin overlying the intended joint should be free of cellulitis. Skin is cleansed with povidone-iodine which should be allowed to air-dry. The intended site should then be cleaned with an alcohol wipe. Skin can be anesthetized with either lidocaine or with ethyl chloride spray. In general, a large-bore needle, 18-G or 19-G, should be used for larger joints such as shoulders and knees while it may be necessary to use a smaller needle for digits.

Traumatic hemarthrosis is associated with intraarticular fracture or ligamentous injury. Aspiration of large effusions may decrease pain and increase range of motion. Treatment is supportive. Spontaneous hemarthrosis may be associated with coagulopathies requiring specific clotting factor replacement. It is usually not recommended to aspirate spontaneous hemarthroses.

TABLE 180-3 Commonly Encountered Organisms in Septic Arthritis in Adolescents and Adults*

Patient/Condition	Expected Organisms	Antibiotic Considerations
Young healthy adults, or patients with risk factors for *Neisseria gonorrhoeae*	*Staphylococcus, N. gonorrhoeae, Streptococcus,* gram-negative bacteria	Vancomycin, 15 mg/kg IV load, if Gram stain reveals gram-positive organisms in clusters. Ceftriaxone, 1 g IV, or imipenem, 500 mg IV, should be used/added if either gram-negative organisms are present or no organisms are present on Gram stain and *N. gonorrhoeae* is suspected (also culture urethra, cervix, or anal canal as indicated).
Adults with comorbid disease (rheumatoid arthritis, human immunodeficiency virus, cancer) or injection drug users	*Staphylococcus*, gram-negative bacilli	Vancomycin, 15 mg/kg IV load, plus cefepime, 2 g IV, or imipenem, 500 mg IV. Meropenem 1 g IV may be used as an alternative agent.
Sickle cell patients	*Salmonella* (increasingly *Staphylococcus*)	Vancomycin, 15 mg/kg IV load, plus ciprofloxacin, 400 mg IV. Imipenem, 500 mg IV, may be used as an alternative agent.

*Recommendations differ from the 2006 British Society of Rheumatology treatment guidelines due to the rising incidence of methicillin-resistant *Staphylococcus aureus* septic arthritis.

Crystal-induced synovitis generally affects middle-age to elderly patients. Gout involves deposition of uric acid crystals, typically affecting the great toe, tarsal joints, and knee, whereas pseudogout involves deposition of calcium pyrophosphate crystals, typically affecting the knee, wrist, ankle, and elbow. Pain with gout usually evolves over hours, whereas the pain associated with pseudogout occurs over a day or more. Either condition may be precipitated by trauma, surgery, significant illness, dietary or alcohol indiscretions, or certain medications. The synovial fluid is inflammatory with negative birefringent needle-shaped crystals in gout, and weakly positive birefringent rhomboid crystals in pseudogout. Treatment is with nonsteroidal anti-inflammatory drugs such as **ibuprophen** 400 to 800 mg three times daily for 3 to 5 days and opioid analgesics. Although not routinely necessary, **colchicine** 0.6 mg/h orally until resolution of symptoms or intolerable gastrointestinal side effects may be used as a complementary therapy.

Osteoarthritis is a chronic, symmetric, polyarticular destruction of joints distinguished by a lack of constitutional symptoms. Patients may present with acute monoarticular exacerbations with small, noninflammatory synovial fluid collections and characteristic joint space narrowing on radiographs. Treatment involves rest and analgesics.

Lyme arthritis is a monoarticular or symmetric oligoarticular arthritis, especially of the large joints, with brief exacerbations followed by complete remission occurring weeks to years after the primary infection. Synovial fluid is inflammatory, typically with negative cultures. Treatment with appropriate antibiotics such as **doxycycline**, **erythromycin**, or **amoxicillin** for 3 to 4 weeks is effective.

Gonococcal arthritis is an immune-mediated infectious arthritis that typically affects adolescents and young adults. Fever, chills, and a migratory tenosynovitis or arthralgias typically precede mono- or oligoarthritis. Vesiculopustular lesions on the distal extremities are characteristic. Synovial fluid is usually inflammatory and often culture negative; cultures of the pharynx, urethra, cervix, and rectum increase the culture yield. The patient should be admitted for pain control and parenteral antibiotic therapy. Orthopedic consultation is advised.

Reiter's syndrome is a seronegative reactive spondyloarthropathy characterized by acute asymmetric oligoarthritis, especially of the lower extremities, preceded 2 to 6 weeks prior by an infectious illness such as urethritis caused by *Ureaplasma* or *Chlamydia*, or enteric infection caused by *Salmonella* or *Shigella*. The classic triad of arthritis, conjunctivitis, and urethritis is not required for the diagnosis. Synovial fluid is inflammatory. Treatment is symptomatic, and antibiotics have not been found to be useful.

Ankylosing spondylitis is a seronegative spondyloarthropathy that primarily affects the spine and pelvis and may be associated with morning stiffness and constitutional symptoms such as fatigue and weakness. Hereditary predilection, with HLA-B27 antigen or absence of rheumatoid factor, is significant. Radiographic findings include sacroiliitis and squaring of the vertebral bodies, known as bamboo spine. Treatment is symptomatic.

Rheumatoid arthritis is a chronic, symmetric, polyarticular joint disease, with sparing of the distal interphalangeal joints and associated with morning stiffness, depression, fatigue, and generalized myalgias. Pericarditis, myocarditis, pleural effusion, pneumonitis, and mononeuritis multiplex may occur. Synovial fluid is inflammatory. Treatment of an acute exacerbation involves immobilization, nonsteroidal anti-inflammatory drugs, and, occasionally, corticosteroids. Antimalarials, immunosuppressants, disease-modifying antirheumatic drugs, and cytotoxic agents are used for long-term therapy.

Bursitis refers to an inflammatory process involving any of the more than 150 bursae throughout the human body and may be caused by infection, trauma, rheumatologic diseases, or crystal deposition. Certain repetitive activities may also precipitate bursitis: prepatellar bursitis, known as "carpet layer's knee" or olecranon bursitis, known as "student's elbow." A suspicion for septic bursitis, especially in olecranon bursitis, necessitates aspiration of bursal fluid. Septic bursal fluid characteristically is purulent in appearance, with more than 1500 leukocytes/mm^3 and positive culture. Treatment principles include drainage, rest, compressive dressing, analgesics, and antibiotics for septic bursitis. Septic bursitis generally responds well to oral antibiotics, with emphasis on coverage of *Staphylococcus*, including methicillin-resistant *Staphylococcus aureus* and *Streptococcus* species.

FURTHER READING

For further reading in *Tintinalli's Emergency Medicine: A Comprehensive Study Guide*, 8th ed., see Chapter 284, "Joints and Bursae," by John H. Burton and Timothy J. Fortuna.

CHAPTER 181

Emergencies in Systemic Rheumatic Diseases

Nicholas Genes

Patients who present to the ED with systemic rheumatic disease manifestations are often at risk for pain and discomfort, organ damage, infection, adverse drug events, and significant morbidity or mortality, especially if their disease presentation is not properly recognized and managed. A new diagnosis of rheumatic disease is usually not possible in an ED visit, but may be completed in the outpatient or inpatient setting, depending on the severity of symptoms. Given the various emergent manifestations, this chapter approaches systemic rheumatic diseases by pertinent organ systems affected (Table 181-1).

TABLE 181-1 Common Features and Complications of Systemic Rheumatic Diseases

Disorder	Common and Characteristic Clinical Features	Complications
Antiphospholipid syndrome	Multiple and recurrent venous and arterial thromboses, recurrent abortions. Secondary form is associated with systemic lupus erythematosus, rheumatoid arthritis, systemic sclerosis, and Sjögren's syndrome. Thrombophlebitis and deep vein thrombosis, thrombocytopenia, hemolytic anemia, microangiopathic hemolytic anemia, livedo reticularis, stroke, transient ischemic attack, eye vascular complications. Coronary, renal, mesenteric, and cerebral vascular occlusion.	ARDS, pulmonary embolism, ischemic complications of vascular occlusion, bleeding, severe anemia, vision loss, catastrophic antiphospholipid syndrome.
Ankylosing spondylitis	Chronic inflammatory disease of the axial skeleton, with progressive stiffness of the spine. Young adults (peak at 20 and 30 years old). Back pain (improves with exercise), buttock, hip, or shoulder pain, systemic complaints (fever, malaise, fatigue, weight loss, myalgias), uveitis, and restrictive pulmonary failure due to costovertebral rigidity, ILD, renal impairment, fracture of the ankylosed spine, asymptomatic ileal and colonic mucosal ulcerations. Secondary amyloidosis.	Acute spinal cord or nerve compression, subluxation of the atlantoaxial joint, aortic regurgitation.
Adult Still's disease	Inflammatory disorder (similar to systemic onset juvenile rheumatoid arthritis). Systemic complaints (fever, malaise, fatigue, weight loss, myalgia), arthritis, myalgia, evanescent rash, pharyngitis, lymphadenopathy, splenomegaly, anemia, thrombocytopenia. Pericarditis, myocarditis, pleurisy.	ARDS, arrhythmias, heart failure, fulminant hepatic failure, red cell aplasia, disseminated intravascular coagulation, microangiopathic hemolytic anemia.

(Continued)

TABLE 181-1 Common Features and Complications of Systemic Rheumatic Diseases (Continued)

Disorder	Common and Characteristic Clinical Features	Complications
Behçet's disease	Chronic, relapsing, inflammatory disease. Systemic vasculitis involving arteries and veins of all sizes (carotid, pulmonary, aortic, and inferior extremity vessels are most commonly involved, with aneurysm, dissection, rupture, or thrombosis). Systemic complaints (fever, malaise, fatigue, weight loss, myalgia), recurrent painful skin and mucosal lesions; asymmetric, nondeforming arthritis of the medium and large joints; thrombophlebitis and deep vein thrombosis; ocular complications. Neuropsychiatric manifestations. Pericarditis, myocarditis.	Hypopyon, retinal vasculitis, optic neuritis, eye vascular complication. Dural sinus thrombosis, aseptic meningitis and encephalitis. Arrhythmias. Superior and inferior vena cava syndrome. Abdominal aorta or pulmonary artery emergencies. Bowel perforation.
Churg–Strauss syndrome	Vasculitis with a multisystemic involvement. Systemic complaints (fever, malaise, fatigue, weight loss, myalgia), allergic rhinitis, nasal obstruction, recurrent sinusitis, asthma, and peripheral blood eosinophilia. Systemic hypertension, pericarditis, abdominal pain, peripheral symmetric neuropathy; skin lesions and rash.	Heart failure, acute myocardial infarction, acute and constrictive pericarditis, GI bleeding, bowel perforation.
Dermatomyositis/polymyositis	Idiopathic inflammatory myopathies. Muscle weakness, myalgia, and muscle tenderness. Elevated serum creatine kinase. Systemic complaints (fever, malaise, fatigue, weight loss, myalgia), Raynaud phenomenon, nonerosive inflammatory polyarthritis, esophageal dysfunction, ILD, aspiration lung infections.	ARDS. Respiratory failure and arrest due to diaphragmatic or chest wall muscle weakness, alveolar hemorrhage, and ILD. Heart failure, arrhythmias, and conduction disturbances.
Giant cell arteritis (temporal arteritis)	Chronic vasculitis of large- and medium-sized vessels. Elderly (mean age at diagnosis: 70 years old). Associated with polymyalgia rheumatica in 50% of cases. Localized headache of new onset, tenderness of the temporal artery, and biopsy revealing a necrotizing arteritis. Temporal artery may be normal on clinical examination. Gradual onset, systemic complaints, jaw or tongue claudication, eye complaints and visual loss. Aortic regurgitation and aortic arch syndrome. Neurologic complications due to carotid and vertebrobasilar vasculitis.	Ischemic optic neuropathy, eye vessel occlusion. Aortitis (especially the thoracic tract) and aortic emergencies. Stroke.
Henoch–Schönlein purpura	Systemic vasculitis associated with immunoglobulin A deposition, generally in children. Frequently, acute presentation follows an upper respiratory infection. Palpable purpura (in patients with neither thrombocytopenia nor coagulopathy), arthritis/arthralgia, abdominal pain, and renal impairment (adult), ILD.	Respiratory failure and alveolar hemorrhage. Seizures, intracranial bleeding, GI hemorrhage, bowel ischemia or perforation, acute pancreatitis, intussusception (children). Acute scrotum.

(Continued)

TABLE 181-1 Common Features and Complications of Systemic Rheumatic Diseases (Continued)

Disorder	Common and Characteristic Clinical Features	Complications
Microscopic polyangiitis	Small-vessel systemic vasculitis, characterized by rapidly progressive glomerulonephritis and pulmonary involvement. Lung complications differentiate microscopic polyangiitis from polyarteritis nodosa. Systemic complaints (fever, malaise, fatigue, weight loss, myalgia), arthralgias, skin lesions, hemoptysis, abdominal pain, renal impairment, systemic hypertension.	Rapidly progressive glomerulonephritis, severe lung hemorrhage, GI bleeding.
Polyarteritis nodosa	Systemic necrotizing vasculitis of the medium-sized muscular arteries. Systemic complaints (fever, malaise, fatigue, weight loss, myalgia), arthralgias, skin lesions, abdominal pain, renal impairment, systemic hypertension, peripheral mononeuropathy typically with both motor and sensory deficits, eye complications, leukocytosis, and normochromic anemia.	Acute scrotum, ischemic and hemorrhagic stroke, acute coronary syndrome, heart failure, peripheral artery ischemia, mesenteric ischemia and bowel perforation, GI bleeding, acute pancreatitis, malignant hypertension.
Relapsing polychondritis	Immune-mediated condition. Ears (violaceous and erythematous auricula), nose (saddle nose deformity), and other cartilaginous structures inflammation (especially joints and respiratory tract). One-third of cases associated with other systemic rheumatic diseases. Sternoclavicular, costochondral, and manubriosternal arthritis, upper airway involvement, aortic or mitral valvular regurgitation, pericarditis, renal impairment, peripheral neuropathies, ocular complications.	Airway obstruction. Acute renal failure, aortitis and aortic emergencies, heart block, ACS, scleritis, peripheral ulcerative keratitis, and acute scrotum.
Rheumatoid arthritis	Chronic, systemic, inflammatory disorder. Symmetric and potentially destructive arthritis. Systemic symptoms (fever, malaise, fatigue, weight loss, myalgia), skin lesions, splenomegaly. Cervical spine involvement, pleuritis, ILD, pericarditis, myocarditis, and aortitis. Cricoarytenoid arthritis with potential for airway obstruction, ocular involvement. Peripheral artery disease, Sjögren's syndrome, vasculitis, and renal impairment. Abdominal pain. Anemia, leukopenia, thrombocytosis, and Felty's syndrome. Increased risk of lymphoproliferative diseases, particularly non-Hodgkin's lymphoma.	Airway obstruction, obliterative bronchiolitis, acute respiratory failure. ACS, heart failure, thoracic aorta dissection, arrhythmias and conduction disturbances, subluxation of the atlantoaxial joints, bowel ischemia and perforation. Septic arthritis. Scleritis.

(Continued)

TABLE 181-1 Common Features and Complications of Systemic Rheumatic Diseases (Continued)

Disorder	Common and Characteristic Clinical Features	Complications
Systemic lupus erythematosus	Systemic autoimmune disease, characterized by relapses and remissions, and affecting virtually every organ. Systemic complaints (fever, malaise, fatigue, weight loss, myalgia), symmetric and polyarticular arthritis (small joints of the hands, wrists, and knees), butterfly rash, mucocutaneous manifestations, oral and/or nasal ulcers, Raynaud's phenomenon. Neuropsychiatric manifestations, pleurisy, lupus pneumonitis, shrinking or vanishing lung syndrome, ILD, and pulmonary hypertension. Libman–Sacks endocarditis, pericarditis, myocarditis, endocarditis. GI nonspecific complaints. Renal impairment, leukopenia, mild anemia, and thrombocytopenia. Antiphospholipid syndrome. Ocular complications.	Airway obstruction, ARDS, respiratory failure and arrest, alveolar hemorrhage, ACS, cardiac tamponade, heart failure, arrhythmias, pulmonary embolism, stroke, acute renal failure, Guillain–Barré like syndrome, transverse myelitis, seizures. Bowel ischemia and perforation, GI bleeding, acute pancreatitis. Hemolytic anemia, thrombotic microangiopathic hemolytic anemia.
Sjögren's syndrome	Autoimmune disease. May be primary; secondary form is mostly associated with rheumatoid arthritis, systemic lupus erythematosus, polymyositis, or dermatomyositis. Xerophthalmia and xerostomia, systemic symptoms, arthralgia, skin lesions, Raynaud's phenomenon. ILD, pulmonary hypertension, pericarditis, neuropsychiatric manifestations, peripheral neuropathy, hepatic abnormalities, renal impairment, increased risk of non-Hodgkin's lymphoma.	Hypokalemic respiratory arrest. Heart block, pulmonary embolism, ischemic stroke, transverse myelitis, optic neuritis, renal tubular acidosis, acute pancreatitis.
Systemic sclerosis (scleroderma)	Inappropriate and excessive accumulation of collagen and matrix in a variety of tissue; widespread vascular lesions with endothelial dysfunction, vascular spasm, thickening of the vascular wall and narrowing of the vascular lumen. Systemic complaints (fever, malaise, fatigue, weight loss, myalgia), skin lesions (fingers, hands, and face), carpal tunnel syndrome, Raynaud's phenomenon. ILD, renal impairment, GI dysmotility, gastroesophageal reflux (aspiration pneumonitis), chronic esophagitis and stricture formation. Vascular ectasia in the stomach ("watermelon stomach").	Scleroderma renal crisis. Respiratory failure, ARDS, aspiration pneumonitis, pulmonary hypertension, alveolar hemorrhage, heart failure, arrhythmias, and conduction disturbances.

(Continued)

TABLE 181-1 Common Features and Complications of Systemic Rheumatic Diseases (Continued)

Disorder	Common and Characteristic Clinical Features	Complications
Takayasu's arteritis	Chronic vasculitis, young women, predominantly Asians. Systemic complaints (fever, malaise, fatigue, weight loss, myalgia), arthralgias, skin lesions, abdominal pain and diarrhea. Aorta and its primary branches, and pulmonary artery involvement. Neurologic manifestations, syncope, subclavian steal syndrome, extremity ischemia. Renovascular hypertension. Normochromic normocytic anemia.	ACS, bowel ischemia and perforation, GI bleeding, stroke.
Wegener's (granulomatosis with polyangiitis)	Multiple organ system vasculitis and necrotizing granulomas. Respiratory tract manifestations in approximately 100% of cases, with nose, oral cavity, upper trachea, external and middle ear, and orbit inflammations. Upper airway and pulmonary manifestations. Constitutional symptoms, arthralgias, glomerulonephritis and small vessel vasculitis (scleritis and episcleritis, palpable purpura or cutaneous nodules, peripheral neuropathy, deafness). Systemic hypertension. Pericarditis, myocarditis. Renal impairment. Anemia, leukocytosis, and thrombocytosis.	Airway obstruction, subglottic stenosis, bronchiolitis obliterans organizing pneumonia, and alveolar hemorrhage. ACS, arrhythmias. Rapidly progressive glomerulonephritis.

Abbreviations: ACS, acute coronary syndrome; ARDS, adult respiratory distress syndrome; ILD, interstitial lung disease.

CLINICAL FEATURES

Airway Emergencies

Cricoarytenoid joint arthritis, seen in rheumatoid arthritis (RA), systemic lupus erythematosis (SLE), and relapsing polychondritis (RP), can present with throat pain, a fullness in the throat, voice changes, and tenderness over cartilaginous structures. More severe cases lead to dyspnea and stridor, leading to acute upper airway obstruction. Evaluate using CT imaging or fiber optic laryngoscopy; initial treatment consists of high-dose steroids, such as **methylprednisolone** 250 mg IV.

Endotracheal intubation is often difficult in patients with systemic rheumatic disease; thus, consider "dual setup" preparation for cricothyrotomy. Moreover, neck hyperextension should be avoided in patients with advanced rheumatoid arthritis or ankylosing spondylitis due to the risk of cervical fractures, subluxation and dislocation, and spinal cord compression.

Pulmonary Emergencies

Systemic sclerosis, RA, SLE, Wegener's granulomatosis, and polymyositis can cause chronic pulmonary symptoms through processes such as interstitial lung disease or acute complications such as alveolar hemorrhage. The risk of pneumonia is elevated due to disease processes and immunosuppression. Pleural effusions are seen in RA and SLE. Systemic rheumatic diseases place patients at higher risk of pulmonary embolism.

Distinguishing pneumonia from alveolar hemorrhage can be difficult, as fever and x-ray infiltrates are common in both conditions. Anemia is often sensitive for alveolar hemorrhage. Bronchoscopy can confirm the diagnosis, but treatment in the ED is high-dose glucocorticoids in patients with alveolar hemorrhage versus antibiotics for patients with pneumonia.

Cardiovascular Emergencies

Systemic rheumatic disease can injure the heart through several mechanisms. Accelerated coronary atherosclerosis is seen in SLE, antiphospholipid syndrome, and RA, and are considered risk factors for coronary artery disease.

Pericarditis can occur in RA and SLE, and pancarditis is a feature of acute rheumatic fever.

Aortitis and aortic aneurysms can be seen in patients with a history of giant cell (temporal) arteritis, Takayasu's arteritis, and Behçet's disease, leading to rupture, dissection, neurologic symptoms, or coronary syndromes.

Neurologic and Ophthalmologic Emergencies

Vascular inflammation and accelerated vascular disease, as well as direct involvement from systemic rheumatologic disease, can lead to neurologic and ophthalmologic emergencies. Ischemic and hemorrhagic stroke symptoms are usually not subtle, but vertebrobasilar circulation lesions may present as vertigo, hearing loss, or ataxia.

Sudden blindness is associated with giant cell (temporal) arteritis; patients may also present with signs of jaw and tongue claudication. Temporal artery biopsy can confirm the diagnosis; however, high-dose steroids should be administered empirically.

Excessive tearing, redness, vision changes, and pain can be manifestations of systemic rheumatic disease.

Renal Emergencies

Almost all systemic rheumatic disease can involve the kidney. SLE, Wegener's granulomatosis, and systemic vasculitis can lead to nephritis. Distal renal tubular acidosis, with associated hypokalemia, occurs in 30% of patients with Sjogrën's syndrome and presents as a progressive weakness. Other rheumatic processes can progress to rhabdomyolysis and acute renal failure.

Gastrointestinal Emergencies

GI manifestations of systemic rheumatic disease are the most commonly vasculitides, from giant-cell arteritis affecting larger vessels to SLE affecting small vessels. These processes present with abdominal pain, ileus, or obstruction, and can lead to bowel ischemia.

OTHER ORGAN SYSTEMS

Anemia, leukopenia, and thrombocytopenia are commonly observed in systemic rheumatic disease. Antiphospholipid disease can present with thrombotic thrombocytopenic purpora. Hemolytic anemia is observed in SLE and systemic sclerosis.

Malignant hypertension can be seen with systemic sclerosis, antiphospholipid syndrome, and polyarteritis nodosa. Hypertension is also a complication of rheumatic processes (and medications) that involve the kidney.

Dermatologic manifestations of rheumatic disease include rash, ulcers, and cellulitis, as well as Raynaud's phenomenon.

Orchitis is commonly seen in polyarteritis nodosa and Henoch–Schonlein purpura. Ultrasound should be performed as the presentation mimics testicular torsion.

Infectious Emergencies/Immunosuppression

Systemic rheumatic diseases themselves cause direct immunosuppression, as do many of the medications to treat them. Anatomic changes resulting from disease progression can also predispose to infection. Opportunistic species as well as typical causative agents are seen.

Empiric antibiotics are indicated for patients with apparent infections; procalcitonin levels greater than 0.5 ng/mL are specific for sepsis in autoimmune disease.

Septic arthritis is more common in patients with RA on steroids or biologic agents, and often presents with a less impressive exam than patients not taking these medications. The clinician should have a low threshold for arthrocentesis.

Adverse Drug Reactions

Stressors or abrupt withdrawal from steroids can trigger adrenal insufficiency. Patients will present with hypotension; hyponatremia, hypoglycemia, and hyperkalemia are commonly seen. **Hydrocortisone 100 mg IV** is the emergent treatment.

Hypertension and renal insufficiency are seen in many patients taking biologic agents to treat rheumatic disease, as well as NSAIDs and cyclophosphamide.

Some biologic agents are associated with increased risk of zoster lesions, particularly zoster ophthalmicus.

FURTHER READING

For further reading in *Tintinalli's Emergency Medicine: A Comprehensive Study Guide*, 8th ed., see Chapter 282, "Systemic Rheumatic Diseases," by R. Darrell Nelson.

CHAPTER 182

Nontraumatic Disorders of The Hand

Michael P. Kefer

Drainage of pus, immobilization, elevation, and antibiotics are the mainstays of treatment for many conditions of the hand. This helps to decrease inflammation, avoid secondary injury, and prevent extension of any infection. Optimal splinting is in the position of function: wrist in 15° to 30° extension, metacarpophalangeal (MCP) joints in 50° to 90° flexion, and the interphalangeal joints in 10° to 15° flexion.

HAND INFECTIONS

Cellulitis is a superficial infection presenting with localized warmth, erythema, and edema. Absence of tenderness on deep palpation and nonpainful digit range of motion help to exclude deep space involvement.

Flexor tenosynovitis is a surgical emergency diagnosed on examination (Table 182-1).

Deep space infections involve the thenar, web, or midpalmar space, or the radial or ulnar bursa. Infection occurs from spread of a flexor tenosynovitis or a penetrating wound. The palm is tender to palpation and range of motion of the digits is painful where the flexor tendons course through the area of infection. Swelling from web space infection causes separation of the affected digits. Deep space infections often require operative drainage.

Closed fist injury is essentially a bite wound to the MCP joint that results from a punch to the teeth. There is high risk of infection to the skin, tendon, joint, bone, and deep space. Wounds penetrating the skin require exploration, irrigation, prophylactic antibiotics, and healing by secondary intention. Wounds with established signs of infection require IV antibiotics and hand surgery consult for consideration of operative intervention.

Paronychia is an infection of the lateral nail fold. If there is no pus, treat with warm soaks, elevation, and antibiotics if warranted. A paronychia is drained by lifting the nail fold with a flat blade. If pus is seen beneath the nail, a portion of the nail may need removal and packing placed for adequate drainage. Recheck within 48 hours, pull the packing, and begin warm soaks.

Felon is an infection of the pulp space of the fingertip. Incision and drainage are by the lateral approach to protect the neurovascular bundle. Do not incise the distal end of the finger pad. Do not extend the incision proximally to the flexor crease of the distal interphalangeal joint. More extensive through-and-through or "hockey stick" incisions are not indicated.

TABLE 182-1 Kanavel's Four Cardinal Signs of Flexor Tenosynovitis

Percussion tenderness	Tenderness over the entire length of the flexor tendon sheath
Uniform swelling	Symmetric finger swelling along the length of the tendon sheath
Intense pain	Intense pain with passive extension
Flexion posture	Flexed posture of the involved digit at rest to minimize pain

Bluntly dissect the septae to ensure complete drainage. If there is a pointing volar abscess, a longitudinal volar incision is used. Pack the wound. Splint the finger. Recheck within 48 hours, pull the packing, and begin warm soaks.

Herpetic whitlow is a viral infection of the distal finger. It may present similar to a felon, but vesicles are present. Immobilize, elevate, and protect with a dry dressing to prevent transmission. Antiviral agents may shorten the duration.

Table 182-2 summarizes antibiotic therapy for common hand infections.

TABLE 182-2 Initial Antibiotic Coverage for Common Hand Infections

Infection	Initial Antimicrobial Agent(s)	Likely Organisms	Comments
Cellulitis	*For mild to moderate cellulitis:* TMP-SMX double strength, 1–2 tablets twice per day PO for 7–10 days.* *Plus/minus* cephalexin, 500 mg PO four times per day for 7–10 days, *or* dicloxacillin, 500 mg PO four times daily for 7–10 days. *For severe cellulitis:* Vancomycin, 1 g IV every 12 h.	*Staphylococcus aureus* (MRSA) *Streptococcus pyogenes*	Clindamycin is an option, but increasing MRSA resistance to clindamycin has been reported. Consider vancomycin for injection drug abusers.
Felon/ paronychia	TMP-SMX double strength, 1–2 tablets twice per day PO for 7–10 days.* *Plus/minus* cephalexin, 500 mg PO four times per day for 7–10 days,* *or* dicloxacillin, 500 mg PO four times daily for 7–10 days.* *Consider* addition of clindamycin or amoxicillin-clavulanate to TMP-SMX (rather than cephalexin) if anaerobic bacteria are suspected.	*S. aureus* (MRSA), *S. pyogenes*, anaerobes, polymicrobial	Antibiotics indicated for infections with associated localized cellulitis, otherwise drainage alone may be sufficient, culture recommended by hand surgeons.
Flexor tenosynovitis	Ampicillin-sulbactam, 1.5 g IV every 6 h, *or* cefoxitin, 2 g IV every 8 h, *or* piperacillin-tazobactam, 3.375 g IV every 6 h. *Plus:* Vancomycin, 1 g IV every 12 h, if MRSA is prevalent in community.	*S. aureus*, streptococci, anaerobes, gram negatives	Parenteral antibiotics are indicated; consider ceftriaxone for suspected *Neisseria gonorrhoeae*.
Deep space infection	Ampicillin-sulbactam, 1.5 g IV every 6 h, *or* cefoxitin, 2 g IV every 8 h, *or* piperacillin-tazobactam, 3.375 g IV every 6 h. *Plus:* Vancomycin, 1 g IV every 12 h, if MRSA is prevalent in community.	*S. aureus*, streptococci, anaerobes, gram negatives	Inpatient management.

(Continued)

TABLE 182-2 Initial Antibiotic Coverage for Common Hand Infections (Continued)

Infection	Initial Antimicrobial Agent(s)	Likely Organisms	Comments
Animal bites (including human)	If no visible signs of infection: amoxicillin/clavulanate, 875/125 mg PO twice daily for 5 days. For signs of infection: Ampicillin-sulbactam, 1.5 g IV every 6 h, *or* cefoxitin, 2 g IV every 8 h, *or* piperacillin-tazobactam, 3.375 g every 6 h. For penicillin allergy, use clindamycin plus moxifloxacin or TMP-SMX and metronidazole.	*S. aureus*, streptococci, *Eikenella corrodens* (human), *Pasteurella multocida* (cat), anaerobes, and gram-negative bacteria	All animal bite wounds should receive prophylactic oral antibiotics.
Herpetic whitlow	Acyclovir, 400 mg PO three times daily for 10 days.	Herpes simplex	No surgical drainage is indicated.

*While many sources recommend 7–10 days of therapy, the Infectious Disease Society of America recommends 5 days of therapy if symptoms resolve, continue therapy if symptoms persist.

Abbreviations: MRSA, methicillin-resistant *Staphylococcus aureus*; TMP-SMX, trimethoprim-sulfamethoxazole.

NONINFECTIOUS CONDITIONS

Tendonitis and tenosynovitis are usually due to overuse. Examination reveals tenderness over the tendon and pain with activation or passive stretch. Treat with immobilization and nonsteroidal anti-inflammatory drugs (NSAIDs).

Trigger finger is a tenosynovitis of the flexor sheath. Inflammation or scarring results in impingement and snap release of the tendon as the finger is extended from a flexed position. Steroid injection may be effective. Definitive treatment is surgery.

DeQuervain tenosynovitis involves the extensor pollicis brevis and abductor pollicis tendons. Pain occurs at the radial aspect of the wrist and radiates into the forearm. The Finkelstein test is diagnostic: the patient grasps the thumb in the fist and deviates the hand ulnarly, reproducing the pain. Treat with a thumb spica splint, NSAIDs, and referral.

Carpal tunnel syndrome results from compression of the median nerve by the transverse carpal ligament. The cause is usually edema from overuse, pregnancy, or congestive heart failure. Pain in the median nerve distribution tends to be worse at night. The pain may be reproduced by tapping over the nerve at the wrist (Tinel's sign) or by holding the wrist flexed maximally for >1 minute (Phalen's test). Treat with a wrist splint, NSAIDs, and referral.

Dupuytren contracture results from fibrous changes in the subcutaneous tissues of the palm which may lead to tethering and joint contractures. Refer to a hand surgeon.

Ganglion cyst is a collection of fluid from synovial tissue that herniates from a joint capsule or tendon sheath. Treat with NSAIDs and referral.

FURTHER READING

For further reading in *Tintinalli's Emergency Medicine: A Comprehensive Study Guide*, 8th ed., see Chapter 283, "Nontraumatic Disorders of the Hand," by Carl A. Germann.

CHAPTER 183

Soft Tissue Problems of The Foot

Gavin R. Budhram

CORNS AND CALLUSES

Calluses represent a dermatologic reaction to focal pressure. They are protective and should not be treated unless they are painful. Ongoing pressure may cause calluses to develop into corns. Corns have a central hyperkaratotic core that is often painful. Hard corns can resemble warts, but can be differentiated with incision; warts will bleed, corns will not. The differential diagnosis includes syphilis, psoriasis, lichen planus, rosacea, arsenic poisoning, basal cell nevus syndrome, and malignancy. Treatment for corns often includes paring with a scalpel to include removal of central keratin plug, but topical salicylic acid treatments may be more effective.

PLANTAR WARTS

Plantar warts are common, contagious, and caused by the human papillomavirus. The diagnosis is clinical and the differential includes corns and undiagnosed melanoma. Topical treatment with 15% to 20% salicylic acid is most effective. Nonhealing lesions should be referred to a dermatologist or podiatrist.

ONYCHOCRYPTOSIS (INGROWN TOENAIL)

Onychocryptosis is characterized by increased inflammation or infection of the lateral or medial aspects of the toenail. This occurs when the nail plate penetrates the nail sulcus and subcutaneous tissue (usually in the great toe). Patients with underlying diabetes, arterial insufficiency, cellulitis, ulceration, or necrosis are at risk for amputation if treatment is delayed. Treatment depends on the type of inflammation. If the toenail is uninfected, sufficient results will often be obtained with elevation of the nail with a wisp of cotton between the nail plate and the skin, daily foot soaks, and avoidance of pressure on the area. A second option (requiring digital block) is to remove a spicule of the nail and debride the nail groove (Fig. 183-1). If granulation tissue or infection is present, partial removal of the nail is indicated. If the toenail is infected, perform digital block and cut one-fourth or less of the nail, including beneath the cuticle, with a longitudinal incision (Fig. 183-2). A nonadherent bulky dressing should be placed and the wound should be checked in 24 to 48 hours.

BURSITIS

Calcaneal bursitis causes pain over the posterior heel in contrast to Achilles tendinopathy that causes pain and tenderness 2 to 6 cm superior to the posterior calcaneus. Pathologic bursae of the foot are categorized as follows: (1) noninflammatory, (2) inflammatory, (3) suppurative, and (4) calcified. Noninflammatory bursae become painful as a result of

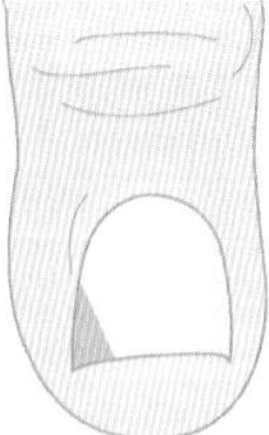

FIGURE 183-1. Partial toenail removal. This method is used for small nail fold swellings without infection. After antiseptic skin preparation and digital nerve block, an oblique portion of the affected nail is trimmed about one-third to two-thirds of the way back to the posterior nail fold. Use scissors to cut the nail; use forceps to grasp and remove the nail fragment.

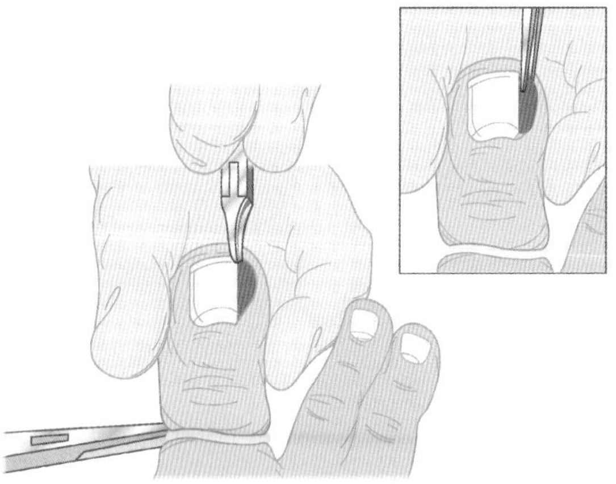

FIGURE 183-2. Partial toenail removal (infection present). This method is used for onychocryptosis in the setting of significant granulation tissue or infection.

direct pressure and resolve with simple measures including comfortable footwear, rest, ice, and nonsteroidal anti-inflammatory drugs (NSAIDs). Inflammatory bursitis results from gout, syphilis, or rheumatoid arthritis. Suppurative bursitis results from spread of pyogenic organisms (often *Staphylococcus aureus*) from adjacent wounds. Complications include hygroma, calcified bursae, fistula, and ulcer formation. Treatment for septic bursitis is discussed in Chapter 180, "Acute Disorders of the Joints and Bursae."

PLANTAR FASCIITIS

The plantar fascia is connective tissue anchoring the plantar skin to the bone. Plantar fasciitis is the most common cause of heel pain due to overuse. Patients have pain on the plantar surface of the foot that is worse when initiating walking and point tenderness over the anterior–medial calcaneus that is worsened by dorsiflexion of the toes. The presence of heel spurs on radiography is of no diagnostic value because many patients without plantar fasciitis have this finding. Treatment includes rest, ice, and NSAIDs. Most of the cases are self-limited and resolve spontaneously within 12 months. Plantar stretch exercises, including using the hands to dorsiflex the ankle and toes are helpful in the acute phase. Glucocorticoid injections are *not* indicated in the ED. Patients with severe cases may require a short-leg walking cast and should be referred to a podiatrist or orthopedist.

NERVE ENTRAPMENT SYNDROMES

Tarsal Tunnel Syndromes

Tarsal tunnel syndrome involves heel and foot pain due to compression of the posterior tibial nerve as it courses inferior to the medial malleolus. Causes include running, restrictive footwear, edema of pregnancy, post-traumatic fibrosis, ganglion cysts, osteophytes, and tumors. Symptoms include numbness or burning of the sole and may be limited to the heel. Pain is worse at night and after running or standing, in contrast to plantar fasciitis which is worse upon morning standing. Typically, pain is located at the medial malleolus, the heel, the sole, and the distal calf.

The differential diagnosis includes plantar fasciitis and Achilles tendonitis. Percussion inferior to the medial malleolus yields pain radiating to the medial or lateral plantar surface (Tinel sign), and eversion and dorsiflexion worsen symptoms. Treatment includes NSAIDs, rest, and possible orthopedic referral.

Deep Peroneal Nerve Entrapment

Entrapment of the deep peroneal nerve occurs most frequently where it courses beneath the extensor retinaculum at the anterior aspect of the ankle. Recurrent ankle sprains, soft tissue masses, and restrictive footwear represent the most common causes. Symptoms include dorsal and medial foot pain as well as sensory hypoesthesia at the first web space. Prolonged entrapment may cause loss of the ability to hyperextend the toes.

Pain and tenderness can be elicited by plantar flexion during inversion of the foot. Treatment includes NSAIDs, rest, and possible orthopedic referral.

GANGLIONS

A ganglion is a benign synovial cyst attached to a joint capsule or tendon sheath near the anterolateral ankle. Typically a firm, nontender, cystic lesion is found on examination. The diagnosis is clinical, but MRI or ultrasound can be used if in doubt. Treatment includes aspiration and injection of glucocorticoids, but most require surgical excision.

TENDON LESIONS

Tenosynovitis and Tendinitis

Tenosynovitis and tendonitis are usually due to overuse and present with pain over the involved tendon. The flexor hallucis longus, posterior tibialis, and Achilles tendon are most commonly involved. Treatment includes ice, rest, and NSAIDs.

Tendon Lacerations

Tendon lacerations in the foot are complex, and orthopedic consultation is needed. After repair, extensor tendons are immobilized in dorsiflexion and flexor tendons in equinus.

Tendon Ruptures

Spontaneous rupture of the Achilles tendon is common, but rupture of the other tendons of the foot can occur. Age and chronic corticosteroid and fluoroquinolone use are risk factors for spontaneous rupture. *Achilles tendon* rupture presents with pain and a palpable defect in the area of the tendon. Patients have an inability to stand on tiptoes and an absence of plantar flexion with squeezing of the calf (Thompson test). Treatment is generally surgical in younger patients and conservative (casting in equinus) in the elderly. *Anterior tibialis tendon* rupture results in a palpable defect and mild foot drop. In most cases surgery is not necessary. *Posterior tibialis tendon* rupture is usually chronic and presents with a flattened arch and swelling over the medial ankle. Examination may show weakness on inversion, a palpable defect, and inability to stand on tiptoes. *Flexor hallucis longus* rupture presents with loss of plantar flexion of the great toe. The need for surgical repair depends on the patient's occupation and lifestyle. *Disruption of the peroneal retinaculum* occurs after a direct blow during dorsiflexion and causes localized pain behind the lateral malleolus; there is clicking during walking, as the tendon is subluxed. Treatment is surgical.

PLANTAR INTERDIGITAL NEUROMA (MORTON NEUROMA)

Neuromas are thought to occur from entrapment of the plantar digital nerve proximal to its bifurcation due to tight-fitting shoes; the third interspace is most commonly affected. Patients often present with burning, cramping, or aching over the affected metatarsal head, and numbness in the toe. Pain is easily reproduced upon palpation of the area and at times a mass is felt. Diagnosis is clinical, but ultrasound or MRI may be helpful. Conservative treatment includes wide shoes and glucocorticoid injections. Local glucocorticoid injections may be curative. Surgical neurolysis is occasionally required.

COMPARTMENT SYNDROMES OF THE FOOT

The foot has nine compartments. Compartment syndromes in the foot are associated with high-energy crush injuries. Other causes include bleeding disorders and postischemic swelling after arterial injury, foot and ankle fractures (especially calcaneal and Lisfranc's fracture/dislocation), burns, and chronic overuse. Pain out of proportion to injury is one of the early findings. Additional symptoms include pain that is worsened on active and passive movement, paresthesias, and neurovascular deficits. Absent pulse and complete anesthesia are late findings.

At-risk patients must have compartment pressures checked. Any difference of less than 30 mm Hg between the Stryker STIC Device (Stryker,

Kalamazoo, MI) and diastolic blood pressure is considered positive. Prompt consideration of emergent fasciotomy is indicated.

MALIGNANT MELANOMA

Melanoma of the foot, which accounts for 15% of all cutaneous melanomas, may present as atypical nonpigmented or pigmented lesions; the nail may be included. Vigilance is key as these lesions often mimic more benign conditions. The differential diagnosis includes fungal infections, plantar warts, and foot ulcers. Because prognosis is directly related to early diagnosis, all atypical or nonhealing lesions should be referred for biopsy.

FURTHER READING

For further reading in *Tintinalli's Emergency Medicine: A Comprehensive Study Guide*, 8th ed., see Chapter 285, "Soft Tissue Problems of the Foot," by Mitchell C. Sokolosky.

SECTION 21

Psychosocial Disorders

Clinical Features of Behavioral Disorders

Leslie S. Zun

INCIDENCE

Mental illness affects 26.2% of the population of the world's adult population in any given year.

DEMENTIA

Dementia is a disorder consisting of a pervasive disturbance in cognition that impairs memory, abstraction, judgment, personality, and higher critical functions such as language. Its onset is typically gradual, and the patient's normal level of consciousness is maintained. The presence of global cognitive impairment can be detected by using a bedside screening test such as the Mini-Mental State Exam or the Clock Drawing Test. Potentially reversible causes of dementia should be sought including metabolic and endocrine disorders, adverse drug effects and interactions, and depression.

Delirium

Delirium is characterized by acute development of impairment in cognitive function, diminished level of consciousness, inattention, and sensory misperceptions that fluctuate over the course of hours. Visual hallucinations are common. Delirium is frequently missed in the ED and is associated with a high mortality rate. The causes of delirium should be sought and treated. Causes include infection, electrolyte abnormalities, toxic and medication ingestion, and head injury

Amnestic Disorders

Amnestic patients cannot learn new information or recall previously learned information. Amnesia may be due to brain trauma, stroke, anoxic brain injury, substance abuse, and chronic nutritional deficiencies.

Substance-Use Disorders

Intoxication is an exogenous substance-induced syndrome that results in maladaptive behavior and impaired cognitive functioning and psychomotor activity. Judgment, perception, attention, and emotional control may be affected. Substance withdrawal symptoms may develop when the amount ingested is reduced or stopped. The symptoms and timing of withdrawal depend on the substance of abuse.

Schizophrenia and Other Psychotic Disorders

Schizophrenia is a chronic disease characterized by positive symptoms such as hallucinations, delusions, disorganized speech or behavior, or catatonic behavior and negative symptoms such as blunted affect, emotional withdrawal, lack of spontaneity, anhedonia, or impaired attention. Chronic illness is distinguished by cognitive impairment with loose associations or incoherence and the relative absence of a mood disorder. Patients may present to the emergency department for worsening psychosis, suicidal ideations, crisis, bizarre or violent behavior, or adverse medication events. Typical antipsychotic medications, such as haloperidol, effectively treat the positive symptoms, and newer atypical antipsychotic medications, such as aripiprazole, quetiapine, olanzapine, risperidone, ziprasidone, and clozapine, effectively treat positive and negative symptoms. The diagnosis of schizophreniform disorder is made when an individual experiences symptoms and demonstrates signs consistent with schizophrenia for less than 6 months. A brief psychotic disorder is a psychosis that lasts less than 4 weeks in response to a traumatic life experience, such as sexual assault, natural disaster, combat, or death of a loved one. Schizophrenia is treated with antipsychotic medications.

Mood Disorders

Major Depression

Major depression is characterized by a persistent dysphoric mood or a pervasive loss of interest and pleasure in usual activities (anhedonia) that lasts longer than 2 weeks. Associated psychological symptoms include feelings of guilt over past events, self-reproach, worthlessness, hopelessness, and recurrent thoughts of death or suicide. Physiologic symptoms include loss of appetite and weight, sleep disturbances, fatigue, inability to concentrate, and psychomotor agitation or retardation. The diagnosis should be entertained in any patient presenting with multiple vague complaints. The lifetime risk of suicide in patients with this disorder is 15%. All patients suspected of having major depression should be questioned about suicidal thoughts. Depression is typically treated with SSRIs.

Bipolar Disorder

Bipolar disorder is characterized by recurrent, cyclic episodes of manic and depressive symptoms, with depressive episodes being more common than manic episodes. Manic individuals experience an elated mood that can quickly deteriorate to irritability and hostility. They appear energetic and expansive, with a decreased need for sleep, poor impulse control, racing thoughts, auditory hallucinations, grandiose ideas and pressured speech. Complications may include suicide, substance abuse, and marital and occupational disruptions. Bipolar illness is treated with lithium and valproate.

Anxiety Disorders

Panic disorder consists of recurrent episodes of severe anxiety and sudden, extreme autonomic symptoms. It is a diagnosis of exclusion as these symptoms can also occur in life-threatening cardiovascular and pulmonary disorders. The diagnosis of generalized anxiety disorder can be made when a patient experiences persistent worry or tension without discrete panic attacks for at least 6 months. Phobias consist of symptoms of anxiety, recognized as excessive by the person, prompted by the exposure to, or the anticipated exposure to, a specific stimulus. Posttraumatic stress disorder is an anxiety reaction to a severe, psychosocial stressor, typically perceived as life threatening. The individual experiences repetitive, intrusive memories of the event. Nightmares, feelings of guilt and depression, and substance abuse are common. Individuals with obsessive-compulsive disorder experience intrusive thoughts or images that create anxiety (obsessions). To control these thoughts and anxiety, the individual engages in repetitive behaviors or rituals (compulsions). Anxiety disorders may be treated with benzodiazepines.

PERSONALITY DISORDERS

Individuals with a personality disorder exhibit a lifelong pattern of maladaptive behavior that is not limited to periods of illness. Personality disorders include paranoid, schizoid, schizotypal, antisocial, borderline, histrionic, narcissistic, avoidant, dependent, and obsessive-compulsive. Personality disorders are difficult to treat.

EMERGENCY DEPARTMENT CARE AND DISPOSITION

1. Many of the patients with psychiatric illnesses presenting to the ED do not need immediate treatment. Delirium is one exception where identification and treatment of the cause of delirium in the ED is essential.
2. The most common treatment in the ED is for the agitation associated with psychiatric illness (Fig. 184-1). Many patients have multiple psychiatric, substance use and medical diagnoses making treatment in the ED more complicated.
3. Disposition depends on the patient's ability to function, risk of suicide and homicidal intent.

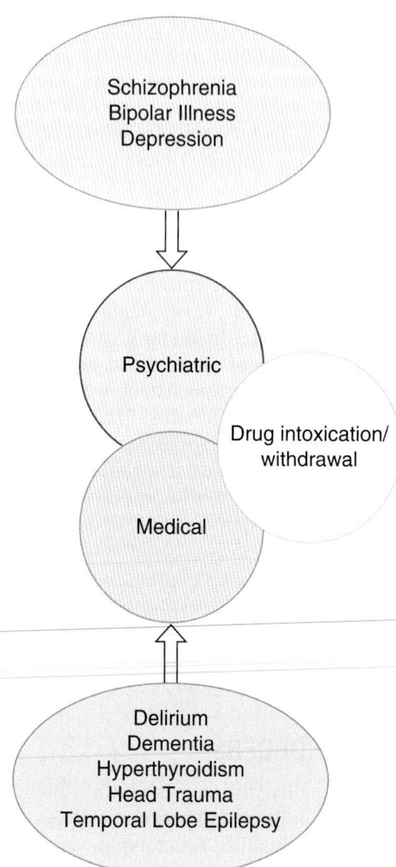

FIGURE 184-1. Diagram of frequent medical, substance use and psychiatric illness in the ED.

FURTHER READING

For further reading in *Tintinalli's Emergency Medicine: A Comprehensive Study Guide*, 8th ed., see Chapter 286, "Mental Health Disorders: ED Evaluation and Disposition," by Leslie S. Zun.

CHAPTER 185

Emergency Assessment and Stabilization of Behavioral Disorders

Leslie S. Zun

INCIDENCE

In the last two decades, mental health-related visits to emergency departments (EDs) in the United States increased by 38% to 23.6 per 1000 population.

CLINICAL FEATURES

Psychiatric patients present to EDs with various complaints including agitation, depression, suicide ideation, mania, or other abnormal behaviors. Some patients have overt psychiatric presentations while some may present with less obvious presentations such as panic disorders, depression, or suicidal ideation.

DIAGNOSIS AND DIFFERENTIAL

The role of the emergency physician is to determine whether the psychiatric presentation is due to a medical or psychiatric etiology in order to decide on an appropriate patient disposition. This differentiation is made more difficult because approximately 50% of these patients have concomitant medical illnesses, most frequently hypertension, diabetes, asthma, and substance use disorder. Some psychiatric patients need treatment for agitation prior to evaluation in order to obtain vital signs, pulse oxygenation, and glucose assessment. The evaluation process includes a detailed medical and psychiatric history, medication history, social history, and a physical examination, including a thorough neurologic and mental status evaluation. The "red flags" for medical illness include initial presentation over the age of 45, abnormal vital signs, focal neurologic deficit, exposure to drugs or toxins, abnormal physical exam findings, and cognitive deficit. Some of the elements of the mental status examination are routinely assessed as part of the history and physical exam: appearance, behavior and attitude, and mood and affect. A number of items need to be specifically tested such as disorders of thought inquiring about suicidal and homicidal ideation, insight and judgment about their illness, disorders of perception such as hallucinations, and cognitive impairment using the Mini Mental State Exam or the clock drawing test. Factors associated with high risk of suicide include male gender, unmarried or recent loss of relationship, family history of suicide, substance abuse, history of depression or psychosis, hopelessness, frequent and pervasive thoughts of suicide, previous attempts, availability of a lethal method, and poor social support. Laboratory testing and imaging of psychiatric patients should be clinically driven rather than rote. Patients with new onset of psychiatric symptoms and patients with chronic mental illness and a new psychiatric presentation need such testing. The testing may include

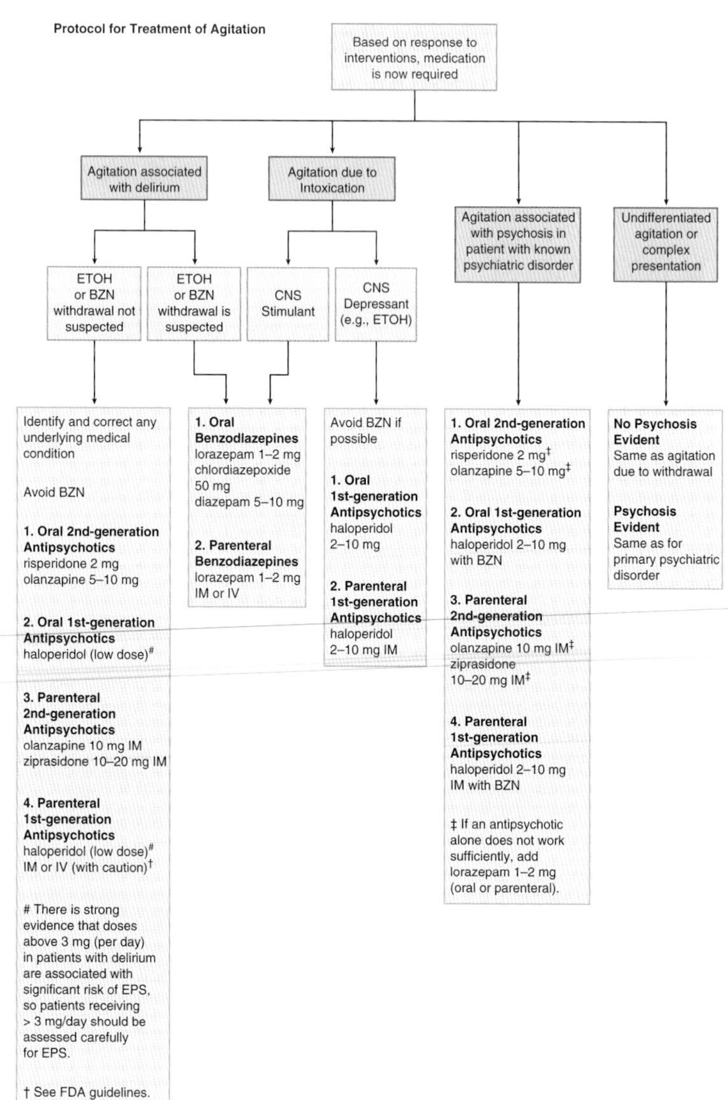

FIGURE 185-1. Suggested algorithm for the ED management of agitated patients. Reproduced with permission from Wilson MP, Pepper D, Currier GW, et al: The psychopharmacology of agitation: consensus statement of the american association for emergency psychiatry project Beta psychopharmacology workgroup, West J Emerg Med. 2012 Feb;13(1):26-34.

complete blood count, serum electrolytes, liver function tests, urinalysis, urine drug screen, alcohol levels, and head CT scan. Elderly patients may need thyroid function testing, ECG, and CXR. Medical illnesses that may masquerade as psychiatric illness include hypoglycemia, hyperthyroidism, and delirium. Delirium has a high rate of mortality and is frequently missed in the ED. It has a fluctuating course with change in consciousness and alertness as well as confusion. Tests of delirium such as the Confusion Assessment Method may be useful to identify these patients.

EMERGENCY DEPARTMENT CARE AND DISPOSITION

1. The first priority is safety and stabilization, including attention to airway, breathing, and circulation.
2. All psychiatric patients need to disrobe and be placed in a gown. The medical and psychiatric evaluations should proceed quickly to determine the need for treatment and admission.
3. Agitation treatment begins with verbal de-escalation. Agitation may lead to violence and require medications and/or restraints to avoid self-injury and the harm to others.
4. The choice of the treatment of agitation depends on the level of agitation and underlying causation, if known.
5. Severely agitated patients associated with a psychiatric illness may need restraints and intramuscular haloperidol and lorazepam or an atypical antipsychotic given IM (Fig. 185-1). The goal of treatment is to calm without over-sedation and to remove restraints as soon as possible. Treat moderate and mild agitation with oral medications, if possible. Treat severely agitated patients with alcohol withdrawal or stimulant intoxication with a benzodiazepine.
6. Patients judged to be at high risk of harming themselves or others or those who are unable to care for themselves require admission to a psychiatric facility.
7. Patients with moderate suicide potential need a psychiatric consultation. Patients with low risk for suicide may go home.
8. All psychiatric patients need close psychiatric follow-up and can benefit from a referral to community mental health resources. Ensure that discharged patients have someone safe with whom to stay.

FURTHER READING

For further reading in *Tintinalli's Emergency Medicine: A Comprehensive Study Guide*, 8th ed., see Chapter 286, "Mental Health Disorders: ED Evaluation and Disposition," by Leslie S. Zun.

CHAPTER 186

Panic and Conversion Disorders

Kimberly Nordstrom

PANIC DISORDER

Panic disorder manifests with a wide variety of symptoms that mimic other major medical problems.

Clinical Features

Panic disorder is defined as recurrent panic attacks followed by 1 month or more of persistent worry of future episodes or maladaptive changes in behavior related to the attack. Episodes begin unexpectedly; severity peaks within 10 minutes and symptoms last for up to 1 hour. Symptoms of panic attacks include palpitations, sweating, shortness of breath, trembling or shaking, choking sensation, chest pain or discomfort, nausea or abdominal distress, dizziness or light-headedness, paresthesias, chills or hot flashes, fear of losing control, fear of dying, and derealization or depersonalization.

Diagnosis and Differential

Panic disorder is a diagnosis of exclusion because its symptoms and signs mimic those of many potentially life-threatening disorders. A thorough history and physical examination and, when indicated, other tests help rule out these life-threatening disorders. The differential diagnosis of panic attacks is listed in Table 186-1.

TABLE 186-1 Medical Differential Diagnosis of Panic Attacks

Cardiovascular	Neurologic	Drug withdrawal
Angina	Migraine headache	Alcohol
Myocardial infarction	Ménière disease	Barbiturates
Mitral valve prolapse	Complex partial seizures	Benzodiazepines
Congestive heart failure	Transient ischemic attacks	Opiates
Tachyarrhythmias: premature atrial contractions, supraventricular tachycardia	Drug induced	β-Antagonists
Pulmonary	Caffeine	Psychiatric
Hyperventilation	Cocaine	Posttraumatic stress disorder
Asthma	Sympathomimetics	Depressive disorders
Pulmonary embolus	Theophylline	Other anxiety disorders
Endocrine	Thyroid preparations	Psychosocial
Hyperthyroidism	Selective serotonin reuptake inhibitors	Partner violence
Hypoglycemia	Cannabis	Sexual abuse or assault
Hyponatremia	Corticosteroids	Other situational stressors
Pheochromocytoma	β-Agonists	
Carcinoid syndrome	Triptans	
Cushing's syndrome	Nicotine	
	Yohimbine	
	Hallucinogens	
	Anticholinergics	

Emergency Department Care and Disposition

1. After excluding life-threatening causes of symptoms, educate and reassure the patient that panic disorder is an illness that can be treated effectively.
2. Benzodiazepines, such as **alprazolam** 0.25 to 1 mg PO or **lorazepam** 0.5 to 1 mg PO/IV, are used to control acute symptoms. Antidepressants, such as selective serotonin reuptake inhibitors (SSRI) and serotonin-norepinephrine reuptake inhibitors (SNRI), are preferred for maintenance therapy. Ideally, follow up should be in place if sending the patient out with a benzodiazepine or SSRI/SNRI prescription. Caution should be used in prescribing benzodiazepines to certain populations, such as drug abusers, geriatric patients, and those with respiratory disorders.
3. Ask the patient about suicidal thoughts, as the patient may require psychiatric consultation and hospitalization.
4. Most patients can be discharged. Refer to outpatient psychiatry for continuation or initiation of pharmacotherapy.

CONVERSION DISORDER

Clinical Features

Patients with conversion disorder develop voluntary motor or sensory function deficits. The symptoms are not consciously produced by the patient and are usually in response to a stressor or conflict. The symptoms or deficits are not explained by a known organic etiology or culturally sanctioned response pattern. Organic disease may be concurrently present.

Diagnosis and Differential

Other medical or mental illnesses must be excluded before the diagnosis of conversion disorder can be made. The differential diagnosis is broad and includes stroke, multiple sclerosis, polymyositis, infectious disorders, as well as drug ingestions or poisonings. The examination techniques listed in Table 186-2 may help test for true neurologic deficits.

TABLE 186-2 Testing Techniques for Conversion Disorder

Function	Technique
Sensation	
Yes/no test	Patient closes eyes and responds *yes* or *no* to touch stimulus. *No* response in numb area favors conversion disorder.
Bowlus and Currier test	Patient extends and then crosses the arms, with thumbs pointed down and palms facing together. Fingers (but not thumbs) are then interlocked, and then the hands are rotated inward toward chest. Sharp stimuli are applied to each finger in turn and the patient is asked to indicate normal or abnormal sensation in each digit. Patients with conversion disorder make mistakes and are inconsistent with responses.
Strength test	Patient closes eyes. Test "strength" by touching finger to be moved. True lack of sensation would not allow patient to ascertain finger to be moved.

(Continued)

TABLE 186-2 Testing Techniques for Conversion Disorder (Continued)

Function	Technique
Pain	
Gray test	With abdominal pain due to psychological factors, the patient will close eyes during palpation. In pain of organic basis, the patient is more likely to watch the examiner's hand to anticipate pain.
Motor	
Drop test	When a patient with paralysis of nonorganic etiology lifts a thumb, the affected limb will drop more slowly or fall with exaggerated speed as compared with the unaffected limb. In addition, an extremity dropped from above the face will miss it.
Thigh adductor test	Examiner places hands against both inner thighs of the patient who is told to adduct the "good" leg against resistance. With pseudoparalysis, the adductor muscles of "bad" leg will also adduct.
Hoover test	Examiner's hands cup both heels of the patient who is asked to elevate the "good" leg. With pseudoparalysis the "bad" leg will push downward. When the patient is asked to lift the "bad" leg, if there is no downward pressure in the "good" leg, the patient is not trying.
Sternocleidomastoid test	Contraction of normal sternocleidomastoid muscle causes face to rotate away from side of the contracted muscle. Patient with conversion hemiplegia cannot turn head to the weak side.
Coma	
Corneal reflex	Corneal reflexes remain intact in an awake patient.
Bell phenomenon	Eyes divert upward when lids are opened, whereas eyes remain in neutral position in true coma.
Lid closing	In true coma, lids when opened close rapidly initially and then more slowly as lids descend. Awake patients will have lids stay open, snap shut, or flutter.
Seizures	
Corneal reflex	Usually intact in pseudoseizure.
Abdominal musculature	Palpation of abdominal musculature reveals lack of contractions with pseudoseizure.
Blindness	
Opticokinetic drum	Rotating drum with alternating black and white stripes or piece of tape with alternating black and white sections pulled laterally in front of a patient's open eyes will produce nystagmus in a patient with intact vision.

Emergency Department Care and Disposition

1. Direct confrontation is not helpful and can be harmful to the patient. After excluding an organic cause for symptoms, gently reassure the patient that a serious medical illness has not been identified.
2. Suggest to the patient that symptoms often resolve spontaneously.
3. Consult with a neurologist or psychiatrist if symptoms do not resolve and preclude discharge. Otherwise, refer for outpatient psychiatric treatment as repetitive reassurance or other forms of therapy may be beneficial.

FURTHER READING

For further reading in *Tintinalli's Emergency Medicine: A Comprehensive Study Guide*, 8th edition, see Chapter 289, "Mood and Anxiety Disorders," by Tracy M. DeSelm.

SECTION 22

Abuse and Assault

Child and Elderly Abuse

Jonathan Glauser

CHILD ABUSE

Child maltreatment includes physical abuse, sexual abuse, emotional abuse, neglect, parental substance abuse, and Munchausen syndrome by proxy.

Clinical Features

Child neglect in early infancy results in the syndrome of failure to thrive. These children are frequently brought to the ED because of other medical problems, such as skin infections, severe diaper dermatitis, or acute gastroenteritis. Infants may have little subcutaneous tissue, protruding ribs, or occipital alopecia from lying on their back all day. They are wide eyed, wary, and difficult to console. They may have increased muscle tone in their lower extremities. Weight gain in the hospital is thought to be diagnostic of failure to thrive.

Children over the age of 2 with environmental neglect are termed psychosocial dwarfs. They exhibit short stature, bizarre and voracious appetites, and are hyperactive with unintelligible or delayed speech.

Physical abuse is suggested by a history that is inconsistent with the nature of the injuries. The history of the event given by the caretaker may keep changing, or may be different from that given by the child.

The following findings suggest physical abuse: bruises over multiple areas, bites with an intercanine diameter >3 cm, lacerations of the frenulum or oral mucosa from force-feeding, burns of an entire hand or foot, or burns of the buttocks or genitalia from toilet training punishment, cigarette burns, spiral fractures caused by twisting of long bones, metaphyseal chip fractures, periosteal elevation from new bone formation at sites of previous microfractures, multiple fractures at different stages of healing, fractures at unusual sites such as lateral clavicle, ribs, sternum, vomiting, irritability, seizures, change in mental status, apnea, or retinal hemorrhages from intracranial hemorrhage (shaken baby syndrome). Vomiting, abdominal pain, and tenderness with diminished bowel sounds or abdominal distention may be due to a duodenal hematoma, as evidenced by a "double-bubble" sign on abdominal x-ray films.

Munchausen syndrome by proxy is a synonym for medical child abuse. A parent fabricates illness in a child in order to secure prolonged contact with health care providers. Complaints may be numerous and agents such as ipecac or warfarin may have been given to precipitate these complaints. Parents typically encourage more diagnostic tests, and are happy if they are positive.

Sexual abuse is suggested with complaints referable to the anogenital area, such as bleeding, discharge, or the presence of a sexually transmitted disease. Clefts or concavities in the hymen typically present in the 6 o'clock position. Victims of child abuse may be overly compliant with painful medical procedures, overly protective of the abusing parent, or overly affectionate to medical staff.

Diagnosis and Differential

Any serious injury in a child under the age of 5 should be viewed with suspicion. Parents and caregivers may appear to be under the influence of drugs or alcohol and refuse diagnostic studies. Victims of neglect may appear dirty, improperly clothed, and may be unimmunized.

A skeletal survey of the long bones will help detect evidence of physical abuse. See Chapter 157, "Trauma in Children," for further workup of traumatic injuries.

Inspect the genital area carefully for injury. Speculum examination in the preadolescent is not needed unless perforating vaginal trauma is suspected. Absence of physical findings does not rule out abuse.

Laboratory testing for sexual abuse should include cultures of the throat, vagina, and rectum for gonorrhea and chlamydia. Rapid antigen assays are **not** reliable forensic evidence in prepubescent children. Perform testing for syphilis if clinical concern exists. Test for HIV if clinically concerned and appropriate counseling is available. Syphilis, gonorrhea, and *C trachomatis* infections are considered presumptive evidence for sexual abuse, as is HIV, if not acquired perinatally or by transfusion.

Rarely, conditions such as leukemia, aplastic anemia, and osteogenesis imperfecta can mimic physical abuse.

Emergency Department Care and Disposition

Address all medical issues and injuries. Infants suspected of suffering from failure to thrive and children with suspected Munchausen syndrome by proxy should be admitted to the hospital. Involve social services during the ED visit. Ensure a safe environment for each child. Every state requires reporting of suspected cases of child abuse. The law protects physicians from legal retaliation from parents.

ELDERLY ABUSE

Elderly abuse is an act or omission resulting in harm to the health or welfare of an elderly person.

Clinical Features

Physical abuse is the most easily recognized form of elderly abuse, although chemical restraint such as intentional overmedication may be subtle. *Caregiver neglect*, defined as failure of a caregiver to provide basic care, goods and services such as food, clothing, hygiene, medical care, and shelter, accounts for the majority of cases of elder abuse. Financial abuse is the second commonest form of abuse, and occurs when family members take control of or steal assets, checks, or pensions for personal gain.

Emotional abuse entails inflicting anguish, emotional pain, or distress. Verbal threats, social isolation, and harassment can contribute to depression and other mental health problems. Self-neglect includes those behaviors of an elderly person that threaten his or her own safety: failure to provide adequate food, medical care, hygiene, clothing, or shelter. The spectrum of sexual abuse ranges from unwanted touching or indecent exposure to rape itself.

Caretakers may give a conflicting report of an injury or illness. The patient may be fearful of his or her companion. The caretaker may seem indifferent or angry toward the patient, or may be overly concerned with costs of treatment needed by the patient.

Diagnosis and Differential

Risk factors for elder abuse may be associated with caregivers, perpetrators, or with the elders. Patient characteristics include (a) cognitive impairment, (b) female sex, (c) physical dependency, (d) alcohol abuse, (e) developmental disability, (f) special medical or psychiatric needs, (g) lack of social support, and (h) limited experience managing finances.

Risk factors for or characteristics of perpetrators of abuse include (a) history of violence within or outside of the family, (b) excessive dependence on the elder for financial support, (c) history of mental illness or substance abuse.

Patients should be interviewed in private. Screening questions for elder abuse are available. Areas of concern include whether anyone has touched or hurt them, forced them to do things, taken something of theirs without asking, threatened them, or made them feel afraid.

The following findings on physical examination are suggestive of abuse: bruising or trauma, poor general appearance and inappropriate hygiene or soiled clothing, malnutrition and dehydration, contusions and lacerations to normally protected areas of the body—inner thighs, mastoid, palms, soles, buttocks, unusual burns or multiple burns in different stages of healing, rope or restraint marks on ankles or wrists, spiral fractures of long bones, midshaft ulnar (nightstick) fractures from attempts to shield blows, multiple deep/uncared for ulcers.

Emergency Department Care and Disposition

Elder abuse is widely underreported and underrecognized. Treatment entails three key components:

1. Address medical and psychosocial needs.
2. Ensure patient safety.
3. Adhere to local reporting requirements.

Medical problems and injuries may be best managed with hospital admission. If neglect is unintentional, educate the caregiver. All 50 states have reporting requirements for elder abuse and neglect. Requirements for reporting within one's practice area are available at www.nceaaoa.gov.

FURTHER READING

For further reading in *Tintinalli's Emergency Medicine: A Comprehensive Study Guide*, 8th ed., see Chapter 148, "Child Abuse and Neglect," by Margaret Colbourne and Michelle S. Clarke; Chapter 295, "Abuse of the Elderly and Impaired," by Jonathan Glauser and Frederic M. Hustey.

CHAPTER 188 Sexual Assault and Intimate Partner Violence and Abuse

Mary Hancock

Not all individuals who are sexually assaulted sustain an injury. Lack of injury does not mean that an assault did not occur. Often the perpetrator is known to the assault survivor.

Intimate partner violence and abuse is defined as a pattern of assaultive behavior that may include physical injury, sexual assault, psychological abuse, stalking, deprivation, intimidation, and threats. Intimate partner violence and abuse occurs in every race, ethnicity, culture, geographic region, and religious affiliation and occurs in gay, lesbian, and heterosexual relationships.

CLINICAL FEATURES

Elements of the sexual assault history are listed in Table 188-1. The history for intimate partner violence and abuse can be more difficult to obtain. Risk factors for intimate partner violence and abuse include female sex, age between 18 and 24 years, low socioeconomic status,

TABLE 188-1 Assault History

Who? Did the assault survivor know the assailant? Was it a single assailant or multiple assailants? Can the survivor recall any identifying features of the assailant (height, build, age, race, tattoos, scars, birthmarks, etc.)? (Document in the medical records.)
What happened? Was the patient physically assaulted? With what (e.g., gun, bat, or fist) and to what part of the body? Was there actual or attempted vaginal, anal, or oral penetration? Did ejaculation occur? If so, where? Was a foreign object used? Was a condom used?
When? When did the assault occur? (Emergency contraception is most effective when started within 72 hours of the assault.)
Where? Where did the assault occur? (Corroborating evidence may be found based on the location of the assault.)
Suspicion of drug-facilitated rape? Was there a period of amnesia? Is there a history of being out drinking and then suddenly feeling very intoxicated? Is there a history of waking up naked or with genital soreness?
Douche, shower, or change of clothing? Did the patient douche, shower, or change clothing after the assault? (Performing any of these activities prior to seeking medical attention may decrease the probability of sperm or acid phosphatase recovery, as well as recovery of other bits of trace evidence.)

separated relationship status, and residence in rental housing. Injuries inconsistent with the patient's history, multiple injuries in various stages of healing, delay in the time of injury occurrence and presentation, a visit for vague complaints without evidence of injury, or suicide attempts should trigger suspicions of intimate partner violence and abuse. Patients may complain initially of chronic pain syndromes, gynecologic or psychiatric difficulties, and alcohol and substance abuse. The patient also may appear frightened when the partner is present or the partner may be hostile, defensive, aggressive, or overly solicitous. Recent and remote abuse, including dates, locations, details of abuse, and witnesses, should be documented. Patients need to be asked about any suicidal or homicidal ideation and plans and get appropriate, immediate evaluation.

Physical Examination

Perform a general medical examination including vital signs, appearance and demeanor. Focus head-to-toe inspection on defensive injury areas, such as the extremities, and potential areas of injury, such as the oral cavity, breasts, thighs, and buttocks. Record all the signs of trauma, new and old, in detail using a body map. Speculum examination should note any trauma, discharge, abrasions, including on the cervix. If anal penetration is reported, the rectum should be examined for abrasions and lacerations. Use of anoscopy in male patients increases detection of trauma.

Characteristic injuries of intimate partner violence and abuse include fingernail scratches, bite marks, cigarette burns, rope burns, and forearm bruising or nightstick fractures, suggesting a defensive posture. Abdominal injuries are common in the pregnant intimate partner violence and abuse patient (Table 188-2).

Evidence Examination

Evidence collection in sexual assault is performed only within the first 72 hours after the assault. Informed consent is required. Most hospitals have a prepackaged rape kit. Chain of custody of the evidence must be maintained and the kit should never be left unattended. Not every part of the forensic evidence kit needs to be used every time. Tailor the evidence collection to the specifics of the assault, if known. If >72 hours have elapsed or the patient declines an evidentiary examination, perform a history and physical examination, document injuries, and provide prophylaxis for pregnancy and sexually transmitted infections. Label evidence clearly with the patient's name, type and source of evidence, date and time, and name of the examiner collecting the evidence. If there is high suspicion of drug-facilitated rape, a urine sample can be sent to a laboratory for toxicologic testing.

DIAGNOSIS AND DIFFERENTIAL

Sexual assault is a legal determination, not a medical diagnosis. The legal definition contains three elements: carnal knowledge, nonconsent, and compulsion or fear of harm. Because of the legal considerations, careful documentation and evidence collection are important.

TABLE 188-2 Signs Suggestive of Intimate Partner Violence

Findings	Comments
Injuries characteristic of violence	Fingernail scratches, broken fingernails, bite marks, dental injuries, cigarette burns, bruises suggesting strangulation or restraint, and rope burns or ligature marks may be seen.
Injuries suggesting a defensive posture	Forearm bruises or fractures may be sustained when individuals try to fend off blows to the face or chest.
Injuries during pregnancy	Up to 45% of women report abuse or assault during pregnancy. Preterm labor, placental abruption, direct fetal injury, and stillbirth can occur.
Central pattern of injury	Injuries to the head, neck, face, and thorax and abdominal injuries in pregnant women may suggest violence.
Extent or type of injury inconsistent with the patient's explanation	Multiple injuries at different anatomic sites inconsistent with the described mechanism of injury. The most common explanation of injury is a "fall." Embarrassment, evasiveness, or lack of concern with the injuries may be noted.
Multiple injuries in various stages of healing	These may be reported as "accidents" or "clumsiness."
Delay between the time of injury and the presentation for treatment	Victims may wait several days before seeking medical care for injuries. Victims may seek care for minor or resolving injuries.
Visits for vague or minor complaints without evidence of physiologic abnormality	Frequent ED visits for a variety of injuries or illnesses including chronic pelvic pain and other chronic pain syndromes.
Suicide attempts	Women who attempt or commit suicide often have a history of intimate partner violence.

Many experts recommend routine screening for intimate partner violence and abuse for all adolescent and adult women who present to the ED and for mothers of children. Providers educated about the dynamics of intimate partner violence and abuse should conduct screening in a safe and private environment. Document all the findings, interventions, referrals, and required reporting.

EMERGENCY DEPARTMENT CARE AND DISPOSITION

Address life-threatening injuries and the psychological needs. Treating critical injuries are the initial priority of the ED physician. A social worker or trained advocate should counsel the patient in the ED. Ensure the safety of the patient and any children involved while they are in the ED. Be familiar with reporting laws in your state.

SEXUAL ASSAULT

Emergency Contraception

1. Obtain a pregnancy test.
2. Offer emergency contraception. **Levonorgestrel** only, 1.5 mg PO in a single dose (available OTC) OR **ulipristal acetate** 30 mg PO single

dose (requires prescription) OR commonly prescribed contraceptive pills, ie. **Ovral** 2 pills once, repeat 2 pills in 12 hours (each dose contains **levonorgestrel** 0.5 mg and **ethinyl estradiol** 100 mcg).

STD Prophylaxis

Recommended regimens for infection prophylaxis include a single dose of **ceftriaxone** 250 mg IM OR single dose of **cefixime** 400 mg PO PLUS a single dose of **metronidazole** 2 g PO PLUS a single dose of **azithromycin** 1 g PO, OR **doxycycline** 100 mg PO twice a day for 7 days.

STD Treatment

1. Gonorrhea: **Ceftriaxone** 250 mg IM single dose or **cefixime** 400 mg PO single dose.
2. Chlamydia: **Azithromycin** 1 g PO as single dose OR **doxycycline** 100 mg PO twice per day for 7 days (do not use doxycycline during pregnancy).
3. Trichomonas and bacterial vaginosis: **metronidazole** 2 g PO in single dose (do not use during first trimester of pregnancy).
4. Syphillis: **Penicillin G benzathine** 2.4 million IU IM. Use **erythromycin** 500 mg PO four times per day for 15 days if penicillin allergic.

Hepatitis Prophylaxis

Administer vaccine at the time of initial exam if patient has not been previously vaccinated. Follow-up doses of vaccine should be administered 1 to 2 months and 4 to 6 months after the first dose

HIV: Prophylaxis and Counseling

Rates of human immunodeficiency virus (HIV) seroconversion are low but occur from sexual assault or sexual abuse. Circumstances should guide the decision to administer postexposure prophylaxis. An assailant known to be infected with HIV, high viral load exposure, vaginal trauma, and ejaculate on membranes increase the risk for HIV seroconversion. Post-HIV exposure recommendations are posted on the Centers for Disease Control and Prevention (CDC) website (www.cdc.gov). Additional assistance may be obtained by calling the 24-hour National HIV/AIDS Post Exposure Hotline at 1-888-448-4911. Routine prophylaxis is not recommended, and counseling and follow-up should be provided.

INTIMATE PARTNER VIOLENCE AND ABUSE

1. An attempt to leave an abusive relationship is often the most dangerous time.
2. Assess for potentially lethal situations. These include increasing frequency or severity of violence, the threat or use of weapons, obsession with the patient, taking hostages, stalking, homicidal or suicidal threats, and substance abuse by the assailant, especially with crack cocaine or amphetamines.
3. Hospital admission is an option in high-risk situations if a safe location cannot be established before discharge.

TABLE 188-3 Hotlines for Patients

National Domestic Violence Hotline: 24 hours; links caller to help in her (or his) area—emergency shelter, domestic violence shelters, legal advocacy and assistance programs, social services	800-799-SAFE (7233) 800-787-3224 (TTY)
Rape, Abuse, and Incest National Network: 24 hours; automatically transfers caller to nearest rape crisis center anywhere in the nation	800-656-HOPE (4673) http://www.rainn.org

Follow-up Care

Follow-up care often requires the coordinated efforts of physicians, law enforcement, survival advocates, and counselors. Some communities and hospitals use the Sexual Assault Nurse Examiner (SANE) programs; others have rape crisis centers, and 24-hours safe rooms. National hotlines are available (Table 188-3). Know the resources available in your community.

FURTHER READING

For further reading in *Tintinalli's Emergency Medicine: A Comprehensive Study Guide*, 8th ed., see Chapter 293, "Female and Male Sexual Assault," by Lisa Moreno-Walton; Chapter 294, "Intimate Partner Violence and Abuse," by Mary Hancock.

SECTION 23

Special Situations

CHAPTER 189 Palliative Care

Kate Aberger

The goal of palliative care is to relieve suffering of patients and families who live with serious illness. It is imperative to ascertain goals of care while concurrently stabilizing or temporizing the patient clinically and treating symptoms. We need to then compassionately communicate diagnosis, prognosis, and treatment alternatives and guide the formulation of a therapeutic plan.

IDENTIFYING PATIENTS FOR PALLIATIVE CARE

It is important to recognize when patients have unmet palliative needs and have a rapid palliative approach to these patients. See Table 189-1. Patient and family expectations can be managed by expert formulation and communication of prognosis. Prognosis will also guide treatment options. The most important factor in formulating a prognosis is functional ability. Generally, components of functional status which herald a poor prognosis and may indicate that the patient is on the dying trajectory are loss of the ability to care for oneself, unintentional weight loss, inability to ambulate, inability to maintain oral intake, and declining level of consciousness.

EMERGENCY DEPARTMENT CARE AND DISPOSITION

1. While decision-making capacity and goals of care are being sorted out, symptoms must be aggressively managed.
2. Identify who is making decisions for the patient. If the patient can make their own decisions, they should guide their own care. If their symptom burden is too high for them to participate, or they otherwise lack decisional capacity, the patient's advance directive should be accessed and the named surrogate decision maker should be contacted as soon as possible. If no written advanced directives or POLST/MOLST forms exist, have they expressed their wishes to a proxy? Even if there is no legal proxy, the closest family members can offer information.
3. Use medical information coupled with the patient's functional status to formulate a prognosis.
4. Conduct an abbreviated family meeting to discuss the approach to care. Communicate prognosis in terms of chunks of time: hours to days, days

TABLE 189-1 Common Diagnoses and Key Findings of Patients Who May Benefit from Palliative Care

Diagnosis	Key Findings
Solid organ neoplasm	Widespread metastasis unresponsive to treatment
End-stage heart failure	Significant symptoms at rest despite therapy
End-stage COPD	Significant symptoms at rest despite therapy
Advanced dementia	Impaired mobility and inability to communicate health needs
Degenerative neurologic disease	Inability to complete ADLs or communicate health needs
End-stage AIDS	Multiple opportunistic infections and/or AIDS dementia
End-stage renal disease	Patient no longer willing or able to undergo dialysis
End-stage liver disease	Repeated episodes of hepatic encephalopathy, bleeding, or symptomatic ascites resistant to medical therapy
End-stage rheumatologic disease	Inability to complete ADLs without significant discomfort
Multisystem trauma	Nonsurvivable injury
Burn	When age plus percent burn exceeds or nears 140
Multiorgan failure	When two or more key body systems fail
Any chronic, progressive, debilitating disease	Whenever symptom burden exceeds resources and the ability of the patient and/or family to cope with medical condition; Caregiver and/or family distress or conflict

Abbreviations: ADLs, activities of daily living; AIDS, acquired immunodeficiency syndrome; COPD, chronic obstructive pulmonary disease.

to weeks, weeks to months, months to years. Communication skills are essential. Families often vividly remember this interaction, and the conversation can have a tremendous impact on decision making and bereavement. (See Table 189-2).

5. Consult palliative care services if available. Consultation is appropriate to continue conversations begun in the ED, or when symptom relief, medical decision making, or disposition and coordination of care are beyond your expertise or available time. Alert the patient's physician of the consultation.
6. Disposition should be to the appropriate level of care that reflects the patient's goals of care.
7. Patients are eligible for hospice if they decide to take a palliative approach and they have a life expectancy of 6 months or less. Hospice referrals can be made from the emergency department, allowing patients to be sent home, to an extended care facility, or to an inpatient unit.
8. The most important task while temporizing and treating symptoms in patients already enrolled in hospice care is to contact the hospice coordinator to gather information needed to understanding patient goals and guide in treatment. The three most common reasons that patients already enrolled in hospice care present to the emergency department are acute symptom crisis, injury or illness unrelated to the hospice diagnosis, and family/caregiver distress or conflict. Usually, hospice is continued, and the coordinator will help guide in the disposition of the patient. The patient may be admitted under hospice if symptoms are not manageable at home, or be treated and sent back home with continued hospice care.

TABLE 189-2 Key Communication Phrases

Determining Decision-Making Capacity Will you describe your current condition? Tell me about the treatment options we have just discussed. Explain to me why you feel that way.
Quality of Life What symptoms bother you the most? What concerns you the most?
Prognosis Has anyone talked to you about what to expect? Do you have any sense of how much time is left? Is this something you would like to talk about?
Talking with Surrogate Decision Makers These decisions are very hard; if [the patient] was sitting with us today, what do you think [he/she] would say? Can you tell me why you feel that way? It is not a question of whether we *will* care for your [loved one], but *how* we will care for them. Then we will do everything possible to keep your [loved one] comfortable, but we won't be providing ineffective and burdensome therapies such as CPR or intubation.
Discussing Palliative Care or Hospice Referral To meet the goals we've discussed, I've asked the palliative care team to visit with you; they are experts in treating the symptoms you are experiencing. They can help your family deal with the changes brought on by your illness.
Breaking Bad News—Death Pronouncement I wish there is more we could have done, your loved one has died; I'm very sorry for your loss. This has to be really difficult for you. Is there anyone I can call to be with you now?

9. In the case of imminent patient death, notify family members and the primary physician, and try to reach agreement to offer comfort measures only. Continuous **opiate infusions** plus intermittent or infused **midazolam** may be initiated and titrated to patient comfort. Delirium therapy can be directed to underlying cause (pain, fever) or, if not known or reversible, treated with IV haloperidol. **Atropine ophthalmic drops**, 2 drops sublingual every 6 hours, can relieve the sound of terminal secretions, which have not been shown to be distressing to the patient, but can be very upsetting to the family. Place patient in a relatively calm quiet bed in the ED, allow all family at bedside, offer chaplain support and attempt to maintain dignity and regard for patient's dying process.

SYMPTOM MANAGEMENT

Pain

Introduction

Any validated pain scale can be used to assess pain and track response to treatment. Remember to evaluate as you would for any pain complaint: location, character, duration, quality, alleviating/exacerbating factors. Asking what pain level is tolerable to them and their baseline pain score can be helpful. Do not judge malignant pain based on outward appearance or vital signs.

To begin to treat the pain, first find out if the patient is opiate naïve or opiate tolerant. If patient is opiate naïve, the starting dose of **morphine** is

0.1 mg/kg IV. For opiate tolerant patients, consider starting with **hydromorphone** 1 or 2 mg IV. Opiates reach maximum therapeutic levels and have peak effects/side effects at 6 to 10 minutes. Therefore, IV pain medications can be safely re-dosed every 15 minutes until relief is reached. The biggest obstacle to aggressive pain management with opiates is the fear of respiratory depression. Respiratory depression is not a sudden occurrence, but instead is part of a progression that starts with sedation, somnolence, and finally respiratory depression. A patient can be safely dosed and re-dosed until the symptoms are palliated, as long as level of consciousness is monitored.

Dyspnea

While identifying the cause of dyspnea and treating the underlying pathology, treatment should also be offered to palliate the symptoms. Opioids are extremely beneficial in treating the agitation and anxiety provoked by dyspnea. For an opioid-naïve patient, start with a dose of **morphine** 0.05 mg/kg IV (half the starting dose used for pain), and monitor for sedation and hypoventilation. Use a goal of maintaining a respiratory rate of at least 10 to 12 breaths per minute

Nausea/Vomiting

The underlying cause of nausea can help identify the class of antiemetic drugs most likely to be therapeutic. For chemotherapy-induced nausea, high doses of serotonin 5-hydroxytryptamine-3 antagonists such as **ondansetron** 8 mg IVP or corticosteroids such as **dexamethasone** 10 mg IVP are helpful. Steroids can improve symptoms caused by increased intracranial pressure and bowel obstruction from cancer. For refractory nausea, try a dopamine antagonist such as **haloperidol** 0.5 to 4 mg IVP. **Metoclopramide** 10 mg in 100 mL NS IV is excellent for the symptoms of diabetic gastroparesis or compression of the stomach due to tumor or ascites, or small bowel obstruction, as it increases motility.

Agitation/Delirium

Patients with terminal illness may become agitated, with or without delirium. The causes of this agitation are multifactorial, including pain, anxiety, terminal restlessness, breathlessness, fecal impaction, and mental anguish. The indicated class of medications varies depending on the situation but includes antipsychotics such as **haloperidol** 1 to 5 mg IV, anxiolytics such as **midazolam** 1 to 4 mg IV, and opiates such as **morphine** 2 to 10 mg IV.There is no evidence that these palliative interventions hasten death.

Constipation

Constipation is a universal side effect for patients on opiates. These patients need a concurrent 2-drug bowel regimen, including an osmotic agent, such as **lactulose** 30 mL every 24 hours or **propylene glycol** 17 g powder in 8 oz of water every 24 hours, along with a stimulant laxative, such as **senna** 2 tabs every evening or **bisacodyl** 5 to 15 mg × 1 dose.

FURTHER READING

For Further reading in *Tintinalli's Emergency Medicine: A Comprehensive Study Guide*, 8th ed., see Chapter 299, "Palliative Care," by Robert J. Zalenski and Erin Zimny.

Index

Note: Page numbers followed by *f* indicate figures, page numbers followed by *t* indicate tables.

A

AAAs. *See* abdominal aortic aneurysms (AAAs)
ABCD scoring system, 773–774, 773*t*
abciximab, 134*t*, 137
abdominal aortic aneurysms (AAA), 181–182, 182*f*
abdominal emergencies, in neonates, 364–365
abdominal injuries, 909–913
  diaphragmatic, 910
  hollow visceral, 909
  retroperitoneal, 909–910
  solid organ, 909
abdominal pain
  acute, 217–221, 218*f*, 220*t*
  in children, 400–404, 401*t*
abdominal trauma, 870, 874, 877
abduction relief sign, 971*t*
aberrant drug-related behaviors, 79–80, 79*t*
ABIs. *See* ankle-brachial indexes (ABIs)
abnormal uterine bleeding (AUB), 320
abortion
  induced, 351–352, 352*t*
  and threatened abortion, 325–326
abscess
  anorectal, 268, 269*f*
  brain, 809–810, 810*t*
  cutaneous, 494–495
  epidural, 810–811
  masticator space, 829
  periodontal, 840
  peritonsillar, 377–378, 845–846
  psoas, 979
  retropharyngeal, 377, 847
absence seizures, 792
abuse
  child, 1013–1014
  elderly, 1014–1015
  intimate partner, 1016–1017, 1018*t*, 1019–1020
  sexual, 1014
accelerated idioventricular rhythms (AIVRs), 14, 14*f*
ACE inhibitors. *See* angiotensin-converting enzyme (ACE) inhibitors
acetaminophen, 557*t*
  for acute mountain sickness, 670
  for acute otitis media, 366
  for acute pain control, 67
  for fever, 356
  for headache, 413
  for orofacial pain, 838
  for pericoronitis, 839
  for pulpitis, 839
  for stomatitis, 370
  for thyrotoxicosis, 713–714
  toxicity, 278, 593–595, 593*t*, 595*f*, 596*t*
  for varicella, 447
acetazolamide
  for acute mountain sickness, 670
  for glaucoma, 823
  for headache, 762
acetic acid, 683*t*
  for otitis externa, 831
acid
  See also nucleic acid amplification
  burns, 683*t*–684*t*
  folinic, 583
  hydrofluoric, 684*t*
  tranexamic, 320, 728, 835, 901
  valproic, 441, 557*t*
acid-base disorders, 53–59
  clinical features, 53
  defining nature of, 54, 54*f*–55*f*
  diagnosis and differential, 53–54
  metabolic acidosis, 56–58, 56*t*, 57*t*
  metabolic alkalosis, 58
  respiratory acidosis, 58–59
  respiratory alkalosis, 59
acid-fast staining, for TB, 205–206
acidosis
  metabolic, 56–58, 56*t*, 57*t*
  respiratory, 58–59
acquired bleeding disorders
  coagulation defects, 727–728
  disseminated intravascular coagulation, 727–728
  due to circulating anticoagulants, 728
  in immune thrombocytopenia, 726–727
  liver disease, 727
  platelet defects, 726
  renal disease, 727
acquired coagulation defects, 727–728
acquired platelet defects, 726
acromioclavicular joint injuries, 943–944, 943*t*–944*t*
ACS. *See* acute coronary syndromes (ACS)
activated charcoal, 560*t*, 561, 561*t*–562*t*
  for acetaminophen toxicity, 593
  for anticholinergic toxicity, 565
  for antidepressants, 566
  for antihypertensive toxicity, 611
  for aspirin toxicity, 592
  for barbiturate overdose, 575

activated charcoal (*Continued*)
for β-blocker toxicity, 606
for benzodiazepine overdose, 576
for calcium channel blocker toxicity, 608
for digitalis glycoside toxicity, 603
for herbicide poisoning, 629
for MAOI toxicity, 570
for mirtazapine toxicity, 568
for phentoin toxicity, 614
for SNRI toxicity, 568
for SSRI toxicity, 568
for trazodone, 567
for vitamin toxicity, 645
for xanthine toxicity, 600
acute abdominal pain, 217–221, 218*f*, 220*t*
in children, 400–404
laboratory studies for, 235*t*
neuromuscular junction disorders, 799
acute allergic reactions, 64–66
acute angle closure glaucoma, 823–825, 823*t*
acute aortic dissection, 177*t*
acute appendicitis, 252–255
acute bacterial sinusitis, 368–369
acute chest syndrome (ACS), 456–457, 736*t*
acute coronary syndromes (ACS), 128*t*, 131–137, 132*t*, 134*t*–135*t*, 177*t*, 178
evaluation process for, 142*t*
low-probability, 141–145
acute gastroenteritis, 395, 396*t*–397*t*, 398
acute glomerulonephritis, 288*t*, 470–471
acute heart failure, 149–151, 151*f*
acute hepatitis, 275–278, 276*t*
acute infectious diarrhea, 226–228, 227*t*
acute interstitial nephritis, 288*t*
acute ischemia, 143*t*
acute ischemic stroke, 177*t*, 179
acute kidney injury (AKI), 287–291, 288*t*, 289*f*, 468–469, 468*t*
acute lymphoblastic leukemia (ALL), 461–463
acute mastoiditis, 832
acute mountain sickness (AMS), 670–671
acute myelogenous leukemia (AML), 461
acute myocardial infarction (AMI), 125, 126, 127*t*, 132*t*
evaluation process for, 142*t*
acute necrotizing ulcerative gingivitis (ANUG), 840
acute-on-chronic heart failure, 149
acute otitis media (AOM), 366–368, 367*f*
acute pain management, 67–68
acute pericarditis, 129, 164–165
acute perioperative hypertension, 177*t*
acute peripheral neurological lesions, 796–799
Bell's palsy, 797–798
CNS, 796*t*
focal mononeuropathies, 798
Guillain-Barré syndrome, 796–797, 797*t*
peripheral nervous system, 796*t*
plexopathies, 798–799
acute prostatitis, 308
acute pulmonary edema, 177–178, 177*t*
acute renal failure, 177*t*, 178, 287–291, 288*t*
acute respiratory distress syndrome (ARDS), 484
acute rheumatic fever (ARF), 440–441
acute septic arthritis, 439
acute sequestration crises, 458–459
acute urinary retention, 303–305, 304*t*
acute vertigo, 784–791, 784*t*, 785*t*
acyclovir
for eczema herpeticum, 445–446
for encephalitis, 809
for herpes simplex, 478, 499–500
for herpes zoster, 857
for HSV, 816
for HZO, 817
for posttransplant infections, 549
for varicella, 447, 501
adalimumab, for Crohn's disease, 230
adenocoticotropin hormone (ACTH), 715
adenosine
for dysrhythmias, 34
for paroxysmal supraventricular tachycardia, 22
for pediatric pulmonary resuscitation, 33*t*
adhesive capsulitis, 977
adhesive tape, 92, 94*f*–95*f*
admission, for TB, 207
adrenal crisis, 753–754
adrenal insufficiency, 715–717, 716*t*–717*t*
adult epiglottitis, 846
adults
seizures in, 792–795
trauma in, 865–868, 866*t*
adult Still's disease, 988*t*
advanced airway support, 1–9
basic airway management, 1–2
extraglottic devices, 2–3
impending/actual cardiac arrest, 1
intubation, 4
mask ventilation, 2, 3*f*
noninvasive positive pressure ventilation, 2
orotracheal intubation, 4–7, 5*f*
rapid airway assessment, 1
RSI induction, 4
surgical airway, 7–8, 8*f*, 9*f*
adverse drug reactions, 994
Aeromonas hydrophila, 528
Aeromonas species, 530*t*, 531*t*

African sleeping sickness, 544
African trypanosomiasis, 544
agitation, 1024
AIDS. *See* human immunodeficiency virus (HIV)/AIDS
airborne isolation, for TB, 207
airway assessment, rapid, 1
airway devices, complications of, 849–850
airway emergencies, 992
airway foreign body, 375–377
airway management, 1–2
  for cardiogenic shock, 139
  in children, 869
  clinical factors for aggressive, 898*t*
  for neck injuries, 901
airway obstruction, 751
airways
  See also advanced airway support; bilevel positive airway pressure
  securing, 29
  in shock, 62
  surgical, 7–8, 8*f*, 9*f*
AIVRs. *See* accelerated idioventricular rhythms (AIVRs)
AKA. *See* alcoholic ketoacidosis (AKA)
albendazole
  for ascariasis, 545
  for enterobiasis, 545
  for hookworm, 545
albumin, for nephrotic syndrome, 470
albuterol
  for anaphylaxis, 65
  for asthma, 380, 383*t*
  for bronchitis, 200
  for HAPE, 672
  for hyperkalemia, 45*t*
  for stings, 658
  for tumor lysis syndrome, 754
albuterol sulfate
  for asthma, 214
  for COPD, 214
alcoholic ketoacidosis (AKA), 709–710, 709*t*
alcoholic liver disease, 276
alcohols
  ethanol, 580
  ethylene glycol, 581–583
  isopropanol, 580–581
  methanol, 581–583
alkalis, 684*t*
alkalosis
  metabolic, 58
  respiratory, 59
allergic conjunctivitis, 816
allergic contact dermatitis, 859–860
allergic reactions, 64–66
  to local anesthesia, 74
aloe vera, for frostbite, 650
alprazolam, for panic disorder, 1011
ALS. *See* amyotrophic lateral sclerosis (ALS)
ALTE. *See* apparent life-threatening event (ALTE)
alteplase
  for STEMI, 134*t*
  for venous thromboembolism, 174
altered mental status (AMS), 413–416, 414*t*–415*t*
  delirium, 775–776, 776*t*
  dementia, 776–777
aluminum acetate, for contact dermatitis, 860
amebiasis, 545
American trypanosomiasis, 544
AMI. *See* acute myocardial infarction (AMI)
aminoglycosides, in pregnancy, 333*t*
amiodarone
  for atrial fibrillation, 20
  for pediatric pulmonary resuscitation, 33*t*
  for ventricular fibrillation, 25
  for ventricular tachycardia, 23–24
amitriptyline, for chronic pain, 78
ammonia, 637*t*, 639
amnestic disorders, 1003
amniotic fluid embolism, 339
amoxicillin
  for acute bacterial sinusitis, 369
  for acute otitis media, 367
  for leptospirosis, 543
  for Lyme arthritis, 986
  for Lyme disease, 535–536
  for odontogenic abscess, 847
  for otitis media, 832
  for peri-implantitis, 840
  for stomatitis, 370
  for UTIs, 408
amoxicillin-clavulanate
  for acute bacterial sinusitis, 369
  for acute otitis media, 367
  for animal bites, 118
  for cervical lymphadenitis, 371
  for epistaxis, 835
  for facial injuries, 895
  for otitis media, 832
  for peritonsillar abscess, 378
  for pneumonia, 202
  for tracheostomy site infection, 849
  for UTIs, 301
amoxicillin-clavulanic acid, for preseptal cellulitis, 813
amphetamines, 585–587
amphotericin B
  for fungal infection, 548
  for sporotrichosis, 496
ampicillin
  for animal bites, 118
  for cholecystis, 251

ampicillin (*Continued*)
 for meningitis, 809
 for pneumonia, 387*t*
 for SBI, 354
 for ulcerative colitis, 232
 for urologic stone disease, 314
 for UTIs, 408
ampicillin/sulbactam
 for abortion, 326
 for appendicitis, 255
 for bacterial tracheitis, 375
 for odontogenic abscess, 847
 for peritonsillar abscess, 378
 for PID, 348*t*
 for postseptal cellulitis, 813
 for retropharyngeal abscess, 377
AMS. *See* altered mental status (AMS)
amyotrophic lateral sclerosis (ALS), 800–801
anal fissures, 266
analgesia, levels of, 68*t*
analgesics
 See also specific types
 acetaminophen, 593–595
 for acute mountain sickness, 670
 aspirin, 591–592
 for dysbarism, 674
 for intubation, 31*t*
 NSAIDs, 595–597
 for peri-implantitis, 840
 salicylates, 591–592
anal tags, 265
anaphylaxis, 64–66
anaplasmosis, 533*t*
α-napthyl-thiourea, 630*t*
androgenic steroids, in pregnancy, 333*t*
anemia
 See also sickle cell anemia
 bleeding and, 719–725
 childhood leukemia and, 462
 in children, 465–466
 evaluation of, 721*f*
anesthesia
 local, 74–76
 regional, 74–76
 for wound care, 82
aneurysms
 abdominal aortic aneurysms, 181–182, 182*f*
 nonnarcotic large-artery aneurysms, 183*t*
angina, 127*t*
 Ludwig's, 847
 unstable, 131–137
angioedema, 64–66
angiotensin-converting enzyme (ACE) inhibitors, 610*t*
 in pregnancy, 333*t*
 toxicity, 611
angiotensin II receptor antagonists, toxicity, 612
angiotensin receptor blockers, 610*t*
 in pregnancy, 333*t*
animal bites, 117–118
 antibiotics for, 997*t*
 infections from, 118–119
anion gap metabolic acidosis, 56*t*
anions, 37*t*
anistreplase, for STEMI, 134*t*
ankle-brachial indexes (ABIs), 921
ankle injuries, 109, 438, 961–962, 963*t*
ankylosing spondylitis, 986, 988*t*
anoplura, 662
anorectal abscesses, 268, 269*f*
anorectal disorders, 265–272
anorectal tumors, 270
anterior cruciate ligament (ACL) tears, 959
anthrax, 537–538
antibiotics
 See also specific types
 for bite wounds, 118–119, 119*t*
 for bursitis, 980
 for corneal foreign bodies, 820
 for diverticulitis, 257*t*
 for facial infections, 826*t*, 827*t*
 for hand infections, 996*t*–997*t*
 for infectious diarrhea, 227*t*
 for marine fauna trauma, 667–668, 668*t*
 for osteomyelitis, 981*t*–982*t*
 for pneumonia, 387*t*
 prophylactic, 84, 116, 121, 122*t*
 for SCD, 737
 for sepsis, 487*t*–489*t*
anticholinergics, 556*t*
 for vertigo, 789*t*
anticholinergic toxicity, 564–565, 564*t*
anticoagulants
 bleeding due to circulating, 728
 oral, 745–747
anticonvulsants, 614–615
 phenytoin, 613–614, 613*t*, 614*t*
 in pregnancy, 333*t*
 second-generation, 616
 valproate, 615–616
 for vertigo, 790*t*
antidepressants
 atypical, 567
 cyclic, 566
antidiuretic hormone (ADH), inappropriate secretion of, 39, 39*t*
antiemetics, 528, 756*t*, 789*t*
antihistamines, 789*t*
antihypertensives, toxicity, 608, 609*t*–610*t*, 611
antimalarials, 526, 526*t*
antimicrobial therapy, for diabetic foot ulcers, 708*t*
antimuscarinic effect, 564*t*
antiperistaltic agents, for hemolytic-uremic syndrome, 472

antiphospholipid syndrome, 988*t*
antiplatelet agents, 134*t*, 747
antipsychotics, 570–572
antiretrovirals, 505–506, 512
anti-RH (D) immunoglobulin, 324, 326
  for ITP, 466–467
anti-staphylococcal penicillin, for cellulitis, 116
antithrombins, for STEMI, 134*t*
antithrombotic therapy, 745–750
  complications of, 748, 748*t*–750*t*
antithyroid agents, in pregnancy, 333*t*
antivenom, 665
antivirals, for vertigo, 790*t*
anxiety disorders, 1005
AOM. *See* acute otitis media (AOM)
aortic aneurysms, abdominal, 181–182, 182*f*
aortic balloon counterpulsation, for mitral regurgitation, 155
aortic dissection, 127*t*, 128, 128*t*, 177, 184–186, 185*f*
aortic regurgitation, 153*t*, 156–157
aortic stenosis, 153*t*, 155–156
Apgar scores, 341
aphthous stomatitis, 840
apixaban, for venous thromboembolism, 173, 173*t*
aplastic episodes, 459
apparent life-threatening event (ALTE), 363
appendicitis, 252–255
apraclonidine, for glaucoma, 823
arboviral infections, 502–503, 541–542
arm injuries, 101–107
arrhythmias, sinus, 10, 10*f*
arsenic, 629*t*
arsenic poisoning, 632–633
artemether-lumefantrine, for malaria, 525*t*
arterial occlusion, 187–189, 189*t*
artesunate, for malaria, 526*t*
artesunate-admodiaquine, for malaria, 525*t*
atherosclerosis, 125
arthritis, 983*t*
  acute septic, 439
  gonococcal, 986
  juvenile idiopathic, 441–442
  Lyme, 986
  osteoarthritis, 986
  post-infectious reactive, 441
  rheumatoid, 986–987
  septic, 985, 985*t*
artificial tears, for conjunctivitis, 815, 816
artificial urinary sphincters, complications of, 318
ASA. *See* aspirin and salicylates (ASA)
ascariasis, 545
ascites, 280–281, 280*f*
aspiration pneumonitis, 202–203
aspirin
  for ACS, 133
  for acute rheumatic fever, 441
  for arterial occlusion, 188
  avoidance, in children, 68
  for cardiogenic shock, 140
  for low-probability ACS, 144
  for prosthetic valve disease, 159
  for STEMI, 134*t*
  for stroke, 772
  for TIA, 772
  toxicity, 591–592, 591*t*
assisted reproductive technology, 352
asthma, 213–216
  in infants and children, 379–381
  medication dosages, 383*t*–384*t*
  in pregnancy, 332
asymptomatic bacteriuria (ABU), 299
asystole (cardiac standstill), 27
ataxia, 781–783, 782*t*
atenolol, for STEMI, 135*t*
ATIII. *See* antithrombin III
atopic dermatitis, 858*t*
atovaquone-proguanil, for malaria, 525*t*
atrial fibrillation (Afib), 19–20, 19*f*, 20*f*
atrial flutter, 18–19, 18*f*
atrioventricular blocks, 15–17
atrioventricular bypass tracts, 21
atrophic vaginitis, 346
atropine
  for AV block, 16–17
  for calcium channel blocker toxicity, 608
  for cardiac transplantation, 550
  for clonidine toxicity, 611
  for digitalis glycoside toxicity, 603
  for intubation, 31
  for junctional rhythms, 14
  for MAOI toxicity, 570
  for organophosphate poisoning, 627–628
  for pediatric pulmonary resuscitation, 33*t*
  for sinus bradycardia, 13
atropine ophthalmic drops, 1023
atypical antidepressants, 567
automated internal cardiac defibrillators (AICDs), 28
AV block. *See* atrioventricular block
Avitene, 840
AVRT. *See* atrioventricular bypass tracts
axillary artery thrombosis, 977
azathioprine
  for Crohn's disease, 230
  for myasthenia gravis, 801
azithromycin
  for acute chest syndrome, 457
  for acute otitis media, 367
  for bronchitis, 199
  for cat-scratch disease, 119

azithromycin (*Continued*)
- for chancroid, 478
- for chlamydial infection, 474
- for folliculitis, 495
- for gonococcal pharyngitis, 371
- for gonorrhea, 474, 475
- for otitis media, 832
- for pneumonia, 202
- for STD prophylaxis, 1019
- for urethritis, 310

B

babesiosis, 533*t*
back pain, 77*t*, 969–974, 971*t*
bacterial conjunctivitis, 814–815
bacterial endocarditis, 516*t*
bacterial gastroenteritis, 395, 396*t*–397*t*
bacterial infections, 448–451
bacterial sinusitis, 368–369
bacterial tracheitis, 375
bacterial vaginosis, 344
bactitracin, for folliculitis, 495
balanoposthitis, 308–309
barbiturates, 574–575
bariatric surgery, complications of, 285
barium carbonate, 629*t*
Bartholin gland cyst/abscess, 346, 494–495
Barton fractures, 932
β-blockers
- for ACS, 137
- avoidance of, 26
- toxicity, 604–606, 604*t*, 605*f*, 605*t*
- for vertigo, 790*t*

beclomethasone, for ulcerative colitis, 232
bed bugs, 663
bee stings, 658–659
behavioral disorders
- amnestic, 1003
- anxiety disorders, 1005
- assessment and stabilization of, 1007–1009, 1008*f*
- delirium, 1003
- dementia, 1003
- incidence, 1003
- mood disorders, 1004–1005
- personality disorders, 1005
- psychotic disorders, 1004
- schizophrenia, 1004
- substance abuse, 1004

Behcet's disease, 989*t*
Bell's palsy, 768*t*, 797–798, 829
bending fractures, 434–435
benign neonatal sleep myoclonus, 363
benign paroxysmal positional vertigo (BPPV), 785, 787, 787*t*, 791
benodiazepines, for sympathetic crisis, 178
bentonite, 629
benzathine penicillin
- for acute rheumatic fever, 441
- for pharyngitis, 845
- for secondary syphilis, 861
- for stomatitis, 370
- for syphilis, 476, 477

benznidazole, for Chagas disease, 544
benzodiazepines
- for antidepressants, 566
- for antipsychotic toxicity, 570, 572
- for bupropion toxicity, 567
- for lithium toxicity, 573
- overdose, 575–576
- for serotonin syndrome, 569
- for SNRI toxicity, 569
- for SSRI toxicity, 568
- for TBI, 884
- for vertigo, 788, 789*t*

β-hCG, *see* β–human chorionic gonadotropin
bicarbonate
- for congenital adrenal hyperplasia, 424
- for diabetes, 426
- for metabolic acidosis, 57, 57*t*
- for rhabdomyolysis, 294
- for tumor lysis syndrome, 754

biceps tendon ruptures, 934
bilevel positive airway pressure (BPAP), 2
biliary colic, 284
biliary tract emergencies, 248–251
bipolar disorder, 1004–1005
bisacodyl, for constipation, 234, 1024
bismuth, 635*t*
bismuth subsalicylate, 228
bites and stings
- bed bugs, 663
- bees, 658–659
- bite wounds, 84, 119*t*
  - antibiotics for, 122*t*
  - human, 119–120
  - infections from, 118–119
  - mammalian, 117–118
  - rodents, livestock, exotic, and wild animals, 120
- black widow spider, 660
- brown recluse spider, 659–660
- chiggers, 662
- fleas, 662
- Gila monster, 665
- hobo spider, 660
- kissing bugs, 663
- lice, 662
- scabies, 661
- scorpions, 661
- snakes
  - coral, 664–665
  - pit viper, 663–664
- stinging ants, 658–659
- tarantulas, 660
- ticks, 661–662
- wasps, 658–659

bivalirudin, for ACS, 133

black cohosh, 644*t*
black widow spider, 660
bladder injuries, 918
bleeding
  See also acquired bleeding disorders
  anemia and, 719–725
  gastrointestinal, 237–238, 404, 405*t*, 406
  hemophilias, 729–732
  postextraction, 840
  posttonsillectomy, 848–849
  vaginal, 319–320, 337–338
blocks. *See specific blocks*
blood pressure (BP)
  elevated, 175–180
  in shock, 60–61
blood transfusion, for shock, 63
blunt eye trauma, 820–821
body lice, 662
Boerhaave's syndrome, 128–129
bone/articular derangements, 981–982
bone metastases, 751
Boston criteria, 355*t*
botulism, 799
boutonniere deformity, 930
bowel obstruction, 259–261, 259*t*
bowing fractures, 434–435
BPPV. *See* benign paroxysmal positional vertigo (BPPV)
brachial plexus injuries, 947–948, 947*f*, 977
brachioradial delay, 155–156
bradycardia
  sinus, 12–13
  toxicologic causes of, 605*t*
bradydysrhythmias, 12–15
brain
  anterior and posterior circulation of the, 767*t*
  injuries, 871*t*–872*t*, 880–885
brain abscess, 809–810, 810*t*
brain neoplasm, 768*t*
brain tumors, 761
breast surgery, complications of, 284
breathing
  in children, 869
  in neonates, 362
breech presentation, 343
brief resolved unexplained event (BRUE), 363
bromethalin, 630*t*
bromo-benzodifuranyl-isopropylamine, 589*t*
bromocriptine, for antipsychotic toxicity, 572
bronchiolitis, 381–383
bronchitis, 199–200
brown recluse spider, 659–660
Brucella canis, 531*t*
brucellosis, 542
Brugada syndrome, 26–27, 27*f*
buckle fractures, 436
budesonide, for viral croup, 372
bullous impetigo, 449, 449*f*
bullous myringitis, 832–833
bumetanide, for acute heart failure, 150
bupivacaine, for local anesthesia, 74
bupropion, 567
buried dermal sutures, 88–89, 88*f*
burns
  chemical, 682–685, 682*t*, 683*t*–685*t*, 822
  depth, 679, 680*t*–681*t*
  thermal, 678–682, 678*f*, 679*f*, 680*t*–681*t*
Burrow's solution, for EM, 852
bursae, acute disorders of, 983–987
bursitis, 980, 980*t*, 987, 998–999
buspirone, 577
butoconazole, for *Candida* vaginitis, 345
buttock trauma, 915
button battery ingestion, 243

C

C1 esterase inhibitor (human), for angioedema, 65
C1 esterase inhibitor replacement, for angioedema, 65
CAD. *See* coronary artery disease (CAD)
cadmium, 635*t*
calcitonin, for hypercalcemia, 51, 753
calcium antagonists, for vertigo, 789*t*
calcium channel blockers
  avoidance of, 26
  toxicity, 605*t*, 606–608, 607*f*
calcium chloride
  as antidote, 558*t*
  for β-blocker toxicity, 606
  for calcium channel blocker toxicity, 608
  for hyperkalemia, 45*t*
  for hypermagnesemia, 48
  for hypocalcemia, 48
  for pediatric pulmonary resuscitation, 33*t*, 34
calcium gluconate
  as antidote, 558*t*
  for β-blocker toxicity, 606
  for calcium channel blocker toxicity, 608
  for caustic toxicity, 625
  for congenital adrenal hyperplasia, 424
  for hyperkalemia, 45*t*
  for seizures, 411
calcium hydroxide paste, 841
calluses, 998
campylobacter, 396*t*
CA-MRSA. *See* community-acquired methicillin-resistant *Staphylococcus aureus* (CA-MRSA)

Canadian cervical spine rule, 889*t*
cancer, oral, 841
Candida vaginitis, 344–345
cannabis, 589*t*
Capnocytophaga, 531*t*
captopril, for hypertensive urgency, 179
carbamazepine, 557*t*
  in pregnancy, 333*t*
  toxicity, 614–615
  for trigeminal neuralgia, 829
carbamide peroxide otic, for cerum impaction, 833
carbon monoxide, 557*t*
carbon monoxide poisoning, 692–694, 692*t*, 693, 694*t*
cardiac arrest
  airway support, 1
  interventions for toxin-induced, 558*t*
cardiac medications
  ACE inhibitors, 611
  angiotensin II receptor antagonists, 612
  antihypertensives, 608, 609*t*–610*t*, 611
  calcium channel blockers, 606–608, 607*f*
  clonidine, 611
  digitalis glycosides, 602–604, 602*t*, 603*t*
cardiac monitoring, for SCD, 737
cardiac pacemakers, 28
cardiac rhythm disturbances, 10–28
  atrioventricular blocks, 15–17
  bradydysrhythmias, 12–15
  dysrhythmia-associated conduction abnormalities, 25–27
  fascicular blocks, 17–18
  narrow complex tachycardias, 18–23
  nontachycardiac irregular dysrhythmias, 10–12
  preterminal rhythms, 27
  wide complex tachycardias, 23–25
cardiac risk factors, 125–126
cardiac standstill, 27
cardiac tamponade, 165–166
cardiac transplantation, 549–550
cardiac troponin (cTn), 127
cardiogenic shock, 138–140, 149
cardiomegaly, 392
cardiomyopathies, 392
  with diastolic dysfunction, 163–166
  dilated cardiomyopathy, 160–161
  hypertrophic, 163
  restrictive, 164
  with systolic and diastolic dysfunction, 160–163
cardiothoracic injuries
  chest wall, 904–905
  diaphragmatic, 905–906
  esophageal, 907
  great vessels, 907, 907*t*
  heart, 905–906
  lung, 903–904, 903*t*
  penetrating cardiac, 906
  pericarditis, 907
  pneumomediastrinum, 905
  thoracic duct, 907
  tracheobronchial, 905
cardiovascular diseases
  acute heart failure, 149–151
  aortic aneurysms, 181–182
  aortic dissection, 184–186, 185*f*
  arterial occlusion, 187–189, 189*t*
  cardiogenic shock, 138–140
  cardiomyopathies, 160–166
  chest pain, 125–130
  congenital heart disease, 365
  hypertension, 175–180
  low-probability acute coronary syndrome, 141–145
  pediatric, 388–394
  syncope, 146–148
  valvular emergencies, 152–159
  venous thromoembolism, 167–174
cardiovascular emergencies, 993
cardiovascular shock, 388*t*, 389–391
cardiovascular syncope, 417–419, 419*t*
cardioversion, in children, 34–35
carisoprodol, 577
Carnett sign, 218
carpal bone fractures, 932, 932*t*
carpal tunnel syndrome, 798, 998
cat bites, 118–119, 119*t*
catheter-associated urinary tract infection (CA-UTIs), 316
cations, 37*t*
cat-scratch disease, 119
caustics, 624–625
cavernous sinus thrombosis, 839
cavitary tuberculosis, 206*f*
cefazolin
  for ankle fracture, 962
  for cellulitis, 493
  for marine fauna trauma, 667
cefdinir, for UTIs, 408
cefepime
  for childhood leukemia, 462
  for epidural abscess, 811
  for pneumonia, 202
  for urologic stone disease, 314
  for UTIs, 408
cefixime
  for gonorrhea, 475
  for STD prophylaxis, 1019
cefotaxime
  for adult epiglottitis, 846
  for altered mental status, 416
  for cholecystis, 251
  for epiglottitis, 375
  for intestinal obstruction, 261
  for meningococcemia, 451, 854

for pneumonia, 548
for SBI, 354
for sepsis, 358
for UTIs, 408
cefotetan, for PID, 348*t*
cefoxitin
for hernia, 264
for postpartum endometritis, 339
for retropharyngeal abscess, 847
cefpodoxime
for acute bacterial sinusitis, 369
for acute otitis media, 367
for CA-UTIs, 316
for urologic stone disease, 314
for UTIs, 300
ceftazidime, for childhood leukemia, 462
ceftotaxime
for acute chest syndrome, 457
for marine fauna trauma, 667
ceftriax-carbapenem, for intestinal obstruction, 261
ceftriaxone
for acute chest syndrome, 457
for acute mastoiditis, 832
for acute otitis media, 367
for altered mental status, 416
for bacterial tracheitis, 375
for chancroid, 478
for cholecystis, 251
for conjunctivitis, 815
for epididymitis, 307
for epiglottitis, 375
for esophageal perforation, 241
for gonococcal pharyngitis, 371
for gonorrhea, 474
for infection, 460
for lateral sinus thrombosis, 832
for leptospirosis, 543
for Lyme disease, 536
for malignant otitis externa, 831
for marine fauna trauma, 667
for meningitis, 809
for meningococcemia, 451, 854
for neutropenia, 467
for pneumonia, 202, 203
for postseptal cellulitis, 813
for retropharyngeal abscess, 377
for SBI, 354
for STD prophylaxis, 1019
for typhoid fever, 542
for urethritis, 310
for UTIs, 301, 408
cefuroxime
for acute bacterial sinusitis, 369
for epiglottitis, 375
for Lyme disease, 536
for otitis media, 832
for postseptal cellulitis, 813
cellulitis, 116, 451, 493
facial, 826–827, 826*t*
hand, 995, 996*t*
postseptal, 813
preseptal, 813
centamicin, for PID, 348*t*
Centor criteria, 370
central nervous system (CNS)
spinal infections and
brain abscess, 809–810, 810*t*
encephalitis, 806–809
epidural abscess, 810–811
meningitis, 806–809, 807*f*, 808*t*
tumors, 463
central retinal artery occlusion, 824
central retinal vein occlusion, 824
central transtentorial herniation, 882
central vertigo, 784, 784*t*, 788
cephalexin
for balanoposthitis, 309
for CA-MRSA, 491
for cellulitis, 451, 493
for folliculitis, 495
for impetigo, 449
for inflammatory lymph nodes, 848
for lid lacerations, 820
for marine fauna trauma, 667
for mastitis, 339
for orbital blowout fracture, 821
cephalosporin, for cellulitis, 116
cephalothin, for peritoneal dialysis complications, 298
cerebellar hemorrhage, 788
cerebellar infarction, 788
cerebellotonsillar herniation, 882
cerebral contusion, 881
cerebral salt-wasting syndrome, 39
cerebral venous thrombosis, 761
cerebrospinal fluid (CSF), diagnostic evaluation of, 808*t*
cerumen impaction, 833
cervical lymphadenitis, 371
cervical radiculopathy, 970*t*
cervical spine injuries, 633*t*, 874, 884
cetazidime, for epidural abscess, 811
cetriaxone, for gonorrhea, 475
Chagas disease, 544
chalazion, 813–814
chancroid, 478–479, 479*f*
cheeks
anatomy, 100*f*
lacerations, 100
chelation therapy
for arsenic poisoning, 633*t*
for lead poisoning, 632*t*
for mercury poisoning, 634*t*
chemical burns, 682–685, 682*t*, 683*t*–685*t*
ocular, 822
chemotherapeutic agents, extravastion of, 757

chest pain, 125–130
in ACS, 131
clinical features, 125–126
common causes of, 127–130, 127*t*
diagnosis and differential, 126–130
ER care and disposition, 130
of esophageal origin, 240–243
life-threatening causes of, 128*t*
in pregnancy, 335
prognosis-based classification systems for, 143*t*
chest radiography, 126
chest trauma
in children, 870
in elderly, 874
chest wall injuries, 904–905
CHF. *See* congestive heart failure (CHF)
chicken pox, 446–447, 446*f*
chiggers, 662
chikungunya, 541–542
child abuse, 1013–1014
fractures associated with, 435
childhood hypertensive emergencies, 179–180
childhood leukemia, 461–463
child neglect, 1013
children
abdominal pain in, 400–404, 401*t*
acute kidney injury in, 468–469
altered mental status in, 413–416, 414*t*–415*t*
appendicitis in, 255
diabetes in, 425–427
drug dosages in, 32
dysrhythmias in, 34
fever in, 353–357, 355*t*, 356*t*, 357*t*
fluid and electrolyte therapy in, 428–431, 430*t*–431*t*
headache in, 412–413
hematologic-oncologic emergencies in, 461–467
hypoglycemia in, 420–421, 423*t*, 424*t*
musculoskeletal disorders in, 432–442
pneumonia in, 385–387
PSA in, 71
rashes in, 443–454
resuscitation of, 29–35
seizures in, 409–411
sickle cell anemia in, 455–460
trauma in, 869–872
brain injuries, 871*t*–872*t*
UTIs in, 407–408
vomiting and diarrhea in, 395–399, 400
wheezing in, 379–384
chlamydial infection, 473–474
Chlamydophila psittaci, 531*t*
chloral hydrate, 577
chloramphenicol, for plague, 539
chlorhexidine mouth rinses, 841
chloride-responsive alkalosis, 58
chlorine, 637*t*, 638–639
chlorohexidine
for ANUG, 840
for aphthous stomatitis, 840
chloroquine, for malaria, 524
chlorpromazine, for headache, 762
cholecalciferol, 630*t*
cholecystitis, 248–251, 250*f*, 284
cholestryramine, for Crohn's disease, 230
cholinergics, 556*t*
chondroitin, 644*t*
chromic acid, 683*t*
chromium, 635*t*
chronic back pain, 77*t*
chronic constipation, 233–236, 234*t*
chronic hypertension, 335
chronic liver failure, 279–281
chronic neurologic disorders
amyotrophic lateral sclerosis, 800–801
Lambert-Eaton myasthenic syndrome, 803
multiple sclerosis, 802–803
myasthenia gravis, 801, 802*t*
Parkinson's disease, 803–804
poliomyelitis, 804–805
postpolio syndrome, 804–805
chronic obstructive pulmonary disease (COPD), 213–216
chronic pain, 77–80, 77*t*
aberrant drug-related behaviors and, 79–80, 79*t*
clinical features, 77–78
diagnosis and differential, 78
management of, 78*t*
chronic systemic hypertension, 175
Churg-Strauss syndrome, 989*t*
ciclopirox, for fungal infection, 448
cimetidine
for methemoglobinemia, 647
for PUD, 245
for xanthine toxicity, 599
ciprofloxacin, 814*t*
for anthrax, 538
for cat-scratch disease, 119
for CA-UTIs, 316
for cellulitis, 116
for chancroid, 478
for conjunctivitis, 815
for corneal abrasion, 819
for Crohn's disease, 230
for foodborne diseases, 528
for meningococcemia, 451
for odontogenic abscess, 847
for otitis externa, 831
for peritoneal dialysis complications, 298
for plague, 539
for prostatitis, 308
for tularemia, 537
for typhoid fever, 542

for urologic stone disease, 314
for UTIs, 300, 301
for vaginal cuff cellulitis, 350
for waterborne diseases, 528
circulation, in children, 869
cirrhosis, 279–281
clarithromycin, for marine fauna trauma, 668
clavicle fracture, 435, 942–943
clenched fist injuries, 102, 119–120, 995
clevidipine
for acute renal failure, 178
for childhood hypertensive emergencies, 180
for hypertensive encephalopathy, 178
for subarachnoid hemorrhage, 179
clindamycin
for abortion, 326
for bacterial tracheitis, 375
for bacterial vaginosis, 344
for bullous impetigo, 449
for CA-MRSA, 491
for cellulitis, 116, 451, 493
for cervical lymphadenitis, 371
for childhood leukemia, 462
for cholecystis, 251
for eczema herpeticum, 446
for esophageal perforation, 241
for impetigo, 449
for malaria, 525*t*, 526*t*
for mastitis, 339
for neck and upper airway masses, 848
for necrotizing soft tissue infections, 492
for odontogenic abscess, 847
for pericoronitis, 839
for periodontal abscess, 840
for peritonsillar abscess, 378, 846
for PID, 348*t*
for pneumonia, 203
for postpartum endometritis, 339
for posttransplant infections, 549
for pulpitis, 839
for retropharyngeal abscess, 377, 847
for scarlet fever, 451
for STSS, 483
for TSS, 481
for vaginal cuff cellulitis, 350
clonidine, 605*t*
for hypertensive urgency, 179
for opioid toxicity, 585
for tetanus, 518
toxicity, 611
clopidogrel
for ACS, 133
for low-probability ACS, 145
for STEMI, 134*t*
for TIA, 772
Clostridium difficile associated diarrhea, 228–229
clotrimazole
for balanoposthitis, 308–309
for *Candida* vaginitis, 345
for fungal infection, 448
for tinea infection, 859
cluster headaches, 762
CNS. *See* central nervous system (CNS)
coagulation defects, 727–728
coagulation factor VIIA (recombinant), 743
cobalt, 635*t*
cocaine, 585–587
cocaine abuse, 125
coccyx fracture, 950*t*
codeine, cautions, 68
coin ingestion, 242–243
colchicine
for acute pericarditis, 165
for crystal-induced synovitis, 986
cold injuries
frostbite, 649–650
hypothermia, 650–653, 651*t*–652*t*, 653*f*
nonfreezing, 649
colitis, 228–229
Colles fractures, 932
colonoscopy, 285
Colorado tick fever, 533*t*
coma, 777–780, 778*t*, 779*t*
myxedema, 711–712
community-acquired methicillin-resistant *Staphylococcus aureus* (CA-MRSA), 491–492
community acquired pneumonia (CAP), 200
compartment syndrome, 931, 966–967, 966*t*, 1001–1002
complete abortion, 325
complete spinal cord lesions, 886
complex regional pain types I and II, 77*t*
complex seizures, 793
complicated migraine, 768*t*
complications of, psychogenic, 778
computed tomography (CT)
for abdominal injuries, 911, 911*t*
for acute abdominal pain, 219
for appendicitis, 253, 254*f*
for cholecystis, 250
for pancreatitis, 247
concussions, 841
condylar fractures, 435–436
congenital adrenal hyperplasia, 365, 423–424
congenital heart disease, 365, 388–394, 388*t*
congestive heart failure (CHF), 388*t*, 391–394, 392*t*
See also acute pulmonary edema
conjugated estrogen, for vaginal bleeding, 320

conjunctivitis
allergic, 816
bacterial, 814–815
viral, 815–816
constipation, 233–236, 234*t*
in children, 403*f*
management of, 1024
constrictive perdicarditis, 166
contact dermatitis, 859–860
contact vulvovaginitis, 346
continuous (running) percutaneous sutures, 86–87, 87*f*
continuous positive airway pressure (CPAP), 2, 215
continuous renal replacement therapies, for poisoning, 562*t*–563*t*
continuous subcuticular sutures, 89, 89*f*
conversion disorder, 768*t*, 1011–1012, 1011*t*–1012*t*
cooling techniques, for heat emergencies, 657*t*
COPD. *See* chronic obstructive pulmonary disease (COPD)
copper, 635*t*
coprofloxacin
for corneal ulcer, 818
for malignant otitis externa, 831
for marine fauna trauma, 667
for pancreatitis, 248
for urologic stone disease, 314
coprofloxacin with hydrocortisone, for otitis externa, 368
coral snake bites, 664–665
cord prolapse, 342
corneal abrasion, 819
corneal foreign bodies, 819–820
corneal ulcer, 817–818
corns, 998
coronary artery disease (CAS), 125–126, 131
corticosteroids
for bronchiolitis, 382–383
for vertigo, 790*t*
cortisol, 715
cough, 195, 196*f*
Coxiella burnetii, 531*t*
coxsackle viruses, 443
CPAP. *See* continuous positive airway pressure (CPAP)
Crimean-Congo hemorrhagic fever, 543
Crohn's disease, 229–231
crossed leg test, 971*t*
crying, in neonates, 362
cryoprecipitate, 742
for ACS, 136
for hematologic complications, 297
for renal disease, 727
for vWD, 732
cryptitis, 266
crystal-induced synovitis, 986
crystalloid fluids, 37
for abdominal injuries, 912
for ACS, 136
for TBI, 884
for trauma, 871
CT. *See* computed tomography (CT)
CTCA. *See* computed tomography coronary angiography (CTCA)
cuff cellulitis, 350
culture, for TB, 206
Cunningham technique, 946
cutaneous abscesses, 494–495
CXR, for TB, 205
cyanide, 640–641, 640*t*, 641*t*
cyanide antidote kit, 558*t*, 640*t*, 641*t*
cyanoacrylate (super glue, crazy glue) exposure, 823
cyanosis, 197, 197*t*, 365, 388*t*, 389–391
cyclic antidepressants, 566
cyclopentolate, 814*t*
for blunt eye trauma, 821
for chemical ocular injury, 822
for corneal abrasion, 819
for corneal ulcer, 818
for HZO, 817
cycloplegics
for corneal abrasion, 819
for corneal foreign bodies, 820
cyproheptadine, for serotonin syndrome, 569
cysticercosis, 544
cystitis, 299
in pregnancy, 332
cysts
ganglion, 998
ovarian, 321
cytomegalovirus (CMV), 507
cytoxic agents, in pregnancy, 333*t*

D

D5 0.45NS IV, for AKA, 710
D5NS IV, for AKA, 710
dabigatran, 746–747
for venous thromboembolism, 173, 173*t*
dalteparin, for venous thromboembolism, 173*t*
dantrolene
for antipsychotic toxicity, 572
for MAOI toxicity, 570
DCM. *See* dilated cardiomyopathy (DCM)
debridement, wounds, 83
decompression sickness (DCS), 673–674
decongestants, for dysbarism, 674
deep peroneal nerve entrapment, 1000
deep space infections, 995, 996*t*
deep vein thrombosis (DVT), 167
antithrombotic therapy for, 173*t*
diagnostic algorithm for, 170*f*

in pregnancy, 330, 335
Wells' Score for, 169*t*
deferoxamine, for iron toxicity, 618, 619
defibrillation, in children, 34–35
dehydration, 398, 428–429
assessment in children, 428*t*
clinical dehydration score, 395*t*
delirium, 775–776, 775*t*, 776*t*, 1003, 1024
delivery. *See* labor and delivery
dementia, 775*t*, 776–777, 1003
demyelinating disease, 768*t*
dengue fever, 541
dental anatomy, 838*f*
dental avulsion, 842–843, 843*t*
dental block, 839
dental caries, 839
dental fractures, 841
deoxylamine with pyridoxine, for nausea and vomiting, 326–327
depression, 1004
DeQuervian tenosynovitis, 998
dermatologic disorders
allergic contact dermatitis, 859–860
atopic dermatitis, 858*t*
common papulosquamous eruptions, 858*t*–859*t*
herpes zoster, 856–857
hidradenitis suppurativa, 862, 863*f*
HSV infection, 857, 857*t*
lichen planus, 858*t*
molluscum contagiosum, 861–862, 862*f*
photosensitivity, 860
pityriasis rosea, 858*t*
pityriasis versicolor, 858*t*
psoriasis, 858*t*
scabies, 859*t*
seborrheic dermatitis, 858*t*
secondary syphilis, 859*t*, 860–861, 861*f*
sunburn, 860
tinea infections, 857–859, 858*t*
dermatologic emergencies
erythema multiforme, 851–852, 852*f*
meningococcemia, 853–854
pemphigus vulgaris, 854–855, 854*f*
TEN, 852–853, 853*f*
dermatomyositis, 989*t*
desmopressin
for hematologic complications, 297
for hemophilia, 732
for renal disease, 727
for vascular access complications, 298
for vWD, 732
dexamethasone
for acute mountain sickness, 671
for adrenal crisis, 754
for adrenal insufficiency, 717
for asthma, 380, 384*t*
for central nervous system tumors, 463
for coma, 780
for epiglottitis, 375
for HACE, 672
for headache, 762
for meningitis, 809
for nausea and vomiting, 1024
for neck and back pain, 973
for preterm labor, 338
for retropharyngeal abscess, 377
for SCV syndrome, 752
for thyrotoxicosis, 714
for typhoid fever, 542
for viral croup, 372
dextrose solutions, 37, 328
as antidote, 558*t*
for adrenal insufficiency, 717
for alcohol poisoning, 583
for altered mental status, 416
for altered mental status, 416
for ethanol overdose, 580
for hypoglycemia, 420
for hypoglycemia, 420, 701
for hypothermia, 652
for inborn errors of metabolism, 422
for seizures, 410
for seizures, 410
for sepsis, 358
DHE. *See* dihydroergotamine (DHE)
diabetes
in children, 425–427
in pregnancy, 328
diabetic emergencies
diabetic ketoacidosis, 702–705, 702*t*, 704*f*
foot ulcers, 706, 707*t*–708*t*
HHS, 705, 706*f*
hypoglycemia, 701–702, 702*t*
diabetic foot ulcers, 706, 707*t*–708*t*
diabetic ketoacidosis (DKA), 425–427
as medical emergency, 702–705, 702*t*, 704*f*
diabetic neuropathy, 77*t*
diagnostic imaging
See also computed tomography (CT); magnetic resonance imaging (MRI); ultrasonography
in pregnancy, 334
diagnostic peritoneal lavage, 911–912, 911*t*
dialysis, 291
complications of, 296–298, 298
peritoneal, 298
3,4-diaminopyridine, for Lambert-Eaton myasthenic syndrome, 803
diaper dermatitis, 452–453
diaper rash, 364
diaphragmatic injuries, 905–906, 910
diaphyseal fractures, 436–437
diarrhea, 225–232
acute infectious, 226–228, 227*t*
in AIDS patients, 509
in children, 400

diarrhea (Continued)
  Clostridium difficile associated, 228–229
  in infants and children, 395–399
  traveler's, 226–228
diazepam, for drug abuse, 586, 587
dicloxacillin
  for cellulitis, 493
  for folliculitis, 495
  for mastitis, 339
digital blocks, 75
digoxin, 557*t*, 605*t*
  as antidote, 558*t*
  for congestive heart failure, 393
digoxin-specific Fab, for digitalis glycoside toxicity, 603
dihydroergotamine (DHE), for headache, 762
dilated cardiomyopathy, 160–161
diltiazem
  for aortic dissection, 177
  for drug abuse, 586
dimercaprol
  for arsenic poisoning, 633
  for mercury poisoning, 634
DIP. *See* distal interphalangeal joint dislocation (DIP)
diphenhydramine
  for anaphylaxis, 65
  for EM, 852
  for foodborne diseases, 528
  for headache, 413
  for insecticide poisoning, 628
  for stings, 658
  for varicella, 447
  for vertigo, 788
  for vitamin toxicity, 645
  for waterborne diseases, 528
diphenoxylate, for Crohn's disease, 230
diphenoxylate and atropine, for diarrhea, 228
DIP joint dislocation, 930
direct laryngoscopy (DL), 4, 5*f*
dislocations. *See* joint dislocation
dislocation of the mandible, 829–830
disorders. *See specific disorders*
disseminated intravascular coagulation (DIC), 727–728
distal phalanx fractures, 931
diuretics, 609*t*
  loop, 608
  potassium-sparing, 611
diverticulitis, 256–258, 257*t*
diving complications, 673–674
dizziness, pharmacotherapy for, 789*t*–790*t*
DKA. *See* diabetic ketoacidosis (DKA)
dobutamine
  for aortic regurgitation, 157
  for cardiac transplantation, 550
  for cardiogenic shock, 140
  for congestive heart failure, 393
  for MAOI toxicity, 570
  for pulmonary hypertension, 180
  for shock, 63
docusate sodium/sennosides, for constipation, 234
dog bites, 118–119, 119*t*
dopamine
  for aortic regurgitation, 157
  for barbiturate overdose, 575
  for cardiac transplantation, 550
  for cardiogenic shock, 140
  for congestive heart failure, 393
  for sepsis, 358
  for shock, 63
  for sinus bradycardia, 13
dorsal forearm laceration, 102
doxazosin, for urologic stone disease, 314
doxycycline
  for anthrax, 538
  for brucellosis, 542
  for chlamydial infection, 474
  for ehrlichiosis, 536
  for epididymitis, 307
  for gonorrhea, 474, 475
  for leptospirosis, 543
  for Lyme arthritis, 986
  for Lyme disease, 535, 536
  for malaria, 525*t*, 526*t*
  for marine fauna trauma, 667
  for PID, 348*t*
  for plague, 539
  for pneumonia, 202
  for rickettsial spotted fever, 543
  for RMSF, 534
  for STD prophylaxis, 1019
  for syphilis, 477
  for tularemia, 537
DPL. *See* diagnostic peritoneal lavage
dressings, 121
drowning
  even algorithm, 676*f*
  near, 675–677
drugs
  See also medications; *specific drugs*
  of abuse
    amphetamines, 585–587
    cocaine, 585–587
    hallucinogens, 587, 588*t*–589*t*
    opioids, 584–585
drug therapy, postoperative complications, 283
drug toxicity, 768*t*
dry socket, 839–840
DUB. *See* dysfunctional uterine bleeding (DUB)
ducosate sodium, for constipation, 234
Duke criteria, 514*t*, 515*t*
duloxetine, for chronic pain, 79
DUMBELS effects, 626, 626*t*

dupuytren contracture, 998
DVT. *See* deep vein thrombosis (DVT)
dysbarism, 673–674
dysfunctional uterine bleeding, 320
dyshemoglobinemias, 646–648
dysphagia, 239
dyspnea, 191–192
  common causes of, 192*t*
  management of, 1024
dysrhythmia-associated conduction abnormalities, 25–27
dysrhythmias, 388*t*, 389, 418*t*
  bradydysrhythmias, 12–15
  hyperkalemia and, 43
  in infants and children, 34
  nontachycardiac irregular, 10–12
  in pregnancy, 329

E

e-aminocaproic acid (EACA)
  for hemophilia, 732
  for vWD, 733
ears
  See also facial injuries
  acute mastoiditis, 832
  cerumen impaction, 833
  foreign bodies in, 833
  lacerations, 98–99, 98*f*
  lateral sinus thrombosis, 832
  otitis externa, 831
  otitis media, 831–832
  trauma to, 833
  tympanic membrane perforation, 833–834
ebola virus, 503–504
ecallantide, for angioedema, 65
echocardiography
  for mitral stenosis, 153
  for right-sided valvular heart disease, 158
  for tamponade, 752
echoviruses, 443
eclampsia, 177*t*, 336–337, 793
econazole, for tinea infection, 859
Ecstasy, 588*t*
ectopic pregnancy, 323–325
eczema herpeticum, 445–446, 445*f*
edrophonium, for myasthenia gravis, 801
EGDs. *See* extraglottic devices (EGDs)
Ehrlichia specia, 531*t*
ehrlichiosis, 533*t*, 536
elbow dislocations, 935–938, 936*f*, 937*f*, 938*f*
elbow fractures, 938–939
elderly
  abuse, 1014–1015
  acute abdominal pain in, 219
  appendicitis in, 254–255
  PSA in, 71
  trauma in, 873–876
electrical injuries, 686–689, 686*t*–689*t*
electrocardiography (ECG)
  for ACS, 131–132, 132*t*
  of Afib, 19
  for aortic regurgitation, 157
  for aortic stenosis, 156
  of atrial flutter, 18
  of Brugada syndrome, 26–27
  for cardiogenic shock, 138–139
  for chest pain, 126
  with hyperkalemia, 44*t*
  of idioventricular rhythm, 14
  for mitral stenosis, 152
  of multifocal atrial tachycardia, 21
  for SCD, 737
  of sinus bradycardia, 12
  of sinus tachycardia, 18
  for syncope, 148
  of ventricular fibrillation, 24
  of ventricular tachycardia, 23
electrolyte disorders
  hypercalcemia, 49–51, 50*t*, 51*t*, 431*t*
  hyperkalemia, 43–45, 44*t*–45*t*, 430*t*
  hypermagnesemia, 47–48, 47*t*, 431*t*
  hypernatremia, 40–42, 41*t*, 430*t*
  hyperphosphatemia, 53, 53*t*
  hypocalcemia, 48, 49*t*, 431*t*
  hypokalemia, 42–43, 42*t*, 43*t*, 430*t*
  hypomagnesemia, 45–47, 46*t*, 47*t*, 431*t*
  hyponatremia, 38–40, 39*t*, 430*t*
  hypophosphatemia, 51–52, 51*t*, 52*t*
  in infants and children, 430*t*–431*t*
electrolytes, concentrations in fluids, 37*t*
electrolyte therapy, 428–431, 430*t*–431*t*
electronic control devices, injuries from, 689
elemental metals, 684*t*
EM. *See* erythema multiforme (EM)
embolism
  See also pulmonary embolism (PE); thromboembolism; venous thromboembolism
  amniotic fluid, 339
emergencies. *See specific emergencies*
emergency contraception, 1018–1019
emergency delivery, 340–343
  breech presentation during, 343
  cord prolapse, 342
  postpartum care, 343
  procedure for, 341
  shoulder dystocia, 343
enalaprilat, for acute pulmonary edema, 178
encephalitis, 768*t*, 806–809
endocarditis, 152
endometriosis, 322
endophthalmitis, 818–819
endoscopic procedures, complications of, 350
endotracheal intubation

for adult epiglottitis, 846
for barbiturate overdose, 575
poisoning and, 557
for TBI, 884
endrophonium, for myasthenia gravis, 801
end-stage renal disease (ESRD), 296–298
enemas, for constipation, 234
enoxaparin
for low-probability ACS, 145
for STEMI, 134*t*
for venous thromboembolism, 173*t*
enteric fever, 542
enterobiasis, 545
enterovirus, 443
envenomation
from marine fauna, 666–669
from snake bites, 663–665
environmental injuries
cold injuries, 649–654
heat emergencies, 655–657
ephedra, 644*t*
epidemic Louse-Borne typhus, 543
epididymitis, 307
epidural abscess, 810–811
epidural hematoma, 768*t*, 882
epiglottitis, 373–375, 374*f*
epinephrine
See also L-epinephrine; norepinephrine; racemic epinephrine
for anaphylaxis, 65
for antidepressants, 566
for asthma, 380
for β-blocker toxicity, 606
for calcium channel blocker toxicity, 608
for COPD and asthma, 215
for hypotension, 391
for local anesthesia, 74
for neonate resuscitation, 36
for pediatric pulmonary resuscitation, 32, 33*t*
for pulseless electrical activity, 27
for shock, 63
for sinus bradycardia, 13
for stings, 658
for ventricular fibrillation, 25
epinephrine autoinjector, 66
epinephrine autoinjector injuries, 117
episiotomy, 341
epistaxis, 834–835
Epley maneuver, 791
Epstein-Barr virus (EBV), 370, 501–502
eptifibatide, for STEMI, 134*t*
erectile dysfunction devices, complications of, 318
erysipelas, 493–494, 826*t*, 827
erythema multiforme (EM), 453–454, 851–852, 852*f*
erythemia infectiosum, 444–445, 444*f*
erythemia toxicum, 452
erythromycin, 814*t*
for acute rheumatic fever, 441
for chancroid, 478
for chemical ocular injury, 822
for chlamydial infection, 474
for corneal abrasion, 819
for HSV, 817
for HZO, 817
for lid lacerations, 820
for Lyme arthritis, 986
for stye, 813–814
erythromycin estolate, in pregnancy, 333*t*
escharotomy, for burns, 682
Escherichia coli, 397*t*, 527
esmolol
for aortic dissection, 177
for childhood hypertensive emergencies, 180
for great vessel injuries, 907
for hypertension, 185
for subarachnoid hemorrhage, 179
esomeprazole, for PUD, 245
esophageal emergencies
chest pain of esophageal origin, 240–243
dysphagia, 239
esophageal injuries, 898, 907
esophageal perforation, 241
esophageal rupture, 127*t*, 128–129, 128*t*
esophagitis, 241
ESRD. *See* end-stage renal disease (ESRD)
ethanmbutol, for TB, 207
ethanol, 557*t*, 580
ethylene glycol, 557*t*, 581–583
ethynyl estradiol
for emergency contraception, 1019
for vaginal bleeding, 320
etomidate
for intubation, 6, 31*t*
for sedation, 70*t*, 71, 72*t*
Ewing's sarcoma, 465
exanthem subitum, 447
exchange transfusion, for SCD, 737
exertional rhabdomyolysis, 295
extended-release dipyridamole, for TIA, 772
extensor tendon lacerations, 102–103, 103*f*
external rotation (Kocher's) technique, 946
extracranial solid tumors, 463–465
extraglottic devices (EGDs), 2–3
extravasation of chemotherapeutic agents, 757
extremities, trauma to, 920–922, 920*t*, 921*f*
extrusive luxations, 841
eye burr, 820

eye emergencies
acute visual reduction/loss, 823–825
infections and inflammation, 813–819
ocular ultrasonography for, 825
transfusion therapy
chemical ocular injury, 822
cyanoacrylate (super glue, crazy glue) exposure, 823
penetrating or ruptured globe, 821–822
trauma
blunt, 820–821
corneal abrasion, 819
corneal foreign bodies, 819–820
hyphema, 821
lid lacerations, 820
orbital blowout fractures, 821
ultraviolet keratitis, 819
eyelid lacerations, 97
eyes
See also facial injuries
eye complaints, in neonates, 364

F

FabAV. *See* polyvalent Crotalidae Immune Fab (FabAV)
F(ab) equine antivenom, 661
face lacerations, 100
facial infections
cellulitis, 826–827, 826*t*
erysipelas, 826*t*, 827
impetigo, 826*t*, 827–828
facial injuries, 892–896
facial space infections, 839
factor replacement, 743, 743*t*
for hemophilia, 730, 730*t*, 731*t*
falls, 873, 951
false labor, 340
famciclovir
for Bell's palsy, 798
for herpes simplex, 478, 499–500
for herpes zoster, 501
for HZO, 817
famotidine, for PUD, 245
fascicular blocks, 17–18
fasciotomy, 847
FAST. *See* focused assessment with sonography for trauma (FAST)
febrile neutropenia, 754–755, 755*t*
febrile seizure, 411
feeding, neonatal, 361–362
felbamate, 616
felon, 995–996, 996*t*
femoral fracture, 437
femoral nerve block, 76
femoral shaft fractures, 955
femure fracture, 952*t*, 953*t*
fenoldopam
for acute renal failure, 178
for hypertensive encephalopathy, 178
fentanyl
for acute pain control, 68
for appendicitis, 255
for intubation, 5, 31*t*
for sedation, 69, 70*t*, 73*t*
fever
acute rheumatic, 440–441
in children, 353–357, 355*t*, 356*t*, 357*t*
Crimean-Congo hemorrhagic, 543
in neonates, 363
postoperative, 282
rickettsial spotted, 542–543
scarlet, 450–451, 450*f*
with surgical procedures, 282
typhoid, 542
yellow, 543
FFP. *See* fresh frozen plasma (FFP)
fibrinogen concentrate, 742
for DIC, 728
fibrinolytics, 747–748, 748*t*
contraindications to, 136*t*
for STEMI, 134*t*, 135
fibromyalgia, 77*t*
fifth disease, 444–445, 444*f*
fight bites, 102, 119–120
finger
fingertip injuries, 106
injuries, 106
mallet, 929
trigger, 998
first-degree atrioventricular (AV) block, 15
fishing hooks, removal of, 114
fistula in ano, 268
fistulas, 285
flank trauma, 914
flashover, 689
fleas, 662
flexor hallucis longus, 1001
flexor tendon lacerations, 105–106
flexor tendons, 105*t*
flexor tendon sheath digital nerve block, 75
flexor tenosynovitis, 995, 995*t*, 996*t*
floaters, 825
flouroquinolone, for marine fauna trauma, 667
fluconazole
for balanoposthitis, 309
for *Candida* vaginitis, 345
for fungal infection, 548
fluid replacement, for shock, 62–63
fluid resuscitation
for burns, 681
Parkland formula for, 681*t*
fluids
See also amniotic fluid embolism
crystalloid, 37
electrolyte concentrations of, 37*t*
electrolyte therapy and, 428–431, 430*t*–431*t*
isotonic, 382, 754, 756

fluids (*Continued*)
  for shock, 32
  for volume replacement, 37
flumazenil
  for altered mental status, 416
  as antidote, 558*t*
  for benzodiazepine overdose, 576, 576*t*
fluocinolone cream, for cold injuries, 649
fluoroquinolones
  for adult epiglottitis, 846
  for otitis externa, 368
  in pregnancy, 333*t*
flurosemide, for congestive heart failure, 393
focal mononeuropathies, 798
focused assessment with sonography for trauma (FAST), 874, 910–911, 910*t*
folate, 644*t*
Foley catheter, for AKI, 469
Foley retention balloon, nondeflation of, 316–317
folinic acid
  for methanol poisoning, 583
  for posttransplant infections, 549
folliculitis, 495
fomepizole, for alcohol poisoning, 582, 582*t*
fondaparinux
  for ACS, 133
  for STEMI, 134*t*
  for venous thromboembolism, 173, 173*t*
foodborne diseases, 527–530, 529*t*
food impaction, 242
foot
  See also hand, foot, and mouth disease (HFMD)
  compartment syndrome of, 1001–1002
  injuries, 109–110, 438, 963–965, 964*t*
  lacerations, 108–111
  soft tissue problems of, 998–1002
forearm compartment, 105*t*
forearm fractures, 939–940, 940*t*–941*t*
forearm injuries, 436
forefoot injuries, 965
forehead lacerations, 96–97
foreign bodies
  airway, 375–377
  corneal, 819–820
  in ear, 833
  nasal, 836
  rectal, 270–271
  in soft tissues, 112–114
    imaging modalities for detection of, 113*t*
  swallowed, 241–242
  urethral, 311
  vaginal, 346
formic acid, 684*t*
fosfomycin, for UTIs, 300
fosphenytoin
  for sedation, 410–411
  for seizures, 794
  for TBI, 884
FOUR (Full Outline of UnResponsiveness) score, 777
Fournier gangrene, 308
fractures, 950*t*
  ankle, 962
  associated with child abuse, 435
  Barton, 932
  buckle, 436
  carpal bone, 932, 932*t*
  from child abuse, 435
  classification of, 926*f*
  clavicle, 435, 942–943
  condylar, 435–436
  dental, 841
  of distal femoral physis, 437–438
  elbow, 938–939
  femoral, 437
  femoral shaft, 955
  forearm, 939–940, 940*t*–941*t*
  frontal sinus, 894
  greenstick, 434
  hip, 874, 951–953, 952*t*, 953*t*
  humerus, 946–947
  immobilization devices, 927*t*–928*t*
  knee, 956, 957*f*, 957*t*
  leg, 956, 957*t*
  line orientation, 925*f*
  mandible, 896
  midfacial, 895
  nasal, 835
  naso-orbito-ethmoid, 894–895
  orbital blowout, 821, 895
  pathologic, 751
  plastic deformities, 434–435
  of radial and ulnar shafts, 436–437
  Salter-Harris, 432*f*, 433–434, 433*f*, 438, 926*f*, 926*t*
  scapula, 942–943
  skull, 881
  Smith, 932
  supracondylar, 435
  tibia, 438
  torus, 434, 436
  tripod, 895
  ulnar styloid, 933
  wrist, 437, 932–933
  zygoma, 895
Francisella tularensis, 532*t*
frank shock, 32
fresh frozen plasma (FFP), 742
  for ACS, 136
  for angioedema, 65
  for coagulation defects, 727–728
  for DIC, 727
  for iron toxicity, 618
frontal sinus fractures, 894

frostbite, 649–650
fuller's earth, 629
fungal infections, 448, 548
furosemide
  for acute heart failure, 150
  for cardiovascular complications, 296
  for hypercalcemia, 51
  for hyperkalemia, 45*t*
  for hyponatremia, 753
  for nephrotic syndrome, 470

G

G6PD. *See* glucose-6-phosphate dehydrogenase deficiency (G6PD)
gabapentin, 79, 616
GABHS. *See* group A β-hemolytic *Streptococcus* (GABHS)
gait disturbances, 781–783, 782*t*
gallstones, 248–251
ganciclovir, for CMV, 549
ganglion cyst, 998
ganglions, 1000
ganiclovir, for encephalitis, 809
garlic, 644*t*
gastric lavage, for iron toxicity, 618
gastritis, 244–246
gastroenteritis, 395, 396*t*–397*t*, 398
gastroesophageal reflux disease (GERD), 240
gastrointestinal bleeding, 237–238, 404, 405*t*, 406
gastrointestinal emergencies, 993
  acute abdominal pain, 217–221, 218*f*, 220*t*
  constipation, 233–236
  diarrhea, 225–232
  diverticulitis, 256–258
  gastrointestinal bleeding, 237–238
  nausea and vomiting, 222–224
gastrointestinal pain, 129–130
gastrointestinal surgery, complications of, 284–285
GBS. *See* Guillain-Barré syndrome (GAS)
GCS. *See* Glasgow Coma Scale (GCS)
Gelfoam, 840
generalized seizures, 792
genital problems. *See* male genital problems
genitourinary complications, postoperative, 282
genitourinary injuries, 916–919, 917*t*
genitourinary trauma, 870
gentamicin
  for abortion, 326
  for acute abdominal pain, 221
  for brucellosis, 542
  for childhood leukemia, 462
  for cholecystis, 251
  for epidural abscess, 811
  for peritoneal dialysis complications, 298
  for plague, 539
  for postpartum endometritis, 339
  for SBI, 354
  for tularemia, 537
  for urologic stone disease, 314
  for UTIs, 408
  for vaginal cuff cellulitis, 350
  for vascular access complications, 298
GERD. *See* gastroesophageal reflux disease (GERD)
germ cell tumors, 464
gestational hypertension, 335
gestational trophoblastic disease (GTD), 325
giant cell arteritis, 825, 989*t*
Gila monster bites, 665
gingko, 644*t*
ginseng, 644*t*
Glasgow Coma Scale, 777, 778*t*, 864, 880*t*
glass ionomer cement, 841
glaucoma, acute angle closure, 823–825, 823*t*
glenohumeral joint dislocation, 944–946
Global Registry of Acute Coronary Events, 130
glucagon
  for anaphylaxis, 65
  as antidote, 558*t*
  for β-blocker toxicity, 606
  for calcium channel blocker toxicity, 608
  for diabetes, 328
  for food impaction, 242
  for hypoglycemia, 420, 701
glucocorticoids, for hypercalcemia, 753
glucose
  for hyperkalemia, 45*t*
  for pediatric pulmonary resuscitation, 33*t*
  for tumor lysis syndrome, 754
glucose-6-phosphate dehydrogenase deficiency (G6PD), 738
glycerin rectal suppositories, for constipation, 234–235
glycoprotein IIb/IIIa antagonists, for ACS, 137
glycoprotein IIb/IIIa inhibitors, for STEMI, 134*t*
glycopyrrolate, for insecticide poisoning, 628
golfer's elbow, 934–935
gonococcal arthritis, 986
gonococcal infection, 474–475
gonococcal pharyngitis, 370, 371
gonorrhea, 474–475
graft-versus-host disease, 553–554, 553*f*

grand mal seizures, 792
great vessels injuries, 907, 907*t*
greenstick fractures, 434
griseofulvin
  for fungal infection, 448
  for tinea infection, 859
group A β-hemolytic *Streptococcus* (GABHS), 369–370
Guillain-Barré syndrome, 796–797, 797*t*
gunshot wounds, 915
gynecological procedure complications, 350–352
  assisted reproductive technology, 352
  endoscopic procedures, 350
  hysteroscopy, 350
  induced abortion, 351–352, 352*t*
  laparoscopy, 350
  postconization bleeding, 351
  postembolization syndrome, 352
  postoperative wound infections, 351
  septic pelvic thrombophlebitis, 351
  ureteral injury, 351
  vaginal cuff cellulitis, 350
  vesicovaginal fistula, 351

H
HACE. *See* high-altitude cerebral edema (HACE)
hair apposition, 92–93
hair-thread tourniquet syndrome, 110
hallucinogens, 587, 588*t*–589*t*
haloperidol
  for agitation/delirium, 1024
  for delirium, 776
  for nausea and vomiting, 1024
hand
  boutonniere deformity, 930
  compartment syndrome, 931
  cutaneous nerve supply of, 929*f*
  distal phalanx fractures, 931
  high-pressure-injection injuries, 931
  infections of, 995–996, 995*t*, 996*t*–997*t*
  injuries, 101–107, 929–931
  joint dislocation
    DIP, 930
    MCP, 930
    PIP, 930
    thumb IP, 930
    thumb MCP, 930
  lacerations, 102, 104
  mallet finger, 929
  noninfectious conditions, 998
  proximal and middle phalanx fractures, 931
  surgery consultation guidelines, 930*t*
  thumb MCP ulnar collateral ligament rupture, 931
hand, foot, and mouth disease (HFMD), 369–371, 443
Hank's balanced salt solution, 842
HAPE. *See* high-altitude pulmonary edema (HAPE)
HCM. *See* hypertrophic cardiomyopathy (HCM)
headaches, 759–764
  brain-tumor associated, 761
  in children, 412–413
  cluster, 762
  high-risk features for, 759*t*
  migraine, 761, 763*t*
  migraine headaches, 768*t*
  in pregnancy, 332
head injury
  See also traumatic brain injury (TBI)
  in children, 869–870
  in elderly, 873–874
head lice, 662
head trauma, 880–885
health care-associated pneumonia (HCAP), 200
hearing loss, 834
heart
  See also congestive heart failure; left ventricular heart failure; pediatric heart disease
  injuries
    blunt, 906
    penetrating, 906
  transplantation, 549–550
heart failure, acute, 149–151, 151*f*
heart murmur, 388*t*
  comparison of, 153*t*
  newly discovered, 152, 153*f*
heat cramps, 655
heat edema, 655
heat emergencies, 655–657
heat rash, 655
heat stroke, 655, 656
heat syncope, 655
heliox
  for asthma, 380
  for viral croup, 373
helium-oxygen (Heliox), for asthma, 380
HELLP syndrome, 177*t*, 336
hematological crises, 458–459
hematologic-oncologic emergencies, in children, 461–467
  anemia, 465–466
  central nervous system tumors, 463
  childhood leukemia, 461–463
  extracranial solid tumors, 463–465
  hemophilia, 465
  idiopathic thrombocytopenic purpura, 466–467
  lymphoma, 463
  neutropenia, 467
hematology consultation, for anemia, 720
hematoma block, 76
hematopoietic stem cell transplant (HSCT), 553–554

hematuria, 301–302
hemodialysis
  for barbiturate overdose, 575
  complications of, 297
  for hyperkalemia, 45*t*
  for hypernatremia, 42
  for lithium toxicity, 573
  for poisoning, 562*t*
  for renal disease, 727
hemolytic anemia, 466
hemolytic crises, 459
hemolytic-uremic syndrome, 471–472
hemoperfusion, for poisoning, 562*t*
hemophilias, 465, 729–732, 730*t*
hemoptysis, 211–212
hemorrhage
  cerebellar, 788
  intracerebral, 760–761, 765, 773, 881
  postpartum, 338–339
  subarachnoid, 177*t*, 178–179, 768*t*, 881
hemorrhagic fevers, 503–504, 543
hemorrhoids, 265–266, 267*f*
hemostatis
  tests for, 722*t*–725*t*
  with wounds, 83
hemothorax, 904
Henoch-Schönlein purpura (HSP), 404, 439, 453, 989*t*
heparin, 747
  for cardiogenic shock, 140
  for low-probability ACS, 145
  for peritoneal dialysis complications, 298
hepatic disorders, 275–281
hepatitis, 273, 275–278, 276*t*
  See also acute hepatitis
hepatitis A, 275
hepatitis B virus (HBV), 275
hepatitis C virus (HCV), 275
hepatitis D, 275
hepatitis E, 275
hepatitis prophylaxis, 1019
hepatomegaly, 509
herbals, toxicities of, 643–645, 644*t*–645*t*
herbicides, 628–629, 628*t*
hereditary spherocytosis, 738
hernia, 262–264, 262*f*, 263*f*, 264*f*
herniation, of brain, 882
herpangina, 369–371, 443
herpes simplex gingivostomatitis, 369
herpes simplex virus (HSV) infection, 369–371, 477–478, 477*f*, 498–500, 816–817, 816*f*, 857, 857*t*
herpes zoster, 500–501, 856–857, 856*f*
herpes zoster ophthalmicus (HZO), 817
herpetic whitlow, 996, 997*t*
HFMD. *See* hand, foot, and mouth disease (HFMD)
HHS. *See* hyperosmolar hyperglycemic state (HHS)
hiccups, 196–197
hidradenitis suppurativa, 495, 862, 863*f*
high-altitude cerebral edema, 672
high-altitude disorders
  acute mountain sickness, 670–671
  HACE, 672
  HAPE, 671–672
high-altitude pulmonary edema (HAPE), 671–672
high-flow nasal cannula (HFNC) therapy, for bronchiolitis, 382
high-output failure, 149
high-pressure-injection injuries, 117, 931
hindfoot injuries, 963
hip
  bursitis, 980, 980*t*
  dislocations, 954–955, 954*f*
  fracture, 874, 951–953, 952*t*, 953*t*
  overuse syndrome, 980*t*
  pain, 979–982, 979*t*
Hirschsprung's disease, 402
hirudins, 747
HIV. *See* human immunodeficiency virus (HIV)/AIDS
HIV-associated sensory neuropathy, 77*t*
hobo spider, 660
Hodgkin's lymphoma, 463
Hoffman's sign, 971*t*
hollow visceral injuries, 909
homatropine, 814*t*
hookworm, 545
horizontal half-buried mattress sutures, 90–91, 92*f*
horizontal mattress sutures, 90, 91*f*
hotlines, 1020*t*
HRIG. *See* human rabies immunoglobulin (HRIG)
HSCT. *See* hematopoietic stem cell transplant (HSCT)
HSP. *See* Henoch-Schönlein purpura (HSP)
human bites, 119–120
human botulism immunoglobulin, 799
human immunodeficiency virus (HIV)/AIDS, 125, 505–512
  clinical features, 505–506
  cutaneous manifestations, 509–510
  diagnosis and differential, 506–510
  febrile illnesses with, 507
  gastrointestinal complications, 509
  neurologic complications, 508–509
  ophthalmologic manifestations, 509
  opportunistic illnesses in, 506*t*, 507
  prophylaxis, 1019
  pulmonary complications, 508
  treatment recommendations, 510*t*–512*t*
human rabies immunoglobulin (HRIG), 521–522
humerus fractures, 946–947
hydantoins, in pregnancy, 333*t*

hydralazine
for childhood hypertensive emergencies, 180
for eclampsia, 336
for hypertension, 330t
for preeclampsia, 178
hydrocarbons, 621–623, 621t
burns from, 684t
toxicity, 622t
hydrochlorothiazide, for hypertension, 179, 330t
hydrocodone
for pericoronitis, 839
for pulpitis, 839
for sickle cell pain crises, 456
hydrocortisone
for adrenal crisis, 754
for adrenal insufficiency, 717
for adverse drug reactions, 994
for anaphylaxis, 65
for congenital adrenal hyperplasia, 423
for Crohn's disease, 230
for hypercalcemia, 51
for hypoglycemia, 421
for myxedma coma, 712
for otitis externa, 831
for phimosis, 309
for thyrotoxicosis, 714
for ulcerative colitis, 232
hydrofluoric acid, 684t
hydrogen peroxide
for cerum impaction, 833
for otitis externa, 831
hydrogen sulfide, 641–642
hydromorphone
for acute pain control, 68
for pain management, 1024
for sickle cell pain crises, 456
for urologic stone disease, 314
hydroxocobalamin, as antidote, 558t
hydroxybutyrate (GHB), 577–578
hyperbaric oxygen, 674
hyperbaric oxygen therapy
for burns, 682
for carbon monoxide poisoning, 693t
hyperbilirubinemia, 273–274
hypercalcemia, 49–51, 50t, 51t, 294, 431t
hypercalcemia of malignancy, 753
hypercapnia, 194
hypercyanotic episodes, 390, 391
hyperinsulinemia-euglycemia (HIE)
for β-blocker toxicity, 606
for calcium channel blocker toxicity, 608
hyperkalemia, 43–45, 44t–45t, 294, 430t
hyperleukocytosis, 463
hypermagnesemia, 47–48, 47t, 431t
hypernatremia, 40–42, 41t, 430t
hyperosmolar hyperglycemic state (HHS), 705, 706f
hyperosmotic coma, 768t
hyperphosphatemia, 53, 53t, 294
hypertension, 388t
childhood hypertensive emergencies, 179–180
chronic, 335
classification of, 175t
in pregnancy, 328–329, 330t, 335
pulmonary, 180
systemic, 175–179
hypertensive acute heart failure, 149
hypertensive emergency, 175, 177t
hypertensive encephalopathy, 177t, 178, 768t
hypertensive retinopathy, 177t
hypertensive urgency, 175, 179
hyperthermia, 655, 656
hyperthyroidism, in pregnancy, 328, 329t
hypertonic saline
for hyponatremia, 39, 753
for TBI, 884
hypertrophic cardiomyopathy, 163
hyperviscosity syndrome, 755–756
hypervitaminosis, 643–644
hypervolemia, 37–38
hypervolemic hyponatremia, 39t
hyphema, 820, 821
hypnotics, 574–579
hypocalcemia, 48, 49t, 294, 431t
hypoglycemia, 420–421, 423t, 424t, 701–702, 702t, 768t
hypokalemia, 42–43, 42t, 43t, 430t
hypomagnesemia, 45–47, 46t, 47t, 431t
hyponatremia, 38–40, 39t, 40t, 430t, 768t
due to syndrome of inappropriate anti-diuretic hormone, 753
hypophosphatemia, 51–52, 51t, 52t, 294
hypotension, 32
systemic arterial, 60
hypotensive patient, 60–63
See also shock
hypothermia, 650–653, 651t–652t, 653f
hypovolemia, 37–38
hypovolemic shock, 429
hypoxemia, 192–193
hypoxia, 192–193
hysteroscopy, 350
HZO. *See* herpes zoster ophthalmicus (HZO)

I

iatrogenic pneumothorax, 210
ibuprofen
for acute otitis media, 366
for acute pain control, 67
for acute pericarditis, 165
for crystal-induced synovitis, 986
for fever, 356
for headache, 413
for HSP, 453

for otitis externa, 368
for pericoronitis, 839
for pulpitis, 839
for sickle cell pain crises, 456
for stomatitis, 370
or transient synovitis, 440
for vaginal bleeding, 320
ibutilide, for atrial fibrillation, 20
icatibant, for angioedema, 65
idarucizumab, 745
idiopathic intracranial hypertension, 761
idiopathic thrombocytopenic purpura (ITP), 466–467
idioventricular rhythm, 14, 14*f*
IGRA. *See* interferon gamma release assay (IGRA)
iliac wing fracture, 950*t*
imipenem
for Fournier gangrene, 308
for liver transplantation, 553
for marine fauna trauma, 667
for pneumonia, 548
for posttransplant infections, 548
imipenem-cilastatin
for pancreatitis, 248
for vaginal cuff cellulitis, 350
immune thrombocytopenia, 726–727
immunoglobulin, 797
See also anti-RHO (D) immunoglobulin
for Guillain-Barré syndrome, 797
for thrombocytopenia, 727
immunosuppresion, 994
immunosuppressive agents, complications of, 549
impetigo, 448–449, 448*f*, 826*t*, 827–828
impingement syndrome, 976
inborn errors of metabolism, 365, 421–423, 422*f*
incomplete spinal cord lesions, 886
induced abortion, 351–352, 352*t*
induction agents, for intubation, 31*t*
industrial toxins
ammonia, 639
chlorine, 638–639
cyanide, 640–641, 640*t*, 641*t*
hydrogen sulfide, 641–642
nitrogen dioxide, 639
phosgene, 638
respiratory toxins, 637–638
inevitable abortion, 325
infants
See also neonatal problems
abdominal pain in, 401–403
acute kidney injury in, 468–469
fever in, 353–357, 356*t*, 357*t*
fluid and electrolyte therapy in, 428–431, 430*t*–431*t*
pneumonia in, 385–387
vomiting and diarrhea in, 395–399
wheezing in, 379–384
infarction
See also acute myocardial infarction (AMI)
infected epidermoid and pilar cysts, 495
infection
See also specific types
from animal bites, 118–119
bacterial, 448–451
childhood leukemia and, 462
CNS and spinal, 806–811
eye, 813–819
facial space, 839
fungal, 448
hand, 996*t*–997*t*
hand lacerations, 995–996, 995*t*
from human bites, 119–120
from needle stick, 116–117
postoperative, 351
posttransplant, 546, 546*t*–547*t*, 548–549
respiratory, 203
sepsis, 358, 484–490
sexually transmitted, 473–479
sickle cell anemia and, 459–460
soft tissue, 491–496
tinea, 857–859
urinary tract, 299–301, 316
viral, 443–447, 497–504
zoonotic, 531–539
infectious emergencies, 994
infective endocarditis, 513–516, 514*t*, 515*t*, 516*t*
infestations, scabies, 451–452
inflammatory bowel disease (IBD), 229–231
infliximab
for Crohn's disease, 230
for ulcerative colitis, 232
influenza, 497–498
ingrown toenail, 998
injuries, 963–965
See also trauma; *specific injuries*
abdominal, 909–913
ankle, 961–962, 963*t*
to arm, hand, fingertip, and nail, 101–107, 104*f*, 107*f*
brachial plexus, 947–948
brain, 871*t*–872*t*
cardiothoracic, lung, 903–904
cervical spine, 874, 884
chest wall, 904–905
electrical, 686–689
electronic control devices, 689
epinephrine autoinjector, 117
facial, 892–896, 892*t*–893*t*, 895*f*
foot, 964*t*
genitourinary, 916–919, 917*t*
hand, 929–931
head, 869–870, 873–874
high-pressure-injection, 117

injuries (*Continued*)
  kidney, 287–291, 289*f*, 468–469
  leg, 959–960
  lightning, 689–691, 690*t*
  neck, 897–902, 897*t*, 900*f*
  needle-stick, 116–117
  orthopedic, 874–875
  overuse, 960
  pelvic, 949–951
  shoulder and humerus, 942–948
  soft tissue, 934–935
  spine, 870, 886–891, 890*t*
  wrist, 931–933
insecticides, 626–628, 626*t*, 627*t*, 628*t*
insulin
  for β-blocker toxicity, 606
  for hyperkalemia, 45*t*
  for tumor lysis syndrome, 754
intercostal nerve block, 75–76
interferon gamma release assay (IGRA), 204, 206–207
international normalized ration (INR), 745, 746*f*
intestinal colic, 362
intestinal obstruction, 259–261, 259*t*
intimate partner violence and abuse, 1016–1017, 1018*t*, 1019–1020
intraabdominal abscesses, 284
intracerebral hemorrhage, 760–761, 765, 773, 881
intracranial hemorrhage, 177*t*, 179
intracranial hypotension, 761
intrauterine pregnancy (IUP), 324
intravenous (IV) crystalloid infusion, for iron toxicity, 618
intravenous immunoglobulin (IVIG), for ITP, 466, 467
intravenous lipid emulsion therapy (ILET), for poisoning, 563*t*
intrinsic renal failure, 288
intubation, 4, 7*f*
  See also rapid sequence intubation (RSI)
  orotracheal, 4–7, 5*f*
  poisoning and, 557
  RSI, 4, 29, 30*t*–31*t*, 31
Intubrite, 5*f*
intussusception, 402–403, 403*f*
ipratropium
  for asthma, 332, 380
  for COPD and asthma, 215
ipratropium bromide
  for anaphylaxis, 65
  for asthma, 384*t*
iritis, 818, 818*t*
iron, 557*t*
  toxicity, 617–620, 618*t*, 619*f*
iron deficiency anemia, 465–466
iron therapy, 466
irrigation
  See also whole-bowel irrigation (WBI)
ischemia, 288*t*
ischemic stroke, 765, 766*t*, 771*t*
  acute, 769*t*–770*t*
ischial tuberosity, 950*t*
ischium body fracture, 950*t*
isoniazid, for TB, 207
isopropanol, 580–581
isoproterenol
  for β-blocker toxicity, 606
  for ventricular tachycardia, 24
isotonic crystalloid, for altered mental status, 416
isotonic fluids
  for bronchiolitis, 382
  for hyperviscosity syndrome, 756
  for tumor lysis syndrome, 754
isotretinoin, in pregnancy, 334*t*
isproterenol, for MAOI toxicity, 570
istonic saline, for hypernatremia, 41
ITP. *See* idiopathic thrombocytopenic purpura (ITP)
itraconazole, for sporotrichosis, 496
IV β-blockers, for sedative overdose, 578
ivermectin
  for ascariasis, 545
  for scabies, 661
IV fat emulsion, for calcium channel blocker toxicity, 608
IV fluids, for asthma, 380
IVIG. *See* intravenous immunoglobulin (IVIG)
IV immunoglobulin, for TSS, 481
IV iopanoic acid, for thyrotoxicosis, 714
IV lipid emulsion, as antidote, 559*t*
IV pyelogram (IVP), 313

J

jaundice, 273–274
  neonatal, 363–364
jellyfish stings, 668
joint dislocation, 954*f*
  ankle, 962
  DIP, 930
  glenohumeral, 944–946
  hip, 954–955
  knee, 958
  MCP, 930
  PIP, 930
  thumb IP, 930
  thumb MCP, 930
joint replacement, 981
joints
  See also temporomandibular joint dysfunction
  acute disorders of, 983–987
joint space injection, 977
JRA. *See* juvenile rheumatoid arthritis (JRA)
jumper's knee, 960
junctional rhythms, 13–14, 13*f*

juniper, 644*t*
juvenile idiopathic arthritis (JIA), 441–442

K
Kaposi sarcoma, 509
Kawasaki's disease, 453
KCl, 43
keraunoparalysis, 691
ketamine
for asthma, 216, 380, 384*t*
for intubation, 6, 31*t*
for sedation, 69, 70*t*, 71, 73*t*
for seizures, 794
ketoacidosis
alcoholic, 709–710
diabetic, 702–705, 702*t*, 704*f*
ketoconazole
for fungal infection, 448
for tinea infection, 859
ketorolac, 815*t*
for cholecystis, 251
for headache, 413
for urologic stone disease, 314
ketorolac ophthalmic solution, for corneal abrasion, 819
ketorolae, for sickle cell pain crises, 456
kidney injury, 289*f*, 917
acute, 287–291, 468–469
kidney stones, 312–315, 313*t*
kidney transplant, 551–552
kidney-ureter bladder film (KIB), 313
kissing bugs, 663
knee
bursitis, 980, 980*t*
fractures, 956, 957*f*, 957*t*
injuries, 109, 437–438
dislocations, 958
mechanisms of, 957*t*–958*t*
overuse, 960, 980*t*
pain, 979–982
pain crises, 979*t*
Kocher's technique, 946

L
LA. *See* local anesthesia
labetalol
for acute ischemic stroke, 179
for aortic dissection, 177
for childhood hypertensive emergencies, 180
for eclampsia, 336
for hypertension, 185, 329, 330*t*
for hypertensive encephalopathy, 178
for hypertensive urgency, 179
for intracranial hemorrhage, 179
for preeclampsia, 178
for stroke, 771
for subarachnoid hemorrhage, 179
labetaolol, for tetanus, 518
labor, preterm, 338
labor and delivery
emergency delivery, 340–343
false labor, 340
movements of normal, 342*f*
postpartum care, 343
labyrinthitis, 768*t*, 787
lacerations
See also specific lacerations
cheeks, 100
dorsal forearm, wrist, and hand, 102
ear, 98–99, 98*f*
extensor tendon, 102–103, 103*f*
eyelid, 97, 820
face, 100
finger, 106
flexor tendon, 105–106
leg and foot, 108–111
lips, 99, 99*f*
nasal, 98
palm, 104–105
scalp and forehead, 96–97
tendon, 1001
tongue, 844
volar forearm, wrist, and hand, 104
lacosamide, 616
lacrimators, 685*t*
Lacrodectus antivenom, 660
lactation, 334*t*
Lacted Ringer's solution, 37, 41
lactulose, for constipation, 234, 1024
Lambert-Eaton myasthenic syndrome, 803
lamotrigine, 79, 616
lansoprazole, for PUD, 245
laparoscopic procedures, complications of, 285
laparoscopy, 350
laparotomy, 912*t*, 915
laryngectomy patients, 850
laryngotracheal injuries, 898
laryngotracheobronchitis, 372–373
lateral epicondylitis, 934–935
lateral medullary infarction of brainstem, 789*t*–790*t*
lateral sinus thrombosis, 832
lavage
See also gastric lavage
L-carnitine, for valproate toxicity, 616
lead poisoning, 631–632, 631*t*, 632*t*
Le Fort injury, 895–896, 895*f*
left ventricular assist devices (LVADs), 162–163
Legg-Calvé-Perthes disease, 440
leg injuries, 959–960
leg lacerations, 108–111
leiomyomas, 322
L-epinephrine
for epiglottitis, 374
for viral croup, 372–373
Leptospira species, 532*t*
leptospirosis, 543

lesions
  See also acute peripheral neurological lesions
leucovorin, for methanol poisoning, 583
leukemia, childhood, 461–463
leukopheresis, for hyperviscosity syndrome, 756
levetiracetam, 616
  for seizures, 411, 794
levofloxacin
  for CA-UTIs, 316
  for chlamydial infection, 474
  for epididymitis, 307
  for foodborne diseases, 528
  for marine fauna trauma, 667
  for odontogenic abscess, 847
  for PID, 348*t*
  for pneumonia, 202
  for urologic stone disease, 314
  for UTIs, 300
  for waterborne diseases, 528
levonorgestrel, for emergency contraception, 1018, 1019
levothyroxine (T4), for hypothyroidism, 712
Lhermitte's sign, 802, 971*t*
lice, 452, 662
lichen planus, 858*t*
lid lacerations, 820
lidocaine
  for β-blocker toxicity, 606
  for delivery, 341
  for dysbarism, 674
  for EM, 852
  for epistaxis, 834
  for foreign bodies in ear, 833
  for local anesthesia, 74
  for MAOI toxicity, 570
  for marine fauna trauma, 668
  for nasal foreign bodies, 836
  for nasal septal hematoma, 836
  for paraphimosis, 310
  for pediatric pulmonary resuscitation, 33*t*
  for tongue lacerations, 844
  for ventricular fibrillation, 25
lidocaine, epinephrine, and tetracaine (LET), 74–75
lidocaine and prilocaine (EMLA), 74, 75
ligamentous injuries, 959–960
lightning injuries, 689–691, 690*t*
limaprost, for cold injuries, 649
linezolid
  for anthrax, 538
  for pneumonia, 202
  for posttransplant infections, 548
  for TSS, 481
liothyronine, for hypothyroidism, 712
lipid emulsion therapy, for drug abuse, 586
lip lacerations, 99, 99*f*
lisinopril, for hypertension, 179
lithium, 557*t*, 572–573
  in pregnancy, 334*t*
lithium carbonate, for thyrotoxicosis, 714
lithotripsy, complications of, 317
liver cirrhosis, 279–281
liver disease, bleeding in, 727
liver transplant, 552–553
livestock bites, 120
LMA. *See* laryngeal mask airway (LMA)
LMWH. *See* low-molecular-weight heparin (LMWH)
local anesthesia, 74–76
locked knee, 960
long-QT syndrome, 26–27
loop diuretics, 608
loperamide
  for Crohn's disease, 230
  for foodborne diseases, 528
  for hemolytic-uremic syndrome, 472
lorazepam
  for anticholinergic toxicity, 565
  for delirium, 776
  for drug abuse, 586, 587
  for intubation, 31*t*
  for nicotine toxicity, 601
  for panic disorder, 1011
  for seizures, 410, 794
  for tetanus, 518
  for xanthine toxicity, 599
losartan, for hypertensive urgency, 179
lower extremity injuries, 437
lower GI (LGI) bleeding, 404, 405*t*, 406
low-molecular-weight heparin (LMWH), 747
  for ACS, 133
  for venous thromboembolism, 173, 173*t*
low-probability acute coronary syndrome, 141–145
Ludwig's angina, 839, 847
lugol solution, for thyrotoxicosis, 714
lumbar puncture, 807*f*
lumbar radiculopathies, 971*t*
lung injuries, 903–904, 903*t*, 904*t*
lung transplantation, 550–551
luxations, 841
LVH. *See* left ventricular hypertrophy (LVH)
Lyme arthritis, 986
Lyme disease, 533*t*, 534–536
lymphoma, 463
lysergic acid diethylamide, 588*t*

M

magnesium, for anaphylaxis, 65
magnesium citrate, for constipation, 234
magnesium sulfate
  for antidepressants, 566
  for asthma, 215, 380, 384*t*
  for β-blocker toxicity, 606

for eclampsia, 336
for hypomagnesemia, 46
for MAT, 21
for seizures, 411, 794
for tetanus, 518
for trazodone, 567
for ventricular fibrillation, 25
for ventricular tachycardia, 24
magnetic resonance imaging (MRI)
for appendicitis, 254
for back pain, 972
major depression, 1004
malaria, 523–526, 525*t*, 526*t*
male genital problems
acute prostatitis, 308
epididymitis, 307
orchitis, 307
penis, 308–310
scrotum, 308
testicular torsion, 306–307
urethra, 310–311
malignancy emergencies
adrenal crisis, 753–754
airway obstruction, 751
bone metastases, 751
extravasation of chemotherapeutic agents, 757
febrile neutropenia, 754–755, 755*t*
hypercalcemia, 753
hyperviscosity syndrome, 755–756
hyponatremia, due to SIADH, 753
nausea and vomiting, 756
pathologic fractures, 751
pericardial effusion, 751–752
spinal cord compression, 751, 752*t*
superior vena cava syndrome, 752
thromboembolism, 756
tumor lysis syndrome, 754
malignant heat illnesses, 655, 656
malignant melanoma, 1002
malignant otitis externa, 831
malignant pericardial effusion, 751–752
mallet finger, 929
malrotation of the intestine, 401–402
mammalian bites, 117–118
infections from, 118–119
mandible disorders, 829–830
mandible fractures, 896
mannitol
for cerebral edema, 426
for coma, 780
for DKA, 705
for glaucoma, 823
for TBI, 884
MAOIs. *See* monoamine oxidase inhibitors (MAOIs)
marijuana, 589*t*
marine fauna trauma and envenomation, 666–669, 668*t*–669*t*
mask ventilation, 2, 3*f*
massive transfusion, 740
masticator space abscess, 829
masticato space infection, 826*t*
mastitis, 339
mastoiditis, 367
MAT. *See* multiple atrial tachycardia (MAT)
MC fractures. *See* metacarpal fractures
MCP. *See* metacarpal phalangeal (MCP) joint dislocation
McRoberts maneuver, 343
measles, 443–444, 502
mebendazole
for ascariasis, 545
for enterobiasis, 545
for hookworm, 545
meclizine
for nausea and vomiting, 223
for vertigo, 788
medial epicondylitis, 934–935
median nerves, 935*t*
medication-induced syncope, 147
medications
See also specific medications
cardiac, 602–612
ophthalmic, 814*t*–815*t*
in pregnancy and lactation, 333, 333*t*, 334*t*
for PSA, 72*t*–73*t*
rapid sequence intubation, 31*t*
medroxyprogesterone, for vaginal bleeding, 320
melanocyte stimulating hormone (MSH), 715
melanoma, 1002
melatonin, 578
Ménière's disease, 768*t*, 787
meningitis, 358–360, 358*t*–359*t*, 768*t*, 806–809, 807*f*, 808*t*
meningococcemia, 451, 853–854
meniscal injuries, 959–960
meprobamate, 577
6-mercaptopurine, for Crohn's disease, 230
mercury poisoning, 633–634, 634*t*
meropenem
for Fournier gangrene, 308
for intestinal obstruction, 261
for necrotizing soft tissue infections, 492
for pancreatitis, 248
for pneumonia, 548
for posttransplant infections, 548
for STSS, 483
merpenem, for anthrax, 538
mertonidazole, for vaginal cuff cellulitis, 350
mesalamine
for Crohn's disease, 230
for ulcerative colitis, 232

mescaline, 588*t*
metabolic acidosis, 56–58, 56*t*, 57*t*
metabolic alkalosis, 58
metabolic disorders, 421–423, 422*f*
metabolism. *See* inborn errors of metabolism
metacarpal phalangeal (MCP) joint dislocation, 930
metal and metalloid poisoning
  arsenic, 632–633
  lead, 631–632, 631*t*, 632*t*
  mercury, 633–634, 634*t*
  miscellaneous metals, 634, 635*t*–636*t*
metal phosphides, 630*t*
metaphyseal fractures, 436
methanol, 557*t*, 581–583
methemoglobin, 557*t*
methemoglobinemia, 646–648, 646*t*, 647*t*
methicillin-resistant *Staphylococcus aureus* (MRSA), 491–492, 831
methimazole, for thyrotoxicosis, 714
methlenedioxymethamphetamine (Ecstasy), 588*t*
methohexital, for sedation, 70*t*, 72*t*
methotrexate, 557*t*
  in pregnancy, 333*t*
methotrexta, in pregnancy, 334*t*
methyldopa, for hypertension, 329, 330*t*
methylene blue
  as antidote, 559*t*
  for methemoglobinemia, 647
methylenedioxymethamphetamine (MDMA), 39
methylnatrexone, for constipation, 235
methylpredisolone
  for adrenal crisis, 754
  for adult epiglottitis, 846
  for airway emergencies, 992
  for anaphylaxis, 65
  for asthma, 384*t*
  for cardiac transplantation, 550
  for COPD and asthma, 215
  for epiglottitis, 375
  for HSCT, 554
  for ITP, 467
  for MS, 803
  for nausea and vomiting, 327
  for SCV syndrome, 752
  for stings, 658
  for temporal arthritis, 825
  for ulcerative colitis, 232
methylprednisolone
  for liver transplantation, 552
  for lung transplantation, 551
  for renal transplantation, 552
methylxanthine, 599*t*
metochlopramide
  for foodborne diseases, 528
  for waterborne diseases, 528
metoclopramide
  for acute abdominal pain, 221
  for GERD, 240
  for headache, 413, 762
  for nausea and vomiting, 223, 326, 1024
  for urologic stone disease, 314
metoprolol
  for atrial fibrillation, 20
  for hypertension, 179
  for STEMI, 135*t*
metronidazole
  for acute abdominal pain, 221
  for amebiasis, 545
  for ANUG, 840
  for bacterial vaginosis, 344
  for childhood leukemia, 462
  for cholecystis, 251
  for Crohn's disease, 230
  for diarrhea, 229
  for esophageal perforation, 241
  for lateral sinus thrombosis, 832
  for liver transplantation, 553
  for pancreatitis, 248
  for peri-implantitis, 840
  for PID, 348*t*
  for posttransplant infections, 548
  for STD prophylaxis, 1019
  for tetanus, 518
  for *Trichomonas* vaginitis, 345
  for trichomoniasis, 475
  for ulcerative colitis, 232
metroprolol, for low-probability ACS, 145
MG. *See* myasthenia gravis (MG)
MI. *See* myocardial infarction (MI)
miconazole
  for *Candida* vaginitis, 345
  for fungal infection, 448
microscopic polyangiitis, 990*t*
midazolam
  for agitation/delirium, 1024
  for intubation, 31*t*
  for palliative care, 1023
  for sedation, 69, 70*t*, 72*t*, 73*t*
  for seizures, 410, 411, 794
Middle East respiratory syndrome (MERS), 203
midfacial fractures, 895
midfoot injuries, 963, 965
migraine headaches, 761, 763*t*, 768*t*
Milch technique, 946
milk of magnesia, for constipation, 234
milrinone
  for cardiogenic shock, 140
  for congestive heart failure, 393
  for pulmonary hypertension, 180
miltefosine, for visceral leishmaniasis, 544
mineral oil
  for burns, 683
  for cerum impaction, 833
mineral oil enemas, for constipation, 234

mineral oil suppositories, for constipation, 235
mirtazapine, 568
misoprostol, for abortion, 326
missed abortion, 325
mitral regurgitation, 153*t*, 154–155
mitral stenosis, 152–154, 153*t*
mitral valve prolapse, 153*t*, 155
modified Hippocratic technique, 945
Modified Pediatric Glasgow Scale, 869, 869*t*
molluscum contagiosum, 861–862, 862*f*
monoamine oxidase inhibitors (MAOIs), 569–570
mood disorders, 1004–1005
morphine
  for acute abdominal pain, 220
  for acute heart failure, 151
  for acute pain control, 68
  for agitation/delirium, 1024
  for appendicitis, 255
  for cholecystis, 251
  for dyspnea, 1024
  for intubation, 31*t*
  for low-probability ACS, 144
  for pain management, 1023–1024
  for pancreatitis, 248
  for STEMI, 134*t*
  for trauma, 871
  for urologic stone disease, 314
morphine sulfate
  for angioedema, 133
  for cardiogenic shock, 140
  for hypercyanotic spells, 391
  for tetanus, 518
Morton neuroma, 1001
MS. *See* multiple sclerosis (MS)
multi-drug resistant (MDR) TB, 207
multifocal atrial tachycardia (MAT), 21, 21*f*
multiple sclerosis (MS), 802–803
mumps, 828
Munchausen syndrome by proxy, 1013–1014
mupirocin
  for bullous impetigo, 449
  for impetigo, 828
musculoskeletal causes, of chest pain, 129
musculoskeletal disorders, in children, 432–442
  childhood patterns of injury, 432–435
  fractures associated with child abuse, 435
  nontraumatic, 439
  pediatric injuries, 435–438
musculoskeletal disorders, nontraumatic
  acute disorders of joints and bursae, 983–987
  hip pain, 979–982
  knee pain, 979–982
  neck and back pain, 969–974
  shoulder pain, 975–978
mushroom poisoning, 695, 696*t*
myasthenia gravis, 801, 802*t*
Mycobacterium marinum, 527, 530*t*
myocardial infarction, 131–137, 132*t*
myocarditis, 161–162, 392–393
myodascial syndromes, 981
myonecrosis, 481
myscarinic effect, 564*t*
myxedema coma, 711–712

N
N-3-pyridylmethyl-N-p-nitrophenyl, 629*t*
N-acetylcysteine (NAC)
  for acetaminophen toxicity, 593, 596*t*
  for herbal toxicity, 645
nafcillin
  for cellulitis, 493
  for lateral sinus thrombosis, 832
  for TSS, 481
NaHCO3, for hyperkalemia, 45*t*
nail and nail bed injuries, 106–107, 107*f*
nail injuries, 106–107
naloxone
  for acute abdominal pain, 220
  for altered mental status, 416
  as antidote, 559*t*
  for clonidine toxicity, 611
  for opioid toxicity, 584
  for pediatric pulmonary resuscitation, 33*t*
naphazoline, 814*t*
naphazoline/pheniramine, for conjunctivitis, 815, 816
naproxen, for vaginal bleeding, 320
narcotic ingestion, 243
narrow complex tachycardias, 18–23
nasal emergencies, 834–837
nasal foreign bodies, 836
nasal fractures, 835
nasal lacerations, 98
nasal septal hematoma, 836
nasal suctioning, for bronchiolitis, 382
naso-orbito-ethmoid fractures, 894–895
National Domestic Violence Hotline, 1020*t*
nausea, 222–224
  as malignancy emergency, 756
  management of, 1024
  of pregnancy, 326–327
near drowning, 675–677
nebulized epinephrine, for bronchiolitis, 382
neck
  injuries, 897–902, 897*t*, 900*f*
  pain, 969–974, 970*t*, 971*t*
  zones of, 899*f*

neck and upper airway disorders
  adult epiglottitis, 846
  complications of airway devices, 849–850
  masses, 848, 848*t*
  odontogenic abscess, 847
  peritonsillar abscess, 845–846
  pharyngitis, 845
  posttonsillectomy bleeding, 848–849
  retropharyngeal abscess, 847
  tonsillitis, 845
necrotizing enterocolitis, 402
necrotizing soft tissue infections, 492–493
needle-stick injuries, 116–117
Neisseria gonorrhoeae, 369
neonatal acne, 452
neonatal problems, 361–365
  abdominal catastrophes, 364–365
  abdominal pain, 401–402
  abnormal movements, 362–363
  ALTE, 363
  breathing and crying, 362
  congenital adrenal hyperplasia, 365
  congenital heart disease, 365
  cyanosis, 365
  diaper rash, 364
  eye complaints, 364
  fever, 363
  inborn errors of metabolism, 365
  intestinal colic, 362
  jaundice, 363–364
  nonaccidental trauma, 365
  oral thrush, 364
  seizures, 362–363
  sepsis, 363
  weight gain, feeding, and stooling, 361–362
neonatal resuscitation, 35–36
neostigmine, for myasthenia gravis, 801
nephrolithiasis, 315*t*
nephrotic syndrome, 469–470
nephrotoxins, 288*t*
nerve entrapment, 979, 980*t*, 1000
neuroblastoma, 463–464
neurogenic shock, 886
neuroleptic malignant syndrome, 571*t*
neurologic emergencies, 993
neurologic injuries, 898
neurologic lesions. *See* acute peripheral neurological lesions
neurologic syncope, 147
neuromuscular junction disorders, 799
neurosurgical consultation, 884
neutropenia, 467
  See also febrile neutropenia
New Orleans criteria, 883*t*
NEXUS criteria, 889*t*
niacin, 643*t*
nicardipine
  for acute ischemic stroke, 179
  for acute pulmonary edema, 178
  for acute renal failure, 178
  for aortic dissection, 177
  for childhood hypertensive emergencies, 180
  for hypertension, 186
  for hypertensive encephalopathy, 178
  for intracranial hemorrhage, 179
  for stroke, 771–772
  for subarachnoid hemorrhage, 178–179
  for sympathetic crisis, 178
nicotine, 600–601, 601*t*
nifedipine
  for cold injuries, 649
  for HAPE, 672
  for hypertension, 329, 330*t*
nifurtimox, for Chagas disease, 544
nimodipine
  for stroke, 773
  for subarachnoid hemorrhage, 179
NIPPV. *See* noninvasive positive pressure ventilation (NIPPV)
nitrates, for mitral regurgitation, 155
nitric acid, 684*t*
nitrofurantoin
  for cystitis, 332
  for UTIs, 300, 301
nitrogen dioxide, 637*t*, 639
nitroglycerin
  for acute coronary syndromes, 178
  for acute heart failure, 150
  for acute pulmonary edema, 178
  for angina, 133
  for cardiogenic shock, 140
  for low-probability ACS, 144
  for STEMI, 134*t*
  for sympathetic crisis, 178
nitroprusside
  for acute heart failure, 150
  for aortic regurgitation, 157
  for childhood hypertensive emergencies, 180
  for drug abuse, 586, 587
  for hypertension, 186
  for MAOI toxicity, 570
nitrous oxide, for sedation, 69, 70*t*, 73*t*
nizatidine, for PUD, 245
nonaccidental trauma, 365
nonnarcotic large-artery aneurysms, 183*t*
nonbenzodiazepine sedatives, 577–578
noninvasive positive pressure ventilation (NIPPV), 2
  for COPD, 215
noninvasive ventilation, for asthma, 381
non-STEMI (NSTEMI), 131, 132–133, 137
nonsteroidal anti-inflammatory drugs (NSAIDs)
  for acute pain control, 67–68

adverse effects of, 68
for concussion, 841
for pelvic pain, 322
in pregnancy, 334*t*
for regional nerve entrapment syndromes, 979
toxicity, 595–597, 596*t*, 597*f*
for vaginal bleeding, 320
nontachycardiac irregular dysrhythmias, 10–12
premature atrial contractions, 10–11
premature atrial contractions (PACs), 11*f*
premature ventricular contractions, 11–12, 12*f*
for shoulder pain, 977
sinus arrhythmia, 10, 10*f*
nontraumatic cardiac tamponade, 165–166
norbormide, 630*t*
norepinephrine
for antidepressants, 566
for antihypertensive toxicity, 611
for antipsychotic toxicity, 572
for barbiturate overdose, 575
for β-blocker toxicity, 606
for calcium channel blocker toxicity, 608
for cardiogenic shock, 140
for clonidine toxicity, 611
for MAOI toxicity, 570
for pulmonary hypertension, 180
for sepsis, 358, 487
for shock, 63
for trazodone, 567
norethindrone, for vaginal bleeding, 320
normal saline (NS), 37
for AKI, 469
for anaphylaxis, 65
for bronchiolitis, 382
for dehydration, 398
for hypercalcemia, 50
for nephrotic syndrome, 470
for sepsis, 358
normovolemic hyponatremia, 39*t*
norovirus, 226
nose
See also facial injuries
lacerations to, 98
novel respiratory infections, 203
NSAIDs. *See* nonsteroidal anti-inflammatory drugs (NSAIDs)
NSTEMI. *See* non-STEMI (NSTEMI)
NTG. *See* nitroglycerin
nursemaid's elbow, 436
nutmeg, 644*t*
nystatin
for balanoposthitis, 308
for diaper rash, 453

O
octreotide
for gastrointestinal bleeding, 238
for hypoglycemia, 701
ocular ultrasonography, 825
odontogenic abscess, 847
OE. *See* otitis externa (OE)
ofloxacin, 815*t*
for chlamydial infection, 474
for corneal abrasion, 819
for corneal ulcer, 818
for otitis externa, 368, 831
for prostatitis, 308
olopatadine, 814*t*
omeprazole
for GERD, 240
for PUD, 245
ondansetron
for acute abdominal pain, 221
for acute mountain sickness, 670
for cholecystis, 251
for foodborne diseases, 528
for iron toxicity, 618
for nausea and vomiting, 223, 326, 1024
for nicotine toxicity, 601
for pancreatitis, 248
for vertigo, 788
for vomiting, 399
for waterborne diseases, 528
for xanthine toxicity, 599
onychocryptosis, 998
ophthalmic medications, 814*t*–815*t*
ophthalmic moisturizing ointment, 798
ophthalmologic emergencies, 993
ophthalmology consultation, 817, 821, 823
opiates
for acute pain control, 68
for palliative care, 1023
opioid analgesia, for corneal abrasion, 819
opioids, 584–585
for chemical ocular injury, 822
for chronic pain, 78
for SCD, 737
optic neuritis (ON), 824
oral anticoagulants, 745–747
oral calcium therapy, for hypocalcemia, 48
oral cancer, 841
oral candidiasis, 509
oral cavity, soft tissue lesions of, 840–841
oral intubation, for COPD, 215
oral rehydration solution (ORS), 398, 429
oral thrush, 364
oral trauma, 844
orbital blowout fractures, 821, 895
orchitis, 307

organophosphates, 605*t*, 626–628, 627*t*
orofacial pain, 838–840
orofacial trauma, 841–844
orogastric lavage (OG)
  for poisoning, 559
  for posttransplant infections, 560*t*, 561
orotracheal intubation, 4–7, 5*f*, 870
orthopedic injuries, 874–875, 963*t*
  See also fractures
  ankle, 961–962
  compartment syndrome, 966–967
  foot injuries, 963–965, 964*t*
  forearm and elbow, 934–941
  hand, 929–931
  hip dislocations, 954–955, 954*f*
  hip fractures, 951–953
  initial evaluation and management of, 923–928
  knee and leg, 956–960
  pelvic, 949–951
  shoulder and humerus, 942–948
  wrist, 931–933
orthostatic syncope, 146
oseltamivir, for influenza, 498
Osgood-Schlatter disease, 440
osteitis pubis, 982
osteoarthritis, 977, 986
osteomyelitis, 116, 981, 981*t*–982*t*
osteonecrosis, 981
osteosarcoma, 465
otitis externa, 368, 831
otitis media, 366–368, 831–832
  See also acute otitis media (AOM)
otologic emergencies
  acute mastoiditis, 832
  bullous myringitis, 832–833
  cerumen impaction, 833
  foreign bodies in ear, 833
  hearing loss, 834
  lateral sinus thrombosis, 832
  otitis externa, 831
  otitis media, 831–832
  tinnitus, 834
  trauma, 833
  tympanic membrane perforation, 833–834
ototoxicity, 787–788
Ottawa ankle rules, 962*f*
Ottawa knee rules, 957*t*
ovarian cysts, 321
ovarian torsion, 321
overuse injuries, 960
overuse syndrome, 934–935, 981
ovral, for emergency contraception, 1019
oxacillin, for TSS, 481
oxalic acid, 684*t*
oxcarbazepine, 616
oxiconazole, for fungal infection, 448
oxycodone/acetaminophen, for pelvic pain, 322
oxygen
  for acute heart failure, 150
  for acute mountain sickness, 670
  for altered mental status, 416
  for asthma, 380
  for bronchiolitis, 382
  for burns, 681
  for carbon monoxide poisoning, 693*t*
  for COPD, 214
  for HAPE, 671
  for headache, 413
  for low-probability ACS, 144
  for pneumothorax, 209
oxymetazoline
  for epistaxis, 834
  for nasal foreign bodies, 836
  for sinusitis, 837
oxytocin
  for postpartum care, 343
  for postpartum hemorrhage, 339

P

packed red blood cells (PRBCs), 739–740
  for anemia, 720
  for trauma, 871, 875
PACs. *See* premature atrial contractions (PACs)
pain
  acute abdominal, 217–221, 218*f*, 220*t*, 400–404
  back, 969–974
  chronic, 77–80
  control of acute, 67–68, 123
  hip, 979–982, 979*t*
  knee, 979–982, 979*t*
  management of, 1023–1024
  neck, 969–974, 970*t*
  orofacial, 838–840
  pelvic, 321–322
  postextraction, 839–840
  responses to, 67
  shoulder, 975–978
pain crises, 455–456
palliative care, 1021–1023, 1022*t*, 1023*t*
palm lacerations, 104–105
pamidronate, for hypercalcemia, 753
pancoast tumor, 977
pancreatitis, 247–248, 284
panic disorder, 1010–1011, 1010*t*
pantoprazole
  for gastrointestinal bleeding, 238
  for PUD, 245
paralytics, for intubation, 31*t*
paraphimosis, 309*f*, 310
paraquat, 557*t*
Parkinson's disease, 803–804
paronychia, 995, 996*t*
paroxysmal supraventricular tachycardia (PSVT), 21–23, 22*f*
partial seizures, 792, 793

patellar dislocations, 438, 958
patellar tendonitis, 960
pathologic fractures, 751
patiromer, for hyperkalemia, 45*t*
PCEV. *See* purified chick embryo cell culture vaccine (PCEV)
PCI. *See* percutaneous coronary intervention (PCI)
pediatric abdominal emergencies, 400–406
pediatric cardiopulmonary resuscitation, 29–35
  defibrillation and cardioversion, 34–35
  drugs, 32, 33*t*, 34
  dysrhythmias, 34
  fluids, 32
  rapid sequence intubation, 29, 30*t*–31*t*, 31
  securing airway, 29
  vascular access, 32
pediatric heart disease, 388–394
pediatric rheumatologic disorders, 439–442
pediatric trauma center, transfer to, 872*t*
pediatric urinary tract infections, 407–408
pelvic fractures, 951*f*
pelvic inflammatory disease (PID), 347–349, 348*t*, 349*t*
pelvic injuries, 949–951
pelvic pain, 321–322
pemphigus vulgaris, 854–855, 854*f*
penetrating buttock trauma, 915
penetrating cardiac injuries, 906
penetrating flank trauma, 914
penicillin
  for acute rheumatic fever, 441
  for animal bites, 118
penicillin G
  for cellulitis, 451
  for leptospirosis, 543
penicillin G bezathine, for STD prophylaxis, 1019
penicillin V
  for scarlet fever, 451
  for stomatitis, 370
penicillin VK
  for acute rheumatic fever, 441
  for odontogenic abscess, 847
  for pericoronitis, 839
  for periodontal abscess, 840
  for peritonsillar abscess, 846
penile entrapment, 310
penile fracture, 310
penis, 308–310
penis injuries, 918–919
pennyroyal, 644*t*
pentamidine
  for African sleeping sickness, 544
  for posttransplant infections, 549
pentobarbital
  for sedation, 70*t*
  for seizures, 794
  for xanthine toxicity, 599
pentoxifyline, for cold injuries, 649
peptic ulcer, 128*t*
peptic ulcer disease (PUD), 244–246
peramivir, for influenza, 498
percutaneous endoscopic gastrostomy, 285
percutaneous nephrostomy, complications of, 317
perforated peptic ulcer, 128*t*
perforation. *See* esophageal perforation
pericarditis, 128*t*, 393, 907
  See also acute pericardial tamponade
  acute, 164–165
  constrictive, 166
pericoronitis, 838–839
peri-implantitis, 840
perilunate and lunate dislocations, 931–932
perilymph fistula, 787
periodontal abscess, 840
perionychium, 106*f*
periorbital anatomy, 97*f*
peripheral nerves
  motor testing of, 101*t*
  sensory testing of, 101*t*
peripheral neurologic lesions. *See* acute peripheral neurological lesions
peripheral vertigo, 784, 784*t*, 787–788
peritoneal dialysis, 298
peritonsillar abscess, 377–378, 845–846
permethrin
  for lice, 452
  for scabies, 452
personality disorders, 1005
pesticides, 626–630, 626*t*, 627*t*, 628*t*, 629*t*, 630*t*
petit mal seizures, 792
peyronie disease, 310
phantom limb pain, 77*t*
pharyngeal injuries, 898
pharyngitis, 369–371, 845
phenazopyridine, for UTIs, 301
phencyclidine (angel dust), 589*t*
pheniramine, 814*t*
phenobarbital, 557*t*
  for antidepressants, 566
  for bupropion toxicity, 567
  for drug abuse, 586
  for lithium toxicity, 573
  for seizures, 410, 794
  for xanthine toxicity, 599
phenol, 683*t*
phentolamine
  for childhood hypertensive emergencies, 180
  for drug abuse, 586, 587
  for MAOI toxicity, 570
  for sympathetic crisis, 178

phenylephrine
for antipsychotic toxicity, 572
for epistaxis, 834
for sinusitis, 837
phenytoin, 557*t*
for seizures, 794
toxicity, 613–614, 613*t*, 614*t*
for xanthine toxicity, 599
pheumothorax, 128*t*
Philadelphia Protocol, 355*t*
phimosis, 309, 309*f*
phlebotomy, for hyperviscosity syndrome, 756
phlegmasia alba dolens, 167
phlegmasia cerulea dolens, 167, 174
phosgene, 637*t*, 638
phosphodiesterase-5 inhibitors, for pulmonary hypertension, 180
photosensitivity, 860
physical abuse, of child, 1013–1014
physostigmine, for anticholinergic toxicity, 565
PID. *See* pelvic inflammatory disease (PID)
pilocarpine, for glaucoma, 823
pilonidal abscess, 495
pilonidal sinus, 271–272
pinworm, 545
PIP. *See* proximal interphalangeal joint dislocation
piperacillin, for malignant otitis externa, 831
piperacillin/tazobactam
for acute abdominal pain, 221
for appendicitis, 255
for buttock trauma, 915
for childhood leukemia, 462
for Crohn's disease, 230
for flank trauma, 914
for hernia, 264
for intestinal obstruction, 261
for liver transplantation, 553
for neck and back pain, 973
for necrotizing soft tissue infections, 492
for peritonsillar abscess, 846
for pneumonia, 202, 203, 548
for posttransplant infections, 548
for prostatitis, 308
for sepsis, 358
for STSS, 483
for tracheostmy site infection, 849
for ulcerative colitis, 232
for urologic stone disease, 314
for UTIs, 301
piperonyl butoxide/pyrethrum, for lice, 452
PIP joint dislocation, 930
PIRA. *See* postinfectious reactive arthritis (PIRA)
Pittsburgh knee rules, 956, 957*f*
pit viper bites, 663–664
pityriasis rosea, 858*t*
pityriasis versicolor, 858*t*
placental abruption, 337
placenta previa, 337–338
plague, 538–539
plantar fasciitis, 999–1000
plantar interdigital neuroma, 1001
plantar puncture wounds, 122*t*
plantar warts, 998
plant poisoning, 697, 697*t*–699*t*
plasmapheresis
for Guillain-Barré syndrome, 797
for hyperviscosity syndrome, 756
plastic deformities, 434–435
platelet disorders, 726
platelets, 740
See also acquired platelet defects
platelet transfusion, 740
for DIC, 727
for ITP, 467
for renal disease, 727
pleural effusion, 198
plexopathies, 798–799
pneumomediastrinum injuries, 905
pneumonia, 127*t*, 128*t*, 200–203, 201*f*
with HIV/AIDS, 508
in infants and children, 385–387, 385*t*, 387*t*
posttransplant, 548
pneumothorax
iatrogenic, 210
spontaneous, 129, 208–210
poisoning, 555–563, 557*t*, 558*t*
See also toxicity
alcohol, 580–583
antidotes, 558*t*–559*t*
arsenic, 632–633
carbon monoxide, 692–694, 692*t*, 693*t*, 694*t*
common toxidromes, 556*t*
enhanced elimination procedures, 561*t*–562*t*
extracorporeal removal techniques, 562*t*–563*t*
gastrointestinal decontamination procedure, 560*t*
iron, 617–620
lead, 631–632
lead poisoning, 631*t*, 632*t*
mercury, 633–634, 634*t*
mushroom, 695, 696*t*
organophosphates, 626–628, 627*t*
plants, 697, 697*t*–699*t*
poliomyelitis, 804–805
polioviruses, 443
polyarteritis nodosa, 990*t*
polyethylene glycol
for constipation, 234
for drug abuse, 586

for iron toxicity, 618
for poisoning, 561
polymyositis, 989*t*
polysaccharides, 747
polyvalent Crotalidae Immune Fab (FabAV), for snake bites, 664
poperacillin/tazobactam, for esophageal perforation, 241
Portland cement, 684*t*
positive end-expiratory pressure (PEEP), 2
postconization bleeding, 351
postembolization syndrome, 352
postextraction alveolar osteitis (dry socket), 839–840
postextraction bleeding, 840
postextraction pain, 839–840
postherapeutic neuralgia, 77*t*
postictal paralysis, 768*t*
post-infectious reactive arthritis (PIRA), 441
postoperative complications, 282–285, 351
postpartum care, 343
postpartum endometritis, 339
postpartum hemorrhage, 338–339
postpolio syndrome, 804–805
postrenal azotemia, 288
postrenal failure, 290–291
postrepair wound care, 121–124
postseptal (orbital) cellulitis, 813
postseptal hemorrhage, 820
poststroke pain, 77*t*
posttonsillectomy bleeding, 848–849
posttransplant infections, 546, 546*t*–547*t*, 548–549
potassium, for aspirin toxicity, 592
potassium-sparing diuretics, 611
prasugrel, for STEMI, 134*t*
praziquantel
for cysticercosis, 544
for schistosomiasis, 545
for tapeworm, 545
prednisolone
for asthma, 380
for ulcerative colitis, 232
prednisolone acetate, 815*t*
for blunt eye trauma, 821
for HZO, 817
prednisone
for acute rheumatic fever, 441
for asthma, 332, 380, 384*t*
for Bell's palsy, 797
for COPD and asthma, 215
for Crohn's disease, 230
for EM, 852
for headache, 762
for HSCT, 554
for HSP, 453
for hypercalcemia, 51
for stings, 658
for temporal arthritis, 825
for thrombocytopenia, 726
for ulcerative colitis, 232
preeclampsia, 177*t*, 178, 336
pregabalin, 79, 616
pregnancy
See also labor and delivery
amniotic fluid embolism in, 339
appendicitis in, 255
asthma in, 332
chest pain in, 335
comorbid diseases in, 328–334
cystitis in, 332
diabetes in, 328
diagnostic imaging in, 334
dysrhythmias in, 329
eclampsia in, 336–337, 793
ectopic, 323–325
emergencies in, 335–339
headaches in, 332
HELLP syndrome, 336
hypertension in, 328–329, 330*t*, 335
hyperthyroidism in, 328, 329*t*
for ITP, 466
medications in, 333, 333*t*, 334*t*
nausea and vomiting during, 222–223, 326–327
preeclampsia in, 336
preterm labor, 338
pyelonephritis in, 332
seizure disorders in, 333, 793
sickle cell disease in, 332
substance abuse in, 333
threatened abortion and abortion, 325–326
thromboembolic disease of, 335
thromboembolism in, 330, 331*t*
trauma in, 877–879
vaginal bleeding in, 337–338
premature atrial contractions (PACs), 10–11, 11*f*
premature rupture of membranes (PROM), 338
premature ventricular contractions, 11–12, 12*f*
prerenal failure, 290
preseptal (periorbital) cellulitis, 813
preterminal rhythms, 27
preterm labor, 338
priapism, 310, 458
PRICE, 961
primaquine, for posttransplant infections, 549
primaquine phosphate, for malaria, 525*t*
procainamide
for atrial fibrillation, 20
for MAOI toxicity, 570
for paroxysmal supraventricular tachycardia, 23
for WPW syndrome, 26

procedural sedation and analgesia (PSA), 67, 68–73
in children, 71
in elderly, 71
medications for, 72*t*–73*t*
preparation for, 68–69
sedation agents, 69, 70*t*, 71
sedation management, 69
prochlorperazine
for cholecystis, 251
for headache, 413, 762
for nausea and vomiting, 223
for pancreatitis, 248
proctitis, 268–270
PROM. *See* premature rupture of membranes (PROM)
promethazine
for iron toxicity, 618
for nausea and vomiting, 223, 326
proparacaine, 814*t*
for corneal abrasion, 819
for corneal foreign bodies, 819–820
prophylactic antibiotics
for postrepair wound care, 121, 122*t*
for puncture wounds, 116
for wounds, 84
propofol
for drug abuse, 586
for intubation, 6, 31*t*
for sedation, 70*t*, 71, 72*t*, 73*t*
for seizures, 411, 794
propranolol
for sedative overdose, 578
for thyrotoxicosis, 714
propylene glycol, for constipation, 1024
propylthiouracil (PTU), for hyperthyroidism, 328
prostagladnin E1, for cardiovascular shock, 391
prostanoids, for pulmonary hypertension, 180
prostatitis, 308
prosthetic valve disease, 158–159
protamine, for vascular access complications, 298
protective eye shield, 821
prothrombin complex concentrate (PCC), 742
proximal and middle phalanx fractures, 931
pruritus ani, 271
pryridostigmine, for myasthenia gravis, 801
pseudocoma, 778
pseudojyperkalemia, 44*t*
Pseudomonas aeruginosa, 530*t*
psilocybin, 588*t*
psoas abscess, 979
psoriasis, 858*t*
PSVT. *See* paroxysmal supraventricular tachycardia (PSVT)
psychiatric disorder, 775*t*
psychogenic coma, 778
psychopharmacologic agents
antipsychotics, 570–572
atypical antidepressants, 567
bupropion, 567
cyclic antidepressants, 566
lithium, 572–573
MAOIs, 569–570
mirtazapine, 568
serotonin reuptake inhibitors, 567
SNRIs, 568–569
SSRIs, 568
traza, 567
psychosocial disorders
behavioral disorders, 1003–1009
conversion disorder, 1011–1012
panic disorder, 1010–1011
psychotic disorders, 1004
psyllium
for constipation, 234
for ulcerative colitis, 232
PTU, for thyrotoxicosis, 714
public lice, 662
PUD. *See* peptic ulcer disease (PUD)
pulmonary contusions, 904
pulmonary edema, 149
pulmonary embolism (PE), 127–128, 127*t*, 128*t*, 167–168, 172*f*
antithrombotic therapy for, 173*t*
in pregnancy, 330, 331*t*, 335
rule-out criteria rule, 168*t*, 171*f*
Wells' Score for, 168, 169*t*
Pulmonary Embolism Rule-Out Criteria (PERC) rule, 168, 171*f*
pulmonary emergencies, 992–993
pulmonary hypertension, 180
pulpitis, 839
pulseless electrical activity, 27
puncture wounds, 115–116
indications for imaging in, 115*t*
plantar, 122*t*
PVCs. *See* premature atrial contractions (PACs)
pyelonephritis, in pregnancy, 332
pyloric stenosis, 402
pyrantel pamoate
for enterobiasis, 545
for hookworm, 545
pyrazinamide, for TB, 207
pyridoxine
as antidote, 559*t*
for methanol poisoning, 583
for TB, 207
toxicity, 643*t*
pyrimethamine, for posttransplant infections, 549

Q
qualitative platelet disorders, 726
quantitative platelet disorders, 726
quinidine gluconate, for malaria, 526*t*
quinine sulfate, for malaria, 525*t*

R
rabeprazole, for PUD, 245
rabies, 518–522, 519*t*, 521*t*
rabies vaccine, 521–522
racemic epinephrine
  for epiglottitis, 374
  for viral croup, 372
radial head subluxation, 436
radial nerves, 935*t*
radial styloid fractures, 932, 933*t*
radiographs, 910
ramelteon, 578
ranitidine
  for anaphylaxis, 65
  for GERD, 240
  for PUD, 245
Rape, Abuse, and Incest National Network, 1020*t*
rapid airway assessment, 1
rapid sequence intubation (RSI), 4
  of children, 29, 30*t*–31*t*, 31
rashes, heat, 655
rashes, in children, 443–454
  bacterial infections, 448–451
  common neonatal, 452–453
  diaper, 364, 452–453
  fungal infections, 448
  other etiologies, 453–454
  scabies, 451–452
  viral infections, 443–447
raxibacumab, for anthrax, 538
reactivation TB, 204–205
recombinant tissue plasminogen activator (rtPA), 772
recompression therapy, 674
rectal foreign bodies, 270–271
rectal prolapse, 270
rectal surgery, 285
red blood cell infusion, for ACS, 136
red squill, 630*t*
reducing agents, 684*t*
regional anesthesia, 74–76
regional blocks, 74–75
regional nerve entrapment syndromes, 979, 980*t*
regurgitation, 361
rehydration, for SCD, 737
Reiter's syndrome, 986
relapsing polychondritis, 990*t*
renal disease
  See also end-stage renal disease (ESRD)
  bleeding in, 727
renal emergencies, 993
renal emergencies, in infants and children
  acute glomerulonephritis, 470–471
  acute kidney injury, 468–469, 468*t*
  hemolytic-uremic syndrome, 471–472
  nephrotic syndrome, 469–470
renal failure, 287–291, 288*t*
  See also acute renal failure
  cardiovascular complications, 296
  emergencies in, 296–298
  gastrointestinal complications, 297
  hematologic complications, 297
  neurologic complications, 296–297
renal hypovolemic hyponatremia, 39*t*
renal stones, 312–315, 313*t*
renal transplant, 551–552
replacement factor products
  See also factor replacement
  for hemophilia, 730, 730*t*
respiratory acidosis, 58–59
respiratory alkalosis, 59
respiratory complications, postoperative, 282
respiratory distress, 191–198
  cough, 195, 196*f*
  cyanosis, 197, 197*t*
  dyspnea, 191–192
  hiccups, 196–197
  hypercapnia, 194
  hypoxemia, 192–193
  hypoxia, 192–193
  pleural effusion, 198
  wheezing, 194–195
respiratory infections, 203
respiratory toxins, 637–638, 637*t*
restrictive cardiomyopathy, 164
resuscitation
  neonatal, 35–36
  pediatric cardiopulmonary, 29–35
  poisoning and, 557
reteplase
  for ACS, 135
  for STEMI, 134*t*
retinal detachment, 825
retinal floaters, 825
retinoblastoma, 464–465, 464*f*
retroglottic, dual-balloon devices, 2
retroperitoneal injuries, 909–910
retropharyngeal abscess, 377, 847
Reye syndrome, 68
Rh (D) immune globulin, 338, 352
rhabdomyolysis, 292–295, 292*t*, 293*t*
rhabdomyosarcoma, 465
rheumatic diseases. *See* systemic rheumatic disease emergencies
rheumatoid arthritis, 986–987, 990*t*
rhinosinusitis, 836–837
ribavirin, for Crimean-Congo hemorrhagic fever, 543
riboflavin, 643*t*
rickettsial spotted fevers, 542–543

Rickettsia rickettsii, 532*t*
rifampin
for brucellosis, 542
for cat-scratch disease, 119
for ehrlichiosis, 536
for meningococcemia, 451
for TB, 207
rifampin plus ethambutol, 668
rifaximin, for Crohn's disease, 230
right heart failure, 149
right-sided valvular heart disease, 157–158
Ringer lactate, for chemical ocular injury, 822
ring tourniquet syndrome, 107
rivaroxaban, 747
for venous thromboembolism, 173, 173*t*
Rochester criteria, 355*t*
Rocky Mountain spotted fever (RMSF), 532, 533*t*, 534
rocuronium, for intubation, 6, 31*t*
rodent bites, 120
rodenticides, 629, 629*t*–630*t*
Romberg test, 781
roseola infactum, 447, 447*f*
rotator cuff tears, 976–977
rotator cuff tendonitis, 976
RSI. *See* rapid sequence intubation (RSI)
rt-PA. *See* recombinant tissue plasminogen activator (rtPA)
rubella, 444
rufinamide, 616
rule of 6s, 32
Rule of Nines, 678, 678*f*
Rumack-Matthew nomogram, 594*f*
Rutherford Criteria for acute limb ischemia, 188, 189*t*

S
sacral fracture, 950*t*
SAH. *See* subarachnoid hemorrhage (SAH)
salbutamol, for asthma, 383*t*
salicylates, 557*t*
toxicity, 591–592, 591*t*
saline boluses, for congenital adrenal hyperplasia, 423
saline drops, for bronchiolitis, 382
salivary gland disorders, 828–829
salmonella, 396*t*
Salmonella, 527
Salmonella enterica, 532*t*
Salter-Harris fracture, 926*t*
classification of, 926*f*
type I, 433, 438
type II, 432*f*, 434, 438
type III, 433*f*, 434, 438
type IV, 434
type V, 434
SA node. *See* sinoatrial node
SARS. *See* severe acute respiratory syndrome (SARS)
SBI. *See* serious bacterial illness (SBI)
SCA. *See* sickle cell anemia
scabies, 451–452, 661, 859*t*
scalp, layers of, 96*f*
scalp lacerations, 96–97
scapholunate dissociation, 931
scapula fracture, 942–943
scapular manipulation technique, 945–946
scarlet fever, 450–451, 450*f*
SCD. *See* sickle cell disease (SCD)
SCFE. *See* slipped capital femoral epiphysis (SCFE)
schistosomiasis, 544–545
schizophrenia, 1004
SCIs. *See* spinal cord injuries (SCIs)
scleroderma, 991*t*
scorpions, 661
scrotal abscesses, 308
scrotum, 308
injuries to, 918
seaworm, 545
seborrheic dermatitis, 452, 858*t*
secondary syphilis, 859*t*, 860–861, 861*f*
second-degree Mobitz I (Wenckebach) AV block, 15–16, 15*f*
second-degree Mobitz II AV block, 16–17, 16*f*
second-generation anticonvulsants, 616
sedation
agents, 69–71, 70*t*
levels of, 68*t*
procedural sedation and analgesia, 68–73
sedatives, 574–579
for intubation, 31*t*
seizures, 768*t*
absence, 792
in adults, 792–795
in children, 409–411, 410*t*
common causes of, 792*t*
generalized, 792
guidelines for management of, 795*f*
in neonates, 362–363
partial, 792, 793
in pregnancy, 333, 793
status epilepticus and, 792–795
tonic-clonic, 792
selective-serotonin reuptake inhibitors (SSRIs), 568
selenium sulfide
for fungal infection, 448
for tinea infection, 859
senna, for constipation, 1024
sepsis, 358, 363, 484–490, 486*t*, 487*t*–489*t*
sickle cell anemia and, 459–460
septic abortion, 325
septic arthritis, 985, 985*t*
septic pelvic thrombophlebitis, 351

serious bacterial illness (SBI), 353–357, 355*t*
serotonin-norepinephrine reuptake inhibitors (SNRIs), 568–569
serotonin reuptake inhibitors, 567
serotonin syndrome, 567, 569
serum markers, for acute myocardial infarction, 127
severe acute respiratory syndrome (SARS), 203
sexual abuse, 1014
sexual assault, 1016–1019, 1016*t*
sexually transmitted infections (STIs)
  chancroid, 478–479, 479*f*
  chlamydial infection, 473–474
  general recommendations, 473
  gonococcal infection, 474–475
  herpes simplex infection, 477–478, 477*f*
  prophylaxis, 1019
  syphilis, 475–477, 476*f*
  trichomoniasis, 475
sharp objects, ingestion of, 243
shigella, 396*t*
shingles, 500–501, 856–857, 856*f*
shock, 32, 60–63
  See also hypotensive patient
  cardiogenic, 138–140, 149
  cardiovascular, 388*t*, 389–391
  clinical features, 60–61
  diagnosis and differential, 61–62
  emergency department care and disposition, 62–63
  hypovolemic, 429
  medications and, 63
  neurogenic, 886
  spinal, 886
short-acting β-adrenergic agonists (SABAs), for COPD and asthma, 214–215
shoulder
  anatomy, 975*f*, 976*f*
  injuries, 942–948
  pain, 975–978
shoulder dystocia, 343
SIADH. *See* syndrome of inappropriate anti-diuretic hormone (SIADH)
sialolithiasis, 828
sickle cell anemia, in children
  acute central nervous system events, 457–458
  acute chest syndrome, 456–457
  acute sequestration crises, 458–459
  aplastic episodes, 459
  in children, 455–460
  hematological crises, 458–459
  hemolytic crises, 459
  infections, 459–460
  pain crises, 455–456
  priapism, 458
  variants of, 460
  vasoocclusive crises, 455–456
sickle cell β-thalassemia, 460
sickle cell disease (SCD), 734–737
  in pregnancy, 332
  variants of, 737–738
sickle cell-hemoglobin C disease, 460
sickle cell trait, 460
sickle trait, 734
sick sinus syndrome, 15
sigmoid volvulus, 260*f*
silver, 636*t*
silver nitrate
  for epistaxis, 834
  for postectraction bleeding, 840
  for tracheostmy site bleeding, 849
simple interrupted percutaneous sutures, 85–86, 86*f*
simple seizures, 793
sinus arrhythmia, 10, 10*f*
sinus bradycardia, 12–13
sinusitis, 836–837
  acute bacterial, 368–369
sinus tachycardia, 18
siphonaptera, 662
Sjögren's syndrome, 991*t*
skin disorders. *See* dermatologic disorders; dermatologic emergencie
skull fractures, 881
sleeping, neonates, 362–363
slipped capital femoral epiphysis (SCFE), 437
SLUDGE effects, 626, 626*t*
small bowel obstruction (SBO), 259
Smith fractures, 932
smoking-related cough, 195
snake bites, 663–665
snowbird technique, 945
SNRIs. *See* serotonin/norepinephrine reuptake inhibitors (SNRIs)
sodium bicarbonate
  for AKA, 710
  for anticholinergic toxicity, 565
  for antidepressants, 566
  as antidote, 559*t*
  for antipsychotic toxicity, 572
  for aspirin toxicity, 592
  for cerum impaction, 833
  for methanol poisoning, 583
  for neonate resuscitation, 36
  for pediatric pulmonary resuscitation, 33*t*, 34
  for shock, 63
  for SNRI toxicity, 569
  for SSRI toxicity, 568
sodium chloride, for seizures, 411
sodium fluroacetate, 629*t*

sodium nitroprusside
for acute ischemic stroke, 179
for acute pulmonary edema, 178
for aortic dissection, 177
for cardiogenic shock, 140
for great vessel injuries, 907
sodium polystyrene sulfonate
for hyperkalemia, 45*t*
for lithium toxicity, 573
sodium stibogluconate, for visceral leishmaniasis, 544
soft tissues
of foot, problems with, 998–1002
foreign bodies in, 112–114
imaging modalities for detection of, 113*t*
removal of, 113–114
infections of
CA-MRSA, 491–492
cellulitis, 493
cutaneous abscesses, 494–495
erysipelas, 493–494
necrotizing, 492–493
sporotrichosis, 495–496
injuries to, 934–935
oral cavity lesions, 840–841
trauma, 844
solid organ injuries, 909
sorbitol
for cardiovascular complications, 296
for constipation, 234
speech devices, 850
spider bites, 659–660
spinal cord compression, 751, 752*t*
spinal cord syndromes, 888*t*
spinal infections, 806–811
spinal shock, 886
spine injuries, 884, 890*t*
in children, 870
spine trauma, 886–891, 887*f*
splinters, removal of, 114
spontaneous pneumothorax, 129, 208–210
sporotrichosis, 495–496
Spurling's sign, 971*t*
SSRIs. *See* selective-serotonin reuptake inhibitors (SSRIs)
staphylococcal toxic shock syndrome (TSS), 480–483, 480*t*
staples, 91, 93*f*
status epilepticus, 409–411, 795*f*
See also seizures
in adults, 792–795
ST-elevation myocardial infarction (STEMI), 131–137, 132*t*, 134*t*–135*t*
stenosis. *See* aortic stenosis; mitral stenosis
sternoclavicular sprains and dislocations, 942
steroid injection, for bursitis, 980
steroids, for Bell's palsy, 829
Stevens-Johnson syndrome, 851–852
Stimson technique, 945
stinging ants, 658–659
stings. *See* bites and stings
STIs. *See* sexually transmitted infections (STIs)
St. John's wort, 644*t*
stomatitis, 369–371
stool, in infants, 361–362
straight leg test, 971*t*
strangulation, 898
streptococcal toxic shock syndrome (STSS), 481, 481–483, 482*t*
Streptococcus iniae cellulitis, 532*t*
streptokinase
for ACS, 136
for STEMI, 134*t*
streptomycin
for brucellosis, 542
for plague, 539
for tularemia, 537
stretomycin, in pregnancy, 334*t*
stroke, 765–774
ABCD scoring system, 773–774, 773*t*
acute ischemic, 177*t*, 179
classification of, 766*t*
hemorrhagic intracerebral, 765, 766*t*
ischemic, 765
acute, 769*t*–770*t*, 771*t*
ischemic stroke, 766*t*
mimics, 768*t*
strychnine, 629*t*
STSS. *See* streptococcal toxic shock syndrome (STSS)
stye, 813–814
subacromial bursitis, 976
subarachnoid hemorrhage (SAH), 177*t*, 178–179, 765, 768*t*, 881
subdural hematoma, 760, 768*t*, 882
substance abuse, 1004
in pregnancy, 333
succimer
for arsenic poisoning, 633
for mercury poisoning, 634
succinylcholine, for intubation, 6, 31*t*
sudden death, in children and adolescents, 417–419
suldadiazine, for posttransplant infections, 549
sulfacetamide sodium, 814*t*
sulfasalazine, for Crohn's disease, 230
sulfonamides, in pregnancy, 334*t*
sumatriptan, for headache, 413, 762
sunburn, 860
sundowning, 775
superior vena cava (SVC) syndrome, 752
suppurative parotitis, 826*t*, 828
supracondylar fractures, 435, 938–939, 939*t*

supraglottic devices, 2
supraglottitis, 846
supraventricular tachycardia (SVT), 21–23, 22*f*, 34
surgical airway, 7–8, 8*f*, 9*f*
surgical complications, 282–285
  acute complications arising from stomas, 285
  bariatric surgery, 285
  breast surgery, 284
  colonoscopy, 285
  drug therapy, 283
  fever, 282
  gastrointestinal surgery, 284–285
  genitourinary complications, 282
  laparoscopic procedures, 285
  percutaneous endoscopic gastrostomy, 285
  rectal surgery, 285
  respiratory complications, 282
  specific considerations, 284–285
  tetanus, 285
  transabdominal feeding tubes, 285
  vascular, 283
  wounds, 282–283
Surgicel, 840
sutures, 85–91, 86*f*, 87*f*, 88*f*, 89*f*, 90*f*, 91*f*, 92*f*
SVT. *See* supraventricular tachycardia (SVT)
swallowed foreign bodies, 241–242
sympathetic crisis, 177*t*, 178
sympatholytics, 609*t*
symptom management
  agitation, 1024
  constipation, 1024
  delirium, 1024
  dyspnea, 1024
  nausea and vomiting, 1024
  pain crises, 1023–1024
synchronized cardioversion, 34
syncope, 146–148, 388*t*, 417–419, 418*t*, 419*t*, 768*t*
syndrome of inappropriate anti-diuretic hormone (SIADH), 39, 39*t*, 753
synovial fluid, 984*t*
synthetic cannabinoids, 589*t*
synthetic cathinone derivatives (bath salts), 589*t*
syphilis, 475–477, 476*f*
systemic arterial hypotension, 60
systemic β-agonists, for asthma, 380
systemic corticosteroids, for asthma, 380
systemic hypertension, 175–179
systemic lupus erythematosus, 991*t*
systemic rheumatic disease emergencies, 988*t*–992*t*
  adverse drug reactions, 994
  airway, 992
  cardiovascular, 993
  gastrointestinal, 993
  infectious, 994
  neurologic, 993
  ophthalmologic, 993
  pulmonary, 992–993
  renal, 993
systemic sclerosis, 991*t*

T

tachy-brady syndrome, 15
tachycardias
  multifocal atrial, 21, 21*f*
  narrow complex, 18–23
  paroxysmal supraventricular, 21–23, 22*f*
  sinus, 18
  supraventricular, 34
  ventricular, 23–24, 23*f*, 24*f*
  wide complex, 23–25
tachypnea, 385*t*
Takayasu's arteritis, 992*t*
tamponade, 752
tamsulosin, for urologic stone disease, 314
tapeworm, 545
tarantulas, 660
tarsal tunnel syndrome, 1000
tasimelteon, 578
TB. *See* tuberculosis (TB)
TBI. *See* traumatic brain injury (TBI)
TB-specific nucleic acid amplification tests (NAATs), 206
temporal arteritis, 761, 761*t*, 989*t*
temporal arteritis (TA), 825
temporomandibular joint dysfunction, 829
TEN. *See* toxic epidermal necrolysis (TEN)
tendinitis, 1000
tendon injuries, 929, 959–960
tendonitis, 998
tendon lacerations, 1001
tendon lesions, 1000–1001
tendon ruptures, 1001
tenecteplase
  for ACS, 136
  for STEMI, 134*t*
tennis elbow, 934–935
tenosynovitis, 1000
terazosin, for urologic stone disease, 314
terbinafine
  for fungal infection, 448
  for tinea infection, 859
terbutaline
  for asthma, 380
  for COPD and asthma, 215
terbutaline sulfate, for asthma, 332
terconazole, for *Candida* vaginitis, 345
tervinafine, for tinea infection, 859
testicular injuries, 918
testicular torsion, 306–307
tetanus, 285, 517–518
tetanus immune globulin, 518

tetanus immunization, 113
tetanus prophylaxis, 122, 122*t*, 878
tetanus toxoid, 518
tetanus vaccination, 529
tetracaine, 814*t*
tetracycline
  in pregnancy, 334*t*
  for syphilis, 477
tetratology of Fallot, 390, 392*t*
tet spells, 390
thalassemias, 737–738
thalidomide, in pregnancy, 334*t*
thallium, 630*t*, 636*t*
theophylline, 557*t*
thermal burns, 678–682, 678*f*, 679*f*, 680*t*–681*t*
thiamine
  for AKA, 710
  as antidote, 559*t*
  for ataxia, 783
  for ethanol overdose, 580
  for methanol poisoning, 583
  toxicity, 643*t*
thiazides, 608
third-degree (complete) AV block, 17, 17*f*
Thompson test, 110*f*
thoracic duct injuries, 907
threatened abortion, 325–326
thrombin, for vascular access complications, 298
thrombocytopenia, 462
thromboembolectomy, 174
thromboembolic disease of pregnancy, 335
thromboembolism
  as malignancy emergency, 756
  in pregnancy, 330, 331*t*
Thrombosis in Myocardial Infarction (TIMI) risk score, 130
thromolytic therapy, for venous thromboembolism, 173–174, 173*t*
thumb
  joint dislocation
    IP, 930
    MCP, 930
  MCP ulnar collateral ligament rupture, 931
thunderclap headache, 760*t*
thyroid disease emergencies
  hypothyroidism, 711–712, 711*f*
  myxedema coma, 711–712
  thyroid storm, 712–714
  thyrotoxicosis, 712–714, 713*t*
thyroid storm, 328, 329*t*, 712–714
thyrotoxicosis, 712–714, 713*t*
tiagabine, 616
tibia fractures, 438
ticagrelor, for STEMI, 134*t*
ticarcillin-clavulanic acid, for urologic stone disease, 314
tick-borne diseases, 532, 533*t*, 534–536, 542–543, 661–662
tick-borne relapsing fever, 533*t*
timolol, for glaucoma, 823
tinea corporis, 858*t*
tinea infections, 448, 857–859
Tinel's sign, 798
tinidazole
  for *Trichomonas* vaginitis, 345
  for trichomoniasis, 475
tinnitus, 834
tinzaparin, for venous thromboembolism, 173*t*
tioconazole, for *Candida* vaginitis, 345
tircarcillin-clavulanate, for intestinal obstruction, 261
tirofiban, for STEMI, 134*t*
tissue adhesives, 92
tissue plasminogen activator (tPA), for ACS, 135
TMD. *See* temporomandibular disorder (TMD)
TMJ. *See* temporomandibular joint dysfunction
TMP-SMX DS, for UTIs, 300–301
TOA. *See* tubo-ovarian abscess (TOA)
tobramycin, 814*t*
  for conjunctivitis, 815
  for corneal abrasion, 819
  for malignant otitis externa, 831
  for urologic stone disease, 314
tocolytics, for trauma in pregnancy, 878
toddler's fracture, 438
Todd's paralysis, 768*t*, 793
toenail removal, 999*f*
tolnaftate, for fungal infection, 448
tongue lacerations, 844
tonsillitis, 845
tooth eruption, 838–839, 842*f*
topical anesthetics, 74–75, 822
topical antibiotics
  for bacterial conjunctivitis, 814
  for corneal abrasion, 819
topiramate, 616
torsemide, for acute heart failure, 150
torus fractures, 434, 436
total anomalous pulmonary venous return, 392*t*
toxic epidermal necrolysis (TEN), 852–853, 853*f*
toxicity
  ACE inhibitors, 611
  angiotensin II receptor antagonists, 612
  antihypertensives, 608–611
  β-blockers, 604–606
  calcium channel blockers, 606–608
  carbamazepine, 614–615
  caustics, 624–625
  clonidine, 611
  digitalis glycosides, 602–604, 602*t*, 603*t*

gerb, 643–645
herbals, 644*t*–645*t*
hydrocarbons, 621–623, 621*t*, 622*t*
industrial toxins, 637–642
iron, 617–620, 618*t*
metal and metalloids, 631–636
pesticides, 626–630
phenytoin, 613–614
valproate, 615–616
vitamins, 643–645, 643*t*–644*t*
volatile substances, 621–623
toxic shock syndrome, 480–483, 480*t*
toxic synovitis, 439–440
toxidromes, 556*t*
tPA. *See* tissue plasminogen activator (tPA)
tracheal stenosis, 850
tracheobronchial injuries, 905
tracheostomy tubes
with airway obstruction, 849
cannulas and, 849
changing, 850
dislodgement of, 849
site bleeding, 849–850
site infection, 849
tramadol, 68
tranexamic acid
for DIC, 728
for epistaxis, 835
for neck injuries, 901
for vaginal bleeding, 320
transabdominal feeding tubes, 285
transcutaneous cardiac pacing, for sinus bradycardia, 13
transformed migraine, 77*t*
transfusion reactions, 741*t*
transfusion therapy
See also platelets
coagulation factor VIIA (recombinant), 743
complications of, 743–744
cryoprecipitate, 742
factor replacement therapy, 743, 743*t*
fresh frozen plasma, 742
massive transfusion, 740
packed red blood cells, 739–740
platelets, 740
transfusion reactions, 741*t*
whole blood, 739
transient ischemic attack (TIA), 765, 772
transient neonatal pustular melanossis, 452
transient synovitis of the hip, 439–440
transplant patient complications, 546–554
cardiac, 549–550
fibrinogen concentrate, 742
HSCT, 553–554
of immunosuppressive agents, 549
liver, 552–553
lung, 550–551
posttransplant infections, 546, 546*t*–547*t*, 548–549
renal, 551–552
transposition of the great arteries, 392*t*
transtentorial herniation, 882
trauma
See also injuries
abdominal, 909–913
in adults, 865–868, 866*t*
buttock, 915
cardiothoracic, 903–908
in children, 869–872
abdominal, 870
airway management, 870
breathing, 870
chest, 870
circulation, 870
disability, 870
exposure, 870
genitourinary, 870
head injury, 869–870
spine injuries, 870
in elderly, 873–876
abdominal, 874
cervical spine injuries, 874
chest, 874
head injury, 873–874
orthopedic injuries, 874–875
to extremities, 920–922, 920*t*, 921*f*
facial, 892–896, 892*t*–893*t*, 895*f*
flank, 914
genitourinary, 916–919, 917*t*
head, 880–885
neck, 897–902, 897*t*, 900*f*
in pregnancy, 877–879
spine, 886–891, 887*f*
traumatic brain injury (TBI), 871*t*–872*t*, 880–885
cerebral contusion, 881
CT scanning for, 883*t*
epidural hematoma, 882
herniation, 882
intracerebral hemorrhage, 881
penetrating injuries, 882–883
skull fractures, 881
subarachnoid hemorrhage, 881
subdural hematoma, 882
traumatic hemarthrosis, 985
traumatic subarachnoid hemorrhage, 881
traveler's diarrhea, 226–228, 227*t*
traveler's diseases, 540–545, 540*t*–541*t*
trazodone, 567
Trendelenburg position, 62
Treponema pallidum, 475–477
triamcinolon acetonide dental paste, 840
triamcinolone, for shoulder pain, 977
triceps tendon ruptures, 934
Trichomonas vaginitis, 345
trichomoniasis, 475
tricuspid atresia, 392*t*

trifluorothtymidine, for HSV, 817
trifluridine, 815*t*
trigeminal neuralgia, 829
trigger finger, 998
trimethoprim-sulfamethoxazole
for bullous impetigo, 449
for CA-MRSA, 491
for cat-scratch disease, 119
for cellulitis, 116, 451
for eczema herpeticum, 446
for epididymitis, 307
for impetigo, 449
for posttransplant infections, 549
for sinusitis, 837
tripod fractures, 895
trivalent botulinum antitoxin, 799
trombiculidae, 662
tropical illnesses, 540–545, 540*t*–541*t*
tropicamide, 814*t*, 818
trumethoprim, in pregnancy, 334*t*
truncus arteriosus, 392*t*
TSS. *See* toxic shock syndrome (TSS)
TSTs. *See* tuberculin skin tests (TSTs)
TTE. *See* transthoracic ethocardiography
tuberculin skin tests (TSTs), 204, 206
tuberculosis (TB), 204–207, 508
cavitary, 206*f*
extrapulmonary, 205
primary, 204
reactivation, 204–205
tube thoracostomy, 674, 904
tularemia, 533*t*, 537
tumor lysis, 462
tumor lysis syndrome, 754
tumors
anorectal, 270
central nervous system, 463
of eighth cranial nerve, 788
extracranial solid, 463–465
"2-finger" technique, 36
"2 thumbs-encircling hands" technique, 36
tympanic membrane perforation, 833–834
typhoid fever, 542

U
UA. *See* unstable angina (UA)
UFH. *See* unfractionated heparin (UFH)
ulcer
corneal, 817–818
diabetic foot, 706, 707*t*–708*t*
peptic ulcer disease, 244–246
ulcerative colitis, 231–232
ulipristal acetate, for emergency contraception, 1018–1019
ulnar nerves, 935*t*
ulnar styloid fractures, 933
ultrasonography
for abdominal injuries, 910–911, 910*t*
for appendicitis, 253–254
for chest wall injuries, 905
for cholecystis, 250, 250*f*
for hernia, 263*f*
ocular, 825
for urologic stone disease, 313*t*
ultraviolet keratitis, 819
undifferentiated wide complex tachycardia, 24
unfractionated heparin (UFH), 747
for ACS, 133
for arterial occlusion, 188
for STEMI, 134*t*
for venous thromboembolism, 173, 173*t*
unstable angina, 127*t*, 131–137
upper GI (UGI) bleeding, 404, 405*t*, 406
upper respiratory emergencies
airway foreign body, 375–377
bacterial tracheitis, 375
epiglottitis, 373–375, 374*f*
peritonsillar abscess, 377–378
retropharyngeal abscess, 377
viral croup, 372–373
ureteral injury, 351, 917–918
ureteral stents, complications of, 317–318
urethra, 310–311
urethra injuries, 918
urethral foreign bodies, 311
urethral stricture, 310–311
urethritis, 299, 310
urinalysis, 299–300
urinary alkalinization, 561*t*
urinary catheters, complications of, 316–317
urinary retention, 304*t*
acute, 303–305
urinary tract infections (UTIs), 299–301
catheter-associated, 316
pediatric, 407–408
urine culture, 300
urine dipstick, 299, 300
urologic stone disease, 312–315, 313*t*
urticaria, 64
UTIs. *See* urinary tract infections (UTIs)

V
vaginal bleeding, 319–320
in pregnancy, 337–338
vaginal cuff cellulitis, 350
vaginal foreign bodies, 346
valacyclovir
for Bell's palsy, 798
for herpes simplex, 478, 499–500
for herpes zoster, 501, 857
for posttransplant infections, 549
valproate
in pregnancy, 333*t*
toxicity, 615–616
valproic acid, 557*t*
for sedation, 411

valvular emergencies, 152–159
 aortic regurgitation, 153*t*, 156–157
 aortic stenosis, 153*t*, 155–156
 mitral regurgitation, 153*t*, 154–155
 mitral stenosis, 152–154
 mitral valve prolapse, 153*t*, 155
 newly discovered murmur, 152, 153*f*
 prosthetic valve disease, 158–159
 right-sided valvular heart disease, 157–158
vancomycin
 for acute mastoiditis, 832
 for adult epiglottitis, 846
 for altered mental status, 416
 for bacterial tracheitis, 375
 for CA-MRSA, 491
 for childhood leukemia, 462
 for diarrhea, 229
 for epidural abscess, 811
 for epiglottitis, 375
 for Fournier gangrene, 308
 for meningitis, 809
 for neck and back pain, 973
 for necrotizing soft tissue infections, 492
 for peritoneal dialysis complications, 298
 for pneumonia, 202, 203
 for posttransplant infections, 548
 for sepsis, 358
 for STSS, 483
 for tracheostomy site infection, 849
 for TSS, 481
 for vascular access complications, 298
varicella, 446–447, 446*f*
varicella-zoster immunoglobulin, 447
varicella zoster virus (VZV), 500–501
vascular access, 32
 complications of, 297–298
vascular complications, postoperative, 283
vascular injuries, 897–898, 897*t*, 898*t*
vasodilators, 610*t*
 for vertigo, 790*t*
vasoocclusive crises, 455–456, 734, 735*t*
vasopressin, for sepsis, 487
vasopressors
 for adrenal insufficiency, 717
 for shock, 63
 for TBI, 884
venous thromboembolism (VTE), 167–174, 169*t*, 170*f*
ventilation bags, 29
ventricular fibrillation (VF), 24–25, 25*f*
ventricular tachycardia, 23–24, 23*f*, 24*f*
verapamil, for atrial fibrillation, 20
vertebral artery dissection, 788
vertebrosbasilar insufficiency, 788
vertical mattress sutures, 89–90, 90*f*
vertigo, 786*f*
 acute, 784–791, 784*t*, 785*t*
  central, 784, 784*t*, 788
  peripheral, 784, 784*t*, 787–788
  pharmacotherapy for, 789*t*–790*t*
vesicants, 684*t*
vesicovaginal fistula, 351
vestibular neuronitis, 787
vestubular ganglionitis, 787
Vibrio vulnificus, 530*t*
video laryngoscopy (VL), 4
violence. *See* abuse
viral conjunctivitis, 815–816
viral croup, 372–373
viral infections, 443–447
 arboviral, 502–503
 ebola, 503–504
 eczema herpeticum, 445–446, 445*f*
 enterovirus, 443
 Epstein-Barr virus, 501–502
 erythemia infectiosum, 444–445, 444*f*
 herpes simplex virus, 498–500
 herpes zoster, 500–501
 influenza, 497–498
 measles, 443–444, 502
 roseola infactum, 447, 447*f*
 rubella, 444
 serious, 497–504
 varicella, 500–501
viral parotitis (mumps), 828
visceral leishmaniasis, 544
vitamins
 A, 643*t*
 B1, 643*t*
 B2, 643*t*
 B3, 643*t*
 B6, 643*t*
 B12, 643*t*
 C, 644*t*
 D, 643*t*
 E, 643*t*
 K, 618, 629, 643*t*, 728
 toxicities of, 643–645, 643*t*–644*t*
volar forearm lacerations, 104
volatile substances, 621–623
volvulus, 259–261, 260*f*, 401–402
vomiting, 222–224
 in children, 400
 in infants, 361
 in infants and children, 395–399
 as malignancy emergency, 756
 management of, 1024
 of pregnancy, 326–327
von Willebrand disease (vWD), 732–733
von Willebrand factor (vWF), 732
VT. *See* ventricular tachycardia (VT)
VTE. *See* venous thromboembolism (VTE)
vulvovaginitis, 344–346
vWF. *See* von Willebrand factor (vWF)
VZV. *See* varicella zoster virus (VZV)

W

warfarin, in pregnancy, 334*t*
warfarin-induced coagulopathy, 746*f*
warts, plantar, 998
wasp stings, 658–659
waterborne diseases, 527–530, 530*t*
Wegener's, 992*t*
weight gain, neonatal, 361–362
welder's keratitis, 819
Wells' scores, 168, 169*t*
Wernicke's encephalopathy, 768*t*
West Nile virus, 502–503
wheezing, 194–195
  in infants and children, 379–384
white phosphorus, 629*t*, 685*t*
whole blood transfusion, 739
whole-bowel irrigation (WBI)
  for arsenic poisoning, 633
  for lead poisoning, 632
  for lithium toxicity, 573
  for poisoning, 560*t*, 561
wide complex tachycardias, 23–25
wild animal bites, 120
Wilms tumor, 464
Wolff-Parkinson-White (WPW) syndrome, 19, 20*f*, 25–26, 26*f*
Woods corkscrew maneuver, 343
world travelers, 540–545
wormwood, 645*t*
wounds
  anesthesia for, 82
  bite, 84, 117–118
  clinical features, 81–82
  closure of
    non-suture techniques for, 91–95, 93*f*, 94*f*, 95*f*
    sutures for, 85–91, 86*f*, 87*f*, 88*f*, 89*f*, 90*f*, 91*f*, 92*f*
  debridement, 83
  diagnosis and differential, 82
  evaluating and preparing, 81–84
  foreign body and hair removal from, 83
  hemostasis with, 83
  infection and, 81–82
  irrigation of, 82
  lacerations. *see* lacerations
  marine fauna, 666–669
  postoperative complications, 282–283, 351
  postrepair care of, 121–124
    cleansing, 123
    drains, 123
    dressings, 121
    follow-up, 123–124
    pain control, 123
    patient education about long-term cosmetic outcome, 124
    patient positioning for, 121
    prophylactic antibiotics, 121, 122*t*
    tetanus prophylaxis, 122, 122*t*
  prophylactic antibiotics for, 84
  puncture, 115–116
  soft tissue foreign bodies, 112–114
  sterile technique for, 83
WPW syndrome. *See* Wolff-Parkinson-White (WPW) syndrome
wrist fractures, 437
wrist injuries, 931–933
  carpal bone fractures, 932, 932*t*
  Colles, Smith, and Barton fractures, 932
  perilunate and lunate dislocations, 931–932
  radial styloid fractures, 932, 933*t*
  scapholunate dissociation, 931
  ulnar styloid fractures, 933
wrist lacerations, 102, 104

X

Xa inhibitors, 747
xanthines, 598–600, 599*t*

Y

yellow fever, 543
yersinia, 397*t*
Yersinia pestis, 532*t*
yohimbine, 645*t*

Z

zaleplon, 578
zanamivir, for influenza, 498
zika virus, 542
zinc, 636*t*
zoledronic acid, for hypercalcemia, 51, 753
zolpidem, 578
zonisamide, 616
zoonotic infections, 531–539
  anthrax, 537–538
  common, 531*t*–532*t*
  ehrlichiosis, 536
  Lyme disease, 533*t*, 534–536
  plague, 538–539
  Rocky Mountain spotted fever, 532, 533*t*, 534
  tick-borne, 532, 533*t*, 534–536
  tularemia, 537
zopiclone, 578
zygoma fractures, 895